Textbook of

Onco-Anesthesia and Critical Care

Textbook of

Onco-Anesthesia and Critical Care

Editors

Atul Prabhakar Kulkarni
MD FISCCM PGDHHM FICCM
Professor and Head
Division of Critical Care Medicine
Department of Anesthesiology, Critical Care and Pain
Tata Memorial Hospital
Homi Bhabha National Institute
Mumbai, Maharashtra, India

Sohan Lal Solanki
MD PDCC MAMS FOAPM
Professor
Department of Anesthesiology, Critical Care and Pain
Tata Memorial Hospital
Homi Bhabha National Institute
Mumbai, Maharashtra, India

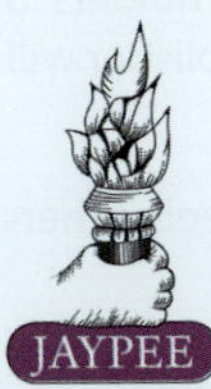

JAYPEE BROTHERS MEDICAL PUBLISHERS
The Health Sciences Publisher
New Delhi | London

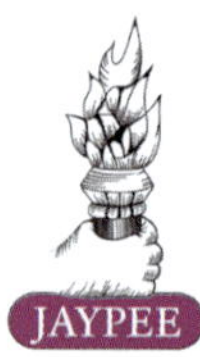

Jaypee Brothers Medical Publishers (P) Ltd

Headquarters
Jaypee Brothers Medical Publishers (P) Ltd
EMCA House, 23/23-B
Ansari Road, Daryaganj
New Delhi 110 002, India
Landline: +91-11-23272143, +91-11-23272703
+91-11-23282021, +91-11-23245672
Email: jaypee@jaypeebrothers.com

Corporate Office
Jaypee Brothers Medical Publishers (P) Ltd
4838/24, Ansari Road, Daryaganj
New Delhi 110 002, India
Phone: +91-11-43574357
Fax: +91-11-43574314
Email: jaypee@jaypeebrothers.com

Overseas Office
JP Medical Ltd.
83, Victoria Street, London
SW1H 0HW (UK)
Phone: +44 20 3170 8910
Fax: +44 (0)20 3008 6180
Email: info@jpmedpub.com

Website: www.jaypeebrothers.com
Website: www.jaypeedigital.com

Inquiries for bulk sales may be solicited at: jaypee@jaypeebrothers.com

Textbook of Onco-Anesthesia and Critical Care

First Edition: **2025**

ISBN: 978-93-6616-840-1

Printed at: Sterling Graphics Pvt. Ltd.

Dedicated to

The newer and bolder breed of doctors,
the practitioners of onco-anesthesia.

Contributors

Aafreen Siddique MD
Consultant Anesthesiologist
Department of Anesthesiology and Pain Medicine
Kokilaben Dhirubhai Ambani Hospital and Medical Research Institute
Mumbai, Maharashtra, India

Aanchal Kakkar MD MAMS
Professor
Department of Anesthesia
Atal Bihari Vajpayee Institute of Medical Sciences and Dr Ram Manohar Lohia Hospital
New Delhi, India

Aditi Suri MD DM DNB PDCC
Assistant Professor
Department of Anesthesia, Pain and Critical Care
All India Institute of Medical Sciences
New Delhi, India

Aditi Tilak MD DNB FRCA
Consultant
Department of Onco-Anesthesia
Nanavati Max Superspeciality Hospital
Mumbai, Maharashtra, India

Aditya Kunte MCh
Consultant
Department of HPB Surgery and Pancreas, Intestine and Liver Transplantation
Gleneagles Hospital
Mumbai, Maharashtra, India

Aishwarya Ramkrishnan
MD DNB MBA
Consultant Anesthesiologist
Department of Anesthesia
PD Hinduja Hospital and Medical Research Centre
Mumbai, Maharashtra, India

Ajit Kumar DA MD
Professor and In-charge (Pain Medicine and Onco-Anesthesiology)
Department of Anesthesiology
All India Institute of Medical Sciences
Rishikesh, Uttarakhand, India

Akankshya Sarangi
DNB (Anesthesiology)
Senior Clinical Fellow in Anesthesia and Day Surgery
Department of Anesthesia
Oxford University Hospitals NHS Foundation Trust
Oxford, UK

Akhil Agarwal MD
Additional Director
Department of Hepato-Biliary and Gastro-Intestinal Anesthesia
Fortis Escorts Hospital
Jaipur, Rajasthan, India

Amit Jain MD MBA
Staff Physician
Department of Anesthesiology
Integrated Hospital Institute
Cleveland Clinic
Abu Dhabi, UAE
Clinical Professor
Department of Anesthesiology
Cleveland Clinic Lerner College of Medicine
Case Western Reserve University
Cleveland, Ohio, USA

Amit Kumar Mittal MD
Senior Consultant
Department of Anesthesia
Rajiv Gandhi Cancer Institute and Research Centre
New Delhi, India

Anil Kumar Jain MD
Chairperson
Institute of Anesthesiology, Pain and Perioperative Medicine
Sir Ganga Ram Hospital
New Delhi, India

Anjali Pingle DA DNB FRCA
Consultant Anesthesiologist
Department of Anesthesia
PD Hinduja Hospital and Medical Research Centre
Mumbai, Maharashtra, India

Anjana Sagar Wajekar
DNB Fellowship in Neuro-Anesthesiology
FAIMER Fellow
Professor
Department of Anesthesiology, Critical Care and Pain
Advanced Centre for Treatment, Research and Education in Cancer (ACTREC)
Tata Memorial Centre
Homi Bhabha National Institute
Navi Mumbai, Maharashtra, India

Anju Grewal MD
Professor and Head
Department of Anesthesiology
All India Institute of Medical Sciences
Bathinda, Punjab, India

Anju Gupta MD CCEPC EDRA IDRA
Associate Professor
Department of Anesthesiology, Pain and Critical Care
All India Institute of Medical Sciences
New Delhi, India

Anjum Shabbar Khan Joad
MD DNB MNAMS Grad Certificate Pall Care (Flinders) Dip Pall Med (Cardiff)
Director
Department of Anesthesia and Palliative Medicine
Bhagwan Mahaveer Cancer Hospital and Research Centre
Jaipur, Rajasthan, India

Ankita Kadam MD
Senior Resident
Department of Anesthesiology, Critical Care and Pain
Tata Memorial Hospital
Homi Bhabha National Institute
Mumbai, Maharashtra, India

Anne Poornachand MD
Consultant
Department of Onco-Anesthesia, Critical Care, Pain, and Palliative Medicine
Basavatarakam Indo-American Cancer Hospital and Research Institute
Hyderabad, Telangana, India

Anupama Gill Sharma DNB IDCCM
Professor
Department of Anesthesia
Atal Bihari Vajpayee Institute of Medical Sciences and Dr Ram Manohar Lohia Hospital
New Delhi, India

Aparna Sanjay Chatterjee
MD FCARCSI (Dublin)
Professor and Head
Division of Pain
Department of Anesthesiology Critical Care and Pain
Tata Memorial Centre
Homi Bhabha National Institute
Mumbai, Maharashtra, India

Arun Muthukumar MD
Resident
Department of Anesthesiology Pain Management and Perioperative Medicine
Henry Ford Health
Detroit, MI, USA

Arupratan Maiti
MD DNB DESAIC FNB FIACTA FTEE FASE EACTA/EACVI
Fellowship in Freeman Hospital, UK
Senior Consultant
Department of Cardiac Anesthesia and Intensive Care
Apollo Multispecialty Hospital
Kolkata, West Bengal, India

Asako Shida BSc MBCHB MCEM FRCA
Consultant
Department of Anesthesia and Perioperative Medicine
The Royal Marsden NHS Foundation Trust
London, SW3 6JJ, UK

Ashish Mani Tripathi MD
Associate Consultant
Department of Critical Care
Regency Hospital
Kanpur, Uttar Pradesh, India

Ashwini Rane
DNB Fellowship in Pediatric Anesthesia
Associate Professor
Department of Anesthesiology, Critical Care and Pain
Advanced Centre for Treatment Research and Education in Cancer (ACTREC)
Tata Memorial Centre
Navi Mumbai, Maharashtra, India

Atul Prabhakar Kulkarni
MD FISCCM PGDHHM FICCM
Professor and Head
Division of Critical Care Medicine
Department of Anesthesiology, Critical Care and Pain
Tata Memorial Hospital
Homi Bhabha National Institute
Mumbai, Maharashtra, India

Babita Ghai
MD DNB Fellowship in Pain Management (London)
Professor
Department of Anesthesia and Intensive Care
Postgraduate Institute of Medical Education and Research
Chandigarh, India

Basanth Kumar Rayani DA DNB MBA
Chief Anesthesiologist
Department of Onco-Anesthesia, Critical Care, Pain, and Palliative Medicine
Basavatarakam Indo-American Cancer Hospital and Research Institute
Hyderabad, Telangana, India

Bhuvaneswari Balasubramanian
MD PDCC (Pediatric Anesthesia) IDRA
Associate Professor
Department of Anesthesia, Critical Care and Pain
All India Institute of Medical Sciences
Nagpur, Maharashtra, India

Bindiya G Salunke MD
Professor
Department of Anesthesiology, Critical Care and Pain
Tata Memorial Hospital
Homi Bhabha National Institute
Mumbai, Maharashtra, India

Carlos Eduardo Guerra-Londono
MD
Staff Anesthesiologist and Medical Co-Director
Division of Anesthesia Research
Department of Anesthesiology, Pain Management, and Perioperative Medicine
Henry Ford Health
Detroit, MI, USA

Darshil Ashok Julasana MD
Fellow of Onco-Anesthesia and Pain
Department of Anesthesiology, Critical Care and Pain
Tata Memorial Hospital
Homi Bhabha National Institute
Mumbai, Maharashtra, India

Debashree Pradipta Lahiri
DNB (Anesthesiology)
PDF in Neuroanesthesiology
Assistant Professor
Department of Anesthesiology, Critical Care and Pain
Tata Memorial Hospital
Homi Bhabha National Institute
Mumbai, Maharashtra, India

Deepa Chandramohan
MD MRCP FCCM DNB
Senior Consultant and Head
Department of Critical Care Medicine
MVR Cancer Centre and Research Institute
Kozhikode, Kerala, India

Deepti Gupta MD DNB
Consultant Pathologist
Department of Pathology
Regency Hospital
Kanpur, Uttar Pradesh, India

Devendra Gupta
MD PDCC (Neuroanesthesia and Neurointensive Care)
Professor
Department of Anesthesiology
Sanjay Gandhi Postgraduate Institute of Medical Sciences
Lucknow, Uttar Pradesh, India

Dileep Damodaran MS MCh
Clinical Director and Senior Consultant
Department of Critical Care Medicine
MVR Cancer Centre and Research Institute
Kozhikode, Kerala, India

Divya Dabholkar MD
Senior Resident
Department of Anesthesia, Critical Care and Pain
Tata Memorial Hospital
Homi Bhabha National Institute
Mumbai, Maharashtra, India

Donal J Buggy
DSc MD MSc FRCPI FFSEM FRCA FESA-IC FCAI
Professor
Department of Anesthesia and Perioperative Medicine
Mater Misericordiae University Hospital
Dublin, Ireland

Gauri Raman Gangakhedkar
DA DNB
Associate Professor
Department of Anesthesiology, Critical Care and Pain
Advanced Centre for Treatment Research and Education in Cancer (ACTREC)
Tata Memorial Centre
Homi Bhabha National Institute
Navi Mumbai, Maharashtra, India

Girija Prasad Rath MD DM
Professor
Department of Neuro-anesthesiology and Neurocritical Care
Neurosciences Centre
All India Institute of Medical Sciences
New Delhi, India

Indubala Maurya MD DNB
Associate Professor
Department of Anesthesiology
Kalyan Singh Super Specialty Cancer Institute and Hospital
Lucknow, Uttar Pradesh, India

Jagdeep Sharma MD DNB DESAIC
Assistant Professor
Department of Anesthesiology, Critical Care and Pain
Homi Bhabha Cancer Hospital and Research Centre
Tata Memorial Centre
New Chandigarh, India

Jayanth Ranganathan Seshan
MD DM
Assistant Professor
Department of Anesthesiology and Critical Care
Jawaharlal Nehru Institute of Postgraduate Medical Education and Research
Puducherry, India

Jeson R Doctor
MD DNB MNAMS FOAPM
Professor
Department of Anesthesiology, Critical Care and Pain
Tata Memorial Hospital
Homi Bhabha National Institute
Mumbai, Maharashtra, India

Jesto Kurian MD MBA
Associate Staff Physician
Department of Anesthesiology
Integrated Hospital Institute
Cleveland Clinic
Abu Dhabi, UAE
Clinical Associate Professor
Department of Anesthesiology
Cleveland Clinic Lerner College of Medicine
Case Western Reserve University
Cleveland, Ohio, USA

Jigeeshu V Divatia MD FCCM FICCM
Head
Department of Critical Care Medicine
Lilawati Hospital and Research Centre
Mumbai, Maharashtra, India

Juan Jose Guerra-Londono MD
Resident
Department of Anesthesiology, Pain Management and Perioperative Medicine
Henry Ford Health
Detroit, MI, USA

Jyoti Sharma MD (Anesthesiology)
Associate Professor
Department of Anesthesiology
All India Institute of Medical Sciences
Bathinda, Punjab, India

Jyotirmay Kirtania
MD (Anesthesiology)
Professor and Head
Department of Anesthesiology, Critical Care and Pain
Mahamana Pandit Madan Mohan Malviya Cancer Centre
Homi Bhabha National Institute
Varanasi, Uttar Pradesh, India

Jyotsna Goswami MD
Consultant
Department of Onco-Anesthesia
Tata Medical Center
Kolkata, West Bengal, India

Kalpana Balakrishnan
DA DNB NFPM (National Fellow in Palliative Medicine)
Director and Head
Department of Anesthesia, Pain and Palliative Care
Cancer Institute (WIA)
Chennai, Tamil Nadu, India

Karthik AR MD DNB DM
Assistant Professor
Department of Anesthesia
Pain and Palliative Care
Cancer Institute (WIA)
Chennai, Tamil Naud, India

Kshama Balakrishna
MD (Anesthesia) Fellowship in Solid Organ Transplant
Fellow, Transplant Anesthesia
Department of Anesthesia and Critical Care
Amrita Institute of Medical Sciences
Kochi, Kerala, India

Laboni Sarkar
MD (Medicine) DM (Medical Oncology)
Assistant Professor
Department of Medical Oncology
Tata Memorial Hospital
Mumbai, Maharashtra, India

Lakshmi Kumar MD (Anesthesia)
Professor and Head
Department of Anesthesia
and Critical Care
Amrita Institute of Medical Sciences
Kochi, Kerala, India

Lalit Gupta DA DNB MNAMS SEFM
Professor
Department of Anesthesia and
Intensive Care
Maulana Azad Medical College
New Delhi, India

Lalita Gouri Mitra DA MD DNB FICCM
Professor and Officer In-charge
Department of Anesthesiology, Critical
Care and Pain
Homi Bhabha Cancer Hospital and
Research Centre
Tata Memorial Centre
Homi Bhabha National Institute
New Chandigarh, India

Lovenish Bains MS FNB FACS FRCS
Professor
Department of Surgery
Maulana Azad Medical College
New Delhi, India

Malini P Joshi MD (Anesthesia)
Professor
Department of Anesthesiology, Critical
Care and Pain
Advanced Centre for Treatment
Research and Education in Cancer
(ACTREC), Tata Memorial Centre
Homi Bhabha National Institute
Mumbai, Maharashtra, India

Mamta Dubey MD
Senior Consultant
Department of Anesthesia
Rajiv Gandhi Cancer Institute and
Research Centre
New Delhi, India

Manbir Kaur MD DNB (Anesthesiology)
Assistant Professor
Department of Anesthesiology
and Critical Care
All India Institute of Medical Sciences
Jodhpur, Rajasthan, India

Manisha Hemrajani MD
Senior Consultant
Department of Anesthesia
and Palliative Medicine
Bhagwan Mahaveer Cancer
Hospital and Research Centre
Jaipur, Rajasthan, India

Manju Sengar MD DM
Professor
Department of Medical Oncology
Tata Memorial Hospital
Homi Bhabha National Institute
Mumbai, Maharashtra, India

Manoj Kamal MD
Professor
Department of Anesthesiology and
Critical Care
All India Institute of Medical Sciences
Jodhpur, Rajasthan, India

Mary Thomas
DA DNB FOAPM
Additional Professor and Head
Department of Anesthesia
Regional Cancer Centre
Thiruvananthapuram, Kerala, India

Massimo Lamperti
MD MBA
Staff Physician and Institute Chair
Department of Anesthesiology
Integrated Hospital Institute
Cleveland Clinic
Abu Dhabi, UAE
Clinical Professor
Department of Anesthesiology
Cleveland Clinic Lerner College
of Medicine
Case Western Reserve University
Cleveland, Ohio, USA

Meenakshi V Venketeswaran
DA MD DNB NFPM (National Fellow
in Palliative Medicine)
Associate Professor
Department of Anesthesia,
Pain and Palliative Care
Cancer Institute (WIA)
Chennai, Tamil Nadu, India

Minhaj Akhter
MD (PMR) Post Doctoral Fellowship in Pain and
Palliative Care FIPM CCEPC
Assistant Consultant
Department of Anesthesia and
Palliative Medicine
Bhagwan Mahaveer Cancer
Hospital and Research Centre
Jaipur, Rajasthan, India

Mira Sudam Wagh
DNB (General Surgery)
DNB (Surgical Oncology)
Associate Professor
Division of Surgical Oncology
Department of Surgical Services
Regional Cancer Centre
Thiruvananthapuram, Kerala, India

Mithilesh Kumar Mishra
DNB FIPM FIAPM NFPM
Senior Consultant
Institute of Anesthesiology,
Pain and Perioperative Medicine
Sir Ganga Ram Hospital
New Delhi, India

Mohd Shazrul M Ramly
MB BCh BaO FCAI FJFICMI
Research Fellow
Department of Anesthesia
Mater Misericordiae University Hospital
Dublin, Ireland

Mounika Yallala
DNB (Medicine) DM (Medical Oncology)
Assistant Professor
Department of Medical Oncology
Tata Memorial Hospital
Mumbai, Maharashtra, India

Muralidhar Kanchi
MD FIACTA FICA MBA FASE PhD
Director (Academic), Senior Consultant
and Professor
(Anesthesia and Intensive Care)
Department of Cardiac Anesthesia and
Intensive Care
Narayana Institute of Cardiac Sciences,
Narayana Health City
Bengaluru, Karnataka, India
Professor of International Health
University of Minnesota, USA

Nairita Das MD (Anesthesiology) EDAIC
Assistant Professor
Department of Anesthesia, Pain and Palliative Care
Cancer Institute (WIA)
Chennai, Tamil Nadu, India

Namrata Ranganath MD
Professor
Department of Anesthesiology and Pain Relief
Kidwai Memorial Institute of Oncology
Bengaluru, Karnataka, India

Nebu Abraham George
MS MNAMS FRCS DNB (Surgical Oncology)
Additional Professor
Division of Surgical Oncology
Department of Surgical Services
Regional Cancer Centre
Thiruvananthapuram, Kerala, India

Neha Desai DA DNB
Consultant
Department of Onco-Anesthesia
Tata Medical Center
Kolkata, West Bengal, India

Nishkarsh Gupta
MD CCEPC Fellowship in Palliative Medicine
Professor
Department of Onco-Anesthesia and Palliative Medicine
All India Institute of Medical Sciences
New Delhi, India

Nitika Goel MD
Associate Professor
Department of Anesthesia and Intensive Care
Postgraduate Institute of Medical Education and Research
Chandigarh, India

Nitya Reddy R
MD FOACCP (ICA) NFPM
Consultant
Department of Onco-Anesthesia, Critical Care, Pain, and Palliative Medicine
Basavatarakam Indo-American Cancer Hospital and Research Institute
Hyderabad, Telangana, India

NK Vinod
MD PDCC (Cardiac Anesthesia) FOAPM
Head and Chief Consultant
Department of Anesthesiology
Critical Care, Pain and Palliative Care
Sri Shankara Cancer Hospital and Research Centre
Bengaluru, Karnataka, India

Pascal Owusu-Agyemang MD
Professor
Department of Anesthesiology and Perioperative Medicine
The University of Texas MD Anderson Cancer Center
Houston, TX, USA

Pooja Natarajan
MD FNB FIACTA FICCC FTEE FASE EACVI-TOE
Fellow Cardiac Anesthesia and Intensive Care (UK)
Senior Consultant, Cardiac Anesthesiologist
Department of Cardiothoracic and Vascular Surgery Anesthesia
Sri Madhusudan Sai Institute of Medical Sciences and Research
Sri Sathya Sai Sarla Memorial Hospital
Mavahalli, Karnataka, India

Pradeep Kumar Bhatia MD
Professor and Head
Department of Anesthesiology and Critical Care
All India Institute of Medical Sciences
Jodhpur, Rajasthan, India

Pragya Gupta
MD PDAF (Neuroanesthesia and Neurointensive Care)
Consultant
Department of Anesthesia and Intensive Care
Divine Life Hospital
Kutch, Gujarat, India

Pralay Shankar Ghosh
MD DM EDICM
Senior Consultant
Department of Critical Care Medicine
Tata Medical Center
Kolkata, West Bengal, India

Pramila Madhu Chandan
MD DrNB (Critical Care Medicine)
Senior Resident
Division of Critical Care Medicine
Department of Anesthesiology
Critical Care and Pain
Tata Memorial Hospital
Homi Bhabha National Institute
Mumbai, Maharashtra, India

Prasanna Vani MD DNB
Assistant Professor
Department of Anesthesia, Pain and Palliative Care
Cancer Institute (WIA)
Chennai, Tamil Nadu, India

Pratishtha Yadav
MD DNB DM (Onco-Anesthesia) MNAMS
Consultant
Department of Onco-Anesthesia and Critical Care
Tata Medical Centre
Kolkata, West Bengal, India

Preethy J Mathew MD
Professor
Department of Anesthesia and Intensive Care
Postgraduate Institute of Medical Education and Research
Chandigarh, India
Visiting Professor
Department of Anesthesia and Perioperative Care
University of California
San Francisco, USA

Pritha Raj MD (Anesthesiology)
Assistant Professor
Department of Anesthesia, Pain and Palliative Care
Cancer Institute (WIA)
Chennai, Tamil Nadu, India

Priya Ranganathan MD
Professor
Department of Anesthesiology
Critical Care and Pain
Tata Memorial Hospital
Homi Bhabha National Institute
Mumbai, Maharashtra, India

Priyanka Sethi MD DNB MNAMS
Additional Professor
Department of Anesthesiology and Critical Care
All India Institute of Medical Sciences
Jodhpur, Rajasthan, India

Punitha Chockalingam DNB DESA
Associate Professor
Department of Anesthesia, Pain and Palliative Care
Cancer Institute (WIA)
Chennai, Tamil Nadu, India

Rachana ND DNB
Associate Professor
Department of Anesthesiology and Pain Relief
Kidwai Memorial Institute of Oncology
Bengaluru, Karnataka, India

Rajiv Chawla
MD MNAMS FISNACC FOAPM
Director and Head
Department of Anesthesiology
Rajiv Gandhi Cancer Institute and Research Centre
New Delhi, India

Rakesh Garg
MD DNB FICCM FICA PGCCHM MNAMS CCEPC
Fellowship in Clinical Research Methodology & Evidence-based Medicine
Professor
Department of Onco-Anesthesia and Palliative Medicine
Dr BR Ambedkar Institute Rotary Cancer Hospital and National Cancer Institute
All India Institute of Medical Sciences
New Delhi, India

Ram Gopal Maurya
MD PDCC (Critical Care)
Assistant Professor
Department of Anesthesiology and Critical Care
King George's Medical University
Lucknow, Uttar Pradesh, India

Rashmi NR MD
Associate Professor
Department of Anesthesiology and Pain Relief
Kidwai Memorial Institute of Oncology
Bengaluru, Karnataka, India

Ravishankar Rao Baikady
DA DNB FRCA
Consultant
Department of Anesthesia and Perioperative Medicine
The Royal Marsden NHS Foundation Trust
London, SW3 6JJ, UK

Reshma Ambulkar MD DA FRCA DHHM
Professor and Head
Department of Anesthesiology, Critical Care and Pain
Advanced Centre for Treatment Research and Education in Cancer (ACTREC)
Tata Memorial Centre
Homi Bhabha National Institute
Mumbai, Maharashtra, India

Ruchi Pathak MD (Anesthesiology)
Neuroanesthesia Fellow
Department of Anesthesiology and Critical Care
All India Institute of Medical Sciences
Jodhpur, Rajasthan, India

Ruma Thakuria MD
Assistant Professor
Department of Anesthesiology
All India Institute of Medical Sciences
Rishikesh, Uttarakhand, India

Rupesh Yadav MD
Professor
Department of Anesthesiology
Atal Bihari Vajpayee Institute of Medical Sciences and Dr Ram Manohar Lohia Hospital
New Delhi, India

S Ramkiran DA DNB
Consultant
Department of Anesthesiology
Critical Care, Pain and Palliative Care
Sri Shankara Cancer Hospital and Research Centre
Bengaluru, Karnataka, India

Sagar Joshi MD
Assistant Professor
Department of Anesthesiology, Critical Care and Pain
Tata Memorial Hospital
Homi Bhabha National Institute
Mumbai, Maharashtra, India

Sanika Patil MD FRCA
Specialty Registrar Anesthetics/Intensive Care Medicine
Department of Anesthesia
Cambridge University Hospital, UK

Sanjay Agrawal MD PDCC
Professor and Head
Department of Anesthesiology
All India Institute of Medical Sciences
Rishikesh, Uttarakhand, India

Satish Vishnu Sarode
MD FNB (Critical Care Medicine)
In-charge
Department of Critical Care Medicine
Sahyadri Superspeciality Hospital
Pune, Maharashtra, India

Shagun Bhatia Shah
DNB DA MNAMS FIMSA FRIOASD FOAPM
Senior Consultant
Department of Anesthesiology
Rajiv Gandhi Cancer Institute and Research Centre
New Delhi, India

Shalini Saksena
MD DA FIPP
Consultant and Head
Department of Onco-Anesthesia
Nanavati Max Superspeciality Hospital
Mumbai, Maharashtra, India

Shardul Diliprao Joshi
DNB (Anesthesia)
Fellow HPB and Gastrointestinal Anesthesia
Department of Anesthesiology, Critical Care and Pain
Tata Memorial Hospital
Homi Bhabha National Institute
Mumbai, Maharashtra, India

Sharmishtha Pathak MD DM
Assistant Professor
Department of Anesthesiology
Pain Medicine and Critical Care
Jai Prakash Narayan Apex Trauma Center
All India Institute of Medical Sciences
New Delhi, India

Shashank Umesh Paliwal MD (Anesthesiology) DM (Neuroanesthesia)
Assistant Professor
Department of Anesthesiology
All India Institute of Medical Sciences
Bathinda, Punjab, India

Shayak Roy MD DM
Assistant Professor
Department of Anesthesiology and Critical Care
Institute of Medical Sciences
Banaras Hindu University
Varanasi, Uttar Pradesh, India

Sheetal Gaikwad MD
Professor
Department of Anesthesiology
Critical Care and Pain
Tata Memorial Hospital
Homi Bhabha National Institute
Mumbai, Maharashtra, India

Sheila Nainan Myatra
MD FICCM FCCM
Professor
Department of Anesthesiology, Critical Care and Pain
Tata Memorial Hospital
Homi Bhabha National Institute
Mumbai, Maharashtra, India

Shikha Sachan
MD IDCCM EDICM FECMO
Principal Consultant
Department of Critical Care
Regency Hospital
Kanpur, Uttar Pradesh, India

Shilpushp J Bhosale
DM (Critical Care) Fellowship (SickKids, Toronto)
Professor and Head
Division of Critical Care Medicine
Department of Anesthesiology
Critical Care and Pain
Advanced Centre for Treatment Research and Education in Cancer (ACTREC)
Tata Memorial Centre
Homi Bhabha National Institute
Mumbai, Maharashtra, India

Shreyasi Ray
MD (Anesthesiology) MBA (Healthcare Services)
Professor
Department of Anesthesiology
Critical Care and Pain
Mahamana Pandit Madan Mohan Malviya Cancer Centre
Homi Bhabha National Institute
Varanasi, Uttar Pradesh, India

Shruti Gairola
MD DM (Onco-Anesthesia)
Assistant Professor
Department of Anesthesiology, Critical Care and Pain
Tata Memorial Hospital
Homi Bhabha National Institute
Mumbai, Maharashtra, India

Siddharth Chavali MD DM
Clinical Assistant Professor
Department of Anesthesia
Carver College of Medicine
University of Iowa
Iowa, USA

Snany Surendran A
MSc (Clinical Nutrition) Dietetics Fellowship in Nutrition Oncology UGC NET Scholar in Home Science
Head
Department of Nutrition Oncology
MVR Cancer Centre and Research Institute
Kozhikode, Kerala, India

Sofia Jaswal MD
Assistant Professor
Department of Anesthesiology, Critical Care and Pain
Homi Bhabha Cancer Hospital and Research Centre
Tata Memorial Centre
Homi Bhabha National Institute
New Chandigarh, India

Sohan Lal Solanki
MD PDCC MAMS FOAPM
Professor
Department of Anesthesiology, Critical Care and Pain
Tata Memorial Hospital
Homi Bhabha National Institute
Mumbai, Maharashtra, India

Sonali Banwait MD PDCC (Critical Care)
Associate Professor
Department of Anesthesia
Vardhman Mahavir Medical College and Safdarjung Hospital
New Delhi, India

Soumi Pathak MD
Consultant
Department of Anesthesia
Rajiv Gandhi Cancer Institute and Research Centre
New Delhi, India

Sravya Adda
MD DNB FOACCP (Fellowship in Onco-Anesthesia, Critical Care and Pain)
Consultant
Department of Onco-Anesthesia
Critical Care, Pain, and Palliative Medicine
Basavatarakam Indo-American Cancer Hospital and Research Institute
Hyderabad, Telangana, India

Sudeep Goyal DA DNB
Consultant
Institute of Anesthesiology, Pain and Perioperative Medicine
Sir Ganga Ram Hospital
New Delhi, India

Sudhindran Surendran MS FRCS
Professor and Head
(Liver Transplant Services)
Department of GI Surgery
Amrita Institute of Medical Sciences
Kochi, Kerala, India

Sudipta Mukherjee
MD IDCCM FNB EDICM FOAPM
Senior Consultant and Head
Department of Critical Care Medicine
Tata Medical Center
Kolkata, West Bengal, India

Sudivya Sharma MD DNB EPIC PGDHHM
Professor
Division of Critical Care
Department of Anesthesiology
Critical Care and Pain
Tata Memorial Hospital
Homi Bhabha National Institute
Mumbai, Maharashtra, India

Suhail Sarwar Siddiqui
MD Fellowship in Critical Care DM (Critical Care Medicine) EDIC
Associate Professor
Department of Critical Care Medicine
King George's Medical University
Lucknow, Uttar Pradesh, India

Sukhada Savarkar MD
Associate Professor
Division of Critical Care Medicine
Department of Anesthesiology, Critical Care and Pain
Tata Memorial Hospital
Homi Bhabha National Institute
Mumbai, Maharashtra, India

Sumitra Bakshi MD
Professor
Department of Anesthesiology, Critical Care and Pain
Tata Memorial Hospital
Homi Bhabha National Institute
Mumbai, Maharashtra, India

Surendra Kumar Pingoliya
MD (Anesthesiology)
Resident
Department of Palliative Medicine
Sawai Man Singh Medical College
Jaipur, Rajasthan, India

Sushan Gupta
MD
Fellow
Department of Pulmonary and Critical Care Medicine
Medical College of Wisconsin Affiliated Hospitals
Milwaukee, Wisconsin, USA

Swapnil Parab
MD (Anesthesiology) Fellowship in Onco-Anesthesia and Pain
Professor
Department of Anesthesiology Critical Care and Pain
Tata Memorial Hospital
Homi Bhabha National Institute
Mumbai, Maharashtra, India

Swati Chhabra
MD DNB Fellowship Neuroanesthesia (University of Toronto)
Additional Professor
Department of Anesthesiology and Critical Care
All India Institute of Medical Sciences
Jodhpur, Rajasthan, India

Thendral Ramasamy
DA MSc (Pall Med) (Cardiff, UK)
Assistant Professor
Department of Anesthesia, Pain and Palliative Care
Cancer Institute (WIA)
Chennai, Tamil Nadu, India

Uddalak Chattopadhyay
MD (Anesthesiology) DNB (Anesthesiology)
Associate Professor
Department of Anesthesiology, Critical Care and Pain
Mahamana Pandit Madan Mohan Malviya Cancer Centre
Homi Bhabha National Institute
Varanasi, Uttar Pradesh, India

Uma Hariharan
DNB MNAMS FIMSA FSNCC DESA FICA PGDHM CCEPC FIAMS FRIOASD
Professor
Department of Critical Care Medicine
Atal Bihari Vajpayee Institute of Medical Sciences and Dr Ram Manohar Lohia Hospital
New Delhi, India

Unmesh Pramod Bedekar MD DrNB
Assistant Professor
Department of Anesthesia Critical Care and Pain
Seth GS Medical College and King Edward Medical College
Mumbai, Maharashtra, India

Usha Yadav
MS (Obstetrics and Gynecology) FICOG FMAS
Senior Specialist
Department of Obstetrics and Gynecology
Deen Dayal Upadhyay Hospital
New Delhi, India

Vandana Agarwal
MD FRCA (London)
Professor
Department of Anesthesiology, Critical Care and Pain
Tata Memorial Hospital
Homi Bhabha National Institute
Mumbai, Maharashtra, India

Veena Asthana MD
Professor
Department of Anesthesiology
Himalayan Institute of Medical Sciences
Dehradun, Uttarakhand, India

Veer D Thakkar
MD (Anesthesiology)
Assistant Professor
Department of Anesthesiology Critical Care and Pain
Tata Memorial Hospital
Homi Bhabha National Institute
Mumbai, Maharashtra, India

Vibhavari Naik
MD DNB FOAPM Honorary Fellowship in Pediatric Anesthesia (IAPA)
Consultant
Department of Onco-Anesthesia Critical Care, Pain, and Palliative Medicine
Basavatarakam Indo-American Cancer Hospital and Research Institute
Hyderabad, Telangana, India

Vighnesh Ashok MD FRCA
Assistant Professor
Department of Anesthesia and Intensive Care
Postgraduate Institute of Medical Education and Research
Chandigarh, India

Vijaya P Patil
MD Dip (Hospital Admin)
Professor and Head
Department of Anesthesiology, Critical Care and Pain
Tata Memorial Hospital
Homi Bhabha National Institute
Mumbai, Maharashtra, India

Vikas Gupta
MD (Anesthesiology)
Assistant Professor
Department of Palliative Medicine
Jawahar Lal Nehru Medical College
Ajmer, Rajasthan, India

Viplab Patro
DNB MNAMS EPGDHA
Consultant
Department of Onco-Anesthesia
Tata Medical Center
Kolkata, West Bengal, India

Yogendra Singhal MD (Anesthesiology)
Professor
Department of Palliative Medicine
Sawai Man Singh Medical College
Jaipur, Rajasthan, India

Yukti Sharma MD
Senior Resident
Department of Onco-Anesthesia and Palliative Medicine
Dr BR Ambedkar Institute Rotary Cancer Hospital and National Cancer Institute
All India Institute of Medical Sciences
New Delhi, India

Preface

परिवर्तनमेव स्थिरमस्ति ॥

(Change is constant)

Cancer is a dreaded word, even among the specialists treating it on a daily basis. Cancer, when detected late, is often not amenable to treatment, but with advancing frontiers in imaging, biomarkers, and increasing awareness about screening tests, early detection has become possible. Improvement in surgical techniques, neoadjuvant therapies, and progressive and ever-increasing safe boundaries of anesthesia means lesions which were deemed unresectable only a decade or two back can now be safely resected, with training in the management of these patients postoperatively, where complex physiological changes occur owing to the resected cancer and neoadjuvant therapies. This, however, means a specially trained anesthesiologist at the head end, who can face the challenges presented by elderly patients with comorbidities, and technically difficult surgeries, head on. This has birthed a new superspecialty in anesthesiology—onco-anesthesia.

We, therefore, felt a need for a comprehensive textbook for the students and the practitioners in this new superspecialty. The challenges are great—the duration of surgeries is getting longer, many physiological changes happen, and the old foes continue to bamboozle such as massive blood loss and massive fluid shifts. For helping the newbies and assure the old hands, this book therefore contains chapters authored by stalwarts in the field of onco-anesthesia, who have utilized their years of experience to share their insights and expertise in this new superspecialty. There are many new areas to train in, new techniques to get used to, and newer challenges to tackle. A prime example is the resurgence of cytoreductive surgery coupled with heated intraperitoneal chemotherapy (CRS-HIPEC).

This is just one example of what awaits you in this book. We hope you enjoy reading it as much as we loved putting this together for you.

We are grateful to the *Adiyogi Mahadev* for his blessings and to our families for their support. We await, as usual, the honest opinion and constructive criticism from all our readers.

Atul Prabhakar Kulkarni
Sohan Lal Solanki

Acknowledgments

We wish to thank the experienced and senior practitioners of the art of onco-anesthesia for making a scholarly contribution to this book, to make it impactful. They have given valuable time, a very precious commodity, which does not come back and dealt very patiently with our impatient pestering to work within the limits of the time frame. We hope we get a critical, constructive, and positive feedback from discerning and learned practitioners and the new entrants in the specialty.

Many thanks go to our families, who stood by us to support us in these time-consuming endeavors and tolerate our mental and sometimes physical absence and eccentric behavior, which may have nothing to do with our work on the book, anyway.

We are especially thankful to Shri Jitendar P Vij (Group Chairman), Mr Ankit Vij (Managing Director), Mr MS Mani (Group President), and Ms Somoshri Banerji (Development Editor) of M/s Jaypee Brothers Medical Publishers (P) Ltd, New Delhi, India, for helping us in every way possible to bring out this book.

Last but not least, our prayers and thanks go to the *Adiyogi Mahadev* for blessing us in this task.

Contents

SECTION 11 BONE AND SOFT TISSUE ONCO-ANESTHESIA

SECTION 12 ONCOCRITICAL CARE

SECTION 13 CANCER PAIN MANAGEMENT

SECTION 14 PALLIATIVE CARE MEDICINE

SECTION 15 MISCELLANEOUS

SECTION 1

Onco-Anesthesia: General

Cancer Epidemiology and Onco-Anesthesiology as Emerging Specialty

Sohan Lal Solanki, Jigeeshu V Divatia

INTRODUCTION

Cancer epidemiology studies the worldwide cancer burden, including risk factors, incidence patterns, and inequalities in disease occurrence. Increasing incidence has driven the development of early detection, precision medicine, and multimodal therapy strategies. Onco-anesthesiology has developed as a subspecialty field for managing the complicated perioperative requirements of cancer patients, incorporating optimized recovery pathways, opioid-sparing strategies, and immunomodulatory anesthetic strategies. There is emerging evidence that anesthetic selection and perioperative management may affect cancer recurrence and long-term survival. This chapter discusses the interaction between cancer epidemiology and onco-anesthesiology, emphasizing their contribution to enhancing global cancer care.

CANCER EPIDEMIOLOGY: A GLOBAL PERSPECTIVE

Cancer remains a major global health challenge, being one of the leading causes of morbidity and mortality worldwide. The latest estimates from the Global Cancer Observatory (GLOBOCAN 2020) report approximately 19.3 million new cancer cases and 10 million deaths due to cancer in a single year.[1] Projections suggest that by 2040, new cancer cases could rise to 28.4 million annually, primarily driven by population growth, aging, and lifestyle changes. Among the most commonly diagnosed cancers are breast cancer, accounting for over 2.2 million cases, followed by lung, colorectal, prostate, and stomach cancers. However, the global distribution of cancer types varies significantly, with lung cancer being predominant in developed regions, while cervical and liver cancers are more prevalent in low- and middle-income countries (LMICs).[2] These disparities reflect differences in exposure to risk factors, healthcare access, and the availability of preventive and diagnostic services. The epidemiological patterns highlight the urgent need for comprehensive cancer control programs that include prevention, early detection, and treatment strategies tailored to regional and cultural contexts.

CANCER EPIDEMIOLOGY IN INDIA

India's cancer burden is growing at an alarming pace, with an estimated 1.4 million new cases and 850,000 deaths annually. The Indian Council of Medical Research (ICMR) predicts that these numbers could increase significantly in the coming years, driven by demographic shifts, urbanization, and the adoption of unhealthy lifestyle habits. The cancer profile in India reveals notable gender and regional disparities. Among women, breast cancer is the leading malignancy, with over 178,000 cases diagnosed annually, often presenting at advanced stages due to lack of awareness and delayed screening.[3] In men, cancers of the oral cavity, lung, and esophagus are most prevalent, largely attributed to tobacco use in various forms. Tobacco-related cancers account for over 30% of the country's cancer burden.[4] Additionally, cervical cancer remains a significant concern among women in rural and underserved regions, despite being largely preventable through vaccination and regular screening. Socioeconomic inequalities further widen the gap in cancer care, with rural populations often lacking access to specialized oncology centers, diagnostic facilities, and treatment options. These factors emphasize the need for strengthened public health policies, including nationwide cancer screening programs, tobacco control initiatives, and equitable access to advanced cancer care.

INTEGRATING CANCER EPIDEMIOLOGY WITH ONCO-ANESTHESIOLOGY

The evolving cancer epidemiological landscape has profound implications for the field of onco-anesthesiology, a specialized discipline focused on the perioperative management of cancer patients. With cancer surgeries forming a substantial component of oncological treatment, anesthesiologists play a pivotal role in optimizing outcomes through preoperative risk assessment, intraoperative management, and postoperative care. Epidemiological data serve as a critical foundation for understanding the burden and distribution of cancer types, thereby informing tailored perioperative strategies. For instance, the high prevalence of tobacco-related cancers in India necessitates preoperative interventions addressing respiratory and cardiovascular complications associated with chronic tobacco use. Similarly, the rising incidence of breast and gastrointestinal cancers calls for enhanced recovery protocols, multimodal analgesia, and measures to mitigate long-term complications such as chronic pain and opioid dependence.

Furthermore, onco-anesthesiologists are increasingly involved in addressing cancer-related pain syndromes, managing complications of chemotherapy and radiotherapy, and ensuring adequate care for high-risk populations such as the elderly and those with comorbidities. The integration of epidemiological insights with perioperative care practices allows for personalized, evidence-based approaches that improve surgical outcomes, reduce complications, and enhance the quality of life for cancer patients. Onco-anesthesiology, thus, stands at the intersection of epidemiology, oncology, and perioperative medicine, contributing to the holistic management of the growing cancer burden both globally and in regions like India.

ONCO-ANESTHESIOLOGY SPECIALTY

Onco-anesthesiology, an emerging subspecialty, addresses the perioperative care of cancer patients. With advancements in oncology and early cancer detection, increasing numbers of patients with cancer are undergoing surgical interventions. Providing perioperative care for these patients demands specialized knowledge of cancer biology, the effects of chemotherapeutic agents on the body, and how these factors influence anesthesia management and postoperative recovery. This subspecialty plays a crucial role in improving surgical outcomes for cancer patients.

Cancer surgery is often required for diagnostic, therapeutic, or palliative purposes. Over time, advancements in perioperative care have led to improved postoperative outcomes and the establishment of onco-anesthesiology as a distinct and essential specialty within anesthesiology.

SPECIFIC CONCERNS IN ONCO-SURGERIES

Onco-anesthesiology

The subspecialty of onco-anesthesiology focuses on managing the perioperative needs of critically ill cancer patients, addressing acute postoperative pain, and managing chronic cancer pain **(Fig. 1)**.

Evidence suggests that anesthesia drugs and techniques can influence oncological outcomes following cancer surgery. For instance, anesthetic methods may impact the perioperative risk of tumor spread and the activation of micrometastases.

Techniques such as total intravenous anesthesia (TIVA), which may exhibit anti-inflammatory effects, and inhalational anesthetics, which can be immunogenic, highlight the importance of anesthetic choices. Other options, including central neuraxial blocks (which block the adrenergic system), and adjuncts like non-steroidal anti-inflammatory drugs, opioids, and beta-adrenergic blockers, may also play a role in influencing outcomes.

A well-established onco-anesthesiology service can enhance recovery after cancer surgery, reduce treatment costs by minimizing intensive care and hospital stays, and alleviate patient suffering through multimodal pain management and palliative care techniques. Additionally,

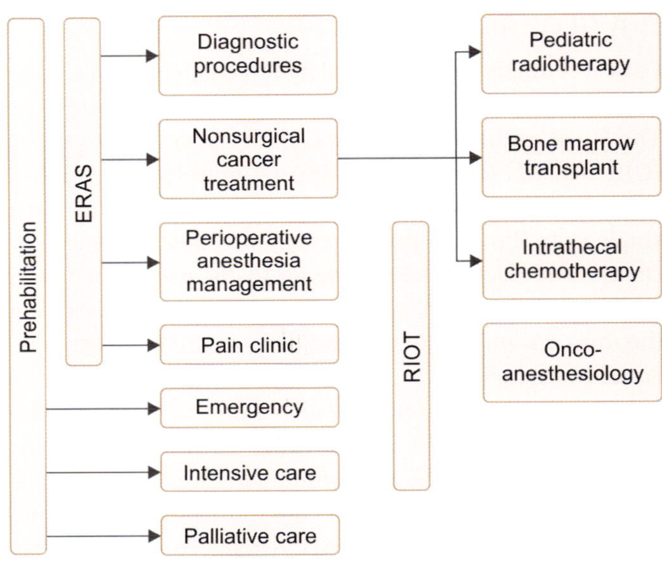

Fig. 1: The onco-anesthesiology. (ERAS: enhanced recovery after surgery; RIOT: return to intended oncological treatment)

it may contribute to improved disease-free survival and overall survival rates.

Postoperative complications can delay the return to intended oncological treatment (RIOT), adversely affecting survival. Therefore, the goal of perioperative management should be a comprehensive and holistic approach to patient care, aimed at optimizing surgical and oncological outcomes while minimizing the risks of locoregional recurrence and distant metastasis.

Patients Factors

Managing cancer patients presents unique challenges to perioperative physicians due to the intricate nature of their physiological disturbances. These complexities arise from the cancer itself, pre-existing medical conditions, the cumulative effects of chemotherapy or radiation on various organ systems, and the demands of extensive and often lengthy surgical procedures. Additionally, effective pain management in the postoperative period is crucial.

Pain may already be present before surgery due to the underlying disease, and many of these patients may be on preoperative opioids for pain relief. As a result, they often require higher-than-usual doses of opioids during and after surgery, which increases the risk of opioid-related adverse drug events (ORADEs). Moreover, cancer imposes a significant psychosocial burden, necessitating psychological support and counseling as an essential component of preoperative care.

Need for Onco-anesthesia and Onco-critical Care

Cancer surgeries demand dedicated perioperative physicians from the moment the decision to operate is made. Prehabilitation should commence at this stage, focusing on respiratory and physical training, nutritional optimization, emotional support, and counseling. Enhancing physical fitness, implementing respiratory exercises, and improving nutrition before surgery can significantly contribute to better perioperative outcomes. Strength and cardiovascular exercises improve physical capacity, which is vital for patients undergoing major resections and chemotherapy. Poor physical fitness correlates with higher rates of postoperative complications, morbidity, and mortality. Moreover, physical activity may also enhance oncological outcomes. Psychological and cognitive-behavioral interventions form essential components of prehabilitation, alongside medical optimization and nutritional support.

Nutritional therapy aims to restore adequate nutrient reserves before surgery, helping to mitigate the catabolic response associated with the surgical process. Malnutrition increases the risk of complications, infections, prolonged hospital stays, mortality, and readmission. Integrating preoperative nutritional support with exercise training has shown a reduction in postoperative stay, particularly in colorectal surgeries. To achieve optimal nutritional status preoperatively, it is crucial to begin interventions early.

The time available for prehabilitation, from cancer diagnosis to surgery, is often limited. Hence, systemic comorbidities, including cardio-respiratory optimization and preoperative anemia management, must be addressed promptly under the supervision of a perioperative physician.

Complex surgical procedures unique to oncology, such as cytoreductive surgery (CRS) combined with hyperthermic intraperitoneal chemotherapy (HIPEC), pressurized intraperitoneal aerosolized chemotherapy (PIPAC), and ischemic limb perfusion (ILP) with chemotherapeutic agents, require specialized perioperative management.[5] For example, CRS-HIPEC involves administering heated chemotherapeutic drugs into the abdomen via a specialized pump following tumor removal, while PIPAC delivers aerosolized chemotherapy into the abdominal cavity using a pneumoperitoneum.

Other challenging surgeries, such as head and neck cancer surgeries with or without microvascular free tissue transfer, extensive gynecological cancer surgeries, and cases involving the inferior vena cava thrombus or other major vessels, present unique anesthetic and surgical challenges. Onco-anesthesiologists managing such cases must employ advanced techniques, including hemodynamic monitoring, precise fluid management, core temperature regulation, coagulation assessment, and acid-base monitoring.

A dedicated onco-anesthesia team has been shown to improve outcomes in these complex cancer procedures. The enhanced recovery after surgery (ERAS) protocol has also demonstrated significant benefits in postoperative outcomes across various surgeries. Expanding the implementation of ERAS principles in cancer surgeries remains a critical focus of global research.[6]

CHEMOTHERAPY AND ITS IMPLICATIONS

Chemotherapeutic agents used in cancer treatment can cause a wide range of multisystem side effects, including severe toxicities and organ damage, which significantly influence perioperative management. Onco-anesthesiologists play a vital role in addressing these complications. Patients who have undergone chemotherapy require a comprehensive preoperative assessment and meticulous perioperative care.

Chemotherapy may be administered as neoadjuvant therapy before surgery, adjuvant therapy during or after surgery, or as palliative care to improve quality of life. Onco-anesthesiologists must possess a thorough understanding of the mechanisms of action, side effects, and toxicities of commonly used chemotherapeutic drugs.[7-9]

For example, bleomycin is known to cause subacute pulmonary damage that can progress to pulmonary fibrosis. During the perioperative period, high oxygen concentrations can exacerbate this condition. Therefore, patients with a history of bleomycin therapy should be ventilated with minimal oxygen concentrations, and the use of positive end-expiratory pressure (PEEP) may help reduce oxygen requirements.[7-9]

Anthracyclines such as doxorubicin and epirubicin directly affect cardiac myocytes and can lead to progressive drug-induced cardiomyopathy. It is essential to assess cardiac contractile function preoperatively in patients with a history of anthracycline use. Invasive cardiac monitoring may also be necessary during surgery for these individuals.[7-9]

Additionally, chemotherapeutic drugs frequently cause gastrointestinal toxicities, including nausea, vomiting, mucositis, and diarrhea. These patients benefit from preoperative hydration, and care must be taken during laryngoscopy to avoid mucosal injury and bleeding due to mucositis.[9]

UNDERSTANDING RADIOTHERAPY AND ITS IMPLICATIONS IN PERIOPERATIVE MANAGEMENT

Radiotherapy, often administered alongside or independently of chemotherapy, plays a significant role in cancer treatment. Perioperative anesthesiologists managing cancer surgeries must be aware that radiotherapy generates free oxygen radicals, which can lead to cellular damage. Radiation to the neck may cause skin induration and stiffness, potentially resulting in a challenging laryngoscopy and intubation.

Additionally, tissue damage caused by radiotherapy can impair postoperative wound healing. When combined with chemotherapy, radiotherapy increases the risk of complications such as myocarditis, pneumonitis, and pulmonary fibrosis.[10]

THROMBOSIS

Cancer patients face an elevated risk of venous thromboembolism (VTE), arterial thrombosis, and chronic disseminated intravascular coagulation. Cancer is a significant risk factor for VTE, alongside conditions such as obesity, prolonged immobilization, and hormone therapy. The risk of VTE increases substantially in obese cancer patients undergoing prolonged surgery and extended periods of inactivity. The incidence of VTE in cancer patients is approximately 0.5%, compared to 0.1% in those without cancer. Moreover, VTE is responsible for 20% of deaths in cancer patients, making it the second leading cause of mortality after cancer itself.[11]

Evidence from the Framingham Heart Study and the Global Anticoagulant Registry in the Field (GARFIELD)-VTE registry highlights that cancer-associated thrombosis (CAT) is linked to poorer survival rates among VTE patients.[11-13] Perioperative physicians and onco-anesthesiologists should be well-versed in the clinical implications, management, and treatment strategies for CAT.[11]

While the principles of managing CAT align with those for non-cancer-related VTE, the safety and efficacy of anticoagulant therapies differ between these groups. Cancer patients are at a higher risk of VTE recurrence (20.7% compared to 6.8% in non-cancer patients) and major bleeding complications (12.4% vs. 4.9% in non-cancer patients).[14]

AIRWAY MANAGEMENT

Head and neck cancer patients are often presumed to have a difficult airway due to the location and size of their tumors. Tumors that are fungating or bleeding, particularly those on the lips or cheeks, can complicate mask ventilation. Furthermore, prior neck radiation can cause restricted neck extension, making laryngoscopy and intubation challenging.

Anesthesiologists managing such cases must be adept at handling difficult airways and proficient in fiberoptic intubation techniques, especially for patients with oral cavity tumors or trismus. This expertise is essential to ensure safe and effective airway management in this high-risk population.[10]

ANESTHETIC TECHNIQUE AND CANCER RECURRENCE

Cancer patients frequently undergo elective surgical procedures for diagnostic, curative, or palliative purposes. During these surgeries, circulating tumor cells can be released and disseminated, potentially increasing the risk of metastasis and recurrence. Cancer surgery, along with perioperative stress, anesthetics, and analgesics, can alter immune surveillance mechanisms and host defenses, potentially creating a pro-tumorigenic microenvironment.

Volatile anesthetic agents have demonstrated significant immunosuppressive effects compared to intravenous agents such as propofol, which has been shown to inhibit cancer cell activity. Opioids, meanwhile, suppress natural killer (NK) cell function and inhibit T and B lymphocyte activity through both direct and indirect mechanisms.[15-23]

The choice of anesthesia, analgesia, and anesthetic techniques is recognized to influence cancer outcomes. Thoracic epidural analgesia, often used in thoracic and upper abdominal surgeries, offers superior pain control, opioid-sparing benefits, and reduced inflammatory and adrenergic responses to circulating catecholamines, thereby minimizing postoperative immunosuppression.[24-25]

Research indicates that volatile anesthetics and opioid analgesics may be associated with reduced disease-free and overall survival after cancer surgeries. Conversely, in CRS-HIPEC procedures for high-volume appendiceal tumors, the use of volatile anesthetics with opioids has been linked to longer survival compared to total intravenous anesthesia (TIVA).[5,26]

Recent randomized trials in breast cancer surgeries, as well as thoracic, abdominal, and colorectal cancer procedures, have not demonstrated significant advantages of epidural or regional anesthesia over general anesthesia.[27-29] However, ongoing randomized controlled trials are expected to provide further insights into the influence of anesthetic techniques on cancer recurrence and progression.

USES OF OPIOIDS

Opioids are commonly used for managing preoperative pain in cancer patients and as postsurgical analgesia following cancer surgeries. However, their widespread and routine use has been reevaluated, particularly after the opioid crisis was declared in the United States in 2017 due to the misuse of these drugs.[30,31] While opioids remain essential for effective cancer pain management, prolonged or unnecessary use can lead to ORADEs.

In India, the use of opioids for managing both cancer and non-cancer pain remains limited. Many physicians lack formal training in pain management, and insufficient awareness about opioid-related policies further impede their prescription. The absence of clear guidelines on perioperative opioid usage and stringent regulatory restrictions on the medical use of opioids are significant barriers to their prescription.

Despite being one of the largest global producers of opioids, India has not experienced the issues of overuse commonly seen elsewhere. In fact, opioid consumption in India for pain management, including end-of-life care, remains relatively low and does not present a significant public health burden.[32-34]

Opioid Free Anesthesia/Opioid-sparing Anesthesia

Opioid-free anesthesia (OFA) refers to the complete exclusion of opioids in any form—systemic, neuraxial, or intracavitary—during the perioperative period. In contrast, opioid-sparing anesthesia (OSA) allows for the use of limited intravenous opioids intraoperatively. OFA has been associated with a reduction in the incidence of ORADEs, potentially leading to improved postoperative outcomes and supporting enhanced recovery programs.[35-37]

Some studies and laboratory data suggest that opioids might contribute to cancer recurrence and metastasis. Therefore, onco-anesthesiologists, in their role as perioperative physicians, should be well-versed in OFA techniques. They can incorporate locoregional anesthesia and utilize non-opioid medications such as gabapentinoids, alpha-2 agonists, N-methyl-D-aspartate (NMDA) antagonists, beta-blockers, paracetamol, and non-steroidal anti-inflammatory drugs (NSAIDs) as part of a multimodal analgesia approach. When applied judiciously, multimodal analgesia that combines opioid analgesics with non-opioid and regional techniques can provide superior postoperative pain relief while minimizing ORADEs.[38-42]

MANAGEMENT OF ACUTE POSTOPERATIVE PAIN

Cancer patients are increasingly receiving surgical treatment, contributing to longer lifespans. As the population ages, many cancer survivors will require redo surgeries or reconstructive procedures. Cancer surgeries often involve extensive resections and prolonged procedures, which demand effective postoperative pain management to reduce complications, shorten hospital stays, and lower overall treatment costs.

Uncontrolled acute postoperative pain can result in persistent pain and mood disturbances. Moreover, inadequate pain management in the postoperative phase may activate the sympathetic nervous system, increase inflammatory cytokines, and potentially promote tumor growth and metastasis. Therefore, managing acute postoperative pain effectively could, in theory, lead to better long-term survival outcomes. This suggests that onco-anesthesiologists may play a role in influencing cancer-related outcomes.[43-47]

ONCO-CRITICAL CARE

As cancer treatments continue to advance, more patients are living with cancer, and many of these individuals will require critical care at some point in their lives. Onco-anesthesiologists must be trained to manage patients in an oncologic ICU, as critical care is an essential component of modern cancer care, both for surgical and non-surgical patients.

While the principles of critical care remain consistent for both cancer and non-cancer patients, cancer patients present unique challenges. Issues such as venous thromboembolism (VTE), tumor lysis syndrome, febrile neutropenia, pancytopenia, superior vena cava syndrome, and hypercalcemia are common in the cancer population and necessitate specialized expertise in oncological critical care. This requires not only a deep understanding of critical care but also knowledge of oncology and palliative medicine.[48]

COMMUNICATION SKILLS

Communication skills are both cognitive and emotional abilities that physicians use to help patients and their families understand the nature and severity of cancer, treatment options, and make informed decisions about care. Effective communication between patients, onco-anesthesiologists, onco-intensivists, and their families is crucial for managing care in both hospital and ICU settings. Evidence suggests that several factors contribute to improving communication, including—the patient-physician relationship, handling medical information effectively, managing patient and family emotions, system-level communication, and educational interventions for physicians, patients, and their families.[49]

Delivering bad news is one of the most studied communication tasks in cancer care. Throughout the diagnosis and treatment process, patients and their families often experience a range of emotions, from fear and shock to sadness and eventual acceptance of the diagnosis.[50] Many cancer centers have established protocols for delivering bad news, but while it is important for physicians to be straightforward in communicating the diagnosis, they must also be sensitive and empathetic in their approach.[51-53]

MANAGEMENT OF CHRONIC PAIN AND PALLIATIVE CARE

Pain, particularly severe pain, is one of the most feared and distressing symptoms of cancer, affecting between 53 and 64% of cancer patients, with almost one-third experiencing moderate-to-severe pain.[54] Cancer pain is often multifactorial, arising from factors such as nerve or bone compression by the tumor, side effects of anticancer treatments, cancer-related debility, prolapsed intervertebral discs, osteoarthritis, or psychological causes triggered by the diagnosis.[55] Chronic pain following oncological surgery is also common, particularly after procedures such as thoracotomy, breast surgery, limb amputation, radical nephrectomy, neck dissection, and inguinal lymph node dissection. Post-thoracotomy and post-mastectomy pain are particularly prevalent, leading to ongoing physical, psychological, and emotional distress for patients, often lasting months or even years after surgery. Onco-surgeons, onco-anesthesiologists, and pain specialists should educate patients about the potential for chronic postsurgical pain and discuss treatment options and management plans.[56]

In addition to surgery, radiotherapy can cause painful conditions such as plexopathies, myelopathies, peripheral nerve entrapments, and more often manifesting months or even years after treatment. Radiation-induced brachial plexopathy and lumbosacral plexopathy are common, with a delayed onset that can range from 6 months to 30 years after radiotherapy. Onco-anesthesiologists need to be aware of these conditions and should be trained in managing chronic cancer-related pain.[56]

Palliative care, which is the fourth pillar of oncology alongside medical, radiation, and surgical care, should be discussed with patients from the point of diagnosis.

Anesthesiologists play a key role in palliative care due to their expertise in medicine, anesthesia, sedation, and critical care. Integrating pain management and palliative care models requires that onco-anesthesiologists be well-versed in providing pain and palliative care to cancer patients.[57-61]

CAREER AND TRAINING IN ONCO-ANESTHESIOLOGY

Onco-anesthesiology is an emerging and rapidly growing specialty, offering diverse career opportunities. Many dedicated cancer centers and cancer wings within multispecialty hospitals now provide advanced training programs, including DM (Doctorate of Medicine) courses in onco-anesthesiology, as well as 2 years fellowships in onco-anesthesiology, pain management, palliative care, and perioperative medicine. The Society of Onco-Anesthesiology and Perioperative Care (SOAPC) offers a fellowship in onco-anesthesia and perioperative medicine.

Professionally trained onco-anesthesiologists have a wide range of job opportunities, including roles in dedicated cancer centers, national cancer centers, and hospitals affiliated with the National Cancer Grid. This expanding field underscores the growing recognition of the importance of specialized anesthetic and perioperative care in oncology.

CONCLUSION

In conclusion, onco-anesthesiology is a fast-growing specialty, driven by the increasing global burden of cancer. With approximately 19.3 million new cancer cases and nearly 10 million cancer-related deaths reported annually worldwide, advancements in diagnostic modalities and early detection have led to a significant rise in cancer diagnoses. This has resulted in more patients requiring cancer-specific surgeries and interventions. There is a growing need for trained onco-anesthesiologists, not only in the field of onco-anesthesiology but also in onco-critical care, acute and chronic cancer pain management, and palliative medicine, to provide comprehensive care for this expanding patient population.

REFERENCES

1. Sung H, Ferlay J, Siegel RL, Laversanne M, Soerjomataram I, Jemal A, et al. Global Cancer Statistics 2020: GLOBOCAN Estimates of Incidence and Mortality Worldwide for 36 Cancers in 185 Countries. CA Cancer J Clin. 2021;71(3):209-49.
2. Brenner DR, Carbonell C, O'Sullivan DE, Ruan Y, Basmadjian RB, Bu V, et al. Exploring the Future of Cancer Impact in Alberta: Projections and Trends 2020-2040. Curr Oncol. 2023;30(11):9981-95.
3. Mehrotra R, Yadav K. Breast cancer in India: Present scenario and the challenges ahead. World J Clin Oncol. 2022;13(3):209-18.
4. Gallaway MS, Henley SJ, Steele CB, Momin B, Thomas CC, Jamal A, et al. Surveillance for Cancers Associated with Tobacco Use - United States, 2010-2014. MMWR Surveill Summ. 2018;67(12):1-42.
5. Bray F, Jemal A, Grey N, Ferlay J, Forman D. Global cancer transitions according to the human development index (2008–2030): a population-based study. Lancet Oncol. 2012;13:790-801.
6. Thota RS, Garg R, Ramkiran S, Divatia JV. Onco-anaesthesiology as an emerging sub-specialty domain: Need of the hour! Indian J Anaesth. 2020;64:69-71.
7. Ahmad A, Ormiston-Smith N, Sasieni P. Trends in the lifetime risk of developing cancer in Great Britain: Comparison of risk for those born from 1930 to 1960. Br J Cancer. 2015;112:943-7.
8. Wigmore T, Gottumukkala V, Riedel B. Making the Case for the Subspecialty of Onco-Anesthesia. Int Anesthesiol Clin. 2016;54:19-28.
9. Solanki SL, Mukherjee S, Agarwal V, Thota RS, Balakrishnan K, Shah SB, et al. Society of Onco-Anaesthesia and Perioperative Care consensus guidelines for perioperative management of patients for cytoreductive surgery and hyperthermic intraperitoneal chemotherapy (CRS-HIPEC). Indian J Anaesth. 2019;63:972-87.
10. Bugada D, Bellini V, Fanelli A, Marchesini M, Compagnone C, Baciarello M, et al. Future perspectives of ERAS: A narrative review on the new applications of an established approach. Surg Res Pract. 2016;2016:3561249.
11. Ewer M, Benjamin R. Perry M. Cardiotoxicity of Chemotherapeutic Drugs, The Chemotherapy Source Book. London: Williams and Wilkins; 1996. pp. 649-59.
12. Pinder MC, Duan Z, Goodwin JS, Hortobagyi GN, Giordano SH. Congestive heart failure in older women treated with adjuvant anthracycline chemotherapy for breast cancer. J Clin Oncol. 2007;25:3808-15.
13. van der Pal HJ, van Dalen EC, Hauptmann M, Kok WE, Caron HN, van den Bos C, et al. Cardiac function in 5-year survivors of childhood cancer: a long-term follow-up study. Arch Intern Med. 2010;170:1247-55.
14. Gudaitytė J, Dvylys D, Šimeliūnaitė I. Anaesthetic challenges in cancer patients: current therapies and pain management. Acta Med Litu. 2017;24:121-7.
15. Fernandes CJ, Morinaga LTK, Alves JL Jr, Castro MA, Calderaro D, Jardim CVP, et al. Cancer-associated thrombosis: the when, how and why. Eur Respir Rev. 2019; 28:180119.

16. Puurunen MK, Gona PN, Larson MG, Murabito JM, Magnani JW, O'Donnell CJ. Epidemiology of venous thromboembolism in the Framingham Heart Study. Thromb Res. 2016;145:27-33.
17. Ageno W, Farjat A, Haas S, Weitz JI, Goldhaber SZ, Turpie AGG, et al. Provoked versus unprovoked venous thromboembolism: Findings from GARFIELD-VTE. Res Pract Thromb Haemost. 2021;5:326-41.
18. Prandoni P, Lensing AW, Piccioli A, Bernardi E, Simioni P, Girolami B, et al. Recurrent venous thromboembolism and bleeding complications during anticoagulant treatment in patients with cancer and venous thrombosis. Blood. 2002;100:3484-8.
19. Dunn GP, Old LJ, Schreiber RD. The Immunobiology of Cancer Immunosurveillance and Immunoediting. Immunity. 2004;21:137-48.
20. Tavare AN, Perry NJ, Benzonana LL, Takata M, Ma D. Cancer recurrence after surgery: direct and indirect effects of anesthetic agents. Int J Cancer. 2012;130:1237-50.
21. Tsuchiya Y, Sawada S, Yoshioka I, Ohashi Y, Matsuo M, Harimaya Y, et al. Increased surgical stress promotes tumor metastasis. Surgery. 2003;133:547-55.
22. Boomsma MF, Garssen B, Slot E, Berbee M, Berkhof J, Meezenbroek Ede J, et al. Breast cancer surgery-induced immunomodulation. J Surg Oncol. 2010;102:640-8.
23. Camara O, Kavallaris A, Nöschel H, Rengsberger M, Jörke C, Pachmann K. Seeding of epithelial cells into circulation during surgery for breast cancer: the fate of malignant and benign mobilized cells. World J Surg Oncol. 2006;4:67.
24. Divatia JV, Ambulkar R. Anesthesia and cancer recurrence: What is the evidence? J Anaesthesiol. Clin Pharmacol. 2014;30:147-50.
25. Heaney A, Buggy DJ. Can Anaesthetic and analgesic techniques affect cancer recurrence or metastasis? British J Anaesth. 2012;109(S1):I17-28.
26. Melamed R, Bar-Yosef S, Shakhar G, Shakhar K, Ben-Eliyahu S. Suppression of natural killer cell activity and promotion of tumor metastasis by ketamine, thiopental, and halothane, but not by propofol: mediating mechanisms and prophylactic measures. Anesth Analg. 2003;97:1331-9.
27. Mammoto T, Mukai M, Mammoto A, Yamanaka Y, Hayashi Y, Mashimo T, et al. Intravenous anesthetic, propofol inhibits invasion of cancer cells. Cancer Lett. 2002;184:165-70.
28. Wigmore TJ, Mohammed K, Jhanji S. Long-term survival for patients undergoing volatile versus IV anesthesia for cancer surgery: A retrospective analysis. Anesthesiology 2016;124:69-79.
29. Wu ZF, Lee MS, Wong CS, Lu CH, Huang YS, Lin KT, et al. Propofol-based total intravenous anesthesia is associated with better survival than desflurane anesthesia in colon cancer surgery. Anesthesiology. 2018;129:932-41.
30. Cata JP, Nguyen LT, Ifeanyi-Pillette IC, Van Meter A, Dangler LA, Feng L, et al. An assessment of the survival impact of multimodal anesthesia/analgesia technique in adults undergoing cytoreductive surgery with hyperthermic intraperitoneal chemotherapy: A propensity score matched analysis. Int J Hyperthermia. 2019;36:369-75.
31. Sessler DI, Pei L, Huang Y, Fleischmann E, Marhofer P, Kurz A, et al; Breast Cancer Recurrence Collaboration. Recurrence of breast cancer after regional or general anaesthesia: a randomised controlled trial. Lancet. 2019;394:1807-15.
32. Du YT, Li YW, Zhao BJ, Guo XY, Feng Y, Zuo MZ, et al; Peking University Clinical Research Program Study Group. Long-term Survival after Combined Epidural-General Anesthesia or General Anesthesia Alone: Follow-up of a Randomized Trial. Anesthesiology. 2021;135:233-45.
33. Falk W, Magnuson A, Eintrei C, Henningsson R, Myrelid P, Matthiessen P, et al. Comparison between epidural and intravenous analgesia effects on disease-free survival after colorectal cancer surgery: a randomised multicentre controlled trial. Br J Anaesth. 2021;127:65-74.
34. Platt S, Raedle J. The opioid crisis in the USA: a public health emergency. Lancet. 2017;390:2016.
35. Shen C, Thornton JD, Gu D, Dodge D, Zhou S, He W, et al. Prolonged Opioid Use After Surgery for Early-Stage Breast Cancer. Oncologist. 2020;25:e1574-82.
36. Thota RS, Jain P, Bakshi SG, Dhanve CN. Opioid-prescribing Practices in Chronic Cancer Pain in a Tertiary Care Pain Clinic. Indian J Palliat Care. 2011;17:222-6.
37. Choudhary N, Sahi MS. A Cross-Sectional Web-Based Survey of Medical Practitioners in India to Assess their Knowledge, Attitude, Prescription Practices, and Barriers toward Opioid Analgesic Prescriptions. Indian J Palliat Care. 2019;25:567-74.
38. Cleary J, Simha N, Panieri A, Scholten W, Radbruch L, Torode J, et al. Formulary availability and regulatory barriers to accessibility of opioids for cancer pain in India: a report from the Global Opioid Policy Initiative (GOPI). Ann Oncol. 2013;24 Suppl11:xi33-40.
39. Kamdar NV, Hoftman N, Rahman S, Cannesson M. Opioid-free analgesia in the era of enhanced recovery after surgery and the surgical home: implications for postoperative outcomes and population health. Anesth Analg. 2017;125:1089-91.
40. White PF. What are the advantages of nonopioid analgesic techniques in the management of acute and chronic pain? Expert Opin Pharmacother. 2017;18:329-33.
41. Piegeler T, Hollmann MW, Borgeat A, Lirk P. Do amide local anesthetics play a therapeutic role in the perioperative management of cancer patients? Int Anesthesiol Clin. 2016;54:e17-32.
42. Siu EY, Moon TS. Opioid-free and opioid-sparing anesthesia. Int Anesthesiol Clin. 2020;58(2):34-41.
43. Elkassabany NM, Mariano ER. Opioid-free anaesthesia–what would Inigo Montoya say? Anaesthesia. 2019;74:560-3.
44. Kumar K, Kirksey MA, Duong S, Wu CL. A review of opioid-sparing modalities in perioperative pain management: methods to decrease opioid use postoperatively. Anesth Analg. 2017;125:1749-60.

45. Thota RS, Ramkiran S, Garg R, Goswami J, Baxi V, Thomas M. Opioid free onco-anesthesia: Is it time to convict opioids? A systematic review of literature. J Anaesthesiol Clin Pharmacol. 2019;35:441-52.
46. Veyckemans F. Opioid-free anaesthesia: Still a debate? Eur J Anaesthesiol. 2019;36:245-6.
47. Cata JP, Corrales G, Speer B, Owusu-Agyemang P. Postoperative acute pain challenges in patients with cancer. Best Pract Res Clin Anaesthesiol. 2019;33:361-71.
48. Peters CL, Shirley B, Erickson J. The effect of a new multimodal perioperative anesthetic regimen on postoperative pain, side effects, rehabilitation, and length of hospital stay after total joint arthroplasty. J Arthroplast. 2006;21:132-8.
49. Caumo W, Broenstrub JC, Fialho L, Petry SM, Brathwait O, Bandeira D, et al. Risk factors for postoperative anxiety in children. Acta Anaesthesiol Scand. 2000;44:782-9.
50. Cata JP, Bauer M, Sokari T, Ramirez MF, Mason D, Plautz G, et al. Effects of surgery, general anesthesia, and perioperative epidural analgesia on the immune function of patients with non-small cell lung cancer. J Clin Anesth. 2013;25:255-62.
51. Missair A, Cata JP, Votta-Velis G, Johnson M, Borgeat A, Tiouririne M, et al. Impact of perioperative pain management on cancer recurrence: an ASRA/ESRA special article. Reg Anesth Pain Med. 2019;44:13-28.
52. Shimabukuro-Vornhagen A, Böll B, Kochanek M. Critical care of patients with cancer. CA Cancer J Clin. 2016;66:496-517.
53. Back A. Patient-physician communication in oncology: what does the evidence show? Oncology (Williston Park). 2006;20:67-74; discussion 77-8, 83.
54. Butow PN, Kazemi JN, Beeney LJ, Griffin AM, Dunn SM, Tattersall MH. When the diagnosis is cancer: Patient communication experiences and preferences. Cancer. 1996;77:2630-7.
55. Baile WF, Buckman R, Lenzi R, Glober G, Beale EA, Kudelka AP. SPIKES-A six-step protocol for delivering bad news: Application to the patient with cancer. Oncologist. 2000;5:302-11.
56. Girgis A, Sanson-Fisher RW. Breaking bad news. 1: Current best advice for clinicians. Behav Med.2000;24:53-9.
57. Wenrich MD, Curtis JR, Shannon SE, Carline JD, Ambrozy DM, Ramsey PG. Communicating with dying patients within the spectrum of medical care from terminal diagnosis to death. Arch Intern Med. 2001;161:868-74.
58. van den Beuken-van Everdingen MH, de Rijke JM, Kessels AG, Schouten HC, van Kleef M, Patijn J. Prevalence of pain in patients with cancer: a systematic review of the past 40 years. Ann Oncol. 2007;18:1437-49.
59. Bhatnagar S, Gupta M. Integrated pain and palliative medicine model. Ann Palliat Med. 2016;5:196-208.
60. Levy MH, Chwistek M, Mehta RS. Management of chronic pain in cancer survivors. Cancer J. 2008;14:401-9.
61. Jain P, Balkrishanan K, Nayak S, Gupta N, Shah S. Onco-Anaesthesiology and palliative medicine: Opportunities and challenges. Indian J Anaesth. 2021;65:29-34.

CHAPTER 2

Systemic Effects of Cancer Therapy

Laboni Sarkar, Mounika Yallala, Manju Sengar

INTRODUCTION

Significant advances have been made in treatment of cancer to optimize the disease control or cure rates. The type and sequence of cancer therapy may vary widely depending on the type of cancer, stage, and host characteristics. It includes modalities for local disease control such as surgery and radiotherapy, and systemic therapy such as chemotherapy, targeted therapy, hormonal therapy, and immunotherapy including cellular therapy. Due to the limitations of conventional chemotherapy including broad-spectrum toxicities and development of resistance, there has been a shift in recent decades toward personalized therapy specific to genetic and molecular characteristics of the tumor type.[1] Compared to conventional chemotherapy, these targeted agents have improved outcomes in specific cancer subtypes and have different toxicity profiles. Toxicities may be class-mediated, specific to the individual drugs or classes of drugs, and non-specific, due to cytotoxic effects on normal cells undergoing division.[2] These may range from mild toxicities to potentially life-threatening conditions.

PATHOPHYSIOLOGY OF TOXICITY

- *Chemotherapy:* In addition to effects on cancer cells, these agents also target rapidly dividing cells, interfering with the normal cell cycle process and resulting in non-specific side effects, such as myelosuppression, mucositis, and alopecia. Additionally, class-specific toxicities include ifosfamide-induced hemorrhagic cystitis[3] and anthracycline-mediated cardiotoxicity.[4]
- *Immunotherapy:* These agents alter immunological homeostasis, affecting both cancer cells and normal cells by a combination of pathways involving autoreactive T cells, autoantibodies, and cytokines which can trigger immune-related adverse events (iRAEs).
- *Targeted therapy:* These include agents active against various targets such as vascular endothelial growth factor (VEGF) receptors (bevacizumab, lenvatinib, sunitinib, and sorafenib), epidermal growth factor receptor (EGFR) receptor (cetuximab, panitumumab, gefitinib, and erlotinib), and human epidermal growth factor receptor 2 (HER 2) receptors (trastuzumab and lapatinib). By various mechanisms including off-target effects on healthy cells, metabolic disruption, vascular effects, and toxic metabolites, these agents can lead to a wide spectrum of side effects.[5]
- *Cellular therapy:* This rapidly evolving field includes stem cell therapy, chimeric antigen receptor (CAR) T-cell therapy, tumor-infiltrating lymphocytes (TIL cells), therapies derived from other cell lines (such as antigen presenting cell/dendritic cells). These therapies activate tumor-reactive T cells, leading to response in tumor tissues, however immune-mediated adverse events may also result, ranging in severity from mild to potentially life-threatening.[6]

A system-wise approach to identifying and managing commonly encountered toxicities of anticancer therapy in the practice of critical care is enumerated below.

- Cardiotoxicity
- Pulmonary toxicity
- Neurological toxicity
- Gastrointestinal toxicity
- Renal toxicity
- Myelosuppression
- Cutaneous toxicity
- Endocrine toxicity
- Systemic Inflammatory Response Syndrome
- Long-term toxicities

CARDIOTOXICITY

Causative Agents and Mechanism of Toxicity

Various classes of systemic anticancer agents have varying mechanisms of cardiotoxicity, although management strategies are broadly similar[7] **(Table 1)**.

TABLE 1: Classes of potentially cardiotoxic systemic anti-cancer therapy and mechanisms of action.	
Class of therapeutic agent	***Mechanism of cardiotoxicity***
Anthracyclines (e.g., doxorubicin)	• Type I cardiomyopathy • Free radical formation • Interference with topoisomerase II leading to DNA damage • Dose dependent • Permanent and irreversible
Anti-HER 2 (human epidermal growth factor receptor 2) therapy (e.g., trastuzumab)	• Type II cardiomyopathy • Inhibition of Erbb signaling • Reversible
Alkylating agents (e.g., cyclophosphamide)	Formation of toxic metabolites affecting cardiac tissues
Antimetabolites (e.g., 5-fluorouracil)	Coronary vasospasm and endothelial dysfunction
Taxanes (e.g., paclitaxel)	Mitochondrial dysfunction leading to myocardial damage
Platinum-based drugs (e.g., cisplatin)	Direct damage to myocardial cells
Vinca alkaloids (e.g., vincristine)	Peripheral neuropathy with autonomic dysfunction
Etoposide	Induction of apoptosis in cardiac cells
Immune checkpoint inhibitors	Autoimmune-mediated myocarditis
Arsenic trioxide	QTc prolongation and arrhythmias

Clinical Presentation

- *Conventional chemotherapy:* Cardiotoxicity is a dose-limiting adverse effect of *anthracycline* therapy. Acute cardiotoxicity occurs within 1 week of cancer therapy, while that which develops thereafter is labeled as chronic cardiotoxicity. Acute anthracycline-related cardiotoxicity is rare, impacting <5% of patients. The clinical presentation includes electrocardiogram (ECG) changes and arrhythmias, ranging from sinus tachycardia to supraventricular tachycardia, heart block, and ventricular arrhythmias, leading to palpitations, syncope, and even cardiac arrest. Acute declines in cardiac function can be seen, resulting in signs and symptoms of heart failure. Additionally, some patients develop pericarditis, with chest pain and shortness of breath.[8]

  5-FU-induced or capecitabine-induced cardiotoxicity results from coronary vasospasm leading to myocardial ischemia and angina. In addition, arrhythmias including bradycardia or ventricular arrhythmias may result. An increased risk of thromboembolism has also been observed.[9]

  Cyclophosphamide is classically associated with myocarditis, particularly at doses >270 mg/kg for 1–4 days or doses of $\geq$1.55 g/m^2, typically used in conditioning regimens for stem cell transplant, are considered to be associated with a substantial risk of cardiotoxicity.[10] This may present as tachyarrhythmias with heart failure in more advanced stages.
- *Targeted therapies:* Studies revealed an incidence of trastuzumab-related cardiotoxicity of 15–20% and of heart failure (HF) of <5%.[11] Importantly, in contrast to anthracycline-related cardiac damage, cardiotoxicity due to trastuzumab is reversible.[12] Other HER2-directed therapies, such as lapatinib, pertuzumab, and trastuzumab-emtansine, are associated with a lower risk of cardiotoxicity than trastuzumab.

  Other cardiovascular side effects involve various mechanisms, such as vascular effects resulting from action against the VEGF receptor, electrophysiological effects by prolonging QT interval and metabolic disruption of cardiomyocytes.[7] The clinical presentation includes:
  - *Hypertension:* Sunitinib, sorafenib, lenvatinib, bevacizumab, and ramucirumab.
  - *Thromboembolic events:* Bevacizumab, lenalidomide, ponatinib, and nilotinib
  - *Heart failure:* Carfilzomib, sunitinib, and ponatinib
  - *Arrhythmias:* Ibrutinib
- *Immunotherapy:* Cytotoxic T-lymphocyte–associated antigen 4 (*CTLA4) inhibitors (such as ipilimumab, tremelimumab)* are generally associated with higher incidence of immune-related adverse events, with the highest risk (>50%) with *combined CTLA4 and programmed death ligand 1 (PDL1) inhibition (e.g., nivolumab-ipilimumab)*. The clinical presentation includes myocarditis, associated with the highest mortality (up to 40%), presenting as decompensated

HF, cardiogenic shock, and sudden cardiac death.[13] ECG changes noted include various forms of conduction block, ventricular ectopy, and ventricular tachycardia (VT), and elevation of circulating cTn levels. Cardiac biomarkers such as circulating brain natriuretic peptide (BNP) and amino-terminal pro-BNP levels are useful in the diagnosis of myocarditis.

Risk Factors[7]

- Age
- Comorbidities, including diabetes, hypertension and pre-existing cardiovascular disease
- Higher cumulative dose
- Concomitant cardiotoxic therapy (such as anthracyclines with trastuzumab)
- Renal insufficiency
- Prolonged infusion rate [e.g., continuous administration of 5-FU (over 2 days) than with bolus infusion (over 3 hours)]

Prevention

According to most standard guidelines, all patients should undergo a baseline assessment of cardiac function before starting any potentially cardiotoxic therapy, including echocardiography (3D echocardiography or 2D contrast echocardiography), with estimation of global longitudinal strain (GLS), and cardiac troponin levels.[14]

Monitoring and Treatment

Diagnosis involves the use of ECG, imaging modalities such as echocardiography, cardiac magnetic resonance imaging (MRI), and computed tomography (CT) coronary angiography, and cardiac biomarkers such as troponins and natriuretic peptides. Management includes drug interruption, the use of cardioprotective agents [e.g., beta blockers, angiotensin-converting enzyme (ACE) inhibitors, angiotensin receptor blockers, and statins] based on clinical judgment, dexrazoxane for anthracycline-mediated cardiotoxicity, and interventions such as angioplasty when indicated.[7] Implantable cardioverter-defibrillator (ICD) placement is indicated for the primary prevention of arrhythmias and sudden cardiac death in patients and survivors with reduced left ventricular (LV) function.[15] For 5-FU mediated vasospasm, calcium-channel blockers (e.g., diltiazem or long-acting and nifedipine) are efficacious. For immunotherapy-mediated cardiotoxicity, immunosuppressive therapies including steroids and other immunosuppressants such as mycophenolate mofetil, infliximab, and antithymocyte globulin based on severity have been recommended for all acutely life-threatening scenarios.[13]

PULMONARY TOXICITY

Causative Agents and Mechanism

Etiology and mechanism of pulmonary toxicity due to chemotherapeutic agents are enumerated in **Table 2.**[16] Targeted and immunotherapeutic agents implicated in pulmonary toxicity are detailed in **Table 3.**[17,18]

Clinical Presentation

Clinical presentation may vary in severity, ranging from mild impairment in effort tolerance to severe symptoms, including dyspnea, hypoxemia and respiratory failure requiring intensive care and mechanical ventilation. Symptoms include cough, chest pain, fever, and shortness of breath.

Risk Factors[16-18]

- High cumulative dose (bleomycin >400 mu/m^2)
- *Pre-existing lung disease:* Chronic obstructive pulmonary disease (COPD), interstitial lung disease (ILD), bronchial asthma, bronchiectasis, history of pulmonary tuberculosis, prior radiation to chest, previous lung resection, and concomitant fungal infection.
- Concomitant radiation therapy
- *Older age:* >50 years

Prevention

Careful selection of patients for therapy with potential for pulmonary toxicity. This may be done by risk assessment (history of smoking, obstructive airway disease, and prior chest irradiation), evaluation of effort tolerance, and pulmonary function tests if indicated for agents such as bleomycin.

Patients with prior bleomycin exposure need to be flagged during preoperative work-up to avoid exposure to high oxygen concentration which can exacerbate the pulmonary toxicity.

Management

Diagnostic evaluation includes imaging modalities such as CT chest, bronchoscopy, and bronchoalveolar lavage.

TABLE 2: Chemotherapy-related pulmonary toxicities.

Manifestation	***Drugs***	***Mechanism***	***Imaging and other features***	***Differentiation from other causes***
Interstitial pneumonitis	Bleomycin, methotrexate, cyclophosphamide, carmustine, gemcitabine, paclitaxel, and docetaxel	Oxidative stress, direct cytotoxicity, inflammation, and immune response	• Ground-glass opacities, reticular patterns on HRCT • Consider recent history of chemotherapy	• Rule out infections (negative cultures) • No evidence of cardiac dysfunction on echocardiography
Pulmonary fibrosis	Bleomycin, methotrexate, busulfan, paclitaxel, and docetaxel	Chronic inflammation—fibroblast activation and collagen deposition	Honeycombing, reticular opacities on HRCT chest	• Chronicity and progressive nature • Lack of acute infectious signs • Exclude other fibrotic lung diseases (e.g., IPF)
Non-cardiogenic pulmonary edema	Gemcitabine and cytarabine	Capillary leak syndrome—increased pulmonary capillary permeability	Bilateral pulmonary infiltrates on imaging	• No signs of left ventricular dysfunction • Normal BNP levels • Absence of volume overload on physical examination
Hypersensitivity pneumonitis	Methotrexate, bleomycin, paclitaxel, and docetaxel	Immune-mediated response—inflammatory infiltrates in alveoli and interstitium	• *Imaging:* Ground-glass opacities, nodular infiltrates • *Bronchoalveolar lavage:* Lymphocytosis—temporal association with drug exposure	• Temporal association with drug exposure • Exclude infections (negative cultures) • Improvement after drug discontinuation
Pulmonary hemorrhage	High dose cyclophosphamide	• Endothelial damage • Capillary leak—coagulopathy	Diffuse alveolar hemorrhage pattern on HRCT	• Rule out infectious causes (negative cultures) • Coagulation profile • Bronchoscopy may be needed to confirm diagnosis

(BNP: brain natriuretic peptide; HRCT: high-resolution computed tomography; IPF: idiopathic pulmonary fibrosis)

TABLE 3: Targeted agents and immunotherapy causing pulmonary toxicity.

Class	***Drugs***	***Pulmonary toxicity***
EGFR inhibitors	Erlotinib, afatinib, gefitinib, and osimertinib	ILD and pneumonitis
VEGF inhibitors	Bevacizumab, sorafenib, sunitinib, and axitinib	Pulmonary hemorrhage, hypertension-related pulmonary edema, and thromboembolism
ALK inhibitors	Crizotinib, certinib, and alectinib	ILD and pneumonitis
mTOR inhibitors	Everolimus and temsirolimus	ILD and pneumonitis
BRAF inhibitors	Vemurafenib and dabrafenib	Pneumonitis and sarcoid-like reactions
Immunotherapy	• CTLA4 inhibitors (ipilimumab) • PD1 inhibitors (nivolumab, pembrolizumab) • PDL1 inhibitors (durvalumab, atezolizumab)	• Organizing pneumonitis (65%) Non-specific interstitial pneumonitis (15%) • Hypersensitivity pneumonitis (10%)

(CTLA4: cytotoxic T-lymphocyte–associated antigen 4; EGFR: epidermal growth factor receptor; ILD: interstitial lung disease; mTOR: mammalian target of rapamycin; PDL1: programmed cell death ligand 1; VEGF: vascular endothelial growth factor)

- *General Principles of Treatment*[18,19]
  - *Early identification:* Regular monitoring of symptoms and pulmonary function tests during chemotherapy.
  - *Prompt discontinuation:* Stop the offending chemotherapeutic agent immediately upon suspicion of pulmonary toxicity.
  - *Corticosteroids:* Mainstay of treatment for most inflammatory pulmonary complications in the early phase. However, this may not be helpful in bleomycin related toxicity.
    - *Grade 1-2:* Oral pulse dose of prednisolone 1 mg/kg/day for 5–7 days followed by maintenance for 8–12 weeks
    - *Grade 3-4:* Intravenous methylprednisolone 1 g/day follow followed by maintenance for 8–12 weeks
    - Repeat HRCT lung—after 4–6 weeks of oral steroid maintenance in case of mild toxicity and after 8–12 weeks of oral steroid maintenance in case of moderate-severe ILD
  - *Supportive care:* Ensure adequate oxygenation, consider mechanical ventilation for severe respiratory distress, and employ pulmonary rehabilitation for chronic conditions.
  - *Multidisciplinary approach:* Involve pulmonologists, oncologists, and critical care specialists for comprehensive management.
- *Specific management strategies:*
  - *Bleomycin:* Provide supplemental oxygen to maintain adequate oxygenation, but avoid high concentrations of oxygen to reduce the risk of exacerbating lung injury
    - *Mechanical ventilation:* In severe cases, consider non-invasive strategies [e.g., low tidal volume, high positive end-expiratory pressure (PEEP)].
  - *Immunotherapy:* Management is done as per the Common Terminology Criteria for Adverse Events (CTCAE) grading. High dose corticosteroids are the first-line treatment. Immunosuppressive drugs such as infliximab [anti-tumor necrosis factor-α (TNF-α)], mycophenolate mofetil, and cyclophosphamide are considered if there is no improvement with steroids. Case studies indicate higher mortality rate due to infections such as sepsis in patients treated with anti-TNF drugs. Pneumocystis prophylaxis is to be considered during long-term immunosuppression to avoid secondary infection and worsening of compromised lung function.

NEUROTOXICITY

Causative Agents and Mechanism

Neurotoxicity resulting from anticancer therapy may occur due to various mechanisms, either direct effects on the nervous system or indirectly from drug-related metabolic alterations, vascular pathology, or immune-mediated damage.

Neurologic syndromes described with the use of anticancer therapy are as follows:

- *Peripheral neuropathy:*[20]
  - Oxaliplatin (acute dysesthesia and/or paresthesias presenting as cold-induced involuntary muscle contractions in limbs and jaw, or cumulative distal sensory neuropathy)
  - Cisplatin (predominantly sensory peripheral neuropathy, typically only after a cumulative dose of 300 mg/m^2)
  - Taxanes (paclitaxel, docetaxel—predominantly sensory neuropathy, taxane acute pain syndrome)
  - Vincristine (peripheral sensory neuropathy and autonomic neuropathy)
  - Thalidomide (peripheral predominantly sensory neuropathy)
  - Proteasome inhibitor (bortezomib—predominantly sensory neuropathy
  - Eribulin (sensory or motor neuropathy, polyneuropathy, and paresthesias)
- *Aseptic meningitis* after intrathecal chemotherapy (cytarabine, methotrexate, and thiotepa, topotecan)[21]
- *Encephalopathy*
  - *Ifosfamide-induced encephalopathy:*[21] It can manifest between hours to days after the start of infusion. Metabolism of ifosfamide leads to formation of active metabolites, including chloroacetaldehyde and acrolein which are neurotoxic.
  - *Methotrexate:*[21] High doses, particularly when given intrathecally, can lead to encephalopathy. Symptoms appear approximately 2–14 days after drug administration, may last up to 72 hours, and usually spontaneously resolve without sequelae.
  - *Drugs causing posterior reversible encephalopathy syndrome (PRES):* Causative agents include cyclosporine, tacrolimus, cyclophosphamide,

bevacizumab, and sunitinib. Blood pressure rises so rapidly that the autoregulation of blood flow is lost, leading to excessive blood flow which damages the blood brain barrier.[22] As a consequence, blood can leak into interstitium causing cerebral edema.
    - *Immune effector-cell associated neurotoxicity syndrome (ICANS):* Caused by immunotherapy, typically with chimeric antigen receptor-T (CAR-T) cell therapy, and is further elaborated in the section on immunotherapy-related toxicity.[23]
- *Cerebellar dysfunction/ataxia:*[21] Most common agent is high dose cytarabine, usually cumulative doses >36 g/m^2 secondary to loss of Purkinje cells in cerebellum. Procarbazine, 5-fluorouracil, and capecitabine may also lead to cerebellar toxicity.
- *Cerebrovascular disease:*[21]
    - *L-asparaginase:* It may lead to venous sinus thrombosis, presenting as headache or seizures or neurological deficit.
    - Cyclosporine, methotrexate, doxorubicin, and platinum agents may also lead to cerebrovascular events.
    - Bevacizumab may increase the risk of cerebrovascular thrombosis as well as intracranial hemorrhage.
    - Tamoxifen
- *Pseudotumor cerebri:* All-trans-retinoic acid, bevacizumab, and steroids

Clinical Presentation

Symptoms depend on the mechanism of neurotoxicity. Peripheral neuropathy may be sensory (numbness or paresthesias), motor (limb weakness, difficulty in coordination, or balance) or autonomic (variations in blood pressure or heart rate). Encephalopathy usually presents as somnolence, confusion, disorientation, and seizures. Meningitis results in headache, vomiting, or seizures.

Risk Factors

Pre-existing neuropathy due to diabetes mellitus, nutritional deficiencies, and high cumulative doses is a risk factor for peripheral neuropathy.

Precipitating factors for ifosfamide encephalopathy are as follows:[24]

- Serum albumin level <3.5 g/dL
- Renal dysfunction
- Hyponatremia
- Cumulative dose
- Previous central nervous system (CNS) disorders
- Concurrent use of aprepitant
- Previous treatment with cisplatin
- Dehydration and hypovolemia

Prevention

In patients who are at risk of developing the toxicities, dose modification and management of reversible factors are important.

Monitoring and Treatment

In most cases the diagnosis is based on the clinical examination and temporal course. In some cases, nerve conduction studies and electromyography for peripheral neuropathy may be needed to confirm. For patients with CNS manifestations imaging with contrast enhanced computerized tomography (CECT) or MRI brain, and cerebrospinal fluid (CSF) analysis is required to rule out other etiologies. General treatment strategies include discontinuation of drug (e.g., cytarabine induced cerebellar toxicities, L-asparaginase-induced cerebral venous sinus thrombosis) or dose modification if not severe (vincristine or bortezomib neuropathy), supportive, care. and specific treatment strategies.

- *Peripheral neuropathy:* Amitriptyline, duloxetine, and gabapentin
- *Ifosfamide encephalopathy*[21]
    - *Methylene blue:*
        - *Mechanism:* It inhibits plasma and extrahepatic monoamine oxidases, acts as an alternative electron acceptor in the mitochondrial respiratory chain, and oxidizes NADH, reducing the negative effects on aldehyde dehydrogenation.
        - *Dosage:* 50 mg of 1% aqueous solution IV over 5 minutes, repeated six times daily.
        - *Considerations:* Potential side effects include hemolytic anemia and blue-green discoloration of urine and feces at higher doses (>4 mg/kg).
    - *Thiamine (vitamin B1):*
        - *Mechanism:* It addresses neurotoxicity similar to Wernicke encephalopathy, potentially caused by severe thiamine deficiency.
        - *Dosage:* 100 mg IV diluted in 100 mL of normal saline over 10 minutes, every 4 hours until symptoms resolve or significantly improve.

- *Supportive measures:*
  - *IV albumin:* It binds to chloroacetaldehyde (CAA) and may prevent its passage across the blood-brain barrier.
  - *Hemodialysis:* It is used to enhance clearance of ifosfamide and its metabolites in patients with severe renal impairment, potentially reversing encephalopathy.
  - *Glucose infusion:* It can be beneficial in treatment, likely by providing energy support to the brain and mitigating neurotoxic effects.
- *Methotrexate encephalopathy:* Some case studies suggest benefits with aminophylline and dextromethorphan.[25]
- *Posterior reversible encephalopathy syndrome:* Management includes control of blood pressure and antiepileptics.
- *Cerebrovascular events:* Anticoagulation for thrombotic events.

GASTROINTESTINAL TOXICITY

Causative Agents and Mechanism

Gastrointestinal toxicity can often be a dose-limiting complication, leading to cessation of treatment with potentially life-threatening implications. Systemic therapeutic agents leading to gastrointestinal toxicity are enumerated in **Table 4**.

Clinical Presentation

Clinical presentation includes mucositis, diarrhea, ileus, pancreatitis, and transaminitis, as detailed in **Table 4**.[26]

Risk Factors

- Low albumin
- Renal dysfunction
- Drug interactions causing increasing dose levels (azoles and antitubercular therapy)
- Comorbidities (chronic liver disease and viral hepatitis)

TABLE 4: Causes, pathogenesis, and management strategies of systemic anticancer agents causing gastrointestinal toxicity.

Class of anti-cancer therapy	*Gastrointestinal toxicity*	*Mechanism*	*Associated drugs*	*Management considerations*
Chemotherapy				
	Mucositis	Inflammation and ulceration of mucous membranes	• Chemotherapy (e.g., fluorouracil, methotrexate, and melphalan) • Radiation therapy to head and neck	• *Oral care:* Gentle mouth rinses, avoid alcohol-based mouthwashes. • *Pain management:* Topical analgesics (e.g., lidocaine), and systemic analgesics as needed • *Nutritional support:* Soft diet, nutritional supplements and total parenteral nutrition for severe grade toxicity
	Nausea and vomiting	Stimulation of chemoreceptor trigger zone and gastrointestinal (GI) tract by chemotherapy agents	Highly emetogenic chemotherapy (e.g., cisplatin, doxorubicin)	• *Prophylactic antiemetics:* 5-HT3 receptor antagonists (e.g., ondansetron), neurokinin 1 (NK 1) receptor antagonists (e.g., aprepitant) • *Supportive care:* Small, frequent meals; hydration and electrolyte correction, and total parenteral nutrition if indicated
	Diarrhea	Direct damage to intestinal mucosa by chemotherapy	- Irinotecan and 5-fluorouracil	• *Antidiarrheal agents:* Loperamide, diphenoxylate/atropine • *Fluid and electrolyte management:* Oral rehydration solutions, and monitor for dehydration • *Dietary adjustments:* Low-fiber, easy-to-digest foods. • Total parenteral nutrition if indicated

Contd...

Contd...

Class of anti-cancer therapy	*Gastrointestinal toxicity*	*Mechanism*	*Associated drugs*	*Management considerations*
Chemotherapy				
	Constipation	Decreased GI motility due to direct effect of chemotherapy, autonomic neuropathy and dyselectrolytemia leading to paralytic ileus in severe cases	• Opioid-based chemotherapy (e.g., oxaliplatin) • Vinca alkaloids (e.g., vincristine)	• *Laxatives:* Bulk-forming, osmotic, or stimulant laxatives as appropriate • *Hydration:* Adequate fluid intake • Supportive management including enema, parenteral nutrition and nasogastric tube decompression if indicated
	Pancreatitis	Not well described	L-asparaginase	Supportive management (analgesics, hydration)
	Hepatotoxicity	Direct effect on hepatocytes	Paclitaxel, methotrexate, and vincristine	Drug interruption and dose modification
		Veno-occlusive disease	Busulfan, high dose cyclophosphamide in conditioning regimens for stem cell transplant	• *Supportive care:* Management of fluid overload • Defibrotide (6.25 mg/kg every 6 hours) • Tissue plasminogen activator • Urso-deoxycholic acid for prophylaxis
Targeted therapy				
	Diarrhea	Off-target effects on gastrointestinal epithelium	Tyrosine kinase inhibitors, (sunitinib, sorafenib, lenvatinib, imatinib, bosutinib, pertuzumab, and trastuzumab-deruxtecan	• Antidiarrheals • Hydration and electrolyte management
	Hepatotoxicity	Off-target effects on hepatocytes	Pazopanib, nilotinib, and brentuximab vedotin	• Supportive management • Drug discontinuation and monitoring
Immune checkpoint inhibitors[27]				
	Diarrhea, colitis, hepatotoxicity	Activation of immune response leading to inflammation and damage in the gastrointestinal tract and liver	More common with CTLA4 inhibitors (ipilimumab)	• Corticosteroids or other immunosuppressive agents (e.g., infliximab) • Antidiarrheals • Monitor liver function tests • Supportive care (e.g., hydration, electrolyte management)

Prevention

Avoid hepatotoxic drugs, dose reduction if indicated (low albumin or creatinine clearance)

Monitoring and Treatment

Management is mainly supportive, as detailed in **Table 4**.

RENAL TOXICITIES

Causative Agents and Mechanism

Renal toxicities of systemic anticancer therapy may result from effects on the glomerulus, tubules, interstitium, or microvasculature by different mechanisms with varied clinical presentations ranging from asymptomatic derangement of creatinine levels to dyselectrolytemia to dysfunction requiring hemodialysis. The mechanisms and implicated drugs of chemotherapy-mediated renal toxicity are detailed in **Table 5**.[28] Renal effects of targeted therapy and causative drugs are enumerated in **Table 6**.

Clinical Presentation

Based on the type of renal injury as detailed in **Tables 5 and 6**, nephrotoxicity may manifest as hypertension, fluid retention, oliguria, hematuria, proteinuria, azotemia, and dyselectrolytemia.

TABLE 5: Mechanism, agents, and management strategies of chemotherapy-mediated renal toxicity.

Type of renal toxicity	*Chemotherapy drug*	*Management strategies*
Acute tubular necrosis: Direct tubular toxicity through oxidative stress and apoptosis of renal tubular cells	• Cisplatin • Ifosfamide • Pemetrexed	Hydration before, during, after chemotherapy to promote renal perfusion and drug excretion[29]
Interstitial nephritis: Immune-mediated inflammatory response in renal interstitium	• Methotrexate • Cyclophosphamide • Streptozosin	• Corticosteroids • Hydration
Hemorrhagic cystitis: Toxic metabolite, such as acrolein, causes bladder irritation and hematuria	• Ifosfamide • High-dose cyclophosphamide[30]	*Mesna:* It binds acrolein and detoxifies it *Hydration:* For dilution of urine and excrete toxic metabolites and continuous bladder irrigation
Glomerular injury: Endothelial damage in the glomeruli, leading to microangiopathic hemolytic anemia and acute renal failure	• Mitomycin-C • Gemcitabine	• Supportive care for blood pressure, electrolyte imbalance, renal function • Plasmapheresis • Dialysis
Crystalluria and tubular obstruction	Methotrexate	• Hydration to prevent crystal formation • *Alkalinization:* Sodium bicarbonate infusion for prevention • Dialysis—may not be helpful

TABLE 6: Nephrotoxicity resulting from targeted therapy.[31]

Class of drugs	*Drugs*	*Type of renal injury*
VEGF inhibitors	Bevacizumab, ramucirumab, sunitinib, sorafenib, axitinib, regorafenib, nintedanib, cabozantinib, and pazopanib	Hypertension, proteinuria, and thrombotic microangiopathy
EGFR inhibitors	Cetuximab, panitumumab, erlotinib, gefitinib, and afatinib	Renal magnesium wasting
mTOR inhibitors	Everolimus and temsirolimus	Hypertension, hypophosphatemia, hyponatremia, and proteinuria
BRAF inhibitors	Dabrafenib and vemurafenib	Granulomatous nephritis and hypophosphatemia
ALK inhibitors	Crizotinib	Renal cysts
Other thyrosine kinase inhibitors	Imatinib	Fluid retention, periorbital edema, and glomerular injury (rare)

(ALK: anaplastic lymphoma kinase; EGFR: epidermal growth factor receptor; mTOR: mammalian target of rapamycin; VEGF: vascular endothelial growth factor)

Risk Factors

- Elderly age
- Pre-existing renal dysfunctions
- Nephrotoxic drugs [nonsteroidal anti-inflammatory drugs (NSAIDs), angiotensin-converting enzyme inhibitors (ACEIs)]
- Hypovolemia (sepsis and gastrointestinal losses)

Prevention

- Adequate hydration (for prevention of cisplatin toxicity)
- Pre-treatment evaluation with diethylenetriamine pentaacetic acid (DTPA) glomerular filtration rate (GFR) in elderly patients
- Avoidance of nephrotoxic drugs
- Specific nephroprotective agents (e.g., mesna for ifosfamide and cyclophosphamide)

Monitoring and Treatment

- *General principles for acute kidney injury*:
  - Adequate hydration for good renal perfusion
  - Monitoring of renal function tests and proteinuria

- Blood pressure control
- Diuretics for fluid retention
- Hemodialysis if indicated
- *Specific treatment strategies*
    - Corticosteroids for immune-related nephritis[32]

TUMOR LYSIS SYNDROME

Causative Agents and Mechanism

Tumor lysis syndrome (TLS) is an oncological emergency resulting from lysis of cancer cells which leads to release of intracellular components into blood. It may result spontaneously or due to treatment such as chemotherapy in highly chemosensitive tumors such as germ cell tumors and lymphomas, or steroids in acute lymphoblastic leukemia (ALL).

Clinical Presentation

The diagnostic criteria (Cairo-Bishop criteria) involve laboratory and clinical TLS. Laboratory TLS is defined by the presence of two or more laboratory changes within 3 days before or 7 days after cytotoxic therapy.[33] These include:

- Uric acid >8 mg/dL or 25% increase from baseline
- Calcium <7 mg/dL mmol/L or 25% decrease from baseline
- Phosphorus >1.45 mmol/L, or 25% increase from baseline
- Potassium >6.0 mmol/L or 25% increase from baseline

Clinical TLS involves laboratory TLS plus one or more of the following:

- Renal insufficiency [creatinine increase >1.5 times of upper limit of normal (ULN)]
- Cardiac arrhythmias
- Seizures

Risk Factors

Risk factors for TLS are detailed in **Table 7**.

Prevention

- *Hydration:* Maintain high urine output (3–5 L/day) to promote renal excretion of metabolites
- *Allopurinol:* Inhibits xanthine oxidase, decreasing uric acid production
- *Rasburicase:* Recombinant urate oxidase that converts uric acid to allantoin, which is more soluble.

TABLE 7: Risk factors for tumor lysis syndrome.

Characteristic	*Risk factor*
Tumor burden/extent of disease	• Bulky disease (>10 cm) • Elevated LDH (>2 times ULN) • Elevated WBC (>25,000/mL)
Tumor type	• Diffuse large B-cell lymphoma • Burkitt's lymphoma • ALL • Lymphoblastic lymphoma • ALL • Solid tumors (typically highly proliferative, chemosensitive tumors)
Renal failure	• Pre-existing renal failure • Oliguria

(ALL: acute lymphoblastic leukemia; LDH: lactate dehydrogenase; ULN: upper limit of normal; WBC: white blood cells)

- *Alkalinization:* Controversial, due to risk of calcium phosphate precipitation.
- Avoid potassium containing foods.

Monitoring and Treatment

The management strategies of TLS are detailed in **Table 8**.[33]

MYELOSUPPRESSION

Myelosuppression is a common side effect of chemotherapy, resulting from reduction in hematopoiesis, leading to anemia, thrombocytopenia, and neutropenia. Of these, neutropenic complications including febrile neutropenia and fungal pneumonia are potentially life-threatening and are, hence, described in detail below.

Febrile Neutropenia

Febrile neutropenia (FN) is defined as an oral temperature of >38.3°C or two consecutive readings of >38.0°C for 2 hours and an absolute neutrophil count (ANC) of $<0.5 \times 10^9$/L, or expected to fall $<0.5 \times 10^9$/L. It is an important cause of morbidity and leads to interruptions in treatment and inability to maintain dose density.[34]

Causative Agents and Mechanism

Any chemotherapy regimen may cause febrile neutropenia based on patient characteristics, comorbidities, and disease status. Commonly implicated regimens

TABLE 8: Management of tumor lysis syndrome.

Abnormality	*Recommendation*
Hyperphosphatemia	Avoid IV phosphate administration Administration of phosphate binder *Severe:* Dialysis
Hypocalcemia	*Asymptomatic:* No therapy *Symptomatic:* Calcium gluconate 50–100 mg/kg IV slowly with cardiac monitoring
Hyperkalemia	*Moderate and asymptomatic, >6.0 mmol/L:* • Avoid IV and oral potassium • ECG and cardiac rhythm monitoring sodium polystyrene sulphonate *Severe (>7.0 mmol/L) and/or symptomatic:* • Same as above, plus: • Calcium gluconate 100–200 mg/kg slow infusion for life-threatening arrhythmias • Regular insulin (0.1 U/kg IV) + D25 (2 mL/kg) • IV sodium bicarbonate (1–2 mEq/kg IV push) • Dialysis
Renal dysfunction (uremia)	Fluid and electrolyte management Uric acid and phosphate management Adjust renally excreted drug doses Dialysis (hemo- or peritoneal) Hemofiltration

include combinations containing alkylating agents (cyclophosphamide and platinum agents), anthracyclines (doxorubicin), and topoisomerase inhibitors (etoposide).

In recent years, antibiotic-resistant strains are increasingly isolated, such as extended spectrum beta-lactamase (ESBL)—producing gram-negative bacteria, vancomycin-resistant enterococci (VRE) and methicillin-resistant *Staphylococcus aureus* (MRSA). There is also an increased incidence of infections with fluconazole-resistant *Candida* strains (e.g., *Candida krusei* and *Candida glabrata*).[35]

Clinical Presentation

The onset of neutropenia is usually around 8–10 days after the start of chemotherapy and most recover by the 3rd week. The risk of febrile neutropenia depends on the underlying cancer, type of chemotherapy, and age. Based on the site of infection, the clinical manifestation varies.

Risk Factors

- Age
- Advanced disease
- History of prior FN
- Mucositis
- Poor performance status and/or
- Cardiovascular disease

Prevention

Most guidelines recommend prophylactic granulocyte colony-stimulating factor (G-CSF) for regimens with >20% risk of febrile neutropenia.

Approach to febrile neutropenia:

- Thorough examination of all systems including respiratory, abdominal examination, perianal examination, examination of catheter sites, for the focus of infection
- At least two sets of blood cultures should be collected for all patients, including simultaneous blood cultures from each lumen of the central venous catheter (CVC) if applicable, in addition to a peripheral vein site. Difference in time between positivity of results between catheter culture and peripheral blood culture, termed as differential time to positivity (DTTP), of 2 hours or more is a highly sensitive and specific indicator of catheter-related bacteremia.
- Initiation of broad-spectrum antibiotics within 60 minutes of presentation is crucial.
- Risk stratification may be done by clinical assessment and the use of tools such as the MASCC score (Multinational Association for Supportive Care in Cancer risk index).[36]
- High-risk patients (defined as those with anticipated severe neutropenia with ANC <500/mm^3 lasting for >7 days, hypotension, altered mental status, multiple comorbidities, and MASCC score <21) are usually treated with combination of an antipseudomonal beta-lactam agent and aminoglycosides.
- *Specific indications for alternative therapy:*
  - Local antibacterial guidelines should be considered.
  - Empirical initiation of antifungal therapy is recommended in patients with non-responding fever after 3–7 days of broad-spectrum antibiotics
  - For catheter-related infections, a glycopeptide such as vancomycin should be administered

through the line to cover gram-positive organisms. Alternatively, teicoplanin can be administered.

- Removal of the line is indicated in patients with tunnel or implanted port infections, persistent bacteremia despite adequate treatment, atypical mycobacterial infection, and candidemia.
- In patients with pneumonia, treatment for *Pneumocystis jirovecii* including steroids and cotrimoxazole should be considered in patients particularly those with a history of prolonged corticosteroid therapy or immunosuppression.
- Early treatment with a mold-active antifungal agent should be considered in patients with profound prolonged neutropenia and lung infiltrates.
- In patients with a suspicion of invasive aspergillus, such as those with prolonged neutropenia or on induction chemotherapy for acute myeloid leukemia, a high-resolution chest CT scan is indicated, along with serum galactomannan estimation. Classical findings include nodules with halos or ground-glass changes; if found, bronchoalveolar lavage aids in further diagnostic evaluation.
- Treatment for presumed aspergillosis (with typical infiltrates on CT) could consist of either voriconazole or liposomal amphotericin B. Echinocandins may be effective in patients with non-responding infection or candidemia.[37]
- Liposomal amphotericin B and an echinocandin antifungal such as caspofungin are appropriate first-line treatments for patients who develop candidiasis while on azole prophylaxis or if non-albicans *Candida* is isolated. Prolonged antifungal therapy is usually indicated (14–21 days, followed by prophylactic azoles throughout cytotoxic therapy).

CUTANEOUS TOXICITY

Cutaneous toxicity includes rash (commonly due to EGFR inhibitors such as erlotinib and cetuximab), hand-foot syndrome (capecitabine and tyrosine-kinase inhibitors), vitiligo or psoriasis (typically post immunotherapy), and in severe cases, erythema multiforme and Steven–Johnson syndrome.[38] Treatment includes topical corticosteroids and antihistamines for mild toxicity, and systemic steroids and immunosuppressants for non-responding or severe toxicity. Patient education is important in prevention of hand-foot syndrome.

ENDOCRINE TOXICITY

These toxicities result from damage to endocrine glands (thyroid, adrenal, pituitary, and gonads) or hormone-related imbalances due to treatment. Common toxicities include hyper- and hypothyroidism (due to tyrosine kinase inhibitors or immune checkpoint inhibitors), and adrenal insufficiency or hypophysitis (due to immune checkpoint inhibitors).[39] Treatment includes hormonal replacement therapy (e.g., levothyroxine for thyroiditis and glucocorticoids for adrenal insufficiency) and monitoring.

SYSTEMIC INFLAMMATORY RESPONSE SYNDROME

Causative Agents and Mechanism

Agents such as CAR-T cell therapy leads to release of inflammatory cytokines such as interleukin-6 (IL-6), IL-10, and interferon-γ (IFN-γ), producing a range of systemic side effects.[6]

Clinical Presentation

Common clinical presentations include cytokine release syndrome (CRS) and ICANS.

Risk Factors

- High tumor burden
- High-dose infusion of CAR-T cells
- Central nervous system disease (ICANS)
- High peak of CAR-T cell expansion

Prevention

Careful selection of monitoring, close monitoring, and prompt initiation of steroids and tocilizumab if indicated.

Monitoring and Treatment

Clinical monitoring post-infusion is mandatory, via assessment of vitals and immune effector cell (ICE) score. Management of CRS is enumerated in **Table 9**.[23]

Immune effector-cell associated neurotoxicity syndrome: Management includes supportive care, dexamethasone, and for refractory cases, additional therapies such as anakinra, cyclophosphamide, and antithymocyte globulin.[40]

TABLE 9: Cytokine-release syndrome.

Grading	*Treatment*
Grade 1: Mild symptoms (e.g., fever <38°C)	Supportive care with antipyretics and monitoring
Grade 2: Moderate symptoms (e.g., fever ≥38°C) requiring intervention	Tocilizumab (IL-6 receptor blockade) and corticosteroids if severe, intensive supportive care
Grade 3: Severe symptoms (e.g., hypotension requiring low-dose vasopressors) or hypoxia required supplemental oxygen including high-flow oxygen or positive pressure ventilation	Tocilizumab, corticosteroids, and intensive supportive care
Grade 4: Life-threatening complications	

LONG-TERM TOXICITIES

- Cardiotoxicity (anthracycline, trastuzumab, and radiation therapy)
- Secondary malignancies [commonly acute myelogenous leukemia (AML); results from alkylating agents such as cyclophosphamide or topoisomerase inhibitors such as etoposide; or breast cancer after chest irradiation]
- Pulmonary toxicities (bleomycin toxicity)
- Neuropathy (vinca alkaloids and taxanes)
- Gonadal dysfunction and infertility (alkylating agents such as cyclophosphamide and pelvic irradiation)
- Bone health issues (osteoporosis due to hormonal therapy such as aromatase inhibitors)
- Cognitive side effects
- Fatigue and quality of life issues

Management of long-term side effects include surveillance, patient education, lifestyle modifications, symptom management, and multidisciplinary approach.[41]

CONCLUSION

Awareness of toxicities of systemic anticancer therapy and the underlying mechanisms is crucial in the setting of critical care of patients with cancer for timely recognition and management. As the armamentarium of systemic anticancer therapy keeps expanding, it is important to stay updated with potential side effects of novel drugs and long-term toxicities. By actively monitoring patients and addressing systemic side effects, clinicians can improve treatment tolerability and enhance patient outcomes, ultimately contributing to a more holistic approach to cancer care. The field continues to evolve, aiming for even more effective and less toxic treatments in the future.

REFERENCES

1. Zhong L, Li Y, Xiong L, Wang W, Wu M, Yuan T, et al. Small molecules in targeted cancer therapy: advances, challenges, and future perspectives. Signal Transduct Target Ther. 2021;6(1):201.
2. Basak D, Arrighi S, Darwiche Y, Deb S. Comparison of Anticancer Drug Toxicities: Paradigm Shift in Adverse Effect Profile. Life (Basel). 2021;12(1):48
3. Korkmaz A, Topal T, Oter S. Pathophysiological aspects of cyclophosphamide and ifosfamide induced hemorrhagic cystitis; implication of reactive oxygen and nitrogen species as well as PARP activation. Cell Biol Toxicol. 2007;23(5):303-12.
4. Bayles CE, Hale DE, Konieczny A, Anderson VD, Richardson CR, Brown KV, et al. Upcycling the anthracyclines: New mechanisms of action, toxicology, and pharmacology. Toxicol Appl Pharmacol. 2023;459:116362.
5. Liu S, Kurzrock R. Toxicity of targeted therapy: Implications for response and impact of genetic polymorphisms. Cancer Treat Rev. 2014;40(7):883-91.
6. Jin Y, Dong Y, Zhang J, Sun J, Liu Y, Chen Y. The toxicity of cell therapy: Mechanism, manifestations, and challenges. J Appl Toxicol. 2021;41(5):659-67.
7. Herrmann J. Adverse cardiac effects of cancer therapies: cardiotoxicity and arrhythmia. Nat Rev Cardiol. 2020; 17(8):474-502.
8. Henriksen PA. Anthracycline cardiotoxicity: an update on mechanisms, monitoring, and prevention. Heart. 2018; 104(12):971-7.
9. Polk A, Vistisen K, Vaage-Nilsen M, Nielsen DL. A systematic review of the pathophysiology of 5-fluorouracil-induced cardiotoxicity. BMC Pharmacol Toxicol. 2014;15:47.
10. Morandi P, Ruffini PA, Benvenuto GM, Raimondi R, Fosser V. Cardiac toxicity of high-dose chemotherapy. Bone Marrow Transplant. 2005;35(4):323-34.
11. Farolfi A, Melegari E, Aquilina M, carpi E, Ibrahim T, Maltoni R, et al. Trastuzumab-induced cardiotoxicity in early breast cancer patients: a retrospective study of possible risk and protective factors. Heart. 2013;99(9):634-9.
12. Ewer MS, Lippman SM. Type II chemotherapy-related cardiac dysfunction: time to recognize a new entity. J Clin Oncol. 2005;23(13):2900-2.
13. Stein-Merlob AF, Rothberg MV, Holman P, Yang EH. Immunotherapy-Associated Cardiotoxicity of Immune Checkpoint Inhibitors and Chimeric Antigen Receptor T Cell Therapy: Diagnostic and Management Challenges and Strategies. Curr Cardiol Rep. 2021;23(3):11.
14. Plana JC, Galderisi M, Barac A, Ewer MS, Ky B, Scherrer-Crosbie M, et al. Expert consensus for multimodality imaging

evaluation of adult patients during and after cancer therapy: a report from the American Society of Echocardiography and the European Association of Cardiovascular Imaging. J Am Soc Echocardiogr. 2014;27(9):911-39.
15. Bianco CM, Al-Kindi SG, Oliveira GH. Advanced Heart Failure Therapies for Cancer Therapeutics-Related Cardiac Dysfunction. Heart Fail Clin. 2017;13(2):327-36.
16. Dhamija E, Meena P, Ramalingam V, Sahoo R, Rastogi S, Thulkar S. Chemotherapy-induced pulmonary complications in cancer: Significance of clinicoradiological correlation. Indian J Radiol Imaging. 2020;30(1):20-6.
17. Barber NA, Ganti AK. Pulmonary toxicities from targeted therapies: a review. Target Oncol. 2011;6(4):235-43.
18. Rashdan S, Minna JD, Gerber DE. Diagnosis and management of pulmonary toxicity associated with cancer immunotherapy. Lancet Respir Med. 2018;6(6):472-8.
19. Limper AH. Chemotherapy-induced lung disease. Clin Chest Med. 2004;25(1):53-64.
20. Staff NP, Grisold A, Grisold W, Windebank AJ. Chemotherapy-induced peripheral neuropathy: A current review. Ann Neurol. 2017;81(6):772-81.
21. Stone JB, DeAngelis LM. Cancer-treatment-induced neurotoxicity–focus on newer treatments. Nat Rev Clin Oncol. 2016;13(2):92-105.
22. Marra A, Vargas M, Striano P, Del Guercio L, Buonanno P, Servillo G. Posterior reversible encephalopathy syndrome: the endothelial hypotheses. Med Hypotheses. 2014;82(5):619-22.
23. Brudno JN, Kochenderfer JN. Current understanding and management of CAR T cell-associated toxicities. Nat Rev Clin Oncol. 2024;21(7):501-21.
24. Lo Y, Shen LJ, Chen WH, Dong YH, Wu FL. Risk factors of ifosfamide-related encephalopathy in adult patients with cancer: A retrospective analysis. J Formos Med Assoc. 2016;115(9):744-51.
25. Bhojwani D, Bansal R, Wayne AS. Managing therapy-associated neurotoxicity in children with ALL. Hematology Am Soc Hematol Educ Program. 2021;2021(1):376-83.
26. Boussios S, Pentheroudakis G, Katsanos K, Pavlidis N. Systemic treatment-induced gastrointestinal toxicity: incidence, clinical presentation and management. Ann Gastroenterol. 2012;25(2):106-18.
27. Samaan MA, Pavlidis P, Papa S, Powell N, Irving PM. Gastrointestinal toxicity of immune checkpoint inhibitors: from mechanisms to management. Nat Rev Gastroenterol Hepatol. 2018;15(4):222-34.
28. Santos MLC, de Brito BB, da Silva FAF, Botelho ACDS, de Melo FF. Nephrotoxicity in cancer treatment: An overview. World J Clin Oncol. 2020;11(4):190-204.
29. Crona DJ, Faso A, Nishijima TF, McGraw KA, Galsky MD, Milowsky MI. A Systematic Review of Strategies to Prevent Cisplatin-Induced Nephrotoxicity. Oncologist. 2017;22(5):609-19.
30. Hadjibabaie M, Alimoghaddam K, Shamshiri AR, Iravani M, Bahar B, Mousavi A, et al. Continuous bladder irrigation prevents hemorrhagic cystitis after allogeneic hematopoietic cell transplantation. Urol Oncol. 2008;26(1):43-46.
31. Launay-Vacher V, Aapro M, De Castro G Jr, Cohen E, Deray G, Dooley M, et al. Renal effects of molecular targeted therapies in oncology: a review by the Cancer and the Kidney International Network (C-KIN). Ann Oncol. 2015;26(8):1677-84.
32. Perazella MA, Shirali AC. Immune checkpoint inhibitor nephrotoxicity: what do we know and what should we do? Kidney Int. 2020;97(1):62-74.
33. Cairo MS, Bishop M. Tumour lysis syndrome: new therapeutic strategies and classification. Br J Haematol. 2004;127(1):3-11.
34. Klastersky J, de Naurois J, Rolston K, Rapoport B, Maschmeyer G, Aapro M, et al. Management of febrile neutropaenia: ESMO Clinical Practice Guidelines. Ann Oncol. 2016;27(suppl 5):v111-8.
35. Feld R. Bloodstream infections in cancer patients with febrile neutropenia. Int J Antimicrob Agents. 2008;32 Suppl 1:S30-3.
36. Innes H, Lim SL, Hall A, Chan SY, Bhalla N, Marshall E. Management of febrile neutropenia in solid tumours and lymphomas using the Multinational Association for Supportive Care in Cancer (MASCC) risk index: feasibility and safety in routine clinical practice. Support Care Cancer. 2008;16(5):485-91.
37. Patterson TF, Thompson GR 3rd, Denning DW, Fishman JA, Hadley S, Herbrecht R, et al. Practice Guidelines for the Diagnosis and Management of Aspergillosis: 2016 Update by the Infectious Diseases Society of America. Clin Infect Dis. 2016;63(4):e1-60.
38. Deutsch A, Leboeuf NR, Lacouture ME, McLellan BN. Dermatologic Adverse Events of Systemic Anticancer Therapies: Cytotoxic Chemotherapy, Targeted Therapy, and Immunotherapy. Am Soc Clin Oncol Educ Book. 2020;40:485-500.
39. Wright JJ, Powers AC, Johnson DB. Endocrine toxicities of immune checkpoint inhibitors. Nat Rev Endocrinol. 2021;17(7):389-99.
40. Sheth VS, Gauthier J. Taming the beast: CRS and ICANS after CAR T-cell therapy for ALL. Bone Marrow Transplant. 2021;56(3):552-66.
41. Lustberg MB, Kuderer NM, Desai A, Bergerot C, Lyman GH. Mitigating long-term and delayed adverse events associated with cancer treatment: implications for survivorship. Nat Rev Clin Oncol. 2023;20(8):527-42.

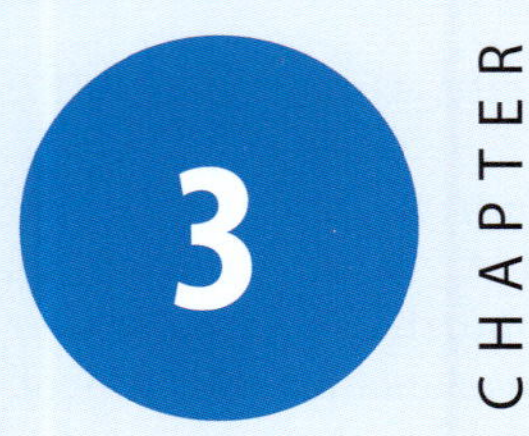

CHAPTER

Chemotherapeutic and Immunotherapy Drugs and Anesthetic Implications

Debashree Pradipta Lahiri, Sohan Lal Solanki

INTRODUCTION

Chemotherapeutic agents are an essential component of treatment of all kinds of cancer.[1] These agents act on rapidly dividing cancer cells leading to apoptosis of these cells.[1] However, they also damage the normally dividing cells leading to various toxicities. Over the past decade, immunotherapy drugs are being increasingly used in treatment of cancer. These immunotherapy agents also lead to pulmonary, cardiac, and endocrine toxicities.[2] Cancer patients on these antineoplastic agents can present for cancer or noncancer surgeries that require anesthesia. Thus, it is of prime importance for an anesthesiologist to have a thorough knowledge of various antineoplastic agents, their effects on patient's physiology and biochemistry, and their toxicities and interactions with anesthetic drugs, if any.

CHEMOTHERAPEUTIC AGENTS

Paul Ehrlich first used these agents to treat ailments in the year 1981.[3] The first use of these drugs for cancer treatment was reported in the year 1940.[4] Chemotherapeutic agents interlope with the protein synthesis and the metabolic processes of deoxyribonucleic acid (DNA) and ribonucleic acid (RNA) of the cancer cells. These agents act by targeting the cancer cell at the various cell cycle phases and also by boosting the immune response of the host by activating various lymphocyte cell receptors in order to reestablish immunosurveillance.[5] These drugs not only cause apoptosis and death of the rapidly dividing cancer cells but also affect the normally dividing noncancer cells producing various chemotherapy-related toxicities including pulmonary, cardiac, neurological, hepatic, renal, and bone marrow damage. Anemia, thrombocytopenia, coagulopathy, and bleeding of the digestive tract are commonly seen. In order to reduce the toxicities, chemotherapy is often administered in cycles. This provides a period of recovery during the treatment. Also, combination of drugs is used to reduce the toxicities. Using drugs with different mechanisms of action reduces the chances of developing resistance to a single agent as well as increases the proportion of cancer cells destroyed. The degree of chemotherapy-related toxicity depends on numerous factors such as the agent, the cumulative dose administered, and comorbidities of the patient.[1]

The use of chemotherapeutic agents can be broadly classified as:[1]

- *Neoadjuvant chemotherapy (NACT)* is administered prior to definitive surgery for tumor or metastasis resection. NACT aims to reduce the need for complex surgeries or to enhance the chances of complete tumor resection and survival.
- *Adjuvant chemotherapy* is administered after surgical resection to decrease the chances of recurrence.
- *Palliative chemotherapy* is administered when definitive cure is not possible. It aims to improve the quality of life and survival.

CLASSIFICATION OF CHEMOTHERAPEUTIC AGENTS

The chemotherapeutic agents are classified based on the mechanism of action as given in **Table 1**.[6]

EFFECTS OF CHEMOTHERAPEUTIC AGENTS ON ORGAN SYSTEMS

The toxic effects of chemotherapy range from acutely occurring hypersensitivity reactions, short-term side effects like hepatic, renal toxicities, and myelosuppression to long-term cardiac and pulmonary toxicities.

Cardiovascular System

Chemotherapy-related cardiovascular toxicity can lead to hypertension, arrhythmias, hypotension, myocardial

TABLE 1: Classification of chemotherapeutic agents and their mechanism of action.

Class of chemotherapeutic agent	***Examples***	***Mechanism of action***
Alkylating agents	• *Nitrogen mustard:* Ifosfamide, bendamustine, and cyclophosphamide • *Nitrosoureas:* Lomustine and carmustine • *Alkyl sulfonate:* Busulfan • *Platinum analogs:* Carboplatin, oxaliplatin, and cisplatin • *Ethyleneimine:* Thiotepa • *Triazenes:* Procarbazine, dacarbazine, and temozolomide	Inhibit transcription and replication of DNA as the alkyl group yielded by these drugs react with the nucleophilic centers of the proteins and nucleic acids
Antimetabolites	• *Folate antagonists:* Pemetrexed and methotrexate • *Cytidine analogs:* Decitabine, azacitidine, gemcitabine, and cytarabine • *Purine analogs:* Cladribine, nelarabine, and clofarabine • *Pyrimidine analogs:* Capecitabine, and 5-fluorouracil (5-FU)	Inhibit DNA replication
Antibiotics	Daunomycin, bleomycin, and actinomycin D	Inhibit DNA and RNA synthesis
Antimicrotubular agents	*Taxanes:* Paclitaxel, docetaxel, and cabazitaxel	Produce abnormal function and disrupts replication of cells by disrupting the equilibrium of polymerization and depolymerization of microtubules, thus leading to apoptosis
	Vinca alkaloids: Vinblastine, vinorelbine, and vincristine	Arrest cell in the metaphase by binding to tubulin and inhibit microtubule formation
	Topoisomerase I inhibitors: Topotecan and irinotecan	Block the release of Top I from the cleavable complex and form a tertiary complex, thus prevent relegation
	Topoisomerase II inhibitors: Anthracyclines like idarubicin, doxorubicin, mitoxantrone, and daunorubicin	Inhibit DNA and RNA synthesis Also, inhibit topoisomerase II, leading to inhibition of repair of DNA
Miscellaneous	Tretinoin (derivative of vitamin A)	Acts on RAR-α promoting cell differentiation
	Arsenic trioxide	Induces differentiation of cell
	Hydroxyurea	Inhibition of ribonucleoside diphosphate reductase

(DNA: deoxyribonucleic acid; RAR: retinoic acid receptor alpha; RNA: ribonucleic acid)

infarction, cardiomyopathy, heart failure, pericarditis, myocarditis, pericardial effusion, and life-threatening tamponade.[7] The underlying mechanisms of these toxicities are not well understood but it is postulated that these agents damage the myocytes producing left ventricular dysfunction and other manifestations.[2] Multiple risk factors for developing cardiotoxicity have been identified. These are age above 70 years, female gender, preexisting cardiac conditions, use of other concurrent chemotherapeutic agents, and current or previous radiation therapy to the mediastinum.[8] Anthracyclines like epirubicin, doxorubicin, and daunorubicin are the most frequently used chemotherapy drugs producing cardiotoxicities, which are irreversible. These agents impair the contractility of myocardium.[9] In spite of restricting the maximum cumulative doses, the incidence of anthracycline-induced cardiotoxicity is reported to be 9–18%.[2] Early acute anthracycline-induced cardiotoxicities include nonspecific ST-T changes, decreased QRS voltage, prolonged QT interval in electrocardiogram (ECG), transient left ventricular dysfunction, and supraventricular arrhythmias while, on a chronic basis, they produce cardiomyopathy.[2] Other chemotherapy drugs that produce cardiotoxicities are

TABLE 2: Effect of drugs on the cardiovascular system (CVS).

Drug	*Effect on CVS*
5-fluorouracil	Coronary spasms and endothelial injury cause myocardial ischemia; recent evidence suggests myocyte toxicity as well
Cyclophosphamide	Endocardial damage, hemorrhagic myocarditis, pericarditis, cardiomyopathy, and heart failure
Bleomycin	Cardiomyopathy and acute pericarditis
Paclitaxel and docetaxel	Asymptomatic to severe bradycardia, tachyarrhythmias, ventricular fibrillation, asystole, and myocardial infarction
Cisplatin[10]	Sinus bradycardia, arrhythmias like atrial fibrillation, supraventricular tachycardia, complete atrioventricular block, angina, myocarditis, and pericarditis
Busulfan	Atrial fibrillation, cardiomyopathy, and heart failure

docetaxel, cyclophosphamide, cisplatin, paclitaxel, 5-fluorouracil, and bleomycin. The effects of these drugs on cardiovascular system (CVS) are described in **Table 2**.[2,3,7,9]

Anesthetic Implications

During the preanesthesia workup of a patient who has received chemotherapy, it is necessary for the anesthesiologist to be aware of the potential cardiac toxicities. A thorough history taking and clinical examination is essential to identify signs or symptoms of cardiac dysfunction. In addition to routine investigations including ECG, patients who have received potential cardiotoxic chemotherapeutic agents should undergo an echocardiography for the assessment of left ventricular ejection fraction, cardiac wall contractility, and presence of pericardial effusion.[7] Left ventricular ejection fraction <45% and diastolic dysfunction on the echocardiography may be considered as early signs of anthracycline toxicity. Patients with suspected chemotherapy-induced cardiotoxicity should be referred to a cardiologist.[11] One study has concluded that in patients with chemotherapy-induced cardiotoxicity, troponin T or I can detect myocardial ischemia early as well as predict heart failure.[12] This is, however, not standard of care yet. There is evidence to suggest the role of beta-blockers and angiotensin-converting enzyme inhibitors in treating chemotherapy-related cardiac toxicities.[13,14] If necessary and deemed safe, stress testing of cardiac functions may be needed. In patients with hemodynamically significant arrhythmias, cardiologist opinion on the need for implantable devices should be taken.[1]

An anesthesia plan depends upon the preexisting comorbidities and the findings of the abovementioned investigations. Previous exposure to chemotherapy agents exacerbates the myocardial depressant effect of the anesthetic agents, even in patients with normal cardiac function. These patients intraoperatively can develop acute left ventricular failure refractory to β-adrenergic receptor agonists.[11] Thus, these patients should be considered high risk for major adverse cardiac events under anesthesia. It would be wise to use 5-lead ECG monitoring intraoperatively. In patients with significant cardiac dysfunction or those undergoing major surgeries, invasive arterial pressure and cardiac output monitoring are deemed necessary. Drugs causing QT-interval prolongation should be avoided. Hypothermia should be prevented. Similar monitoring and care should be maintained in the postoperative phase.

Respiratory System

Pulmonary complaints seen in patients undergoing chemotherapy can be due to metastatic disease, pulmonary embolism, infection or drug-induced pulmonary toxicity.[7] 75–90% of the pulmonary complications occur because of infections such as pneumonia.[9] The clinical presentation may range from subtle cough with no physiological compromise, cough with breathlessness on exertion to bronchospasm, pneumothorax, pleural effusion, hypoxemia, and severe pulmonary fibrosis.[15] Bibasal crepts or rhonchi may be present. Chest radiograph commonly reveals unilateral or bilateral reticular markings or consolidation. High-resolution computerized tomogram is a sensitive but not specific tool for pulmonary finding.[10] It may also show reticular patterns with ground-glass opacities and consolidation.[2] Pulmonary function testing shows decreased diffusing capacity for CO_2, forced vital capacity, and total lung capacity.[2] Common chemotherapeutic agents producing pulmonary toxicity are bleomycin, mitomycin, cyclophosphamide, busulfan, nitrosoureas, cytarabine, and methotrexate.[7,4] The underlying mechanism of chemotherapy-related pulmonary toxicity is not well understood. It is said that chemotherapy-induced pulmonary toxicity occurs within weeks to months of starting chemotherapy and is usually a diagnosis of exclusion.[2]

Bleomycin-induced Pulmonary Toxicity

Bleomycin is commonly used for treatment of Hodgkin's disease and germ cell tumors. Bleomycin-induced lung toxicity occurs 10 weeks to 6 months after starting treatment.[2,3] About 40% of patients receiving bleomycin develop pulmonary toxicity, 30% develop pulmonary fibrosis while 10% patients can have ARDS-related mortality.[3] Risk factors for developing bleomycin pulmonary toxicity are cumulative dose of >400 units, old age, baseline poor pulmonary reserves, uremia, radiotherapy, higher inspired oxygen concentrations, and concomitantly administered other chemotherapeutic agents like cisplatin.[9] The mechanism of bleomycin-induced lung injury is thought to be the direct cytotoxic effect of bleomycin. This causes damage to the respiratory epithelial cells leading to metaplasia from squamous epithelium to cuboidal epithelium. If the exposure continues, the affected cells will not undergo reversion. Thus, the defective immune response leads to macrophage invasion producing an inflammatory response and pulmonary fibrosis.[1] The symptoms are often nonspecific like dry cough and breathlessness. Patients can also complain of fever and pleuritic chest pain. They can also present with pneumomediastinum and pneumothorax. It has been suggested that bleomycin produces free radicals that effect the DNA homeostasis leading to cell death.[1] This is of concern in patients who have received bleomycin and are undergoing surgery as exposure to oxygen in the perioperative period can induce as well as exacerbate bleomycin-induced lung injury.[7] Thus, for safety, it is recommended to avoid high concentrations of inspired oxygen in the perioperative period.[2] For hypoxic patients, it is best to titrate the inspired oxygen concentration to maintain oxygen saturation of 88–92%.[2]

Other chemotherapeutic agents producing pulmonary toxicities are listed in **Table 3**.[2,9]

TABLE 3: Effect of drugs on the respiratory system.

Drug	Effect on respiratory system
Mitomycin C	Bronchospasm, acute respiratory distress syndrome, and interstitial pneumonitis
Gemcitabine	Interstitial pneumonitis, diffuse alveolar hemorrhage, noncardiogenic pulmonary edema, and pleural effusion
Busulfan	Pulmonary alveolar lipoproteinosis and pulmonary fibrosis
Methotrexate	Pleurisy with acute chest pain, hypersensitivity pneumonitis, noncardiogenic pulmonary edema, and pulmonary fibrosis
Paclitaxel and docetaxel	Interstitial pneumonitis

Anesthetic Implications

Patients who have received bleomycin or other chemotherapeutic agents known to produce lung toxicities should undergo a detailed preanesthesia checkup to understand the degree of lung toxicity caused. It is essential to elicit history of any exertional dyspnea or dyspnea at rest in order to further evaluate the lung functions of the patient. Investigations such as chest radiograph, room air arterial blood gas analysis, pulmonary function tests including carbon monoxide diffusion capacity, and computed tomography of the chest are needed to evaluate the lung functions.[7] Preoperative optimization may be essential for some patients. In patients with progressive pulmonary fibrosis, very little can be done to optimize the chest conditions.[1] For these patients, it is necessary to have a multidisciplinary discussion among the anesthetist, surgeon, oncologist, chest physician, and physiotherapist to risk stratify the patient and chalk out the perioperative plan. These patients are at increased risk of postoperative pulmonary complications and need ventilatory support. Though, antibiotics and inhaled steroids are not generally used prophylactically in the perioperative period, there is some evidence to suggest the role of antibiotics, inhaled bronchodilators, inhaled steroids, and mucolytics combined with physical rehabilitation to prevent postoperative pulmonary complications.[16,17] Intraoperatively, lung-protective ventilation with positive end-expiratory pressure (PEEP) and inspired oxygen concentration titrated to achieve oxygen saturation between 88% and 92% should be used.[2,7] Cautious fluid administration should be instituted.[7] If indicated, stress dose of glucocorticoids may have to be given.[2] Adequate postoperative analgesia, chest physiotherapy, and early mobilization reduce the risk of pulmonary complications in these patients undergoing thoracic and upper abdominal surgeries.[4]

Renal System

Chemotherapeutic drugs are excreted by the kidney and thus can lead to acute kidney injury. These injuries are usually reversible and dose-related. Acute kidney injury occurs due to proximal tubular injury, which is characterized by proteinuria, phosphate wasting, Fanconi syndrome (hypophosphatemia, hypokalemia, proteinuria, and glycosuria), and magnesium wasting.[2] Also many of these agents are themselves nephrotoxic leading to acute and chronic kidney failure.[7] Platinum-based chemotherapy agents like carboplatin, cisplatin, and oxaliplatin commonly lead to renal tubular and glomerular injury resulting in reduction of glomerular filtration rate and increased serum creatinine. On an average, 20% of patients receiving cisplatin develop nephrotoxicity.[18] Cisplatin-induced acute kidney injury can present as early as 5–7 days after starting the drug or even earlier in patients with preexisting kidney disease. Various risk factors of chemotherapy-related nephrotoxicity have been identified, which include elderly female patients, smoking, hypoalbuminemia, history of hypertension, total cisplatin dose of more than 100 milligrams, dehydration, concomitant administration of paclitaxel, and other nephrotoxic drugs like nonsteroidal anti-inflammatory analgesics.

Other chemotherapeutic agents producing renal toxicities are listed in **Table 4**.[2,7,9]

Anesthetic Implications

Preoperative evaluation should include renal function tests like urea, creatinine, and serum electrolytes, which help anesthetist gauge the extent of kidney damage caused by various nephrotoxic chemotherapy drugs.[2] Any electrolyte imbalance should be addressed preoperatively. In these patients, it is essential to estimate the glomerular filtration rate preoperatively for proper dose adjustments of the drugs.[2] Intraoperatively, it is essential to use a balanced fluid approach to maintain euvolemia and prevent dehydration. Hypotension and hemodynamic instability should be avoided in the perioperative period as they reduce the renal blood flow, which can further aggravate the renal injury.[4] Patients with severe kidney dysfunction will need dose modifications of drugs used intraoperatively like opioids, antibiotics, and muscle relaxants.[3] Nephrotoxic agents like nonsteroidal anti-inflammatory drugs should be avoided.

TABLE 4: Drugs producing renal effects.

Drug	*Renal effect*
Ifosfamide	Nephrogenic diabetes insipidus, Fanconi syndrome, and proximal tubular injury
Cyclophosphamide	Hemorrhagic cystitis
Mitomycin C	Microangiopathic hemolytic anemia and renal failure
Methotrexate	Acute nephrotoxicity due to intratubular drug precipitation

Hepatic and Gastrointestinal System

Chemotherapy-related liver injury leads to damage of liver parenchyma along with fatty change, cholestasis, and eventually hepatocellular necrosis. 85% of patients undergoing chemotherapy suffer from steatosis.[19] Chemotherapy-associated liver injury is usually asymptomatic or sometimes may lead to increases in liver enzymes.[2] However, in severe cases, inflammatory hepatitis, chemotherapy-induced acute steatohepatitis, and end-stage liver disease may occur.[1]

Chemotherapeutic agents producing liver toxicities are listed in **Table 5**.[2,6,7]

Most chemotherapy drugs cause mucositis, nausea, vomiting, and diarrhea leading to electrolyte imbalance and dehydration.

Anesthetic Implications

Preoperative investigations like bilirubin, alanine aminotransferase, aspartate aminotransferase, alkaline phosphatase, gamma-glutamyl transpeptidase, and international normalized ratio help to evaluate the liver function. Usually, general anesthesia is well-tolerated.[3] Hypotension should be avoided as it can impair hepatic blood flow, further aggravating the liver dysfunction. As in patients with hepatic diseases, anesthesia drug doses should be modified and hepatotoxic drugs should be avoided.[7] Cytochrome P450 enzymes are

TABLE 5: Drugs producing liver toxicities.

Drug	*Hepatic toxicity*
5-fluorouracil and alkylating agents	Steatosis and thus increased risk of perioperative blood loss
Methotrexate	Fibrosis and hepatic cirrhosis
Cyclophosphamide	Diffuse hepatocellular destruction
Platinum compounds	Hepatic necrosis
Topotecan and irinotecan	Steatosis, increased transaminases, and severe hepatocellular injury
Vincristine	Transient rise in transaminases

inhibited by chemotherapeutic agents like vinblastine, cyclophosphamide, docetaxel and ifosfamide affecting drug metabolism. Regional anesthesia may be contraindicated if coagulopathy is present.

Nausea, vomiting, and diarrhea cause fluid and electrolyte imbalance, which needs optimization in the preoperative period. Thus, it is essential to closely monitor the fluid status intraoperatively. Hemodynamic monitors like systolic blood pressure variation, pulse pressure variation, and stroke volume variation are useful to achieve optimal fluid status.[3]

In patients with mucositis, trauma due to direct laryngoscopy can cause bleeding making airway visualization difficult.[7]

Central Nervous System

Central and peripheral neurotoxicities are frequently seen as side effects of chemotherapy. Autonomic neuropathy due to chemotherapeutic agents leading to orthostatic hypotension is of concern to anesthesiologist. Chemotherapy-related neurotoxicity depends on the cumulative drug dose and intensities.[2] Risk factors of developing neurotoxicities are preexisting diabetes mellitus, advanced age, prior treatment with neurotoxic chemotherapy.[2] 40% of patients receiving chemotherapy develop peripheral neuropathy.[20,21] Various chemotherapy drugs affect sensory neurons leading to peripheral neuropathy, which may manifest clinically as tingling and numbness in hand and foot.[2] Chemotherapy-induced central neurotoxicity may clinically present as posterior reversible encephalopathy syndrome, acute cerebellar syndrome, hemiparesis, aseptic meningitis, cognitive deficits, and progressive dementia.[2]

Chemotherapeutic agents producing central nervous system (CNS) toxicities are listed in **Table 6**.[2,7,9]

Anesthetic Implications

A thorough preoperative examination with clear documentation of the existing neurodeficits is warranted in patients who have chemotherapy-related neurotoxicities. Regional anesthesia is not contraindicated in these patients; however, it is essential to properly document the existing neurological abnormalities.[2]

TABLE 6: Drugs producing central nervous system (CNS) toxicities.

Drugs	*CNS toxicities*
Vincristine	Muscle pain, peripheral neuropathy, cranial neuropathy, and seizures
High-dose methotrexate	Hemiparesis, confusion, seizures, and reversible coma
Ifosfamide	Encephalopathy
Oxaliplatin and paclitaxel	Peripheral neuropathy
Cytarabine	Peripheral neuropathy, seizures, myelopathy, cerebellar dysfunction, and pseudobulbar palsy
Procarbazine	Peripheral neuropathy and lethargy

TABLE 7: Effect of drugs on the hematopoietic and immune system.

Drug	*Effect on hematopoietic and immune system*
Platinum-based agents	Myelosuppression, thrombocytopenia, and enhanced T-cell activation by dendritic cells
Alkylating agents	Impaired proliferative or effector function of peripheral T cells and bone marrow suppression
Protein kinase inhibitors	Impaired proliferative or effector function of peripheral T cells
Anthracyclines	Bone marrow suppression
Vincristine	Bone marrow suppression
Antimetabolites	Bone marrow suppression

Hematopoietic and Immune System

Chemotherapy causes myelosuppression.[7] The synthesis of various blood components may be hampered. Thus, leading to anemia and decreased leukocyte production.[1] The European Cancer Anemia Survey found an increase in the incidence of anemia from 19.5% to 46.7% between first and fifth cycles of chemotherapy.[22] Leukocyte counts are at nadir usually 7–14 days after chemotherapy. Serious systemic infections leading to life-threatening sepsis can occur. Thrombocytopenia is also commonly seen after chemotherapy. The myelosuppression is usually reversed within 6 weeks of stopping chemotherapy.

Chemotherapy affects both the adaptive and innate immunity. The degree of immunosuppression depends on the type of cancer and the chemotherapy drug used. Both cancer and chemotherapy produce an inflammatory response leading to decrease in anticoagulant factors and a procoagulant state leading to venous thrombosis.[3]

Chemotherapeutic agents affecting hematopoietic and immune systems are listed in **Table 7**.[1-3]

Anesthetic Implications

In the perioperative period, there is a decrease in the oxygen-carrying capacity with an increased risk of opportunistic infection and hemorrhage. Thus, a detailed assessment of the bone marrow functions is essential. In cancer, anemia is multifactorial. Patient blood management program with its three pillars is an useful tool for the anemia management in the perioperative period.[23] There is some evidence to support the role of tranexamic acid to reduce intraoperative blood loss and blood transfusion.[24,25] Intraoperatively, acidemia and hypothermia should be prevented as they may worsen the coagulopathy. Point-of-care viscoelastic testing helps to identify and appropriately treat coagulopathy.[1] Strict aseptic technique should be applied particularly when invasive arterial or intravenous lines are placed and perioperative antibiotic prophylaxis should be as per the local or institutional protocol. These patients should be monitored closely for infections in the postoperative period as well. Thrombocytopenia, if present, can be a contraindication for regional anesthesia techniques. Therapeutic anticoagulation for venous thrombosis can interfere or need careful timing of neuraxial blockade. In neutropenic patients, nonemergency surgery should be postponed whenever possible as risk of life-threatening opportunistic infection may outweigh the benefits of surgical intervention. If prolonged neutropenia delays time-critical surgery, a multidisciplinary discussion with surgeon, hematologist, and anesthetist can be done for giving granulocyte colony-stimulating factors.

TIMING OF SURGERY AFTER CHEMOTHERAPY

The optimal time for surgery after neoadjuvant chemotherapy is usually around 4–6 weeks.[2] This allows recovery of the cytotoxic effects of the chemotherapy. Also, this time duration reduces the disease volume and helps in optimizing the conditions for surgical resection. The ERAS Society consensus guidelines recommend a time to esophagectomy of 3–6 weeks following neoadjuvant chemotherapy.[26] However, the optimal time for surgery is unknown in many cases. There is evidence to suggest that delayed surgery worsens survival. A time to surgery of 4–6 weeks also gives sufficient time for effective prehabilitation. A randomized control trial in patients with esophageal cancer could not demonstrate any difference in short-term postoperative outcomes between 4–6 weeks and 10–12 weeks of time to surgery after neoadjuvant chemotherapy.[27]

INTERACTIONS WITH ANESTHETIC DRUGS

Some of the chemotherapeutic agents interact with the medications administered in the perioperative period. This is because the chemotherapeutic agents alter the pharmacodynamics and pharmacokinetics of commonly used anesthetic drugs. Significant anticholinesterase activity of cyclophosphamide persists up to 3–4 weeks after administration. This increases the risk of prolonged neuromuscular blockade and respiratory depression when succinylcholine is given.[1] Similarly, the anticholinesterase effects of alkylating agents can cause prolonged respiratory depression with succinylcholine.[9] Procarbazine, which is a monoamine oxidase inhibitor, and ephedrine, an indirect sympathomimetic, produce an exaggerated blood pressure response.[28] Nonsteroidal anti-inflammatory drugs compete with methotrexate for the same renal tubule receptor, and thus reduce the excretion of methotrexate, which may lead to fatal side effects.[1]

There is now some evidence that indicates that chemotherapy causes central and peripheral nervous system sensitization to anesthetic agents.[1,29] Studies have shown that, in breast cancer patients who have received chemotherapy, lower than usual doses of propofol are required to elicit unconsciousness and maintain anesthesia.[30,31] Similarly, some studies have demonstrated that the minimum alveolar concentrations of sevoflurane required for maintenance of anesthesia is less in patients who have received chemotherapy and are undergoing gastrectomy[32] and hepatic resections[33] as compared to those who have not received chemotherapy. Further research needs to be conducted to understand the effects of chemotherapeutic agents on the drugs used perioperatively.

IMMUNOTHERAPY

Immunotherapy acts on the host's immune system and reactivates the host's antitumor response.[3] Immunotherapy can be molecular targeted or cell-targeted. Molecular-targeted therapy acts on molecules like growth factors, receptors, and surface antigens, as well as on signal transduction pathways that regulate cell cycle and progression of disease and death. Thus, these are also known as monoclonal antibodies or checkpoint inhibitors. Cell-based therapies comprise the genetically manipulated T-cell lymphocytes with T-cell receptors, which recognize tumor-specific antigens. These are also known as cell-based immunotherapy, chimeric antigen receptor T-cell (CAR T-cell) therapy, or adaptive cell therapy (ACT).

Immune Checkpoint Inhibitors

Immune checkpoint inhibitors (ICI) have effective antitumor response. Some examples of ICIs used commonly are as follows:[34]

- Ipilimumab, an antibody against cytotoxic T-lymphocyte-associated protein 4 (CTLA-4), is used for colorectal cancer, metastatic melanoma, and renal cell carcinoma.
- Nivolumab and pembrolizumab are antiprogrammed cell death-1 (PD-1) agents and are used in late-stage lung cancer, hepatocellular carcinoma, Hodgkin's lymphoma, metastatic urothelial carcinoma, and esophageal and gastric and tumors.
- Atezolizumab, avelumab, and durvalumab are also anti-PD-1 agents and are used for metastatic triple-negative breast cancer, metastatic urothelial carcinoma, lung cancer, and Merkel cell carcinoma.

Immune checkpoint inhibitors are considered to be safe in the perioperative period with a low incidence of grade III or IV Clavien-Dindo postoperative complications. They are not stopped before surgery.[35] The incidence of neurological toxicities is as low as 1–5%. However, if present, it is associated with significant morbidity and mortality. ICI-related neurotoxicity produces myasthenia gravis-like symptoms, peripheral neuropathies such as Guillain–Barré syndrome and meningoencephalitis. Treatment includes discontinuation of ICI, supportive care, and high-dose steroids. ICI-related acute kidney injury occurs due to immune-related acute tubular nephritis. Cardiac complications of ICI are rare with reported incidence of <1%.[36] ICI-related cardiotoxicity manifests as myocardial fibrosis, cardiomyopathy, heart failure, conduction abnormalities, myocarditis, and pericarditis. Myocarditis is the most common adverse cardiac toxicity with an incidence of 1.14%.[36] Symptoms can vary from nonspecific features like fatigue to more specific symptoms such as dyspnea and chest pain. Patients with a grade-3 ICI-related cardiac toxicity may have elevated brain natriuretic peptide (BNP) and troponins along with new ECG findings such as QTc prolongation or ST-T changes, which may require a cardiologist's consultation. ICI-related endocrinopathies lead to adrenal insufficiency, hypophysitis, and thyroiditis. Pulmonary toxicity can present as pneumonitis and pneumonia or it can be as severe as hypoxia and ARDS. ICIs are also associated with diarrhea, colitis, and raised transaminases levels. ICI-related vasculitis is rare but a potentially life-threatening condition.

Anesthetic Implications

During the preanesthetic checkup, a detailed history to assess the cardiovascular functioning and common ICI-related toxicities is essential. Investigations such as complete blood count, renal function tests, liver function tests, serum electrolytes are mandatory. Apart from these, investigations like levels of free T4, thyroid stimulating hormone (TSH), glycosylated hemoglobin (HbA1c), cortisol, adrenocorticotropic hormone (ACTH), and cortisol-stimulation test may be required in patients suspected to have ICI-related endocrinopathy. Preoperative ECG, baseline BNP, troponins, and transthoracic echocardiography should be done for patients who develop myocarditis. If patient has overt signs of heart failure, elective surgery should be postponed till the patient is optimized and a cardiologist consultation is warranted.[36] For major surgery involving blood loss and fluid shifts, intraoperatively invasive arterial pressure monitoring should be done. Intraoperative transesophageal echocardiography can also be done to monitor contractility and guide fluid management. Patients who are on chronic steroid therapy should receive stress dose steroids in the perioperative period to prevent an adrenal crisis.[36] In patients with pulmonary toxicities, it is necessary to assess the lung functions preoperatively with a pulmonary function test, 6-minute-walk test, room-air oxygen saturation, chest radiograph, or computerized tomogram. If needed, a chest physician's advise should be taken for optimization of the lung functions. Intraoperatively, it is essential to use lung protective ventilation strategies and prevent fluid overload.[36] For the management of patients with endocrinopathy, an endocrinologist should be involved in the perioperative period for adequate steroid and hormone replacement. In the perioperative period, adrenal insufficiency can present as persistent hyponatremia and hypotension. An adrenal crisis should be suspected if the patient develops treatment-resistant hypotension (fluid resuscitation, vasopressors, and optimizing depth of anesthesia), which should be treated with hydrocortisone supplementation. Hypopituitarism should also be treated as it is associated with major complications in the perioperative period. In patients having moderate-to-severe hypothyroidism, elective surgeries should be postponed till euthyroid status is achieved. Untreated hypothyroidism may lead to hypothermia, bradycardia, low cardiac output, impaired respiratory drive, and delayed emergence.[37] In some severe cases, patients develop myxedema coma, which can be life-threatening. If myxedema coma is diagnosed, it is recommended to initially administer either 200–400 mg of intravenous levothyroxine (T4) followed by 100 μg/day or 10–25 mg of intravenous triiodothyronine (T3) every 8 hourly. Dosing needs to be carefully monitored in cardiac patients.[38] Corticosteroid should also be administered because myxedema coma may have a concomitant diagnosis of adrenal insufficiency. Hyperthyroidism caused by ICI is rare but if left untreated, can precipitate life-threatening thyroid storm intraoperatively. Treatment is usually supportive with inotropes, hydration, cooling, steroids, and intravenous beta-blockers.[39] Iodine is reserved as a rescue therapy. The pancreatic exocrine functions are also affected. It is, thus, important to monitor the blood sugar levels in the perioperative period.

Cytokines

High-dose interleukin-2 (HDIL-2) is approved for treatment of metastatic renal cell cancer and melanoma. It leads to thrombocytopenia, hypotension, pulmonary edema, myocarditis, renal insufficiency, and vascular leak syndrome.[34,40]

There is some evidence of use of interleukin-15 (IL-15) in the treatment of leukemia, metastatic melanoma, and lung cancers. IL-15 causes fever, thrombocytopenia, hypotension, and less extensive capillary leak syndrome as compared to HDIL-2.

Unconjugated Monoclonal Antibodies

Unconjugated monoclonal antibodies (mABs) are used in various hematological malignancies as well as solid tumors. Rituximab was the first FDA-approved mAB used in the treatment of non-Hodgkin B-cell lymphoma. Other available unconjugated mABs are bevacizumab for colorectal cancer, trastuzumab for breast cancer, daratumumab, and isatuximab for multiple myeloma, etc.

Anesthetic Implications

Bevacizumab delays wound healing and also leads to thromboembolic events. It should be discontinued 6–8 weeks before surgery and restarted >28 days after surgery.[41]

Trastuzumab is associated with cardiac toxicity. It causes cardiomyopathy characterized by contractile dysfunction and reduced left ventricular systolic function.[42] The risk of cardiac toxicity increases with history of previous radiation, low baseline left ventricular ejection fraction, high body mass index, and concomitant administration of anthracycline.[3] In patients who have received mABs, it is necessary to perform a thorough preoperative check to elucidate signs and symptoms of cardiovascular pathology. Additional preoperative testing in these patients such as complete blood count, complete blood metabolic panel including serum magnesium, potassium, calcium, ECG, and echocardiogram should be done. In the perioperative period, high vigilance for cardiovascular complications should be kept.[34]

Many of the mABs like rituximab and trastuzumab produce pulmonary toxicity including pneumonitis and interstitial lung disease, which increase the risk of pulmonary complications in the postoperative period. Thus, proper preoperative optimization may be needed. Perioperative management is similar to patients with lung diseases such as using protective lung ventilation strategies, avoiding fluid overload, and oxygenation monitoring.[34]

Neurotoxicities are also seen in patients who are treated with mABs. These include seizures, progressive multifocal leukoencephalopathy, cerebrovascular accidents, cerebellar changes causing abnormal coordination and balance, aseptic meningitis, and posterior reversible encephalopathy syndrome which presents as headaches, vision changes, and seizures.[34] Some of them cause neuropathic pain needing opioids. These agents cause hypomagnesemia-related cramps, fatigue, and somnolence. The incidence of perioperative neurologic complications is seen more in patients treated with these agents.[34] Preoperatively, it is necessary to carry out a detailed neurological examination, review the imaging, and properly document the deficits. Electrolyte abnormalities like hypomagnesemia should be treated preoperatively. Anticonvulsants should be continued preoperatively. Anesthetic management should aim at prompt recovery of mental status, and thus facilitate postoperative neurologic assessment.[34]

Some of the mABs like alemtuzumab and moxetumomab pasudotox have boxed warnings for autoimmune reactions (including antiglomerular basement membrane disease) and hemolytic uremic syndrome, respectively. Cytokine release and tumor lysis syndrome associated with mABs cause severe kidney injury. mABs also can cause interstitial nephritis, nephrotic syndrome, and thrombotic microangiopathy. Preoperative kidney functions should be assessed. Perioperative concerns are renal dose adjustments, avoidance of nephrotoxic drugs, and meticulous blood pressure and fluid management.

Hepatotoxicities associated with mABs are high-grade transaminitis and increased risk of hepatic veno-occlusive diseases. Elective surgeries should be delayed till normalization of liver functions.

Hematologic toxicities such as cytopenia are commonly seen with mABs. Preoperatively, correction of cytopenia may be needed. mABs like daratumumab cross react with red blood cells and interfere with cross matching leading to false-positive indirect antiglobulin tests. Neutralizing agents against CD38 mAB are added during crossmatch. Thus, it is important to notify the blood bank if the patient is on these agents and closely monitor them for any reactions during the transfusion.[34]

Adaptive Cell Therapy

These are cell-based immunotherapy also known as CAR T-cell therapy. The host's immune system is manipulated by genetically engineered T-cell lymphocytes, which target a specific antigen.[3] These genetically engineered T-cell lymphocytes are custom-tailored for each patient. CAR T-cell therapy has been used in various childhood and adult hematological malignancies like acute lymphoblastic leukemia, non-Hodgkin lymphoma, mantle cell lymphoma, follicular lymphoma, and multiple myeloma. Their adverse effects include cardiomyopathy, neurotoxicity, pancytopenia, and life-threatening cytokine-release syndrome.[3] Cytokine-release syndrome usually manifests as vasodilatory shock, fever, and respiratory failure, which usually needs intensive care management.

Anesthetic Implications

Patients on CAR T-cell therapy usually present for vascular access or any emergency surgeries. These patients should not be scheduled for any elective surgery. There are no guidelines for the perioperative management of these patients. The perioperative team should be aware of the side effects of the CAR T-cell therapy. An important thing to consider is that corticosteroids, which are frequently used perioperatively for postoperative nausea and vomiting or as adjuvants in regional anesthesia, should be avoided within 30 days of treatment.[43] This is because corticosteroids inhibit T-cell function, and hence, counteract the effect of CAR T-cell therapy. Antibiotic prophylaxis is important as these patients are lymphodepleted and highly prone to infections.[34]

Oncolytic Viruses

Oncolytic viruses are engineered immuno-oncology drugs that replicate and enhance the host's immune system to selectively attack and destroy cancerous cells.[3] These viruses attack the transcription process of the tumor cells, act as immunomodulators, and enhance the cytotoxic activity. They also have a reporter gene that checks the pharmacokinetics of the virotherapy. The time of administration of the oncolytic viruses is an important factor.

Anesthetic Implications

Perioperative period: Oncolytic viruses when administered in the perioperative period have been shown to improve survival by preventing surgical stress-induced suppression of NK cells.[3] Talimogene approved in treatment of brain tumors and malignant melanoma, leads to flu-like symptoms or more severe and life-threatening tumor lysis syndrome.[3] Safety and feasibility are the main barriers to administration of oncolytic viruses in the perioperative period.[44]

Cancer Vaccines

These vaccines activate host's cellular and humoral responses to selectively destroy cancerous cells.[3] Cancer vaccines contain DNA, RNA, and viral tumor antigens, which activate the host's immune response. Few examples are Bacillus Calmette–Guérin vaccine used for treatment of bladder cancers and Sipuleucel-T for prostate cancer patients who are not responsive to hormone therapy.[3]

Anesthetic Implications

There is some evidence to suggest that cancer vaccines administered in the perioperative period can increase the production of natural killer cells and CD8 T-cells directed at tumor antigens.[45,46] This can help in reducing the tumor burden.[3] However, presently there are no standard guidelines on the use of cancer vaccines in the perioperative period. Viral spread to the perioperative team involved in the care of the patient is an important concern.[3] More evidence is needed to understand the efficacy and safety of cancer vaccines in the perioperative period.

CONCLUSION

Neoadjuvant therapy with chemotherapeutic or immunotherapy agents produces cardiac, pulmonary, neurologic, hepatic, and gastrointestinal toxicities. The perioperative physician should have a detailed knowledge of the short-term and long-term side effects of these agents. These adverse effects can have significant effect on the perioperative management. During preoperative assessment, it is essential to obtain a detailed history and perform a comprehensive physical examination and investigations to detect various toxic adverse effects of these agents. Optimization and multimodal prehabilitation are essential before surgery to reduce the incidences of postoperative complications.

REFERENCES

1. Barnes TC, Navaneetham S, Jones C. Neo-adjuvant chemotherapy and its anaesthetic implications for surgery—a narrative review. Dig Med Res. 2021;4:55.
2. Groenewold MD, Olthof CG, Bosch DJ. Anaesthesia after neoadjuvant chemotherapy, immunotherapy or radiotherapy. BJA Educ. 2022;22(1):12-9.
3. Dabo-Trubelja A, Gottumukkala V. Review of cancer therapies for the perioperative physician. Perioper Med (Lond). 2023;12(1):25.
4. Lacerda MA. Chemotherapy and Anesthesia. Rev Bras Anestesiol. 2001;51(3):250-70.
5. Galluzzi L, Buqué A, Kepp O, Zitvogel L, Kroemer G. Immunological effects of conventional chemotherapy and targeted anticancer agents. Cancer Cell. 2015;28(6):690-714.
6. Amjad MT, Chidharla A, Kasi A. Cancer Chemotherapy. In: StatPearls [Internet]. Treasure Island (FL): StatPearls Publishing; 2025. Available from https://pubmed.ncbi.nlm.nih.gov/33232037/ [Last accessed January, 2025]
7. Allan N, Siller C, Breen A. Anaesthetic implications of chemotherapy. BJA Education. 2012;2:52-56.
8. Pinder MC, Duan Z, Goodwin JS, Hortobagyi GN, Giordano SH. Congestive heart failure in older women treated with adjuvant anthracycline chemotherapy for breast cancer. J Clin Oncol. 2007;25(25):3808-15.
9. Gehdoo RP. Anticancer chemotherapy and it's anaesthetic implications (Current Concepts). Indian J Anaesth. 2009;53(1):18-29.
10. Dugbartey GJ, Peppone LJ, de Graaf IA. An integrative view of cisplatin-induced renal and cardiac toxicities: Molecular mechanisms, current treatment challenges and potential protective measures. Toxicology. 2016;371:58-66.
11. Zeien J, Qiu W, Triay M, Dhaibar H.A, Cruz-Topete D, Cornett EM, et al. Clinical implications of chemotherapeutic agent organ toxicity on perioperative care. Biomed Pharmacother. 2022;146:112503.
12. Colombo A, Cipolla C, Beggiato M, Cardinale D. Cardiac toxicity of anticancer Agents. Curr Cardiol Rep. 2013;15(5):362.
13. Cardinale D, Colombo A, Sandri MT, Lamantia G, Colombo N, Civelli M, et al. Prevention of high-dose chemotherapy-induced cardiotoxicity in high-risk patients by angiotensin-converting enzyme inhibition. Circulation. 2006;114 (23):2474-81.
14. Kalay N, Basar E, Ozdogru I, Cetinkaya Y, Er O, Dogan A, et al. Protective effects of carvedilol against anthracycline-induced cardiomyopathy. J Am Coll Cardiol. 2006;48(11):2258-62.
15. Mayet S. A practical approach to the patient receiving chemotherapy and anaesthesia. SAJAA. 2018;24(3):S38-42.
16. Gao S, Barello S, Chen L, Chen C, Che G, Cai K, et al. Clinical guidelines on perioperative management strategies for enhanced recovery after lung surgery. Transl Lung Cancer Res. 2019;8(6):1174-87.
17. Zhu X, Zhang P, Lou C, Wu J. Perioperative inhaled corticosteroids treatment is associated with decreased length-of-stay and direct medical costs in high-respiratory-risk surgeries. J Med Econ. 2020;23(3):280-6.
18. Yao X, Panichpisal K, Kurtzman N, Nugent K. Cisplatin nephrotoxicity: A review. Am J Med Sci. 2007;334(2):115-24.
19. Ramadori G, Cameron S. Effects of systemic chemotherapy on the liver. Ann Hepatol. 2010;9(2):133-43.
20. Pachman DR, Barton DL, Watson JC, Loprinzi CL. Chemotherapy-induced peripheral neuropathy: Prevention and treatment. Clin Pharmacol Ther. 2011;90(3):377-87.
21. Kopp SL, Jacob AK, Hebl JR. Regional anesthesia in patients with preexisting neurologic disease. Reg Anesth Pain Med. 2015;40(5):467-78.
22. Ludwig H, Van Belle S, Barrett-Lee P, Birgegård G, Bokemeyer C, Gascón P, et al. The European Cancer Anaemia Survey (ECAS): A large, multinational, prospective survey defining the prevalence, incidence, and treatment of anaemia in cancer patients. Eur J Cancer. 2004; 40(15):2293-306.
23. Goodnough LT, Shander A. Patient blood management. Anesthesiology. 2012;116(6):1367-76.
24. Roberts I, Shakur H, Coats T, Hunt B, Balogun E, Barnetson L, et al. The CRASH-2 trial: A randomised controlled trial and economic evaluation of the effects of tranexamic acid on death, vascular occlusive events and transfusion requirement in bleeding trauma patients. Health Technol Assess. 2013;17(10):1-79.
25. Shakur H, Elbourne D, Gülmezoglu M, Alfirevic Z, Ronsmans C, Allen E, et al. The WOMAN Trial (World

Maternal Antifibrinolytic Trial): Tranexamic acid for the treatment of postpartum haemorrhage: An international randomised, double blind placebo-controlled trial. Trials. 2010;11:40.

26. Low DE, Allum W, De Manzoni G, Ferri L, Immanuel A, Kuppusamy M, et al. Guidelines for perioperative care in esophagectomy: Enhanced recovery after surgery (ERAS®) society recommendations. World J Surg. 2019;43(2): 299-330.
27. Nilsson K, Klevebro, F, Rouvelas I, Lindblad M, Szabo E, Halldestam I, et al. Surgical morbidity and mortality from the multicenter randomized controlled NeoRes II Trial: Standard versus prolonged time to surgery after neoadjuvant chemoradiotherapy for esophageal cancer. Ann Surg. 2020;272(5):684-9.
28. Armand JP, Ribrag V, Harrousseau JL, Abrey L. Reappraisal of the use of procarbazine in the treatment of lymphomas and brain tumors. Ther Clin Risk Manag. 2007;3(2):213-24.
29. He ZJ, Hu YH, Fan ZY. Median effective effect-site concentration of intravenous anesthetics for loss of consciousness in neoadjuvant chemotherapy patients. Chin Med J (Engl). 2011;124(4):504-8.
30. Tan JT, Xu HM, Jia L, Xing Y, Wang Y, Qiu D. Effect of chemotherapy on sedation with propofol in breast cancer patients. Chin J Anesthesiol. 2014;34:395-7.
31. Wu G, Fu G, Zhang L, Zhang Z, Wang X. Effects of neoadjuvant chemotherapy on the depth of total intravenous anesthesia in patients with breast cancer undergoing unilateral modified radical mastectomy: A prospective observational study. Medicine (Baltimore). 2018;97(51):e13776.
32. Du W, Li C, Wang H, Zhao A, Shen J, Yong F, et al. Effect of neoadjuvant chemotherapy on sevoflurane MAC-BAR value of patients undergoing radical stomach carcinoma surgery. Int J Clin Exp Med. 2015;8(4):5649-57.
33. Zhang L, Zuo M, Ma X, Dong Y. Effects of neoadjuvant chemotherapy on minimum alveolar concentration values of sevoflurane and desflurane in patients with hepatocellular carcinoma complicated with jaundice. Oncol Lett. 2018;16(1):388-94.
34. Ackerman RS, Muncey AR, Aldawoodi NN, Kotha R, Getting REG. Cancer immunotherapies: What the perioperative physician needs to know. Curr Oncol Re. 2022;24(4):399-414.
35. Elias AW, Kasi PM, Stauffer JA, Thiel DD, Colibaseanu DT, Mody K, et al. The feasibility and safety of surgery in patients receiving immune checkpoint inhibitors: A retrospective study. Front Oncol. 2017;7:121.
36. Lewis AL, Chaft J, Girotra M, Fischer GW. Immune checkpoint inhibitors: A narrative review of considerations for the anaesthesiologist. Br J Anaesth. 2020;124(3):251-60.
37. Palace MR. Perioperative management of thyroid dysfunction. Health Serv Insights. 2017; 10:1178632916689677.
38. Bennett-Guerrero E, Kramer DC, Schwinn DA. Effect of chronic and acute thyroid hormone reduction on perioperative outcome. Anesth Analg. 1997;85(1):30-6.
39. Farling PA. Thyroid disease. Br J Anaesth. 2000;85(1):15-28.
40. Conlon KC, Miljkovic MD, Waldmann TA. Cytokines in the treatment of cancer. J Interferon Cytokine Res. 2019;39(1):6-21.
41. Libert N, Tourtier JP, Védrine L, Chargari C. Inhibitors of angiogenesis: New hopes for oncologists, new challenges for anesthesiologists. Anesthesiology. 2010;113(3):704-12.
42. Peshin S, Modi S, Namburu L, Rathod M. Unpacking trastuzumab-induced cardiomyopathy: A cardiac conundrum. Hearts. 2024;5(2):246-52.
43. Rohaan MW, Wilgenhof S, Haanen JBAG. Adoptive cellular therapies: The current landscape. Virchows Arch. 2019;474(4):449-61.
44. Tai LH, Zhang J, Scott KJ, de Souza CT, Alkayyal AA, Ananth AA, et al. Perioperative influenza vaccination reduces postoperative metastatic disease by reversing surgeryinduced dysfunction in natural killer cells. Clin Cancer Res. 2013;19(18):5104-15.
45. Bakos O, Lawson C, Rouleau S, Tai LH. Combining surgery and immunotherapy: Turning an immunosuppressive effect into a therapeutic opportunity. J Immunother Cancer. 2018;6(1):86.
46. Jarahian M, Watzl C, Fournier P, Arnold A, Djandji D, Zahedi S, et al. Activation of natural killer cells by newcastle disease virus hemagglutinin-neuraminidase. J Virol. 2009;83(16):8108-21.

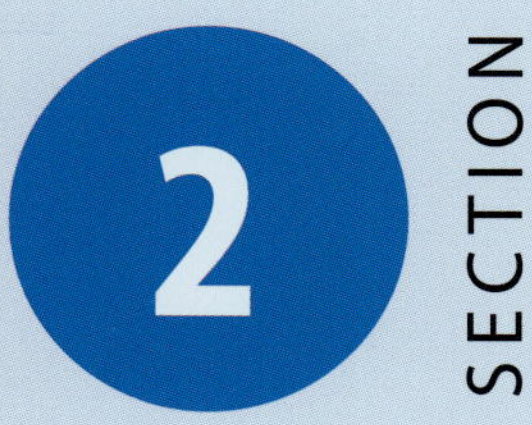

SECTION

Preoperative Preparation and Prehabilitation

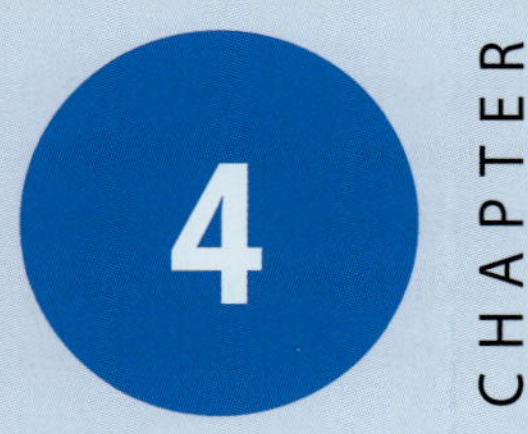

CHAPTER

Risk Stratification Tools and Outcomes Assessment in Major Cancer Surgeries

Sohan Lal Solanki, Sagar Joshi

INTRODUCTION

Major cancer surgeries are invariably associated with significant morbidity and mortality. These surgeries are often complex and high-risk, requiring meticulous preoperative evaluation, including risk stratification, to ensure optimal patient outcomes. Given the intricacies associated with these surgeries, such as tumor staging, patient comorbidities, and the potential for perioperative complications, stratifying risk and predicting postoperative outcomes accurately becomes vital. The use of risk stratification tools and outcome assessment frameworks has evolved to assist clinicians in tailoring patient management, minimizing complications, and improving survival rates.

In this chapter, we aim to explore the various risk stratification tools and outcome assessment measures employed in the context of major cancer surgeries. We will review specific scoring systems, the role of multidisciplinary team involvement, and the importance of patient-specific factors. Additionally, we will assess how these tools have been applied in different cancer types and surgical settings, with a focus on their predictive accuracy and clinical utility.

UNDERSTANDING RISK STRATIFICATION IN CANCER SURGERIES

Definition and Importance

Risk stratification refers to the process of categorizing patients based on their likelihood of experiencing adverse outcomes, such as perioperative complications, postoperative mortality, or recurrence of cancer. It is a critical component in the decision-making process for major cancer surgeries. Surgeons, anesthesiologists, and oncologists often need to balance the potential benefits of surgery with the risks associated with extensive procedures, particularly in cases involving advanced-stage tumors or patients with significant comorbidities.

Risk stratification enables personalized medical care, ensuring that high-risk patients receive appropriate care tailored to their needs. For example, a frail elderly patient with multiple comorbidities may require a more conservative surgical approach compared to a younger, healthier patient. Moreover, by identifying high-risk patients, we can focus on prehabilitation, i.e., optimizing preoperative conditions, such as managing comorbidities, improving nutritional status, and enhancing overall physical fitness.

Furthermore, stratifying risk helps inform patients about the potential benefits and drawbacks of undergoing surgery, facilitating shared decision-making and enabling informed consent. This is particularly crucial in cancer surgery, where the risks of complications must be weighed against the potential for improved survival and disease control.

Risk stratification also helps in meaningful comparison of surgical outcomes among service providers and helps in service evaluation and clinical audits.

Key Components of Risk Stratification

Risk stratification tools in cancer surgeries integrate various clinical and nonclinical factors. These include:

- *Patient factors:* Age, gender, overall health, and presence of comorbidities (e.g., cardiovascular disease and diabetes) are essential factors that contribute to surgical risk.
- *Tumor characteristics:* Tumor size, grade, and stage, along with molecular markers, play a significant role in determining prognosis and surgical complexity.
- *Surgical considerations:* The complexity of the procedure, duration, and potential for blood loss are critical in estimating the perioperative risk.
- *Functional status and frailty:* Functional status, as measured by tools like the Karnofsky Performance Scale (KPS) or the Eastern Cooperative Oncology

Group (ECOG) performance status, has a direct impact on outcomes, especially in elderly cancer patients.

Evolution of Risk Stratification Tools

Over the past few decades, numerous risk assessment tools have been developed and validated to predict the risks associated with major surgeries. Initially, these tools were generalized for noncancer surgeries but have since been refined to address the specific challenges of cancer surgery.

- The American Society of Anesthesiologists (ASA) Physical Status Classification System, which categorizes patients into six classes based on their preoperative health, has been one of the most commonly used tools. It ranges from ASA I (healthy patient) to ASA V (moribund patient unlikely to survive without surgery) and ASA VI (brain-dead patient for organ donation). Higher ASA scores are associated with increased risk of postoperative complications and mortality **(Tables 1 and 2)**.[1]
- *Lee's revised cardiac risk index (RCRI):* The RCRI is revised Goldman's cardiac risk index, developed by Lee et al. in 1999. It was designed for perioperative cardiac risk assessment before elective major noncardiac and vascular surgeries. It uses six clinical risk predictors, and patients are categorized into four classes depending on 0, 1, 2, and ≥3 risk predictors with 3.9%, 6%, 10.1%, and 15% risk of major adverse cardiac events (MACE), respectively **(Table 3)**.[2]
- *Surgical risk scale (SRS):* SRS integrated 3 scales with 3–14 variables. Each procedure was allocated a score on the basis of the Confidential Enquiry into Perioperative Deaths (CEPOD), British United Provident Association (BUPA), and ASA grades. Mortality at 1 month and 1 year after emergency surgery was predicted **(Table 4)**.[3]
- *Physiological and operative severity score for the enumeration of mortality and morbidity (POSSUM):* It is a comprehensive risk assessment tool that incorporates physiological and operative factors to predict morbidity and mortality after surgery. It includes variables such as age, cardiac and respiratory function, blood pressure, and intraoperative blood loss **(Table 5)**.
- *Estimation of physiologic ability and surgical stress (E-PASS):* It is made up of three scores: Preoperative risk score (PRS), surgical stress score (SSS), and comprehensive risk score (CRS) **(Fig. 1)**.[4]

However, the growing complexity of cancer surgery has necessitated the development of more detailed, surgery-specific tools.

Some of these tools include:

- *Charlson Comorbidity Index (CCI):* Originally developed to predict mortality by classifying or weighting comorbid conditions, the CCI has been adapted for cancer surgery to evaluate long-term outcomes **(Table 6)**.[5]

TABLE 1: ASA physical status classification system.

P1: Normal and healthy
P2: Mild systemic disease
P3: Severe systemic disease
P4: Severe systemic disease that is a constant threat to life
P5: Moribund and not expected to survive without operation
P6: Brain dead, whose organs are being removed for donation

(ASA: American Society of Anesthesiologists)

TABLE 2: ASA classification.

ASA class	*Definition*	*Pooled mortality (%)*
I	Healthy	0–0.3
II	Mild systemic disease with no functional limitation	0.3–1.4
III	Severe systemic disease with functional limitation	1.8–5.4
IV	Severe systemic disease constant threat to life	7.8–25.0
V	Moribund patient—unlikely to survive 24 hour with or without operation	9.4–57.8
E	Suffix added to denote emergency operation	

(ASA: American Society of Anesthesiologists)

TABLE 3: Lee's revised cardiac risk index.

Number of risk predictors	*Risk of MACE*
0	3.9% (2.8–5.4%)
1	6.0% (4.9–7.4%)
2	10.1% (8.1–12.6%)
≥3	15% (11.1–20.0%)

Note: MACE defined as death, myocardial infarction, or cardiac arrest at 30 days after noncardiac surgery
Source: Duceppe 2017

TABLE 4: Surgical risk scale.

Description		***Score***
CEPOD		
• Elective	• Routine booked nonurgent case, e.g., varicose veins or hernia	1
• Scheduled	• Booked admission, e.g., cancer of the colon or AAA	2
• Urgent	• Cases requiring treatment within 24–48 hours of admission, e.g., obstructed colon	3
• Emergency	• Cases requiring immediate treatment, e.g., ruptured AAA	4
BUPA		
• Minor	• Removal of sebaceous cyst, skin lesions, and esophagogastric duodenoscopy	1
• Intermediate	• Unilateral varicose veins, unilateral hernia repair, and colonoscopy	2
• Major	• Appendicectomy and open cholecystectomy	3
• Major plus	• Gastrectomy, any colectomy, and laparoscopic cholecystectomy	4
• Complex major	• Carotid endarterectomy, AAA repair, limb salvage, anterior resection, and esophagectomy	5
ASA		
• I	• No systemic disease	1
• II	• Mild systemic disease	2
• III	• Systemic disease affecting activity	3
• IV	• Serious disease but not moribund	4
• V	• Moribund, not expected to survive	5
The Surgical Risk Scale score was calculated for each procedure by adding the CEPOD, ASA, and BUPA scores.		

(AAA: abdominal aortic aneurysm; ASA: American Society of Anesthesiologists; BUPA: British United Provident Association; CEPOD: confidential enquiry into perioperative deaths)

TABLE 5: Physiological and operative severity score for the enumeration of mortality and morbidity (POSSUM).

POSSUM physiological Score	***1***	***2***	***4***	***8***
Age (years)	<60	61–70	>71	
Cardiac signs + CXR	No failure	Diuretic, digoxin, and antianginal/ antihypertensive	Dyspnea on exertion and moderate COPD	Resting dyspnea, RR > 30/min, fibrosis, and consolidation
Systolic BP (mm Hg)	110–130	131–170 or 100–109	>171or 90–99	<90
Heart rate (beats/min)	50–80	81–100 or 40–49	101–120	>121 or <40
GCS	15	12–14	9–11	<8
Hemoglobin (g/dL)	13–16	11.5–12.9 or 16.1–17.0	10.0–11.4 or 17.1–18.0	<9.9 or >18.1
WBC ($\times 10^9$/L)	4–10	10.1–20.0 or 3.1–4.0	>20.1 or <3.0	>15.1
Urea (mmol/L)	< 7.5	7.5–10.0	10.1–15.0	>15.1
Sodium (mmol/L)	>136	131–135	126–130	<125
Potassium (mmol/L)	3.5–5.0	3.2–3.4 or 5.1–5.3	2.9–3.1 or 5.4–5.9	<2.8 or >6.0
ECG	Normal		Atria fibrillation (rate 60–90/min)	Any abnormal rhythm, >5 ectopics/min, Q waves, ST/T wave changes
POSSUM Operative Severity Score				
Severity score	Minor	Moderate (colectomies)	Major (APR)	Major +
Multiple procedures	1		2	>2

Contd...

Contd...

POSSUM Operative Severity Score				
Blood Loss (mL)	<100	100–500	501–999	>999
Contamination	None	Minor (Serous)	Local pus	Free bowel content, pus, or blood
Presence of Ca	None	Primary	Nodal metastasis	Distant metastasis
Mode of surgery	Elective		Urgent	Emergency (Immediate <2 hours)

$x = (0.16 \times \text{physiologic score}) + (0.19 \times \text{operative score}) - 5.91$

Predicted morbidity rate $= 1/(1+e^{(-x)})$

$y = (0.13 \times \text{physiologic score}) + (0.16 \times \text{operative score}) - 7.04$

Predicted mortality rate $= 1/(1+e^{(-y)})$

(APR: abdominoperineal resection BP: blood pressure; CXR: chest X-ray: COPD: chronic obstructive pulmonary disease; ECG: electrocardiogram; GCS: Glasgow Coma Scale; RR: relative risk; ; WBC white blood cells)

Evaluation

Are you evaluating a surgical patient's perioperative risk? Yes No

Age of the patient — years

Body weight — kilograms

Does the patient have a severe cardiac arrhythmia? Yes No

Pulmonary vital capacity as percent of predicted (enter from 0 to 100)

FEV1 as percent of predicted (enter from 0 to 100)

Does the patient have diabetes mellitus? Yes No

Blood loss — grams

Operating room time — hours

Select an appropriate answer for each finding

Extent of skin incision at surgery — Select

Heart failure — Select

ECOG performance status — Select

ASA class — Select

Reset Submit

Fig. 1: Estimation of physiologic ability and surgical stress (E-PASS). (ASA: American Society of Anesthesiologists; ECOG: Eastern Cooperative Oncology Group; FEV1: forced expiratory volume in one second)

TABLE 6: Charlson comorbidity index (CCI).

Comorbid conditions	***cCCI weights***	***uCCI weights***
Myocardial infarction	1	0
Congestive heart failure	1	2
Peripheral vascular disease	1	0
Cerebrovascular disease	1	0
Dementia	1	2
Chronic pulmonary disease	1	1
Rheumatic disease	1	1
Peptic ulcer disease	1	0
Mild liver disease	1	2
Diabetes without chronic complication	1	0
Diabetes with chronic complication	2	1
Hemiplegia or paraplegia	2	2
Renal disease	2	1
Any malignancy without metastasis	2	2
Leukemia	2	
Lymphoma	2	
Moderate or severe liver disease	3	4
Metastatic solid tumor	6	6
AIDS (excluded asymptomatic infection	6	4
Maximum comorbidity score	33	24

(AIDS: acquired immunodeficiency syndrome; cCCI: classical Charlson comorbidity index; uCCI: updated Charlson comorbidity index)

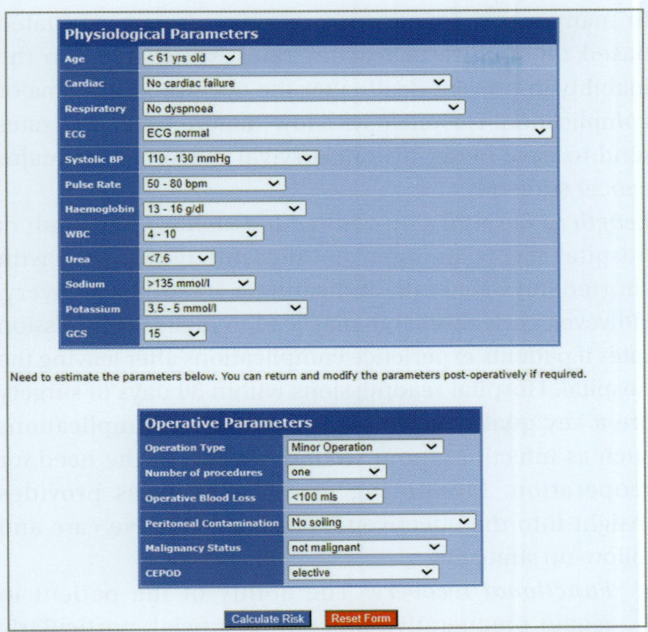

Fig. 2: Portsmouth-Physiological and Operative Severity Score for the Enumeration of Mortality and Morbidity (P-POSSUM). (BP: blood pressure; CEPOD: confidential enquiry into perioperative deaths; ECG: electrocardiogram GCS: Glasgow Coma Scale; WBC: white blood cells)

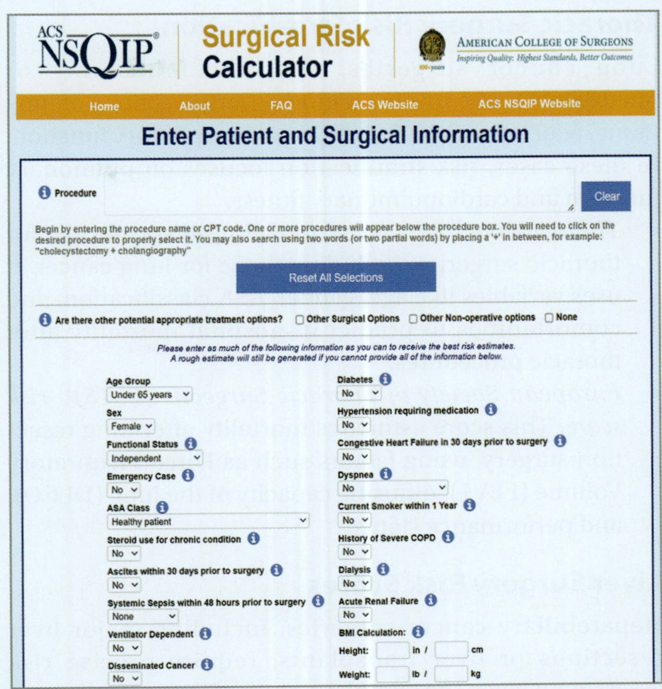

Fig. 3: American College of Surgeons National Surgical Quality Improvement Program (ACS-NSQIP). (BMI: body mass index; COPD: chronic obstructive pulmonary disease)

- *Portsmouth-Physiological and Operative Severity Score for the Enumeration of Mortality and Morbidity (P-POSSUM):* This system is used to estimate morbidity and mortality following surgery and has been applied to various types of cancer surgeries **(Fig. 2)**[6]
- *Cancer-specific risk scores:* For certain cancers, such as esophageal, lung, and colorectal cancers, more specialized scores have been developed. Examples include the Mayo Risk Score for liver transplant patients with hepatocellular carcinoma and the Thoracoscore for thoracic cancer surgeries.

MAJOR RISK STRATIFICATION TOOLS USED IN CANCER SURGERY

Preoperative Assessment of Cancer Surgery Risk[7]

The American College of Surgeons National Surgical Quality Improvement Program (ACS-NSQIP) **(Fig. 3)** provides one of the most widely used databases for predicting the risk of postoperative complications. The ACS-NSQIP includes a preoperative risk calculator that integrates a range of patient characteristics, including demographics, comorbidities, and surgical variables, to provide individualized risk predictions. For cancer surgery, the tool is valuable because it is based on a large, real-world dataset and offers predictions for various outcomes, including mortality, morbidity, and length of stay. It is particularly useful for high-risk procedures, such as esophagectomies and pancreatectomies, where complications are common.

Colorectal Cancer-specific Tools

Colorectal cancer surgery, especially in advanced stages, carries significant risks of complications such as anastomotic leakage, infections, and reoperation. Risk assessment tools tailored to colorectal cancer include:

- *CR-POSSUM:*[8] It is a variation of the general POSSUM score that specifically addresses the risks associated with colorectal surgeries. It incorporates both physiological and operative variables to provide an estimate of postoperative morbidity and mortality.
- *ColoRectal anastomotic leak score (CRALS):*[9] It is designed to predict the risk of anastomotic leaks following colorectal surgery, which is a major complication that can significantly affect patient outcomes.

Thoracic Surgery Risk Stratification

Lung cancer surgeries, such as lobectomy or pneumonectomy, involve removing large sections of lung tissue, which can significantly impact respiratory function. In these cases, risk stratification focuses on pulmonary function and cardiopulmonary fitness.

- *Thoracoscore:*[10] It is a risk model used specifically for thoracic surgeries, including those for lung cancer. It uses variables like age, gender, ASA classification, and comorbidities to predict in-hospital mortality after thoracic procedures.
- *European Society of Thoracic Surgeons (ESTS)*[11] *risk score:* This score estimates mortality after lung resection surgery, using factors such as Forced Expiratory Volume (FEV1), diffusing capacity of the lung (DLCO), and performance status.

Liver Surgery Risk Scores

Hepatobiliary cancer surgeries, including major liver resections or liver transplants, require precise risk assessment given the complex nature of liver function and regeneration.

- *Mayo Risk Score for Hepatocellular Carcinoma (HCC):*[12] This score predicts postoperative mortality for patients undergoing liver transplantation for HCC. It incorporates variables like tumor size, number of tumors, and alpha-fetoprotein (AFP) levels.
- *Albumin-Bilirubin (ALBI) Score:* This is a noninvasive tool for assessing liver function in patients with hepatocellular carcinoma. It provides prognostic information regarding surgical risk and long-term survival outcomes.

OUTCOME ASSESSMENT IN CANCER SURGERY

Key Outcome Measures

Outcome assessment following major cancer surgery includes a variety of short-term and long-term metrics:

Perioperative morbidity and mortality: These are the most immediate and critical outcomes after cancer surgery. Morbidity encompasses complications such as infection, bleeding, anastomotic leaks, and organ dysfunction, while mortality rates provide an overall measure of survival post-surgery. Mortality is typically assessed within 30 days of surgery (early mortality) and long-term survival is measured in years. Both morbidity and mortality are critical metrics for evaluating the safety and efficacy of major cancer surgeries.

In many cases, cancer surgery outcomes are evaluated based on "failure to rescue" rates, which refer to the inability to prevent death after the occurrence of a major complication. Hospitals with low "failure to rescue" rates tend to have better overall survival outcomes for major cancer surgeries.

Length of hospital stay and readmission rates: Length of hospital stay is an important measure of recovery, with shorter stays generally indicating a smoother recovery. However, early discharge may lead to higher readmission rates if patients experience complications after leaving the hospital. Hospital readmissions within 30 days of surgery are a key quality metric, often reflecting complications such as infections, poor wound healing, or the need for reoperation. Monitoring readmission rates provides insight into the effectiveness of postoperative care and follow-up strategies.

- *Functional recovery:* The ability of the patient to regain preoperative function is crucial, particularly in elderly patients or those undergoing extensive procedures. Tools like the Karnofsky Performance Status (KPS) and the Eastern Cooperative Oncology Group (ECOG) Performance Status are used to assess functional outcomes **(Tables 7 and 8)**. A standard way

TABLE 7: Karnofsky Performance Scale (KPS).

Able to carry on normal activity and work; no special care needed	100	Normal no complaints; no evidence of disease
	90	Able to carry on normal activity; minor signs or symptoms of disease
	80	Normal activity with effort; some signs or symptoms of disease
Unable to work; able to self care at home for most personal needs; varying amount of assistance needed	70	Cares for self; unable to carry on normal activity or to do active work
	60	Requires occasional assistance, but is able to care for most of his personal needs
	50	Requires considerable assistance and frequent medical care
Unable to care for self; requires equivalent of institutional or hospital care; disease may be progressing rapidly	40	Disabled; requires special care and assistance
	30	Severely disabled; hospital admission is indicated although death not imminent
	20	Very sick; hospital admission necessary; active supportive treatment necessary.
	10	Moribund: fatal processes progressing rapidly
	0	Dead

TABLE 8: Eastern Cooperative Oncology Group (ECOG) Scale.

ECOG scale value	*Definition*
0	Fully active and able to carry on all predisease performance without restriction
1	Restricted in physically strenuous activity but ambulatory and able to carry out work of a light or sedentary nature (e.g., light housework and office work)
2	Ambulatory and capable of all self-care but unable to carry out any work activities; up and about more than 50% of waking hours
3	Capable of only limited self-care; confined to bed or chair more than 50% of waking hours
4	Completely disabled; cannot carry on any self-care; totally confined to bed or chair
5	Death

of measuring the ability of cancer patients to perform ordinary tasks, the KPS scores range from 0 to 100. A higher score means the patient is better able to carry out daily activities. KPS may be used to determine a patient's prognosis, to measure changes in a patient's ability to function, or to decide if a patient could be included in a clinical trial. Physical function, cognitive function, and independence in daily activities are commonly assessed as part of functional recovery.

- *Quality of life (QoL):*[13] It is a multidimensional concept that encompasses physical, emotional, social, and functional well-being. In cancer surgery, QoL assessments are critical, as the physical and psychological impact of surgery can significantly affect patients' overall well-being. Health-related QoL can be assessed using validated questionnaires like the EORTC QLQ-C30 (European Organization for Research and Treatment of Cancer Quality of Life Questionnaire), Short Form Health Survey (SF-36), and the Functional Assessment of Cancer Therapy (FACT) questionnaire are used to measure QoL in cancer patients.
- *Cancer-specific survival:* This refers to survival outcomes directly related to cancer recurrence and progression. Disease-free survival (DFS) and overall survival (OS) are commonly used metrics in oncology.

Methods of Outcomes Assessment

Various methods and tools are used to assess outcomes following major cancer surgeries. These range from clinical data collection to patient-reported outcomes (PROs) to the use of predictive modeling to forecast long-term outcomes.

- *Clinical outcome registries:* Clinical registries, such as the National Cancer Database (NCDB) or NSQIP, collect data on surgical outcomes across hospitals and practices. These registries provide valuable benchmarks for evaluating individual hospital performance and identifying areas for improvement.
- *PROs:* These are increasingly being recognized as vital measures of success in cancer surgery. PROs capture the patient's perspective on their health status, symptoms, and overall well-being. Instruments like the patient-reported outcomes measurement information system (PROMIS) questionnaire allow clinicians to track recovery in real time and adjust treatment plans accordingly.
- *Predictive models and machine learning:* Advances in predictive modeling and machine learning have allowed for more sophisticated analyses of cancer surgery outcomes. Machine learning algorithms can analyze large datasets to identify patterns and predictors of complications or poor outcomes. Predictive models are also being used to forecast long-term survival and recurrence, helping to guide follow-up care.
- *Risk-adjusted outcome measures:* These account for differences in patient populations when comparing surgical outcomes across hospitals or surgeons. They ensure that comparisons are fair and meaningful, as some hospitals may treat sicker, more complex patients than others. Tools like the NSQIP risk calculator and the ACS operative risk calculator adjust for patient and procedure-related factors when reporting outcomes.

Predictive Accuracy and Limitations

While risk stratification tools provide valuable insights into perioperative risks, their predictive accuracy can be limited by several factors:

- *Patient variability:* Every cancer patient is unique, with variations in genetics, tumor biology, and response to therapy. This can make it challenging for standardized tools to fully capture individual risk.
- *Surgeon expertise:* The skill and experience of the surgical team can significantly influence outcomes, especially for complex cancer resections. Thus, risk scores may not adequately reflect this variable.
- *Evolving treatment paradigms:* Advances in cancer therapy, including minimally invasive

surgery, immunotherapy, and targeted treatments, continuously alter the risk landscape. Many risk tools may not be updated to reflect these changes.

FUTURE DIRECTIONS IN RISK STRATIFICATION AND OUTCOMES ASSESSMENT

Personalized Medicine and Genomic Risk Profiling

As precision medicine continues to advance, the integration of genomic data into risk stratification tools offers the potential for more personalized risk predictions. By analyzing the molecular and genetic profile of both the tumor and the patient, clinicians can better estimate surgical risks and tailor postoperative therapies accordingly.

Machine Learning and Artificial Intelligence

The use of artificial intelligence (AI) and machine learning algorithms in healthcare is growing rapidly. AI-driven risk models, capable of analyzing large datasets and incorporating numerous variables, are expected to improve the accuracy of risk stratification and outcomes prediction in cancer surgery. Machine learning models have already shown promise in predicting surgical outcomes and identifying patients at risk of complications based on complex data patterns.

CONCLUSION

Risk stratification and outcomes assessment are indispensable components of the surgical management of cancer patients. Through the use of various tools and frameworks, clinicians can make informed decisions regarding patient eligibility for surgery, predict potential complications, and optimize postoperative care. However, as cancer care continues to evolve, the integration of novel technologies, personalized medicine, and enhanced care protocols will be crucial in improving patient outcomes and further refining the precision of risk stratification.

REFERENCES

1. Ahmed SMG, Ahmad Alali M, Gaviola Atuel KLG, Hussein MIH. American Society of Anesthesiologists Physical Status Classification System: History, Development, Reliability, and Its Future. In: Sözen S. Surgical Recovery. London, UK: IntechOpen; 2020.
2. Lee TH, Marcantonio ER, Mangione CM, Thomas EJ, Polanczyk CA, Cook EF, et al. Derivation and prospective validation of a simple index for prediction of cardiac risk of major noncardiac surgery. Circulation. 1999;100(10):1043-9.
3. Sutton R, Bann S, Brooks M, Sarin S. The Surgical Risk Scale as an improved tool for risk-adjusted analysis in comparative surgical audit. Br J Surg. 2002;89(6):763-8.
4. Haga Y, Ikei S, Ogawa M. Estimation of physiologic ability and surgical stress (E-PASS) as a new prediction scoring system for postoperative morbidity and mortality following elective gastrointestinal surgery. Surg Today. 1999;29(3):219-25.
5. Charlson ME, Carrozzino D, Guidi J, Patierno C. Charlson comorbidity index: A critical review of clinimetric properties. Psychother Psychosom. 2022;91(1):8-35.
6. Prytherch DR, Whiteley MS, Higgins B, Weaver PC, Prout WG, Powell SJ. POSSUM and Portsmouth POSSUM for predicting mortality. Physiological and Operative Severity Score for the enUmeration of Mortality and morbidity. Br J Surg. 1998;85(9):1217-20.
7. American College of Surgeons. (2025), ACS NSQIP Surgical Risk Calculator. [online]. Available from: https://riskcalculator.facs.org/RiskCalculator/ [Last accessed February 2025].
8. Tekkis PP, Prytherch DR, Kocher HM, Senapati A, Poloniecki JD, Stamatakis JD, et al.; Evidencio. CR-POSSUM: ColoRectal physiological and operative severity score for the enumeration of mortality and morbidity. [online] Available from: https://www.evidencio.com/models/show/1775 [Last accessed February, 2025].
9. Ozata IH, Bozkurt E, Sucu S, Karahan SN, Camci F, Cetin F, et al. A novel scoring system for the early detection of anastomotic leakage: Bedside leak score—a pilot study. Front Surg. 2023;10:1204785.
10. Falcoz PE, Conti M, Brouchet L, Chocron S, Puyraveau M, Mercier M, et al. The Thoracic Surgery Scoring System (Thoracoscore): Risk model for in-hospital death in 15,183 patients requiring thoracic surgery. J Thorac Cardiovasc Surg. 2007;133(2):325-32.
11. Brunelli A, Rocco G, Van Raemdonck D, Varela G, Dahan M. Lessons learned from the European thoracic surgery database: The composite performance score. Eur J Surg Oncol. 2010;36(Suppl 1):S93-9.
12. Mayo Clinic. Post-operative Mortality Risk in Patients with Cirrhosis. [online]. Available from: https://www.mayoclinic.org/medical-professionals/transplant-medicine/calculators/post-operative-mortality-risk-in-patients-with-cirrhosis/itt-20434721 [Last accessed February, 2025].
13. Burckhardt CS, Anderson KL. The Quality of Life Scale (QOLS): Reliability, validity, and utilization. Health Qual Life Outcomes. 2003;1:60.

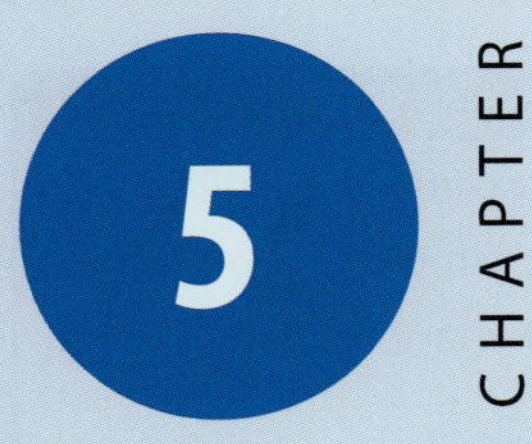

CHAPTER

Cardiopulmonary Exercise Testing and Uses in Cancer Surgical Patients

Asako Shida, Ravishankar Rao Baikady

INTRODUCTION

Cardiopulmonary exercise testing (CPET) has become an established tool in the preoperative evaluation for patients undergoing major surgery. It provides an objective assessment of a patient's fitness and cardiorespiratory function, which aids to predict surgical risk and guides perioperative management. Major surgeries involving hearts, lungs, gastrointestinal tract, or gynecological systems puts significant stress on the cardiovascular and respiratory systems, making CPET a valuable tool for planning safe and effective care.

Many of major surgeries involve cancer surgery. Patients suffering from cancer may suffer from multiple comorbidities, advanced age, and cancer itself has detrimental effect on metabolism causing cachexia and fragility. In addition, chemotherapy, radiotherapy, and immunotherapy induce multiple toxic effects on healthy organs increasing perioperative risks.

This chapter aims to explain the role of CPET in major cancer surgeries.

WHAT IS CARDIOPULMONARY EXERCISE TESTING?

Cardiopulmonary exercise testing is a comprehensive assessment of exercise performance, functional capacity, and function of the heart and lungs during physical exertion. During a symptom-limited exercise test on a bike or treadmill, various physiological parameters are measured. Some of the key components are oxygen consumption (VO_2), carbon dioxide production (VCO_2), heart rate, blood pressure, and ventilation (VE).

Indications of Cardiopulmonary Exercise Testing

Cardiopulmonary exercise testing is used in various clinical settings to assess patient's cardiovascular and respiratory fitness. Its primary role is in evaluating how well a patient's heart, lungs, and muscles work together during exercise, providing comprehensive information about patients' multiple physiological systems.

There are four main indications of CPET use clinically, which are outlined as follows.

1. *Risk assessment for major surgery:* CPET is used to determine perioperative complications for major surgeries including cardiothoracic surgery, abdominal surgery, and complex gynecological or urological surgery.[1,2] CPET identifies any modifiable factors such as problems with perfusion and or ventilations including undiagnosed pulmonary embolism and allows referral to cardiologist to exclude any ischemic heart disease.[1-3] In addition, poor CPET results aid risk stratification for postoperative mortality and morbidity. Results of CPET can be an objective way to share information with patients ahead of major surgery. In addition, it is used to determine and estimate the effect when considering lobectomy for lung disorders or making decisions on when to operate on certain heart conditions such as valve replacements, heart failure, and coronary bypass grafting.[1-3]
2. *Diagnosis of cardiopulmonary disease:* CPET is used in diagnosing and assessing the severity of the heart and lung disorders and differentiating the cause.[1] It is useful in diagnosing or monitoring conditions including heart failure, chronic pulmonary obstructive disorder (COPD), pulmonary hypertension, and interstitial lung disease. CPET helps differentiate between cardiac and pulmonary cause of exercise intolerance.[1]
3. *Assessment in congenital heart disease or lung disease:* Use of CPET is now a common investigation at tertiary lung and heart centers.[1,3] Indications of its use include risk stratification and assessing need for medical or surgical treatment, surveillance of

therapeutic interventions, and being part of physical rehabilitation. Most adult congenital heart patients should be encouraged to take part in physical activities and at times in competitive sports except for very small portion of patients who are prone to malignant arrhythmias.[3,4] Prognostications in interstitial lung disease and congenital heart disease are complicated and not validated and more research is needed.

4. *Assessments in athletes:* CPET is used to optimize the performance of athletes and research studies in assessing fitness levels in healthy populations. It is used to determine athletes' anaerobic and aerobic threshold and overall cardiovascular health, and it is also used when there is a suspicion of cardiopulmonary or cardiovascular disease.[4]

TABLE 1: Absolute and relative contraindications.

Absolute contraindications	*Relative contraindications*
Active myocardial infarction	Severe pulmonary hypertension
Active inflammation within heart	Severe hypertension
Severe aortic stenosis	Complicated pregnancy
Decompensated arrhythmias	Advanced pregnancy
Complete heart block	Uncorrected electrolytes
Trifascicular block	Exacerbation of asthma
Pulmonary edema	ICD that cannot be switched off
Acute desaturation	Pain
Aortic dissection	Large tumor interfering with mobility

Contraindications of Cardiopulmonary Exercise Testing

Cardiopulmonary exercise testing is generally tolerated well; however, there are absolute and relative contraindications to be aware of. Absolute contraindications include active myocardial infarction, active inflammation of heart including myocarditis, pericarditis, endocarditis, severe aortic stenosis potentially rendering patients to have an ischemic cardiac event, decompensated arrhythmias or heart blocks, pulmonary edema, acute desaturations, known aortic dissections, or uncontrolled COPD, or asthma.[1,2] Relative contraindications include severe pulmonary hypertension, severe hypertension with systolic blood pressure greater than 200 mm Hg or diastolic blood pressure greater than 120 mm Hg, advanced or complicated pregnancy, uncorrected electrolyte abnormalities, implanted cardiac defibrillator that cannot be interrogated or temporarily reset, and arrhythmias waiting for pacemaker insertion. Others include impairment of disability that compromises exercise performance including orthopedic conditions, or large intra-abdominal masses, or fluids.[1,2] Summary of contraindications is given in **Table 1**.

PERFORMING CARDIOPULMONARY EXCERCISE TEST

Static spirometry is normally conducted prior to CPET. Forced vital capacity (FVC), forced expired volume (FEV1) in one second, FEV1 FVC ratio, Vital capacity (VC), and minute volume ventilation (MVV) are measured.[1,2]

Cardiopulmonary exercise testing is conducted normally as part of an outpatient investigation and takes approximately 10–20 minutes. Patients are usually asked to have heavy meals prior to the test to avoid errors in respiratory quotient (R/Q). For example, high carbohydrate intake will increase R/Q ratio whereas high fat and protein content will decrease the R/Q causing errors in data obtained.[1-4]

Patient either sits on stationary bike or stands on treadmill with a tight-fitting mask, which measures the oxygen consumption and carbon dioxide production. Other parameters such as blood pressure, electrocardiograms (ECGs), and oxygen are also collected.[1-4]

Initial recording includes pre-exercise blood pressure, oxygen saturations, spirometry, resting ECG, and resting VO_2 mL/min) and VCO_2 mL/min.14 These baseline values are then compared with the values obtained when peak of exercise is reached. The degree of change from baseline to peak as well as time to return to baseline are also collected.[1-4]

Patient will commence exercise over 10–15 minutes aiming to reach maximum intensity of exercise. Patient is encouraged to exercise until they are unable to exercise any longer. Common symptoms for not being able to continue are leg pain and shortness of breath. Attention is needed when patient complains of chest pains or syncope.[1-3] The treadmill or bicycle resistance is set to increase every 2–3 minutes. Data is continuously collected into recovery phase to ensure blood pressure, heart rate, and ECG_S are returned to normal values.

Analysis of Data

A nine-panel plot is commonly used to visualize the results of CPET testing, providing comprehensive overview of the patient's psychological responses to exercise, as shown in **Figure 1**.[2] Each panel represents different parameter allowing for detailed cardiovascular, respiratory, and metabolic changes that occur during exercise.[2]

- *Ventilation over time:* Ventilation over time is measured to display how ventilation increases during exercise. Ventilation is expressed at VE (liters per minute)—volume of air moving in and out of the lungs. On average, resting adults will have VE of 7–9 L/min and can increase up to 200 L/min in athletes.[2,4] As intensity of exercise increases, heart rate, and ventilation increase to take in more oxygen to deliver to muscles.

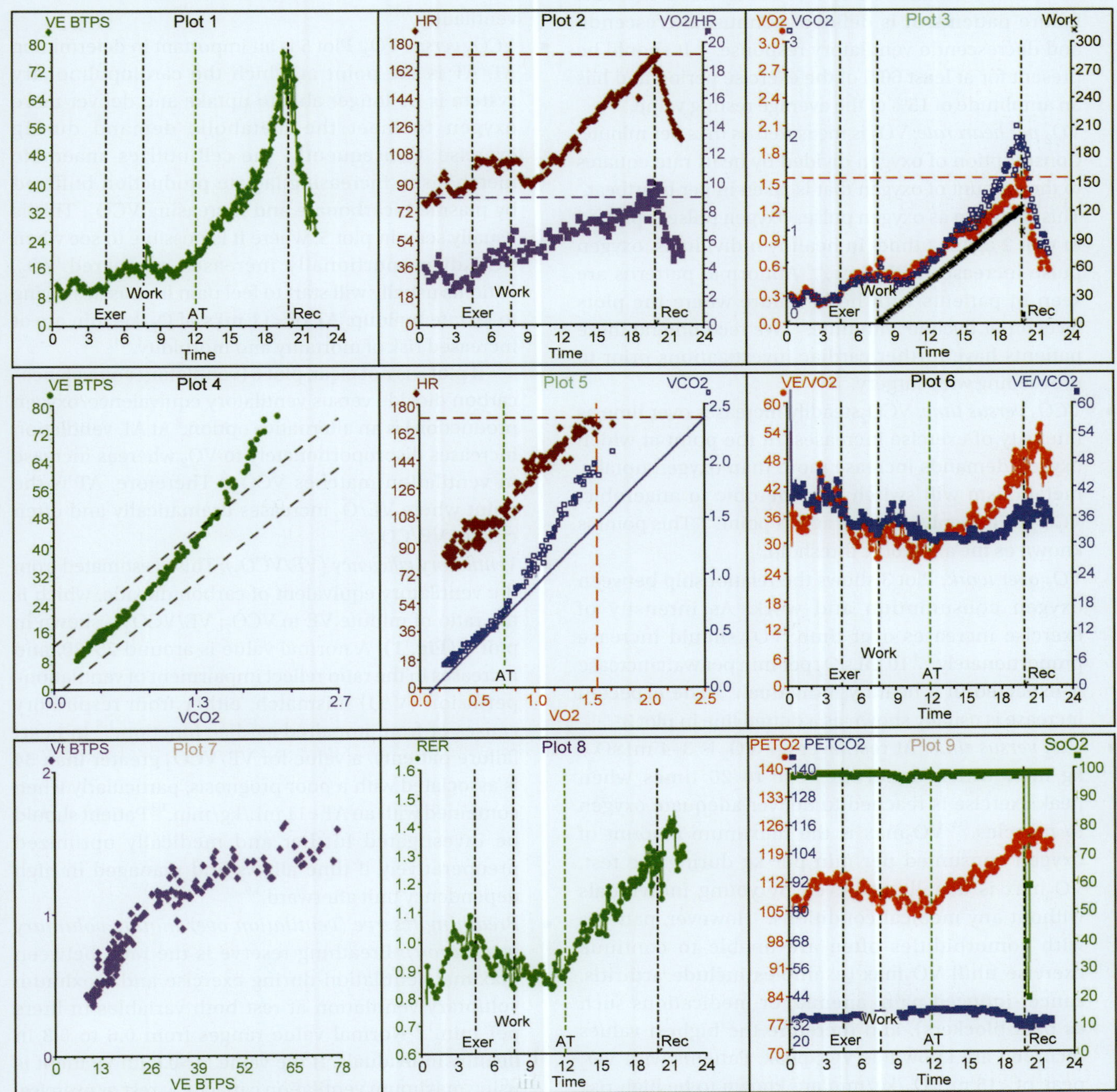

Fig. 1: Nine-panel plot of cardiopulmonary exercise test results.

When limit of oxygen uptake is reached, muscles will rely on anaerobic metabolism and there will be a sharp increase in carbon dioxide production. This steep increase in carbon dioxide production reflects reaching anaerobic threshold.[1-4] As production of carbon dioxide increases, ventilation increases accordingly. Oscillatory ventilation is frequently seen in heart failure patients. It is defined as unusual crescendo and decrescendo ventilatory response.[1-3] It should be present for at least 60% of the exercise period and has an amplitude of 15% of the average resting value.[1-3]

VO_2 per heart rate: VO_2 is measured as mLs per minute. Consumption of oxygen divided by heart rate equates to the amount of oxygen that is taken in per heartbeat.[2] This is known as oxygen pulse. Oxygen pulse is plotted in plot 2 against time. In healthy individuals, oxygen pulse increases with time.[1-3] Abnormal patterns are seen in patients with heart failure where the plots level off or decline with time.[1-4] We recommend these patients have further cardiac investigations prior to proceeding with surgery.

- *VCO_2 versus time:* VCO_2steadily increases over time as intensity of exercise increases. At the point at which oxygen demands increase more than oxygen uptake, metabolism will switch from aerobic to anaerobic. VCO_2 will steeply increase at this point.[1-3] This point is known as the anaerobic threshold.[1-4]

  VO_2 over work: Plot 3 shows the relationship between oxygen consumption and work. As intensity of exercise increases over time, VO_2 should increase proportionately.[1-4] 10 mLs O_2 per min per watt increase is expected in a healthy individual.[1-4] The expected increase is usually shown as a dotted line in plot 3.
- *VO_2 versus time:* At rest, average VO_2 is 3–4 mLsO_2/kg/min, which could increase to 20 times when peak exercise is reached to deliver adequate oxygen to muscles.[1-4] VO_2max is the maximum amount of oxygen consumed per min per kg during the test. VO_2max is usually achieved by young individuals without any medical conditions.[4] However, patients with comorbidities often are unable to continue exercise until VO_2max (examples include arthritis, cancer-induced pain, anemia, or medications such as beta-blockers), and therefore the highest values recorded are known as VO_2 peak. Patients with VO_2 peak of <15 mL/O_2/kg/min are known to be high risk of suffering from perioperative complications.[1-4]
- *Ventilation over VCO_2:* Ventilation response to exercise should be linear in healthy individuals.[4] Even at anaerobic threshold, ventilation should increase proportionately, which is shown in plot 4 where ventilation is steeply increased following anaerobic threshold (AT).[1,4] Patients with lung diseases including COPD, or restrictive lung disease may have reduced ventilation.[1,4]
- *VCO_2 versus VO_2:* Plot 5 is an important in determining AT. AT is the point at which the cardiopulmonary system is no longer able to uptake and deliver more oxygen to meet the metabolic demand during exercise. Consequently, the cell utilizes anaerobic metabolism, increasing lactate production buffered by plasma bicarbonate and increasing VCO_2. This is usually seen in plot 5, where it is possible to see when VCO_2disproportionally increases compared VO_2. Patients usually will start to feel pain in muscles owing to lactate buildup. AT of <11 mLs of O_2/kg/min are at increased risk of mortality and morbidity.[1-4]

  If plot 5 is not clear, plot 6 (ventilatory equivalence/carbon dioxide versus ventilatory equivalence/oxygen production) is an alternative option.[2] At AT, ventilation increases disproportionately to VO_2 whereas increase in ventilation matches VCO_2.[2] Therefore, AT is the point where VE/O_2 increases dramatically and often crosses VE/CO_2.[2]
- *Ventilatory efficiency (VE/VCO_2):* This is estimated from the ventilatory equivalent of carbon dioxide, which is the ratio of minute VE to VCO_2; VE/VCO_2 is shown in plot 6 **(Fig. 1)**. A normal value is around 25–30, and increases in the ratio reflect impairment of ventilation–perfusion (V/Q) mismatch, either from respiratory causes or from impaired cardiac function.[1-5] In heart failure patients, a value for VE/VCO_2 greater than 34 is associated with a poor prognosis, particularly when combined with an AT <11 mL/kg/min.[1,3] Patient should be investigated further and medically optimized preoperatively if time allows and managed in high dependency unit afterward.[1,5]
- *Breathing reserve (ventilation over minute voluntary ventilation):* Breathing reserve is the ratio between maximal ventilation during exercise and maximum voluntary ventilation at rest both variables in liters per min.[1-5] Normal value ranges from 0.6 to 0.8 in healthy individuals. If the value is >0.8, the patient is using maximum ventilation capacity at rest or exercise, which may signify COPD or restrictive lung disease.[1]

Low value indicates lack of full use of ventilation and may have an underlying restrictive lung disease.[1,6]

- *ECG changes:* ECG changes during CPET warrant attention including ST depression of 1 mm in two adjacent leads or 2 mm in single lead, t-wave inversion, left or right bundle branch blocks, or arrhythmias.
- Regular noninvasive blood pressures are recorded during CPET testing. The BP reading will aid diagnosis of hypertension and optimization of BP with medications. There are ongoing research studies looking at heart rate and blood pressure recovery time to understand whether there is a link between autonomic dysfunction and perioperative complications.[6]

EVIDENCE OF PERIOPERATIVE CARDIOPULMONARY EXERCISE TESTING USE

Exercise can mimic some of the physiological effects seen in the perioperative period and therefore cardiopulmonary exercise testing is increasingly becoming a useful tool to risk stratify patients undergoing major or major complex surgery.

Use of perioperative CPET is published in various surgical specialties including aortic aneurysm, hepatobiliary surgery, bariatric surgery, thoracic surgery, radical cystoprostatectomy, and colorectal surgery.[7] West et al. in 2004 studied the use of CPET in 136 colorectal surgical patients. VO_2 at AT of <11.1 mg/kg/min with peak VO_2 below 18.2 mL/kg/min indicated higher risk of morbidity and mortality.[8] CPET did not change the decision to proceed laparoscopically or open.[8] Junejo et al., in 2014, published two papers on preoperative CPET use in patients undergoing Whipple's procedure.[9] It highlights that VE/VCO_2 greater than 34 is predictive of postoperative complications and highlights the importance of surgical risk stratification and patient optimization[9] Another publication from hepatobiliary surgical team published that low AT (<11 mLs/kg/min) is associated with increased mortality and morbidity following Whipple's procedure.[10] Pancreatic leak was present in 45% with low AT versus 19.2% in higher reserve patients ($p < 0.02$), post operative complications (70 vs. 38·5%; $p = 0·013$) and prolonged hospital stay (29·4 vs. 17·5 days; $p = 0·001$).[10] Research study in bariatric surgery suggests reduced cardiorespiratory fitness levels were associated with increased short-term complications after bariatric surgery.[11] Findings include, there were no complications in those with BMI of 45 or less or peak VO_2 of 15.8 mL/kg/min ($p = 0.002$) or above.[11] Recent retrospective study examines the duration of intensive care unit (ICU) stay in 38 patients with aortic aneurysm who had CPET or not had CPET. Mean duration of stay in ICU who had CPET preoperatively was 2.5 ± 2.13 days whilst in non-CPET centers, it was 3.68 ± 4.08 days ($p = 0.05$). However, mortality was not statistically significant whether patient had CPET or not (2.63% vs. 5.26%, respectively).[11]

Systematic review published in 2021 by Steffens et al. summarizes 52 studies to elucidate whether preoperative CPET could predict postoperative outcomes in patients undergoing cancer surgery.[12] Higher preoperative peak VO_2 was associated with absence of postoperative complications [mean difference (MD): 2.28; 95% confidence interval (CI): 1.26–3.29) and no pulmonary complication (MD 1.47; 95% CI: 0.49–2.45).[12] Preoperative AT and V_E/V_{CO_2} also demonstrated some positive trends.[12] None of the included studies reported a negative trend.

To conclude, there are few retrospective studies strongly suggesting that CPET benefits patients on mortality and morbidity across multiple surgical specialties. Prospective studies are needed to strengthen evidence of effectiveness of CPET. We strongly believe that CPET benefits not only patients' outcomes but is also important in sharing information with patients and their families in their decision-making process. In this chapter, obtaining peak VO_2, oxygen pulse, VE/VCO_2, and AT are crucial parameters to risk stratify and plan for appropriate postoperative care.

COST-EFFECTIVENESS OF PERIOPERATIVE CARDIOPULMONARY EXERCISE TESTING USE

There is scanty evidence looking at cost-effectiveness of perioperative CPET use. There is one retrospective study conducted in 2013 that examines 210 patients with aortic aneurysm. The group investigated the mortality and morbidity in patients who had CPET with those who did not have CPET.[13] The study found patients who had CPET had shorter median stays in hospital. For open abdominal aortic aneurysm (AAA) repair, median stay was 10 days for patients who had CPET versus 13 days for patients who did not ($p < 0.01$).[13] For endovascular repair, stays were 4 days versus 6 days, respectively ($p < 0.05$). Nonoperative costs were 5,387 pounds for patients who received CPET versus 9,634 pounds for those who did not receive CPET.[13]

Although promising data, this is the only study published. More studies are required to establish cost-effectiveness across all major surgeries.

LIMITATIONS OF CARDIOPULMONARY EXERCISE TESTING USE

Cardiopulmonary exercise testing requires specialized equipment with trained personnel and appropriate accreditation must be present, which may not be readily available in all centers. Certain patients including morbidly obese and patients with pain or mass in abdomen that impeded mobility may not be able to complete the test. In addition, CPET machines are expensive to buy as well as require regular maintenance. It may not be feasible to adopt CPET services in poorly resourced hospitals.

EVIDENCE OF USE OF CARDIOPULMONARY EXERCISE TESTING IN PREHABILITATION

Prehabilitation is defined as the process of improving the functional capability of patients prior to treatment such as chemotherapy and major surgery.[14,15]

Randomized control trial published by Molenaar et al. in 2023 looks at whether 4 weeks of multimodal prehabilitation reduces postoperative complications in patients who had colorectal cancer surgery and whether it improves functional capacity in 251 patients.[14,16] Baseline CPET values were used to set training programs. Supervised training consisted of 1-hour session of aerobic and strength exercises 3 times per week with rest days in between.[14] Aerobic exercise consisted of 4 intervals of 2 minutes of high-intensity bouts conducted at 85–90% of peak power, alternated with 4 intervals of 4 minutes of moderate-intensity at 30% of peak power.[14] Resistance exercise consisted of 2 series of 10 repetitions targeting major muscles.[14] Baseline 1.5 g per kg per day of protein was advised as well as multivitamins and vitamin D supplements were provided. Overall, 39 of 123 patients (31.7%) in prehabilitation group experienced fewer severe complications. Prehabilitation group also experienced fewer medical complications compared with standard care (19 of 123 (15.4% vs 25 of 128 (27.3%); odds ratio 0.48 (95% CI 0.26–0.89) $p = 0.02$) compared to 54 of 128 (42.2%) in standard care (OR, 0.62 95% CI, 0.37–1.05; $p = 0.07$).[14] Interestingly, there was no difference in 6-minute-walking distance between the 2 groups compared with baseline.[14]

Systematic review published in 2021 analyzes 2 randomized control trials to determine the benefit or harm of prehabilitation on postoperative outcomes in patients undergoing major elective surgery.[17] 178 studies were included for analysis.[17] Inspiratory muscle training (IMT), immunonutrition, and multimodal interventions reduced hospital stay (mean difference vs. usual care: –1.81 days, 95% CI –2.31 to –1.31; –2.11 days, 95% CI –3.07 to –1.15; –1.67 days, 95% CI –2.31 to –1.03, respectively).[17] This systematic review concludes that cessation of smoking as well as provision of immunonutrition also reduces wound infections.[17]

To summarize, prehabilitation encompasses multiple interventions such as aerobic exercise, strengthening exercise, cessation of smoking, immunonutrition, high protein intake, and psychological therapies. Despite few publications, finding out which prehabilitation improves outcomes can be challenging. It is important to highlight that all that is previously mentioned is likely to improve perioperative outcomes and therefore we believe that advising patients to modify lifestyle is essential.

CARDIOPULMONARY EXERCISE TESTING USE IN CANCER TREATMENT

Cancer treatment has improved over the last few decades. Patients may receive multiple cycles of radiotherapy, chemotherapy, and immunotherapy combined with major surgery. This process can last for years. Historically, patients were normally advised to stay quiet when unwell. However, there is growing evidence to suggest that increasing fitness improves outcomes. Exercise not only improves patient's outcomes but improves psychological well-being, which is important when suffering from chronic illness. More than 60% of major cancer surgical patients will require further oncological therapy within 6–12 weeks of major surgical recovery. American Society of Clinical Oncology (ASCO) published guidelines to include exercise as a standard of care during cancer treatment.[18] A systematic review published in 2022 looks at 45 reports of epidemiological studies with several million participants looking at reduced risks of developing bladder, breast, colon, endometrial, esophageal adenocarcinomas, and renal and gastric cancers with physical exercise. The paper concludes relative risk reduction of up to 10–20%.[19] This systematic review also looks at physical activity reducing all-cause and cancer-specific mortality by 40–50% based on 5 meta-analyses and 25 source papers.[19]

As described in the prehabilitation section earlier, the role of CPET in cancer treatment is not only used as marker of fitness perioperatively but can be used as tool to improve outcomes prior to nonsurgical intervention. CPET is deemed to be a safe tool for perioperative use in cancer patients; however, the duration of exercise and type of exercise are yet to be elucidated.[15,20]

Finally, chemotherapy and immunotherapy are known to cause side effects including nausea, vomiting, weight loss, lung injuries, mitochondrial dysfunction, and general reduction in exercise tolerance. For example, doxorubicin is known to cause skeletal muscle cell damage and is toxic to cardiomyocytes.[21] Cisplatin, trastuzumab, and sunitinib all cause reversible mitochondrial dysfunction by interfering with adenosine monophosphate kinase (AMPK) and the mammalian target of rapamycin (mTOR) pathways known to regulate energy metabolism.[21,22] Many immunotherapy agents can affect vital organs causing inflammation. The degree to which these agents affect CPET results remains unknown. Future studies are needed to know the extent to which these anticancer treatments affect CPET results. Question remains on whether we should reduce the peak VO_2 and AT levels from 18 mL/kg/min and 11mLs/kg/min, respectively in this specific group of patients to deem them as high-risk patients.

CONCLUSION

The role of exercise in cancer surgery is increasingly being recognized by healthcare professionals, carers, and patients. The increasing evidence supports CPET in both preoperative and postoperative settings for optimization before and after cancer surgery. Though the current evidence is limited to few single-center studies and retrospective analyses, overall exercise is key to cancer outcomes and better quality of life. Ongoing research continues to improve understanding of exercise intervention in cancer care pathways.

REFERENCES

1. Glaab T, Taube C. Practical guide to cardiopulmonary exercise testing in adults. Respir Res. 202;23(1):9.
2. Chambers DJ, Wisely NA. Cardiopulmonary exercise testing—a beginner's guide to the nine-panel plot. BJA Educ. 2019;19(5):158-64.
3. Razvi Y, Ladie DE. Cardiopulmonary exercise testing. In: StatPearls [Internet]. Treasure Island (FL): StatPearls Publishing; 2025. Available from: https://www.ncbi.nlm.nih.gov/books/NBK557886/ [Last accessed February, 2025].
4. Petek BJ, Gustus SK, Wasfy MM. Cardiopulmonary exercise testing in athletes: Expect the unexpected. Curr Treat Options Cardiovasc Med. 2021;23(7):49.
5. Malhotra R, Bakken K, D'Elia E, Lewis GD. Cardiopulmonary exercise testing in heart failure. JACC Heart Fail. 2016;4(8):607-16.
6. James A, Bruce D, Tetlow N, Patel ABU, Black E, Whitehead N, et al. Heart rate recovery after orthostatic challenge and cardiopulmonary exercise testing in older individuals: Prospective multicentre observational cohort study. BJA open. 2023;8:100238.
7. National Guideline Centre (UK). Preoperative (update) Routine preoperative tests for elective surgery. London: National Institute for Health and Care Excellence (NICE); 2016.
8. West MA, Parry MG, Lythgoe D, Barben CP, Kemp GJ, Grocott MPW, et al. Cardiopulmonary exercise testing for the prediction of morbidity risk after rectal cancer surgery. Br J Surg. 2014;101(9):1166-72.
9. Junejo MA, Mason JM, Sheen AJ, Bryan A, Moore J, Foster P, et al. Cardiopulmonary exercise testing for preoperative risk assessment before pancreaticoduodenectomy for cancer. Ann Surg Oncol 2014;21(6):1929-36.
10. Ausania F, Snowden CP, Prentis JM, Holmes LR, Jaques BC, White SA, et al. Effects of low cardiopulmonary reserve on pancreatic leak following pancreaticoduodenectomy. Br J Surg. 2012;99(9):1290-4.
11. McCullough PA, Gallagher MJ, DeJong AT, Sandberg KR, Trivax JE, Alexander D, et al. Cardiorespiratory fitness and short-term complications after bariatric surgery. Chest. 2006;130(2):517-25.
12. Steffens D, Ismail H, Denehy L, Beckenkamp PR, Solomon M, Koh C, et al. Preoperative Cardiopulmonary Exercise Test Associated with Postoperative Outcomes in Patients Undergoing Cancer Surgery: A Systematic Review and Meta-Analyses. Ann Surg Oncol [Internet]. 2021 Nov 1 [cited 2024 Nov 19];28(12):7120. Available from: https://pmc.ncbi.nlm.nih.gov/articles/PMC8186024/
13. Goodyear SJ, Yow H, Saedon M, Shakespeare J, Hill CE, Watson D, et al. Risk stratification by pre-operative cardiopulmonary exercise testing improves outcomes following elective abdominal aortic aneurysm surgery: A cohort study. Perioperative Med (Lond). 2013;2(1):1-13.
14. Molenaar CJL, Minnella EM, Coca-Martinez M, Ten Cate DWG, Regis M, Awasthi R, et al. Effect of multimodal prehabilitation on reducing postoperative complications and enhancing functional capacity following colorectal cancer surgery: The PREHAB randomized clinical trial. JAMA Surg. 2023;158(6):572-81.
15. Guerra-Londono CE, Cata JP, Nowak K, Gottumukkala V. Prehabilitation in adults undergoing cancer surgery: A comprehensive review on rationale, methodology, and measures of effectiveness. Curr Oncol. 2024;31(4):2185-200.
16. Steffens D, Ismail H, Denehy L, Beckenkamp PR, Solomon M, Koh C, et al. Preoperative cardiopulmonary exercise test associated with postoperative outcomes in

patients undergoing cancer surgery: A Systematic Review and Meta-Analyses. Ann Surg Oncol. 2021;28(12):7120-46.
17. Perry R, Herbert G, Atkinson C, England C, Northstone K, Baos S, et al. Pre-admission interventions (prehabilitation) to improve outcome after major elective surgery: A systematic review and meta-analysis. BMJ Open. 2021; 11(9):e050806.
18. Ligibel JA, Bohlke K, May AM, Clinton SK, Demark-Wahnefried W, Gilchrist SC, et al. Exercise, Diet, and Weight Management During Cancer Treatment: ASCO Guideline. J Clin Oncol. 2022;40(22):2491-507.
19. McTiernan A, Friedenreich CM, Katzmarzyk PT, Powell KE, Macko R, Buchner D, et al. Physical activity in cancer prevention and survival: A systematic review. Med Sci Sports Exerc. 2019;51(6):1252-61.
20. Steins Bisschop CN, Velthuis MJ, Wittink H, Kuiper K, Takken T, Van Der Meulen WJTM, et al. Cardiopulmonary exercise testing in cancer rehabilitation: A systematic review. Sports Med. 2012;42(5):367-79.
21. Gorini S, De Angelis A, Berrino L, Malara N, Rosano G, Ferraro E. Chemotherapeutic drugs and mitochondrial dysfunction: Focus on doxorubicin, trastuzumab, and sunitinib. Oxid Med Cell Longev. 2018;2018:7582730.
22. Waseem M, Parvez S. Mitochondrial dysfunction mediated cisplatin induced toxicity: Modulatory role of curcumin. Food Chem Toxicol. 2013;53:334-42.

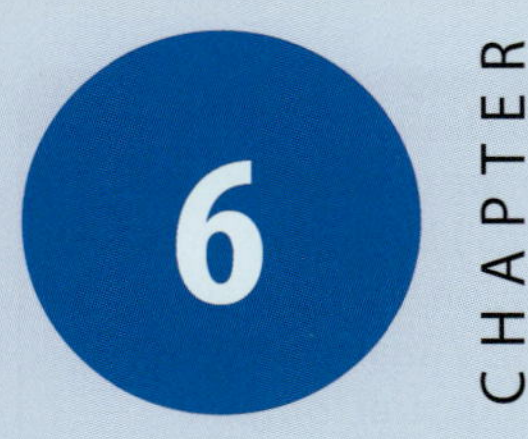

CHAPTER

Preoperative Anemia Management

Amit Jain, Massimo Lamperti

INTRODUCTION

Preoperative anemia is frequent in patients undergoing major surgical procedures. The reported mean prevalence of preoperative anemia is about 35% in elective nononcologic surgical patients.[1] However, due to a high estimated prevalence of anemia of about 30–90% in cancer patients,[2] oncology patients scheduled for various surgeries have a much higher incidence of perioperative anemia. As a high body of evidence exists linking preoperative anemia with an increased risk of morbidity and mortality in surgical patients, a similar or higher incidence of complications can be expected in oncological patients with preexisting anemia.[2] Though anemia can most easily be managed with blood transfusions, anemia treatment with transfusion may not alleviate the perioperative risks but instead appears to deteriorate perioperative outcomes, including morbidity, mortality, and increased length of hospital stay.[2] Transfusion-related infectious complications and or cancer recurrence are other major concerns.[3] Nonetheless, blood transfusions remain one of the costliest treatments in present-day medicine. Implementing perioperative patient blood management (PBM) programs in specific relation to the oncology population can improve recognition and treatment of preoperative anemia and promote safe and evidence-based use of transfusions in the perioperative period, leading to better clinical outcomes and cost savings.[2]

In this chapter, we will first discuss the burden of anemia and its pathophysiology in cancer patients, along with the problems of blood transfusion in general and oncological patients. Subsequently, the current clinical practice guidelines on general anemia management in cancer patients will be discussed briefly. Finally, the perioperative PBM aimed at improving patients' hemoglobin (Hb) through nontransfusion-based modalities, preoperative blood conservation, perioperative blood salvage, and restrictive red blood cell (RBC) transfusion practices would be provided to improve outcomes in surgical oncology.

ANEMIA IN CANCER PATIENTS

Although the Hb level below which diagnosis and treatment of anemia should be considered in cancer patients is not clear, the World Health Organization (WHO) defines anemia as Hb <13 g/dL in males, <12 g/dL in nonpregnant females, and <11 g/dL in pregnant females.[1] Depending on Hb level, anemia is classified as mild, moderate, or severe **(Table 1)**.[1]

The current literature on the prevalence of anemia in cancer patients has a major limitation in using different Hb levels to define anemia.[1-3] Prevalence also varied by cancer type and disease stage. The reported prevalence of anemia in cancer patients ranges widely from 30 to 90%. Nonetheless, 40% of patients have anemia at the time of cancer diagnosis, and this incidence may rise to nearly 80% in patients with advanced cancer disease. **Table 2** shows the reported prevalence of anemia in various cancers with

TABLE 1: World Health Organization (WHO) anemia grading based on hemoglobin levels.[1]

		*Anemia**		
Population	***Nonanemia****	***Mild***	***Moderate***	***Severe***
Men (15 years of age and above)	13 or higher	11–12.9	8–10.9	Lower than 8
Nonpregnant women (15 years of age and above)	12 or higher	11–11.9	8–10.9	Lower than 8
Pregnant women	11 or higher	10–10.9	7–9.9	Lower than 7

*Hemoglobin in g/dL

TABLE 2: Prevalence of anemia by cancer type.[4]

Cancer type	*Prevalence % of anemia**
Lung	8–84
Colon	30–67
Breast	41–82
Prostate	5–32
Head and neck	16–65
Larynx	21
Kidney	39
Ovary	26–85
Cervix/uterus	67–82
Vulva	31

*Based on studies that kept liberal cutoffs of hemoglobin >11 g/dL or hematocrit (Hct) >0.33

the use of liberal cutoffs (Hb ≤ 11g/dL or hematocrit (Hct) ≤ 0.33) for anemia definition.[4]

Further, the prevalence of anemia is also affected by chemotherapy and or radiotherapy treatment. In the prospective European Cancer Anaemia Survey (ECAS)[5] involving 15,367 cancer patients from 24 European countries, >50% developed anemia during anticancer treatment. Another observational study involving 999 patients from 13 Polish oncology centers found anemia in more than half of the patients after treatment completion.[6] Cancer of the female reproductive system, lung cancer, and testicular cancer were the most common cancer types in this study. In one study of colon cancer patients, the prevalence of anemia (defined as a Hb value of <12 g/dL) was 53% before radiation treatment and 67% afterward.[4] Similar effects on anemia prevalence were observed in most of the solid tumors.[4] A rise in anemia prevalence from 41 to 44% following radiation therapy in breast cancer patients and from 9 to 26% after radiation therapy in prostate patients has been reported.[4]

The mechanism of anemia in cancer patients is often multifactorial **(Table 3)**. Abnormal hematopoiesis, hemolysis, and acute or chronic blood loss could decrease Hb levels and RBC counts in the peripheral blood below the normal values **(Table 4)**[7] Cancer and cancer treatments such as chemotherapy and radiotherapy can induce increased release of inflammatory cytokines that may impair erythropoietic activity and disturb iron hemostasis.[1-3] Altered dietary activity in cancer cachexia, abnormal malabsorption, and cancer-related

TABLE 3: Mechanism of anemia in cancer patients.[2,3,7]

Nutritional deficiency	• Iron deficiency (tumor-related bleeding as gastrointestinal (GI) blood loss in GI cancers, malabsorption, functional) • Vitamin B_{12} deficiency [malabsorption disorders (e.g., after gastrectomy, in gastrointestinal neoplasms)] • Folic acid deficiency due to malnutrition
Bleeding	• Intratumor • Internal bleeding (cerebral hemorrhage in brain tumor) • External bleeding (surgical or nonsurgical such as hematemesis, melena, hematuria, and hemoptysis)
Immunological	• Cancer-mediated immune (lymphomas, chronic lymphocytic leukemia, and adenocarcinomas) • Anti-rHuEPO mediated red cell aplasia • Nonimmune hemolysis [e.g., microangiopathic hemolytic anemia (MAHA)] in mucus-producing tumors or prostate cancer—usual reticulocytes below 2%
Bone marrow suppression: Functional	• Aplastic anemia after systemic use of cytotoxic drugs • Nephrotoxic chemotherapy-induced red cell aplasia • Aplastic anemia after irradiation >20% of the bone marrow volume
Bone marrow suppression: Mechanical	Erythropoiesis inhibition due to tumor infiltration of bone marrow

(rHuEPO: recombinant human erythropoietin)

TABLE 4: Reference values of the red cell system.[7]

	Women	*Men*
Hemoglobin level	12.5–15.5 g/dL	13.5–17.5 g/dL
RBC count	4.2–5.4 T/L	4.6–6.2 T/L
Hematocrit	37–47%	40–54%
MCV	80–94 fL	
MCHC	32–38 g/dL	
MCH	27–32 pg	
Reticulocyte percentage	5–15% (28–100 G/L)	
RDW*	11.5–14.5%	
Peripheral blood smear	Normocytic normochromic	

*Coefficient of variation of red blood cell volume size

(MCH: mean corpuscular hemoglobin; MCV: mean corpuscular volume; MCHC: mean corpuscular hemoglobin concentration; RBC: red blood count; RDW: red cell distribution width) gastrointestinal blood loss can be additional mechanisms for iron deficiency (ID) in cancer patients. Though rare, folate and vitamin B_{12} deficiency can be other nutritional deficiencies leading to anemia in cancer patients.

Anemia in cancer patients is associated with fatigue, impaired physical function, decreased quality of life (QoL), and worse performance scores.[1-7] Anemia may be linked to impaired response to cancer treatment, radiation curability, and increased mortality, particularly in patients with lymphomas, head and neck cancers, lung cancer, cervical cancer, and prostate cancer.[7]

DIAGNOSTIC TESTS FOR ANEMIA MANAGEMENT IN CANCER PATIENTS

If the clinical symptomatology allows, before considering any specific treatment method, certain tests should be performed to determine the etiology of anemia and then plan causative treatment and therapy with the lowest risk of adverse reactions. Generally, the following diagnostic tests are recommended:[7]

- Complete blood count
- Reticulocyte count
- Iron concentration, total iron binding capacity (TIBC), transferrin saturation, and ferritin concentration
- Folic acid concentration
- Vitamin B_{12} assay
- Fecal occult blood test (FOBT)
- Renal function tests

Additional tests such as erythropoietin concentration, thyroid-stimulating hormone level, direct antiglobulin test (in myelodysplastic syndromes and prior autoimmune disease), and testing for hemoglobinopathy may be advised based on differential diagnosis.[3,7]

When the cause of anemia in cancer patients is not determined, it is classified as cancer-induced anemia.

INDICATIONS FOR INITIATION OF ANEMIA TREATMENT IN CANCER PATIENTS

Anemia treatment is not only guided by the level of Hb. It should also depend upon the clinical symptomatology, comorbidities, volume status, and rapidity of fall in Hb, as well as on chemotherapy or combined chemoradiotherapy status of the cancer patients.[3] Most patients—even in a severe general state—tolerate Hb levels in the 7–10 g/dL range.[7] In patients with normal volume status, Hb level as low as 6–7 g/dL ensures proper oxygenation of tissues during normal life activities. With Hb <6–7 g/dL, RBC transfusion should be performed even if the patient is asymptomatic. However, if the patient has coexisting cardiorespiratory diseases, a blood transfusion may be considered at a higher threshold of 8 g/dL, even in asymptomatic status. For patients with coexisting cardiorespiratory diseases with symptoms of anemia (angina, tachycardia, dyspnea, orthostatic hypotension, and fatigability), treatment is indicated when the Hb concentration is lower than 10–11 g/dL.[3,7]

IRON DEFICIENCY IN PATIENTS WITH SOLID OR HEMATOLOGICAL MALIGNANCIES

Iron deficiency is characterized by reduced iron availability in the body below the levels necessary for maintaining certain cellular functions. The most important is the synthesis of heme for erythropoiesis.[3] Absolute ID, i.e., the depletion of iron stores, is mainly due to bleeding issues in cancer patients. For example, hematemesis and/or melena are common in gastrointestinal malignancies. At the same time, bladder cancers may present with hematuria, resulting in a direct drop in Hb along with depletion of iron stores. Other factors, such as reduced iron absorption from intestines due to poor nutrition or malabsorption, are usually of minor importance. Functional ID involves failure of iron utilization for heme synthesis despite adequate iron stores. Impaired iron hemostasis is common in malignancy. Mechanisms include increased release of proinflammatory cytokines and raised levels of hepcidin, the main regulator of iron uptake and release. Increased hepcidin levels result in the internalization of ferroportin, the most important transmembrane channel for exporting iron from enterocytes and macrophages into the circulation. This results in reduced iron utilization and functional ID.

IRON STATUS ASSESSMENT

Iron deficiency is reflected by a low transferrin saturation (TSAT) below 20%. This and serum ferritin levels <30 ng/mL characterize absolute ID in noninflammatory states. However, in inflammatory states such as malignancy, ferritin rises parallel to proinflammatory cytokines, and serum ferritin levels are often elevated. As a result, the cut-off for low iron stores is best represented by the threshold of <100 ng/mL.[3,7] Hence, in cancer patients, TSAT <20% with serum ferritin <100 ng/mL is considered an absolute ID. Functional ID is defined as TSAT <20%

and serum ferritin ≥100 ng/mL; ferritin may rise during the inflammatory process and functional ID (adequate iron stores with normal or increased serum ferritin).[8] The ratio of soluble transferrin receptor (sTfR) to log-ferritin (sTfR/log Ft) ≥2 indicates absolute ID. A sTfR/log Ft <1 indicates functional ID. Chemotherapy may reduce sTfR levels, while the use of erythropoietin therapy in patients on chemotherapy can increase sTfR levels. This limits the relevance of sTfR as an indicator of iron status. ID anemia is characterized by hypochromic, microcytic red cells, a low cellular Hb content in reticulocytes (CHr <28 pg), and an increased percentage of hypochromic RBCs (%HYPO >5%).[8]

IRON TREATMENT IN CANCER-INDUCED ANEMIA[5]

In cancer patients, iron treatment should be limited to patients on chemotherapy. Patients receiving ongoing chemotherapy who present with anemia (Hb ≤11 g/dL or Hb decrease ≥2 g/dL from a baseline level ≤12 g/dL) and absolute ID (serum ferritin <100 ng/mL) should receive iron treatment with an IV iron preparation to correct ID. Due to frequently reduced iron absorption from the gastrointestinal tract in cancer patients, therapy with oral iron did not result in better outcomes than control arms with no iron. Conversely, the benefits of IV iron were substantial, with significantly greater hematological response rate improvement than oral iron. Oral iron is to be considered only for patients with ferritin <30 ng/mL and noninflammatory conditions (CRP <5 mg/L).

If erythropoiesis-stimulating agent (ESA) treatment is considered, iron treatment should be given before initiating and/or during ESA therapy in the case of functional ID (TSAT < 20% and serum ferritin > 100 ng/mL). IV iron without additional anemia therapy may sometimes be considered in patients with functional ID. In controlled clinical trials investigating iron supplementation in ESA-treated anemic cancer patients, IV iron supplementation (total doses in the range of 1,000 mg) significantly improved the hematological response to ESA treatment versus ESA alone.[3,9,10] Individual studies also showed additional benefits of IV iron, such as improvement of QoL,[9] reduction of RBC transfusions,[11] and ESA doses.[3] In patients receiving cardiotoxic chemotherapy, IV iron should either be given before or after (not on the same day) administration of chemotherapy or at the end of a treatment cycle.[3,7]

Patients with confirmed functional ID should receive a dose of 1,000 mg iron, given as a single dose or multiple doses, according to the label-available IV iron formulations. Total dose infusion of calculated iron needs was as effective as multiple low-dose infusions,[9] yet, depending on the individual IV iron product's approved maximum infusion doses **(Table 5)**, administering a single 1,000 mg

TABLE 5: Comparison of IV iron preparations.[3,12]

	Standard label maximum single dose	*Minimum infusion dose*	*Risk of HSRs*	*Incidence of HSRs*
Iron dextran (LMW)	1,000 mg	240–360 minutes	High risk	Any HSR: 4.7–5.6% Moderate-to-severe HSR: 0.7%
Ferric gluconate	125 mg	60 minutes	Low risk	Any HSR: 3.9% Moderate-to-severe HSR: 0.4%
Iron sucrose	200–500 mg	30–210 minutes	Low risk	Any HSR: 4.7–5.6% Moderate-to-severe HSR: 0.7%
Ferric derisomaltose (Iron isomaltoside)	20 mg/kg (not to exceed 1,500 mg)	15 minutes	Low-intermediate risk	Any HSR: 8.7% Moderate-to-severe HSR: 0.3–66.4%
Ferric carboxymaltose	*Maximum infusion dose:* †20 mg/kg body weight (up to 1,000 mg iron per week); ‡750 mg for patient ≤50 kg, 15 mg/kg for patient <50 kg	15 minutes	Low risk	Any HSR: 2.1% Moderate-to-severe HSR: 0.7%

†European Society for Medical Oncology (ESMO) clinical practice guideline; ‡Dose recommendation for management of anemia in preoperative settings (followed at authors' institution).
(HSRs: hypersensitivity reactions; LMW: Low molecular weight)

iron dose may be more convenient for patients than multiple lower doses. Patients with confirmed absolute ID should receive IV iron doses according to the approved labels of available products until correction of ID.[9] Iron overload is unlikely in patients with cancer-induced anemia.

Table 5 highlights dosing protocols and the risk and severity of hypersensitivity reactions associated with different IV iron preparations available.[12] IV iron should only be administered in setups where resuscitation facilities to manage anaphylactic and anaphylactoid reactions are immediately available, including the staff trained to diagnose and treat anaphylaxis.[7] Close monitoring of the patient for symptoms of hypersensitivity reactions should be continued for at least 30 minutes after completion of each IV iron dosing.

ERYTHROPOIESIS-STIMULATING AGENTS

Erythropoiesis-stimulating agents promote bone marrow erythropoiesis by direct stimulation of erythropoietin receptors. ESA therapy reduces RBC transfusion requirements and so reduces the risk of post-transfusion adverse reactions and improves anemia symptoms and QoL in patients with chemotherapy-induced anemia (CIA).[2,3,7] In contrast to packed RBC transfusions, ESA has a positive immune response.[7] ESA suppresses the expression of pro-inflammatory cytokine genes such as IL-1β, IL-6, IL-10, and TNF-α, reduces IL-1α and IL-6 levels, and lowers the number of CD8+CD152+ suppressor T-cells.[13-15]

Currently, ESAs such as epoetin (alpha, beta, and theta) and darbepoetin alfa are recommended for the management of symptomatic anemia in cancer patients on chemotherapy or combined radiochemotherapy and present with a Hb level <10 g/dL.[2,3,7] ESA therapy is also recommended for patients with asymptomatic anemia who receive chemotherapy and present with an Hb level <8 g/dL. Cancer patients not on chemotherapy are not candidates for ESA treatment.[3]

In CIA, ESA therapy should be considered after correcting ID and other underlying causes other than the cancer or its treatment.[3,7] When using ESA therapy, the aim is to achieve a stable Hb of 12 g/dL without RBC transfusions. A Hb level of 12 g/dL should not be exceeded. ESA doses should be reduced by approximately 25–50% if the Hb concentration rises to levels preventing RBC transfusions or increases by >2 g/dL within 4 weeks.

Table 6 mentions the doses for different ESAs for CIA treatment.[3] Epoetin theta is usually started in low weekly doses, and its dose may be doubled after 4 weeks if an increase of Hb is <1 g/dL. For all other ESAs, dose escalations and changes from one ESA to another in patients not responding within 4–8 weeks are not recommended. In patients who do not show evidence of at least an initial Hb response at this time, ESA therapy should be stopped. ESA discontinuation is also recommended after a maximum of 4 weeks after chemotherapy completion and in the case of the appearance of neutralizing anti-ESA antibodies.[3,7] The use of ESA in patients with hypersensitivity to the drug and uncontrolled hypertension is not recommended.

Patients should be provided comprehensive information on the purpose of ESA therapy along with the potential adverse reactions associated with the treatment, especially thromboembolic complications and hypertension.

TABLE 6: Approved erythropoiesis-stimulating agents (ESAs) dosing in chemotherapy-induced anemia.[3,7]

Approved erythropoiesis-stimulating agents (ESAs)	*Approved dosing in patients with solid tumors and hematological malignancies*[a,b]
Epoetin alpha	450 IU/kg subcutaneously once weekly or 150 IU/kg subcutaneously 3 times per week
Epoetin beta	30,000 IU subcutaneously (i.e., 450 IU/kg body weight in a 70 kg patient) given once weekly or divided over 3–7 times per week
Epoetin theta	20,000 IU subcutaneously independent of body weight given once weekly, dose may be doubled after 4 weeks if Hb has not increased by at least 1 g/dL
Epoetin zeta	450 IU/kg subcutaneously once weekly, or 150 IU/kg subcutaneously 3 times per week
Darbepoetin alfa	500 µg (6.75 µg/kg body weight) subcutaneously given once every 3 weeks or 2.25 µg/kg body weight subcutaneously once weekly

[a]Epoetin alpha is European Medicines Agency (EMA)-approved for low or intermediate-1 risk myelodysplastic syndromes.
[b]Both originator products and biosimilars approved by the EMA have been shown to have similar safety and therapeutic equivalence in clinical practice.

Thromboembolic Complications

Cancer patients are at higher risk of thromboembolic complications than the general population. ESA use in cancer patients may increase the risk of venous thromboembolic events (VTE) by 1.5 folds. Certain cancer types, such as pancreatic and gastric cancers and multiple myeloma during immunomodulatory treatment, are particularly associated with high-risk of VTEs.[16,17] However, there is no convincing clinical evidence that the use of ESA further increases the risk of thromboembolic events in patients treated with lenalidomide or thalidomide.[18,19] In the absence of prospective randomized clinical trials (RCTs) supporting the use of anticoagulation treatment to reduce the risk of thromboembolic events in ESA-treated patients, current guidelines do not advocate prophylactic anticoagulation therapy in these patients.[3,7]

Hypertension

Cancer patients with chronic renal failure are particularly at risk of developing or worsening hypertension following initiation of ESA therapy.[7]

ERYTHROPOIESIS-STIMULATING AGENTS' IMPACT ON CANCER MORTALITY AND TUMOR PROGRESSION

A meta-analysis and Cochrane review published in the late 2000s linked ESA treatment with increased mortality in cancer patients with Hb ≥12 g/dL.[20] Based on this outcome analysis, the current guidelines recommend Hb target range of 10–12 g/dL for ESA treatment.[3] Additionally, Hb rise >2g/dL over a 4-week period should be avoided. However, several other large studies and metanalysis failed to link ESA treatment with increased mortality in cancer patients.[3,7,21] Similarly, no clinical evidence exists supporting the harmful effects of ESAs on cancer progression or relapse when used within the label and following recommendations for the treatment of CIA.[21]

BLOOD TRANSFUSIONS

Red blood cell transfusions are usually indicated in cancer patients with severe anemia symptoms or bleeding conditions to obtain a rapid increase in Hb and Hct closer to normal laboratory values. However, despite the lack of any supporting evidence for a significant treatment effect, RBC transfusions are a routine practice for the management of cancer-related anemia and CIA, even in the absence of any life-threatening situations.[22,23]

Such a practice of routine, as well as liberal RBC transfusion, is questionable due to multiple reasons. Despite advances in molecular testing for known pathogens and potential donor–recipient incompatibilities, there remains the risk of transmitting unknown or emerging pathogens and an increased risk of infections due to transfusion-related immunosuppression.[24] Transfusion of stored allogeneic blood can induce prothrombotic and proinflammatory responses often referred to as "storage lesions".[25,26] In the oncology surgery setting, cancer patients receiving blood transfusions are found to have a reduced survival time,[2,8,27] early cancer relapse,[7,28-30] and higher mortality due to recurrence of the neoplastic disease.[7,30] A higher incidence of postoperative complications (including infections), prolonged hospital stay, and a higher risk of thromboembolic complications is also reported.[7] Some of the mechanistic explanations for the blood transfusion-related adverse effects are changes that occur during the RBC storage, immunogenicity of blood cells, thrombogenicity of blood components, presence of pathogens and/or leukocytes in blood components, immunomodulation, human error, and using less safe blood concentrates due to lower costs.[2,7] **Table 7** lists immune and nonimmune mediated adverse reactions post-transfusion.[7]

TABLE 7: Transfusion-mediated adverse reactions.[2,3,7]

Post-transfusion immune-mediated adverse reactions	
Early	***Delayed***
Acute hemolytic transfusion reaction (AHTR)	Delayed hemolytic transfusion reaction
Transfusion-related acute lung injury (TRALI)	Transfusion-associated graft-versus-host disease (TA-GvHD)
Febrile nonhemolytic transfusion reactions (FNHTR)	Post-transfusion purpura (PTP)
Anaphylactic reaction	Alloimmunization to blood cell antigens
Urticaria	Immunosuppression
Post-transfusion nonimmune-mediated adverse reactions	
Early	***Delayed***
Nonimmune hemolysis	Hemosiderosis
Transfusion-associated circulatory overload (TACO)	Transmission of viral, bacterial, and protozoal infections
Air embolism	Transmission of prions
Citrate intoxication	
Sepsis	

Liberal versus Restrictive Blood Transfusion Policy

Several meta-analyses of published studies in patients with noncancer surgeries (orthopedic or cardiovascular) demonstrated that the restrictive blood transfusion protocols are associated with significant reductions in the proportions of transfused patients and the numbers of transfused RBC units without negative impact on mortality, morbidity, and functional outcome.[2,31] A restrictive Hb threshold <7 g/dL for blood transfusion showed significant reductions in total and in-hospital mortality, rebleeding, acute coronary syndrome, pulmonary edema, and bacterial infections in comparison with a more liberal strategy (transfusion trigger of Hb concentration <10 g/dL).[32] Based on these findings, RBC transfusions should be reserved primarily for patients with severe anemia symptoms and or active bleeding in need of rapid Hb improvement. Whether a higher transfusion threshold may be warranted in patients with specific conditions and symptomatic cardiopulmonary diseases needs to be investigated.

The recommendations on RBC transfusion strategies in oncology surgery patients are primarily derived from data from noncancer surgery studies. In cancer patients, the lowest "safe" Hb before blood transfusion remains an area of active research.[33] One prospective RCT involving 198 oncology surgical patients found fewer major postoperative complication rates (19.6% vs 35.6%) with liberal RBC transfusion strategy (Hb <9 g/dL) in comparison to restrictive targets (Hb <7g/dL).[34] In contrast to general patients, cancer patients appear to tolerate anemia poorly. It is estimated that for every 1-g decrease in postoperative Hb concentrations below 8 g/dL, the odds of death increase 2.5-fold.[35] Significantly, mortality risk sharply increases if the Hb concentration is <6 g/dL.

In the oncology setting, most anemia treatment guidelines recommend transfusing only the minimum number of RBC units required to relieve severe anemia symptoms or return the patient to a safe Hb range (e.g., 7–8 g/dL in stable, noncardiac inpatients).[3,7]

PATIENT BLOOD MANAGEMENT

The concept of "patient blood management" (PBM) was developed in a nononcology population. It involves taking every reasonable measure to increase and maintain the patient's endogenous RBC mass early on and protect it throughout the entire treatment, thus preempting transfusion.[2] It is based on three pillars; namely (1) optimizing the patient's red cell mass, (2) minimizing blood loss and bleeding, and (3) evaluating the physiological tolerance of anemia.[2,36] It should be accompanied by a comprehensive assessment of a patient's hematological status at the initial presentation and throughout therapy. The **Flowchart 1** provides a schematic approach for general management of anemia in cancer patients.

Anemia in Oncosurgical Patients

Surgery is a routine therapeutic option for most solid tumors. Surgical procedures may be for the curative excision of malignant tumors with or without reconstructive procedures, for cancer diagnosis and staging, for debulking masses, and for palliative care to reduce pain and suffering.[2] The presence of anemia in the perioperative period is associated with increased morbidity and mortality, as well as the need for allogeneic blood transfusions.[1,2] The more severe the anemia, the poorer the outcomes in oncological patients.[2,33,36] The presence of cardiovascular and pulmonary comorbidities with anemia further increases the risk of adverse outcomes in surgical patients with anemia. Often, oncological patients are also on other cancer treatment modalities such as chemotherapy, radiotherapy, target therapy, and hormone therapy that could further increase the risk of anemia and or worsen the severity of preexisting anemia that puts these patients in higher need of allogenic blood transfusions, perioperative morbidity, and mortality.[2,32-35]

With tremendous advancements in surgical techniques and equipment, the number of oncology surgeries has increased overall.[2] As a result, the number of patients with uncorrected anemia coming for major oncological procedures is on the rise, along with the use of allogeneic blood transfusions.

With a greater understanding of the impact of allogeneic blood transfusions for the management of perioperative anemia on increased mortality and poorer longer outcomes for oncology patients, the practice of routine and liberal use of blood transfusions is now being questioned. One study on colon resection surgery in cancer patients showed increased rates of postoperative sepsis and decreased survival.[27] Several other studies in oncological patients advocate a purposeful reduction in perioperative blood transfusions through best-practice PBM protocols.[2]

Flowchart 1: Algorithm for management of anemia in cancer patients.

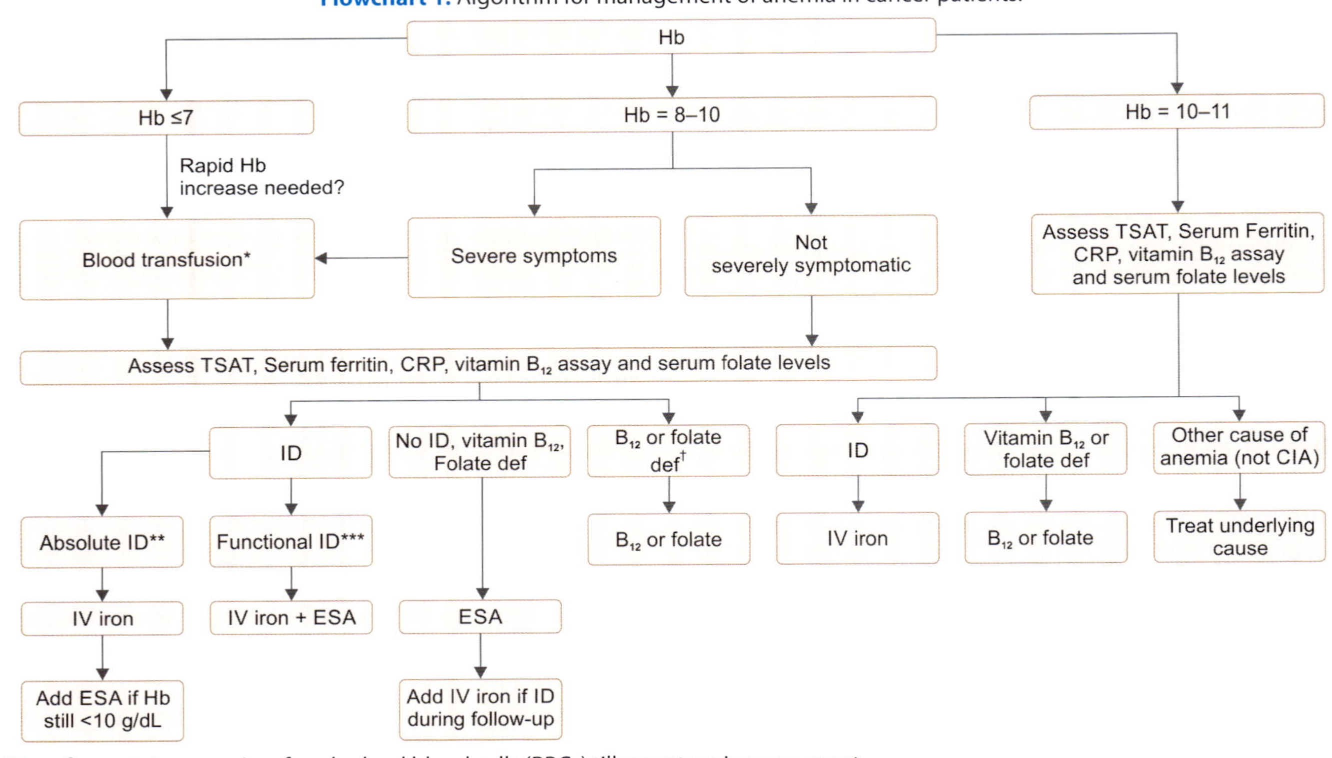

*Transfuse minimum units of packed red blood cells (RBCs) till symptom improvement
***Absolute ID:* TSAT <20% and serum ferritin <100 ng/mL
**** Functional ID:* TSAT <20% and serum ferritin >100 ng/mL
†*Vitamin B_{12} deficiency:* Serum vitamin B_{12} <200 pg/mL; *Folate deficiency:* Serum folate <5ng/mL
(CIA: chemotherapy-induced anemia; CRP: C-reactive protein; def: deficiency; ESA: erythropoiesis-stimulating agent; Hb: hemoglobin; ID: iron deficiency; IV: intravenous; TSAT: transferrin saturation)

Perioperative Patient Blood Management in Oncological Patients

In surgical patients, applying PBM best practice recommendations seeks to reduce the need for blood transfusions in three ways: (1) Treating anemia in the preoperative phase, (2) minimizing blood loss during surgery, monitoring and maintaining hemostasis and physiological functions of the body using nontransfusion-based fluid therapies, (3) and encouraging the appropriate use of blood in the intraoperative and postoperative period.[2]

Patient blood management strategies can be best modified for oncological patients by incorporating the European Society for Medical Oncology (ESMO) current practice guidelines on the management of anemia and ID in cancer patients[3] early in the preoperative phase with the "three pillar model" advocated by Australian National Blood Authority.[36]

Pillar 1 (Optimize Red Blood Cell Mass)

- *Perioperative phase:*
  - *Detect and treat cancer-related anemia, CIA, and iron deficiency.*[2]
    - Optimal timing of cancer surgeries from the time of diagnosis or relative to chemotherapy or radiotherapy is important for the best possible outcomes. In some cases, surgery should be scheduled within weeks of diagnosis of cancer. In many others, surgery must be carefully planned within a specific time interval relative to chemotherapy and radiation. In either case, delaying surgery can result in cancer progression or a reduction in the effectiveness of treatment. This time-sensitive schedule often prevents nontransfusion modalities from reaching peak therapeutic effect. These therapies also carry unique risks for cancer patients.

- The use of ESA treatment to improve Hb in the perioperative period is limited due to the increased risk of VTE and hypertension.
- Intravenous iron therapy is efficacious and safe if surgery is planned for <6 weeks after the diagnosis of ID. The optimal timing for IV iron administration before surgery is yet to be established but should best be administered at least 2 weeks before surgery. However, one study showed the benefit of even a single postoperative dose in improving Hb and reducing blood transfusion needs after surgery.[37] Oncosurgical patients with s-ferritin <100 ng/mL or s-ferritin between 100 ng/mL and 500 ng/mL with TSAT <20% are candidates for IV iron therapy in the preoperative period. We use ferric carboxymaltose, and the doses are based on body weight and Hb level. The usual protocol is to administer 2 doses of IV ferric carboxymaltose 750 mg each, one week apart, to be administered at least 1 week before the surgery **(Flowchart 2)**.
- Anemic patients with folate deficiency (serum folate <5 ng/mL) should be given folic acid 5 mg per day for 1 month. While patients with vitamin B_{12} <200 pg/mL should receive 1 mg vitamin B_{12} tablets for 1 month.
- However, these interventions are appropriate in certain settings and if patients are appropriately educated about the risks. As most cancer surgeries are urgent, an attempt should be made to treat all treatable causes of anemia in all cancer patients within 2–6 weeks before surgery. Intravenous iron is used as the first line.

Flowchart 2: Preoperative anemia treatment algorithm in oncosurgical patients based on PBM protocol.

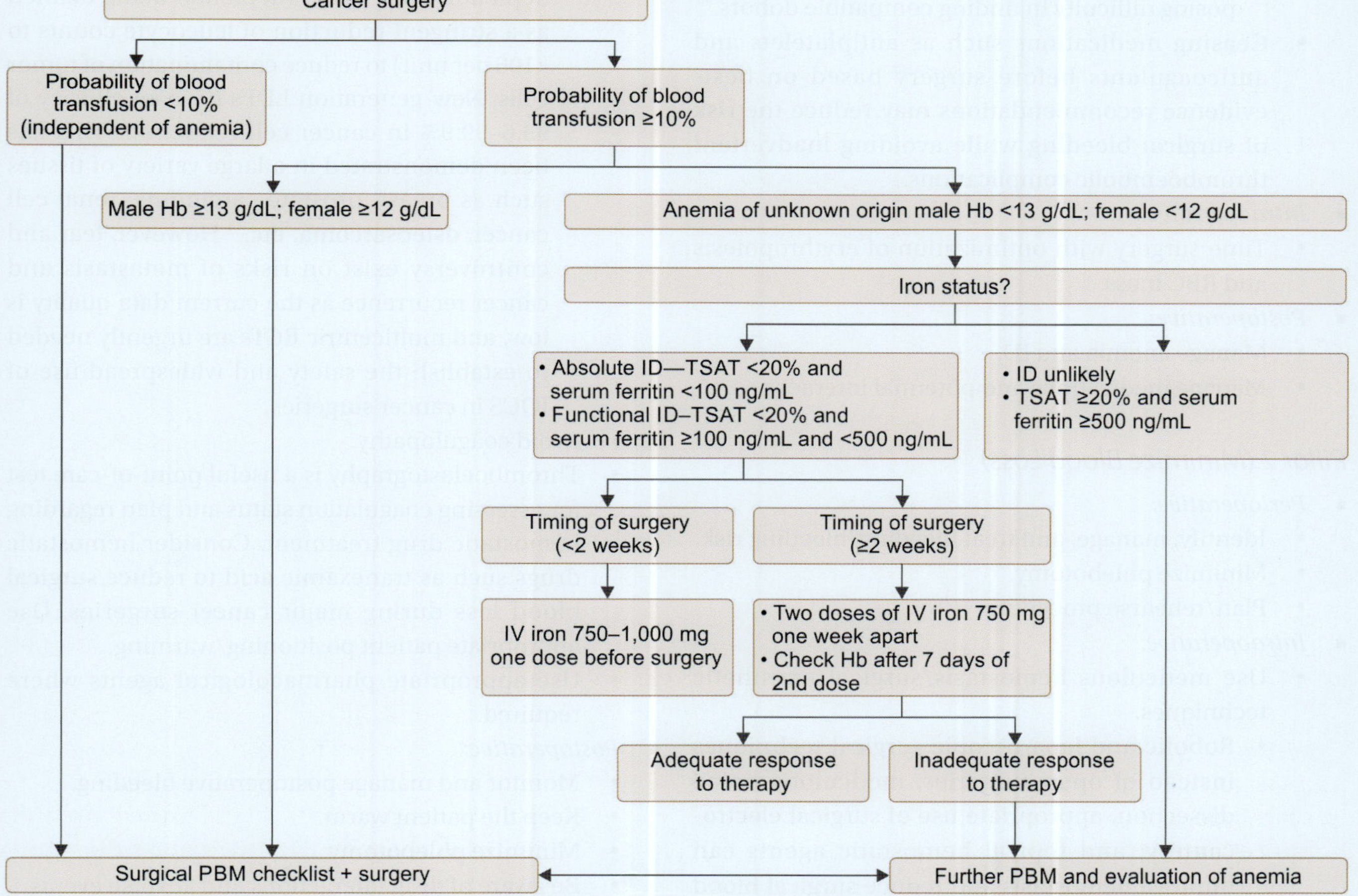

(Hb: hemoglobin; ID: iron deficiency; IV: intravenous; PBM: patient blood management; TSAT: transferrin saturation)

- Optimize hemoglobin. Target Hb about 12 g/dL. For ESA therapy, the target Hb should not be >12 g/dL
    - Preoperative blood conservation, such as acute normovolemic hemodilution (ANH) and preoperative autologous blood donation (PABD), have been studied largely in noncancer surgery patients.[33] Although PABD and ANH effectively reduced the need for allogeneic blood transfusion in the intraoperative period, overall perioperative transfusion volumes remain unaffected. In cancer patients, there exists a paucity of literature on the safety and clinical benefits of these techniques. Additionally, the use of ESA therapy that was often sought to attain target Hb for PABD may result in higher perioperative complication risks and higher costs in oncological patients.[2] One condition wherein ANH and PABD may be advantageous is in patients with multiple blood group antibodies, posing difficulty in finding compatible donors.[33]
- Ceasing medications such as antiplatelets and anticoagulants before surgery based on best-evidence recommendations may reduce the risk of surgical bleeding while avoiding inadvertent thromboembolic complications.

- *Intraoperative:*
    - Time surgery with optimization of erythropoiesis and RBC mass.
- *Postoperative:*
    - Manage anemia and ID.
    - Manage medications and potential interactions.

Pillar 2 (Minimize Blood Loss)

- *Perioperative:*
    - Identify, manage, and treat bleeding/bleeding risk.
    - Minimize phlebotomy.
    - Plan/rehearse procedure.
- *Intraoperative:*
    - Use meticulous hemostasis/surgical/anesthetic techniques.
        - Robotic and laparoscopic surgical techniques instead of open surgeries, meticulous tissue dissection, appropriate use of surgical electrocautery, and topical hemostatic agents can improve hemostasis and reduce surgical blood loss. Anesthesia techniques such as regional anesthesia, especially epidurals, and appropriate patient positioning can also be useful in reducing intraoperative blood loss.
    - Consider using cell salvage techniques.
        - Cell salvage is a technique of autologous blood transfusion wherein blood shed during surgery or the postoperative period is collected from the surgical site via suction drains or postoperative drains, respectively, then processed and prepared for safe return to the patient's circulation immediately or within certain safe time limits. Although the evidence is encouraging and large in support of the benefits of intraoperative cell salvage (IOCS) during major noncancer surgeries, evidence on the risk–benefits of IOCS in cancer surgeries is limited to metanalysis based on observational studies only.[38] The technique involves filtration of autologous blood return using a leukocyte depletion filter (LDF) (depletion being defined as a stringent reduction of leucocyte counts to <106 per unit) to reduce contamination of tumor cells. New-generation LDFs have an efficacy of 99.6–99.9% in cancer cell reduction. This has been demonstrated in a large variety of tissues such as breast, prostate carcinoma, renal cell cancer, osteosarcoma, etc.[38] However, fear and controversy exist on risks of metastasis and cancer recurrence as the current data quality is low, and multicentric RCTs are urgently needed to establish the safety and widespread use of IOCS in cancer surgeries.
    - Avoid coagulopathy.
    - Thromboelastography is a useful point-of-care test for assessing coagulation status and plan regarding hemostatic drug treatment. Consider hemostatic drugs such as tranexamic acid to reduce surgical blood loss during major cancer surgeries. Use appropriate patient positioning/warming.
    - Use appropriate pharmacological agents where required.
- *Postoperative:*
    - Monitor and manage postoperative bleeding.
    - Keep the patient warm.
    - Minimize phlebotomy.
    - Be aware of drug interactions and adverse events.
    - Treat infections promptly.

Pillar 3 (Manage Anemia)

- *Perioperative:*
  - Review and discuss their bleeding history with the patient and develop a management plan.
  - Estimate the patient's tolerance for blood loss.
  - Optimize cardiopulmonary function.
- *Intraoperative:*
  - Optimize hemodynamic parameters.
  - Optimize ventilation and oxygenation.
  - Use restrictive transfusion strategies.
    - In nononcology surgical patients, RBC transfusions are recommended when the patient is profoundly anemic (Hb ≤6 g/dL). With Hb between 6 and 10 gm/dL, the need to transfuse RBCs should be based on potential or actual ongoing bleeding. The rate and magnitude of ongoing bleeding should be considered along with volume status, signs and symptoms of organ ischemia, and baseline cardiopulmonary reserves. However, a higher transfusion threshold of ~7–8 g/dL may be considered in major oncology surgical patients. An Hb trigger of 8–9 g/dL may be appropriate in oncology patients with major cardiac issues. Current PBM guidelines advocate single-unit transfusion approaches for clinically stable patients, with clinical reassessment of patients before subsequent transfusions as the best way to restrict unnecessary transfusions. Normovolemia should be maintained using crystalloids or colloids to avoid hypotension and to ensure good cardiac output and tissue perfusion.
- *Postoperative:*
  - Maximize oxygen delivery.
  - Minimize oxygen use.
  - Treat infections promptly.
  - Optimize tolerance of anemia.
  - Use restrictive transfusion strategies.

Although a growing body of evidence shows a lack of any significant outcomes, benefits, and risk of potential complications of allogenic blood transfusions, blood transfusions can still be lifesaving in many cases, especially in hemodynamically unstable patients with hypovolemia, Hb ≤6–7 gm/dL and or ongoing surgical bleeding. As anesthesia providers need to be prepared for situations of major intraoperative bleeding during complex oncology surgeries, detailed knowledge about the different types of blood preparation is necessary.

Blood Preparation: Leukocyte-depleted[7]

With the growing body of literature on transfusion-related immunomodulation and its pathogenesis[2,33,36] arguments have certainly been raised on the safety of blood transfusions in general and its impact on cancer outcomes in particular. However, overall, evidence is conflicting on the benefits of leukocyte-depleted RBC concentrate transfusions over RBC transfusions without a reduced number of leukocytes during the neoplastic disease. Nonetheless, the presence of leukocytes in RBC concentrates is associated with higher risk of post-transfusion adverse reactions (febrile nonhemolytic transfusion reactions, transfusion-related acute lung injury, alloimmunization, cytomegalovirus (CMV) transmission, and platelet refractoriness). It is advisable to use leukocyte-depleted RBC concentrate in chronically transfused cancer patients who are often immunocompromised from chemotherapy and/or are prospective bone marrow transplant candidates.[7]

Leukocytes in whole blood or RBCs can expose recipients to foreign human leukocyte antigens, which are strongly immunogenic. The American Association of Blood Banks industry standard recommends a white blood cell (WBC) count of $<5 \times 10^6$ in leukocyte-reduced RBCs.[39] As neither buffy coat removal nor washing of the RBCs can adequately meet this standard, it is recommended to use leukocyte filters either at the time of collection or poststorage. Prestorage leukoreduction is preferred, as it reduces inflammatory cytokine accumulation from stored WBCs. While the FDA does not mandate universal leukoreduction, the American Red Cross only provides leukodepleted RBCs.[39]

Blood Preparation: Cytomegalovirus Negative

Cytomegalovirus, a herpes virus, infections in immunocompromised patients such as cancer patients can produce life-threatening disease.[3,7] Usually, transfusion of CMV-infested monocytes has been implicated in transfusion-transmitted CMV (TT-CMV) infections.[40] As a result, leukoreduction is advocated to remove the potential source of this infection for blood transfusion. However, as a newly CMV-infected donor may carry the free virus in the blood, even leukoreduction cannot eliminate the risk of CMV transmission.[41] Blood from CMV-negative donors has been proposed. Unfortunately, even diagnostic techniques such as serology and nucleic acid testing may fail to detect new CMV infections.[40] For this reason, strategies commonly involve using leukoreduced blood alone or combined with blood from CMV-negative donors. Trials are currently underway to identify methods for pathogen inactivation.[39,40]

Blood Preparation: Irradiated Blood Components

Blood transfusions can rarely be associated with fatal transfusion-associated graft-versus-host disease (TA-GVHD) **(Table 8)**.[7,39] The pathogenesis involves the potential replication of donor T cells. The incidence is higher in immunocompromised recipients (such as those receiving chemotherapy, especially fludarabine,[42] and those with myelodysplastic disease, lymphoma, or leukemia). Such gamma-irradiated blood products prevent this rare but usually fatal disease. Gamma irradiation of blood components can render donor lymphocytes incapable of proliferation. The minimum recommended dose is at least 25 Grays for each cellular component.[39] Notably, components containing no viable white cells, such as fresh frozen plasma and cryoprecipitate, do not require irradiation.

TABLE 8: Absolute indications of leukocyte-depleted and or irradiated-packed RBCs.[7]

Absolute indications of leukocyte-depleted packed RBCs	***Absolute indications of irradiated-packed RBCs***
Patients with previous TRALI	Relatedness (1st and 2nd degrees) between donor and recipient
Patients with or suspected to have anti-HLA antibodies	HLA-compatible blood components
Prophylaxis of immunization with erythrocyte antigens	Immunodeficiency (especially with severe T-cell deficiency syndrome)
Multiple recipients (during hematopoietic malignancies or chronic renal failure)	Transfusion of granulocyte concentrates
Prophylaxis of immunization with HLA antigens: Nonhemolytic febrile reactions and platelet transfusion refractoriness	Hematopoietic cell transplant recipients
Prophylaxis of cytomega-lovirus (CMV) infection	Chronic GvHD
	Autologous hematopoietic cells collection and within 7 days prior to collection
	Immunosuppressive treatment
	Hodgkin's disease
	Treatment with purine analogs (e.g., fludarabine and cladribine) or purine antagonists (bendamustine and clofarabine)
	Treatment with alemtuzumab (anti-CD52)

(HLA: human leukocyte antigen; GvHD: graft-versus-host disease; RBCs: red blood cells; TRALI: transfusion-related acute lung injury;)

CONCLUSION

With an increasing number of patients being diagnosed with cancer worldwide, the number of oncology surgery cases is increasing every year. As many oncology patients are anemic in the preoperative period and surgeries in these patients may often be associated with major blood losses, the burden for perioperative blood transfusions is high. Henceforth, it is important to manage anemia in cancer patients as early as possible based on the best practice guidelines and personalized PBM strategies in the perioperative settings to reduce the need and risks of allogenic blood transfusions for overall survival outcomes in oncological patients.

REFERENCES

1. Muñoz M, Gómez-Ramírez S, Campos A, Ruiz J, Liumbruno GM. Pre-operative anaemia: Prevalence, consequences and approaches to management. Blood Transfus. 2015;13(3):370-79.
2. Stephens J, Tano R. Hemoglobin matters: Perioperative blood management for oncology patients. Can Oncol Nurs J. 2021;31(4):399-404.
3. Aapro M, Beguin Y, Bokemeyer C, Dicato M, Gascón P, Glaspy J, et al. Management of anaemia and iron deficiency in patients with cancer: ESMO Clinical Practice Guidelines. Ann Oncol. 2018;29(Suppl 4):iv96-110.
4. Knight K, Wade S, Balducci L. Prevalence and outcomes of anemia in cancer: A systematic review of the literature. Am J Med. 2004;116 Suppl 7A:11S-26S
5. Ludwig H, Van Belle S, Barrett-Lee P, Birgegård G, Bokemeyer C, Gascón P, et al. The European Cancer Anaemia Survey (ECAS): A large, multinational, prospective survey defining the prevalence, incidence, and treatment of anaemia in cancer patients. Eur J Cancer. 2004; 40(15):2293-306.
6. Wojtukiewicz MZ, Sierko E, Rybaltowski M, Filipczyk-Cisarz E, Staroslawska E, Tujakowski J, et al. The Polish Cancer Anemia Survey (POLCAS): A retrospective multicenter study of 999 cases. Int J Hematol. 2009;89:276-84.

7. Radziwon P, Krzakowski M, Kalinka E, Zaucha R, Wysocki R, Kowalski D, et al. Anemia in cancer patients—Expert Group recommendations. Revision 2020. Oncol Clin Pract. 2020;16:261-9.
8. Aapro M, Österborg A, Gascón P, Ludwig H, Beguin Y. Prevalence and management of cancer-related anaemia, iron deficiency and the specific role of i.v. iron. Ann Oncol. 2012;23(8):1954-62.
9. Auerbach M, Ballard H, Trout JR, McIlwain M, Ackerman A, Bahrain H, et al. Intravenous iron optimizes the response to recombinant human erythropoietin in cancer patients with chemotherapy-related anemia: A multicenter, open-label, randomized trial. J Clin Oncol. 2004;22(7):1301-7.
10. Auerbach M, Silberstein PT, Webb RT, Averyanova S, Ciuleanu TE, Shao J, et al. Darbepoetin alfa 300 or 500 μg once every 3 weeks with or without intravenous iron in patients with chemotherapy-induced anemia. Am J Hematol. 2010;85(9):655-63.
11. Bastit L, Vandebroek A, Altintas S, Gaede B, Pintér T, Suto TS, et al. Randomized, multicenter, controlled trial comparing the efficacy and safety of darbepoetin alpha administered every 3 weeks with or without intravenous iron in patients with chemotherapy-induced anemia. J Clin Oncol 2008;26(10):1611-8.
12. Khan H, May P, Kuo E, Pai P, Boles K, McGee A, et al. Safety and efficacy of a single total dose infusion (1020 mg) of ferumoxytol. Ther Adv Hematol. 2021;12:20406207211006022.
13. Zhang J, Zou YR, Zhong X, Deng HD, Pu L, Peng K, et al. Erythropoietin pretreatment ameliorates renal ischaemia-reperfusion injury by activating PI3K/Akt signalling. Nephrology (Carlton). 2015;20(4):266-72.
14. Rong R, Xijun X. Erythropoietin pretreatment suppresses inflammation by activating the PI3K/Akt signaling pathway in myocardial ischemia-reperfusion injury. Exp Ther Med. 2015;10(2):413-8.
15. Li J, Xu J, Yan X, Jin K, Li W, Zhang R. Targeting Interleukin-6 (IL-6) Sensitizes Anti-PD-L1 Treatment in a Colorectal Cancer Preclinical Model. Med Sci Monit. 2018;24:5501-8.
16. Musallam KM, Dahdaleh FS, Shamseddine AI, Taher AT. Incidence and prophylaxis of venous thromboembolic events in multiple myeloma patients receiving immunomodulatory therapy. Thromb Res 2009;123:679-86.
17. Zonder JA. Thrombotic complications of myeloma therapy. Hematology Am Soc Hematol Educ Program. 2006:348-55.
18. Galli M, Elice F, Crippa C, Comotti B, Rodeghiero F, Barbui T. Recombinant human erythropoietin and the risk of thrombosis in patients receiving thalidomide for multiple myeloma. Haematologica. 2004;89(9):1141-2.
19. Knight R, DeLap RJ, Zeldis JB. Lenalidomide and venous thrombosis in multiple myeloma. N Engl J Med. 2006;354(19):2079-80.
20. Bohlius J, Schmidlin K, Brillant C, Schwarzer G, Trelle S, Seidenfeld J, et al. Erythropoietin or darbepoetin for patients with cancer–meta-analysis based on individual patient data. Cochrane Database Syst Rev. 2009;2009(3):CD007303.
21. Tonia T, Mettler A, Robert N, Schwarzer G, Seidenfeld J, Weingart O, et al. Erythropoietin or darbepoetin for patients with cancer. Cochrane Database Syst Rev. 2012;12(12):CD003407.
22. Ludwig H, Aapro M, Bokemeyer C, Glaspy J, Hedenus M, Littlewood TJ, et al. A European patient record study on diagnosis and treatment of chemotherapy-induced anaemia. Support Care Cancer. 2014;22(8):2197-206.
23. Schrijvers D. Management of anemia in cancer patients: Transfusions. Oncologist. 2011;16(Suppl 3):12-8.
24. Murphy GJ, Reeves BC, Rogers CA, Rizvi SI, Culliford L, Angelini GD. Increased mortality, postoperative morbidity, and cost after red blood cell transfusion in patients having cardiac surgery. Circulation. 2007;116(22):2544-52.
25. Isbister JP, Shander A, Spahn DR, Erhard J, Farmer SL, Hofmann A. Adverse blood transfusion outcomes: Establishing causation. Transfus Med Rev. 2011;25(2):89-101.
26. Baek JH, D'Agnillo F, Vallelian F, Pereira CP, Williams MC, Jia Y, et al. Hemoglobin-driven pathophysiology is an in vivo consequence of the red blood cell storage lesion that can be attenuated in guinea pigs by haptoglobin therapy. J Clin Invest. 2012;122(4):1444-58.
27. Aquina CT, Blumberg N, Becerra A, Boscoe F, Schymura M, Noyes K, et al. Association among blood transfusion, sepsis, and decreased long-term survival after colon cancer resection. Ann Surg. 2017;266(2):311-7.
28. Yamamoto J, Kosuge T, Takayama T, Shimada K, Yamasaki S, Ozaki H, et al. Perioperative blood transfusion promotes recurrence of hepatocellular carcinoma after hepatectomy. Surgery. 1994;115(3):303-9.
29. Amato A, Pescatori M. Perioperative blood transfusions for the recurrence of colorectal cancer. Cochrane Database Syst Rev. 2006:2006(1):CD005033.
30. Schiergens TS, Rentsch M, Kasparek MS, Frenes K, Jauch KW, Thasler WE. Impact of perioperative allogeneic red blood cell transfusion on recurrence and overall survival after resection of colorectal liver metastases. Dis Colon Rectum. 2015;58(1):74-82.
31. Freedman J. Transfusion medicine: Time for a change: Patient blood management and the Ontario ONTraC program. JP&CICN. 2016;2:1-9.
32. Salpeter SR, Buckley JS, Chatterjee S. Impact of more restrictive blood transfusion strategies on clinical outcomes: A meta-analysis and systematic review. Am J Med 2014;127(2):124-31.
33. Weber RS, Jabbour N, Martin RC 2nd. Anemia and transfusions in patients undergoing surgery for cancer. Ann Surg Oncol. 2008;15(1):34-45.
34. de Almeida JP, Vincent JL, Galas FR, de Almeida EP, Fukushima JT, Osawa EA, et al. Transfusion requirements in surgical oncology patients: A prospective, randomized controlled trial. Anesthesiology. 2015;122(1):29-38.

35. Cata JP. Perioperative anemia and blood transfusions in patients with cancer: When the problem, the solution, and their combination are each associated with poor outcomes. Anesthesiology. 2015;122(1):3-4.
36. Althoff FC, Neb H, Herrmann E, Trentino KM, Vernich L, Füllenbach C, et al. Multimodal patient blood management program based on a three-pillar strategy: A systematic review and meta-analysis. Ann Surg. 2019;269(5): 794-804.
37. Khalafallah AA, Yan C, Al-Badri R, Robinson E, Kirkby BE, Ingram E, et al. Intravenous ferric carboxymaltose versus standard care in the management of postoperative anaemia: A prospective, open-label, randomised controlled trial. Lancet Haematol. 2016;3(9):e415-25.
38. Frietsch T, Steinbicker AU, Horn A, Metz M, Dietrich G, Weigand MA, et al. Safety of intraoperative cell salvage in cancer surgery: An updated meta-analysis of the current literature. Transfus Med Hemother. 2022;49(3):143-57.
39. McMaster M, Sinha AC. Perioperative anemia management for the onco-surgical patient. In: Garg R, Bhatnagar S (Eds). Textbook of Onco-Anesthesiology. Singapore: Springer; 2021.
40. Ziemann M, Thiele T. Transfusion-transmitted CMV infection-current knowledge and future perspectives. Transfus Med. 2017;27(4):238-48.
41. Wu YY, Zou SM, Cable R, Dorsey K, Tang YL, Hapip CA, et al. Direct assessment of cytomegalovirus transfusion-transmitted risks after universal leukoreduction. Transfusion. 2010;50(4):776-86.
42. Williamson LM, Wimperis JZ, Wood ME, Woodcock B. Fludarabine treatment and transfusion associated graft-versus-host disease. Lancet. 1996;348(9025):472-3.

CHAPTER

Preoperative Nutritional Assessment and Optimization

Rajiv Chawla, Shagun Bhatia Shah, Uma Hariharan, Pratishtha Yadav

INTRODUCTION

One of the leading causes of death worldwide is cancer. 20 million new cases of cancer were reported in the year 2022, and it is expected to rise to 29.9 million per year by 2040. Malnutrition and metabolic derangements frequently seen in cancer patients can limit the response and can even hinder the progress of treatment.

Nutrition is the study of food and how it affects our bodies with special regard to the essential nutrients necessary to support physiological and biochemical processes.[1] European Society for Clinical Nutrition and Metabolism (ESPEN) has defined malnutrition, or undernutrition, as "A state resulting from lack of intake or uptake of nutrition that leads to altered body composition (decreased fat-free mass) and body cell mass leading to diminished physical and mental function and impaired clinical outcome from disease".[2] Malnutrition in cancer differs from simple malnutrition as it is interplay of reduced food intake with tumor- or host-derived metabolic derangements.[3]

Depending on the type, location, grade, and stage of the tumor, tumor spread, and cancer treatment the global incidence of malnutrition in cancer is 30–90%. Approximately 15–50% cancer patients present with nutritional deficiencies, and 43% have overt malnutrition at the time of their diagnosis.[4] This prevalence can rise up to 80% during the course of treatment. Up to 20% of cancer deaths are caused by cancer-related malnutrition and associated cachexia, which is itself a poor predictor of overall survival.[5,6] Malnutrition is also one of the independent predictors of post-operative complications. It has been noted that early nutritional assessment is rarely performed (<50% of patients) with a great number of patients remaining undiagnosed at the time of cancer diagnosis. Almost 65% of the cancer patients remain without any nutritional intervention.[3]

Obesity is the other extreme of malnutrition, which is relatively infrequent in cancer and not discussed in this chapter.

MALNUTRITION IN ONCOLOGY

Malnutrition can be due to a multitude of causes like inadequate intake, local tumor effects, side-effects of cancer treatments (surgery, chemotherapy, and radiotherapy), or other complications pertaining to cancer metabolic derangements and systematic inflammation impairing substrate utilization **(Table 1)**.[7-10]

Cancer can create a state of chronic inflammation leading to complex metabolic derangements like muscle wasting, lipolysis, insulin resistance, anorexia, fatigue, etc. Weight loss,[11] impaired physical performance,[12] and systemic inflammation in cancer patients are independent risk predictors of poor prognosis. Cancer can also lead to a hypermetabolic state.[2] As per literature, 47% of new cancer patients were hypermetabolic with higher predicted Resting Energy Expenditure (REE in Kcal per kg of body weight) as compared to normal population.

TABLE 1: Causes of malnutrition in cancer patients.

Causes of malnutrition	
Decrease intake	Anorexia, smell/taste alteration, and nausea
Difficulty in eating	Dysphagia, vomiting, oral mucositis, and oral tumors
Impaired GI motility/ digestion/absorption	Mucositis, stenosis, obstruction, and diarrhea
Metabolic derangements	Cancer-induced systemic inflammation
Increased energy expenditure	Infection and systemic inflammation

(GI: gastrointestinal)

IMPACT OF CANCER TREATMENT ON NUTRITION

Chemotherapy and radiotherapy are main pillars of cancer treatment, which can have a negative impact on overall nutrition of cancer patients.[13] Numerous mechanisms can aggravate nutritional derangements in patients undergoing radiotherapy and chemotherapy **(Tables 2 and 3)**.

TABLE 2: Micronutrients and chemotherapy

Cytotoxic agent	*Micronutrient deficit*	*Mechanism*
Cisplatin	• L-carnitine • Magnesium • Potassium	Increased renal excretion
Cyclophosphamide	Vitamin D	Increased breakdown to inactive metabolites
Fluorouracil	Vitamin B_1	Inhibition of phosphorylation to active coenzyme
Ifosfamide	L-carnitine	Increased renal excretion
Paclitaxel	Vitamin D	Increased breakdown to inactive metabolites
Methotrexate	Folic acid	Antagonist mechanism

TABLE 3: Radiation therapy and nutrition.[14]

System affected	*Effects*
Central nervous system	Nausea and vomiting
Gastrointestinal system	• Swallowing disorder (dry mouth, mucositis, ulcers, caries, and sensitive teeth) • Anorexia (altered sense of taste and smell) • Esophageal ulcer, fibrosis, perforation, and fistula
Thorax	• Swallowing difficulty • Pain • Nausea and vomiting
Abdomen and pelvis	• Anorexia • Nausea and vomiting • Diarrhea • Acute enteritis, colitis, proctitis, and cystitis • Sphincter dysfunction • Bleeding, obstruction, and fistula • Renal dysfunction

CANCER CACHEXIA[15]

Another extreme manifestation of malnutrition is cancer cachexia, a devastating disorder characterized by nutritional impairment, weakness, and muscle wasting **(Fig. 1)**.

"Cancer cachexia" is a multifactorial syndrome defined by an ongoing loss of skeletal muscle mass (with or without loss of fat mass) that cannot be fully reversed by conventional nutritional support and leads to progressive functional impairment.[16] Cancer cachexia caused by tumor-induced metabolic derangement is termed "Cacobolism".[17-19]

Cancer cachexia not only decreases the quality of life of cancer patients but can also hinder ongoing treatment, overall outcome, and return to intended oncology therapy (RIOT).

IMPACT OF MALNUTRITION IN CANCER PATIENTS

Malnutrition can have a negative impact on the overall survival of cancer patients by:

- Delayed wound healing
- Impaired muscle function
- *Lower tolerance to anticancer treatments:* Increased toxicity, poor compliance, and reduced response to treatment[3]
- Increased incidence of postoperative complications
- *Prolonged intensive care unit (ICU)/hospital stay:* Frequent treatment interruptions

Recent studies have shown that early clinical nutrition interventions can lower incidence of therapy-related

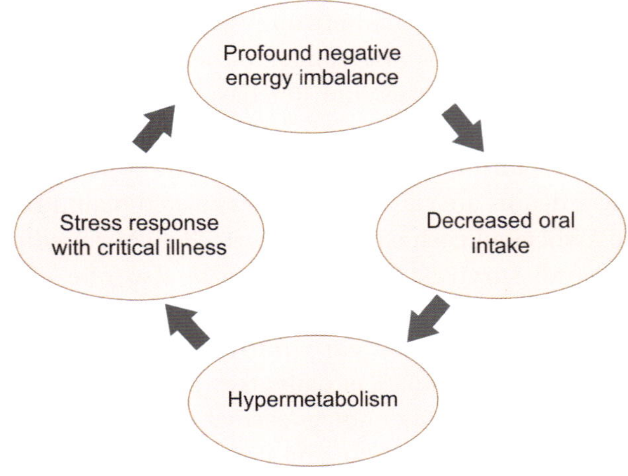

Fig. 1: Cycle of cancer cachexia.

toxicity, with increase in relative dose intensity and fewer delays in cancer treatment. Patients with gastrointestinal (GI) cancers are particularly at risk of malnutrition. A recent review of literature recommended in favor of early nutritional screening and intervention irrespective of the treatment phase in gastric and esophageal cancer patients.

Screening, Assessment, and Diagnosis

Nutritional risk screening is an essential component of the preoperative assessment of oncosurgical patients. Screening tools must be sensitive, specific, and reproducible. They should be applied within 24–48 hours of admission and repeated at regular intervals depending upon nutritional deterioration during hospital stay. It helps create awareness and allows early diagnosis and intervention.

Major screening components include ABCD: *A*nthropometric, *B*iochemical, *C*linical, and *D*ietary history **(Table 4)**.

Apart from above individual tests, there are some validated nutrition screening tools, which are given in **Table 5**.

TABLE 4: ABCD of nutritional screening.

Anthropometric measurement	• Height, weight, and body mass index (BMI) • Mid-arm, abdominal, and thigh circumferences (protein stores) • Skin-fold thickness (fat stores)
Biochemical assessment	• *Routine tests:* Serum electrolytes, blood glucose, lipid profile, LFT, and KFT • *Biomarkers:* Serum albumin, prealbumin, transferrin, urinary creatinine, urinary 3-methyl histidine, insulin-like growth factor-1 (IGF-1), lepton, and blood lymphocyte counts • Micronutrient levels of vitamins and minerals (thiamine, riboflavin, pyridoxine, folic acid, vitamin B_{12}, vitamin A, C, D, E, and K, selenium, and iron levels)
Clinical assessment	*Head-to-toe physical examination:* Reduced hand-grip strength, easy fatiguability, poor oral health, brittle hair/hair loss, thin extremities with swollen abdomen or face, etc
Dietary assessment	Subjective responses to questionnaire

(KFT: kidney function test; LFT: liver function test)

Abnormal screening tests usually lack detailed information that may guide further management. Patients with abnormal screening, therefore, need to undergo detailed assessment to determine specific nutritional and metabolic derangements to help design proper treatment plans. In patients with abnormal screening, ESPEN guidelines recommend objective and quantitative assessment of nutritional intake, nutrition impact symptoms, muscle mass, physical performance, and the degree of systemic inflammation.

There is no consensus on any individual nutrition assessment tool but frequently used tools include subjective global assessment (SGA), patient-generated subjective global assessment (PG-SGA), and minimal nutrition assessment (MNA).

In January 2016, major global clinical nutrition societies came together to develop Global Leadership Initiative on Malnutrition (GLIM).[20] It recommends a two-step approach for the malnutrition diagnosis, i.e., first screening to identify "at risk" status using any validated screening tool, and second, assessment for diagnosis and grading the severity of malnutrition.

The top five ranked criteria are as follows:

- *Three phenotypic criteria*
    - Nonvolitional weight loss

TABLE 5: Nutrition screening tools.

Tool name	*Parameters*	*Oncology specific*	*Population*
Nutrition Risk Screening 2002 (NRS-2002)	• BMI <20.5 • Weight loss • Change in intake • Severity of illness	Nonspecific	Inpatient
Malnutrition Universal Screening Tool (MUST)	• BMI • Unintentional weight loss >5% over 3–6 months • Decreased oral intake >5 days	Oncology	Inpatient
Malnutrition Screening Tool (MST)	• Weight loss • Appetite change	Oncology	Inpatient Outpatient
Mini Nutritional Assessment Short Form-Revised	• Food intake • BMI • Weight loss • Mobility • Neuropsychological stress	Nonspecific	Elderly outpatient

(BMI: body mass index)

- Low body mass index
- Reduced muscle mass
- Two etiological criteria
  - Reduced food intake or assimilation
  - Inflammation or disease burden

Diagnosis: One phenotypic criterion + one etiologic criterion

Phenotypic metrics for grading severity: Stage 1 (moderate) and Stage 2 (severe) malnutrition

PREHABILITATION AND ENHANCED RECOVERY AFTER SURGERY PROGRAMS IN COMBATING MALNUTRITION[3]

Prehabilitation is a continuous process that commences at the time of diagnosis and goes on till the beginning of treatment. Nutrition is one of the four pillars of prehabilitation. It aims at early diagnosis and correction of nutritional deficits and increasing lean muscle mass and amino acid reserve. The recommended target protein intake is 1.2 g/kg body weight/day along with regular exercise program to help gain muscle mass. For example, 30 gm protein in the form of whey protein (leucine-rich) or milk-based protein can be divided over 3 meals a day.

Enhanced recovery after surgery (ERAS) program involves a multidisciplinary approach, which is spread over preoperative, perioperative, and postoperative phases. It emphasizes preoperative nutritional screening, improving the nutritional status, and the correction of specific deficits. The team includes surgeons, anesthesiologists, nurses, dieticians, pharmacists, physiotherapists, and clinical nutritionists. Over the years, the role of nutrition in cancer survival trajectory has been realized and globally, there is a trend toward early detection and improvement of nutritional status through various guidelines. Although initiated for colorectal cancers and other GI surgeries, ERAS guidelines for oncosurgeries are also available now.

CONCEPT OF CALORIE RESTRICTION PROGRAMS IN CANCER CARE

The concept of calorie restriction in cancer patients assumes that starvation-induced autophagy may sensitize cancer cells to chemotherapy by lowering side effects. Theoretically, starvation in normal cells leads to reduction of circulating insulin-like growth factor-1 (IGF-1) and glucose levels, which leads to decreased proliferation and an increase of maintenance and repair pathways, making them resistant to anticancer therapies and causing lower chemotherapy side effects. On the contrary, cancer cells have slower fasting adaptation and continue to proliferate at a high rate, even during caloric reduction. Starvation tends to enhance cancer cells' sensitization to chemotherapy-induced apoptosis, and thus increases efficacy of treatment. The ESPEN recommends against any kind of dietary provisions that might restrict energy intake in patients with or at risk of malnutrition.

CORRECTION OF MALNUTRITION IN CANCER

According to recommendations made by ESPEN expert group, nutritional care for cancer patients should be based on three key aspects, which are (1) early screening, (2) detailed nutritional assessment, followed by (3) multimodal dietary intervention plans.[21] The key aspects of nutrition therapy in cancer patients are summarized in **Figure 2**.

The goal of the diet is to meet the patient's energy requirements, i.e., total energy expenditure (TEE), which is the sum of the REE, physical activity, and diet-induced thermogenesis (minor). There is sufficient evidence that REE is elevated in some cancer patients.[22] It is important to note that although REE is increased, TEE appears to be lower in patients with advanced cancer when compared to predicted values for healthy individuals.[23,24] The probable explanation is the reduction in daily physical activity. Inactivity and systemic inflammation frequently encountered in cancer patients are known to induce decreased responsiveness of protein synthesis

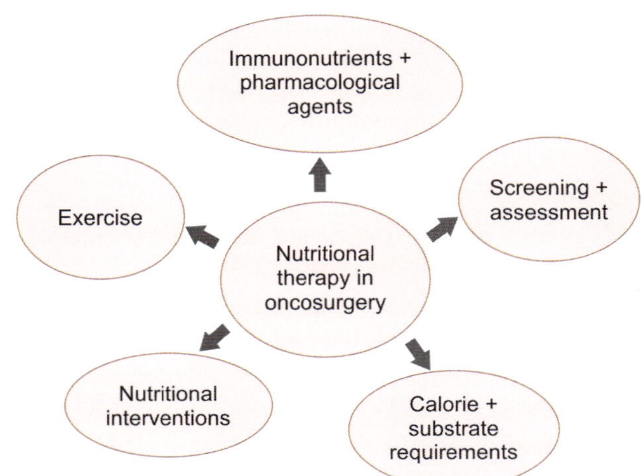

Fig. 2: Nutrition therapy in cancer patients.

TABLE 6: Energy and substrate requirement.

Energy requirements	25 and 30 kcal/kg/day (if not measured individually, assumed to be similar to healthy subjects)
Protein requirement	1 g/kg/day and up to 1.5 g/kg/day
Vitamins and trace elements	Equal to the RDA and discourage the use of high-dose micronutrients in the absence of specific deficiencies

(RDA: recommended dietary allowance)

to anabolic stimuli, also called "anabolic resistance".[25] The optimal nitrogen supply for cancer patients has not been determined but experts recommend a minimum protein supply of 1 g/kg/day with a target supply of 1.2–2 g/kg/day,[26-28] more so if systemic inflammation and inactivity are present.[29] It is recommended to increase the ratio of energy from fat to energy from carbohydrates in weight-losing cancer patients who have insulin resistance. The advantages of replacing glucose with fat are lower glycemic load, reduced incidence of hyperglycemia-induced infectious risks, and deleterious positive water balance.[30,31] ESPEN recommends measures to increase oral intake in cancer patients who are able to eat but are malnourished or at risk of malnutrition **(Table 6)**.

METHODS OF NUTRITION THERAPY[15,32]

After initial screening and assessment, prompt and aggressive nutrition intervention is required for cancer patients, especially at risk of precachexia or cancer cachexia. Nutrition can be administered via oral, enteral, or parenteral route. Irrespective of the route of nutrition, the efforts are to achieve the goals of nutrition therapy listed in **Table 7**.

Individualized approach is recommended based on patient's current nutritional status, symptom severity, and function of the GI tract guided by evidence-based guidelines.

Types of Nutrition

One can provide nutrients orally (normal diet, therapeutic diet, fortified food, oral nutritional supplements), or via enteral or parenteral route. Enteral nutrition (EN) and parenteral nutrition (PN) fall under the category of artificial nutritional support.

Oral Nutrition Supplements

Commercially available oral nutrition supplements (ONS) are often used to improve the nutrient intake. These medically fortified food products serve as supplements for energy, protein, fat, carbohydrates, fibers, vitamins, and minerals. They cannot be the sole source of nutrition. Based on assessment of a patient's clinical condition, comorbidities, nutrition status, nutrient needs, GI function, food preferences, and resources available, recommendations for oral nutrition supplements are individualized.

TABLE 7: Goals of nutrition therapy.

Weight/Nutrition status	***Treatment***
Optimal weight and nutrition status	Maintain lean body mass
	Maintain healthy weight
Malnutrition	
Acute	Support vital organ function
	Preserve host response
	Cater to higher energy and protein demand
Chronic	Maintain and improve lean body mass and fat
Obesity	Maintain lean body mass
	Modest weight reduction (up to 1 kg/week)

Dieticians play a crucial part in the healthcare team, working in coordination with patients, caregivers, and members of the healthcare team to improve compliance and the effectiveness of pharmacotherapy interventions and also counsel patients about behavioral strategies to alleviate nutrition impact symptoms.

High-quality protein supplements are required to maintain and rebuild lean body mass in patients. Pharmaconutrients are specific nutrients that have a modulating effect on the immune and metabolic function, e.g., glutamine, arginine, and omega-3 fatty acids (FA). There is a lack of clear evidence and recommendation for routine supplementation of pharmaconutrients. Perioperative or postoperative administration of specific formula enriched with immunonutrients (arginine, omega-3 FAs, and ribonucleotides) should be given to malnourished patients undergoing major cancer surgery as per ESPEN.

Oral nutrition supplements can cause taste fatigue and decreased compliance with recommendations on long-term use. A systematic review of compliance with ONS suggested that compliance is good, especially with higher-energy-density supplements.[33]

Enteral Nutrition

Enteral nutrition is a treatment modality where nutrition is directly delivered into the GI tract using feeding tube.[34] Enteral feeding can be as efficient as parenteral feeding if intestinal functions are preserved. Nutritional status can be maintained by artificial EN in patients with tumors that impair oral intake or food transport into the upper GI tract.[35,36] If oral intake is <60% of daily requirement despite nutritional interventions per-os, and GI function is preserved then feeding by tube is indicated.

Historically, postoperative initiation of EN was delayed following GI and abdominal vascular surgeries. But now it is a well-established fact that even in postoperative period, GI function returns almost immediately, and it is recommended to start EN as soon as possible as per ERAS guidelines. EN during postoperative period has been associated with:

- Improved anastomotic site healing[17]
- Maintenance of gut integrity
- Decreased length of stay in ICU
- Decreased risk of infection
- Decreased intestinal permeability
- Lower risk of hyperglycemia
- Improved nitrogen balance and weight gain

Choice of the enteral route feeding depends on following factors:

- Anticipated length of need
- Aspiration risk
- Tumor location
- Side effects

When EN is expected to last >4–6 weeks, ostomy is preferred. Jejunostomy or nasojejunal tube is preferred over nasogastric or gastrostomy nutrition, if there is a risk of reflux, gastroparesis, or bronchoaspiration.

Parenteral Nutrition

Parenteral nutrition is the intravenous infusion of nutrients. Overall, whenever possible EN is the preferred technique over PN. PN in cancer patients is undertaken only when oral nutrition strategies are not possible or fail because of tumor location or severe side effects.

Indications for PN includes:[37-39]

- Malfunctioning GI tract (radiation enteritis)
- Malabsorptive conditions
- Mechanical obstructions
- Severe bleeding
- Severe diarrhea
- Intractable vomiting
- Difficult GI fistulas when bypassed with an enteral tube are not easy
- Prolonged ileus and severe enterocolitis

Parenteral nutrition is appropriate for moderately to severely malnourished patients who are unable to ingest and/or absorb nutrients enterally for a period of 7–10 days or greater [American Society for Parenteral and Enteral Nutrition (ASPEN) 2017]. There is a definite benefit of PN over standard isotonic fluids in these groups of patients.[40]

A central venous catheter or peripheral venous access can be employed for PN.

Dextrose (carbohydrate), amino acids (protein), lipids (fat), electrolytes, vitamins, and trace minerals in several combinations comprise PN. Ideally, a multidisciplinary team of clinicians, comprising a registered dietitian, clinical pharmacist, and other experts in the field of nutrition, should manage PN.

Beginning with a 24-hour infusion, PN is usually cycled to an infusion period of over 10–14 hours, especially in home-based care. This is possible after attaining daily macronutrient targets and institution of patient tolerance. In-hospital initiation of PN is advocated unless benefits of home initiation far outweigh the attendant risks, hemodynamic stability, minimal risk of refeeding syndrome, and negative diabetic status being prerequisites. Overuse of the peripheral venous access may lead to thrombophlebitis and sclerosis.

Nutrition support should not be withheld solely based on risk of nutritional supplements stimulating tumor growth and metastasis as there is lack of definitive evidence. However, caution must be taken while delivering PN as it is associated with increased incidence of infections, surgical complications, line-associated complications, and increased cost.

Perioperative administration of pharmaconutrients is upheld by current evidence. The most widely studied formula in this category contains a combination of a mix of arginine, omega-3 FAs, and nucleotides. It is the most extensively explored formula and is associated with reduced incidence of contagious and noncontagious surgical complications leading to a shorter length of hospital stay.

Types of nutrition based on duration are given in **Table 8**.

TABLE 8: Types of nutrition based on duration.

Short-term feeding	*Long-term feeding*
• *Duration:* <2 weeks • *Types:* Tip of tube ending in – Stomach (nasogastric tube) – Duodenum (nasoduodenal tube) – Jejunum (nasojejunal tube)—in patients with aspiration risk	• *Duration:* > 4 weeks • *Direct enteral access:* Percutaneous tubes may be placed endoscopically, surgically, or with fluoroscopy by interventional radiology
• *Via nasoenteric tube:* 5–16F diameter, 30–43 inches long silicone or polyurethane tube with weighted tips	• *Larger diameter of the tube:* 15F–24F, allowing easier and faster passage of formulas and medications
• Higher risk of aspiration	• Lower risk of aspiration
• Immunocompromised patients with mucositis, esophagitis, and/or herpetic, fungal, or candidiasis lesions in the mouth or throat may not be able to tolerate the presence of a nasoenteric tube	• Lower risk of sinusitis or nasoesophageal erosion • More convenient and aesthetically pleasing to patients because they can conceal the tube

METHOD OF DELIVERING NUTRITION: INFUSION METHODS AND FORMULAS

The method of delivering the source of nutrition depends on where the tube terminates in GI tract and the likely side effects.

The infusion methods and considerations for initiation and administration of EN are as follows:

Bolus and Intermittent Feeding

A bolus or intermittent (gravity) drip mimics normal feeding. It should be used when the endpoint of the tube is in the stomach; it should never be used when feedings are delivered into the duodenum or jejunum. Bolus feedings can be offered 3–6 times each day, and as much as 250–500 mL can be given over 10–15 minutes. A gravity drip from a bag or syringe with a slow push can be used to administer the formula. It requires less time and equipment and offers greater flexibility to the patient. Diarrhea is a common side effect of this infusion method but can be controlled with a change in formula and change in the amount of formula given over a finite period.

Continuous or Cyclic Drip Feeding

A slower administration rate is necessary for tubes terminating in the duodenum or jejunum with the help of infusion pump. Feedings via a pump may be administered cyclically (<24 hours per day) or continuously. The target rate and time of drip feeding depend on the nutrient, calorie, and free water demands of the patient.

Probability of gastric retention is reduced by robust enteral feeding pumps with consistent rates of infusion. When no compounding factors are present, feeding into the stomach (25–30 mL/h) can be started at a higher rate than feeding into the jejunum (10 mL/h); infusion rates can be stepped up over 4–6 hours to reach the target rate after ensuring patient tolerance. A cycle of continuous nocturnal feeds followed by diurnal oral or bolus feeds can suffice to meet the calorie and nutrition targets, providing enhanced comfort and a near-normal lifestyle.

In patients with malabsorption or intolerance to standard enteral feeds, semielemental or elemental formulas or specially designed disease-specific formulas may be considered. In lieu of segregated protein, fat, and carbohydrate components, blended whole food has become an attractive option. Both commercial products and recipes for home-made formulas are available but a dietitian's review of nutritional contents in home blenderized formulae is imperative.

DOES NUTRITION FOR CANCER PATIENTS FEED THE TUMOR?

Literature review reveals that certain neoplasms (brain, head–neck, and lung) are glucose-dependent. A normocaloric ketogenic diet can be prescribed to patients with neoplasms displaying elevated fluorodeoxyglucose (18 F-FDG) capitation. A high fat-protein, low-carbohydrate diet appears to better fulfill the nutritional requirements of these cancer patients. But current evidence shows no improvement in tumoral response after restricting patient's caloric intake, whereas malnutrition is acknowledged as an important negative predictive and prognostic factor in all cancer patients.[41]

PRECISION NUTRITION THERAPY

Just as precision or personalized medicine has transformed cancer treatment from a one-size-fits-all to biomarker-guided drug therapy, it is proposed that a similar approach can be applied to nutrition in oncology—*precision nutrition therapy*. By incorporating genetics, nutrition, and the microbiome as factors in cancer therapy, we can dramatically improve treatment outcomes for cancer patients.[42]

NUTRITION IN ADVANCED OR TERMINAL CANCER[15]

Advanced malignancy patients exhibit specific nutrition-related side effects or may experience deterioration of preexisting side effects in course of disease progression or therapy. Four most frequent nutrition-impact symptoms in terminal cancer patients are anorexia, dry mouth, constipation, and giddiness. Other symptoms include bloating, constipation, dysphagia, chewing difficulties, early satiety, mucositis, dysgeusia, and vomiting. Terminal cancer patients on opioids for pain relief may experience one additional side effect—opioid-induced constipation. Management of these symptoms is an important component while dealing with malnutrition in this specter of patients.

Nutrition support in terminally ill patients has been shown to improve quality of life, decrease risk of death due to malnutrition, and lower incidence of physical, cognitive, and psychological problems but it has no effect on overall survival. However, nutrition support in advanced cancer patients can be withheld if:

- Short estimated life expectancy (less than 2–3 months)
- Poor performance status as determined by a Karnofsky Performance Status score (lower than 50) or an Eastern Cooperative Oncology Group Performance Status grade of 3 or 4
- Severe organ dysfunction
- Uncontrolled symptoms
- Patient's choice

Nutrition support, however, may be appropriate in patients who have incurable disease and are undergoing anticancer treatment as stated by ESPEN and the Multinational Association of Supportive Care in Cancer (MASCC) guidelines. These guidelines endorse the use of nutrition support for willing individuals with advanced cancer who cannot ingest or absorb sufficient nutrients, if their survival is for more than 1 month and those who have adequate cognitive and physical abilities.

Goals of Nutrition Therapy in Advanced Cancer

Terminally ill cancer patients may be receiving anticancer treatment, concurrent palliative care, or hospice care. Nutrition goals in this subset of patients should fit in with the overall plan of care after screening for nutrition-specific requirements. PG-SGA focuses on history of weight gain/loss, food intake, symptomology, and physiological condition and has been endorsed for cancer patients.[43] Nutritional targets concentrate on sustaining active therapy and improving treatment results, body composition, and physiological improvement, and symptomatic relief as a part of palliative care.

With a pivotal shift from disease-modifying treatment to hospice care, nutritional goals start leaning toward patient comfort.

CONCLUSION

Clinical nutritional therapy for malignancy requires effectual structural tactics and distinct action plans for tangible results.

Cancer patients exhibiting loss of body weight, a cardinal symptom of malnutrition, display the maximum adverse results after chemotherapy. Tailor-made dietary plans for individual cancer patients can only be materialized by devising a robust tool to secure dietary data for healthcare workers and cancer patients.

Teaching and training to improve clinical awareness and creating a multidisciplinary team incorporating the services of a clinical nutritionist can go a long way in detecting patients at increased malnutrition risk and streamlining their management with timely and relevant interventions.

An abridged version of the ESPN clinical nutrition guidelines for patients with malignancy in the form of user-friendly flowcharts is available.[2] These practical guidelines are pledged to all healthcare workers (physicians, dieticians, nutritionists, and nurses) working in the oncology setup.

Malnutrition has an impact not only on clinical outcomes but also on healthcare expenditures.[4]

Tapping significant dietary and microbiome information in longitudinal cohorts will augment our comprehension and insight into the diet–microbiome interactions in the therapy gamut and streamline our efforts toward precision nutrition therapy for oncological patients.

REFERENCES

1. The School of Health. (2017). What is Nutrition? [online] Available from https://www.schoolofhealth.com/nutrition-courses/what-is-nutrition/ [Last accessed February, 2024].
2. Muscaritoli M, Arends J, Bachmann P, Baracos V, Barthelemy N, Bertz H, et al. ESPEN practical guideline: Clinical Nutrition in cancer. Clin Nutr. 2021;40(5):2898-913.
3. Serón-Arbeloa C, Labarta-Monzón L, Puzo-Foncillas J, Mallor-Bonet T, Lafita-López A, Bueno-Vidales N, et al.

Malnutrition screening and assessment. Nutrients. 2022;14(12):2392.
4. Bossi P, De Luca R, Ciani O, D'Angelo E, Caccialanza R. Malnutrition management in oncology: An expert view on controversial issues and future perspectives. Front Oncol. 2022;12:910770.
5. Fearon K, Strasser F, Anker SD, Bosaeus I, Bruera E, Fainsinger RL, et al. Definition and classification of cancer cachexia: An international consensus. Lancet Oncol. 2011;12(5):489-95.
6. Fukushima H, Nakanishi Y, Kataoka M, Tobisu K, Koga F. Prognostic significance of sarcopenia in patients with metastatic renal cell carcinoma. J Urol. 2016;195:26-32.
7. Walsh D, Donnelly S, Rybicki L. The symptoms of advanced cancer: Relationship to age, gender, and performance status in 1,000 patients. Support Care Cancer. 2000;8(3):175-9.
8. Siemens W, Schönsteiner SS, Orellana-Rios CL, Schaekel U, Kessler J, Eschbach C, et al. Severe symptoms and very low quality-of-life among outpatients newly diagnosed with advanced cancer: Data from a multicenter cohort study. Support Care Cancer. 2020;28(11):5547-55.
9. Elia M, Goren A, Behrens R, Barber RW, Neale G. Effect of total starvation and very low calorie diets on intestinal permeability in man. Clin Sci (Lond). 1987;73(2):205-10. August 1987.
10. Peuhkuri K, Vapaatalo H, Korpela R. Even low-grade inflammation impacts on small intestinal function. World J Gastroenterol. 2010;16(9):1057-62.
11. Dewys WD, Begg C, Lavin PT, Band PR, Bennett JM, Bertino JR, et al. Prognostic effect of weight loss prior to chemotherapy in cancer patients. Eastern Cooperative Oncology Group. Am J Med. 1980;69(4):491-7.
12. Jang RW, Caraiscos VB, Swami N, Banerjee S, Mak E, Kaya E, et al. Simple prognostic model for patients with advanced cancer based on performance status. J Oncol Pract. 2014;10(5):e335-41.
13. Gröber U, Holzhauer P, Kisters K, Holick MF, Adamietz IA. Micronutrients in oncological intervention. Nutrients. 2016;8(3):163.
14. Ströhle A, Zänker K, Hahn A. Nutrition in oncology: The case of micronutrients. Oncol Rep. 2010;24(4):815-28.
15. National Cancer Institute. (2024). Nutrition in Cancer Care (PDQ®–Health Professional Version. Nutrition in Advanced or Terminal Cancer. [online] Available from https://www.cancer.gov/about-cancer/treatment/side-effects/appetite-loss/nutrition-hp-pdq#_210 [Last accessed February, 2025].
16. Lach K, Peterson SJ. Nutrition support for critically ill patients with cancer. Nutr Clin Pract. 2017;32(5):578-86.
17. Coussens LM, Werb Z. Inflammation and cancer. Nature. 2002;420(6917):860-7.
18. Apollonio B, Ioannou N, Papazoglou D, Ramsay AG. Understanding the immune-stroma microenvironment in B cell malignancies for effective immunotherapy. Front Oncol. 2021;11:626818.
19. Baracos VE, Martin L, Korc M, Guttridge DC, Fearon KCH. Cancer-associated cachexia. Nat Rev Dis Primers. 2018;18:17105.
20. Cederholm T, Jensen GL, Correia MITD, Gonzalez MC, Fukushima R, Higashiguchi T, et al. GLIM criteria for the diagnosis of malnutrition–A consensus report from the global clinical nutrition community. Clin Nutr. 2019;38(1):1-9.
21. National Cancer Institute. (2024). Nutrition in Cancer Care (PDQ®–Health Professional Version. Nutrition Therapy. [online] Available from https://www.cancer.gov/about-cancer/treatment/side-effects/appetite-loss/nutrition-hp-pdq#_104 [Last accessed February, 2025].
22. Bosaeus I, Daneryd P, Svanberg E, Lundholm K. Dietary intake, resting energy expenditure in relation to weight loss in unselected cancer patients. Int J Cancer. 2001;93(3):380-3.
23. Moses AW, Slater C, Preston T, Barber MD, Fearon KC. Reduced total energy expenditure and physical activity in cachectic patients with pancreatic cancer can be modulated by an energy and protein dense oral supplement enriched with N-3 fatty acids. Br J Cancer. 2004;90(5):996-1002.
24. Gibney E, Elia M, Jebb SA, Murgatroyd P, Jennings G. Total energy expenditure in patients with small-cell lung cancer: Results of a validated study using the bicarbonate-urea method. Metabolism. 1997;46(12):1412-7.
25. Haran PH, Rivas DA, Fielding RA. Role and potential mechanisms of anabolic resistance in sarcopenia. J Cachexia Sarcopenia Muscle. 2012;3(3):157-62.
26. Nitenberg G, Raynard B. Nutritional support of the cancer patient: Issues and dilemmas. Crit Rev Oncol Hematol. 2000;34(3):137-68.
27. Baracos VE. Meeting the amino acid requirements for protein anabolism in cancer cachexia. In: Mantovani G (Ed). Cachexia and Wasting. A Modern Approach. Milan: Springer; 2006. pp. 631-4.
28. Barrera R. Nutritional support in cancer patients. JPEN J Parenter Enteral Nutr. 2002;26(5 Suppl):563-71.
29. Guadagni M, Biolo G. Effects of inflammation and/or inactivity on the need for dietary protein. Curr Opin Clin Nutr Metab Care. 2009;12(6):617-22.
30. Gamble JL. The Harvey Lectures, Series XLIII, 1946-1947: Physiological information gained from studies on the life raft ration. Nutr Rev. 1989;47(7):199-201.
31. Bloom WL. Inhibition of salt excretion by carbohydrate. Arch Intern Med. 1962;109:26-32.
32. Russell L, Bode AH, Dengler A. A Practical Guide to Nutrition Support in the Oncology Patient: Tips, Tricks, and Ethical Considerations. Curr Treat Options Gastro. 2024;22:279-86.
33. Hubbard GP, Elia M, Holdoway A, Stratton RJ. A systematic review of compliance to oral nutritional supplements. Clin Nutr. 2012;31(3):293-312.

34. Bozzetti F. Nutritional support in patients with oesophageal cancer. Support Care Cancer 2010;18(Suppl 2):S41-50
35. Corry J, Poon W, McPhee N, Milner AD, Cruickshank D, Porceddu SV, et al. Randomized study of percutaneous endoscopic gastrostomy versus nasogastric tubes for enteral feeding in head and neck cancer patients treated with (chemo)radiation. J Med Imaging Radiat Oncol. 2008;52(5):503-10
36. Nugent B, Parker MJ, McIntyre IA. Nasogastric tube feeding and percutaneous endoscopic gastrostomy tube feeding in patients with head and neck cancer. J Hum Nutr Diet. 2010;23(3):277-84.
37. Bozzetti F, Santarpia L, Pironi L, Thul P, Klek S, Gavazzi C, et al. The prognosis of incurable cachectic cancer patients on home parenteral nutrition: A multi-centre observational study with prospective follow-up of 414 patients. Ann Oncol. 2014;25(2):487-93.
38. Brennan MF, Pisters PW, Posner M, Quesada O, Shike M. A prospective randomized trial of total parenteral nutrition after major pancreatic resection for malignancy. Ann Surg. 1994;220(4):436-44.
39. Scolapio JS, Ukleja A, Burnes JU, Kelly DG. Outcome of patients with radiation enteritis treated with home parenteral nutrition. Am J Gastroenterol. 2002;97(3):662-6.
40. Braga M, Ljungqvist O, Soeters P, Fearon K, Weimann A, Bozzetti F. ESPEN guidelines on parenteral nutrition: Surgery. Clin Nutr. 2009;28:378-86.
41. Bozzetti F, Stanga Z. Does nutrition for cancer patients feed the tumour? A clinical perspective. Crit Rev Oncol Hematol. 2020;153:103061.
42. Greathouse KL, Wyatt M, Johnson AJ, Toy EP, Khan JM, Dunn K, et al. Diet-microbiome interactions in cancer treatment: Opportunities and challenges for precision nutrition in cancer. Neoplasia. 2022;29:100800.
43. Balstad TR, Bye A, Jenssen CR, Solheim TS, Thoresen L, Sand K. Patient interpretation of the Patient-Generated Subjective Global Assessment (PG-SGA) Short Form. Patient Prefer Adherence. 2019;13:1391-400.

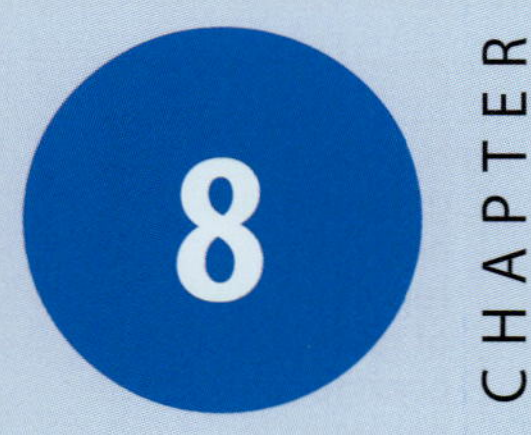

Physical and Pulmonary Assessment and Optimization before Major Onco-Surgery

Aditya Kunte, Sanika Patil, Reshma Ambulkar

INTRODUCTION

Surgery is one of the major components of multimodality cancer treatment and is often associated with significant perioperative morbidity and mortality. In addition, preoperative chemotherapy/radiation can worsen preexisting cancer-related malnutrition and functional detriment, thus further compromising the ability to withstand major oncologic surgery. Consequently, a delayed recovery from surgery decreases the probability of completing intended adjuvant therapies, thus compromising overall cancer care. A dedicated, structured, and individualized program intended to evaluate and optimize the preoperative functional capacity of cancer patients is crucial to ensuring optimal oncologic outcomes.

PREHABILITATION: DEFINITION AND STAGES

Prehabilitation is the first stage in the rehabilitation pathway, otherwise known as preventative rehabilitation, and is followed by conventional rehabilitation, which is comprised of restorative, supportive, and palliative rehabilitation **(Fig. 1)**.[1]

Prehabilitation in the context of cancer care was defined by Silver et al. as "A process on the cancer continuum of care that occurs between the time of cancer diagnosis and the beginning of acute treatment and includes physical and psychological assessments that establish a baseline functional level, identify impairments, and provide interventions that promote physical and psychological health to reduce the incidence and/or severity of future impairments."[2]

Prehabilitation is divided into three stages:

1. Preassessment
2. Prehabilitation regimen
3. Follow-up during and post prehabilitation

The concept of prehabilitation is illustrated in the "prehabilitation diagram" shown in **Figure 2.**

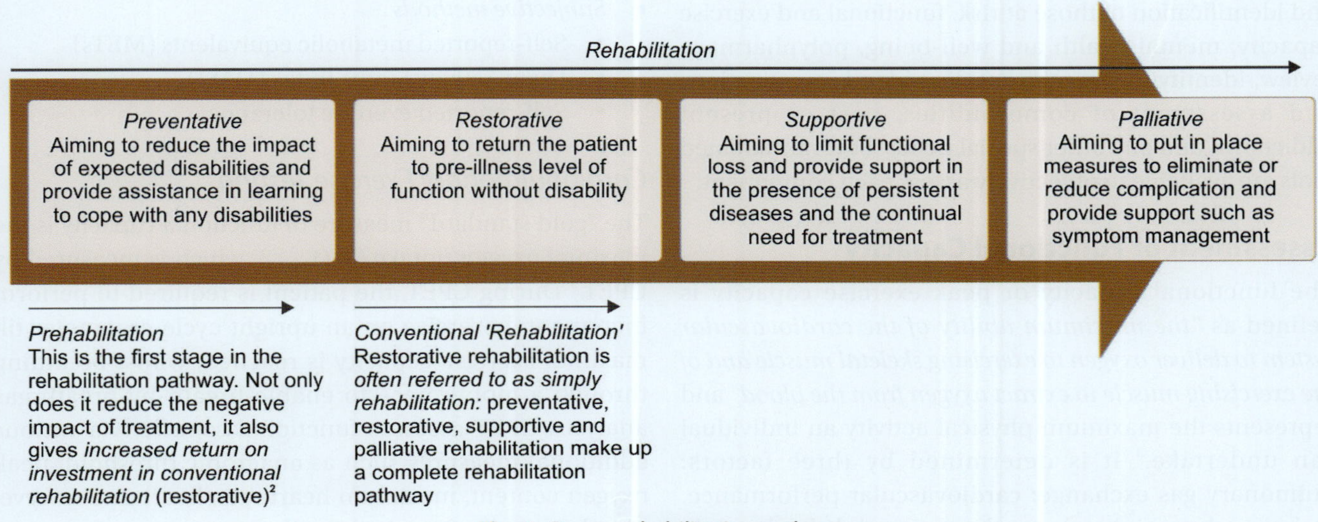

Fig. 1: Cancer rehabilitation pathway.

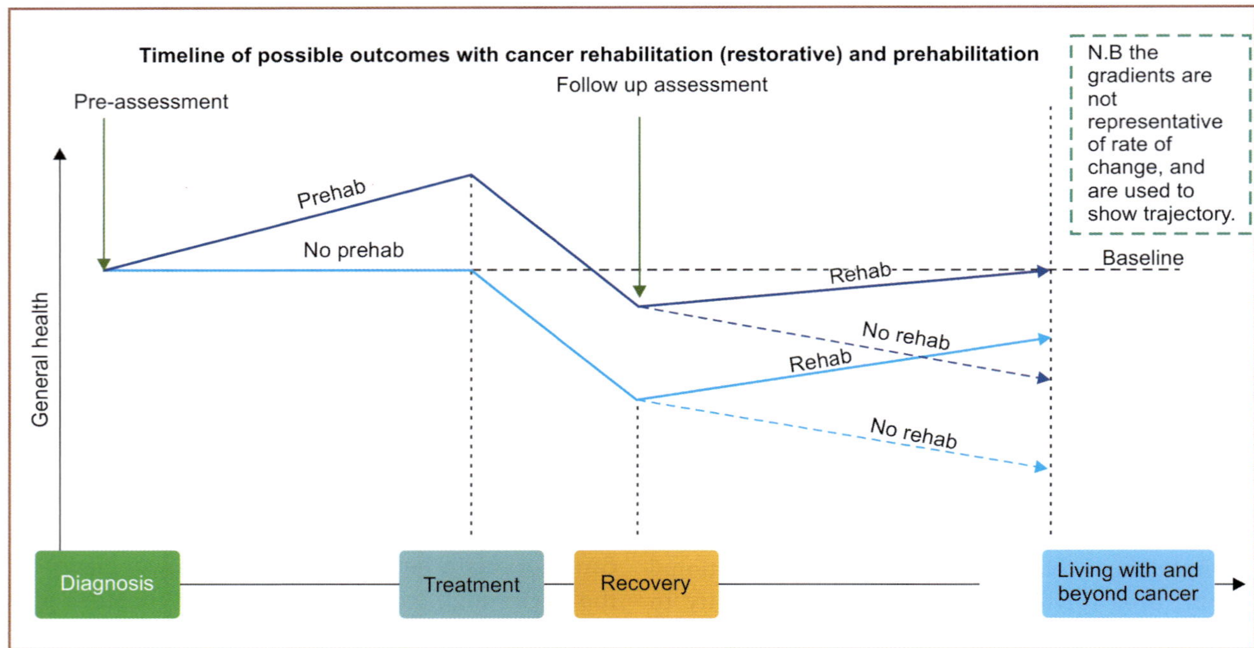

Fig. 2: Prehabilitation diagram: Timeline of cancer prehabilitation and rehabilitation.

PREASSESSMENT

The preassessment phase begins with the diagnosis of cancer and involves assessing the baseline status of patients, including a comprehensive risk-assessment. It is important to involve patients at this stage of care by having joint discussions to establish the goals of treatment and set reasonable and realistic expectations from the intended treatment. Baseline patient assessment should evaluate cardiopulmonary function, nutritional status and identification of those at risk, functional and exercise capacity, mental health and well-being, polypharmacy review, identifying anemia, baseline blood investigations and assessment of comorbidities, past or present addictions, and any other special needs. Several validated tools are available to objectively assess each component.

Assessment of Functional Capacity

The functional capacity or peak exercise capacity is defined as "*the maximum ability of the cardiovascular system to deliver oxygen to exercising skeletal muscle and of the exercising muscle to extract oxygen from the blood*" and represents the maximum physical activity an individual can undertake.[3] It is determined by three factors: Pulmonary gas exchange; cardiovascular performance, including the peripheral vascular tree; and skeletal muscle metabolism. Functional capacity can be assessed by the following methods:

- *Objective methods:*
  - Direct measures
    - Cardiopulmonary exercise testing (CPET)
  - Indirect measures
    - Incremental shuttle walk test (ISWT)
    - 6-minute walk test (6-MWT)
    - Stair-climbing test
- *Subjective methods*
  - Self-reported metabolic equivalents (METs)
  - Duke Activity Status Index (DASI)
  - Self-reported exercise tolerance

Cardiopulmonary Exercise Testing

The "gold standard" measure of functional capacity is the maximal oxygen uptake ($V\text{-}O_{2max}$), which is measured by CPET.[3] During CPET, the patient is required to perform incremental exercise on an upright cycle ergometer till maximal exercise capacity is reached, whilst breathing through a mouthpiece to enable breath-by-breath gas analysis. CPET assesses functional capacity via various additional measures such as anaerobic threshold, peak oxygen content, maximum heart rate, heart rate reserve, blood pressure, O_2 pulse, ventilatory reserve, respiratory

TABLE 1: Normal values of cardiopulmonary exercise testing (CPET) variables.

Variables	*Normal value*
Peak oxygen content (PVO_2)	>84% predicted
Ventilatory anaerobic threshold (VAT)	>40% PVO_2 (4,080)
Maximum heart rate (HRmax)	>90% age predicted
Heart rate reserve (HRR)	<15 beats/min
Blood pressure (BP)	<220/90 mm Hg
O_2 pulse (VO_2/HR)	>80%
Ventilatory reserve (VR)	MVV – VEmax > 11 L or VEmax/MVV × 100 < 85%
Respiratory rate (RR)	<60 breaths/min
Minute ventilation/carbon dioxide output ratio (VE/VCO_2) at VAT	<34

rate, and minute ventilation/CO_2 output ratio. Normal values of CPET variables are detailed in **Table 1**.[3]

The advantage of CPET is that it is a comprehensive and accurate test of the cardiorespiratory capacity that reflects the entire oxygen transport system starting with the lungs and ending with the skeletal muscles. However, its utilization is limited by the need for expensive equipment and trained personnel.

Incremental Shuttle Walk Test

The ISWT requires a subject to walk back and forth between two cones 10 m apart, at speeds that increase every minute by 0.17 m/s in time to audio signals. The test is terminated when the subject fails to reach the next cone before the signal. Measurements obtained include the incremental shuttle walk distance (ISWD), heart rate, oxygen saturation, noninvasive systolic and diastolic blood pressures, and modified Borg dyspnea scale. Normal values for the ISWD vary with age but are usually between 560 and 820 m in healthy individuals. Studies evaluating lung cancer resection and major colorectal surgery have found an ISWD < 250 m to predict an increased risk of major complications and mortality. A disadvantage of ISWT is that the threshold ISWD that predicts postoperative complications varies according to the type of surgery performed.[4]

6-minute Walk Test

The self-paced 6-minute walking test is a submaximal assessment of exercise tolerance. The patient is asked to walk and cover as much distance as possible along a flat, hard-surfaced, 30 m long stretch of corridor for a period of 6 minutes. The primary outcome measure of this test is the total distance covered by the patient in 6 minutes. Oxygen saturation and heart rate are recorded before and after the test. In addition, leg fatigue and Borg dyspnea scale can also be documented.[5] During a 6MWT, healthy subjects can typically walk 400–700 m. In addition to the total distance walked, the magnitude of desaturation and timing of heart rate recovery have been associated with clinical outcomes.[6,7] Although it is a simple and inexpensive, 6MWT involves operator encouragement that may potentially influence the 6MWD.

Stair Climbing Test

There are two variants of the stair climbing test: "Symptom-limited" and "fixed-altitude" tests.

Symptom-limited stair climbing test: This test was described by Brunelli et al.[8] in which patients are asked to climb the maximum number of steps on a staircase at a pace of their choosing and to stop only for exhaustion, limiting dyspnea, leg fatigue, or chest pain. Patients are accompanied by a physician and are encouraged to continue the exercise for as long as they can. A continuous verbal interaction is used between the physician and the patient to assess the degree of exertional dyspnea. A pulse oximeter is used to monitor heart rate and capillary oxygen saturation. The total number of steps climbed, height of each step, and time taken to complete the test are recorded. Patients who were unable to climb to an altitude of at least 12 m were found to have a significantly higher complication rate than those able to climb 14–14 m or more.

Fixed-altitude stair climbing test: Ambrozin et al.[9] and Cataneo et al.[10] described a variation of the symptom-limited stair climbing test in which subjects were required to climb stairs to a fixed altitude of 12.16 m as fast as they could. The postoperative complication rate was 4.3-fold higher in patients who took 50 seconds or longer to complete the test as opposed to those who took 30 seconds or less.[9] However, these findings are applicable only to patients undergoing lung resections as there is limited evidence in literature regarding the ability of this test to predict postoperative outcomes in patients undergoing abdominal surgery. Arruda et al.[11] reported that the test was unable to predict postoperative cardiopulmonary complications whereas Reddy et al.[12] concluded it to be the strongest predictor of perioperative complications after abdominal surgery.

Self-reported METs

A MET represents the resting oxygen consumption of a 40-year-old, 70-kg man, equivalent to a VO_2 of 3.5 mL/kg/min. Questionnaires such as the Veterans Specific Activity Questionnaire (VSAQ)[13] or the MET-REPAIR questionnaires,[14] which estimate METs for various levels of physical activity, are administered to the patients to assess their functional capacity **(Figs. 3A and B)**. An activity level equivalent to <4 METs is considered as poor functional capacity. However, estimating METs solely through a preoperative history of activities of daily living can underestimate the true METs as measured by stress testing. Therefore, METs should not be solely relied upon but rather assist healthcare practitioners in identifying patients who may require further assessment.

Duke Activity Status Index

The DASI is a structured, self-administered questionnaire which was developed to address the limitations of assessing functional capacity by self-reported MET questionnaires[15] **(Fig. 4)**. The DASI questionnaire consists of 12 activities, ranging from daily living tasks to sports activities, with each activity assigned a weight based on its known energy expenditure. The sum of these weights provides a DASI score, which ranges from 0 (equivalent to 2.74 METs, indicating all "no" answers) to 58.2 (approximately 9.89 METs, indicating all "yes" answers).[15] A DASI score below 34 is associated with an increased risk of myocardial infarction, moderate-to-severe complications, and new

European Society of Anaesthesiology ESA

Section 1

Study_ID Date of complection____________

Please mark the appropriate box (☐)

1. Can you do any of the listed activities? Please consider the last month, If you are able of perform **ANY** of the activities listed in each question please check yes)

	Yes	No	MET
• Stair climbing at rapid pace: • Carrying upstairs a suitcase (*10–20 kg/20–40 lb*): • Running	☐	☐	8
♦ Moving furniture, household items ♦ Lifting light loads: ♦ Running, playing laying with children or animals at vigorous effort ♦ Recreational swimming.	☐	☐	5
• Carrying groceries upstairs; • Jogging: • Recreational soccer of tennis	☐	☐	7
♦ Descending stairs; ♦ Marking beds; ♦ Vacuuming or sweeping floors; ♦ Walking the dog for pleasure; ♦ Play with children at moderate effort.	☐	☐	3
• Stair climbing at slow pace; • Hanging laundry; • Cleaning the bathroom; • Mowing lawn (power mower); • Raking lawn or sweeping outside the house; • Leisure bicycling; • Walking for exercise, level, moderate pace.	☐	☐	4
♦ Sitting, reading, watching TV, listening to music	☐	☐	1
• Moving household items upstairs, carrying boxes (upstairs); • Climbing hills carrying ≥ 20 kg/≥40 lb; • Swimming fast.	☐	☐	7.5
♦ Hiking cross country; ♦ Walking for exercise uphill; ♦ Bilking to/from work at self-selected pace; ♦ Scrubbing floors on hands and knees, vigorous effort; ♦ Mowing lawn (hand mower); ♦ Shoveling snow; ♦ Chopping wood, vigorous effort.	☐	☐	6

European Society of Anaesthesiology ESA

• Walk indoors, such as around your house; • *Dressing/undressing.*	☐	☐	2
♦ Carrying loads ≥ 25 kg/50 lb. (e.g. furniture, 2 suitcases) upstairs; ♦ Running 10 km/h. / 6 mph please notice: 10 km/h or 6 mph is faster than a bicycle at leisure pace.	☐	☐	8.5

2. How many floors can you continuously climb without having to stop to rest?

☐ less than 1 ☐ 1 ☐ 2 ☐ 3 ☐ 4 ☐ more than 4

3. How dependent on assistance for activities of daily living are you? (e.g. cooking, dressing, etc.)

☐ fully independent ☐ partially dependent ☐ fully dependent

4. How do you rate your cardiorespiratory fitness compared to your peers?

☐ lower ☐ same ☐ higher

5. Choose one activity category that best describes your usual pattern of daily physical activities, including activities related to house and family care, transportation, occupation, exercise and wellness and leisure or recreational purpose.

☐ Inactive or little activity other than usual daily activities.

☐ Regularly (≥ 1day/week) participate in physical activities requiring low levels of exertion that result in slight increases in breathing and heart rate for at least 10 minutes at a time.

Brisk walking, jogging or running, cycling, swimming, or vigorous sports at a comfortable pace or other activities requiring similar levels of exertion

☐ For 20 to 60 minutes per week

☐ For 1 to 3 hours per per week

☐ For over 3 hours per week

6. Do bone, muscle, or neurological disorders or diseases impair your physical activity?

☐ Yes, bone/muscle ☐ Yes, neurological ☐ No

Section 2

Thank you for completing this questionnaire!

Fig. 3A

Before beginning your exercise test today, we need to estimate what your usual limits are during daily activities. The following is a list of activities which increase in difficulty as you read down the page. Think carefully, then underline the first activity that, if you performed it for a period, would typically cause fatigue, shortness of breath, chest discomfort, or otherwise cause you to want to stop. If you do not normally perform a particular activity, try to imagine what it would be like if you did.

METs
- Eating, getting dressed, working at a desk
- Taking a shower
 -Walking down 8 steps
- Walking slowly on a flat surface for 1 or 2 blocks
 -A moderate amount of work around the house, such as vacuuming, sweeping the floors, or carrying groceries
- Light yard work, that us, raking leaves, weeding, or pushing a power mower
 -Painting or light carpentry
- Walking briskly, that is, 4 mph
 -Social dancing, washing the car
- Play 9-hole golf carrying your own clubs; heavy carpentry, mow lawn with push mower
- Perform heavy outdoor work, that is, digging, spading soil, etc
 -Play tennis (singles), carry 60 lb
- Move heavy furniture
 -Jog slowly, climb stairs quickly, carry 20 lb upstairs
- Bicycling at a moderate pace, sawing wood, jumping rope (slowly)
- Brisk swimming, bicycle up a hill, walking briskly uphill, jog 6 mph.
- 11-Cross-country ski
 -Play basketball (full court)
- Running briskly, continuously (level ground, 8 min/mile)
- Any competitive activity, including those which involve intermittent sprinting
 -Running competitively, rowing, backpacking

Fig. 3B

Figs. 3A and B: (A) MET-Repair questionnaire; (B) Veterans Specific Activity Questionnaire.

Can you...	
1. Take care of yourself, that is eating, dressing, bathing or using the toilet?	2.75
2. Walk indoors, such as around your house?	1.75
3. Walk a block or 2 on level ground?	2.75
4. Climb a flight of stairs or walk up a hill?	5.50
5. Run a short distance?	8.00
6. Do light work around the house like dusting or washing dishes?	2.70
7. Do moderate work around the house like vacuuming, sweeping floors, or carrying in groceries?	3.50
8. Do heavy work around the house like scrubbing floors, or lifting or moving heavy furniture?	8.00
9. Do yardwork like raking leaves, weeding or pushing a power mower?	4.50
10. Have sexual relations?	5.25
11. Participate in moderate recreational activities like golf, bowling, dancing, doubles tennis, or throwing a baseball or football?	6.00
12. Participate in strenuous sports like swimming, singles tennis, football, basketball or skiing?	7.50

Fig. 4: Duke Activity Status Index (DASI) questionnaire.

disability following noncardiac surgery.[16] A modified version of the DASI comprising only five questions has been developed (M-DASI), demonstrating comparable predictive capacity to the original DASI while being more concise and user-friendly.[17]

Self-reported Exercise Tolerance

Reilly et al. reported an increased risk of postoperative cardiovascular complications in patients with poor self-reported exercise tolerance.[18] Poor exercise tolerance was defined as the inability to walk at least four blocks (approximately half a kilometer) or climb two flights of stairs.

Assessment of Pulmonary Function

Pulmonary function tests (PFTs) are usually done in patients undergoing thoracic surgery or those with poorly controlled chronic obstructive pulmonary disease (COPD)/asthma to help guide optimization preoperatively. Assessment of oxygenation and hypercapnia is done by baseline arterial blood gas (ABG) analysis and diffusion studies such as diffusing capacity of the lungs for carbon monoxide/transfer factor of the lungs for carbon monoxide (DLCO/TLCO). ABG is indicated in the presence of resting peripheral capillary saturations < 94%, elevated serum bicarbonate, or severe abnormalities of PFTs. It is not done routinely as part of preoperative assessment for nonthoracic surgeries. The ARISCAT Risk Index[19] and Gupta calculator for postoperative respiratory failure[20] are validated risk scores which predict postoperative pulmonary complications.

Nutritional Assessment

Malnourished surgical patients have significantly higher postoperative mortality, morbidity, length of stay (LOS), readmission rates, and increased hospital costs.[21-23] It is estimated that 24–65% of patients undergoing surgery are at risk of nutrition.[22,24-26] Preoperative nutrition (regardless of the route of administration) in malnourished patients before gastrointestinal (GI) surgery reduces postoperative morbidity by 20%.[27] Screening for malnutrition before major surgery is essential as it can identify patients at risk of malnutrition who may benefit from a nutritional intervention preoperatively. The Subjective Global Assessment (SGA) and Mini Nutritional Assessment (MNA) tools are considered accepted global reference standards against which other malnutrition screening tools are assessed.[28] Several screening tools to identify those at risk have been developed and are summarized in **Table 2**.

A meta-analysis concluded that the Malnutrition Universal Screening Tool (MUST)[29] **(Fig. 5)**, developed by the Malnutrition Advisory Group (MAG), a standing committee of the British Association for Enteral and Parenteral Nutrition (BAPEN), had the highest overall test accuracy performance with a sensitivity and specificity of 86% and 89%, respectively, when compared to the reference standard, i.e., SGA.[30]

TABLE 2: Nutrition screening tools.

Tools specific for elderly population	
NRI[31]	Nutritional Risk Index
MNA[32]	Mini Nutritional Assessment
MNA-SF[33] and mMNA-SF[34]	Short and modified versions of MNA
NUFFE[35]	Nutritional Form for the Elderly
SST I and II[36]	Simple Screening Tools I & II
MEONF-II[37]	Minimal Eating Observation and Nutrition Form-II
NSI[38]	Nutrition Screening Initiative
CNS[38]	Chandra Nutrition Screen
Tools for general adult hospital population	
SGA[39]	Subjective Global Assessment
NSEq[40]	Nutrition Subjective Screening Tool, Nutrition Screening Equation
NRS[41]	Nutrition Risk Screening
MST[42]	Malnutrition Screening Tool
MUST[29]	Malnutrition Universal Screening Tool
MAG-ST[43]	Malnutrition Advisory Group Screening Tools
NST-2002[44]	Nutrition Risk Screening Tool-2002
B-NST[45]	British Nutrition Screening tool
SNAQ[46]	Short Nutritional Assessment Questionnaire
CNR[47]	Chinese Nutrition Risk
G-NST[48]	Glasgow Nutrition Screening tool
PG-SGA[49]	Patient Generated Subjective Global Assessment
INSYST-I and INSYST-II[50]	Imperial Nutrition Screening System
Nutrition tools developed to predict clinical outcome	
GNRI[31]	Geriatric Nutrition Risk Index
MRC[51]	Screening for Malnutrition related Complications
ANS[51]	Automated Nutrition Score
ANS-B[51]	Automated Nutrition Score-Blood measurements
PONS[52]	Perioperative Nutrition Screen
SGA[39]	Subjective Global Assessment
MST[42]	Malnutrition Screening Tool
MUST[41]	Malnutrition Universal Screening Tool
NRS-2002[44]	Nutrition Risk Screening Tool-2002

Psychological Evaluation

Patients should be formally evaluated by a trained clinical psychologist in the preoperative period. Commonly used tools to assess the psychological well-being of patients are as follows:

- Hospital Anxiety and Depression Scale (HADS)
- Beck Anxiety Index
- Zung Anxiety Inventory
- State-Trait Anxiety Inventory (STAI)
- SF-36
- Patient Health Questionnaire (PHQ-4)

PREHABILITATION REGIMEN

There are four important aspects to consider while planning a prehabilitation regimen:

1. *Personalization:* This includes the actual nature of the intervention itself which must be tailored to meet the individual needs of the patient.
2. *Duration:* Although the length of the prehabilitation regimen can vary from 1 week to 2 months, most interventions are typically 4–6 weeks long.

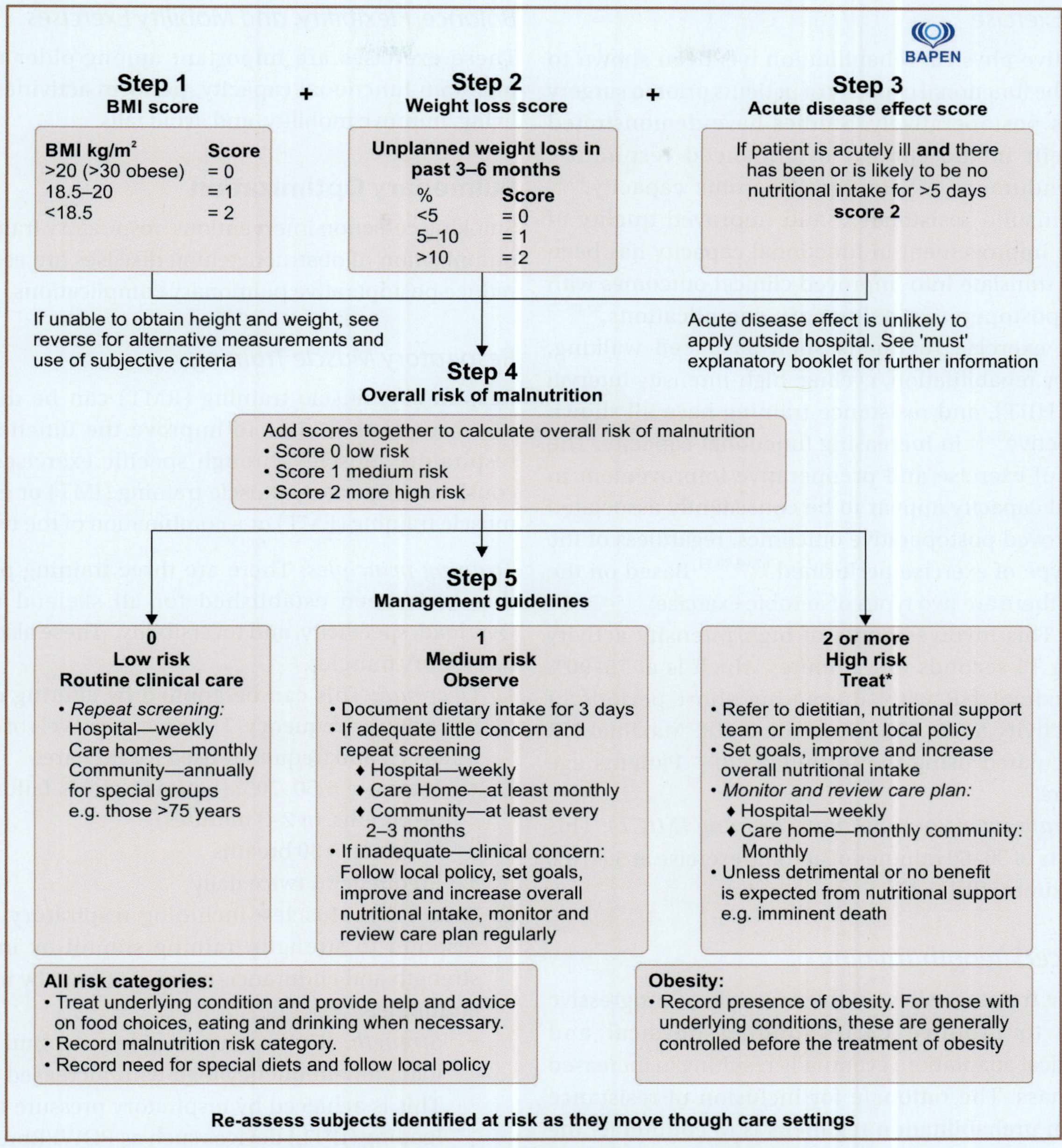

Fig. 5: Malnutrition Universal Screening Tool (MUST).[53]

3. *Setting:* The setting in which the intervention is implemented is largely dependent on the availability and accessibility of facilities. Urban centers may be able to implement a supervised intervention, whereas a home-based intervention may be suitable for more remote areas.
4. *Opt-in/Opt-out model:* There is compelling evidence demonstrating the efficacy of prehabilitation programs in improving functional status, postoperative outcomes, and long-term quality of life to be able to recommend an "opt-out" policy of implementation whenever feasible.[54-61]

Functional Optimization

Physical exercise regimens improve cardiovascular fitness and strength and are an essential component of prehabilitation. Various exercise modalities include the following.

Aerobic Exercise

Preoperative physical rehabilitation has been shown to improve the functional capacity of patients prior to surgery as well as postoperatively. Studies have demonstrated this benefit in the context of enhanced respiratory muscle endurance,[62,63] improved aerobic capacity,[63-67] reduced insulin resistance,[68] and improved quality of life.[65] The improvement in functional capacity has been shown to translate into improved clinical outcomes with reduced postoperative pulmonary complications.[63,69,70] Different exercise regimens such as paced walking, respiratory rehabilitation, cycling, high-intensity interval training (HIIT), and resistance training have all shown to be effective[62-71] in increasing functional capacity. The intensity of exercise and preoperative improvement in functional capacity appear to be consistently associated with improved postoperative outcomes, regardless of the specific type of exercise performed.[67,68,70,71] Based on the intensity, there are two types of aerobic exercise:

1. *HIIT:* This involves bouts of high-intensity activity lasting 15 seconds to 4 minutes which is at 75–90% of maximal HR with alternating short periods of low activity at 40–50% of maximal HR. Maximal HR is calculated using the formula: 220 – Patients age in years.
2. *Moderate-intensity continuous training (MICT):* This consists of 30–60 minutes of aerobic exercise at 50–70% of maximal HR.

Resistance/Strength Training

Resistance training relies on the principle of progressive overload to produce corresponding physical and physiological adaptation, eventually resulting in increased muscle mass. The rationale for inclusion of resistance training in prehabilitation regimens is to counteract the detrimental effects of reduced muscle mass associated with older age, cancer cachexia, and after completion of extensive preoperative cytotoxic chemotherapy and radiation. Various approaches to strength training include bodyweight training, resistance bands, and weight-training machines. However, there is limited evidence in literature regarding the efficacy of resistance training, over and above aerobic exercise, in producing meaningful improvements in postoperative outcomes to recommend their routine inclusion in prehabilitation regimens.[62,72]

Balance, Flexibility, and Mobility Exercises

These exercises are important among older adults to maintain functional capacity, perform activities of daily living, improve mobility, and avoid falls.

Pulmonary Optimization

Smoking cessation interventions, respiratory training, and optimization of obstructive lung diseases are essential to reduce postoperative pulmonary complications.

Respiratory Muscle Training

Respiratory muscle training (RMT) can be defined as a technique that aims to improve the function of the respiratory muscles through specific exercises. It may consist of inspiratory muscle training (IMT) or expiratory muscle training (EMT) or a combination of the two.

Training principles: There are three training principles that have been established for all skeletal muscles: Overload, specificity, and reversibility. These also apply to respiratory muscles.

1. *Overload:* This can be applied by altering duration, intensity, or frequency. The accepted levels of duration, intensity, and frequency used for IMT are:
   - Intensity = 50–70% (typically yields failure within 30 breaths, or 2–3 minutes)
   - Duration = 30 breaths
   - Frequency = twice daily
2. *Specificity:* Muscles, including respiratory muscles, respond to strength-training stimuli by improving strength and endurance-training stimuli by improving endurance.
   - *Strength:* Respiratory muscles respond to high-load, low-frequency load with increased strength. This is achieved by inspiratory pressure threshold loading (IPTL) devices such as POWERbreathe.
   - *Endurance:* Endurance training can be achieved with low-load, high-frequency load. This type of training uses a technique called voluntary isocapnic hyperventilation (VIH) which requires people to maintain high levels of respiration for up to 40 minutes. It utilizes a hyperventilation method that employs a partial rebreathing circuit to prevent hypocapnia.
3. *Reversibility*
   - *Detraining:* Respiratory muscles respond in a similar way to other muscles when the training

stimulus is removed. Most of the losses occur within 2–3 months of the cessation of training.

- *Maintenance:* Improvements in inspiratory muscle function can be sustained with training frequency reduced by as much as two thirds, i.e., 2 days/wk in healthy adults and 3 days/wk in patients with COPD.

Types of RMT

- *Resistance training:* IPTL is a technique wherein a certain inspiratory pressure threshold must be achieved by the patient. Progressive pressure loading of the inspiratory muscles with regular use results in increased strength and endurance of the inspiratory muscles. It is a small handheld device with a mouthpiece and a calibrated spring-loaded valve. The inspiratory pressure threshold can be calibrated from 9 to 41 cm of water.
- *Volume-based training:* Volume-based incentive spirometry requires patients to breathe through a mechanical device which provides visual feedback of the volume of air inspired to the patients to encourage progressive increase in the inspiratory volume. Since this device is volume or flow driven, it helps prevent lung atelectasis and restore lung volumes through slow and sustained deep breathing.
- *Endurance training:* It uses a technique called voluntary isocapnic hyperventilation which requires people to maintain high levels of respiration for up to 40 minutes. It utilizes a hyperventilation method that employs a partial rebreathing circuit to prevent hypocapnia

Smoking Cessation

Preoperative smoking cessation has demonstrated a relative risk reduction of 41% for prevention of postoperative complications.[73] A minimum of 6–8 weeks of smoking abstinence is required to produce meaningful reductions in postoperative pulmonary complications, with a 19% risk reduction with each additional week of smoking cessation prior to surgery.[73] A combination of behavioral therapy and pharmacotherapy such as nicotine replacement, varenicline, bupropion, nortriptyline, and cytosine is used to aid smoking cessation.

Respiratory Optimization in Obstructive Lung Diseases

Perioperative bronchodilator usage should be optimized with appropriate use of long-acting beta agonists, muscarinic antagonists, and inhaled corticosteroids as per symptom severity. Use of mucolytic therapy with inhaled N-acetylcysteine should be used for chronic cough with sputum production.

Anemia Correction

Functional iron deficiency in critically ill patients is associated with an increased duration of systemic inflammatory response syndrome and prolonged intensive care unit (ICU) stay.[74] Anemic patients have higher perioperative transfusion requirements.[75] Low ferritin levels before major orthopedic or abdominal surgery have been associated with increased rates of postoperative infections.[76] **Flowchart 1** shows a suggested diagnostic approach to preoperative anemia.[77]

The Association of Anaesthetists of Great Britain and Ireland (AAGBI) consensus recommendations for screening and treatment of anemia in the preoperative setting are summarized in **Box 1**.[78]

Nutritional Optimization

The ESPEN 2021 guidelines make the following recommendations regarding preoperative nutritional supplementation.[79]

Definition of Malnutrition

The Global Leadership Initiative on Malnutrition (GLIM) proposed criteria for a global consensus for the definition

Flowchart 1: Diagnostic algorithm for preoperative anemia.

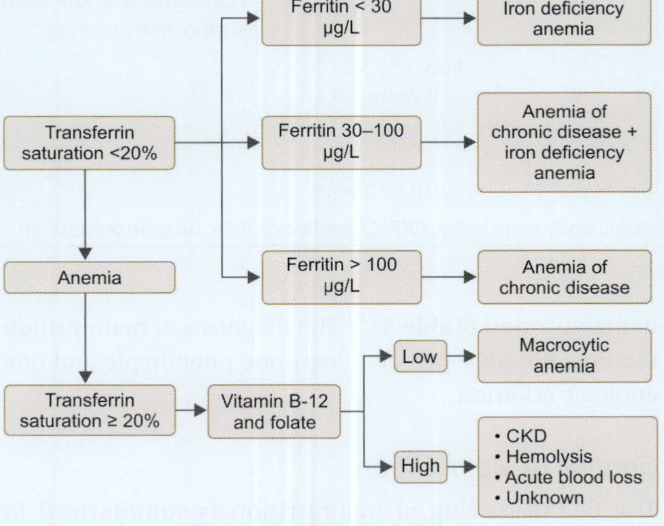

(CKD: chronic kidney disease)

BOX 1: AAGBI consensus recommendations for screening and treatment of anemia prior to major surgery.

- Physicians should consider preoperative anemia and iron deficiency as an indication for a perioperative care pathway that stretches from the decision to operate until complete recovery from surgery
- The presence of anemia should be investigated in all surgical procedures with expected moderate-to-high blood loss (>500 mL)
- Serum ferritin level <30 µg/L is the most sensitive and specific test used for the identification of absolute iron deficiency. However, in the presence of inflammation (C-reactive protein >5 mg/L) and/or transferrin saturation < 20%, a serum ferritin level <100 µg/L is indicative of iron deficiency
- Major, nonurgent surgery should be postponed to allow the diagnosis and treatment of anemia and iron deficiency
- When treating anemia preoperatively, the target hemoglobin concentration should be ≥130 g/L in both sexes, to minimize the risk of transfusion-associated unfavorable outcomes
- Oral iron replacement should be targeted to patients with iron deficiency with or without anemia whose surgery is scheduled 6–8 weeks after diagnosis, preferably by the primary care physician (General Practitioner)
- Daily (40–60 mg) or alternate-day (80–100 mg) treatment with oral iron and nutritional advice should be initiated immediately in patients with iron deficiency and no contraindications
- Sufficient data exist to support intravenous iron as efficacious and safe. Intravenous iron should be used as frontline therapy in patients who do not respond to oral iron or are not able to tolerate it or if surgery is planned for <6 weeks after the diagnosis of iron deficiency
- The diagnosis and treatment of anemia and iron deficiency should commence as early as possible in the perioperative period and ideally as soon as the decision to undertake surgery is made

TABLE 3: GLIM criteria for definition of malnutrition.

Phenotypic criteria			***Etiologic criteria***	
Weight loss (%)	***Low BMI (kg/m²)***	***Reduced muscle mass***	***Reduced food intake or assimilation***	***Inflammation***
>5% within the past 6 months OR	<20 if <70 years, OR	*Body composition methods*: • Dual-energy absorptiometry (DXA) • Bioelectrical impedance analysis (BIA) • CT • MRI	50% of energy requirement >1 week, OR	• Acute disease/ injury or chronic disease-related • CRP used as supportive measure
>10% beyond 6 months	<22 if >70 years	• Physical examination • Mid-arm circumference • Calf circumference • Hand-grip strength used as supportive measure	Any reduction for >2 weeks, OR	
	Asia: <18.5 if <70 years, OR		Any chronic GI condition that adversely impacts food assimilation or absorption	
	<20 if >70 years			

(BMI: body mass index; CRP: C-reactive protein; GI: gastrointestinal)

of malnutrition **(Table 3)**.[80] The diagnosis of malnutrition requires the presence of at least one phenotypic and one etiologic criterion.

Grading of Malnutrition

The GLIM grading of malnutrition is summarized in **Table 4**.[80]

Indications for Preoperative Nutritional Supplementation

- All malnourished cancer patients
- All high-risk patients undergoing major abdominal surgery. To be given for 7–14 days. Postpone surgery if required. Criteria for high risk includes presence of at least one of the following:

TABLE 4: GLIM grading of malnutrition.

	Weight loss (%)	*Low BMI (kg/m²)*	*Reduced muscle mass*
Stage 1 (Moderate malnutrition/low risk) Requires 1 phenotypic criterion that meets this grade	5–10% within the past 6 months OR 10–20% beyond 6 months	<20 if <70 years <22 if ≥70 years	Mild-to-moderate deficit
Stage 2 (Severe malnutrition/high risk) Requires 1 phenotypic criterion that meets this grade	>10% within the past 6 months OR >20% beyond 6 months	<18.5 if <70 years <20 if ≥70 years	Severe deficit

Flowchart 2: Algorithm for nutritional supplementation (ESPEN guidelines).

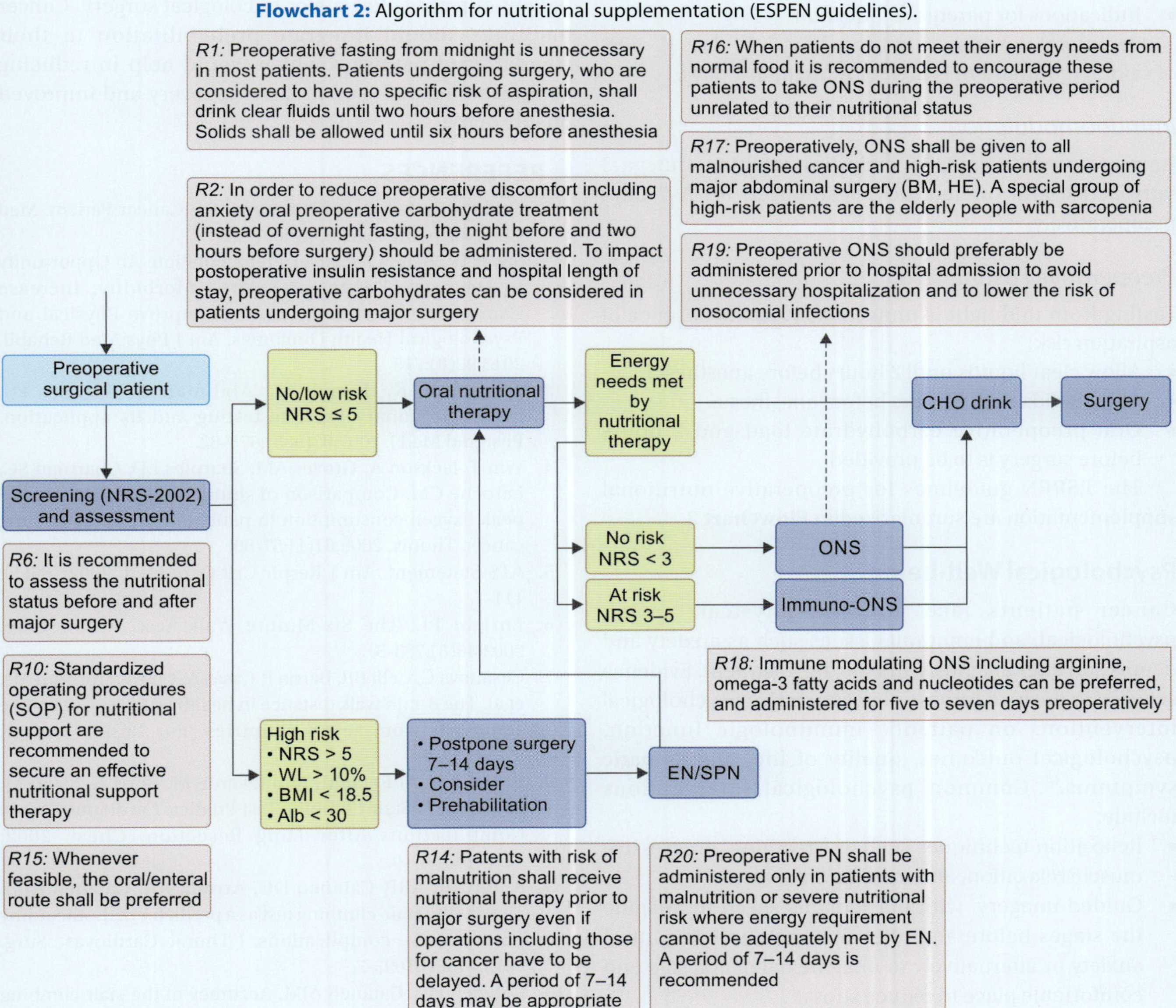

- Severe malnutrition OR
- Nutritional risk score OR
- Subjective Global Assessment Grade C
- Albumin <3 g/dL with no evidence of hepatic or renal dysfunction
- Elderly people with sarcopenia

Route of Nutrition Supplementation

The enteral route should always be preferred except for the following contraindications:

- Intestinal obstruction or ileus
- Severe shock
- Intestinal ischemia
- High-output fistula
- Severe intestinal hemorrhage
- Indications for parenteral nutrition

Parenteral nutrition is indicated for 7–14 days if <50% of caloric requirement is met for more than 7 days.

Immunomodulation

Immune modulating ONS including arginine, omega-3 fatty acids, and nucleotides is preferred for 5–7 days preoperatively.

Preoperative Fasting

Fasting from midnight is unnecessary. In the absence of aspiration risk:

- Allow clear liquids until 2 hours before anesthesia.
- Allow solids until 6 hours before anesthesia.
- Oral preoperative carbohydrate load and 2 hours before surgery is to be provided.

The ESPEN guidelines for preoperative nutritional supplementation are summarized in **Flowchart 2**.

Psychological Well-being

Cancer patients face multiple physical, social, psychological, and emotional issues such as anxiety and depression after diagnosis and during treatment. Evidence suggests a positive impact of preoperative psychological interventions on patients' immunologic function, psychological outcomes, quality of life, and somatic symptoms.[81] Common psychological interventions include:

- Relaxation techniques such as breathing, progressive muscle relaxation, and meditation
- Guided imagery, with participants asked to imagine the stages before and after the operation to control anxiety or alternatively to imagine being at a safe and comfortable place to reduce stress
- Problem solving and coping strategies

FOLLOW-UP POST-TREATMENT

Adequate follow-up after initiation of treatment is essential to ensure patient compliance and monitor progress. Regular follow-up also increases involvement of patients in their own care resulting in greater motivation and earlier return to normal life.

CONCLUSION

A holistic approach to cancer patients in the perioperative period resting on the pillars of preassessment, physical and pulmonary optimization is crucial in improving patient outcome after major oncological surgery. Cancer institutes should integrate prehabilitation in their standardized pathways which would help in reducing complications and lead to faster recovery and improved quality of life.

REFERENCES

1. Herbert Dietz J. Rehabilitation of the Cancer Patient. Med Clin North Am. 1969;53(3):607-24.
2. Silver JK, Baima J. Cancer Prehabilitation: An Opportunity to Decrease Treatment-Related Morbidity, Increase Cancer Treatment Options, and Improve Physical and Psychological Health Outcomes. Am J Phys Med Rehabil. 2013;92(8):715.
3. Albouaini K, Egred M, Alahmar A, Wright DJ. Cardiopulmonary exercise testing and its application. Postgrad Med J. 2007;83(985):675-82.
4. Win T, Jackson A, Groves AM, Sharples LD, Charman SC, Laroche CM. Comparison of shuttle walk with measured peak oxygen consumption in patients with operable lung cancer. Thorax. 2006;61(1):57-60.
5. ATS Statement. Am J Respir Crit Care Med. 2002;166(1):111-7.
6. Enright PL. The Six-Minute Walk Test. Respir Care. 2003;48(8):783-5.
7. Casanova C, Celli BR, Barria P, Casas A, Cote C, Torres JP de, et al. The 6-min walk distance in healthy subjects: reference standards from seven countries. Eur Respir J. 2011;37(1):150-6.
8. Brunelli A, Al Refai M, Monteverde M, Borri A, Salati M, Fianchini A. Stair Climbing Test Predicts Cardiopulmonary Complications After Lung Resection. Chest. 2002;121(4):1106-10.
9. Ambrozin ARP, Cataneo DC, Arruda KA, Cataneo AJM. Time in the stair-climbing test as a predictor of thoracotomy postoperative complications. J Thorac Cardiovasc Surg. 2013;145(4):1093-7.
10. Cataneo DC, Cataneo AJM. Accuracy of the stair climbing test using maximal oxygen uptake as the gold standard. J Bras Pneumol. 2007;33:128-33.
11. Arruda KA, Cataneo DC, Cataneo AJM. Surgical risk tests related to cardiopulmonary postoperative complications: comparison between upper abdominal and thoracic surgery. Acta Cirúrgica Bras. 2013;28:458-66.

12. Reddy S, Contreras CM, Singletary B, Bradford MT, Waldrop MG, Mims AH, et al. Timed Stair Climbing Is the Single Strongest Predictor of Perioperative Complications in Patients Undergoing Abdominal Surgery. J Am Coll Surg. 2016;222(4):559-66.
13. McAuley P, Myers J, Abella J, Froelicher V. Evaluation of a specific activity questionnaire to predict mortality in men referred for exercise testing. Am Heart J. 2006;151(4):890.e1-e7.
14. Jaeger C, Burkard T, Kamber F, Seeberger E, Bolliger D, Pfister O, et al. Quantification of metabolic equivalents (METs) by the MET-REPAIR questionnaire: A validation study in patients with a high cardiovascular burden. J Clin Anesth. 2022;76:110559.
15. Hlatky MA, Boineau RE, Higginbotham MB, Lee KL, Mark DB, Califf RM, et al. A brief self-administered questionnaire to determine functional capacity (The Duke Activity Status Index). Am J Cardiol. 1989;64(10):651-4.
16. Wijeysundera DN, Beattie WS, Hillis GS, Abbott TEF, Shulman MA, Ackland GL, et al. Integration of the Duke Activity Status Index into preoperative risk evaluation: a multicentre prospective cohort study. Br J Anaesth. 2020;124(3):261-70.
17. Riedel B, Li MHG, Lee CHA, Ismail H, Cuthbertson BH, Wijeysundera DN, et al. A simplified (modified) Duke Activity Status Index (M-DASI) to characterise functional capacity: a secondary analysis of the Measurement of Exercise Tolerance before Surgery (METS) study. Br J Anaesth. 2021;126(1):181-90.
18. Reilly DF, McNeely MJ, Doerner D, Greenberg DL, Staiger TO, Geist MJ, et al. Self-reported Exercise Tolerance and the Risk of Serious Perioperative Complications. Arch Intern Med. 1999;159(18):2185-92.
19. Kara S, Küpeli E, Yılmaz HEB, Yabanoğlu H. Predicting Pulmonary Complications Following Upper and Lower Abdominal Surgery: ASA vs. ARISCAT Risk Index. Turk J Anaesthesiol Reanim. 2020;48(2):96-101.
20. Gupta H, Gupta PK, Fang X, Miller WJ, Cemaj S, Forse RA, et al. Development and Validation of a Risk Calculator Predicting Postoperative Respiratory Failure. Chest. 2011;140(5):1207-15.
21. Isabel TD, Correia M, Waitzberg DL. The impact of malnutrition on morbidity, mortality, length of hospital stay and costs evaluated through a multivariate model analysis. Clin Nutr. 2003;22(3):235-9.
22. Bozzetti F, Gianotti L, Braga M, Di Carlo V, Mariani L. Postoperative complications in gastrointestinal cancer patients: The joint role of the nutritional status and the nutritional support. Clin Nutr. 2007;26(6):698-709.
23. Kassin MT, Owen RM, Perez SD, Leeds I, Cox JC, Schnier K, et al. Risk Factors for 30-Day Hospital Readmission among General Surgery Patients. J Am Coll Surg. 2012; 215(3):322-30.
24. Thomas MN, Kufeldt J, Kisser U, Hornung HM, Hoffmann J, Andraschko M, et al. Effects of malnutrition on complication rates, length of hospital stay, and revenue in elective surgical patients in the G-DRG-system. Nutrition. 2016;32(2):249-54.
25. Awad S, Lobo DN. What's new in perioperative nutritional support? Curr Opin Anesthesiol. 2011;24(3):339.
26. Geurden B, Franck E, Weyler J, Ysebaert D. The Risk of Malnutrition in Community-Living Elderly on Admission to Hospital for Major Surgery. Acta Chir Belg. 2015;115(5):341-7.
27. Benoist S, Brouquet A. Nutritional assessment and screening for malnutrition. J Visc Surg. 2015;152:S3-7.
28. Van Bokhorst-de Van Der Schueren MAE, Guaitoli PR, Jansma EP, De Vet HCW. Nutrition screening tools: Does one size fit all? A systematic review of screening tools for the hospital setting. Clin Nutr. 2014;33(1):39-58.
29. Elia PM. Nutritional screening of adults: a multidisciplinary responsibility. [online] Available from https://www.bapen.org.uk/pdfs/must/must-report.pdf [Last accessed January, 2025].
30. Cheung HHT, Joynt GM, Lee A. Diagnostic test accuracy of preoperative nutritional screening tools in adults for malnutrition: a systematic review and network meta-analysis. Int J Surg. 2024;110(2):1090.
31. Wolinsky FD, Coe RM, McIntosh WmA, Kubena KS, Prendergast JM, Chavez MN, et al. Progress in the Development of a Nutritional Risk Index. J Nutr. 1990; 120:1549-53.
32. Guigoz Y, Vellas B, Garry PJ. Mini nutritional assessment : A practical assessment tool for grading the nutritional state of elderly patients. Mini Nutr Assess Pract Assess Tool Grading Nutr State Elder Patients. 1997;15-60.
33. Rubenstein LZ, Harker JO, Salvà A, Guigoz Y, Vellas B. Screening for Undernutrition in Geriatric Practice: Developing the Short-Form Mini-Nutritional Assessment (MNA-SF). J Gerontol Ser A. 2001;56(6):M366-72.
34. Kaiser MJ, Bauer JM, Ramsch C, Uter W, Guigoz Y, Cederholm T, et al. Validation of the Mini Nutritional Assessment short-form (MNA®-SF): A practical tool for identification of nutritional status. JNHA - J Nutr Health Aging. 2009;13(9):782-8.
35. Söderhamn U, Söderhamn O. Developing and testing the Nutritional Form For the Elderly. Int J Nurs Pract. 2001;7(5):336-41.
36. Laporte M, Villalon L, Payette H. Simple nutrition screening tools for healthcare facilities: development and validity assessment. Can J Diet Pract Res Publ Dietit Can Rev Can Prat Rech En Diet Une Publ Diet Can. 2001;62(1):26-34.
37. Westergren A, Norberg E, Vallén C, Hagell P. Cut-off scores for the Minimal Eating Observation and Nutrition Form – Version II (MEONF-II) among hospital inpatients. Food Nutr Res. 2011;55(1):7289.
38. Azad N, Murphy J, Amos SS, Toppan J. Nutrition survey in an elderly population following admission to a tertiary care hospital. CMAJ. 1999;161(5):511-5.

39. Baker JP, Detsky AS, Wesson DE, Wolman SL, Stewart S, Whitewell J, et al. Nutritional Assessment. N Engl J Med. 1982;306(16):969-72.
40. Elmore MF, Wagner DR, Knoll DM, Eizember L, Oswalt MA, Glowinski EA, et al. Developing an effective adult nutrition screening tool for a community hospital. J Am Diet Assoc. 1994;94(10):1113-21.
41. Reilly HM, Martineau JK, Moran A, Kennedy H. Nutritional screening - Evaluation and implementation of a simple Nutrition Risk Score. Clin Nutr. 1995;14(5):269-73.
42. Ferguson M, Capra S, Bauer J, Banks M. Development of a valid and reliable malnutrition screening tool for adult acute hospital patients. Nutrition. 1999;15(6):458-64.
43. Bauer J, Capra S. Comparison of a malnutrition screening tool with subjective global assessment in hospitalised patients with cancer--sensitivity and specificity. Asia Pac J Clin Nutr. 2003;12(3):257-60.
44. Kondrup J, Rasmussen HH, Hamberg O, Stanga Z. Nutritional risk screening (NRS 2002): a new method based on an analysis of controlled clinical trials. Clin Nutr. 2003;22(3):321-36.
45. Elizabeth Weekes C, Elia M, Emery PW. The development, validation and reliability of a nutrition screening tool based on the recommendations of the British Association for Parenteral and Enteral Nutrition (BAPEN). Clin Nutr. 2004;23(5):1104-12.
46. Kruizenga HM, Seidell JC, de Vet HCW, Wierdsma NJ, van Bokhorst-de van der Schueren MAE. Development and validation of a hospital screening tool for malnutrition: the short nutritional assessment questionnaire (SNAQ©). Clin Nutr. 2005;24(1):75-82.
47. Woo J, Chumlea WC, Sun SS, Kwok T, Lui HH, Hui E, et al. Development of the Chinese nutrition screen (CNS) for use in institutional settings. J Nutr Health Aging. 2005; 9(4):203-10.
48. Gerasimidis K, Drongitis P, Murray L, Young D, McKee RF. A local nutritional screening tool compared to malnutrition universal screening tool. Eur J Clin Nutr. 2007;61(7):916-21.
49. Bauer J, Capra S, Ferguson M. Use of the scored Patient-Generated Subjective Global Assessment (PG-SGA) as a nutrition assessment tool in patients with cancer. Eur J Clin Nutr. 2002;56(8):779-85.
50. Tammam JD, Gardner L, Hickson M. Validity, reliability and acceptability of the Imperial Nutritional Screening System (INSYST): a tool that does not require the body mass index. J Hum Nutr Diet. 2009;22(6):536-44.
51. Smith RC, Ledgard JP, Doig G, Chesher D, Smith SF. An effective automated nutrition screen for hospitalized patients. Nutrition. 2009;25(3):309-15.
52. Wischmeyer PE, Carli F, Evans DC, Guilbert S, Kozar R, Pryor A, et al. American Society for Enhanced Recovery and Perioperative Quality Initiative Joint Consensus Statement on Nutrition Screening and Therapy Within a Surgical Enhanced Recovery Pathway. Anesth Analg. 2018;126(6):1883.
53. Malnutrition Universal Screening Tool(https://www.bapen.org.uk/pdfs/must/must_full.pdf)
54. Minnella EM, Awasthi R, Loiselle SE, Agnihotram RV, Ferri LE, Carli F. Effect of Exercise and Nutrition Prehabilitation on Functional Capacity in Esophagogastric Cancer Surgery: A Randomized Clinical Trial. JAMA Surg. 2018;153(12):1081-9.
55. Minnella EM, Awasthi R, Bousquet-Dion G, Ferreira V, Austin B, Audi C, et al. Multimodal Prehabilitation to Enhance Functional Capacity Following Radical Cystectomy: A Randomized Controlled Trial. Eur Urol Focus. 2021;7(1):132-8.
56. Liu Z, Qiu T, Pei L, Zhang Y, Xu L, Cui Y, et al. Two-Week Multimodal Prehabilitation Program Improves Perioperative Functional Capability in Patients Undergoing Thoracoscopic Lobectomy for Lung Cancer: A Randomized Controlled Trial. Anesth Analg. 2020;131(3):840.
57. Li C, Carli F, Lee L, Charlebois P, Stein B, Liberman AS, et al. Impact of a trimodal prehabilitation program on functional recovery after colorectal cancer surgery: a pilot study. Surg Endosc. 2013;27(4):1072-82.
58. Chia CLK, Mantoo SK, Tan KY. 'Start to finish trans-institutional transdisciplinary care': a novel approach improves colorectal surgical results in frail elderly patients. Colorectal Dis. 2016;18(1):O43-50.
59. Molenaar CJL, Minnella EM, Coca-Martinez M, Ten Cate DWG, Regis M, Awasthi R, et al. Effect of Multimodal Prehabilitation on Reducing Postoperative Complications and Enhancing Functional Capacity Following Colorectal Cancer Surgery: The PREHAB Randomized Clinical Trial. JAMA Surg. 2023;158(6):572-81.
60. Bolshinsky V, Li MHG, Ismail H, Burbury K, Riedel B, Heriot A. Multimodal Prehabilitation Programs as a Bundle of Care in Gastrointestinal Cancer Surgery: A Systematic Review. Dis Colon Rectum. 2018;61(1):124.
61. Jain SR, Kandarpa VL, Yaow CYL, Tan WJ, Ho LML, Sivarajah SS, et al. The Role and Effect of Multimodal Prehabilitation Before Major Abdominal Surgery: A Systemic Review and Meta-Analysis. World J Surg. 2023; 47(1):1.
62. Dronkers J, Lamberts H, Reutelingsperger I, Naber R, Dronkers-Landman C, Veldman A, et al. Preoperative therapeutic programme for elderly patients scheduled for elective abdominal oncological surgery: a randomized controlled pilot study. Clin Rehabil. 2010;24(7):614-22.
63. Soares SM de TP, Nucci LB, da Silva MM de C, Campacci TC. Pulmonary function and physical performance outcomes with preoperative physical therapy in upper abdominal surgery: a randomized controlled trial. Clin Rehabil. 2013;27(7):616-27.
64. Barberan-Garcia A, Ubré M, Roca J, Lacy AM, Burgos F, Risco R, et al. Personalised Prehabilitation in High-risk Patients Undergoing Elective Major Abdominal Surgery: A Randomized Blinded Controlled Trial. Ann Surg. 2018;267(1):50-6.

65. Dunne DFJ, Jack S, Jones RP, Jones L, Lythgoe DT, Malik HZ, et al. Randomized clinical trial of prehabilitation before planned liver resection. Br J Surg. 2016;103(5):504-12.
66. West MA, Loughney L, Lythgoe D, Barben CP, Sripadam R, Kemp GJ, et al. Effect of prehabilitation on objectively measured physical fitness after neoadjuvant treatment in preoperative rectal cancer patients: a blinded interventional pilot study. Br J Anaesth. 2015;114(2):244-51.
67. Mayo NE, Feldman L, Scott S, Zavorsky G, Kim DJ, Charlebois P, et al. Impact of preoperative change in physical function on postoperative recovery: argument supporting prehabilitation for colorectal surgery. Surgery. 2011;150(3):505-14.
68. Kaibori M, Ishizaki M, Matsui K, Nakatake R, Yoshiuchi S, Kimura Y, et al. Perioperative exercise for chronic liver injury patients with hepatocellular carcinoma undergoing hepatectomy. Am J Surg. 2013;206(2):202-9.
69. Yamana I, Takeno S, Hashimoto T, Maki K, Shibata R, Shiwaku H, et al. Randomized Controlled Study to Evaluate the Efficacy of a Preoperative Respiratory Rehabilitation Program to Prevent Postoperative Pulmonary Complications after Esophagectomy. Dig Surg. 2015;32(5):331-7.
70. Boden I, Skinner EH, Browning L, Reeve J, Anderson L, Hill C, et al. Preoperative physiotherapy for the prevention of respiratory complications after upper abdominal surgery: pragmatic, double blinded, multicentre randomised controlled trial. BMJ. 2018;360:j5916.
71. Carli F, Charlebois P, Stein B, Feldman L, Zavorsky G, Kim DJ, et al. Randomized clinical trial of prehabilitation in colorectal surgery. Br J Surg. 2010;97(8):1187-97.
72. Ahn KY, Hur H, Kim DH, Min J, Jeong DH, Chu SH, et al. The effects of inpatient exercise therapy on the length of hospital stay in stages I–III colon cancer patients: randomized controlled trial. Int J Colorectal Dis. 2013;28(5):643-51.
73. Mills E, Eyawo O, Lockhart I, Kelly S, Wu P, Ebbert JO. Smoking Cessation Reduces Postoperative Complications: A Systematic Review and Meta-analysis. Am J Med. 2011;124(2):144-54.e8.
74. Patteril MV, Davey-Quinn AP, Gedney JA, Murdoch SD, Bellamy MC. Functional Iron Deficiency, Infection and Systemic Inflammatory Response Syndrome in Critical Illness. Anaesth Intensive Care. 2001;29(5):473-8.
75. Okuyama M, Ikeda K, Shibata T, Tsukahara Y, Kitada M, Shimano T. Preoperative Iron Supplementation and Intraoperative Transfusion During Colorectal Cancer Surgery. Surg Today. 2005;35(1):36-40.
76. Harju E. Empty iron stores as a significant risk factor in abdominal surgery. J Parenter Enter Nutr. 1988;12(3):282-5.
77. Muñoz M, Gómez-Ramírez S, Campos A. Iron Supplementation for Perioperative Anaemia in Patient Blood Management. EMJ Hematol. 2014;1:123-32.
78. Muñoz M, Acheson AG, Auerbach M, Besser M, Habler O, Kehlet H, et al. International consensus statement on the peri-operative management of anaemia and iron deficiency. Anaesthesia. 2017;72(2):233-47.
79. Weimann A, Braga M, Carli F, Higashiguchi T, Hübner M, Klek S, et al. ESPEN practical guideline: Clinical nutrition in surgery. Clin Nutr. 2021;40(7):4745-61.
80. Cederholm T, Jensen GL, Correia MITD, Gonzalez MC, Fukushima R, Higashiguchi T, et al. GLIM criteria for the diagnosis of malnutrition – A consensus report from the global clinical nutrition community. Clin Nutr. 2019; 38(1):1-9.
81. Tsimopoulou I, Pasquali S, Howard R, Desai A, Gourevitch D, Tolosa I, et al. Psychological Prehabilitation Before Cancer Surgery: A Systematic Review. Ann Surg Oncol. 2015;22(13):4117-23.

9

CHAPTER

Enhanced Recovery after Surgery and Outcomes in Oncosurgery

Vandana Agarwal, Shardul Diliprao Joshi

INTRODUCTION

GLOBOCAN 2022 estimated 20 million new cancer cases and 9.7 million deaths every year. It is estimated that one in five men or women develop cancer in a lifetime, and one in 9 men and one in 12 women succumb to it.[1] Enhanced Recovery After Surgery (ERAS) is a multidisciplinary and multimodal perioperative care pathway aimed at improving patient outcomes, reducing complications, and promoting early recovery. The ERAS society has published recommendations for various surgical disciplines. Perioperative ERAS pathway employs multimodal evidence-based components, which hasten recovery and overall patient experience and satisfaction.[2] Often patients with cancer may need postoperative adjuvant cancer treatment depending on the extent of surgical resection, presence of any residual disease and tumor biology. Early postoperative recovery within an ERAS program facilitates earlier return to intended oncological treatment, which in turn may be associated with improved survival.[3] This chapter will cover impact of ERAS pathway following various cancer surgery on short-term postoperative outcomes, patient reported outcomes, and survival.

COMPONENTS OF ENHANCED RECOVERY AFTER SURGERY

The program/pathway incorporates components across the perioperative period, i.e., preoperative, intraoperative, and postoperative in addition there are surgery specific recommendations. Surgery specific recommendations are beyond the scope of this chapter. Reader is encouraged to visit the ERAS society website for surgery site specific recommendations. General components of ERAS are as follows.

- *Preoperative components:*
  - Preoperative optimization of comorbidities such as diabetes, heart disease, or hypertension, anemia correction if any, etc.
  - *Patient education:* Informed patients are more likely to engage in recovery strategies. Patients are educated about surgical process, anesthesia and postoperative pain management plan, benefits of ERAS, and expectations in the postoperative period.
  - Prehabilitation consists of nutritional support, physical, and pulmonary prehabilitation.
    - *Preoperative nutritional supplementation:* Cancer patients are often malnourished and present with considerable weight loss. Often because of weight loss, majority of these patients may need nutritional supplementation. All cancer patients likely to undergo must undergo nutritional screening and considerable number of these patients require nutritional supplementation. Preoperative nutrition supplementation is associated with lower incidence of postoperative complications and length of stay (LOS).[4] Nutritional supplementation along with physical prehabilitation may improve postoperative outcomes, particularly in malnourished patients.
    - Physical therapy should be given consideration if there is time before surgery. It improves the exercise capacity. Multimodal prehabilitation is associated lower odds of developing postoperative pulmonary complications.[5]
    - *Psychological counseling:* It is an important aspect of prehabilitation as it reduces anxiety and stress which may impede recovery.
  - *Preoperative carbohydrate supplementation:* Preoperative treatment with oral carbohydrate increases preoperative insulin level, reduces postoperative insulin resistance, maintains glycogen reserves, decreases protein breakdown, and improves muscle strength. In addition, it reduces

patients' thirst, hunger, and dry mouth. Patients with documented delayed gastric emptying or gastrointestinal (GI) motility disorders and diabetics should not be administered preoperative oral carbohydrate.[6,7]
- Venous thromboembolism prophylaxis reduces the risk of venous thrombosis during the perioperative period and secondary to malignancy.

- *Intraoperative management:*
  - *Minimally invasive techniques:* Whenever possible, laparoscopic or robotic surgery techniques reduce tissue trauma, minimize blood loss, and hasten recovery.
  - *Fluid management:* Goal-directed fluid management to avoid both dehydration and overhydration. *Pain management*: Regional anesthesia, such as neuraxial, nerve blocks and fascial plane block, reduces the need for opioids (which can slow recovery and increase the risk of complications) and hastens recovery.
  - *Preventing hypothermia:* Maintaining normothermia during surgery is important to reduce risk of infection and promotes recovery.
- *Postoperative care:*
  - Early mobilization helps in preventing complications such as venous thromboembolism and pneumonia.
  - Early feeding stimulates gut function and reduces the likelihood of postoperative ileus.
  - *Multimodal analgesia:* Nonopioid pain management strategies, including nerve blocks etc., reduce perioperative opioid use and associated side effects, such as constipation and delayed recovery.

IMPACT OF ERAS ON SHORT-TERM POSTOPERATIVE OUTCOMES

Short-term postoperative outcomes imply postoperative morbidity and mortality. In addition, a very relevant and important short-term outcome is return to intended oncologic therapy (RIOT). It has been proposed as a novel quality indicator in surgical oncology. RIOT rate is the proportion of patients who receive intended postoperative adjuvant therapy (includes second-stage operations, interventional radiology and endoscopic cancer therapies, radiotherapy, biological and hormonal therapies, etc.). It has two components, firstly whether the patient did or did not receive intended oncologic therapy after surgery, and secondly, the duration between surgery and initiation of postoperative adjuvant treatment. Recurrence free survival (RFS) and overall survival (OS) may be compromised if there is a delay beyond 12 weeks (upper limit, some cancers have 8 weeks) for adjuvant chemotherapy after definitive surgery.[8] Therefore, early adjuvant treatment is beneficial. Duration of RIOT is important as it may affect the OS based on the type and histopathological characteristics of tumor. If a patient receives postoperative adjuvant therapy earlier, e.g., within 3 weeks compared to 10 weeks, then the likelihood of favorable response in terms of RFS and OS is greater in patients who receive it earlier.

The ERAS pathway implantation has been associated with improved postoperative outcomes, early discharge and therefore these patients may have shorter duration to RIOT. The following section will cover evidence regarding the impact of ERAS across various surgical disciplines within the context of postoperative outcomes and RIOT.

Marcus et al. conducted a large-scale (2,747 patients) enhanced recovery implementation in multispecialty major oncologic surgery (colorectal, gynecology, thoracic/vascular, hepatobiliary, and urology surgery) utilizing institutional NSQIP database and observed reduction in overall, and severe complication rates, and median hospital LOS with no change in readmission rates. ERAS adherence was associated with improved outcomes and reduced opioid use on subgroup analysis of high-magnitude cases and surgery specific complications.[9]

HEPATOBILIARY AND PANCREATIC SURGERY

A randomized controlled trial (RCT) evaluated efficiency of ERAS pathway in patients undergoing pancreaticoduodenectomy (PD). In comparison to control ERAS group was associated with significantly lower rate of postoperative complications (32.4% vs. 56.8%), LOS (20 vs. 26 days) and readmissions (0% vs. 8.1%).[2] In a before-after cohort study, in patients who underwent PD with high-risk pancreatic anastomosis, ERAS pathway was associated with lower incidence of delayed gastric emptying, respiratory complications, and shorter postoperative LOS.[10] Kuemmerli C et al. conducted a meta-analysis, to investigate the impact of ERAS pathway in elderly (70–79 years septuagenarian's and >80 years octogenarians) compared to conventional care on postoperative outcomes patients undergoing PD. Overall and major complications, readmission rates were similar in both groups. However, LOS was significantly shorter in octogenarians in ERAS group, suggesting it is safe in elderly patients.[11] Agarwal et al. compared quantum of compliance (>80% vs. ≤80%) with enhanced recovery pathway in PD. They reported significantly lower rate of major complications (28.7 vs. 44%), mortality (2.1 vs. 6.8%), and postoperative stay with compliance >80%.[12] In a multicenter, retrospective cohort study in PD, found overall compliance ≥70% was associated with significant reduction in complications and LOS. Independent predictors associated with reduced complications within the ERAS pathway were avoidance of postoperative nasogastric tube, mobilization on day of surgery, and mobilization >6 hours on postoperative day 2.[13] Based on current literature, ERAS is safe, feasible, associated with improved outcomes even in elderly in patients undergoing PD.

Aloia et al. studied the RIOT rate following open and MIS liver resection. With an open approach RIOT rate was 75% whereas it was 100% for MIS. Multiple preoperative chemotherapy regimens, postoperative complications were identified as risk factors for delayed RIOT. Shorter RFS and OS correlated with inability to RIOT.[14] A meta-analysis compared safety and efficacy of ERAS programs and traditional care in patients undergoing open or MIS hepatectomy. ERAS was associated with reduction in blood loss, morbidity, LOS, early functional GI recovery, and cost for both open and MIS approach.[15]

Gall bladder cancer is the sixth most common GI malignancy with poor prognosis. Joshi et al assessed compliance with ERP elements and its impact on postoperative outcomes. Increased adherence (>80%) to ERAS protocol was associated with significantly less major complication (0.8% vs. 6.1%) and shorter LOS (5.8 ± 4.8 vs. 7.5 ± 6.6 days) and earlier functional GI recovery.[16]

COLORECTAL SURGERY

POWER, a multicenter, prospective cohort study of 2,084 patients evaluated the association between compliance with ERAS protocol and postoperative outcomes following elective colorectal surgery. Increased adherence to ERAS protocol was associated with significantly lower overall, and moderate-to-severe complications.[17] Targa et al. studied the impact of ERAS in laparoscopic colorectal surgery and reported lower incidence of complications, shorter LOS, no effect on readmission rate and mortality. Conventional care was identified as the independent predictor of complications.[18] Liu et al. evaluated, role of ERAS in elderly patients (71–92 years) compared to young patients (19–44 years). Elderly patients had significantly earlier tolerance of diet, mobilization, and shorter LOS (compared to younger group and elderly non-ERAS group) with no difference in readmission rates.[19] Adherence to ERAS protocol has been associated earlier functional GI recovery.[20] Thomas et al., in a large prospective study (937 patients) evaluated the role of quantum of compliance on postoperative complications and RIOT in patients undergoing open and minimally invasive colorectal surgery (MIS). Patients with >80% compliance had significantly lower overall surgery-specific complications, shorter postoperative stay, and early functional GI recovery for both open and MIS procedures. RIOT rate was 96.5%. RIOT duration was significantly shorter for open surgery with ≥80% compliance. There was no difference in RIOT duration for MIS irrespective of the compliance. Compliance <80% to ERP was identified as one of the independent predictors for developing postoperative complications.[21] A large, stepped wedge, cluster randomized trial reported significantly shorter LOS with increasing adherence to ERAS protocol.[22] In summary, ERAS protocol has beneficial effects in open and MIS colorectal surgery with reduced overall complications, earlier functional GI recovery, shorter stay, and RIOT duration. In addition, it is safe in elderly patients.

GASTRIC CANCER SURGERY

A multicenter, RCT compared oncological outcomes of ERAS with conventional care for laparoscopic distal gastrectomy. ERAS group had significantly lower overall complications (21% vs. 30.4%), LOS and costs.[23] A single-center prospective study investigated feasibility and safety of laparoscopic radical gastrectomy within ERAS program. They observed significantly earlier functional GI recovery, and shorter LOS. There was no difference in complications and readmission rate.[24] A large before-and-after propensity score matching study (219 patients) compared short-term surgical outcomes. They found shorter LOS in the ERAS group with no difference in complications and readmission rate. Postoperative ileus was significantly higher in the ERAS group (8.6% vs. 0.5%), however, these patients had earlier functional GI recovery suggesting that ileus was insignificant.[25] Similarly, in patients >80 years undergoing elective subtotal or total gastrectomy, ERAS was associated with a trend toward shorter LOS with no difference in complications and readmission rate.[26]

GYNE-ONCOSURGERY

A prospective, interventional randomized clinical trial (PROFAST) compared ERAS with conventional care in women undergoing cytoreductive surgery for suspected or diagnosed advanced ovarian cancer. ERAS was associated with significantly shorter LOS and readmission rate. There was no difference in morbidity, mortality, comprehensive complication index, and reoperations. Authors recommend ERAS should be a standard of care for cytoreductive surgeries.[27] In patients undergoing laparotomy for advanced ovarian cancer (stages IIb-IV), ERAS was associated with reduction in complications and LOS with no difference in readmission.[28] Kugelman et al. evaluated the role of ERAS in major open gynecological surgery in a before-after surgery, ERAS program was associated with significantly shorter LOS, decrease in nausea and opioid use. However, there was no difference in complications, readmission rate.[29] In elderly (≥70 years) women undergoing hysterectomy and/or pelvic or para-aortic lymphadenectomy for gynecological cancer, age was not identified as independent predictor of postoperative LOS. There was no difference in morbidity and readmissions between elderly and <70-year-old women.[30] ERAS protocol was associated with reduction in costs.[31]

THORACIC SURGERY

A systematic review and meta-analysis compared pre-ERAS and post-ERAS outcomes following thoracic surgery and observed reduction in overall complications, LOS by 3 days, and readmission rate with ERAS program.[32]

Overall adherence to ERAS program is associated improved short-term postoperative outcomes and costs across various oncosurgical procedures.

IMPACT OF ERAS ON PATIENT REPORTED OUTCOMES

Takagi et al. in a RCT compared quality of life (QOL) using Japanese version of QoR-40 within ERAS pathway and conventional care in patients undergoing PD. QOL was significantly better QOL in four out of five domains in the ERAS group.[2] In 293 women undergoing open gynecologic surgery patient reported outcome was assessed within an ERAS program and historical control using the MD Anderson Symptom Inventory-Ovarian Cancer (27-item validated tool) preoperatively and on postoperative day 1 and 2. ERAS was associated with significantly lower use of opioids, less fatigue, interference with walking, and total interference (composite score of physical and affective measures) during hospital stay.[33]

Choi et al. conducted a RCT and reported no difference in QOL between ERAS and conventional care group following distal gastrectomy using European Organization for Research and Treatment of Cancer C30 and STO22 QOL questionnaire.[34]

In summary, there are fewer studies which have addressed patient reported outcomes, while there seems improvement in patient reported outcomes. There is heterogeneity in the instruments and time points studied. Therefore, more studies are needed to address the impact of ERAS on patient reported outcomes.

IMPACT OF ERAS ON LONG-TERM POSTOPERATIVE OUTCOMES

A multicenter, RCT comparing oncological outcomes of ERAS with conventional care for laparoscopic distal gastrectomy reported median follow-up of 42 months. The 3-year OS and disease-free survival (DFS) in the ERAS group was significantly higher than conventional care [(86.56% and 80.11%) and (79.57% and 69.57%), respectively] particularly in stage III gastric cancer.[23]

Gustafsson et al. retrospectively explored the relationship between overall and colorectal cancer specific survival and short-term postoperative outcomes within an ERAS program. Patients with ≥70% adherence to ERAS program was associated with 42% lower risk of mortality compared to those with <70% adherence. This was one of the initial studies to explore this relationship, however, adherence to ERAS was not identified as independent predictor of survival.[3] Tidadini et al. reported significantly better 3-year survival (64.4% vs. 73.1%) irrespective of the age following colorectal resection in before-after ERAS groups respectively. In addition, adherence to ERAS was identified as protective factor with reduction in mortality by 30%, independent of other risk factors.[35] In contrast, Gomaa et al. report no difference in RFS and OS at 10 years in a large dataset of 600 patients with a median follow-up of 9.3 years, suggesting the benefits in the above mentioned literature was observed as they evaluated survival at 3 and 5 years.[36]

In PD, one-year survival was similar in ERAS and conventional care group, despite shorter LOS.[10] Similarly, there was no difference in cancer specific 5-year survival following radical cystectomy between ERAS and conventional care (49 vs. 58%).[37] Also, there was no difference in 3-year survival in head and neck cancer patients between ERAS and control group (73% vs. 76%).[38]

In summary, beneficial effect of ERAS on RIOT rate and duration to RIOT may be favorable, its impact on OS and RFS remains uncertain. This may be due to type of cancer, tumor stage at presentation, tumor biology, and completion of adjuvant if indicated. While patients may RIOT, completion of intended therapy is equally important, as it can impact survival. However, this is often not mentioned in the published literature.

CONCLUSION

Enhanced recovery after surgery program is associated with improved short-term and patient reported outcomes following various cancer surgery. It also has a favorable association with early return to intended oncologic treatment, however, its impact on long-term survival remains uncertain.

REFERENCES

1. Bray F, Laversanne M, Sung H, Ferlay J, Siegel RL, Soerjomataram I, et al. Global cancer statistics 2022: GLOBOCAN estimates of incidence and mortality worldwide for 36 cancers in 185 countries. CA Cancer J Clin. 2024;74(3):22963.
2. Takagi K, Yoshida R, Yagi T, Umeda Y, Nobuoka D, Kuise T, et al. Effect of an enhanced recovery after surgery protocol in patients undergoing pancreaticoduodenectomy: A randomized controlled trial. Clin Nutr. 2019;38(1):17481.
3. Gustafsson UO, Oppelstrup H, Thorell A, Nygren J, Ljungqvist O. Adherence to the ERAS protocol is Associated with 5-Year Survival After Colorectal Cancer Surgery: A Retrospective Cohort Study. World J Surg. 2016; 40(7):17417.
4. Loon MM, Goshe M, Rashid M, Shehryar A, Rehman A, Abdallah S, et al. Impact of Preoperative Nutritional Support on Surgical Outcomes in Gastrointestinal Surgeries: A Systematic Review. Cureus. 2024;16(3):e56416.
5. Amirkhosravi F, Allenson KC, Moore LW, Kolman JM, Foster M, Hsu E, et al. Multimodal prehabilitation and postoperative outcomes in upper abdominal surgery: systematic review and meta-analysis. Sci Rep. 2024;14(1):16012.
6. Kumar SM, Anandhi A, Sureshkumar S, Keerthi AR, Raja K, Jha AK, et al. Effect of preoperative oral carbohydrate loading on postoperative insulin resistance, patient-perceived well-being, and surgical outcomes in elective colorectal surgery: a randomized controlled trial. J Gastrointest Surg. 2024;28(10):1654-60.
7. Ljungqvist O. Modulating postoperative insulin resistance by preoperative carbohydrate loading. Best Pract Res Clin Anaesthesiol. 2009;23(4):401-9.
8. Kim BJ, Caudle AS, Gottumukkala V, Aloia TA. The Impact of Postoperative Complications on a Timely Return to Intended Oncologic Therapy (RIOT): the Role of Enhanced Recovery in the Cancer Journey. Int Anesthesiol Clin. 2016;54(4):e33-46.
9. Marcus RK, Lillemoe HA, Rice DC, Mena G, Bednarski BK, Speer BB, et al. Determining the Safety and Efficacy of Enhanced Recovery Protocols in Major Oncologic Surgery: An Institutional NSQIP Analysis. Ann Surg Oncol. 2019; 26(3):782-90.
10. Zhu J, Li X, Li H, Liu Z, Ma J, Kou J, et al. Enhanced recovery after surgery pathways benefit patients with soft pancreatic texture following pancreaticoduodenectomy. Am J Surg. 2020;219(6):1019-23.
11. Kuemmerli C, Balzano G, Bouwense SA, Braga M, Coolsen M, Daniel SK, et al. Are enhanced recovery protocols after pancreatoduodenectomy still efficient when applied in elderly patients? A systematic review and individual patient data meta-analysis. J Hepato-Biliary-Pancreat Sci. 2024;31(5):308-17.
12. Agarwal V, Thomas MJ, Joshi R, Chaudhari V, Bhandare M, Mitra A, et al. Improved Outcomes in 394 Pancreatic Cancer Resections: the Impact of Enhanced Recovery Pathway. J Gastrointest Surg. 2018;22(10):1732-42.
13. Roulin D, Melloul E, Wellg BE, Izbicki J, Vrochides D, Adham M, et al. Feasibility of an Enhanced Recovery Protocol for Elective Pancreatoduodenectomy: A Multicenter International Cohort Study. World J Surg. 2020;44(8):2761-9.
14. Aloia TA, Zimmitti G, Conrad C, Gottumukalla V, Kopetz S, Vauthey JN. Return to intended oncologic treatment (RIOT): A novel metric for evaluating the quality of oncosurgical therapy for malignancy: Return to Adjuvant Therapy Post Cancer Surgery. J Surg Oncol. 2014;110(2):107-14.
15. Wang C, Zheng G, Zhang W, Zhang F, Lv S, Wang A, et al. Enhanced Recovery after Surgery Programs for Liver Resection: a Meta-analysis. J Gastrointest Surg. 2017; 21(3):47286.
16. Joshi R, Thomas M, Patkar S, Gupta AM, Panhale K, Rane PP, et al. Impact of enhanced recovery pathway in 408 gallbladder cancer resections. HPB. 2022;24(1):4756.
17. Ripollés-Melchor J, Abad-Motos A, Zorrilla-Vaca A. Enhanced Recovery After Surgery (ERAS) in Surgical Oncology. Curr Oncol Rep. 2022;24(9):117787.
18. Targa S, Portinari M, Ascanelli S, Camerani S, Verri M, Volta CA, et al. Enhanced Recovery Program in Laparoscopic Colorectal Surgery: An Observational Controlled Trial. J Laparoendosc Adv Surg Tech. 2021;31(4):36370.
19. Liu JY, Perez SD, Balch GG, Sullivan PS, Srinivasan JK, Staley CA, et al. Elderly Patients Benefit From Enhanced

Recovery Protocols After Colorectal Surgery. J Surg Res. 2021;266:5461.

20. Barbieux J, Hamy A, Talbot MF, Casa C, Mucci S, Lermite E, et al. Does enhanced recovery reduce postoperative ileus after colorectal surgery? J Visc Surg. 2017;154(2):7985.
21. Thomas M, Agarwal V, DeSouza A, Joshi R, Mali M, Panhale K, et al. Enhanced recovery pathway in open and minimally invasive colorectal cancer surgery: a prospective study on feasibility, compliance, and outcomes in a high-volume resource limited tertiary cancer center. Langenbecks Arch Surg. 2023;408(1):99.
22. Pagano E, Pellegrino L, Robella M, Castiglione A, Brunetti F, Giacometti L, et al. Implementation of an enhanced recovery after surgery protocol for colorectal cancer in a regional hospital network supported by audit and feedback: a stepped wedge, cluster randomised trial. BMJ Qual Saf. 2024;33(6):36374.
23. Tian Y, Cao S, Li L, Yu W, Ding Y, Zhang G, et al. 3-Year Survival Outcomes of Patients with Enhanced Recovery After Surgery vs. Conventional Care in Laparoscopic Distal Gastrectomy: The GISSG1901 Randomized Clinical Trial. Ann Surg. 2024
24. Mingjie X, Luyao Z, Ze T, YinQuan Z, Quan W. Laparoscopic Radical Gastrectomy for Resectable Advanced Gastric Cancer Within Enhanced Recovery Programs: A Prospective Randomized Controlled Trial. J Laparoendosc Adv Surg Tech. 2017;27(9):95964.
25. Jeong O, Jang A, Jung MR, Kang JH, Ryu SY. The benefits of enhanced recovery after surgery for gastric cancer: A large before-and-after propensity score matching study. Clin Nutr. 2021;40(4):21628.
26. Tankel J, Sticca G, Kammili A, Dehghani M, Sakalla R, Ahmed N, et al. ERAS following Gastrectomy for Octo- and Nonagenarians: A Single-Center Retrospective Analysis. J Laparoendosc Adv Surg Tech. 2024;34(6):4849.
27. Sánchez-Iglesias JL, Carbonell-Socias M, Pérez-Benavente MA, Monreal Clua S, Manrique-Muñoz S, García Gorriz M, et al. PROFAST: A randomised trial implementing enhanced recovery after surgery for advanced ovarian cancer surgery. Eur J Cancer. 2020;136:14958.
28. Agarwal R, Rajanbabu A, P V N, Goel G, Madhusudanan L, U G U. A prospective study evaluating the impact of implementing the ERAS protocol on patients undergoing surgery for advanced ovarian cancer. Int J Gynecol Cancer. 2019;29(3):60512.
29. Kugelman N, Lavie O, Cohen N, Schmidt M, Reuveni A, Ostrovsky L, et al. Enhanced Recovery after Surgery is Feasible and Beneficial and Should Be the Standard in Major Gynecological Surgeries. Isr Med Assoc J IMAJ. 2021;23(11):72530.
30. De Nonneville A, Jauffret C, Braticevic C, Cecile M, Faucher M, Pouliquen C, et al. Enhanced recovery after surgery program in older patients undergoing gynaecologic oncological surgery is feasible and safe. Gynecol Oncol. 2018;151(3):4716.
31. Harrison RF, Li Y, Guzman A, Pitcher B, Rodriguez-Restrepo A, Cain KE, et al. Impact of implementation of an enhanced recovery program in gynecologic surgery on healthcare costs. Am J Obstet Gynecol. 2020;222(1): 66.e166.e9.
32. Khoury AL, McGinigle KL, Freeman NL, El-Zaatari H, Feltner C, Long JM, et al. Enhanced recovery after thoracic surgery: Systematic review and meta-analysis. JTCVS Open. 2021;7:37091.
33. Meyer LA, Lasala J, Iniesta MD, Nick AM, Munsell MF, Shi Q, et al. Effect of an Enhanced Recovery After Surgery Program on Opioid Use and Patient-Reported Outcomes. Obstet Gynecol. 2018;132(2):28190.
34. Choi CI, Park JK, Chung JH, Lee SH, Hwang SH, Jeon TY, et al. The application of enhanced recovery after surgery protocol after distal gastrectomy for patients with gastric cancer: a prospective randomized clinical trial. J Gastrointest Surg. 2024;28(6):7918.
35. Tidadini F, Trilling B, Quesada JL, Foote A, Sage PY, Bonne A, et al. Association between Enhanced Recovery After Surgery (ERAS) protocol, risk factors and 3-year survival after colorectal surgery for cancer in the elderly. Aging Clin Exp Res. 2022;35(1):16775.
36. Gomaa I, Aboelmaaty S, Narasimhan AL, Bhatt H, Day CN, Harmsen WS, et al. The Impact of Enhanced Recovery on Long-Term Survival in Rectal Cancer. Ann Surg Oncol. 2024;31(5):323341.
37. Ziegelmueller BK, Jokisch JF, Buchner A, Grimm T, Kretschmer A, Schulz GB, et al. Long-Term Follow-Up and Oncological Outcome of Patients Undergoing Radical Cystectomy for Bladder Cancer following an Enhanced Recovery after Surgery (ERAS) Protocol: Results of a Large Randomized, Prospective, Single-Center Study. Urol Int. 2020;104(1–2):5561.
38. Kiong KL, Moreno A, Vu CN, Zheng G, Rosenthal DI, Weber RS, et al. Enhanced recovery after surgery (ERAS) in head and neck oncologic surgery: Impact on return to intended oncologic therapy (RIOT) and survival. Oral Oncol. 2022;130:105906.

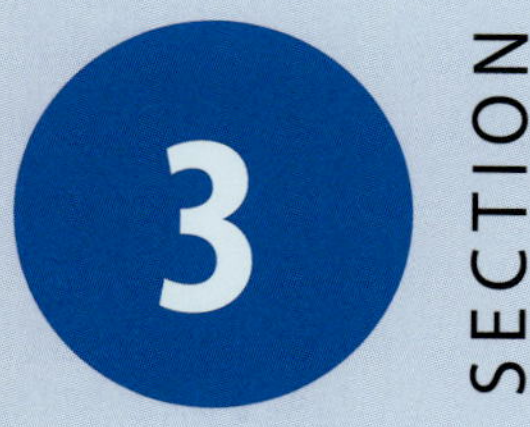

SECTION 3 Head and Neck Onco-Anesthesia

10 CHAPTER

Anesthesia for Robotic Head and Neck Surgeries

Namrata Ranganath, Rashmi NR, Rachana ND

INTRODUCTION

In the surgical field, robots have revolutionized the surgical procedures. Over the last decade, there have been major advances in robotic surgeries and this minimally invasive surgery has become a well-recognized option among patients across various surgical specialties. Transoral robotic surgery (TORS) is the recent surgical technique developed in the mid 2000s that involves a robot to perform minimally invasive surgeries for the treatment of oropharyngeal cancers.[1] TORS is also used for localization of occult primary head and neck tumors and in the treatment of benign conditions such as snoring and obstructive sleep apnea.[2,3] With conventional open surgical techniques, surgeons have limited line of sight in the working space when operating through mouth. The quality of visualization, exposure, and dissection in confined spaces is improved with advanced optics and instrumentation of robotic technology.

The fundamental concept of TORS is "de-intensified treatment" that represents the reduction of chemotherapeutic drug doses and the radiotherapy field of action which could imply on long-term survival benefits and low morbidity for the patients.

With this advancement of minimally invasive head and neck surgery, anesthetic challenges have increased mainly due to the anatomical complexity of oropharynx, sharing of the airway with the surgical team, and restricted patient access.[4]

In this chapter, we discuss in brief about the surgical robots that have been used, the perioperative management of the patient undergoing TORS that includes preoperative evaluation, intraoperative management, and postoperative care, and management of complications.

HISTORY OF ROBOTS

The word robot was first used by Capek in his play Rossum's Universal Robots in 1921. It is derived from the Czech word robota, meaning "forced labor". Robots were first developed by the National Aeronautics and Space Administration (NASA) for use in space exploration.[5]

COMPONENTS OF ROBOTIC SYSTEM

The technology developed in the robotic system is a Master–Slave Manipulator based on the concept developed by NASA to remotely treat orbiting astronauts **(Flowchart 1)**.

The da Vinci system **(Figs. 1A to C)** is the widely used endoscopic robotic system in the surgical field. After Si and X robotic systems, the da Vinci Xi was developed which is the high-end version of the robotic system with enhanced 3D high-definition vision and laser targeting with a scope for adding future technologies.

After several modifications which range from the original da Vinci with the three-arm system to a four-arm system, the da Vinci S with improved vision technology (including 3D HD) and an easier setup, the da Vinci Si with further visual enhancements and upgradeable architecture was developed.

Flowchart 1: Evolution of surgical technology: From stereotaxic to autonomous systems.

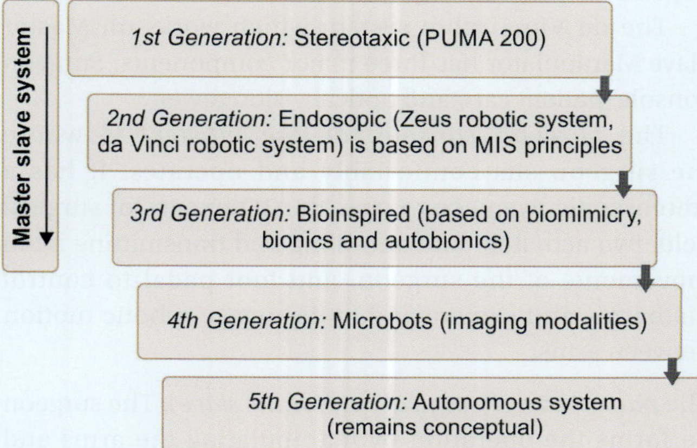

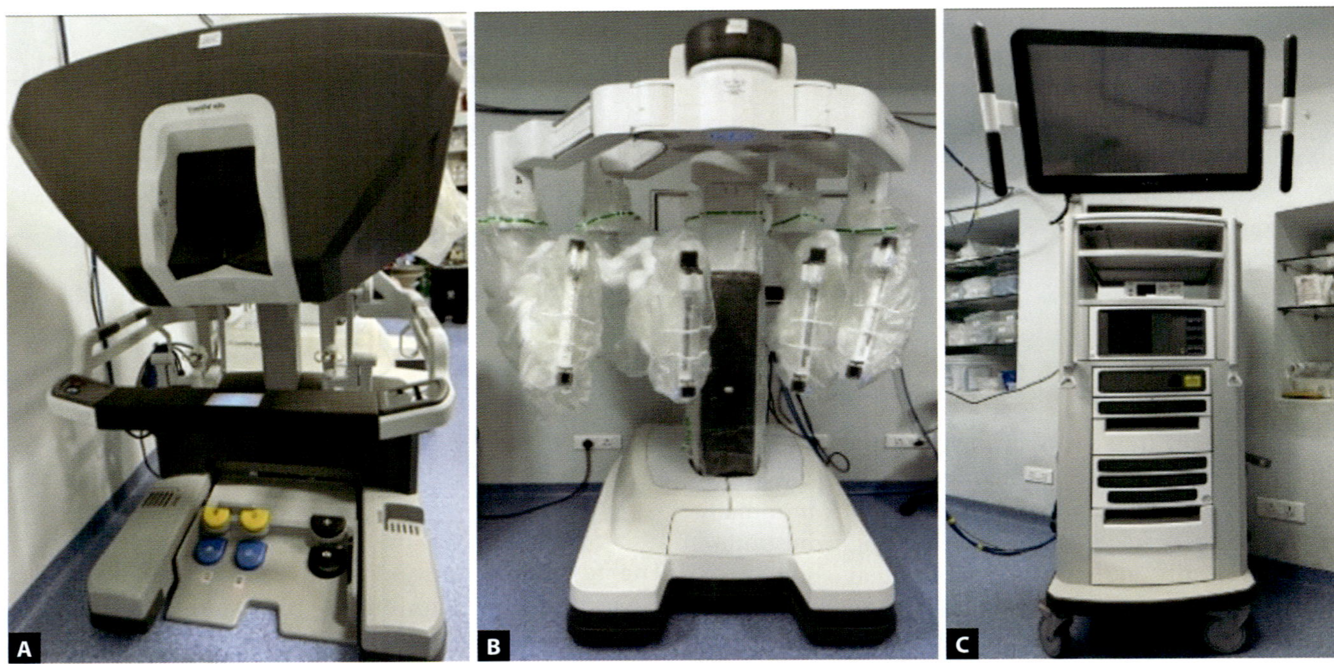

Figs. 1A to C: Components of robotic system: (A) Surgeon console; (B) Patient cart; (C) Optical tower.

The da Vinci system provides a comfortable environment and ergonomic console for a surgeon to operate with a 3D high-dimensional imaging view of the surgical field that offers accurate depth perception with multiple degrees of magnification and two cameras in a single endoscope. This system also has in-line "intuitive" eye–hand control of the instruments at the console.

Movement of the mechanical "endo-wrists" with 7 degrees of freedom beyond that of the human wrist during laparoscopy/thoracoscopy (4 degrees of freedom) will also take care of the physiological tremors of surgeon. Robotic systems also allow access to "hard-to-reach" areas of the body. These features of the da Vinci system makes it popular for usage in surgeries.

The da Vinci robot system which works on Master Slave Manipulator has three major components: Surgeon console, patient cart, and optical vision tower.

The *surgeon console (or the master)* is where the surgeon sits comfortably and operates. It has a stereoscopic eyepiece to view the 3D images of surgical field, two actuators for controlling and transmitting hand movements of the surgeon, and foot pedal to control diathermy and camera and to disengage robotic motion between arms.

The *patient cart or surgical cart (or the slave):* The surgeon performs the operation by manipulating the arms and instruments of the patient cart (slave), which is docked prior to the patient. One arm functions as endoscope arm, left and right arms function as surgeons' arms for manipulators, and fourth arm for surgical assistance. The endoscope consists of dual independent optical channels capable of transmitting digital images to the consoles visual monitor. The cart is bulky and heavy and it has to be moved to the patient's surgical area and docked. Because of the proximity of this bulky cart to the patient, the patient must be guarded against any inadvertent contact and motion.

The *video cart or vision cart or optical tower:* The cart holds an insufflator for creating pneumoperitoneum, has software needed to control the kinematics of the robotic arms, and also will have a display monitor which displays and records the surgical site.

ADVANTAGES OF TORS OVER CONVENTIONAL SURGERY[6]

- Greater precision because of higher magnification
- Elimination of hand tremors and improved maneuvering with 7 degrees of freedom
- Improved kinematics and ergonomics
- Surgeon's comfort
- Minimally invasive so less requirement of intraoperative fluids and perioperative pain medications

- Quicker recovery and early return to normal activity
- Early initiation of adjuvant chemotherapy
- Shorter hospitalization stays
- Reduced risk of long-term swallowing problems that are more commonly seen with chemoradiation or traditional open surgery
- Fewer surgical complications with en bloc tumor removal
- Less scarring
- Less risk of infection
- Less risk of blood transfusion
- TORS avoids need for tracheostomy as compared to routine open surgery

DISADVANTAGES OF TORS OVER CONVENTIONAL SURGERY

- Absence of sensory tactile feedback
- Bulky equipment and hence can lead to collisions with the patient, assistant, or its own arms
- Extra training is required.
- Inaccessibility of the patient once robotic arms are docked due to its bulkiness
- Delay in undocking in case of emergencies
- Any movement of the patient can be catastrophic and time available for weaning of neuromuscular blockade once the robot is undocked is less, if immediate extubation is planned
- The initial cost factor of the robotic system and yearly maintenance fee

INDICATIONS FOR TORS[6,7]

Head and Neck Oncology Conditions

- Base of tongue carcinomas
- Tonsillar surgeries
- Laryngeal and hypopharyngeal lesions
- Parapharyngeal space and infratemporal fossa tumors
- Head and neck reconstructive surgeries
- Thyroid carcinomas
- Sublingual and submandibular gland excision
- Neck dissection
- Parotid surgery
- Retropharyngeal mass excision

Benign Conditions

- Obstructive sleep apnea
- Vallecular cysts
- Foreign body removal
- Thyroid lesions
- Retropharyngeal mass excision
- Sublingual and submandibular gland excision

CONTRAINDICATIONS FOR TORS[8,9]

Oncological contraindications:

- All T4b cancers
- Trismus
- Tumor resection requiring more than 50% resection of tongue and posterior pharyngeal wall
- Tumors with bony invasion and close to carotid artery
- Unresectable neck disease
- Multiple distant metastases

Nononcological contraindications:

- Medical comorbidities which preclude the patient unfit for general anesthesia
- Cervical spine disease that interferes with necessary positioning

OPERATING ROOM AND ROBOT SETUP[10]

Advantages of TORS over open surgery for patients and surgeons are remarkable but also are associated with a different set of challenges to the anesthetist, particularly with respect to the restricted intraoperative access to the patient and patient's airway that is shared with a robot.

This necessitates for meticulous planning and preparation in the perioperative period including the unique operating theater ergonomics and the distinct procedure-specific postoperative requirements and complication.

In the initial years of starting robotic surgeries docking of robot and the surgery both used to take time but with experience the time taken decreases. To have a clear plan for the OR and anesthetic setup, planning and management with the surgical team are very essential. Positioning of the anesthesia machine is very crucial. Anesthesia workstation can be placed either at the foot end of the patient once the patient is induced or at the head end with long breathing circuits connected to the patient's end **(Figs. 2 and 3)**. A surgical retractor such as a Boyle–Davis or Feyh–Kastenbauer type **(Fig. 4)** is inserted into the oral cavity along with the bulky robotic arms in the surgical field and hence an OR setup is important. The bulky robot system is driven into position and the robotic arms are positioned over the patient's chest. The camera endoscope is the center arm and the right and left instruments are inserted

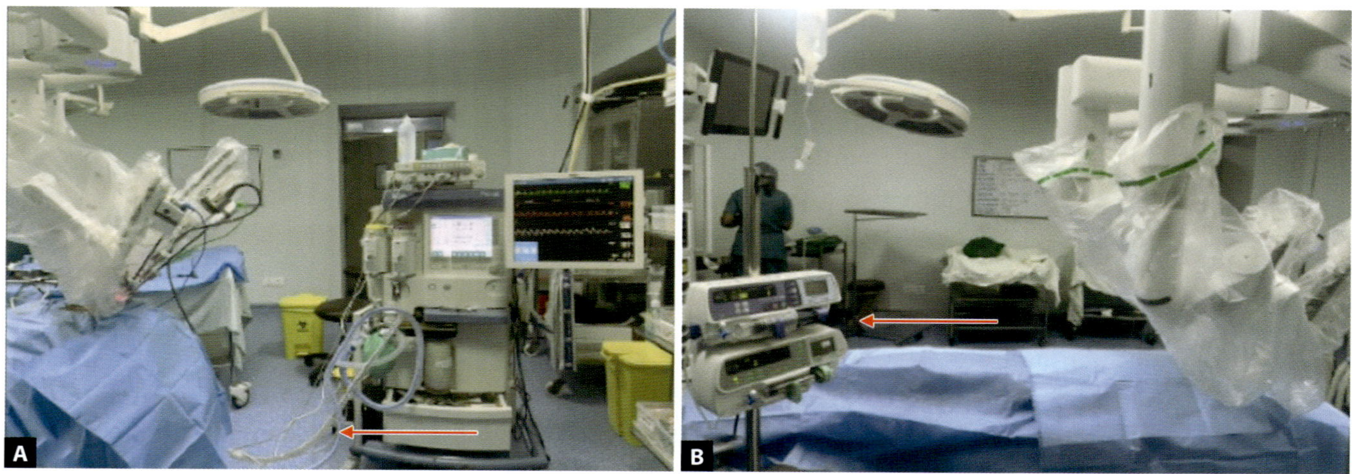

Figs. 2A and B: Operating room setup. (A) Placement of anesthesia workstation with long breathing circuits; (B) Infusion pump placed at the foot end of the table.

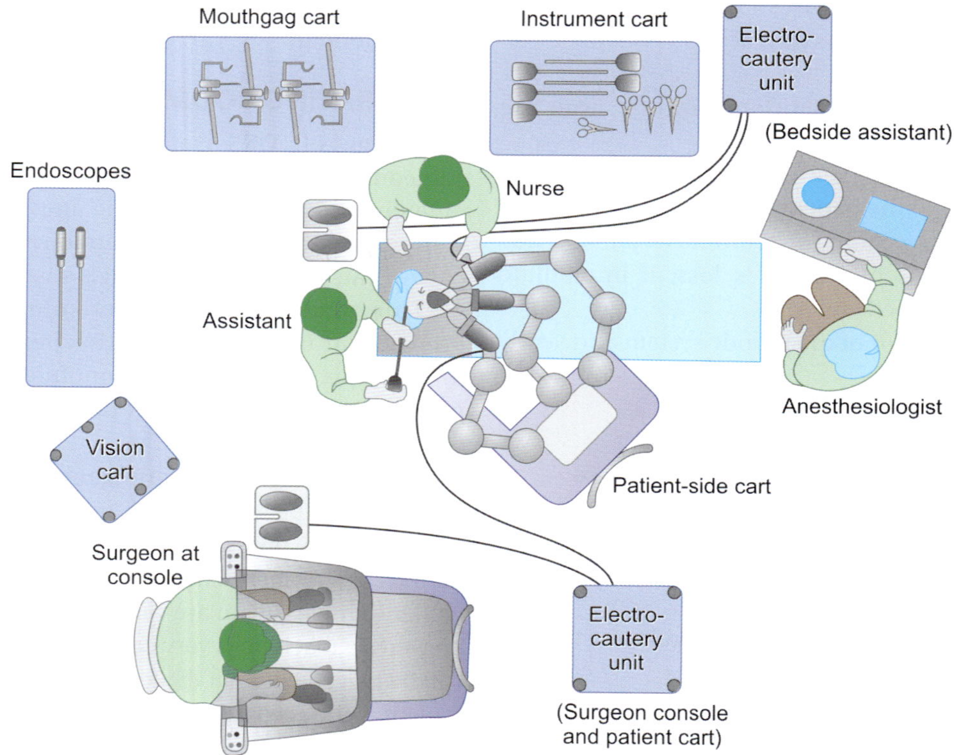

Fig. 3: Operating room setup for transoral robotic surgery.

into other two arms and then the robot is advanced into the mouth and docked. Once docked, the robotic arms are controlled by the surgeon from the console in the OR. After docking access to the airway and chest of patient is very restricted **(Figs. 5A and B)**. In few emergency situations such as airway problems, cardiac arrest, and surgical site hemorrhage that warrants immediate access to the patient, emergency undocking should be done.

PREOPERATIVE ASSESSMENT

The preoperative assessment influences and improves perioperative care. The goals of preoperative assessment are to have a proper planning of the anesthetic technique, ensure patient safety, and mitigate the risks in the perioperative period.

History

Preoperative airway assessment with history of airway obstructive symptoms such as dyspnea at rest or on exertion, stridor, cough, voice changes, and dysphagia indicate airway compromise. Thorough medical history should be taken as alcohol and tobacco are the causative factors of head and neck cancers and can predispose patients to COPD.[1] Information on previous surgical and anesthetic procedures with emphasis on difficult intubation and anesthetic management must be obtained.

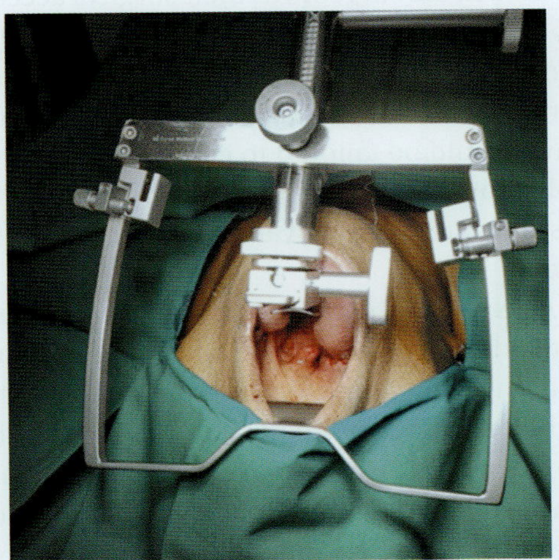

Fig. 4: Boyle–Davis surgical retractor.

History of previous radiation to the airway has to be elicited. In an acute phase, radiation therapy can lead to tissue edema and subsequently to tissue fibrosis and also osteomyelitis and tissue necrosis resulting in a decrease in submental compliance which will lead to distorted airway.[11,12]

Chemotherapy drug history needs to be elicited as chemotherapy drugs are known to have systemic effects which need to be identified and optimized before surgery.[13]

Physical Examination

A systematic and comprehensive examination of the patient's upper airway is mandatory. Routine airway assessment such as modified Mallampati, thyromental and hyomental distances, and assessment of neck movements should be evaluated.

Along with routine airway assessment, the presence of facial defects, facial hair (beard), trismus, condition of dentition, and mobility of tongue should be evaluated. These conditions are known to cause difficulty in mask ventilation and intubation.

Facial defects which can be due to tumor invasion of skin, previous surgery, radiation, and scars are known to cause difficulty in mask ventilation.[14]

Tumors arising from the tongue or oropharynx which may hamper the insertion of a laryngoscope or glottic view must be examined. Ankyloglossia in which protrusion of tongue is restricted because of tumor infiltration makes it

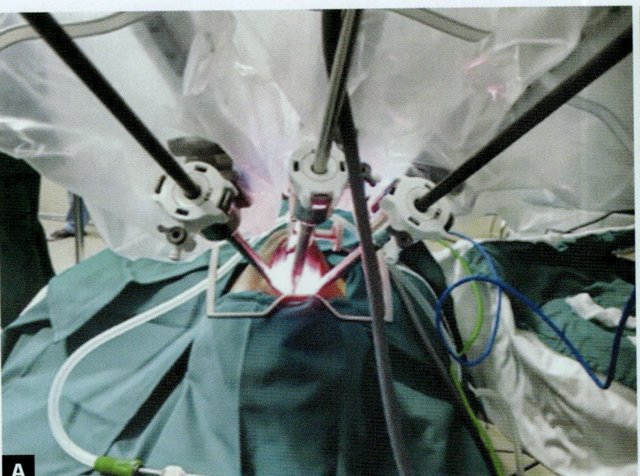

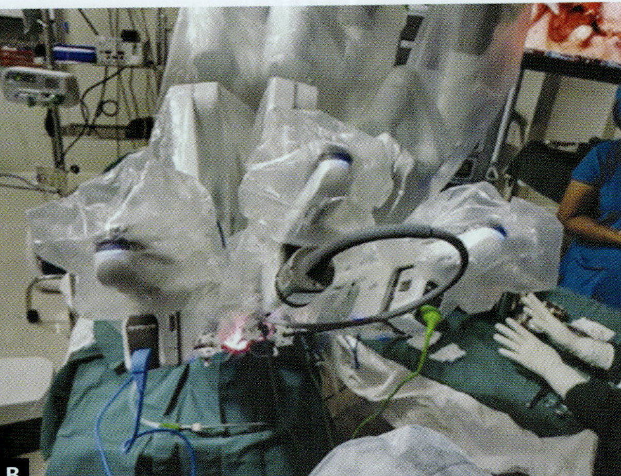

Figs. 5A and B: Robotic arms after docking.

difficult to move the tongue during laryngoscopy and thus can have suboptimal glottic view.

Base of the tongue involvement has a higher risk of bleeding. So, proper evaluation of the tongue lesions for size, extent involvement of the base of tongue, and disease crossing midline will help in planning of the safer option to secure the airway.[14]

Dentition should be examined and documented for destruction or cavitation of tooth or dental decay or loss of tooth which can be due to tobacco chewing or post irradiation. Dental damage is a recognized complication of TORS.

Examination to check for patency of nasal airway is must because most of these patients would undergo nasotracheal intubation.[15] Examination is done by feeling the blast of air during breathing and by evaluating the history regarding the ease of breathing. Findings can be confirmed with CT scan.[16]

Laboratory and Imaging Studies

Laboratory and imaging studies can help in providing additional information before a definitive plan for airway management.

Oral cancer patients are known to have poor general condition and reduced oral intake and hence are known to have anemia which needs to be corrected prior to surgery.[17] Also, chronic bleed from the tumor site can lead to anemia. Hence, complete blood count to look for anemia should be done. Nutritional status should be optimized prior to surgery.[17]

To have an airway plan in head and neck cancer surgery, airway imaging can be very useful. Airway compromise or loss of airway during the procedures can be disastrous; hence, previous imaging is important to assess the extent of the disease and nature of the airway compromise.

CT and MRI help us to assess the extent and location of tumor, carotid encasement, bony erosion, and nature of airway compromise. CT scan can also help us in detecting the intranasal spurs which are known to cause endotracheal tube (ETT) cuff damage which can result in volume loss during ventilation and nasal patency to facilitate anesthesiologists in planning of side of the nostril for nasal intubation.[17,18]

Indirect laryngoscopy, nasendoscopy, and panendoscopy performed by an otolaryngologist may help in disease mapping, anticipation, and planning of difficult airway.

Ultrasonography (USG) of neck helps us in locating cricothyroid membrane, aberrant vessels around, and altered anatomy for emergency cricothyroidotomy.

A newer technique, virtual endoscopy, which gives a 3D reconstructed video of airway anatomy helps us in identifying the difficult airway.[19] In this technique, previous diagnostic CT images are reconstructed into a 3D "fly-though" video of airway anatomy.

AIRWAY PLAN

To make appropriate airway plans, it is important to understand the pathology of the disease and the surgery being considered. Tumors can be anatomically divided into supraglottic, glottic, and subglottic lesions. An appropriate airway plan should be considered after discussion with the surgeon, as their surgical access can be affected by the anesthesiologist's choice of airway route.[1] Clear communication between the two is important to ensure a safe airway plan. The choice of intubation technique should be tailored to each patient individually. Due to the nature of the surgery, tracheal intubation and tracheostomy are the only valid airway strategies during the surgery.

Oral/nasal ETT can be secured in a completely anesthetized patient or in an awake patient using either a videolaryngoscope or a flexible optical bronchoscope (FOB) when there are predictors of difficult ventilation or intubation present. Use of such equipment can also help avoid traumatizing potentially friable airway tumors from multiple intubation attempts, and thus limit bleeding within the oropharynx.[20]

In patients with difficult airway access prior to surgery, including those with poor access to the cricothyroid membrane due to pathology, obesity, or other causes, an elective tracheostomy prior to the robotic procedure should be considered. It ensures optimal access for the surgeon, as well as secures airway patency post operatively.

INTRAOPERATIVE PREPARATION AND MONITORING

American Society of Anesthesiologists (ASA) standard routine monitors—pulse oximeter, electrocardiography (ECG), noninvasive blood pressure device, temperature probe, and end-tidal carbon dioxide ($ETCO_2$) monitor (after securing definitive airway)—are attached. Intravenous (IV) lines have to be placed preferably on the opposite side to the robotic arms to limit the risks of disconnections.

Fluids are given through the fluid warmers in view of maintaining normothermia. A conservative intraoperative fluid regimen is preferred over liberal fluid regimen to reduce the risk of postoperative airway edema.[21]

Invasive monitoring like a central venous catheter (CVC) or an arterial catheter is required, in high-risk surgery or if indicated by the patient's morbid condition. If a CVC is required, femoral access is the preferred route.[1] Use of train-of-four neuromuscular blockade monitoring is highly advantageous as the movement of the patient while docked could be deleterious. The ideal location is the tibial nerve.[1] Bispectral index monitoring is used to guide total IV anesthesia (TIVA) for induction and maintenance of anesthesia. Though TORS is a much less invasive procedure in comparison to the open surgical alternatives and allows patients to mobilize sooner, currently there is little evidence to support lower incidence of venous thromboembolic events. Thus, mechanical thromboprophylaxis should be used during surgery unless contraindicated.[1,10] IV antibiotics (according to the local policy) is administered prior to incision and are continued for 72 hours postoperatively.[22]

SECURING THE AIRWAY, INDUCTION, AND MAINTENANCE OF ANESTHESIA

Anesthetic induction should encompass a technique that is familiar for the anesthesiologist and suitable for the patient. The technique mainly depends on the airway plan—tracheal intubation (nasal/oral) versus tracheostomy and if tracheal intubation, awake versus asleep patient.

Preoxygenation is vital in these patients. Paraoxygenation (apneic oxygenation) is beneficial in patients who have an anticipated difficult airway, where securing the airway may take longer than the expected time with a significant risk of airway loss. Different techniques of doing it are with either NODESAT (Nasal Oxygen During Effort Securing A Tube) using a simple nasal cannula from an auxiliary oxygen source[23] or THRIVE (Transnasal Humidified Rapid-Insufflation Ventilatory Exchange) using high-flow nasal oxygen (HFNO) apparatus.[24]

Nasal intubation is the preferred technique for TORS procedures. The nostril contralateral to the surgical dissection is preferred. It is advisable to keep both the nostrils prepared as at times, unexpected resistance can be encountered for the passage of ETT on the planned side. Prior topicalization with the use of nasal vasoconstrictors and local anesthetic (LA) gel prior to nasal intubation minimizes nasal mucosa injury and bleeding. Cophenylcaine spray is also used in few centers to provide vasoconstriction and local anesthesia.[25]

Anesthetizing the airway for awake intubation needs meticulous preparation of the airway using any of the available methods such as viscous lignocaine gargle, lignocaine nebulization, atomizers, translaryngeal injection of LA, "SprAY as you GO" technique (SAYGO), and airway nerve blocks (glossopharyngeal nerve, superior laryngeal nerve). Anti-sialagogues such as IV glycopyrrolate should be given at least 15 minutes before the procedure to create a dry field that improves visibility for the procedure.[26] Techniques of securing the awake airway could be using a flexible fiberoptic bronchoscope or video laryngoscope depending on the site of lesion and available infrastructure. Once the airway is secured and confirmed using sustained capnography waveform, anesthesia can be induced, using an appropriate anesthetizing agent like IV fentanyl and propofol followed by a muscle relaxant of choice.

For tracheal intubation in an asleep patient, TIVA, IV induction with an agent like propofol, or induction with volatile gases, either alone or in conjunction with a strong opioid such as fentanyl, are the usual available options.[27] Any one of these techniques is followed as per the anesthesiologist's preference or the institutional protocol. Neuromuscular blockade is routinely used to facilitate intubation. None the less, Chi JJ et al.[28] have mentioned not routinely paralyzing their patients before intubation at their institution.

A wire-reinforced ETT is chosen over normal portex ETT **(Figs. 6A to C)** for intubation, as the tube should be resistant to compression from the robotic arms. These tubes resist compression well, but it has to be kept in mind if compressed above their resistance threshold they will buckle and then remain compressed, leading to airway obstruction **(Figs. 7A and B)**. Nasal RAE ETT (north facing) **(Figs. 6A to C)** are used in few centers as this allows optimal access for the robot with minimal obstruction to the surgical field. If the patient is orally intubated, it is advisable to suture the tube to the face to keep it out of the surgical field. Smaller-sized tracheal tubes which are chosen for nasal intubation are also shorter in length. Attention needs to be paid to ensure that the ETT is placed sufficiently deep so as not to be dislodged when the head is extended during surgical positioning and when the surgical instruments are being placed.[1]

If the surgery is near the laryngeal inlet, a double-cuffed tube may be preferable, due to the risk of damage to the cuff.[29] Tumors encroaching on the larynx that require use of a laser during surgery may necessitate the use of a laser-resistant ETT, with the associated essential laser safety measures for the patient and theater personnel.

Once intubated, the ETT should be meticulously secured to avoid inadvertent loss of the airway in the middle of the procedure. Adequate padding has to be placed between the ETT and the forehead to prevent pressure damage. Meticulous care of the patient's eyes with tapes and pads is required to avoid any ocular injury because of the proximity of the robotic instruments to the eyes. Molded dental guards are used to protect the patient from potential dental injury from the robotic instruments. Additional care should be taken for those patients with restricted neck extension, arthritis, or cervical radiculopathy.[25]

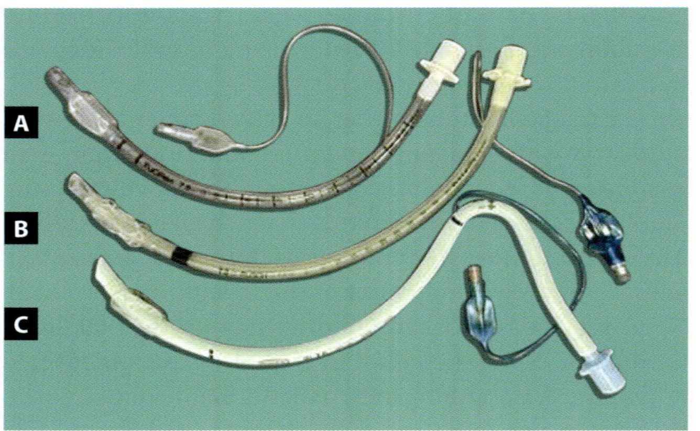

Figs. 6A to C: Endotracheal tubes (ETTs) for TORS. (A) Portex ETT; (B) Wire-reinforced ETT; (C) North facing RAE ETT.

Insertion of the gag or robotic instruments into the oral cavity could be highly noxious stimuli, leading to hemodynamic stress response. This intraoperative sympathetic stimulation from sustained application of the surgical gag can be obtunded with deepening of anesthesia or providing adequate analgesia. Remifentanil target-controlled infusions in conjunction with propofol, clonidine, dexmedetomidine, magnesium, fentanyl, or β-blockers, either as bolus or as infusion, can be used as per the anesthesiologist's choice to combat this sympathetic nervous system stimulation and prevent intraoperative hypertension.[1,30]

The nasogastric tube should be sited under direct vision preferably at the beginning of the surgery or once the surgery is complete but before tracheal extubation. As reinsertion is likely to be problematic, the nasogastric tube may be sutured to the nasal septum.

Maintenance of anesthesia can be with either a TIVA or IV agents such as propofol along with volatile anesthetic agents. Neuromuscular blocker infusions of cisatracurium, vecuronium, or rocuronium are used in order to provide adequate surgical conditions and an immobile patient throughout the intraoperative period, depending on the duration of surgery. Infusions are discontinued after undocking depending on the subsequent reversal plan at the end of surgery.[28]

The intraoperative analgesic regimen is multimodal and includes nonsteroidal anti-inflammatory drugs, paracetamol, and opioids. Judicious use of opiates is advocated due to the risk of oversedation.

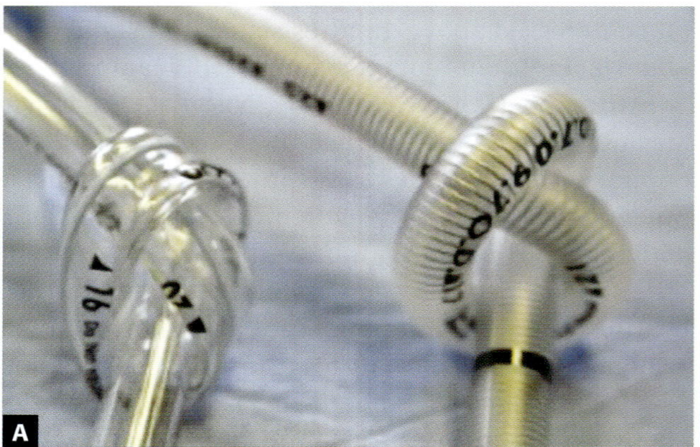

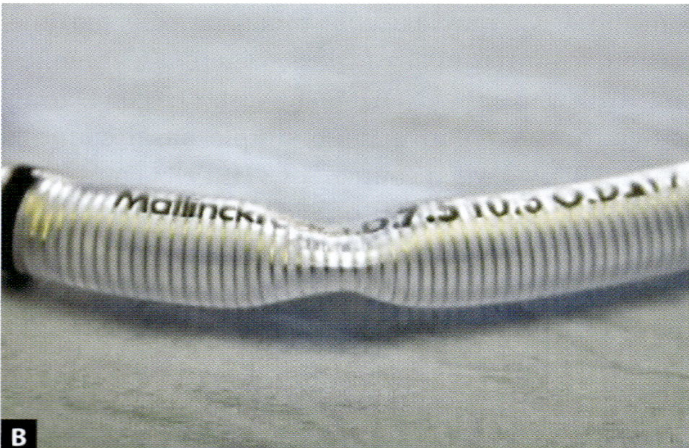

Figs. 7A and B: (A) Kink-resistant wire-reinforced endotracheal tube (ETT); (B) Compressed wire-reinforced tube.

Toward the end of the TORS procedure, the surgeons will request a Valsalva maneuver with normalized blood pressure to ensure that hemostasis has been achieved. This will reduce the chances of postoperative bleeding.

Dexamethasone 10 mg is often used, along with routine antiemetic drugs, because of its additional benefit of reducing laryngeal edema. A short course of postoperative dexamethasone has been shown to reduce pain, improve swallowing, and shorten hospital length of stay after TORS procedures.[22]

DOCKING

The patient has to be safely secured on the operating table and properly positioned before commencing the TORS procedure. The anesthesiologist should ensure that the patient's pressure points are protected, his/her arms wrapped and protected by their side, and the tracheal tube is well secured and away from the operative field. The diathermy mattress or pad needs to be adequately placed.[1] It is important to check all monitors, airway, and IV line connections and tubings before proceeding to dock to prevent potentially devastating consequences. It is important that capnography and airway pressures are monitored closely during the procedure to guarantee that any problems are detected immediately and addressed at the earliest.

As a result of the patient's positioning during TORS, an extra-long breathing circuit is required **(Fig. 2)**. In order to reduce the risk of disconnections or kinking of the tubing, the angle piece is removed when using the nasal route and the breathing circuit is placed in an upward direction over the head end of the operating table with the inspiratory and expiratory circuit limbs slung on the contralateral side to the surgical cart so as to reduce the risk of kinking from the bulky cart.[1]

The operating table is dropped to a low position to accommodate safe placement of the robotic arms which will eventually lie over the chest and torso of the patient.[25]

Infusion pumps are placed at the foot end of the patient, near the anesthetic machine and monitors **(Fig. 8)**. Cables, infusion lines, and circuits should be minimally entangled to ensure that there is no risk of damage or disconnection from the equipment. Robotic arms are docked subsequently.

An airway trolley including advanced airway equipment and a surgical tracheostomy kit, with a variety of tracheostomy tube sizes, must always remain in the theater during surgery should an emergency arise.

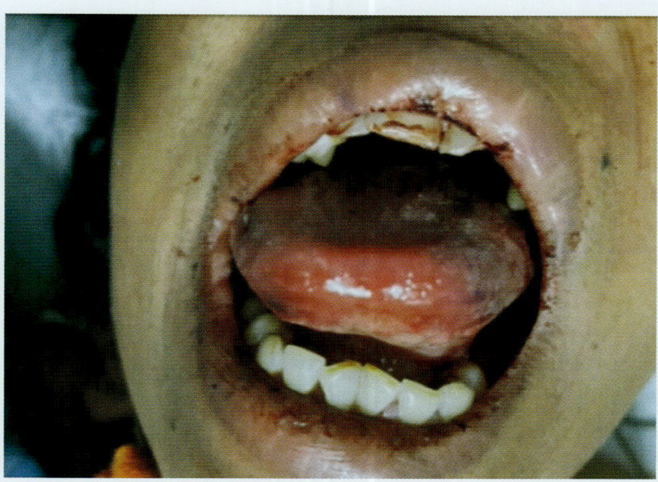

Fig. 8: Tongue edema.

EMERGENCY UNDOCKING

Undocking of the robot is routinely performed at the end of the TORS procedure. But all theater staff should be trained to rapidly undock the robot in case of an emergency. Such emergency undocking should be performed smoothly and should take no less than a minute. Practice drills to help simulate emergency undocking are important amongst multidisciplinary team members along with awareness of the specific special situations associated with TORS cases. These training programs can reduce time to undocking and access to the patient to less than a minute.[31] It is recommended that institutions have a local emergency undocking protocol. Ongoing educational simulation training for robotic emergencies ensure a successful undocking so that the teams are clear of their individual roles.[32,33]

It is crucial that in the event of airway compromise, the anesthetist takes charge and declares loudly, to the entire team, that the robot needs to be undocked immediately to allow adequate access to manage the airway.[1]

EXTUBATION

There is an immediate and a delayed postoperative risk of airway complications. Discussion between the surgical team and anesthesiologist is required to aid decisions regarding an appropriate extubation plan. Knowing from the surgeon about the effect of the performed surgery on airway post operatively prior to extubation will be useful in deciding whether the patient is to remain sedated and intubated, or if a tracheostomy is appropriate.[9,28] The same should be documented in the patient's notes so that the staff handling the patient in the postoperative phase are aware of the situation. The decision is made on a case-by-case basis.

Factors that influence the need for tracheostomy or prolonged invasive ventilation can broadly be categorized into:

- Type of surgery (primary or salvage)
- Anatomical subsite (e.g., extensive tongue base or supraglottic resection)
- Factors related to the patient (obstructive sleep apnea, obesity, known difficult airway management)

Due to duration and nature of airway manipulation during TORS, there is a potential risk of airway edema, bleeding, aspiration, and obstruction of the airway due to blood clots. Tongue swelling **(Fig. 2)** is expected due to mouth gag or surgery. Salvage surgery has an increased complication rate and increased risk of bleeding.

If the airway plan is to keep the patient sedated and intubated with or without assisted ventilation, the metallic reinforced ETT should be exchanged for a portex (PVC) ETT utilizing a tube exchange catheter or under direct vision of the airway, via a fiberoptic scope or cautious use of a videolaryngoscope. It is advisable for the surgeon to be in the OR while performing this tube exchange.

Indications for a tracheostomy would be any resection that involves both the tongue base and a portion of the epiglottis, any patient in whom postoperative emergency intubation is expected to be difficult as assessed at the end of the surgery, or a patient with a pre-existing difficult airway condition (e.g., morbid obesity, previous RT).

If extubation is appropriate, then all sedatives and neuromuscular blockade should be fully reversed, the patient sat up to 30–45°, and undertaken in the presence of the surgical team.[27] If the tube was sutured in place, at the beginning of the procedure, removing the stitches prior to extubation has to be kept in mind. The throat pack if placed has to be removed before attempting extubation.

POSTOPERATIVE ANALGESIA

Away from the surgical site, tongue and nasal septum are other sites of potentially significant postoperative discomfort. The tongue is the most common site for retraction during the procedure and also unintended injury caused by retraction or shearing movements of robot arms **(Fig. 8)**. The nasal septum may also be painful due to the attempted nasal intubation and also if a nasal gastric tube has been sutured to it.[10]

Opioid-based multimodal analgesia with IV fentanyl or morphine via patient-controlled analgesia (PCA) or infusions are most commonly used for the first 24–72 hours.[27,34] Regular paracetamol, nonsteroidal anti-inflammatory drug (NSAID) analgesics, and gabapentinoid are used to reduce strong opioid requirements.

Fentanyl transdermal patch is also used. The transdermal route offers the possibility of delivering consistent plasma levels of strong opioids. The patch is applied immediately postoperatively as it does not deliver minimally effective blood concentrations of fentanyl until after 12 hours, and the time to maximum concentration is approximately 36 hours. Care should be taken while discharging patients on fentanyl patch. The patient must be closely monitored for sedation and respiratory depression.[1]

Ultrasound-guided submental and superficial cervical plexus blocks have been described to supplement analgesia for similar surgical procedures and may provide some benefit in the more difficult cases.[35]

New evidence is emerging that enhanced recovery pathways improve pain scores and reduce postoperative opioids usage.[22,36]

COMPLICATIONS

Reported complications of TORS include skin lacerations, dental damage, mucosal lacerations, mandibular fractures, cervical spine fractures, and ocular injury. Other recognized complications are dehydration, dental damage, laryngeal edema leading to airway obstruction requiring unplanned tracheotomy, pain, nerve injuries (hypoglossal and lingual nerves), and dysphagia-related percutaneous endoscopic gastrostomy (PEG) dependency.[37]

TORS is associated with a 3–8% risk of postoperative bleeding, which can be either minor or major in nature and most commonly occurs around the 10th postoperative day.[3,38] In case bleeding occurs, patients should place their head in a dependent mouth position to prevent aspiration. External pressure should be applied to the neck ipsilateral to the pharyngeal defect. All significant bleeds should be taken back to the theater. It is suggested that these patients should receive closer physiological monitoring in an intensive or high-dependency care setting. Airway management during such events can be particularly difficult and may be associated with significant cardiovascular and respiratory compromise.

Should an extubated TORS patient require reintubation for any reason, in the immediate postoperative phase, it is important to understand that the airway anatomy may have been substantially altered by the surgical procedure. Advanced airway techniques should be considered even if the patient had a straightforward intubation for the initial procedure.

CONCLUSION

TORS has provided a breakthrough in the field of minimally invasive management of head and neck cancers minimizing morbidity and improving functional outcome as compared with open surgical approaches. In the current technologically advanced consumer-focused health care environment, a higher number of well-informed patients are seeking out TORS exclusively because of its benefits. Anesthesiologists have a key role to play in the delivery of safe patient care in this evolving area. It is important that local guidelines are formulated that support high standards of perioperative care and have these guidelines periodically evaluated as per the ongoing research in the field.

REFERENCES

1. Hawkins J, Ahmad I. Anaesthesia for transoral robotic surgery. BJA Educ. 2022;22(3):118-23.
2. Hamilton D, Paleri V. Role of transoral robotic surgery in current head and neck practice. Surgeon. 2017;15:147-54.
3. Grillone GA, Scharukh J. Robotic Surgery of the Head and Neck, 1st ed. New York: Springer; 2015.
4. Vasan N, Sharum M, Rodney JP. Potential of robotic systems in phonosurgery. Robot Surg Auckl. 2019;6:3-8.
5. Ashrafian H, Clancy O, Grover V, Darzi A. The evolution of robotic surgery: surgical and anaesthetic aspects. Br J Anaesth. 2017;119(suppl_1):i72-i84.
6. Rinaldi V, Pagani D, Torretta S, Pignataro L. Transoral robotic surgery in the management of head and neck tumours. Ecancermedicalscience. 2013;7:359.
7. Cammaroto G, Stringa LM, Zhang H, Capaccio P, Galletti F, Galletti B, et al. Alternative Applications of Trans-Oral Robotic Surgery (TORS): A Systematic Review. J Clin Med. 2020;9(1):201.
8. Luginbuhl A, Baker A, Curry J, Drejet S, Miller M, Cognetti D. Preoperative cephalometric analysis to predict transoral robotic surgery exposure. J Robot Surg. 2014;8(4):313-7.
9. Weinstein GS, O'Malley BW, Magnuson JS, Carroll WR, Olsen KD, Daio L, et al. Transoral robotic surgery: a multicenter study to assess feasibility, safety, and surgical margins. Laryngoscope. 2012;122(8):1701-7.
10. Court AA, James E, Dinsmore JE. Anesthetic considerations for transoral robotic surgery (TORS). Anaes TOTW. 2018;386:1-6.
11. Sroussi HY, Epstein JB, Bensadoun RJ, Saunders DP, Lalla RV, Migliorati CA, et al. Common oral complications of head and neck cancer radiation therapy: mucositis, infections, saliva change, fibro- sis, sensory dysfunctions, dental caries, periodontal disease, and osteoradionecrosis. Cancer Med. 2017;6(12):2918-31.
12. Becker M, Schroth G, Zbären P, Delavelle J, Greiner R, Vock P, et al. Long-term changes induced by high- dose irradiation of the head and neck region: imaging findings. Radiographics. 1997;17(1):5-26.
13. Iqbal MS, Chaw C, Kovarik J, Aslam S, Jackson A, Kelly J, et al. Primary concurrent chemoradiation in head and neck cancers with weekly cisplatin chemotherapy: analysis of compliance, toxicity and survival. Int Arch Otorhinolaryngol. 2017;21(2):171-7.
14. Dougherty TB, Clayman GL. Airway management of surgical patients with head and neck malignancies. Anesthesiol Clin North Am. 1998;16(3):547-62.
15. Smith J, Reid A. Identifying the more patent nostril before nasotracheal intubation. Anaesthesia. 2001;56(3):258-62.
16. Thota RS, Doctor JR. Evaluation of paranasal sinuses on available computed tomography in head and neck cancer patients: An assessment tool for nasotracheal intubation. Indian J Anaesth. 2016;60(12):960.
17. Talwar B, Donnelly R, Skelly R, Donaldson M. Nutritional management in head and neck cancer: United Kingdom National Multidisciplinary Guidelines. J Laryngol Otol. 2016;130(S2):S32-40.
18. Prasanna D, Bhat S. Nasotracheal intubation: an overview. J Maxillofac Oral Surg. 2014;13(4):366-72.
19. Ahmad I, Keane O, Muldoon S. Enhancing airway assessment of patients with head and neck pathology using virtual endoscopy. Indian J Anaesth. 2017;61(10):782.
20. Puchner W, Drabauer L, Kern K, Mayer C, Bierbaumer J, Rehak PH, et al. Indirect versus direct laryngoscopy for routine nasotracheal intubation. J Clin Anesth 2011; 23:280-5.
21. Sullivan MJ, Frost EA, Lew MW. Anesthetic care of the patient for robotic surgery. Middle East J Anaesthesiol. 2008;19(5):967-82.
22. Clayburgh D, Stott W, Bolognone R, et al. A randomized controlled trial of corticosteroids for pain after transoral robotic surgery. Laryngoscope. 2017;127:2558-64.
23. Weingart SD, Levitan RM. Preoxygenation and prevention of desaturation during emergency airway management. Ann Emerg Med. 2012;59(3):165-75.
24. Patel A, Nouraei S. Transnasal Humidified Rapid-Insufflation Ventilatory Exchange (THRIVE): a physiological method of increasing apnoea time in patients with difficult airways. Anaesthesia. 2015;70(3):323-9.

25. Jeyarajah J, Ahmad I, Jacovou E. Anaesthesia and Perioperative Care for Transoral Robotic Surgery. ORL J Otorhinolaryngol Relat Spec. 2018;80(3-4):125-33.
26. Myatra SN, Gupta S. Anesthesia for oral cancer surgery. In: Garg R, Bhatnagar S (Eds). Textbook of Onco-Anesthesiology. Singapore: Springer Singapore; 2021. pp. 119-42.
27. Hariharan U, Shah SB, Bhargava AK. Anesthesia for trans-oral robotic surgery: practical considerations. EC Anaesthesia. 2016;2.5:212-6.
28. Chi JJ, Mandel JE, Weinstein GS, O'Malley BW Jr: Anesthetic considerations for transoral robotic surgery. Anesthesiol Clin 2010;28:411–422.
29. Winkel R, Kristensen MS. The airway in anaesthesia for transoral robotic surgery. In: Cook T, Kristensen MS (Eds). Core Topics in Airway Management. Cambridge: Cambridge University Press; 2020. pp. 290-2.
30. Narayanasamy S, Khanna P, Bhalla AP, Singh AK. Perioperative concerns in transoral robotic surgery: initial experience of four cases. J Anaesthesiol Clin Pharmacol. 2012;28:226-9.
31. Irvine M, Patil V. Anaesthesia for robotic-assisted laparoscopic surgery. Contin Educ Anaesth Crit Care Pain. 2009;9:125-9.
32. Ballas DA, Cesta M, Gothard D, Ahmed R. Emergency undocking curriculum in robotic surgery. Cureus. 2019; 11:e4321.
33. O'Sullivan OE, O'Sullivan S, Hewitt M, O'Reilly BA. Da Vinci robot emergency undocking protocol. J Robot Surg. 2016; 10:251-3.
34. Loh KW, Teo LM. Anaesthesia for DaVinci assisted intraoral and tongue base operations. Trends Anaesth Crit Care. 2013;3:342-5.
35. Perisanidis C, Saranteas T, Kostopanagiotou G: Ultrasound-guided combined intermediate and deep cervical plexus nerve block for regional anesthesia in oral and maxillofacial surgery. Dentomaxillofac Radiol. 2013;42:29945724.
36. Ganti A, Eggerstedt M, Grudzinski K et al. Enhanced recovery protocol for transoral robotic surgery demonstrates improved analgesia and narcotic use reduction. Am J Otolaryngol. 2020;41:102649.
37. Hay A, Migliacci J, Karassawa Zanoni D, O Boyle J, Singh B, Wong RJ, et al. Complications following transoral robotic surgery (TORS): a detailed institutional review of complications. Oral Oncol. 2017;67:160-6.
38. Pollei TR, Hinni ML, Moore EJ, Hayden RE, Olsen KD, Casler JD, et al. Analysis of postoperative bleeding and risk factors in transoral surgery of the oropharynx. JAMA Otolaryngol Head Neck Surg. 2013;139:1212-8.

CHAPTER

Anesthesia for Thyroid Cancer Surgeries (With and Without Neuromonitoring)

Shalini Saksena, Aditi Tilak

INTRODUCTION

Thyroid cancer is the uncontrolled growth of thyroid parenchymal cells. The global incidence of thyroid cancer is 1–4% of all malignancies, with a female preponderance of 3:1. While the incidence has been steadily increasing over the last two decades, the mortality has remained stable. This is partly due to more sensitive screening and imaging tools leading to overdiagnosis.[1] Thyroid tumors exhibit varied biological behavior, ranging from slowly growing and localized to highly aggressive metastatic disease.

Surgical resection is the mainstay of treatment of thyroid malignancies followed by radioactive iodine ablation with thyroid hormone suppression. Systemic chemotherapy with radiotherapy is also an option in patients with high-grade malignancies.

CLASSIFICATION

Depending on the cells from which it originates and the histopathological features, thyroid cancer is classified as follows:

- Arising from cells producing thyroid hormone (differentiated thyroid cancer)
    - Follicular cancer
    - Papillary cancer
    - Anaplastic cancer
- Arising from parafollicular C-cells producing calcitonin
    - Medullary cancer
- Thyroid lymphomas and sarcomas

Eighty percent of thyroid malignancies are papillary carcinomas. Ten percent constitute follicular carcinomas. Variants of follicular carcinomas (Hurthle cell carcinoma), anaplastic carcinoma, and medullary carcinoma make the remaining 10%.[2] Thyroid cancers may be accompanied by primary tumors in other organs when they are part of tumor syndromes such as multiple endocrine neoplasia (MEN).

PRESENTATION

Patients usually present with painless neck swelling. Some patients may have symptoms of hypothyroidism or hyperthyroidism but are mostly euthyroid. The frequency of incidentally detected thyroid nodules is increasing with better imaging and diagnostic techniques and growing awareness of screening. Pressure symptoms such as hoarseness of voice, dysphagia, dyspnea or Horner's syndrome are rare but indicate involvement of surrounding structures like the recurrent laryngeal nerve, sympathetic chain, and compression over the esophagus or trachea. Superior vena cava may be compressed in case of retrosternal extension causing engorgement of upper limb and neck veins.

Clinical features which raise suspicion of a malignancy are:[3]

- Sudden increase in size of swelling
- Family history (associated neuroendocrine tumors, MEN)
- History of irradiation to head and neck
- Systemic signs weight loss, fever, anorexia, tiredness
- Firmness, fixed nature of swelling or palpable neck nodes on examination
- Distant metastasis involving brain, lungs, liver, or bones

INDICATIONS OF THYROID SURGERY

Surgery is performed to relieve compressive symptoms due to the enlarged gland, prevent spread of cancer, or achieve metabolic control of the hormonal imbalance. The broad indications for surgery are:

- Symptomatic benign goiter
- Thyroid carcinoma
- Hyperthyroidism refractory to medical management

PREOPERATIVE EVALUATION

History

The evolution of the thyroid swelling over time should be noted in the history. Its duration, increase in size if any, and the presence or absence of pressure symptoms are of significance. Long-standing enlargement is a risk factor for tracheomalacia and postoperative airway obstruction. Pressure symptoms give a clue about the extent of growth and involvement of surrounding structures. Dyspnea in supine position is an indication of potentially difficult intubation, oxygenation, and ventilation under general anesthesia.

Symptoms of uncorrected hypothyroidism (lethargy, fatigue, cold intolerance, constipation) or hyperthyroidism (palpitations, excessive sweating, weight loss, diarrhea) are uncommon in malignancy.

Symptoms suggestive of a second primary may be obvious on history. Pheochromocytoma and parathyroid adenoma accompany medullary thyroid carcinoma in MEN syndrome. Headaches, palpitations, sweating, and abdominal pain could be due to coexisting pheochromocytoma. Parathyroid adenomas are associated with nausea, vomiting, bone pains, fractures, and abdominal pain due to pancreatitis or kidney stones.

Information about other coexisting systemic diseases, their treatment, and the patient's functional status are essential in formulating the anesthesia plan.

Examination

The size, consistency, and extent of enlargement are noted on examination. Malignant thyroid nodules are usually painless. Hard and fixed nature of the swelling is more indicative of malignancy than a soft, supple feel on palpation.[2] Inability to palpate the lower border indicates retrosternal extension. Superior vena cava obstruction causing swelling and flushing of the face and neck with prominent neck veins is a rare feature of substernal thyroid enlargement. Pemberton's sign, where elevation of arms above the head causes facial flushing and shortness of breath, is seen due to latent thoracic inlet obstruction in thyroid swellings extending into the superior mediastinum. The involvement of the cervical sympathetic chain causes ptosis, miosis, anhidrosis, and enophthalmos, described as Horner's syndrome.

Clinical signs of uncorrected hypothyroidism (dry coarse skin, periorbital edema, slow responses) or hyperthyroidism (exophthalmos, resting tachycardia, warm moist skin) are unusual as presenting features in malignancies.

Airway examination is an essential part of any anesthetic pre-evaluation. It is especially important in case of large neck masses where special attention should be paid to neck movements, thyromental distance, and ability to lie supine without developing hypoxia.

Investigations

Routine blood investigations include complete blood count, prothrombin time-international normalized ratio (PT-INR), serum creatinine and electrolytes, serum calcium, thyroid function tests.

Electrocardiogram, X-ray chest, and X-ray neck (anteroposterior and lateral views) to look for tracheal compression and deviation are recommended **(Figs. 1A and B)**. Further tests such as blood sugar and 2D echo are warranted as per associated comorbidities.

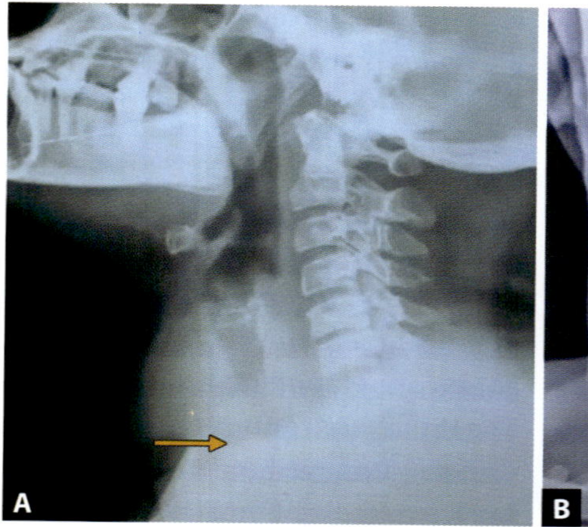

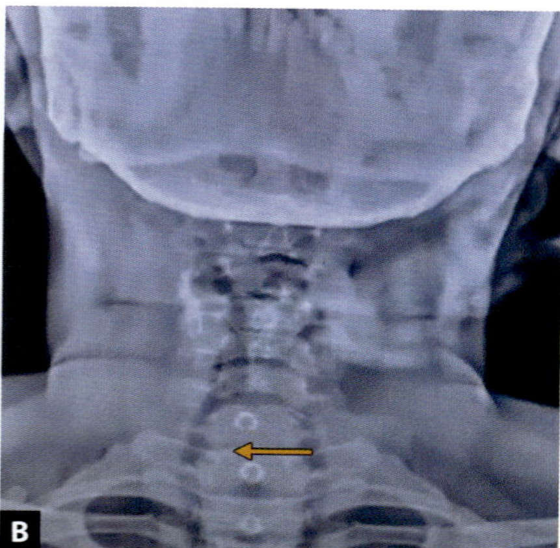

Figs. 1A and B: X-ray neck—lateral and anteroposterior views showing tracheal compression and deviation.

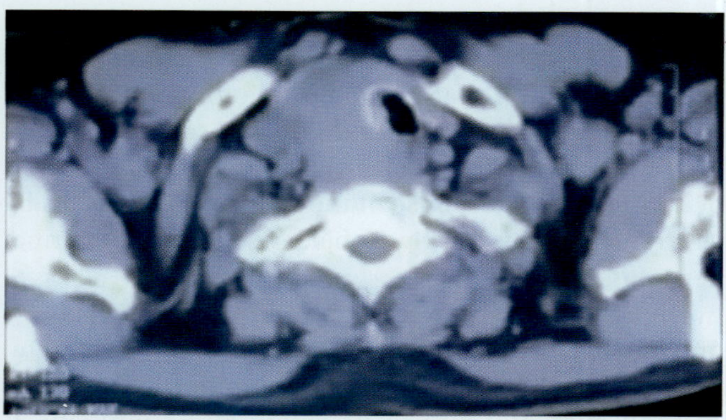

Fig. 2: CT scan showing tracheal deviation and erosion.

Indirect laryngoscopy is often done in an outpatient clinic to assess vocal cord movement and document any preexisting involvement. Pulmonary function tests are not routinely done anymore but are a useful adjunct to detect fixed upper airway obstruction. Radiological investigations such as computerized tomography (CT) scan and magnetic resonance imaging (MRI), which are often done as part of the surgical workup, should be studied carefully in case of large glands and retrosternal extension to delineate the extent of the tumor, presence and degree of tracheal compression, and involvement of surrounding structures **(Fig. 2)**. Bronchoscopy and virtual endoscopy may be useful.

The diagnostic workup of a thyroid swelling starts with ultrasound imaging to assess for high-risk features, look for other nonpalpable nodules, and evaluate for the presence of enlarged neck nodes. Ultrasound-guided fine needle aspiration biopsy is often the next step to get a tissue diagnosis in case of radiologically suspicious lesions. The decision to proceed with surgery is based on the biopsy results and the patient's clinical condition.

OPTIMIZATION

It is important to achieve clinical euthyroid status prior to elective surgery. The stress of surgery in the presence of moderate-to-severe hypothyroidism or hyperthyroidism can precipitate a metabolic crisis intraoperatively or in the immediate postoperative period.

Uncontrolled hyperthyroidism is treated with anti-thyroid medication (methimazole, carbimazole, or propylthiouracil) and beta-blockers like propranolol which control the cardiovascular symptoms of thyrotoxicosis.[4] Antithyroid drugs take 6–8 weeks to take effect as they act by decreasing the synthesis of thyroid hormones. But beta-blockers work in the immediate preoperative period. Historically, Lugol's iodine or saturated solution of potassium iodide (SSKI) was used for 6–8 weeks preoperatively. It helps to achieve euthyroid status and decrease the vascularity of the gland preoperatively.[5] Glucocorticoids decrease the conversion of thyroxine to the biologically active triiodothyronine in a matter of hours and can be used preoperatively and tapered in the postoperative period.[6]

Hypothyroidism is treated with exogenous thyroxine supplementation in a graded manner so as to avoid precipitating cardiac ischemia due to oxygen supply-demand imbalance.[5] Emergency surgery in a severely hypothyroid patient warrants the use of intravenous levothyroxine. Perioperative steroids are required in patients with coexisting adrenal insufficiency.

In emergency surgery of nonoptimized patients, suitable modification of the anesthesia technique with titrated induction is essential to prevent crisis. In hyperthyroid patients, measures should be taken to blunt the laryngoscopy and intubation response with use of potent opioids like fentanyl, bolus of propofol, and lignocaine prior to laryngoscopy.[7] Inadequate control of hyperthyroidism results in a major brunt on the cardiovascular system with tachycardia, atrial fibrillation, other arrhythmias, uncontrolled hypertension, ischemic changes, or heart failure. In hypothyroid patients, avoidance of sedative premedication and use of smaller doses of opioids, inhaled anesthetics, and hypnotics are prudent to avoid delay in extubation and recovery. Adequate time must be allowed for intravenous agents to act in the presence of altered circulatory status in both the conditions. Maintaining normothermia and euvolemia is vital, and advanced hemodynamic monitoring may be considered for these patients.

INTRAOPERATIVE MANAGEMENT

Airway Management of Large Thyroid

Difficult airway in thyroid patients can occur due to anteroposterior compression or lateral deviation of trachea. Difficulty in extension of neck changes the alignment of the axes, and there is reduced mobility of laryngeal structures due to infiltration. Also, surgical access of the airway is difficult. A difficult airway cart with all sizes of endotracheal tubes, videolaryngoscope, and rigid bronchoscope must be ready.

Standard endotracheal intubation after adequate muscle relaxation is the norm for most thyroid surgeries. Even with large neck masses extending retrosternal, this technique ensures a smooth and successful placement of a definitive airway device at the first attempt in majority of patients.[8] However, symptoms such as dyspnea in supine position may warrant an alternate plan. Administration of anesthesia and muscle relaxants without securing the airway carries the risk of complete airway obstruction in such patients. Hence, awake intubation in the propped-up position with placement of the tube beyond the narrowing is the safest way of keeping the airway patent in these cases.[9] Inhalational agents such as sevoflurane can be used to induce anesthesia while maintaining spontaneous respiration followed by check laryngoscopy and placement of endotracheal tube with or without giving a muscle relaxant. In case of inability to mask ventilate, lifting of the thyroid mass by the assistant may help. A rigid bronchoscope is a useful rescue device in case of complete loss of airway in this situation. While front of neck access is technically challenging due to the thyroid enlargement and tracheal distortion, all equipment and an experienced surgeon must be present in the theater for rescue tracheostomy if needed.

If an invasive airway approach is not possible after failed awake intubation attempts, veno-venous extra-corporeal membrane oxygenation (VV-ECMO) which bypasses only the respiratory system is an option.[10,11] The cannulation for VV ECMO can be done under local anesthesia in the operating room.

Neuromonitoring

Surgery for thyroid cancer carries a potentially higher risk of recurrent laryngeal nerve injury than noncancer surgeries.[4] The practice of intraoperative neuromonitoring (IONM) has been introduced to reduce the incidence of this complication. IONM aids in identifying the vagus and recurrent laryngeal nerves during surgery. Also, it tests nerve integrity by electrical stimulation followed by recording the response of the muscle it innervates by electromyography and gives objective evidence of normal nerve function.[12]

Neuromonitoring can be continuous via an implantable electrode in the vagus nerve or intermittent. Intermittent IONM is the most commonly practiced method currently due to its safety and simplicity. It involves using a special flexometallic endotracheal tube with an inbuilt electrode that is placed at the level of the vocal cords **(Figs. 3A and B)**. During surgery, an electrical probe is used to stimulate what is identified as the nerve with a current of 0.5–2 mA. After a latent period, the contraction of the vocalis muscle is detected by the surface electrodes on the endotracheal tube and converted into a visual and auditory electromyographic signal displayed on the neuromonitor. An amplitude of >200 μV at this current intensity is reassuring of normal nerve function. A decrease in amplitude from baseline indicates loss of signal and nerve injury.[13] Stimulation of the vagus nerve and recurrent laryngeal nerve should be carried out before and after surgical resection. The signals are described as V1 and R1, pre resection, and V2 and R2, post resection.

This exercise requires close co-operation between the surgeon, anesthetist, and neurophysiologist. Certain modifications of the anesthesia technique are essential to maintain neuromuscular transmission and the quality of the response.

Of utmost importance is the placement of the endotracheal tube. No lubricant or local anesthetic is

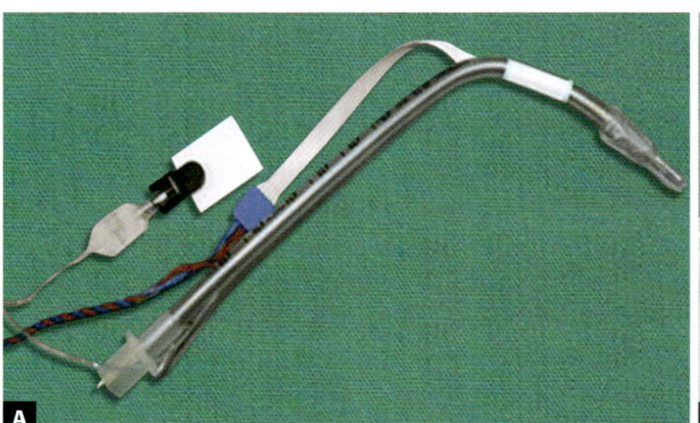

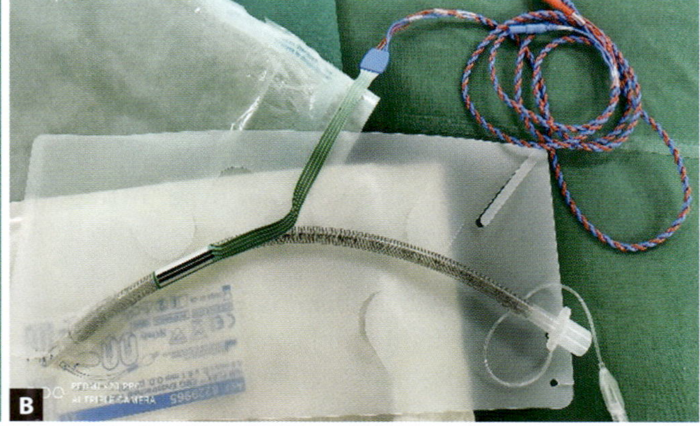

Figs. 3A and B: Neural integrity monitor (NIM) endotracheal tube.

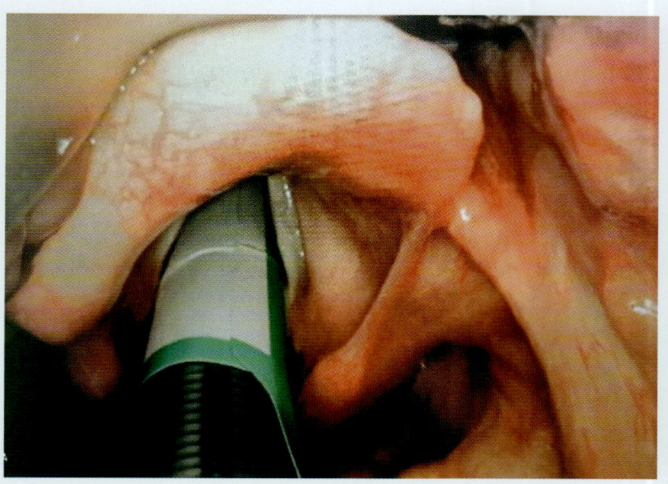

Fig. 4: Laryngoscopic view of an appropriately placed neural integrity monitor (NIM) tube.

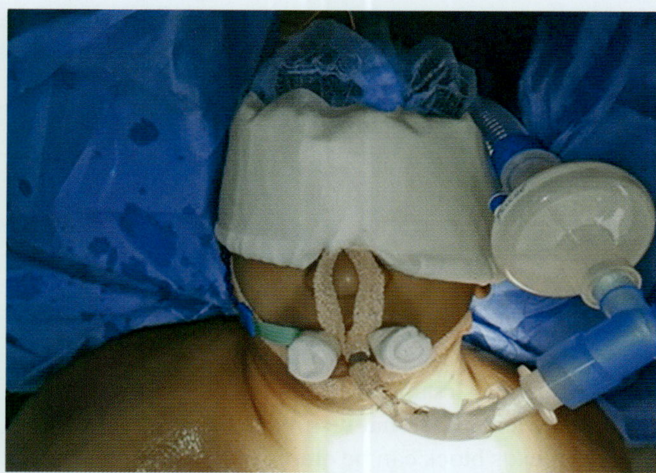

Fig. 5: Tube fixation.

applied on the tube which is introduced with a stylet. The surface electrode is placed at the level of the vocal cords under vision during laryngoscopy and intubation. **(Fig. 4)**. However, since surgical position involves neck extension with placement of bolster under the shoulder, there is a risk of displacement of the electrode at final position as the tube tends to migrate out with neck extension. Videolaryngoscopy for primary intubation, where other team members can confirm appropriate placement of the tube, is recommended.[14] The fixation of the tube should be done after final positioning and rechecking with a videolaryngoscope. Gauze rolls in shape of cigars are placed on either side of the endotracheal tube which is fixed in the center of the mouth to prevent biting and intraoperative displacement resulting in loss of stimulation **(Fig. 5)**. Following this, the neurophysiologist applies the external electrodes and checks the impedance value of the endotracheal electrode, thus confirming good contact with the vocal cords.[12]

Anesthesia drugs have to be chosen carefully as some of them can interfere with the signal quality and be a confounding factor in case of loss of signal. Neuromuscular transmission is vital for eliciting the vocalis muscle response. So, only short-acting muscle relaxants such as suxamethonium or atracurium are used for intubation and none thereafter. The return of normal neuromuscular transmission at the time of nerve stimulation is monitored objectively by train of four response and ratio. Inhalational anesthetics produce a dose-dependent suppression of amplitude of the response.[15] Their use must be limited to low minimum alveolar concentration (MAC) values ≤0.5 if not completely avoidable. All intravenous anesthetic agents, sedatives, and hypnotics are compatible with multimodal neuromonitoring.[15] Total intravenous anesthesia (TIVA) using drugs such as propofol and remifentanil, which have a quick onset of action and short context-sensitive half-times, would be the ideal choice for these surgeries.

Blood pressure, body temperature, and oxygenation also influence the IONM response and its quality and reliability.[15] Maintaining these parameters within a close range of their baseline is part of the anesthesia management to facilitate neuromonitoring.

Maintenance of Anesthesia and Recovery

Patients are positioned supine with neck extension for thyroid surgeries. Adequate padding of pressure points, eye padding, and occipital support must be ensured while providing the optimum position for surgery. Long extensions to airway circuits and intravenous lines maybe needed as the head end is away from the anesthesia machine and arms tucked and adducted.

Without IONM, either inhalational agents or TIVA may be used for maintenance of anesthesia. Muscle relaxants are helpful to prevent coughing and bucking during manipulation of crucial structures. Adequate prophylaxis for postoperative nausea and vomiting with ondansetron and dexamethasone is recommended to avoid straining and retching during recovery. Attention must be given to maintaining normothermia and euvolemia. Being a superficial surgery, not much blood loss or insensible loss is expected in thyroidectomy. Most patients are not catheterized. So, a restrictive strategy with administration of maintenance fluids is appropriate for this procedure.

Infiltration of the surgical incision with local anesthetic must be encouraged prior to incision. Intraoperative analgesia is provided with paracetamol and short-acting opioids such as fentanyl. Nonsteroidal inflammatory agents should be given in the absence of contraindications for the same. Multimodal analgesia is sufficient for most patients in the days following surgery. Opioids can be used as rescue analgesics and are better avoided post head and neck surgeries.[16] Regional techniques such as superficial cervical plexus block can be employed to enhance patient satisfaction in the immediate recovery phase.

At the end of surgery, neuromuscular blockade is reversed and the patient extubated after confirming adequacy of spontaneous respiration. Smooth extubation in a deep plane in an uncomplicated airway, without straining and coughing, is advisable. Administration of a small bolus of lignocaine or fentanyl can help to prevent coughing while allowing extubation.

Suspicion of tracheomalacia requires an extubation plan. The trachea can be extubated over a fiberoptic bronchoscope which can show the presence of expiratory collapse of the tracheal wall in addition to a videolaryngoscope to examine the vocal cord movement.[17] If there is significant tracheomalacia, reintubation or tracheostomy is done. In such cases, cuff leak test and protected extubation with an airway exchange catheter can be considered.

Robotic thyroid surgery: An oral flexometallic tube is required for transaxillary and retroauricular approach with IONM. Nasal intubation with a preformed northpole tube may be needed for transoral robotic-assisted thyroid surgery. Long breathing circuits and intravenous lines with extensions must be in place as the access is quite remote. Absolute immobility is essential after docking of the robot and anesthesia is tailored as per patient and surgical requirements.

POSTOPERATIVE COMPLICATIONS

Thyroidectomy is associated with airway complications in the immediate postoperative period. Although their incidence is low, especially in high-volume centers, they can be life threatening if not diagnosed and treated in a timely manner.

Hematoma

Inadequate hemostasis with collection of blood into the neck can lead to airway compromise due to external compression. This is a devastating complication in the immediate recovery period with an incidence of approximately 0.6% in some studies.[18] Several risk factors have been identified including male gender, old age, use of antiplatelets, revision surgery, increasing duration of surgery, retrosternal goiter, and low-volume centers.[19] Vigilance in the recovery period with attention to the subtle changes in hemodynamic parameters and patient symptoms such as anxiety, difficulty swallowing, neck discomfort, and tachypnea can help identify this complication before full-blown stridor and loss of airway. Stitch cutters must be readily available for such an emergency situation. Opening the wound and releasing the compression over the airway comprise the first step of management. The patient should be intubated and airway secured by the most senior anesthetist available. In case of unsuccessful attempts at intubating, front of neck access may be necessary. While the operation theater is the best place for management of the airway and control of hemorrhage, it may be necessary to open and pack the wound and secure the airway at the bedside in critical situations.

Recurrent Laryngeal Nerve Palsy

Recurrent laryngeal nerve can get injured during surgery due to traction, contusion, partial or complete transection or injury to its blood supply. This results in paralysis of the vocal cords. Bilateral nerve injury leads to the vocal cords remaining in paramedian position causing airway obstruction and stridor immediately on extubation. Sometimes, the presentation may be delayed and the patient may present with stridor at the time of follow-up. Unilateral nerve injury results in hoarseness and change in voice and increased risk of aspiration. In case of bilateral vocal cord paralysis, immediate reintubation is needed to maintain airway patency. Re-exploration of the neck may be considered to rule out treatable causes of nerve injury. If the patient fails the trial of extubation and there is obvious bilateral vocal cord paralysis on fiberoptic examination, tracheostomy is needed for longer term airway management.

Hypocalcemia

Post thyroidectomy hypocalcemia may be transient or permanent. Perioral numbness, twitching, restlessness, and neuromuscular weakness are early signs. Typical signs like Trousseau's sign (carpopedal spasm precipitated by inflation of blood pressure cuff over the arm) and Chvostek's sign (facial spasm caused by tapping the facial nerve over the parotid gland) aid clinical diagnosis. The initial treatment is by oral calcium supplementation. In spite of regular oral treatment, if the patient worsens with appearance of ECG changes, QT prolongation and arrythmias intravenous calcium supplementation is needed along with intensive monitoring.[20]

Tracheomalacia due to chronic pressure causing degeneration of the tracheal cartilage, superior laryngeal nerve injury, and laryngeal edema in case of prolonged and complex surgery are some other airway complications following thyroid surgery. Maintaining airway patency by appropriate interventions is the first step in managing most of these scenarios. But a diagnosis needs to be established to guide definitive treatment. Postoperative pain, nausea, and vomiting are rare with effective intraoperative strategies for the same. However, their presence can mask and make the diagnosis of other airway complications more challenging. Emergency surgery in nonoptimized patients can precipitate metabolic complications such as thyroid storm and myxedema coma. These require intensive care management of airway, breathing, and circulation.

CONCLUSION

Thyroid surgery forms a bulk of head and neck onco-surgical cases. Clear communication with the surgical team is essential, especially in anticipated difficult airway and when IONM is needed. Along with the airway challenges associated with a large neck swelling, injury to recurrent laryngeal nerves is a major concern in thyroid cancer surgery. The use of intraoperative neuromonitoring has reduced the incidence of this complication but requires suitable modification of anesthesia management. A meticulous surgical technique along with vigilance in the postoperative care unit plays a role in enhancing patient outcomes.

REFERENCES

1. Kitahara CM, Schneider AB. Epidemiology of Thyroid Cancer. Cancer Epidemiol Biomarkers Prev. 2022; 31(7):1284-97.
2. Medscape. Thyroid cancer: Practice essentials, overview, clinical presentation. eMedicine. Available from https://emedicine.medscape.com/article/851968-overview#a2 [Last accessed February, 2025].
3. Lee K, Cassaro S. Thyroid Cancer. Treasure Island (FL): StatPearls Publishing; 2021. Available from https://www.ncbi.nlm.nih.gov/books/NBK459299/ [Last accessed February, 2025].
4. Farling PA. Thyroid disease. Br J Anaesth. 2000;85(1):15-28.
5. Bajwa SJ, Sehgal V. Anesthesia and thyroid surgery: The never ending challenges. Indian J Endocrinol Metab. 2013;17(2):228-34.
6. Palace MR. Perioperative management of thyroid dysfunction. Health Serv Insights. 2017;10:1178632916689677.
7. Guzzetti L, Inversini D, Bacuzzi A. Anaesthesia for thyroid and parathyroid surgery. BJA Educ. 2024;24(8):270-6.
8. Sajid B, Rekha K. Airway management in patients with tracheal compression undergoing thyroidectomy: a retrospective analysis. Anesth Essays Res. 2017;11(1):110-6.
9. Dabbagh A, Mobasseri N, Elyasi H, Gharaei B, Fathololumi M, Ghasemi M, Chamkhale IB. A rapidly enlarging neck mass: the role of the sitting position in fiberoptic bronchoscopy for difficult intubation. Anesth Analg. 2008;107(5):1627-9.
10. Tan D, Zhang X. Awake fiberoptic nasotracheal intubation and anesthetic management of a patient with a compressed and deviated airway from a massive thyroid goiter: A case report. Cureus. 2023;15(2):e35278.
11. Jeong YI, Jun IG, Ha SS, Kwon HJ, Lee YM. Extracorporeal membrane oxygenation for the anesthetic management of a patient with a massive intrathoracic goiter causing severe tracheal obstruction with positional symptoms: A case report. Medicine. 2019;98(42):e17650.
12. Medas F, Canu GL, Erdas E, Giorgio P. (2019). Intraoperative neuromonitoring in thyroid surgery. InKnowledges on thyroid cancer. DOI: 10.5772/intechopen.83840
13. Wojtczak B, Sutkowska-Stępień K, Głód M, Kaliszewski K, Sutkowski K, Barczyński M. Current knowledge on the use of neuromonitoring in thyroid surgery. Biomedicines. 2024;12(3):675.
14. Kriege M, Hilt JA, Dette F, Wittenmeier E, Meuser R, Staubitz JI, et al. Impact of direct laryngoscopy vs. videolaryngoscopy on signal quality of recurrent laryngeal nerve monitoring in thyroid surgery: a randomised parallel group trial. Anaesthesia. 2023;78(1):55-63.
15. Wi SM, Lee HJ, Kang T, Chang SY, Kim SM, Chang BS, et al. Clinical significance of improved intraoperative neurophysiological monitoring signal during spine surgery: a retrospective study of a single-institution prospective cohort. Asian Spine J. 2020;14(1):79.
16. Solanki SL, Thota RS, Rajan J, Gangakhedkar GR, Jain P, Gottumukkala V, et al. Multimodal opioid sparing onco-anesthesia: A consensus practice guideline from Society of Onco-Anesthesia and Perioperative Care (SOAPC). J Opioid Manage. 2021;17(5):417-37.

17. Shah SB, Kulkarni A. Thyroid cancer and post thyroidectomy tracheomalacia: algorithm for decoding a diagnostic dilemma! Ain-Shams J Anesthesiol. 2020;12:1-4.
18. Talutis SD, Drake FT, Sachs T, Rao SR, McAneny D. Evacuation of postoperative hematomas after thyroid and parathyroid surgery: an analysis of the CESQIP database. Surgery. 2019;165(1):250-6.
19. Chereau N, Godiris-Petit G, Noullet S, Di Maria S, Tezenas du Montcel S, Menegaux F. Risk score of neck hematoma: how to select patients for ambulatory thyroid surgery? World J Surg. 2021;45:515-21.
20. Malhotra S, Sodhi V. Anaesthesia for thyroid and parathyroid surgery. Continuing Educ Anaesth Crit Care Pain. 2007;7(2):55-8.

12 CHAPTER

Airway Management in Head and Neck Cancer Surgery

Sheila Nainan Myatra, Darshil Ashok Julasana, Sushan Gupta

INTRODUCTION

Head and neck cancers (HNCs) are a heterogeneous group of malignancies extending from the upper aerodigestive tract up to larynx, including carcinomas of the lip, tongue, gingiva, palate, the floor of the mouth, oropharynx, nasopharynx, hypopharynx, and larynx.[1] They account for approximately 4.5% of cancer diagnoses and deaths.[2] In India, HNC is considered to be the most common among all types of cancer.[3] HNC accounted for about 26% of all cancer cases in males and 8% in females.[4]

Considering the current burden of head and neck malignancies and increasing survival, most anesthesiologists would be faced with providing anesthesia to these patients at some point, either for primary surgeries or for nononcological procedures. Anatomical and physiological alterations in these patients often make airway management difficult. Approximately, 30–40% of patients with advanced HNC have some degree of airway difficulty.[1] Globally, the incidence of difficult airway is approximately 15.8%, compared to 2.5% in the general surgical population.[1]

Difficult airway management, intraoperatively shared airway, prolonged duration of the surgery, and postoperative airway management are the main concerns for the anesthesiologist. Lack of cooperation and presurgical planning with the anesthesiology team can make a simple microlaryngoscopy case an airway crisis.[5]

The management of HNC patients is constantly evolving, with respect to the type of surgery, reconstruction, and newer adjuvant therapies. Hence, it is imperative that we understand the anatomical and physiological changes secondary to the HNC itself and its associated therapies. In this chapter, we will discuss the various airway management considerations during HNC surgery. These recommendations should supplement the routine evaluation and airway management strategies of a patient undergoing major surgeries.

APPLIED ANATOMY

Maintenance of a patent airway after surgical resection is one of the major concerns for the anesthesiologists following HNC surgery. It is therefore important to have an understanding of the role of various structures in maintaining a viable and patent airway. The mandible, maxilla, and the tongue form the external boundary of the airway. The genial tubercle over the mandible provides attachment to genioglossus and geniohyoid muscles, which maintain airway patency. Therefore, loss of any of these structures may lead to collapse of the airway, similar to that seen during rapid eye movement sleep.[6,7]

The pharyngeal muscles are crucial in ensuring that the food bolus enters safely into the esophagus. This is accompanied by the simultaneous anterior movement of epiglottis to close the laryngeal inlet. Superior constrictors close the soft palate and the middle and inferior constrictors contract to push food into the esophagus. In addition, pharyngeal muscles also act as sphincters preventing regurgitation of food from the esophagus.[8] The arytenoid cartilages and the vocal cords prevent aspiration. The posterior cricoarytenoid muscle is the only muscle that opens the vocal cords and ensures patency. The thyroid and cricoid cartilages provide structural support to keep the airway open. The glossopharyngeal (CN IX) and the vagus nerve (CN X) regulate airway reflexes while the hypoglossal nerve (CN XII) controls the tongue movements.

CANCER SURGERY

Surgery remains the mainstay of treatment in HNC. Depending on the extent of surgeries and the stage of tumor, radiation or chemotherapy (cisplatin/cetuximab-based) may also be administered.[9] Debulking surgery may be performed for palliation of symptoms and to maintain airway patency.[10] The main goal of surgery is to obtain disease-free margins. Therefore, unlike nononcological procedures, the surgical excision may often be extensive, with accompanying lymph node dissection, and often requires reconstructive procedures.

Neck dissection: The most common site of cancer spread is the cervical group of lymph nodes, which are commonly excised during HNC surgery. The patient may undergo a partial, modified, or radical neck dissection along with removal of the surrounding muscles, nerves, and veins.

Reconstructive procedures: Flap reconstructions are often required for cosmetic purposes and to help with chewing and swallowing. These may be pedicle flaps where the original blood supply of the structure is retained or they may be free-flaps, which require microvascular anastomosis.

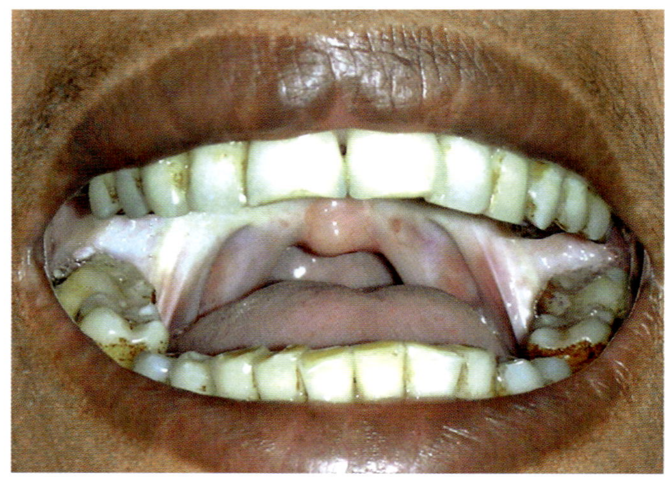

Fig. 1: Fibrous bands in the oral cavity.

PREOPERATIVE AIRWAY ASSESSMENT

Other than the routine assessment and optimization prior to major surgery, there are some special considerations for airway assessment in HNC patients. A careful history of the signs and symptoms related to the airway is vital. The presence of progressive dysphagia, hoarseness of voice, breathlessness, or discomfort on lying supine may be a sign of a compromised airway. Laryngeal cancers may present with stridor and difficulty in breathing. These may present with almost complete obstruction, requiring an immediate tracheostomy.

Apart from routine airway examination like Mallampati grading, thyromental distance, etc., there are special considerations during airway assessment, which are specific to HNC patients that need to be evaluated carefully.

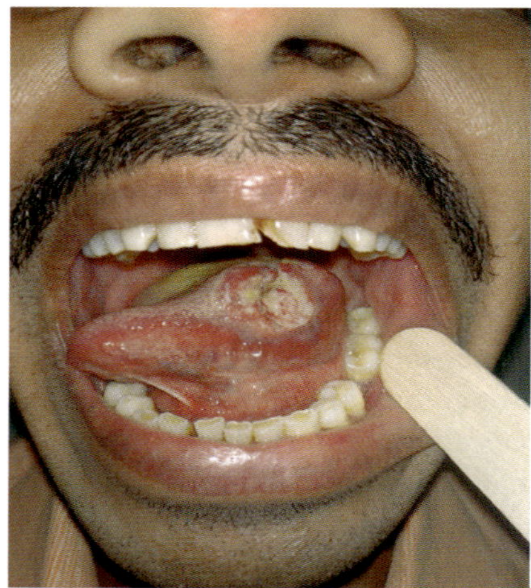

Fig. 2: Cancer of the left lateral border of the tongue.

Primary Tumor

A thorough examination of the oral cavity should be performed to examine the size, location, and extent of oral tumors, in addition to looking at dentition, presence of fibrous bands **(Fig. 1)**, and any other conditions in the oral cavity. It is imperative to assess the extent of the tumor in order to identify the possible difficulties in carrying out the laryngoscopy and the tracheal intubation. **Figure 2** shows a patient with cancer of the lateral border of the tongue.

Proliferative lesions along the airway may add to the difficulty at both bag-mask ventilation and laryngoscopy. These tumors can also bleed during laryngoscopic manipulation, especially tumors involving the base of the tongue and the vallecula.

Facial Defects

Previous surgeries, the external proliferation of tumors, radiation, etc., may lead to improper fit/seal of the face mask, making mask ventilation difficult, and sometimes even lead to bleeding due to manipulation.

Trismus

Fibrosis along the temporomandibular[11] joint due to primary tumor itself, due to radiation, submucous fibrosis due to tobacco chewing, etc. may hinder mouth opening. Unlike trismus secondary to inflammation, this may not be relieved after induction of general anesthesia, thus making orotracheal intubation and supraglottic airway insertion often impossible. Grades of trismus are provided in **Table 1**.[12]

TABLE 1: Grades of trismus.[12]

Grade	Specifics
M1	Interincisal mouth opening up to or >35 mm
M2	Interincisal mouth opening between 25 and 35 mm
M3	Interincisal mouth opening between 15 and 25 mm
M4	Interincisal mouth opening <15 mm

Ankyloglossia

As the tumor infiltrates the root of the tongue, it hinders the protrusion of the tongue. Due to the restricted tongue movement, lateral displacement of the tongue may not be possible during direct laryngoscopy, which may lead to poor glottis view and failed intubation.[13]

Dentition

The tumor, radiation, and tobacco chewing can lead to loosening, weakening, and destruction of the teeth. Both mask-ventilation and laryngoscopy may be difficult in edentulous patients.[13]

Nasal Pathology

The presence of intranasal anomalies like spurs, septal deviation, nasal polyps, concha bullosa, and increased size of the turbinates should be ruled out both clinically and using imaging [computed tomography (CT) scan or anterior/posterior rhinoscopy) to select the more suitable nares for smooth passage of tracheal tube nasally.[14] Patient history and clinical examination should be performed to assess comfort while breathing and feeling the blast of air on the back of the hand while alternately occluding the nares, after administration of a nasal vasoconstrictor. This may also help in preventing trauma during nasal intubation. In case of equal patency, the nostrils opposite to the side of surgery should be selected, especially for maxillectomies where the hard palate will have to be excised. Moreover, if there is no surgical preference, the right nostril should be preferred over left, as in case of right nostril, the bevel of the endotracheal tube (ETT) faces the nasal septum. This reduces the risk of damage to the nasal turbinates.[14-16]

Tracheomalacia

A long-standing large thyroid mass may weaken the tracheal cartilage and longitudinal elastic fibers. The trachea becomes soft and susceptible to collapse in such cases. A narrowing of >50% along the posterior wall is significant and such patients may have a complete collapse of the airway under anesthesia and may require tracheostomy or intra-operative aortopexy/bronchopexy to maintain a patent airway postoperatively.[17] Patients commonly present with asthma-like symptoms, which may be continuous or intermittent. Symptoms include prolonged and labored breathing, wheeze, or coughing. Thorough clinical examination and pulmonary function tests should be performed to rule out respiratory conditions. Bronchoscopy, fluoroscopy, multi-slice helical CT scan or magnetic resonance imaging (MRI) can be used to confirm the diagnosis preoperatively.

Airway Imaging

History and clinical examination should be complemented with reviewing the airway imaging. Most patients with head and neck cancer have some prior airway imaging performed for disease evaluation.

- *X-ray:* It is performed to help screen the site and size of the mass, compression, or deviation of the airway. Further investigations may be required to confirm the findings.
- *CT scan:* It is done to assess the extent of disease and airway compromise to help tailor the best anesthesia plan. The CT scan can also be used to assess the patency of either nostril and the presence of aberrant spurs, which could cause tracheal cuff damage during a nasotracheal intubation.
- *Ultrasonography (USG):* A preoperative ultrasound neck should be performed, especially in patients with difficult airway, to identify cricothyroid membrane, its anatomy, and any associated aberrant vessels. This might be extremely helpful if the need for emergency cricothyroidotomy arises.
- *Dynamic MRI:* It is used in uncommon airway pathologies such as in diagnosis of tracheobronchomalacia in children and in sleep studies for visualization of upper airway dynamics, etc.
- *Three-dimensional (3D) printing:* It can be used in simulation of airway for precision and preoperative planning.
- *Virtual endoscopy:* This is a radiological simulation of the anatomy of the airway extending from the oropharynx up to the carina. Previous CT scan images are reconstructed to create a video (3D "fly-through") of the airway anatomy. This further improves our

interpretation of the two-dimensional (2D) CT scan images and helps better identify a difficult airway to make an appropriate airway management plan.[18]

Diagnostic Airway Procedures

The patient may be subjected to diagnostic procedures prior to major surgeries like an indirect laryngoscopy (IDL) or awake fiber optic laryngoscopy (FOL) performed in the outpatient department to assess the extent of the disease. This may give an important clue regarding the extent of disease and airway compromise and help formulate an airway plan. It is important to note the date on which these procedures or diagnostic investigations were performed, as the disease may have progressed significantly in some patients from the time of the pervious assessment and the airway may be further compromised.

Patients with HNC may also be posted for short diagnostic procedures like direct or microlaryngoscopy usually under general anesthesia, to assess the extent of disease. These are extremely vital procedures that help to delineate the disease and decide on the further course of management. Findings from these procedures will help the anesthesiologists to plan for airway management.

Previous Cancer Therapies

Previous Surgery

The airway should be carefully evaluated in patients who have undergone previous surgery. Presence of flaps, mandibulectomy, previous tracheostomy, airway defects, etc. may make both mask ventilation and tracheal intubation challenging. An awake tracheal intubation may often be required in these cases

Radiation

Radiation can significantly alter the airway making airway management difficult. Radiation can lead to fibrosis of the temporomandibular joint leading to trismus. It also affects dentition leading to loss of teeth. Edema secondary to radiation affects the tongue (glossomegaly and glossitis) and epiglottis. Kheterpal et al. found radiation to neck as an independent risk factor in patients with difficult bag-mask ventilation. Radiation-induced fibrosis in the oropharyngeal region makes tissue extremely rigid and noncompliant, which presents as poor submental compliance. Obtaining a satisfactory glottic view might be difficult in such patients. Patients receiving head and neck radiation may also be associated with limited neck movement. In addition, considering the laryngeal edema and increased risk of bleeding, anesthesiologist should prefer to use smaller sized ETT in these patients.[19,20] These effects of radiation may not always be visible; hence, anesthesiologists should keep these changes in mind while managing such patients. Performing a tracheostomy may also be difficult in a patient with a postradiation neck. **Figure 3** shows a postradiation neck.

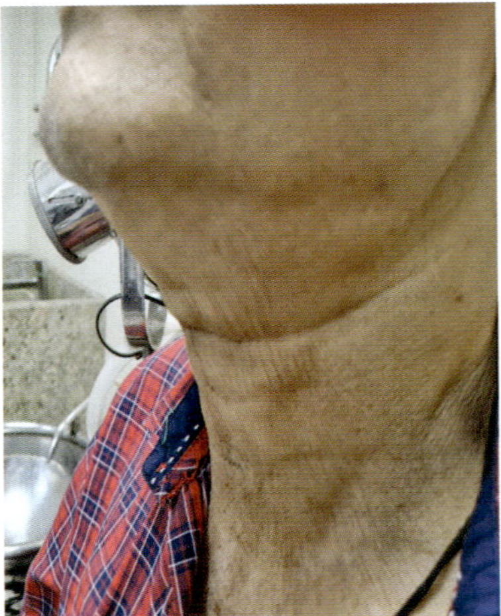

Fig. 3: The neck post radiation.

PATIENT EDUCATION AND COUNSELING

Patient education and counseling should be conducted preoperatively to make them understand the surgery and airway procedures performed. This includes counseling regarding the surgery, anesthesia, and the recovery process including the need for a tracheostomy intraoperatively or postoperatively. This improves patient satisfaction and compliance with recuperation.

INTRAOPERATIVE AIRWAY MANAGEMENT

It is essential to make a plan of airway management prior to induction of anesthesia. The decision of whether to secure the airway awake or asleep is crucial. This planning should include a discussion with the surgeon, careful history and assessment of the airway, and a review of airway imaging. If the airway management is planned under general anesthesia, a backup plan for rescue ventilation in case of inability to perform tracheal intubation, including equipment and preparedness for performing an emergency cricothyroidotomy if complete ventilation failure occurs, should be made in advance. Patent with intraoral surgery usually require a nasal ETT. Skull-base fractures and bleeding disorders (risk of epistaxis) are relative contraindications.

Tracheostomy Under Local Anesthesia

In patients in whom there is a prior plan for tracheotomy, for example, a laryngectomy where the glottic opening is severely reduced or a plan for extensive resection where the airway patency is likely to be compromised post operatively, the patient may undergo tracheostomy under local anesthesia prior to administration of general anesthesia.

Awake Tracheal Intubation

Awake tracheal intubation (ATI) is considered the gold standard in these patients with an anticipated difficult airway. It is prudent to familiarize oneself with various available techniques. The guidelines for ATI in adults help practitioners to better plan, perform, and address complications related to the procedure. A combination of sedation, topicalization, oxygenation throughout the procedure and proper performance of the procedure is the key the to success.[21]

Oxygenation

During ATI, nasal oxygen should be continued throughout the procedure. The use of high-flow nasal cannula oxygen (HFNO), especially when sedation is administered can increase the margin of safety. The use of HFNO during ATI techniques has additional benefits while providing supplemental oxygen. These include improved spread of local anesthetic during airway topicalization, expansion of the caliber of the airway passages that a flexible bronchoscope may pass through, reduced risk of contact bleeding of friable tissues, as well as decreased misting of the scope tip.[22]

Premedication

To reduce the risk of bleeding in case of nasal intubation, topical vasoconstrictor agents like pure alpha-agonist agents (oxymetazoline and xylometazoline) can be used. In addition, anti-sialagogue agents such as glycopyrrolate given intravenously reduce the number of secretions and ensure a dry field for better visibility during the procedure. In addition, these also ensure that local anesthetic used to anesthetize the airway does not get diluted with secretions or suctioned out during intubation using the flexible bronchoscope. Glycopyrrolate, if used, should be administered at least 15 minutes prior to the procedure, giving enough time for its action.[23]

Sedation

Patients with head and neck malignancies might have a compromised airway, and hence anesthesiologists should be judicious with the use of sedation. However, mild sedation helps in tolerating awake intubation and increases the success of the procedure. The most commonly used sedatives for awake intubation include intravenous infusion of dexmedetomidine or remifentanil, mainly due to shorter duration of action, ability to titrate, and increased margin of safety. Proper patient counseling prior to the procedure is paramount and increases patient tolerability, often with no requirement for sedation.

Anesthetizing the Airway

Intranasal 2% lignocaine jelly, viscous lignocaine gargle (2% concentration), pressurized bottles using 10% lignocaine, atomizers can be used to anesthetize parts of the airway for awake intubation. The airway can further be anesthetized using "Spray As You GO (SAYGO)" technique. This is, however, administered while performing fiberoptic bronchoscopy. The local anesthetic is injected through the suction port of the scope either using a syringe or bypassing via an epidural catheter passed through the suction port. It anesthetizes part of the airway distal to scope. More invasive techniques include translaryngeal injection and regional nerve blocks such as the glossopharyngeal nerve block and superior laryngeal nerve block may also be used to anesthetize the airway prior to performing awake intubation. However, these invasive techniques are not routinely recommended or required when good topical anesthesia is used. Largely, the dictum should be a combination of good counseling, effective topicalization, with or without sedation.

Types of Awake Tracheal Intubations

Intubation with the flexible bronchoscope (FB): Most patients, especially with oral pathologies, require a nasal ETT. The FB can be used to intubate these patients nasally. A retromolar technique of insertion may also be used. The ETT is mounted over the scope after adequate lubrication, and the scope is introduced along the base of the nose in case of nasal intubation and between the molars and cheeks in case of retromolar intubation and guided through the vocal cords. This procedure takes time and requires a skilled operator. The passage of the ETT over the scope through the vocal cords is not performed under vision, combining this technique with a VL or direct laryngoscopy can overcome this limitation. Excess secretions, bleeding or difficulty in maneuvering the scope around the tumor may make this procedure challenging. Alternatively, a hybrid technique using an additional device, such as video laryngoscope, may also assist with passing the flexible bronchoscope over the base of tongue.

Awake video laryngoscopy: Awake video laryngoscopy (VL) is gaining popularity as an alternate technique to awake FB intubation because of ease of performance and less time taken. A meta-analysis comparing awake intubation using VL and FB, found VL to be associated with shorter intubation time.[24] There was no reported difference between the two techniques regarding first attempt success rate, rate of complication, and level of patient satisfaction. However, most studies in this meta-analysis did not include patients with trismus or intraoral cancers where use of VL may not always be feasible and FB-guided intubation still remain the gold standard.[25] It is important to note that in the presence of friable tumors susceptible to bleeding on contact, which may cause the airway to deteriorate significantly after airway instrumentation, techniques such as VL are best avoided and intubation using a flexible bronchoscope should be preferred.

Retrograde intubation: This involves the passage of an ETT over a guide (epidural catheter/guidewire) passed in a retrograde manner through the cricothyroid membrane/transtracheal puncture using an epidural needle or intravenous cannula (16/18 G) to allow passage of a retrograde guidewire and advancement of the guidewire in a cephalad direction until it emerges from the upper airway (nasal or oral cavity). This procedure needs patient cooperation and at least 0.5 cm of mouth opening is to retrieve the retrograde guide.[26] Delivery of the tracheal tube into the trachea can be facilitated by using a variety of techniques such as using an airway exchange catheter (AEC) or passing the guidewire through the distal end of the working channel of a flexible bronchoscope or utilization of the guidewire as a visual guide to the laryngeal inlet. Though the intubation is completely blind, the success rate is higher than blind nasal as the ETT is railroaded over a guide present in the trachea. Complications[26] include injury to vocal cords, bleeding secondary to aberrant vessels from superior thyroid artery,[27] and injury to the thyroid gland.

Blind nasal intubation: This involves blindly guiding the ETT through the nose toward the larynx. The ETT passage is guided by the help of the patient's breath sounds or an end-tidal carbon dioxide ($EtCO_2$) trace during spontaneous breathing. This procedure requires skill and experience and has a low success rate. Complications include trauma to oral, pharyngeal, and laryngeal structures as tube is passed blindly into the trachea.

Blind techniques should be discouraged in the era of VL and FB-guided intubations to avoid complications and improve intubation success rates.

Monitoring

American Society of Anesthesiologist (ASA) recommendations for monitoring should be instituted for all the patients prior to the induction of anesthesia. This includes continuous ECG monitoring, pulse oximeter monitoring, $EtCO_2$, and noninvasive blood pressure monitoring. Bispectral index (BIS) monitoring is recommended especially if total intravenous anesthesia (TIVA) is being planned to titrate anesthetic doses. Peripheral nerve stimulator (PNS) is also recommended to titrate muscle relaxant dosing and reversal. More invasive monitoring such as arterial cannulation and central venous cannulation, should be reserved for patients with cardiac conditions or when extensive blood loss is anticipated.

Peri-intubation Oxygenation

- *Preoxygenation:* Patients with HNC are anticipated difficult airways and hence, preoxygenation is vital. One could use a facemask or in some cases, where adequate fitting of facemask is not possible due to facial defects, alternate methods of preoxygenation such as HFNO may be used.
- *Apneic oxygenation:* Apneic oxygenation is a technique to constantly replete oxygen stores during period of apnea. This leverages extra time for an anesthesiologist to secure a definitive airway. Apneic oxygenation can be established by delivering high-flow oxygen using a nasal oxygenation technique called transnasal humidified rapid-insufflation ventilatory exchange (THRIVE)[28] or alternately by supraglottic jet oxygenation and ventilation (SJOV).[29]

General Anesthesia and Tracheal Intubation

Depending on the plan of airway management, the induction of general anesthesia may vary. More commonly used techniques include a complete total intravenous anesthesia (TIVA) or balanced anesthesia using a combination of inhaled and intravenous anesthetics, analgesics such as opioids, and sedatives such as benzodiazepine. Inhalational induction is slow and titratable, with the theoretical advantage of the ability to wake up the patient in case of airway obstruction. However, it's important to note that in case of total obstruction, patient will not be able to exhale gases, and hypoxia will still occur. In addition, it does not provide adequate intubating conditions, making an otherwise normal airway difficult to secure. Muscle relaxants should be used at the time of induction of anesthesia, especially for intubation to improve glottis view during direct laryngoscopy (DL). However, HNC surgeries being surface surgeries, do not require profound relaxation during the further course of the surgery.

Following oral surgery, depending upon the extent of the resection and reconstruction, a decision is made intraoperatively as to whether to perform a delayed extubation (DE)—keep the nasal tube overnight postoperatively, and extubate the next morning or perform a tracheostomy on table. This decision is often subjective. **Figures 4A and 4B** show reconstruction with bulky pedicle flaps. A study including 720 major oral cancer surgeries who underwent DE or on table tracheostomy (TT), a DE strategy after major oral cancer surgery was found to be a safe alternative to TT in a selected group of patients. On multivariable analysis, T1–T2 tumor stage, absence of extensive resection, primary closure or reconstruction using fascio-cutaneous flap, absence of preoperative radiation, no neck dissection or unilateral neck dissection, and shorter duration of anesthesia were independent predictors for a safe DE **(Flowchart 1)**.[30]

Types of Endotracheal Tubes Used

Ring–Adair–Elwyn (RAE) Tubes

The North-pole ETT made of ivory, which curves away from the surgical site is most commonly used ETT used nasal intubation in HNC surgeries.[31] These tubes are much softer than the routine polyvinyl chloride tubes causing less trauma during insertion. RAE tubes maintain a fixed contour similar to the average facial profile, thus, allowing for oral cavity surgery whilst minimizing surgical field interference from bulky connections between the tube and ventilator circuit. However, they are opaque, obscuring any tube blockade and due to the preformed curve, suctioning is not easily performed through the ETT. Moreover, the length, narrower lumen, and preformed curve add to the resistance to spontaneous breathing. Hence, it is recommended to cut these tubes along the prelabeled black mark to reduce airway resistance and facilitate suctioning in the postoperative period.[32] The insertion of north-pole ETT over the flexible bronchoscope is also difficult due to the curvature. The North Pole tube needs to be straightened manually to be loaded over the bronchoscope.

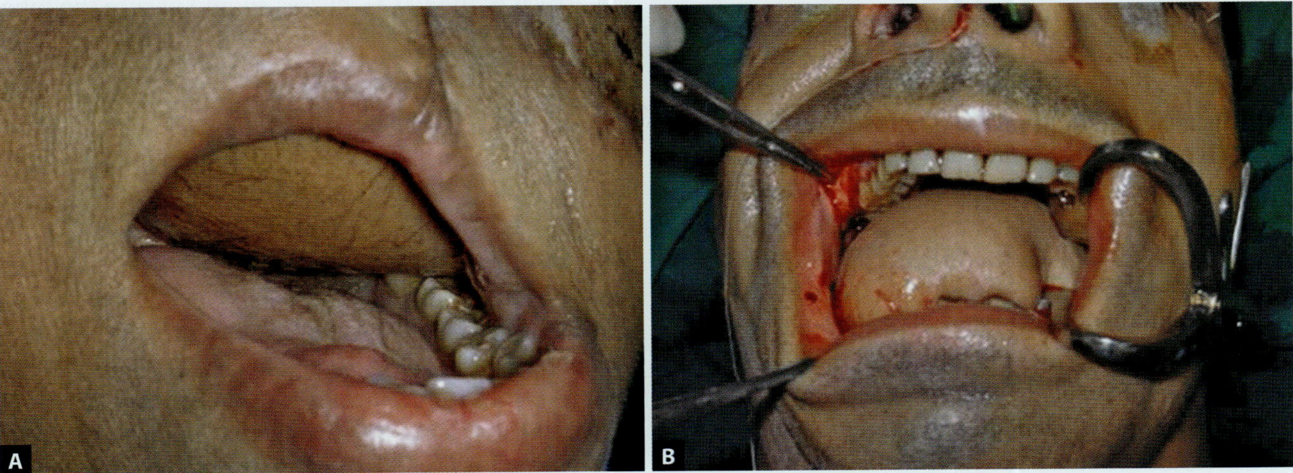

Figs. 4A and 4B: Surgical reconstruction with a bulky oral pedicle flap.

Flexometallic Tubes

The advantage of flexometallic ETT is that it is resistant to kinking and compression, making them particularly suitable for oral cancer surgery since the tube and circuit can be easily secured and draped away from the operating field. They are also less traumatic compared to a conventional polyvinylchloride (PVC) tracheal tube. However, some of these ETT might be opaque and have a floppy nature that makes them difficult to insert.

Parker Flex-Tip Tube

These tubes have a curved, centered, tapered, and flexible distal tip with a posterior facing bevel. These features are intended to decrease the risk of the tube tip impinging on laryngeal structures during railroading by reducing the size of the gap between the introducer device and the inner wall of the tube compared to a conventional PVC tracheal tube.

Electromyographic Tube

Intraoperative nerve monitoring (IONM) is being increasingly used to help identify the nerve. The common indication includes thyroid surgery, partial laryngectomy, neck dissection, carotid endarterectomy, etc. These are standard PVC tubes with conductive silver ink electrodes. There is a dark black crossband that guides in electromyographic (EMG) tube placement. These tubes have a minimum outer diameter of 8.8 mm, and hence, are preferentially used for oral intubation.[33]

POSTOPERATIVE AIRWAY MANAGEMENT PLAN

Tracheostomy versus Endotracheal Tube

Tracheostomy was traditionally considered a safer technique of airway management in patients undergoing HCN surgeries. Postoperative edema, reduced airway caliber, altered anatomy, and postoperative bleeding are main reasons for advocating for tracheostomy. However, recent studies have questioned this practice. They found that the rate of airway complication was much higher in tracheostomy group. The alternative to tracheostomy is the DE strategy in select patients, where the ETT is kept overnight, allowing the edema to settle and patients are extubated next day in the morning. The DE strategy is associated with fewer complications and faster recovery as compared to tracheostomy. However, it carries the risk of airway compromise if not performed in the appropriate patient. Extensive resections crossing the midline, bulky flaps, especially osteocutaneous flaps such as free-fibula flaps are major indications for performing tracheostomy. Gupta et al. suggested that tracheostomy should be preferred if radiation was previously received at the surgical site, bilateral neck dissection was performed or there was extensive resection or the use of bulky flaps.[34]

Flowchart 1: An algorithm to select patients suitable for delayed extubation after major oral cancer surgery.

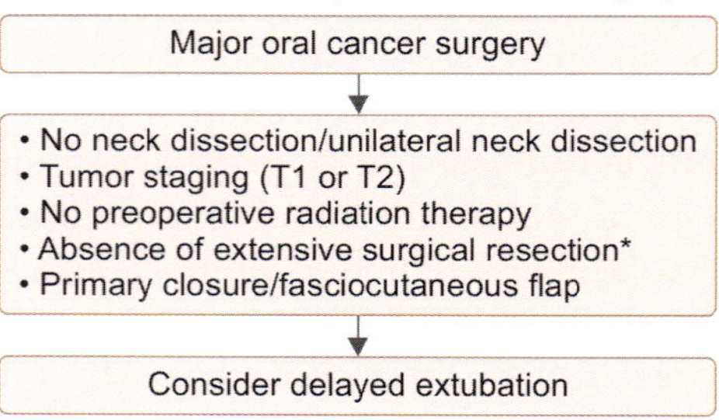

*Extensive surgical resection

- *Tongue resections* crossing midline, which included near-total and total glossectomy
- *Mandibular resections* involving genial tubercle, which included extended and middle one-third mandibulectomy
- *Maxillary resections* crossing the midline or extending into the soft palate

Myatra et al.[30] in a prospective study of 720 patients operated for major oral cancer surgery, identified independent predictors for a safe delayed extubation. **(Flowchart 1)**. Confirm that the throat pack, if used, has been removed prior to transfer to the post anesthesia care unit (PACU).

Airway Monitoring

On arrival in the PACU, nurses should ensure the tube is in proper position, free of secretions, and well-secured. Vigilant monitoring is essential for any airway obstruction, hypoventilation or apnea with sedation or opioids, and bleeding. All patients should be closely monitored for airway patency and tube malposition. Patients can be maintained overnight on T-piece or on a mechanical ventilator with spontaneous breathing using pressure support (PS) ventilation, depending on the available resources. Humidification is must to ensure tube tolerance. Dry oxygen might irritate the airway, causing coughing, sloughing of mucosa, thickening, and retention of secretions with impaired mucociliary clearance, increasing the risk of tube blockage.[35] Humidification may be provided passively using heat and moisture exchanger (HME) filters or actively using nebulizers.[36]

Extubation in Post Anesthesia Care Unit

In addition to a preoperatively difficult airway, laryngopharyngeal edema due to surgical handling, bulky flaps encroaching into oral cavity, and the risk of postoperative bleeding may make resecuring these airways postextubation extremely difficult. Hence, extubation in these patients is considered as high risk.[37] Extubation being an elective procedure, should be performed with careful planning in these patients Airway edema can be checked either by performing laryngoscopy or by doing a cuff-leak test. Steroids can be administered on admission to the recovery unit to reduce airway edema.[38,39] Some centers advocate use of steroids 4 hours prior to extubation. If used, they should be continued at least till 12 hours postextubation.[40] Adrenaline nebulization may also be used to reduce airway obstruction secondary to edema.

Extubation should be performed with a plan to resecure the airway in case of extubation failure, preferably in the daytime and when there is adequate staffing. In case of bleeding from surgical site or severe edema, extubation should be delayed. Once the patient is completely awake with intact airway reflexes, extubation should be attempted. Suctioning of the ETT followed by the oropharynx should be performed prior to extubation.

In borderline cases where there is a high possibility of extubation failure, the surgeon should be present during extubation to perform a tracheostomy if needed.[37] In such cases, extubation may be performed over an AEC or bronchoscope. Care should be taken to keep the AEC well above the carina and no oxygenation/ventilation should be provided through this catheter. The patient may be oxygenated using a facemask or nasal cannula when the AEC is in place. The AEC should be removed as soon as there are no concerns about airway patency.

Reconfirm that the throat pack has been removed prior to extubation. Postextubation, patients should receive oxygen via a simple nasal cannula and be monitored for airway compromise. Patients should be encouraged to take deep breaths and do incentive spirometry, if feasible.

IMMEDIATE AIRWAY COMPLICATIONS: POSTEXTUBATION

Airway patency should be closely monitored following extubation. Common causes of postoperative airway obstruction are listed in **Box 1**.[41] Management of a few commonly occurring causes of post-operative airway obstruction are described as follows:

BOX 1: Common causes of postoperative airway obstruction in head and neck cancer patients.[41]

- Laryngeal spasm
- Laryngeal edema
- Vocal cord paralysis
- Foreign body in the airway (secretions and throat pack)
- Neck hematoma
- Bleeding in the airway
- Inadequate reversal of neuromuscular blockade
- Reduced venous drainage
- Laryngeal or pharyngeal infections
- Obstructive sleep apnea

Stridor

Edema from trauma to the airway is the most common cause of immediate stridor postextubation. This can be managed by sitting the patient up and giving a dose of intravenous steroids. Nebulization with epinephrine may also be considered postextubation.[42] If the stridor persists and the patient is deteriorating, examine the airway under anesthesia to rule out other causes such as a blood clot, secretions, or retained throat pack. Reintubation may be required in some cases.

Laryngeal Compromise

Edema and malfunctions of the glottis cause laryngeal compromise, which can lead to airway obstruction. This usually happens after Ludwig's angina or a dental abscess drainage. It can start with postoperative sore throat and then progress to hoarseness of voice, weak cough, deep throat pain, and odynophagia, finally ending with stridor, usually associated with difficult intubation. Close monitoring and early intervention are the keys to early prediction and successful management of these patients.

Bleeding

In case of major bleeding such as carotid blowout or rapidly expanding hematoma, the patient requires urgent surgical and anesthetic intervention. The removal of surgical skin clips may help to reduce airway deterioration. The patient should be immediately transferred to the operation theatre. Reintubation with a smaller size tracheal tube may be needed.

Postobstructive Negative Pressure Pulmonary Edema

This commonly happens in the immediate postoperative time when the patient is trying to breathe while the airway is closed as he/she is biting on tracheal tube. This will create negative intrathoracic pressures, and this will lead to pulmonary edema. Using bite blocks can reduce this risk. Deflating the cuff of the tube allowing the patient to breathe around it may be helpful. Using continuous positive airway pressure (CPAP) may help; but, if there is significant hypoxia, reintubation should not be delayed. Early management with reintubation and ventilation will help with full recovery.

Laryngospasm

It usually happens due to stimulation during a light plane of anesthesia but may occur due to blood, secretions, or foreign body in the larynx. This can be managed by clearing the oropharynx, applying CPAP with 100% oxygen, followed by deepening the plane of anesthesia using intravenous anesthetic agents. Rapid and short-acting muscle relaxant such as succinylcholine may be needed if laryngospasm persists. Reintubation may be required in certain cases.

Most tracheostomies performed for HNC surgeries are temporary. On the other hand, laryngostoma done for laryngectomies are permanent. Airway complications with tracheostomy include obstructed tube, displaced tube, infection at tracheostomy site, and lower respiratory tract infection.[43] Long-term complications include trachea-cutaneous fistula and a blocked tube.[44] In patients managed with DE, tube-blockade secondary to airway secretions or collected blood and inability to maintain a patent airway post-extubation are the two most important complications. The rate of airway complications is, however, more common with tracheostomy.[43]

CARE OF PATIENT WITH TRACHEOSTOMY

Temporary tracheostomy care includes humidification, secure fixation, and regular cleaning of the inner cannula in a productive chest (4 hours) with an 8-hour gap at night and for mechanically ventilated patients. A separate cannula should be placed at bedside, allowing for a quick change if ventilator parameters suggest. The entire assembly should be changed after 30 days. If the tube is suspected to be blocked, the suction catheter should be passed, failure to do so suggests a possibility of a tube block or misplacement. While changing tube, methods of confirmation like $ETCO_2$ should be readily available. Every ward having patients with a tracheostomy tube should have experienced staff, daily checks at the time of shift change, and clear procedure guidelines in case of emergencies. In case of emergencies of blocked tube, they must be aware that bag-mask ventilation may not be possible, and changing of cannula or suction in case of laryngostoma will most often relieve obstruction. It is always better to replace a partially displaced tube rather than attempt to reposition it. As a bid to buy time, one can deflate the cuff in case of a cuffed tube allowing the patient to breathe around the tube.[45,46] Patients with laryngostomas are neck-only breathers and there should be awareness, patient bands, or signs in patient-care areas to avoid facemask ventilation or oral intubation in these patients during an airway emergency.

SPECIAL CONSIDERATIONS FOR SPECIFIC SURGERIES

Laryngectomy

Total laryngectomy involves en bloc removal of laryngeal structures including epiglottis, hyoid, and variable part of trachea with creation of permanent tracheostomy for breathing.

Preoperative Considerations

Airway assessment should focus on clinical signs related to change in voice, dysphagia, stridor, and difficulty sleeping, which might be clues to a difficult airway and chances of airway obstruction under anesthesia. Patients presenting with stridor may require emergency tracheostomy. Tracheostomy is usually avoided in the elective setting due to concerns of seeding of disease at the stoma sites. Adrenaline nebulization, steroids, and the use of HFNO can help buy time while an airway plan is formulated. HFNO helps to splint the airway open, thereby partially overcoming the obstruction and giving the patient symptomatic relief, while awaiting definitive airway management.

Intraoperative Considerations

Tracheal intubation is usually easy; however, smaller-size ETTs are required due to airway narrowing due to the disease. FB-guided intubation might not be a suitable choice as it may cork an already narrow airway leading to catastrophic occlusion of the narrow laryngeal aperture. When the laryngostoma (end tracheostomy) is created, the oral ETT should be removed and a flexometallic ETT should be placed within the laryngostoma to continue ventilation.

The ETT should be properly secured, preferably with sutures. One should ensure, that the ETT is not pushed inside during surgery, resulting in an endobronchial intubation. The tube should be inserted just enough that cuff is visible at the laryngostoma to avoid leak of gases and air entry on auscultation is bilaterally equal

Postoperative Considerations

A pediatric mask or tracheostomy mask should be placed over laryngostoma for oxygen delivery. A tracheostomy tube should always be available on beside of the patient in the event of the need for emergency ventilation. It should be remembered that the patients with an end stoma (larynx removed) are "neck-only" breathers, therefore, intubation and facemask ventilation should not be attempted in an emergency

Endolaryngeal Vocal Fold Surgery

This is performed with the use of laser or by means of a micro-laryngeal endoscope. Indications include vocal cord nodule, polyp, leukoplakia, etc. In terms of surgery, it is not a morbid procedure, but due to shared airway, it is extremely challenging for the anesthesiologist. There is an added concern of airway fire when these surgeries are performed using laser technique.

Airway Management and Ventilation

Mechanical ventilation can be performed continuously with the use of an ETT with a smaller-diameter like the microlaryngoscopy (ML) tubes, which are of smaller diameter and longer in length with a cuff placed distally to avoid rupture secondary to the surgical instruments. These are good for surgeries of anterior part of vocal cords, as the posterior parts get obscured by the tube. Laser-resistant tubes can also be used during laser surgery with minimal risk of airway fire. Intermittent jet ventilation through a jet catheter or via the side port of the ML scope or intermittent intubation and ventilation are other techniques used for ventilation. A recent method of oxygenation described as a part of tubeless surgery is apneic oxygenation using HFNO called THRIVE. The advantage of this technique is that there is no tube in the field of the surgeon and no interruption for ventilation either. However, during laser surgery, THRIVE should be used only by those experienced in laser surgery and those who understand the fire triangle well. In addition to the type of tubes, recommendations regarding the safety of operating room (OR) personnel and patients and preventing laser fire should be strictly followed in the operation room.

Thyroid Surgery

Anesthesia of thyroid surgery includes preoperative assessment of airway compromise and thyroid function, careful airway management plan in case of retrosternal extension of thyroid, and postoperative management of thyroid functions and serum calcium in addition to understanding the management of complications specifically related to bilateral vocal cord palsy and bilateral hematoma. While the use of intraoperative neuromonitoring has significantly reduced recurrent laryngeal nerve injury, it may still occur due to poor placement of electrodes or inadequate reversal from muscle relaxants at the time of monitoring.

Airway Assessment

Assessment of tracheomalacia is important in case of a long-standing and large-size thyroid mass. In addition, thyroid function needs to be assessed preoperatively. In case of neuromonitoring, the correct placement of ETT electrode is essential with respect to vocal cords. A videolaryngoscope may be of assistance, for vocal cord visualization and documentation of the electrode between the vocal cords. In case of anticipated tracheal collapse due to tracheomalacia, or retrosternal goiter, where collapse of airway might be expected, it is better to maintain spontaneous breathing in patients till a secured airway is established. The use of reinforced tubes is preferred to prevent compression of ETT due to external compression. FB might be used to ensure ETT is pushed beyond the point of extrinsic compression. In case of extrinsic compression, normal-sized tube might be used. But in cases where tumor infiltrates the trachea, it might be a fixed deformity, and smaller-sized tubes might be required. In a consensus statement for the management of tracheomalacia, consensus was for a rigid bronchoscope to always be present in the OR to manage the airway in case of airway collapse.[47]

Postoperative Considerations

Postoperatively, recurrent laryngeal nerve (RLN) palsy may be transient or permanent. Most cases of RLN palsy tend to recover and do not call for intervention unless the patient goes into stridor, in which case one might have to resort to performing a tracheostomy. In case bilateral neck hematoma leading to airway compromise, neck sutures can be removed in an emergency in the PACU itself to relieve airway compression, while the OR is prepared for hemostatic surgery.[48] A smaller size ETT should be considered for reintubation

Surgeries Requiring Neuromuscular Monitoring

The two most common surgeries in head and neck cancer that require neuromonitoring are thyroid surgeries for RLN identification and parotid surgery for facial nerve branch identification.

Thyroid Surgery

Permanent RLN injuries account between 0.5% and 5% and transient injuries account between 1% and 30% following thyroid surgery.[49-51] IONM helps in nerve identification and dissection without causing nerve injury. For anesthesiologist, the induction should be carried out using an intermediate or short-acting muscle relaxant, such that effects of relaxant completely wear off at the time of intraoperative monitoring. Special ETTs with conductive silver ink electrodes are used, which have a dark black cross-band that is positioned between the vocal cords. During the time of dissection and RLN stimulation, the patient should not be under any effect of a muscle relaxant. Muscle relaxants reduce the amplitude of evoked responses, making IONM less sensitive technique to prevent RLN injury. Anesthesia may be maintained using a continuous infusion of intravenous anesthetic agents like propofol, dexmedetomidine, remifentanil, lidocaine, etc. At very high doses, propofol might suppress the compound muscle action potential. Adjuvant agents help to minimize the dose of propofol to maintain anesthesia. Ventilation can be maintained using air and oxygen. Inhalational agents if used should be at a minimum alveolar concentration less than one. The neuromuscular monitor should be used to check the action of adductor pollicis.

Parotid Surgery

Intraoperative nerve monitoring (IONM) is used during parotid surgery to avoid dissection of facial nerve branches, which are closely associated with the parotid gland. The electrodes are placed along the facial nerve distribution on the face. The basic physiology and anesthetic management are very similar to thyroid surgery.

Transoral Robotic Surgeries (TORS)

Minimally invasive robotic surgery may be performed for oropharyngeal tumors. The *Da Vinci* robot is remotely controlled by the surgeon who sits at a console, while one robotic arm holds the camera (endoscope) and the other two hands hold left and right-hand instruments. The surgery is carried out with patient's feet toward the anesthesia machine, and the robot is moved into position, with arms positioned over patient's chest. This limits access to patient's face, neck, and chest. The anesthesia plan is similar to that described earlier. Nasal RAE tubes are preferred. A longer-length anesthesia circuit is required. The face should be well padded, eyes covered using eyeglasses, and adequate muscle relaxation provided to avoid injury due to the robotic arms. If extensive airway edema is suspected, a delayed extubation or tracheostomy may be performed.

CONCLUSION

Airway management in HNC patients is a complex and challenging task due to factors related to tumor obstruction, anatomical alterations, previous radiation or surgeries. Therefore, a careful history taking with thorough preoperative airway assessment using specific tests and radiological imagining can help to anticipate a difficult airway and plan the tracheal intubation. Proper patient counseling, with careful airway management planning, peri-intubation oxygenation and preparedness for rescue ventilation are paramount. Intra-operative concerns include shared airway, risk of airway bleeding, airway obstruction, aspiration and failed tracheostomy. A delayed extubation strategy is a safe alternative to tracheostomy in a select group of patients. In these patients extubation is always considered 'at risk' and should be performed electively with a back up rescue plan. A multi-disciplinary, collaborative approach including the anesthesiologist, onco-surgeon, nurse, operative room and ICU team is essential to improve patient and outcomes.

REFERENCES

1. Shah JP, Gil Z. Current concepts in management of oral cancer: surgery. Oral Oncol. 2009;45(4-5):394-401.
2. Barsouk A, Aluru JS, Rawla P, Saginala K, Barsouk A. Epidemiology, risk factors, and prevention of head and neck squamous cell carcinoma. Med Sci (Basel). 2023;11(2):42.
3. Mehrotra R, Singh M, Gupta RK, Singh M, Kapoor AK. Trends of prevalence and pathological spectrum of

head and neck cancers in North India. Indian J Cancer. 2005;42(2):89-93.
4. Bagal S, Budukh A, Thakur JS, Dora T, Qayyumi B, Khanna D, et al. Head and neck cancer burden in India: an analysis from published data of 37 population-based cancer registries. Ecancermedicalscience. 2023;17:1603.
5. Sofferman RA, Johnson DL, Spencer RF. Lost airway during anesthesia induction: alternatives for management. Laryngoscope. 1997;107(11 Pt 1):1476-81.
6. Wiegand DA, Latz B, Zwillich CW, Wiegand L. Upper airway resistance and geniohyoid muscle activity in normal men during wakefulness and sleep. J Appl Physiol. 1990;69(4):1252-61.
7. Cunningham DP, Basmajian JV. Electromyography of genioglossus and geniohyoid muscles during deglutition. Anat Rec. 1969;165(3):401-9.
8. Albahout KS, Lopez RA. Anatomy, Head and Neck, Pharynx. In: StatPearls [Internet]. Treasure Island (FL): StatPearls Publishing; 2025. Available from: https://www.ncbi.nlm.nih.gov/books/NBK544271/[Last accessed March, 2025].
9. Iglesias Docampo LC, Arrazubi Arrula V, Baste Rotllan N, Carral Maseda A, Cirauqui Cirauqui B, et al. SEOM clinical guidelines for the treatment of head and neck cancer (2017). Clin Transl Oncol. 2018;20(1):75-83.
10. Homer J, Fardy M. Surgery in head and neck cancer: United Kingdom national multidisciplinary guidelines. J Laryngol Otol. 2016;130(S2):S68-70.
11. Gastmeier P, Sohr D, Breier A, Behnke M, Geffers C. Prolonged duration of operation: an indicator of complicated surgery or of surgical (mis) management? Infection. 2011;39(3):211-5.
12. More CB, Das S, Patel H, Adalja C, Kamatchi V, Venkatesh R. Proposed clinical classification for oral submucous fibrosis. Oral oncology. 2012;48(3):200-2.
13. Dougherty TB, Clayman GL. Airway management of surgical patients with head and neck malignancies. Anesthesiol Clin North Am. 1998;16(3):547-62.
14. Prasanna D, Bhat S. Nasotracheal intubation: An overview. J MaxillofacOral Surgery. 2014;13(4):366-72.
15. Smith J, Reid A. Identifying the more patent nostril before nasotracheal intubation. Anaesthesia. 2001;56(3):258-62.
16. Thota RS, Doctor JR. Evaluation of paranasal sinuses on available computed tomography in head and neck cancer patients: An assessment tool for nasotracheal intubation. Indian J Anaesth. 2016;60(12):960-1.
17. Murgu SD, Colt HG. Tracheobronchomalacia and excessive dynamic airway collapse. Respirology. 2006;11(4):388-406.
18. Ahmad I, Keane O, Muldoon S. Enhancing airway assessment of patients with head and neck pathology using virtual endoscopy. Indian J of Anaesth. 2017;61(10):782-6.
19. Sroussi HY, Epstein JB, Bensadoun RJ, Saunders DP, Lalla RV, Migliorati CA, et al. Common oral complications of head and neck cancer radiation therapy: mucositis, infections, saliva change, fibrosis, sensory dysfunctions, dental caries, periodontal disease, and osteoradionecrosis. Cancer Med. 2017;6(12):2918-31.
20. Kheterpal S, Martin L, Shanks AM, Tremper KK. Prediction and outcomes of impossible mask ventilation: a review of 50,000 anesthetics. Anesthesiology. 2009;110(4):891-7.
21. Aziz MF, Kristensen MS. From variance to guidance for awake tracheal intubation. Anaesthesia. 2020;75(4):442-6.
22. Badiger S, John M, Fearnley RA, Ahmad I. Optimizing oxygenation and intubation conditions during awake fibreoptic intubation using a high-flow nasal oxygen-delivery system. Br J Anaesth. 2015;115(4):629-32.
23. Ramkumar V. Preparation of the patient and the airway for awake intubation. Indian J Anaesth. 2011;55(5):442-7.
24. Alhomary M, Ramadan E, Curran E, Walsh S. Videolaryngoscopy vs. fibreoptic bronchoscopy for awake tracheal intubation: a systematic review and meta-analysis. Anaesthesia. 2018;73(9):1151-61.
25. Rosenstock CV, Thøgersen B, Afshari A, Christensen A-L, Eriksen C, Gätke MR. Awake fiberoptic or awake video laryngoscopic tracheal intubation in patients with anticipated difficult airway management. A Randomized Clinical Trial. Anesthesiology. 2012;116(6):1210-6.
26. Dhara SS. Retrograde tracheal intubation. Anaesthesia. 2009;64(10):1094-104.
27. Bennett JD, Guha SC, Sankar AB. Cricothyrotomy: The anatomical basis. J R Coll Surg Edinb. 1996;41(1):57-60.
28. Patel A, Nouraei SA. Transnasal humidified rapid-insufflation ventilatory exchange (THRIVE): a physiological method of increasing apnoea time in patients with difficult airways. Anaesthesia. 2015;70(3):323-9.
29. Wu C, Wei J, Cen Q, Sha X, Cai Q, Ma W, et al. Supraglottic jet oxygenation and ventilation-assisted fibre-optic bronchoscope intubation in patients with difficult airways. Intern Emerg Med. 2017;12(5):667-73.
30. Myatra SN, Gupta S, D'Cruz AK, Rajanala V, Dhar H, Sharma S, et al. Identification of patients for a delayed extubation strategy versus elective tracheostomy for postoperative airway management in major oral cancer surgery: a prospective observational study in seven hundred and twenty patients. Oral Oncol. 2021;121:105502.
31. Chauhan V, Acharya G. Nasal intubation: A comprehensive review. Indian J Crit Care Med. 2016;20(11):662-7.
32. Hall CEJ, Shutt LE. Nasotracheal intubation for head and neck surgery. Anaesthesia. 2003;58(3):249-56.
33. Atlas G, Lee M. The neural integrity monitor electromyogram tracheal tube: Anesthetic considerations. J Anaesthesiol Clin Pharmacol. 2013;29(3):403-4.
34. Gupta K, Mandlik D, Patel D, Patel P, Shah B, Vijay DG, et al. Clinical assessment scoring system for tracheostomy (CASST) criterion: Objective criteria to predict pre-operatively the need for a tracheostomy in head and neck malignancies. J Craniomaxillofac Surg. 2016;44(9):1310-3.
35. Chalon J. Low humidity and damage to tracheal mucosa. Bull N Y Acad Med. 1980;56(3):314-22.

36. American Association for Respiratory Care; Restrepo RD, Walsh BK. Humidification during invasive and noninvasive mechanical ventilation: 2012. Respir Care. 2012;57(5):782-8.
37. Kundra P, Garg R, Patwa A, Ahmed SM, Ramkumar V, Shah A, et al. All India difficult airway association 2016 guidelines for the management of anticipated difficult extubation. Indian J Anaesth. 2016;60(12):915-21.
38. Hartley M, Vaughan RS. Problems associated with tracheal extubation. Br J Anaesth. 1993;71(4):561-8.
39. Kriner EJ, Shafazand S, Colice GL. The endotracheal tube cuff-leak test as a predictor for postextubation stridor. Respir Care. 2005;50(12):1632-8.
40. Jaber S, Jung B, Chanques G, Bonnet F, Marret E. Effects of steroids on reintubation and post-extubation stridor in adults: meta-analysis of randomised controlled trials. Crit Care. 2009;13(2):R49.
41. Batuwitage B, Charters P. Postoperative management of the difficult airway. BJA Educ. 2017;17(7):235-41.
42. Lee CH, Peng MJ, Wu CL. Dexamethasone to prevent post extubation airway obstruction in adults: a prospective, randomized, double-blind, placebo-controlled study. Crit Care 2007;11:R72
43. Coyle MJ, Tyrrell R, Godden A, Hughes CW, Perkins C, Thomas S, et al. Replacing tracheostomy with overnight intubation to manage the airway in head and neck oncology patients: towards an improved recovery. Br J Oral Maxillofac Surg. 2013;51(6):493-6.
44. Anehosur VS, Karadiguddi P, Joshi VK, Lakkundi BC, Ghosh R, Krishnan G. Elective tracheostomy in head and neck surgery: Our experience. J ClinDiagn Res. J Clin Diagn Res. 2017;11(5):ZC36-9.
45. Bodenham A, Bell D, Bonner S, Branch F, Dawson D, Morgan P, et al. Standards for the care of adult patients with a temporary tracheostomy: Standards and Guidelines. Intensive Care Society Standards. 2014;1:3.
46. McGrath B, Bates L, Atkinson D, Moore J; National Tracheostomy Safety Project. Multidisciplinary guidelines for the management of tracheostomy and laryngectomy airway emergencies. Anaesthesia. 2012;67(9):1025-41.
47. Lu IC, Lin IH, Wu CW, Chen HY, Lin YC, Chiang FY, et al. Preoperative, intraoperative and postoperative anesthetic prospective for thyroid surgery: What's new. Gland Surg. 2017;6(5):469-75.
48. Christou N, Mathonnet M. Complications after total thyroidectomy. J Visc Surg. 2013;150(4):249-56.
49. Rosato L, Avenia N, Bernante P, De Palma M, Gulino G, Nasi PG, et al. Complications of thyroid surgery: analysis of a multicentric study on 14,934 patients operated on in Italy over 5 years. World J Surg. 2004;28(3):271-6.
50. Bergenfelz A, Jansson S, Kristoffersson A, Mårtensson H, Reihnér E, Wallin G, et al. Complications to thyroid surgery: results as reported in a database from a multicenter audit comprising 3,660 patients. Langenbecks Arch Surg. 2008;393(5):667-73.
51. Jeannon JP, Orabi AA, Bruch GA, Abdalsalam HA, Simo R. Diagnosis of recurrent laryngeal nerve palsy after thyroidectomy: a systematic review. Int J Clin Pract. 2009;63(4):624-9.

13 CHAPTER

Anesthesia of Airway Procedures and Laser Surgeries

Jyoti Sharma, Shashank Umesh Paliwal, Anju Grewal

INTRODUCTION

Airway procedures are unique as the anesthesiologist and surgeon work in the same field, presenting a significant challenge. Lasers were invented in the 1950s, and medical use began in the 1960s. Since then, their scope has expanded vastly, with applications in airway procedures and other body parts continuing to progress rapidly. In laryngotracheal surgery, carbon dioxide lasers are often preferred for procedures such as cordotomy, tracheal stenosis treatment, and airway tumor resection. They provide precise, bloodless surgical fields, minimal tissue damage and sterile conditions.[1] It requires high coordination among the anesthesia, surgical, and operating theater (OT) teams. The working area is constrained, and the use of lasers introduces hazards such as fire and accidental damage to the patient or OT staff. Operating room personnel must be well-informed about the benefits and risks of medical lasers and adhere to safety protocols. The anesthetist must be skilled and thorough with knowledge in managing airway complications that may arise during laser surgeries. Common laser-assisted procedures include excision of laryngeal cancers and papillomas, removal of vocal cord nodules and cysts, and treatment of tracheal stenosis, obstructive tumors and vocal cord dysfunction. Understanding OT fires' principles, types, hazards, precautions, and management is crucial to successfully conducting laser airway surgery.

This chapter will cover critical aspects of perioperative management in laser airway surgery, focusing on selecting anesthetic techniques, strategies for maintaining adequate ventilation, and understanding the mechanisms behind potential adverse events.

LASER

The first laser, developed by Theodore Maiman in 1960, used a high-powered flash lamp focused on a ruby rod as the active medium, which was later replaced by gases, liquids and other materials. "Laser" is an acronym for Light Amplification by Stimulated Emission of Radiation. A laser generates energy in the form of light, which is in or close to the optical portion of the electromagnetic spectrum. The laser energy is amplified to extremely high intensity by an atomic process called stimulated emission. Laser beams provide a highly focused energy source capable of vaporizing tissue or achieving photocoagulation.[2,3] It acts as a surgeon's scalpel, cutting through tissues but much at a microscopic level, making it precise and bloodless (**Fig. 1**).

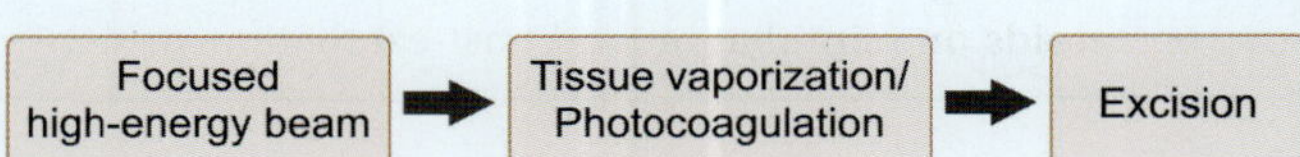

Fig. 1: Mechanism of laser surgery.

Types of Laser

Lasers are categorized by their medium: gas, solid, liquid, or semiconductor. The choice of laser for clinical applications is influenced by factors such as wavelength, tissue absorption characteristics, cost, ease of use, and safety. Lasers differ in their emitted wavelength, output power, mode of operation (pulsed or continuous), and whether they are applied in contact or noncontact mode.

The carbon dioxide (CO_2) laser is the most used in otolaryngology, emitting infrared light at 10,600 nm, which is invisible to the naked eye. Water strongly absorbs this wavelength, leading to significant thermal effects that can cause tissue vaporization or coagulation. Proper eye protection is essential for patients and operating room personnel using clear glass or plastic shields. Other lasers frequently used in medical practice include argon, Nd, potassium titanyl phosphate (KTP), and diode lasers, each with distinct characteristics summarized in the **Table 1**.

TABLE 1: Types of lasers—summary and key features.

Type	*Medium*	*Wavelength (nm)*	*Color*	*Fiberoptic transmission*	*Feature*	*Surgery*
CO_2	Gas	10,600	Invisible	No	High vaporization	Laryngeal, head and neck surgical procedures
Argon	Gas	500	Blue-green	Yes	Transmitted by water, absorbed by hemoglobin	
Ruby	Solid	695	Red	Yes	Pigment tissue absorption is high	
Nd: YAG	Solid	1,060	Invisible	Yes	Coagulation is high	Tracheobronchial lesions, vascular diseases
KTP	Solid	532	Green	Yes		

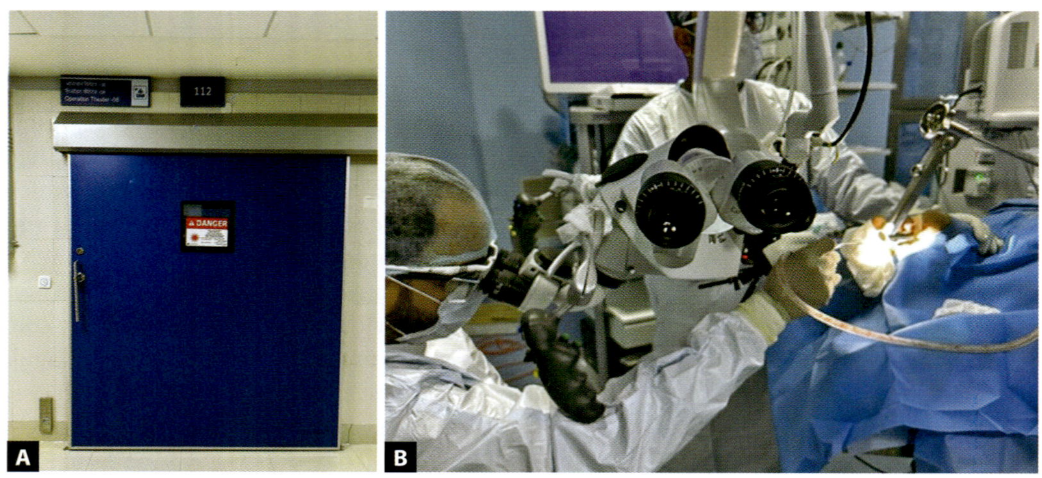

Figs. 2A and B: (A) Laser warning sign at the operation theater door; (B) OT personnel wearing protective goggles.

Laser Hazards

- *Eyes:* Damage in the eyes results from direct exposure of radiant energy amplified to the laser or its reflection. The eye contains several structures that can absorb laser light, acting as chromophores. Wavelengths in the mid-infrared (1,400–3,000 nm) and far-infrared (3,000–10,600 nm) ranges are mainly absorbed by water, a key component of the cornea and lens. Individuals outside the operating room should be warned, as shown in **Figure 2A**, and windows should be covered with opaque material. Laser protective eyewear (LPE) is essential for patients and healthcare providers **(Fig. 2B)** involved in laser procedures.[4]
- *Airway fire:* Laser airway surgery poses a risk of airway fires due to lasers' high energy and combustion potential, as the surgical site is near the airway. A laser directed at an unprotected endotracheal tube (ETT) can ignite it, and a punctured ETT cuff can expose the oxidant-rich gas within the circuit, significantly increasing the risk of a fire or even a blowtorch effect.

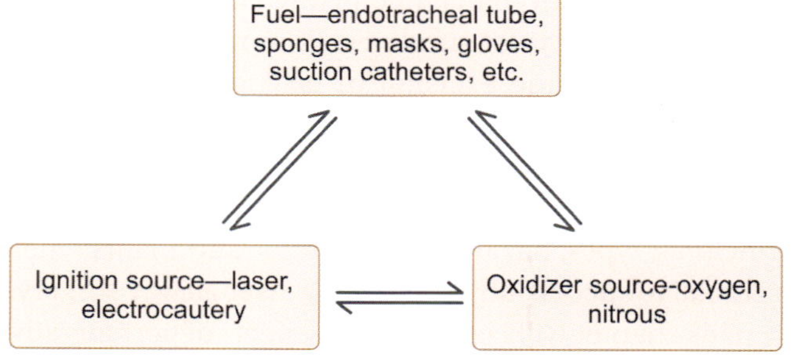

Fig. 3: Fire triad.

In the operating theater, fires can occur when the fire triad—fuel, an oxidant, and an ignition source—is present **(Fig. 3)**. Common fuel sources include

ETTs, volatile anesthetics, sponges, drapes, and gauze. An oxidant-rich environment can develop in closed circuits with high oxygen or nitrous oxide levels or accumulate under drapes or masks. Potential ignition sources in the surgical setting include lasers, electrocautery devices, defibrillator pads, and heated probes.

The American Society of Anesthesiologists has recommended guidelines for managing operating room fires: "*Operating Room Fire Prevention and Management*" is mentioned in **Box 1**.

- *Iatrogenic burns:* These burns are additional to airway fires to other normal parts near the surgical or other body parts such as trachea and pharynx. Applying saline-soaked gauze to the mucosal areas adjacent to the surgery site is an effective preventive measure to prevent such collateral damage.
- Other laser hazards, such as laser plumes, may pose carcinogenic risks. These hazards can be mitigated by using plume scavenging systems and high-efficiency filtering masks.

BOX 1: Operating room fire prevention and management.[5]

Fire prevention:
- *Identify high-risk situations:*
  - Is there a potential for an ignition source (e.g., laser, electrosurgical unit) near an oxidizer-enriched environment (oxygen, nitrous oxide)?
  - *Yes:* Continue to "Prevention Measures"
  - *No:* Continue normal procedures
- *Prevention measures:*
  - Avoid using ignition sources in proximity to oxygen >30% or nitrous oxide
  - Configure surgical drapes to minimize the accumulation of oxidizers
  - Allow sufficient drying time for prep solutions and avoid pooling of alcohol-based skin preps
  - Moisten sponges and gauze when near ignition sources

Fire management:
- *Early warning signs of fire:*
  - Unexpected flash, flame, smoke, or heat
  - Unusual sounds (e.g., "pop", "sizzle" or "from")
  - Unusual movement or discolouration of drapes or breathing circuit
  - Unexpected patient movement or complaints
- *Assess fire presence:*
  - *If fire is not present:* Halt the procedure and assess for prevention steps
  - *If fire is present:* Continue to "Fire Response"
- *Fire Response:*
  - Airway Fire:
    - Remove the endotracheal tube immediately
    - Stop the flow of airway gases
    - Remove flammable materials from the airway
    - Pour saline into the airway
  - Non-airway Fire:
    - Stop the flow of all airway gases
    - Remove drapes and all burning materials
    - Extinguish burning materials
- *If fire persists:*
  - Use a CO_2 fire extinguisher if available
  - Activate the fire alarm, evacuate the patient, close the OR door, and turn off the gas supply to the room

Postfire management:
- *Airway fire:*
  - Re-establish ventilation
  - Avoid oxidizer-enriched atmosphere
  - Examine ETT to see if fragments were left behind
  - Consider bronchoscopy
- *Non-airway fire:*
  - Maintain ventilation
  - Assess for inhalation injury if the patient was intubated
  - Consider bronchoscopy

Preoperative Assessment

The preoperative evaluation aims to identify potential challenges during the perioperative period through a comprehensive airway and general examination. The anesthesiologist should have a clear understanding of the lesion's size, mobility, and location. Recognizing any compromised or anatomically distorted upper airway during this process is crucial—extensive preoperative history with general examination.

The patient population undergoing airway surgery consists of elderly individuals who have coexisting respiratory and cardiovascular conditions, often due to long-term smoking, alcohol consumption, and underlying cardiovascular and respiratory dysfunction. Optimization of these parameters, along with nutritional and metabolic status, should be done. However, in some cases, it may not be possible because of the urgency or palliative nature of the procedure.

- Airway examination should include existing airway obstruction, breathing difficulty, presence of hoarseness of voice, stridor, hemoptysis, dysphagia, odynophagia, and pain caused by cartilage invasion.
- Positional exacerbation due to pedunculated tumor of the glottis: A very mobile lesion may cause increased obstruction after the induction and, if subglottic, may lead to a difficult passage of ETT.
- Presence of stridor
- Indirect laryngoscopy to check cords and assess nerves by the surgeon

- CT scan is used for subglottic or tracheal lesion dimensions and the requirement for a tracheostomy before induction. The size of the lesion will also give information regarding airflow obstruction
- Comorbidities
- Pulmonary function test—spirometry—can determine the type and degree of obstruction. If PFT is abnormal, arterial blood gas analysis can be done.

At the end of the preoperative assessment, the anesthesiologist must be able to predict the difficulty or ease of airway management and be ready with a plan of ventilation mode.

In laryngeal and airway surgeries, the key goals of anesthesia are:

- Ensuring proper oxygenation and effective CO_2 removal is crucial. Since the surgeon and anesthesiologist work within the airway, maintaining patency through various techniques is important for the procedure's safety.
- Ensure smooth induction and maintain anesthesia while keeping the airway secure and minimizing the risk of aspiration.
- Preventing contamination of the tracheobronchial tree is essential. Maintaining a secretion-free airway in an immobile surgical field significantly aids the surgeon.
- Profound muscle paralysis is required to keep the masseter muscle relaxed for the introduction of scope, and other instruments are needed till the end of the surgery.
- Cardiovascular stability during surgical stimulation
- Additionally, maintaining safe conditions, particularly by preventing an airway fire, is crucial due to the flammable materials and equipment used in these surgeries
- Ensuring a smooth emergence with no coughing or bucking and a fully awake patient is critical. The risk of laryngospasm is high since the airway may come into contact with blood and other debris
- Postoperative analgesia with an awake patient who can protect his airway

Premedication

Premedication depends on the severity or potential for airway obstruction, such as in mobile or large lesions such as papillomas. For patients with minor-to-moderate airway obstruction, premedication to reduce secretions and anxiety can be beneficial. Intravenous injections of glycopyrrolate (0.004 mg/kg), fentanyl (1 μg/kg), and midazolam (0.02 mg/kg) may be administered. An opiate, sedative, and anticholinergic combination is generally safe for patients without compromised airways. These drugs should be given in the holding area or the OR once monitors are attached. Antisialogogues such as glycopyrrolate help keep the airway secretion-free during surgery, but since they may thicken secretions and further narrow the airway, they should be used with caution in patients who already have excessive secretions. In cases of compromised airways, opiates or sedative premedication should be avoided.

Airway topicalization involves the application of a local anesthetic to the mucosal surface to achieve localized uptake and neural blockade in the targeted area. This technique can be performed as a part of awake airway management or as an adjunct to general anesthesia (GA).

Induction of Anesthesia

The choice of anesthesia technique is influenced by the patient's clinical condition, the size and location of the lesion, and the surgical plan. In cases without airway obstruction, intravenous or inhalational induction techniques can be used. For selected patients undergoing short endoscopic procedures with a flexible bronchoscope, sedation and topical anesthesia may be sufficient, provided the patient is cooperative. While this approach allows the patient to maintain control of their airway, few procedures can be comfortably tolerated under these conditions.

The anesthesia plan for patients with compromised airways should be carefully coordinated between an experienced anesthesiologist and a surgeon. The specific technique chosen depends on the anesthesiologist's expertise, surgical requirements, available equipment, the type of laser being used, the duration of the procedure, the lesion's type and vascularity, and the need to prevent airway contamination from blood or secretions.

Options include **(Flowchart 1)**:

- *Closed system:* Cuffed laser tracheal tube
- *Open system:* Spontaneous or jet ventilation
- *Laser tube:* One significant concern with regular ETTs is their susceptibility to ignition when exposed to laser beams during surgeries. The endotracheal cuff is particularly vulnerable, which can lead to cuff damage or, in severe cases, an airway fire. Traditionally, to mitigate this risk, the cuff is filled with saline or dye to detect leaks, and the tube is wrapped in metal foil as

Flowchart 1: Selection of anesthesia techniques for airway laser surgery.

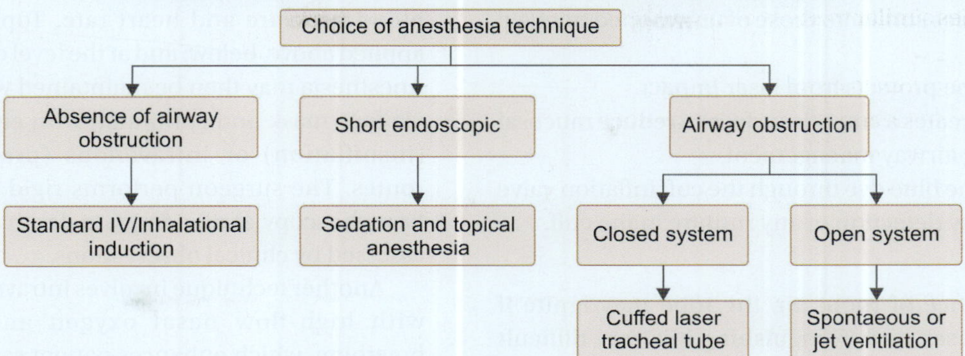

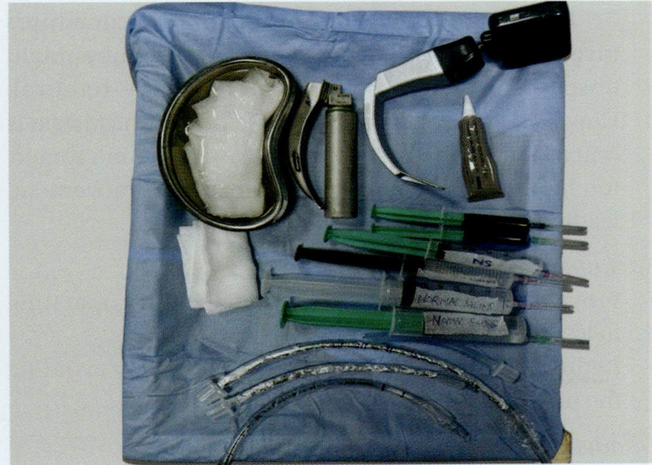

Fig. 4: Airway cart displaying metal foil-wrapped endotracheal tube (ETT).

shown in **Figure 4**. Copper tape is often used because of its high reflectivity for far-infrared wavelengths, although aluminum tape is also effective. However, wrapping the tube with tape poses challenges such as rough edges, the risk of fragments breaking off and being aspirated, or causing injury. Such noncertified metal foil wrapped around ETT is not recommended, and the product liability lies on the physician using it. Additionally, the wrapped tube may kink under compression. Muslin soaked in water was previously used to dissipate laser energy, but this required frequent watering, making the setup bulky and increasing the risk of fire if the muslin dried out.[1]

Various laser-resistant ETTs are available, eliminating the need for traditional metallic tapes. These specialized ETTs are designed for laser surgeries, improving safety and efficiency.[5-7] However, the outer diameter of laser-resistant tubes is larger due to their protective coverings, which can restrict surgical access and reduce the visibility of laryngeal lesions. To ensure adequate exposure for the surgeon, smaller laser tubes are often used, which may result in higher inflation pressures.

- *Laser-flex:* This tube has an airtight, stainless steel corrugated spiral with polyvinyl chloride (PVC) Murphy eye tip and double cuffs, and an uncuffed version is available for pediatric use. It is specifically designed for CO_2 or KTP lasers.

Advantages:
- The metal components are resistant to fire.
- The tube maintains its shape during intubation and resists kinking.
- The proximal cuff protects the distal tracheal cuff.

Disadvantages:
- The metal may reflect the laser onto unintended tissues, potentially causing damage, although this risk is reduced by the matte finish and convex design.
- The cuffed version contains flammable materials, necessitating inflation with saline to minimize the risk of ignition.
- Metal tubes have higher airway resistance than PVC tubes of the same size due to their thicker walls, and their double cuff design requires more time to inflate and deflate than single cuffs.
- Additionally, the metal can transfer heat to adjacent tissues or materials, which may pose further risks.

- Laser-Shield II

  This tube is made of silicone rubber with an outer layer of aluminum-filled silicone.

Advantages:

- It has properties similar to those of unwrapped tracheal tubes.
- A metallic tape protects from laser impact.
- Teflon tape creates a smooth surface to reduce mucosal injury during airway management.
- Dry methylene blue dye through the cuff inflation valve allows for easy detection of any rupture in the cuff.

Disadvantages:

- In the presence of room air, the tube may ignite if struck by a laser, and extinguishing it is very difficult once ignited.
- The proximal and distal ends of the silicone shaft and cuff are unprotected, making them susceptible to laser exposure.
  - *LaserTubus:* This laser-resistant ETT has a soft white rubber shaft and a 17-cm laser guard composed of a Merocel sponge reinforced with corrugated copper foil. It has a double-cuff system, with an inner cuff encased by an outer cuff. The sponge surface should be thoroughly moistened before use to lower the risk of airway fire.
  - *The Sheridan Laser-Trach:* This single-use red rubber ETT includes a spiral-wrapped, nonflammable copper foil that extends from the cuff to the proximal end. An absorbent fabric layer covers the copper foil to help minimize damage to mucosal surfaces and vocal cords. The manufacturer recommends soaking the outer layer with sterile isotonic saline before use and keeping it moist throughout the procedure, as a dry fabric layer increases the risk of ignition if struck by a laser.
- *Spontaneous ventilation technique:* This technique requires the patient to breathe spontaneously, providing a clear view of the glottis. Anesthetic gases can be insufflated through various methods, such as a small catheter in the nasopharynx near the larynx, a shortened tracheal tube or nasopharyngeal airway, or the side channel of a laryngoscope or bronchoscope. While avoiding an endotracheal tube reduces the risk of airway fires, ensuring that insufflation catheters are not advanced too far into the larynx or esophagus is essential.

  Inhalational induction can be done using sevoflurane with 100% oxygen. A laryngoscopy is performed once a suitable depth of anesthesia is achieved, as assessed by clinical indicators such as respiratory rate and depth, pupil size, eye reflexes, blood pressure and heart rate. Topical lidocaine is applied above, below, and at the level of the vocal cords. Anesthesia may then be maintained with 100% oxygen via face mask and continued with either inhalational (insufflation) or intravenous (propofol infusion) routes. The surgeon performs rigid laryngoscopy or bronchoscopy at an adequate depth of anesthesia, as assessed by clinical observations.

  Another technique involves intravenous anesthesia with high-flow nasal oxygen and spontaneous breathing, which enhances patient safety in managing airways compromised by tumors or laryngotracheal stenosis.[8]

  This technique is beneficial for procedures involving the vocal cords, where a laser tube might obscure the lesion, or for foreign body removal. However, achieving the correct depth of anesthesia is crucial—too deep, and the patient may become apneic; too light, and there is a risk of vocal cord movement, leading to laryngospasm or coughing.

Advantages:

- Provides a clear, unobstructed view of the operating field
- Reduces the risk of operating room fires by avoiding the use of an ETT

Disadvantages:

- Limited control over ventilation
- Risk of airway soiling and aspiration
- Operating room pollution from insufflation

  Insufflation techniques are unsuitable for large, soft, or floppy lesions in the supraglottic or glottic areas, as these can obstruct the airway.
- *Intermittent apneic technique:* Following induction of general anesthesia, patients are paralyzed with atracurium or vecuronium, and anesthesia is maintained with halothane or enflurane in 100% oxygen. Small-caliber ETTs are used for intubation. A high-flow nasal cannula (HFNC) may be added to extend the apneic period through continuous respiratory gas delivery, allowing stable, unobstructed views of immobile laryngeal structures.[9] If oxygen saturation decreases, the surgery is paused, and patients are reintubated and hyperventilated with 100% oxygen. Muscle relaxants ensure an immobile surgical field, with sugammadex available for rapid reversal.

Advantages: It provides a clear view and immobility, removing all flammable materials.

Contraindication: Not suitable for patients with difficult laryngeal visualization

- *Jet ventilation:* Jet ventilation involves delivering a high-pressure stream of gas into the upper airway, which minimizes stimulation and provides a clearer surgical view. This technique uses intermittent bursts of air, oxygen, or oxygen-air mixtures, which mix with room air to reduce the overall pressure. Manual jet ventilation can be done with a Sanders-type injector (providing a fixed 4 atm pressure) or the Manujet device (offering a controlled pressure range of 0–4 atm). It is preferable to start with the lowest pressure possible to reduce complications. Some devices also provide humidification. While end-tidal CO_2 ($EtCO_2$) monitoring is unreliable with this technique, it can be measured through a side port.

  In manual jet ventilation, an injector connected to the gas supply delivers the respiratory mixture into the trachea. The removal of gas occurs through passive exhalation, which requires a clear upper airway and sufficient time between jet insufflations to prevent barotrauma. The inflow pressures are regulated by a reducing valve, typically ranging from 1 to 4 atmospheres. Respiratory gas can then be actively insufflated either supraglottically or transglottically or using a transtracheal approach.

  Oxygen delivery and carbon dioxide removal during manual jet ventilation primarily rely on diffusion through the bronchial tree, as lung volume changes are minimal. Ventilation frequency and the positioning of the jet cannula should be adjusted based on the extent of airway obstruction and the lesion's location. High-frequency jet ventilation (HFJV) uses minimal tidal volumes and high respiratory rates (100–150 breaths per minute) to enhance diffusion.

  Potential complications include mucosal dehydration, stomach insufflation, laser burns to the trachea (if no cuff protects distal areas), pneumothorax, and pneumomediastinum. High-pressure jets of air, oxygen, or oxygen-air mixtures entrain room air, reducing the pressure delivered. Specially designed equipment such as catheters, laryngoscopes, bronchoscopes, and ventilators are available, with various techniques offering different benefits. Risks include barotrauma, pneumomediastinum, pneumothorax, and surgical emphysema.[10] Dry jetting gases can lead to mucosal dehydration and thickened secretions. Additionally, measuring $EtCO_2$ is challenging with this technique.[11]

  Jet ventilation can be administered through multiple delivery routes:[12]

  - *Supraglottic:* This method utilizes a tubeless surgical field using a rigid surgical bronchoscope attached to a jet ventilator. The efficacy of ventilation through this setup relies on the precise alignment of the stream of the jet with the patient's airway. Successful alignment allows the jet stream to pass gas through the narrowed glottis, employing the Venturi effect to entrain air. This can lead to a sudden increase in airway pressure, particularly in patients with narrow stenosis.

    Limitations of Supraglottic Jet Ventilation

    There are several limitations associated with this method:

    - *Ventilation efficiency:* Improper alignment of the jet with the airway can result in inadequate ventilation.
    - *Gastric distention and aspiration:* There is a risk of gastric distention and aspiration of surgical debris due to poor ventilation.
    - *Monitoring challenges:* There is either no provision for measuring $EtCO_2$, or it is unreliable, complicating monitoring the patient's ventilation status.
    - *Vocal cord movement:* The movement of the vocal cords during the procedure increases the risk of complications.
    - *Barotrauma risk:* There is an inherent risk of barotrauma due to potential variations in airway pressure during the procedure.

  - In the transglottic/subglottic approach, ventilation is provided below the glottis using a small catheter or specialized tubes, such as the Hunsaker or Benjet, inserted through the glottis into the trachea. This technique allows for the direct delivery of a gas jet into the trachea, minimizing vocal cord movement during the procedure. During expiration, the expiratory airflow drives blood and debris outward, preventing them from entering the tracheobronchial tree. One key advantage of this method is the minimal entrainment of ambient air, allowing for the consistent delivery of a fixed inspired oxygen concentration (FiO_2) and the possibility of monitoring $EtCO_2$. Subglottic jet ventilation is generally more efficient than supraglottic jet ventilation. It results in reduced driving pressures, minimized vocal cord movements, improved surgical field visibility, and the absence of strict time constraints.

Risks: However, a significant consideration is that a fuel source (the catheter) in the trachea poses a higher risk, especially during laser surgery. Therefore, the catheter must be laser-resistant. Additionally, there is an increased risk of barotrauma due to the direct delivery of gas into the trachea.

- *Transtracheal ventilation:* The transtracheal approach may be preferable for patients with anticipated difficulties in intubation, often due to significant laryngeal pathology or upper airway obstruction. A transtracheal or cricothyroid cannula can be inserted in awake patients under local anesthesia or general anesthesia for elective laryngeal surgeries. This approach also provides an immediate route for oxygenation in cases where initial airway management attempts fail and oxygenation deteriorates.

  Risks: The most significant risks associated with the transtracheal approach include barotrauma, subcutaneous emphysema, cannula blockage, kinking, infection, bleeding, and failure to place the catheter correctly.[13,14] Additionally, no commercially available cannula is specifically designed for laser surgery, further complicating the procedure in such cases.
- *High- or low-frequency jet ventilation:* Jet ventilation can be administered using a high-pressure gas source through a narrow cannula, with frequencies below 60 breaths per minute (1 Hz) classified as Low-frequency jet ventilation (LFJV). A metal jet needle or cannula is placed within a laryngoscope or rigid bronchoscope and attached to an oxygen source. A pressure regulator keeps oxygen pressure below 50 psi in adults, with the minimum necessary pressure applied. The tidal volume delivered depends on various factors, including air entrainment, the cannula's length and the size of the laryngoscope, alignment with the trachea, and the patient's lung compliance. The high-velocity gas stream entrains air and expands the generated tidal volume, causing a reduction in the inspired oxygen concentration. This leads to an immobile surgical field, temporarily making it suitable for brief procedures. LFJV is relatively simple to perform and requires only basic anesthetic equipment. Ventilation monitoring via $EtCO_2$ is not feasible; visible chest movements must be observed. Additionally, controlled delivery of inhalational anesthesia is not possible, making total intravenous anesthesia (TIVA) necessary.

  High-frequency jet ventilation (HFJV) delivers 60–150 breaths per minute from a high-pressure source (5–50 psi), with each breath's inspiration phase lasting 20–40% of the cycle. A longer catheter may be placed subglottically or via a cricothyroid cannula, and inspiration is managed by a high-frequency flow interrupter rather than a manual switch. HFJV provides efficient gas exchange and unobstructed visibility at the surgical site, making it especially useful for patients with severe airway obstructions or pulmonary issues, ensuring a stable, immobile field.

  HFJV carries risks such as air trapping and laryngospasm if the depth of anesthesia is inadequate. A combined approach using both low- and high-frequency jet ventilation may enhance oxygenation and CO_2 clearance.[15]
- *Rigid bronchoscopic ventilation:* The rigid bronchoscope has a side port for connecting to anesthetic gases and oxygen. It is an alternative to an ETT during procedures, lowering the risk of airway fires. It helps manage severely obstructing tracheal masses, allowing airway control, evaluating, diagnosing, and treating pediatric respiratory diseases.[16] It provides better surgical field visibility than flexible scopes, but its reach is limited to the trachea and carina.

  Limitations associated with rigid bronchoscopy include higher secretion production, restricted access to the distal airways and upper lobes, and difficulties in patients with jaw ankylosis or a rigid cervical spine, which may obstruct clear visualization of the larynx. General anesthesia with greater depth and opioids for analgesia is often required for rigid bronchoscopy.
- *Flexible bronchoscopy:* Flexible bronchoscopy is advantageous for reaching the distal airways, which can be done under sedation and local anesthesia with an anticholinergic drug as premedication. It can also be conducted under general anesthesia by passing the

bronchoscope through a laryngeal mask airway (LMA) or ETT. Flexible bronchoscopy airway in children is useful and safe in removing airway foreign bodies.[17]

Flexible bronchoscopy can maneuver throughout the entire airway, with the bronchoscope's tip flexing through an arc of up to 220 degrees. It also includes a working channel for suction and instrument passage, though the channel is typically narrow, limiting its use to airway visualization rather than more complex procedures.

MAINTENANCE OF ANESTHESIA

For laser surgery, total intravenous anesthesia (TIVA) using an infusion of propofol in combination with low-dose remifentanil or fentanyl is preferred, particularly in open-system techniques. TIVA offers significant advantages, as it eliminates the need for gas-based anesthesia, which can be difficult to maintain and monitor during tubeless procedures. Additionally, TIVA reduces the risk of airway contamination and minimizes the potential for airway fires associated with laser use. This approach ensures optimal conditions for shared airway surgeries, providing unobstructed access to the surgical field.

EXTUBATION

In most cases, the patient is extubated in the operating room. It is essential to inspect the ETT for any foil or adhesive wrapping remnants to ensure they are not present. The risk of high-risk extubation is significantly increased in laryngotracheal surgeries due to the nature of the pathologies and the complexity of the procedures. For such cases, advanced extubation techniques may be considered, including the use of a LMA exchange, administering remifentanil to facilitate smoother extubation, or leaving an airway rescue device in place, such as an airway exchange catheter, to ensure patient safety.

POSTOPERATIVE CARE

After airway surgery, patients are at risk for laryngospasm, aspiration, or airway obstruction due to edema or hematoma formation. To reduce the risk of laryngospasm, patients should be positioned in a semisitting position, and extubation should be performed either while the patient is fully awake or under deep anesthesia. A LMA can be used to maintain airway patency after deep anesthesia extubation. In case of emergency, a cricothyroid cannula may be kept ready. All necessary equipment for emergency airway access should be available in recovery, and anesthetic and surgical staff must remain nearby until the patient is stable enough to be discharged.

Edema can be managed with intraoperative administration of dexamethasone. If stridor develops, nebulized epinephrine (2–3 mL of 1:1,000) may be helpful. To prevent drying of the oral mucosa and thickening of secretions, all patients should receive humidified oxygen postoperatively. Heliox, a mixture of helium and 21% oxygen, may also be used, though additional oxygen is often necessary.

CONCLUSION

Anesthesia for airway procedures and laser surgeries poses unique challenges due to the shared surgical field, the risk of airway fires, and the need for specialized ventilation techniques. Effective perioperative management requires selecting the appropriate anesthetic technique, ensuring adequate oxygenation and CO_2 removal, and maintaining a secure airway while minimizing airway trauma. The choice of ventilation method, including closed-system techniques with laser-resistant endotracheal tubes (such as Laser-Flex, Laser-Shield II, and LaserTubus), open-system approaches like jet ventilation, and intermittent apneic techniques, depends on the surgical requirements and patient factors. Preventing airway fires remains a critical priority, necessitating adherence to fire safety protocols, the use of specialized ETTs, and minimizing oxidizer-enriched environments. TIVA is preferred in many cases due to its ability to maintain an immobile surgical field while reducing airway fire risks. Postoperative complications, including laryngospasm, airway edema, and aspiration, require vigilant monitoring, with strategies such as dexamethasone administration to reduce airway swelling and nebulized epinephrine for post-extubation stridor. Given the complexity of these procedures, interdisciplinary coordination among anesthesiologists, surgeons, and operating room staff is essential to optimize patient safety. Continuous refinement of airway management strategies and adherence to updated clinical guidelines will further improve perioperative outcomes in laser airway surgeries.

REFERENCES

1. Hermens JM, Bennett MJ, Hirshman CA. Anesthesia for laser surgery. Anesth Analg. 1983;62(2):218.

2. Ta F. The physics of surgical lasers. Lasers in surgery and medicine [Internet]. 1980 [cited 2024 Oct 15;1(1).
3. Lasers in medicine and surgery. Council on Scientific Affairs. JAMA. 1986;256(7):900-7.
4. Wamsley CE, Hoopman J, Kenkel JM. Safety guidelines concerning the use of protective eyewear and gauze during laser procedures. Aesthet Surg J. 2021;41(10):1179-85.
5. Jones TS, Black IH, Robinson TN, Jones EL. Operating room fires. Anesthesiology. 2019;130(3):492-501.
6. Doroshenko M, Guerra A, Vu L. Airway for Laser Surgery. Available from: http://www.ncbi.nlm.nih.gov/books/NBK564406/. [Last accessed February, 2025].
7. Apfelbaum JL, Caplan RA, Barker SJ, Connis RT, Cowles C, Ehrenwerth J, et al. Practice Advisory for the prevention and management of operating room fires: An updated report by the American Society of Anesthesiologists Task Force on Operating Room Fires. Anesthesiology. 2013;118(2):271-90.
8. Courbon C. Spontaneous ventilation with high-flow nasal oxygen for elective suspension microlaryngoscopy. OTO Open. 2023;7(2):e54.
9. Benninger MS, Zhang ES, Chen B, Tierney WS, Abdelmalak B, Bryson PC. Utility of transnasal humidified rapid insufflation ventilatory exchange for microlaryngeal surgery. Laryngoscope. 2021;131(3):587-91.
10. Cook TM, Alexander R. Major complications during anaesthesia for elective laryngeal surgery in the UK: A national survey of the use of high-pressure source ventilation. Br J Anaesth. 2008;101(2):266-72.
11. McRae K. Anesthesia for airway surgery. Anesthesiol Clin North Am. 2001;19(3):497-541.
12. Evans E, Biro P, Bedforth N. Jet ventilation. Continuing education in anaesthesia. Crit Care Pain. 2007;7(1):2-5.
13. Bourgain JL, Desruennes E, Fischler M, Ravussin P. Transtracheal high frequency jet ventilation for endoscopic airway surgery: A multicentre study. Br J Anaesth. 2001;87(6):870–5.
14. Patel A, Randhawa N, Semenov RA. Transtracheal high frequency jet ventilation and iatrogenic injury. Br J Anaesth. 2002;89(1):184; author reply 184.
15. Bacher A, Pichler K, Aloy A. Supraglottic combined frequency jet ventilation versus subglottic monofrequent jet ventilation in patients undergoing microlaryngeal surgery. Anesth Analg. 2000;90(2):460-5.
16. Yavuz S, Sherif A, Saif S, Alzamar A, Alawad D, Abdelwahab A, et al. Indications, efficacy, and complications of pediatric bronchoscopy: a retrospective study at a tertiary center. Cureus. 15(6):e40888.
17. Tang L-F, Xu Y-C, Wang Y-S, Wang C-F, Zhu G-H, Bao X-E, et al. Airway foreign body removal by flexible bronchoscopy: experience with 1027 children during 2000-2008. World J Pediatr. 2009;5(3):191-5.

14 CHAPTER

Anesthesia for Skull Base Surgeries

Anjana Sagar Wajekar, Akankshya Sarangi

INTRODUCTION

The base of the skull is an area densely packed with vital nerves, blood vessels and brain structures. Skull base surgeries are intricate procedures that require a nuanced approach to anesthesia management due to the complex anatomical structures involved and the critical nature of the surgeries. Anesthesia for these surgeries can be a challenging, often requiring a close-knit multidisciplinary teamwork with otolaryngology and neurosurgery to develop a safe and effective neuroprotective strategy.[1] Perioperative collaboration with endocrinology, neuroradiology, critical care, ophthalmology, and radiation oncology encompasses the comprehensive management of these complex disorders.[2] Anesthetists play a crucial role in ensuring patient safety and optimizing surgical outcomes. In this chapter, we look into the various intricacies of these kind of surgeries and outline some key considerations for anesthesia in patients undergoing these procedures.

ANATOMY OF BASE OF SKULL

The base of skull is the bony foundation of the cranial vault. It comprises the following bones—two frontal and temporal bones each, occipital, sphenoid and ethmoid bones. Several apertures dot the skull base, which allow the passage of various neurovascular structures **(Table 1)**.

TABLE 1: Apertures at the skull base and their contents.

Apertures	*Contents*
Optic canal	Cranial nerve II
Superior orbital fissure	Cranial nerve III, IV, V1, VI, superior ophthalmic vein
Foramen rotundum	Cranial nerve V2
Foramen ovale	Cranial nerve V3
Foramen spinosum	Middle meningeal artery
Foramen lacerum	Meningeal branches of the ascending pharyngeal artery
Vidian canal	Vidian artery and nerve
Internal auditory canal	Cranial nerve VII, VIII
Jugular foramen pars nervosa	Cranial nerve IX
Jugular foramen pars vascularis	Cranial nerve X, XI, Internal jugular vein
Carotid canal	Internal carotid artery
Stylomastoid foramen	Cranial nerve VII
Hypoglossal canal	Cranial nerve XII
Foramen magnum	Medulla

SURGICAL APPROACHES

The various approaches to skull base surgery include open, endoscopic, combined open/endoscopic and robotic.[1-5] Larger and more advanced tumors, and tumors with major vascular invasions are generally operated by open approaches. Open approaches include craniofacial, orbitocranial, infratemporal, suboccipital, lateral rectosigmoid, or translabyrinthine depending upon the site of surgery—anterior, middle or posterior skull base surgery. Initially indicated for transsphenoidal hypophysectomy, the expanded oncosurgical indications for endoscopic skull base surgery are given in **Table 2**.[3]

Revision endoscopic or open surgeries may be required for residual tumors, as a planned secondary procedure or to decompress neurovascular structures.

PREOPERATIVE EVALUATION AND RISK STRATIFICATION

General preoperative assessment of these patients follows the common guidelines as other patients posted for

TABLE 2: Indications for endoscopic skull base surgery.

Site	*Tumor type*
Cribriform lesions	• Olfactory groove meningioma • Esthesioneuroblastoma • Adenocarcinoma • Squamous cell carcinoma • Sinonasal undifferentiated carcinoma • Mucosal melanoma
Parasellar lesions	• Meningiomas • Craniopharyngiomas • Pituitary macroadenomas • Other tumors—dermoid, germinoma, metastasis, optic glioma
Clival lesions	• Chordomas • Chondrosarcomas
Spinomedullary junction lesions	Nasopharyngeal carcinoma refractory to radiotherapy
Petrous apex lesions	• Chordomas • Chondrosarcomas • Meningiomas
Pterygopalatine and infratemporal fossa lesions	• Paragangliomas • Schwannomas • Sphenoid wing meningiomas • Juvenile nasopharyngeal angiofibromas

elective surgery, vis-a-vis a comprehensive evaluation of the cardiopulmonary function and the medical comorbidities, including specialty-specific consultations such as cardiology or pulmonology consultations. A detailed neurological evaluation including the preoperative neurodeficits, cranial nerve involvement and signs of raised intracranial pressure, is indicated for all patients with intracranial extension of the tumor.[6]

Radiological assessment of the tumor for location, extent and neurovascular structure involvement is imperative. An angiography is required in cases of vascular tumors such as juvenile nasopharyngeal angiofibromas or to check for cavernous sinus invasion in pituitary tumors.[7] An angiography may also help with assessment of adequacy of intracranial collateral circulation. Angiography can help delineate the tumor vascular supply and embolization of the feeding vessels can help mitigate perioperative hemorrhage. Embolization should be followed by surgical resection within a timeframe of 24–48 hours. Preoperative carotid balloon occlusion testing maybe indicated in cases where the internal carotid artery is at high risk, secondary to tumor encasement, prior radiation, etc.

Specific considerations for pituitary tumors are mentioned in **Table 3**.[6] (6). Adenomas are the most common pituitary tumors. These can be microadenomas (size <10 mm) or macroadenomas. Functional pituitary tumors are the hormone-secreting tumors, commonly the microadenomas.

TABLE 3: Hormones secreted by pituitary microadenomas and their perioperative considerations.

Hormone	*Manifestation*	*Preoperative considerations*
Adrenocorticotropic hormone (ACTH)	Cushing's disease	Centripetal obesity—difficult airway, hypertension, adrenal hyperplasia, glucose intolerance, and osteoporosis
Growth hormone (GH)	Acromegaly	• Hypertension, glucose intolerance, visual loss, hoarseness and dyspnea (laryngeal stenosis from soft-tissue overgrowth), lumbar spinal stenosis, cardiomyopathy • Difficult airway (Ventilation, intubation and extubation)—bone and soft-tissue enlargement in mandible, tongue, lips, nasal turbinates, palate, tonsils, epiglottis, arytenoids, glottis, vocal cord palsy, OSA
Prolactin (PRL)	Prolactinoma	Infertility, amenorrhea, galactorrhea, gynecomastia, and osteoporosis
Thyroid-stimulating hormone (TSH)	Hyper-thyroidism	Tachycardia, electrolyte disturbances, and arrythmias

Nonfunctioning sellar tumors include pituitary macro-adenomas, craniopharyngiomas, and meningiomas. These tend to be large and involve cavernous sinus, internal carotid artery, or suprasellar structures. Opthalmoplegia, diplopia, seizures (due to spread to temporal lobes), and other symptoms depending upon the involvement of perisellar structures may occur. Panhypopituitarism, including hypothyroidism, hypoadrenalism, and hypogonadism, can occur due to compression of normal pituitary gland or disruption of the hypothalamus-pituitary pathways. Hormone replacement with prednisolone and levothyroxine is started preoperatively in such patients. Intraoperative stress dose of steroids is then indicated in these patients.

Diabetes insipidus is a common symptom with craniopharyngiomas and is a known intraoperative and postoperative complication of pituitary surgery. Craniopharyngioma is a benign tumor, which occurs more frequently in pediatric patients. Preoperative assessment of electrolytes and osmolarity is indicated in all cases of craniopharyngiomas.[3]

SURGICAL MANAGEMENT

The surgical approach can either be open craniofacial resection or endoscopic transsphenoidal resection. Preoperative radiological evaluation of the tumor anatomy is essential prior to deciding the approach for surgery. The patient demographic and comorbidities, underlying cancer pathology and extent, all help to define the surgical goal and approach. Endoscopic approaches are usually limited by the tumor spread deep to critical neurovascular structures. Subtotal vascular tumor resections may lead to increased risk of postoperative bleeding and edema, causing mass effect. Despite these limitations, endoscopic resections are increasing multifold due to improved surgical skills and faster recovery after surgery. Stereotactic navigation is frequently used during endoscopic skull base surgery.[3] Intraoperative neurophysiological monitoring is also strongly indicated in complex and high-risk cases due to inherent risk to critical neurovascular structures such as cranial nerves, internal carotid artery, etc. Somatosensory-evoked potentials (SSEP), brainstem auditory-evoked potential (BAEP) are some options. Lumbar drains may also be used in certain cases.

INTRAOPERATIVE ANESTHESIA MANAGEMENT

These surgeries necessitate general anesthesia. Intraoperative anesthesia monitoring for skull base cancer surgeries involves a multifaceted approach to ensure patient safety and successful surgical outcomes. Standard monitoring includes electrocardiography, pulse oximetry, noninvasive blood pressure, end-tidal capnography, depth of anesthesia, temperature, and urine output. In addition, radial artery catheterization is indicated in most patients. Up to 50% of acromegalic patients have incomplete palmer arch and hence, caution is warranted during arterial catheterizations. Coagulation monitoring using point-of-care testing (thromboelastography) may be indicated in cases of anticipated massive blood loss. The patient is positioned supine with head elevation such that it is ergonomic for the surgeons during endonasal endoscopy.[1] This also helps facilitate venous decongestion. There exists a theoretical risk of venous air embolism (VAE) with head elevation of >15°. Preparation for diagnosis of VAE with end-tidal carbon dioxide and precordial Doppler, central line is recommended, especially in cases of cavernous sinus invasion. A minimum of two wide-bore peripheral venous cannulation suffices in most cases.[3] In cases of cavernous sinus invasion, meningiomas, or juvenile nasopharyngeal angiofibromas, central venous access is prudent. Adequate extensions should be attached to all access lines. Antibiotic prophylaxis such as cefuroxime is indicated in all cases although the risk of meningitis is low.[2]

Mucosal surfaces of the nose should be packed with combination of local anesthetic (lignocaine) and vasoconstrictor (adrenaline) prior to endoscopy. Occasional hypertensive response may be observed, especially in hypertensive or cardiac patients and medication to treat must be kept ready. Anesthetic agents should be selected to permit early postoperative neurological and ophthalmic assessment. Anesthesia may be maintained with total intravenous anesthesia with target-controlled infusions of propofol and remifentanil in cases with intraoperative neuromonitoring or a combination of opioid-inhalation anesthetic with muscle relaxants. Use of short-acting agents such as propofol, remifentanil, sevoflurane, and atracurium are popular. Endoscopic surgery may necessitate mild controlled hypotension to improve surgical visibility.[3]

Oral intubation is performed in all the cases. Difficult airway management including difficult mask fit, should be anticipated in patients with acromegaly. Availability of supraglottic airways, videolaryngoscope, and fiberless intubating endoscope is prudent. Throat packing is imperative in all patients to prevent aspiration. As access to the patient's head end is limited, long ventilator circuits are the norm. Additionally, before induction of anesthesia the patients should be warned about postoperative hemostatic nasal packing, especially if the approach is bilateral. The patients should be preemptively informed about the need for postoperative mouth breathing upon awakening. The eyes should be properly taped and eye shields used. All pressure sites must be padded adequately, and graduated compression stockings should be used. Goal-directed fluid therapy (using crystalloids, colloids, and blood products as needed) should be practiced to maintain hemodynamic stability and avoid fluid overload or hypovolemia. Massive blood loss protocols should be in place in cases of juvenile nasopharyngeal angiofibroma, meningiomas, and cavernous sinus invasion.[7]

Valsalva maneuvers advance the pituitary gland toward the surgeon to facilitate the excision of the tumor and examination for any transsellar CSF leak. In events of cavernous sinus injury or internal carotid artery rupture, surgical packing may be done and the patient re-explored after 24–48 hours for pack removal.

In cases of dural opening, reconstructions entail use of fat or fascia from lateral thigh and even pedicled nasoseptal flap in large defects to prevent cerebrospinal leak and its consequences.

Skull base surgeries are often prolonged complex surgeries. There are concerns related to extubations such as airway edema, lower cranial nerve deficits, and pulmonary comorbidities, which may necessitate admission of intubated patients to neurocritical care unit.[8] When transmandibular or transpalatal approaches are used for resection of skull base tumors extending into oral cavity, tracheostomy is advisable.

By employing advanced monitoring techniques and maintaining vigilant oversight, we can effectively manage the unique challenges posed by these complex procedures. However, it should be kept in mind that the above-mentioned monitoring strategies would differ from case to case and also would depend on the facilities/technology available in the different oncocenters.

Postoperative Management

All patients are shifted to postanesthesia care unit. Close monitoring of neurological parameters should be continued for 24–48 hours. Patients are kept in head elevation position to avoid pressure on the skull base reconstructions. Prevention of nausea and vomiting and pain control are paramount. For pituitary pathologies, hourly fluid monitoring supplemented by serial biochemistries to check for diabetes insipidus should be done.[6]

Postoperative Nasal Care

Sinonasal precautions include avoidance of hyperventilation, nasal blowing, nasogastric tube insertion, incentive spirometry, and use of drinking straws.[8] In patients with obstructive sleep apnea, postoperative continuous positive airway pressure (CPAP) may also be withheld in patients with cerebrospinal leaks.[9] Supplemental oxygenation, if required, should be done via humidified face tent rather than direct injection into nasal cavity, to avoid drying of nasal mucosa and the risk of pneumocephalus. Postoperative sinonasal morbidities include decreased olfaction, nasal crusting, obstruction, rhinosinusitis, formation of a mucocele, and cosmetic deformities. Nasal saline (spray/irrigation) has shown benefit to prevent nasal crusting and help with remucosalization in several randomized controlled trials after endoscopic surgery.[9]

Complications

A wide spectrum of complications have been reported after both open and endoscopic skull base surgery. An overall mortality of ≤1% and morbidity of 10–20% is reported in most series.[2,8] The complications are closely related to the indication and approach for surgery. Common postoperative morbidities include ischemic stroke, intracranial hemorrhage, vascular injuries, symptomatic pneumocephaly, postoperative visual loss, CSF leak, endocrine dysfunction, diabetes insipidus, and meningitis. Uncommon complications include wound dehiscence, lacrimal duct obstruction, pseudomeningocele, brain abscess, superficial wound infections, etc. Open surgeries have a higher rate of both surgical and medical complications as compared to endoscopic surgeries.

Cerebrospinal fluid (CSF) rhinorrhea: The overall incidence of CSF leaks is reported to be around 5–10%.[8] Usually, it occurs between postoperative days 2 and 7. They can lead to development of meningitis, pneumocephaly, abducens palsy due to traction, or acute subdural hemorrhage. CSF leaks are classified as low flow or high flow. The high flow leaks are secondary to large dural defects, opening into the ventricle or a cistern. They may require either therapeutic lumbar drains or revision surgeries. Use of lumbar drains may lead to development or exacerbation in pneumocephalus through a one-way valve mechanism where air enters through the CSF drainage as the CSF is removed, especially during inappropriate sinonasal precaution. Careful lumbar drain management and strict adherence to sinonasal precautions help minimize the risk.

Diabetes insipidus (DI): DI affects approximately 20% of transsphenoid hypophysectomy patients.[8] It can occur both intraoperatively and postoperatively. Central DI occurs due to either reduced secretion of antidiuretic hormone (ADH) or destruction of ADH-secreting neurons. There are three postoperative patterns: transient DI, permanent DI, and triphasic DI. Triphasic DI has three phases: an initial phase (first 4–7 days) caused by damage to the ADH-secreting neurons leading to polyuria and hypernatremia, followed by a recovery phase (7–14 days) due to the release of stored ADH from pituitary leading to hyponatremia and increased urine osmolality, followed by the third phase of permanent DI on exhaustion of this stored ADH. DI manifests as polyuria (>3 L/day), polydipsia, hyperosmolality (>320 mOsm/kg), hypernatremia (se Na >150 mEq/L), and dilute urine. Treatment of DI entails calculation of free water deficit (FWD) = Weight (kg) × 0.6 × ([serum Na/140]–1). This deficit should be replaced over 24 hours in addition to maintenance and other losses with hypoosmolar fluids. Correction of hypernatremia should not proceed at a rate greater than 1 mEq/L/h. Pharmacological treatment entails use of desmopressin (DDAVP) 1–2 µg twice or thrice a day intravenously or via nasal spray (2.5–20 µg). Vasopressin 0.2–1 mU/kg/h as an intravenous infusion maybe used but consequent hypertension contraindicates its use in coronary artery disease patients.

CONCLUSION AND FUTURE DIRECTION

A multidisciplinary team is a cornerstone for comprehensive management of such intricate surgeries to ensure patient safety and improved oncological outcomes. A new frontier for the anesthesiologist to conquer would be the recent interest in transoral robotic surgery for anterior skull base surgery.

REFERENCES

1. Jellish WS, Murdoch J, Leonetti JP. Perioperative management of complex skull base surgery: the anesthesiologist's point of view. Neurosurg Focus. 2002;12(5):e5.
2. Hussaini AS, Clark CM, DeKlotz TR. Perioperative Considerations in Endoscopic Skull Base Surgery. Curr Otorhinolaryngol Rep. 2020;8(2):129-35.
3. Lee SC, Senior BA. Endoscopic skull base surgery. Clin Exp Otorhinolaryngol. 2008;1(2):53-62.
4. Porras JL, Rowan NR, Mukherjee D. Endoscopic Endonasal Skull Base Surgery Complication Avoidance: A Contemporary Review. Brain Sci. 2022;12(12):1685.
5. Campbell RG. Robotic surgery of the anterior skull base. Int Forum Allergy Rhinol. 2019;9(12):1508-14.
6. Amorocho MC, Fat I. Anesthetic techniques in endoscopic sinus and skull base surgery. Otolaryngol Clin North Am. 2016;49(3):531-47.
7. Ezri T, Roth Y, Geva D, Konichezky S, Marshak G, Halperin D. Anesthetic management of juvenile nasopharyngeal angiofibroma resection. J Cardiothorac Vasc Anesth. 2003;17(5):622-4.
8. Tien DA, Stokken JK, Recinos PF, Woodard TD, Sindwani R. Comprehensive Postoperative Management After Endoscopic Skull Base Surgery. Otolaryngol Clin North Am. 2016;49(1):253-63.
9. Chaskes MB, Rabinowitz MR. Safety of restarting continuous positive airway pressure (CPAP) therapy following endoscopic endonasal skull base surgery. World J Otorhinolaryngol Head Neck Surg. 2022;8(1):61-5.

15 CHAPTER

Anesthesia for Free Flap Microvascular Surgeries

Mary Thomas, Mira Sudam Wagh, Nebu Abraham George

INTRODUCTION

When an area in the surface of the body needs to be removed due to malignancy or has been destroyed due to burns, we need to reconstruct that area to look like its original self. Tissue flaps consisting of skin, fat, muscle, and bone cartilage are used. Skin along with muscle and fat can be rotated from a nearby area keeping the blood vessels intact and used or for better aesthetics, an area of tissue along with its artery and vein is cut and re-anastomosed with similar sized vessels in the recipient area. Free flap surgery also involves using bowel segments for reconstruction of the gastrointestinal tract.

Anastomosis of the small vessels from donor site to vessels in the recipient site involves microvascular anastomosis under the microscope. The physiology of transplanting a piece of tissue to another part of the body needs care like in organ transplant. The surgery is time consuming and requires great expertise. The surgery carries great morbidity for flap failure and incidence of redo of anastomosis. Anesthetic management during various stages of surgery requires great understanding of the effect of various anesthetics on the physiology of the flap.

TYPES OF FLAPS

Pedicled flaps are transferred from donor to recipient site with the blood supply coming from the donor site to the tissue.

In free flaps, the blood vessels are severed from their original site and anastomosed to vessels of similar caliber in the recipient site under the microscope. Usually, there is only one artery and vein, no lymphatic supply initially and neither any sympathetic nerve supply.[1]

Soft tissue flaps commonly used are—radial forearm free flap, anterolateral thigh free flap, jejunum, and deep inferior epigastric perforator flap.

Composite free flaps include the transfer of multiple types of tissue including muscle, skin, fascia, and bone having a single common blood supply. The commonly used composite flaps are the fibular free flap, deep circumflex iliac free flap, and composite radial free flap.

INDICATIONS

Though free flaps are used for aesthetics and repair of post-traumatic defects, in this chapter, we discuss the use in oncosurgery. Tumor removal requiring full oncological clearance may leave huge defects which cannot be closed by tissue of adjacent area or muscle flaps with blood supply from a nearby site. When the tumor is in the lower jaw, soft tissue and bone are required for reconstruction, while in the breast only soft tissue is required and for oropharynx intestinal segments are used.

Anesthesia is a major determinant in the success of the flap surgery. Maintenance of stable blood pressure (BP) within 20% of the patient's original BP is essential for flap perfusion. Balancing the regional anesthesia to provide pain relief while providing analgesia with regional anesthesia we need to maintain normotension so that regional blood flow and flap perfusion is not compromised. Normothermia is essential to avoid vasoconstriction. Excess fluid would cause flap edema and too less underperfusion. So, adequate fluid maintenance is difficult. Dilution anemia should not compromise oxygenation.

FLAP BIOLOGY

Free flap surgery causes discontinuation of blood circulation and calls for painstakingly accurate microvascular resuturing. Requisite flap perfusion is a complicated interaction between technical factors (the arterial and venous bore diameter and exceptional expertise in resuturing) and intraoperative physiological factors (such as maintenance of appropriate flap vascularity and oxygen supply). The fundamentals of intraoperative stewardship are primarily based on preserving the Hagen–Poiseuille equation which states:[2]

$$\frac{\Delta P \times r^4 \times \pi}{8 \times \eta \times l}$$

Where ΔP is the pressure difference across the vessel anastomosed, r is the radius of the vessel, η is viscosity of the blood flowing through, and l is the length of the vessel.

Sustenance of neocirculation in the flap is affected by BP in the anastomosed vessels, vessel radius and length, and blood consistency. The initial vessel anatomy is influenced by the surgical team, the hemodynamics, vessel diameter, and blood viscidity can be subject to anesthetic management. Not only oxygen delivery but flap survival is definitely influenced by anesthetic stewardship.[2]

Let us discuss in detail the various perioperative precautions and steps of surgery and the interventions needed to be done by the anesthetist.

PREOPERATIVE EVALUATION FOR FREE FLAP SURGERY

Definite Reasons to Avoid Surgery

Thrombophilic states, such as sickling disorder due to hemoglobin S and Osler–Vaquez disease, escalate the probability of clot formation in the area of neovascularization.[3]

Relative Contraindications

- *Severe lung or cardiac disease*
- *Active smokers*
- *Deep vein thrombosis*
- *Atherosclerotic disease:* A research paper with a cohort of around 2,500 patients awaiting surgery for oral cancer found hyperglycemia, atherosclerosis, compromised renal parameters, and history of treatment with radiation to be crucial prognosticators of bad outcome.[4]
- *Body mass index (BMI) >30:* Overweight patients should be encouraged to exercise and diet to reduce weight before surgery to improve surgical outcome.[3]
- Collagen vascular disease
- *Age >65 years:* Increase in age does not have a negative effect on free flap outcome but indirectly increase risk due to the higher incidence of comorbidities.[5]

RISK ASSESSMENT

A thorough understanding of the risk factors predisposing to flap failure will help us to optimize the patient and also help surgeon to decide the feasibility of taking up the patient for such a high-risk procedure. If factors increasing risk of vascular compromise after surgery and need for reanastomosis can be predicted from medical history and comorbidities, surgical plan can be altered accordingly. An index was created linking the pathology of the disease with patients whose BP and sugars are uncontrolled, have cardiac illness and obliterative arteriopathy, and are in the habit of smoking. They were found to have higher morbidity of anastomotic failure. Of all the prognosticators, the statistically significant ones were the American Society of Anesthesiologists (ASA) score and the sort of flap. ASA grade 2 patients were associated with twice the risk of progressing to adverse events after surgery, while the possibility of unfavorable outcome was increased by 2.6 times in ASA 3 patients. Research shows that patients reconstructed with free osteocutaneous fibula flap unfortunately had more than two times likelihood of flap survival issues.[6]

Risk stratification for complex procedures such as microsurgical reconstruction is an important part of preoperative planning and counseling. Frailty index (5-mFI) score is a validated tool for assessing risk in surgical patients.[7]

Cardiopulmonary exercise testing is an emerging tool in perioperative assessment. An anaerobic threshold of <11 mL/min/kg raises concern for significant perioperative morbidity, although this is not an absolute number (Older, 2013).

PREOPERATIVE OPTIMIZATION

Prehabilitation

A systematic review by Loewen et al. (2021) found significant variability in the timing, duration, and outcomes of prehabilitation. Further research is required in this area.

- *Control of diabetes mellitus:* Hemoglobin A1c (HbA1c) to be brought down below 8.5%, 69 mmol/mol, and blood sugars to be brought under tight control.[8] Maintaining blood sugar below 150 mg may decrease surgical site infection.[9]

The uncontrolled sugars can cause vessel thickening and stiffening making microvascular anastomosis risky. The decrease in vessel pliability and oxygenation created by diabetes can raise the risk for flap failure. Peripheral arterial disease is common in diabetics and may increase morbidity. Recently, vascular mapping for assessing the vessels to be used for anastomosis by color Doppler, computed tomography (CT) angiography, or magnetic resonance imaging (MRI) angiography is being adopted.[10]

- *Preoperative chemotherapy:* Bleomycin can cause pulmonary fibrosis and compromise oxygenation. ARISCAT scores assessment and arterial blood gas analysis should be done. Anthracyclines can cause cardiomyopathies. So, these patients should be sent to pulmonologists and cardiologists for screening and optimization. Revised cardiac risk index (RCRI) is used to assess the tolerance to this procedure.
- *Preoperative radiotherapy:* Some studies show that radiation given before surgery might affect the blood vessels and give rise to increase incidence of flap failure.[11] But some show no evidence of it.[12]
- *Hypertension:* Resting hypertension is a relative contraindication for controlled hypotension. Controlled hypotension increases visibility of surgical field. Hence hypertension should be controlled preoperatively.
- Uncontrolled BP also causes hematoma and bleeding. Increased BP and coronary vascular abnormalities can cause problems especially during interventions and extubation.[13]
- *Bronchial asthma and chronic obstructive pulmonary disease (COPD):* Patients should be evaluated optimised with steroids and bronchodilators. History of obstructive sleep apnea should be noted
- *Psychological well-being:* Patients should be assessed and treated (Machiels et al., 2020).
- *Smoking:* The vascular linings become abnormal and nonfunctional due to smoking. This causes decrease in vascular blood flow. Smoking causes a rise in microvascular complications. They can be rectified by cessation of smoking as studied by O'Neill et al.[14]
- Smokers cannot be denied surgery but are counseled to refrain from smoking for a minimum of 1 month prior to the surgical procedure. This reduces the tobacco-induced side effects on the heart and lung. Carbon monoxide generated by smoking causes cellular deoxygenation. Thrombophilia occurs due to platelet clustering. Hence, tobacco users can have issues related to flap survival.[3]

Airway Assessment

Patients with head and neck cancer can be anticipated difficult intubations and airway assessment should be done meticulously. Consent for awake intubation and tracheostomy should be taken preoperatively. Elective postoperative ventilation and ICU admission as a possibility should be explained.

Venous Access and Arterial Cannulation

The need for central venous access will depend on patient and availability of good peripheral venous access. Femoral vein is cannulated as the internal jugular and subclavian vein cannulation can encroach the surgical sites. We should abstain from starting venous and arterial lines in and around flap harvesting areas. Monitor probes should also stay clear of this site. It is crucial to communicate to the surgeon when accessing any artery or vein.

Venous thrombosis should be ruled out via Doppler. Arterial and venous access should be checked before surgery. Allen's test should be performed before arterial cannulation.

PREOPERATIVE INVESTIGATIONS

Routine blood tests include total blood count, coagulation profile, urea and electrolytes, liver function tests, blood grouping HIV, HbSAg screening, and an electrocardiogram. A chest radiograph is not mandatory if patients have a CT, MRI, or positron emission tomography/CT scan of the chest.

Since these surgeries usually go on beyond 5 hours arterial blood gas analysis, pulmonary function tests and echocardiography should be done. Cardiopulmonary exercise testing is considered gold standard in risk analysis. An anaerobic threshold of <11 mL/min/kg raises the probability for acute intraoperative adverse events. But 6-minute walk test or shuttle walk test will also give us a fair estimation.

PERIOPERATIVE MONITORING AND SPECIAL REQUIREMENTS

- *Saturation monitor:* High-flow nasal oxygenation may be used if difficult intubation is anticipated and awake tracheal intubation is planned. Hypoxia can produce adrenaline release and vasoconstriction so meticulous monitoring of saturation must be maintained.
- *Invasive BP:* If radial forearm flap is planned, the arterial cannulation must be put in another site. *Cardiac output monitoring* is done by stroke volume variation (SVV)/pulse pressure variation (PPV)/ plethysmographic variability index (PVI). Noninvasive options of Masimo probe for PVI can also be used.

Warm fluids to be given to maintain values around 13. Esophageal Doppler monitoring can also be used. When a radial forearm free flap is being used for reconstruction, it is wise not to use both radial arteries (in case the side of harvest has to be changed due to unforeseen problems intraoperatively). Dorsalis pedis or femoral arteries are the practical replacements.

- *Fluid management:* It is very important as edema and hypovolemia can compromise flap vascularity. Hence, goal-directed fluid therapy should be practiced.
- *Temperature:* Temperature probe to maintain normothermia of around 36.5°C. Forced air warmers (43°C) or circulating water blankets (40°C) can be used. Prolonged operative time in the operation theater with two surgical sites exposed to cold temperatures with intravenous (IV) fluids which are cooled by the cold temperature often leads to hypothermia. Hypothermia has been connected to numerous postoperative complications such as incomplete or complete flap loss, prolonged wound healing, vessel spasm, raised hematocrit causing decreased blood flow, coagulation failure leading to hematoma formation, and surgical site infections. Patient wakes up and shivers to compensate for the hypothermia leading to higher oxygen demand, desaturation, arrhythmias, and adverse cardiac events.[15]
- Fluid warmers are useful to a certain extent only, especially if a restrictive fluid administration policy is incorporated. Warmed fluids do help in decreasing hypothermia during the intraoperative period.
- *Muscle blockade:* Acceleromyograph can be used to assess the depth of muscle paralysis. As patient needs to be completely immobile during anastomosis. Muscle relaxant infusions are given to maintain absolute immobility. The return of muscle function should be documented using quantitative train of four ratios.
- *Depth of anesthesia monitoring:* If total intravenous anesthesia (TIVA) is used for maintenance of Bispectral index, entropy or any monitoring for the drop in awareness under anesthesia becomes mandatory. The UK Fifth National Anaesthesia Project 5 (NAP5) advocates inadvertent awareness surveillance whenever TIVA is used, particularly if muscles are paralyzed for surgery. Monitoring of processed electroencephalography (pEEG) can also be done by connecting sensors on the forehead prior to initiation of anesthesia, for continuous monitoring throughout the duration of TIVA.[16]
- *End tidal CO_2 ($EtCO_2$) monitor:* Hypocapnia can produce vasoconstriction and hence $EtCO_2$ must be maintained between 35 and 40 mm Hg. Hypercapnia can produce tachycardia and hypertension.
- *Hemoglobin estimation:* Hematocrit is another major factor influencing microvascular flow and blood viscosity. Higher packed cell volumes (PCVs) cause a rise in viscosity and decrease blood flow in the microcirculation.[17]
- Isovolemic hemodilution increases blood flow in smaller vessels, causes muscle reperfusion injury, and increases the patency of capillaries that minimizes tissue death. PCV value of 30% is associated with the best equilibrium between viscosity and oxygen delivery. Giving blood for the sustenance of hemoglobin around 10 gm% had no consequence on the end result of the flap. Neither PCV nor blood administration had a negative impact on flap viability.[13]
- *Positioning:* As these surgeries are prolonged, care should be taken to protect pressure areas to avoid nerve and compression soft tissue injury. Eyes and bony prominences should be padded.
- *Deep vein thrombosis prophylaxis:* Patients should have thromboembolic prevention devices. Pressure graded stockings and pneumatic compression devices can be used.
- *Nasogastric (NG) tube/percutaneous endoscopic gastrostomy (PEG):* All patients should be seen by a dietician and have a calculated nutritional schedule charted out after preoperative discussion by team members. Postoperative enteral nutrition may be given via a PEG or NG tube at the earliest.

SURGICAL FACTORS

Time under general anesthesia (GA) has been shown to be positively correlated with postoperative adverse events and delay in discharge from hospital.[18]

Multiple operating surgeons may have adverse consequences. Better results are seen when preoperative patient optimization and postoperative care are done under the care of a single surgeon.[5]

ANESTHETIC TECHNIQUE

Venous Access

At least two peripheral venous cannulae (PVCs) are always secured. If TIVA is the chosen method of induction and maintenance of anesthesia, double check the cannula site for leaks and confirm adequate flow through the PVC, as any failure of TIVA delivery could result in accidental awareness under GA. Customized TIVA sets should be utilized to ameliorate security. Propofol and remifentanil are currently the best medications for use in target-controlled infusions (TCI). In case, various drugs which cannot be mixed together are needed a central vein cannula that is more applicable and more pertinent if patient requires hemodynamic support with inotropes or vasoconstrictors. The femoral or subclavian vein is customarily used, inserted conventionally after the patient anesthetized except in case of emergency when there is an uncertainty about the hemodynamic condition.

Mention Induction

Standard anesthetic practice may be followed for induction. If the patients airway assessment predicts difficult airway, airway topicalization and awake securement of airway are planned. Previously blind nasal intubation was practiced but with the advent of flexible intubating scopes into airway management, this technique has become popular. Tracheostomy is not usually a preferred method of airway securement unless in emergency. Postoperatively, elective tracheostomy may be done in head and neck surgery to prevent coughing on the endotracheal tube which needs to be retained postoperatively to prevent respiratory distress as the surgical area is edematous. Usually, a nasotracheal tube is used to provide an optimum oropharyngeal access to the surgeons—permitting unlimited view at the beginning just after induction of anesthesia to insert the PEG feeding tube and enhancing the approachability for the elective tracheostomy. A preformed Ring, Adair, and Elwin tube or a reinforced flexometallic tracheal tube is used. The endotracheal tube is inserted after a nasal vasoconstrictor application like xylometazoline (to reduce the risk of epistaxis). Nasal xylocaine 10% spray also helps to reduce the stress of intubation. The endotracheal tube should be softened with sterile warm water to prevent bruising during placement. If tube positioning is achieved via direct or video laryngoscopy, Magill's forceps is extremely useful to lift and guide the glottic end of the tracheal tube to pass through the vocal cord. One should take care not to injure the cuff during the procedure. Bilateral air entry should be equal and tube secured firmly as further access will not be easy.

Maintenance

General Anesthesia (GA)

- Inhalational anesthesia with air—oxygen and inhalation agent—sevoflurane or isoflurane may be used.[3] Isoflurane has peripheral vasodilatory effects and maintains microcirculation. Sevoflurane before ischemia can cause preconditioning and after reperfusion can cause postconditioning. Hence, it is protective for the flap. Reperfusion injury is the cell damage and death caused by sudden blood flow in the previously ischemic piece of tissue. Not much has been studied about the effect of desflurane on free flap surgery though early recovery after a prolonged surgery is an advantage.
- *Inhalation anesthesia* has the advantage of producing less nausea and vomiting. Propofol and remifentanil is a popular combination. Remifentanil renders good analgesia, adequate vasodilatation, and stable hemodynamics.[3]

  Chang et al. compared the technique of anesthetizing with IV drugs only with standard GA using sevoflurane or desflurane and concluded that the TIVA group needed minimal intraoperative fluids and was associated with lesser pulmonary complications.[19]
- *Dexmeditomidine usage* is controversial. IV dexmedetomidine can also be used as an infusion for postoperative pain relief in the postoperative care area. The disagreement about the use of this α2-adrenoreceptor agonist in free flap surgeries is that there is a possibility of constriction of blood vessels compromising blood supply leading to flap failure.[20] On the contrary, it is also seen that dexmedetomidine maintains stable hemodynamics without any increase in flap failure. It also has the advantage of allaying postoperative anxiety.[21] Ventilator settings are adjusted to avoid both hyperoxia and hypocarbia as they can stimulate arteriolar vasoconstriction.[22]
- *Neuromuscular blocking agents:* Since surgery is of long duration, the relaxant of choice is rocuronium, as at a dose of 1 mg/kg. It can be used for intubation in 60 seconds for difficult intubation or mask ventilation cases as immediate reversal is possible with sugammadex in case intubation attempt fails. It acts for 45 minutes. The long duration of action also makes it easier for the subsequent insertion of PEG or Ryle's tube and elective tracheostomy. Further bolus doses will be needed and can be tailored according

to quantitative neuromuscular monitoring to give appropriate relaxation and immobility. Quantitative neuromuscular monitoring has become standard of care. Train of four is used to confirm that the reversal of neuromuscular blocking drug (NMBD) can be performed and post-tetanic count is checked to prevent patient from suddenly coming out of relaxation and establishing absolute immobility during microvascular anastomosis. It is also used when the surgeon wants intraoperative nerve monitoring of facial or recurrent laryngeal nerve.

Fluid Management

The most popular central venous catheter access is the subclavian vein and should be cannulated in these patients for recommendations in calculating fluid administration. Goal-directed fluid therapy is now the gold standard and leads to adequate hydration during the intraoperative period.[23] Cardiac output measurement, cardiac index (CI), and stroke volume index (SVI) may be monitored intraoperatively with the arterial pulse contour device.

Fluid overload with crystalloids (more than 7 L) leads to tissue edema and low colloid oncotic pressure. This may exacerbate with tissue handling.[5]

Vasoactive drugs: Medications used for vasoconstriction during hypotension during anesthesia have been believed to be a source of hypoperfusion to the anastomosed tissue.[24]

Nevertheless, there are research papers that show that the type (dopamine, noradrenaline, and metaraminol) or dosage of vasoconstrictors could not be proved to be a cause of flap failure directly and the probability that vasoconstrictors such as noradrenaline can be favorable by sustaining perfusion.[25,26]

Sodium nitroprusside ameliorates circulation in the free flap on application topically at the anastomotic site. It is preferred over α-blocker (labetalol), as it produces intense vasodilation in the free flap which has lost its sympathetic supply without an adverse effect on the entire sympathetic nervous system.[27]

A retrospective study of around 250 free flap breast reconstructions studied intraoperative vasopressor use and deduced that phenylephrine and/or ephedrine use did not adversely affect the flap outcome.[26]

Antithrombotic therapy: Aspirin, dextran 40, and unfractionated heparin decrease platelet aggregation, enhance blood flow, or impede blood viscosity. Statins are said to be vasoprotective and prevent inflammation but their role in intercepting thrombosis in the surgical site vasculature is yet to be proved.[28]

Dextran infusion was used to enhance flow in the free flap vessels.[29] Unlike in the past, the regular administration of dextran has been abandoned as a result of unfavorable events such as anaphylaxis, respiratory failure, cardiac failure, bleeding, and renal failure. The success rates using dextran for free flap vessel anastomosis and the absence of clot occlusions were not worthy of attention.

Analgesia

Analgesia in free flap surgery is required for two sites separately:

1. *Harvesting site:* Since harvesting sites are usually extremities, regional anesthesia techniques such as epidural or local nerve blocks with perineural catheter are commonly used. Regional anesthetic techniques commonly used are epidural for lower extremities and brachial plexus block for upper extremities. Peripheral nerve catheters have been used without any complications to inject local anesthetic into the fibular donor site.[30] Continuous infusions via elastomeric pumps, patient-controlled analgesia pumps, or intermittent bolus by staff are effective.

   Mini-catheters have also been used without any adverse report to inject local anesthetic into the abdominal donor site.[31]
2. *Free flap surgery site:* The studies done on the effect of regional anesthesia on microvascular free flap surgery have not revealed any definite result. Spinal or epidural anesthesia producing hypotension >20% from basal value can be deleterious for flap blood flow. Erni et al. have studied the free vascularized tissue and displayed a reduction in blood flow by using laser flow velocimetry after epidural anesthesia.[32]

Regional Anesthesia

Epidural local anesthetics cause sympathetic block. This can cause vasodilatation and better flap survival but it cannot prevent vasospasm which is caused by surgical manipulation.[13,22]

Sodium nitroprusside infusion could be useful. We should also remember that the vessels used for anastomosis are sympathetically denervated and so the neo-revascularized tissue may not be perfused due to a steal phenomenon.

Plane Blocks

High thoracic paravertebral block with local anesthetic proven to increase hemodynamics of maxillofacial free flap surgery.[33] In deep inferior epigastric perforator (DIEP) reconstruction surgeries, the two surgical sites are in the torso—the thorax and the lower abdomen. Surprisingly when mastectomy is done and reconstructed with a free flap, there is less postoperative pain as the flap has no sensory supply and it prevents the skin at the edges from being stretched for primary closure. Therefore, in comparison the mastectomy wound causes less distress than the abdominal wound. Usually intravenous drugs deal with the pain but transverse abdominal plane blocks are efficient in decreasing the discomfort and have an opioid-sparing capacity up to 48 hours after surgery.[34] Ultrasound guidance can be used to place catheters in the right plane by the anesthetist at induction or surgeons can also do it intraoperatively under direct vision.

Nerve Blocks for Head and Neck Surgery

A nerve block performed preoperatively does not impart much postoperative pain relief due to the long duration of surgery by which time the effect would have worn off. However, the head and neck region meets the requirement for local anesthetic nerve blocks given under the skin or mucous membrane which can have favorable effects in decreasing inhalation agent usage and therefore minimizing cognitive disorders and narcotic demand after the long surgery. A superficial or deep cervical plexus block may be given for pain relief of neck dissection. Some surgeons request infiltration of larger volumes of diluted local anesthetic along with adrenaline at the surgical site to decrease local bleeding. There is lack of evidence justifying an advantage of regional anesthesia on cancer recurrence.[35]

Multimodal Analgesia

The approach used for postsurgical pain relief includes multimodal analgesia. Paracetamol if liver functions are not very abnormal and nonsteroidal anti-inflammatory drugs (NSAIDs) if renal function is within normal limits. Opioids are delivered by bolus IV doses, IV infusion, patient-controlled analgesia, patch application on the skin, or as tablets or syrups.[3] Paramount importance has to be given to providing adequate analgesia after the patient is awake not only for well-being but also to avoid pain-induced stimulation of sympathetic activity which could adversely affect the morbidity of the free flap.

REVERSAL

When the patient is reversed from muscle relaxant and awakened from GA or TIVA at the end of surgery, care has to be taken not to allow the patient to struggle with the endotracheal tube in the throat. This causes raised venous pressure and compromise in flap perfusion; hence, smooth simultaneous initiation of reversal and arousal from anesthesia culminating in a peaceful extubation should be provided.[3] Many methods are used to ensure an uneventful extubation. Remifentanil infusion is used to prevent bucking on the tube. Deep extubation is the practise of removing the endotracheal tube after the patient has started breathing but before being awake. This technique carries a risk of aspiration and so should be performed only by senior anesthetists. The Baileys method is recommended—replacing the tracheal tube for a supraglottic airway device (SGAD) before reversal under anesthesia. The patient is reversed with the SGAD in situ and allowed to awaken and then the device is removed. Most head and neck reconstructions with free flap require the endotracheal tube to be retained overnight as they develop edema in the oral cavity. Morphine as bolus dose is very effective in assisting tube tolerance and to prevent coughing on the tube. Most surgeons perform elective tracheostomy to avoid the risk of postoperative tube intolerance and agitation which can compromise the success of flap survival.

STAGES OF FREE FLAP SURGERY[36]

Removal of tumor just before reconstruction procedure if not removed earlier

Phases of Free Flap Surgery

- The phases of free flap surgery are:
  - *Flap preferment* and cessation of blood flow in vessels by applying clamps
  - *Primary ischemia:* Due to ischemia as a consequence of inadequate blood flow and oxygen delivery after clamp application, anaerobic intracellular metabolism increases in proportion to the duration before release of clamp after anastomosis.
  - *Reperfusion injury:* Occurs as soon as both the artery and vein are sutured and the clamps removed. Secondary ischemia is a consequence of compromised circulation of the flap (curtailed by congruous patient care by the anesthetist).[3]

Flap Elevation and Clamping of Vessels

Dissection and raising the flap through the muscle and scrupulously isolating the minute blood vessels supplying the graft is the first stage. It is of prime importance that the flap should be maintained at normal body temperature before it is dissected out (before the initiation of "warm ischemia" time). This stage of microscopic surgery is usually linked with decreased anesthetic depth requirement as there is no major surgical stimulus (unless dual sites are being addressed). During this interval, the anesthetist has time to optimize hemodynamic conditions for the next stage of graft reperfusion and absolute immobility is crucial in all these stages.

Primary Ischemia

Primary ischemia of the flap occurs as circulation comes to a halt due to vessel clamping, during the time, the flap is transferred for anastomosis. The free flap is taken out after halting the blood supply and then the pivotal step of microanastomosis begins under the microscope. The category of flap modifies the time endurance of "warm ischemia"—free flaps which have increased muscle bulk have a higher metabolic rate and do not tolerate extended duration of warm ischemia. This induces anaerobic cellular metabolism. Lactate levels rise, intracellular pH falls with escalating levels of calcium and cytokines, chemokines, histamine, prostaglandins, and leukotrienes. The intensity of the injury brought about by the initial ischemia is equivalent to the time span of hypoperfusion. The cutaneous oxygen uptake by is quintuple below muscle fibers at rest (0.2 and 1 mL min^{-1} per 100 g of tissue, respectively). The time depends on the expertise of the surgeon but is usually around 60–90 minutes.

Reperfusion

Restoration of blood flow is the subsequent predominant stage in free flap surgery and starts with removal of vessel clamps after culmination of microvascular suturing. Classically, the flow restarts and countermands the transitory functional disturbances activated by temporary halt of local circulation. However, the short duration during which the tissue did not receive blood supply followed by restoration of circulation may cause injury if some aspects are not conducive, such as extended duration of hypoperfusion or insufficient BP. In such situations, reperfusion injury takes place when restoration of circulation permits the inflow of leukotrienes, prostaglandins, platelet activating factors, and cytokines that may eventually result in flap anastomotic failure.[3]

The Classic Physiological Environment

The classic physiological environment to enhance perfusion of the freshly anastomosed flap encompasses a number of factors such as normothermia, a fairly hyperdynamic circulation with a wide pulse pressure, and a PCV between 30 and 35%—ideal blood viscosity to increase blood flow, without making concessions on oxygen delivery, and keep in mind the patients' comorbidities.

Fall in temperature causes constriction of blood vessels to conserve heat which is an unfavorable event preceding the harvesting of flap and also subsequent to the anastomosis, as this causes compromise in blood circulation within the flap. Free flaps have no nerve supply and hence have deficient autonomic protective response to maintain blood flow (by vasodilation and constriction) and so they depend on stable hemodynamic parameters for pressure-dependent flow. Therefore, at the time of flap reperfusion by releasing the clamp, the patients' BP should be raised to the preinduction level. As a matter of fact, the more the number, size, and anatomy of the vessels used for anastomosis, the anesthetist should ensure to maintain a higher than normal perfusion pressure. A point to be kept in mind is that a supranormal BP can cause increased bleeding in the harvested site and at the anastomotic site, which can cause clot formation, wound dehiscence, and, more critically, flap failure. BP should be managed with vigilant IV fluid input (optimal preload) and prudent use of vasopressors (ideal afterload). Nevertheless, we must remember that the direct action of vasopressors on the tiny arteries supplying (and within) the flap can produce an adverse effect. In the same way, venous anastomosis can also get constricted and engorge within the flap and decrease flap blood outflow. This obstruction to flap blood flow from the flap can cause interstitial edema, exacerbating any venous clogging, which may be further harmed by enthusiastic IV fluid administration (due to deficiency of lymphatic system in the free flap). Therefore, a cautious titrated fluid strategy to achieve predetermined targets is vital. Continuous esophageal Doppler monitoring is impractical as the site is not accessible during surgery. Central lines are not essential as a routine. Arterial pulsed contour analysis is easiest and practical option of monitoring trends (PPV, SVV, etc.). Prime importance should be given to clear communication between anesthetic and surgical teams in optimizing all stages of flap surgery.

Flap circulation may also be ensured by imaging after the flap has been isolated, using indocyanine green near-infrared video angiography (ICG-NIR-VA). This method is performed to evaluate the caliber of flap vessels and "run off" before the flap is removed for anastomosis. IV ICG is given intravenously by the anesthetist as per protocol. Any past history of unpleasant reactions to ICG or iodine must be ruled out. Patients' urine may turn green due to the dye in the circulation.

POSTOPERATIVE FACTORS

Postoperative care should give importance to maintain normal temperature, normal BP, PCV not <30%, urine output of at least 1 mL $kg^{-1}$and h^{-1}, and arterial oxygen saturation (SaO_2) >94% for the first 24 hours. Pulmonary complications such as pulmonary edema, pneumonia, or atelectasis may occur in these patients.[18]

Evaluation of flap color is done by checking the capillary refill time, skin turgor, temperature, and presence of bleeding on pinprick.

Grafts should be vigilantly inspected for 24 hours for arterial spasm, graft congestion, and venous occlusion.[22] Reanastomosis of the graft vessels may be necessary if manifestation of compromise of blood flow occurs. Graft edema can be minimized by elevation of the anastomotic site. A bolus dose of dexamethasone (40 mg) and mannitol 10% (0.5 g/kg) will help to reduce the edema. Regular administration of IV heparin and dextran infusion is not followed as a protocol due to high incidence of rebleed.

The flap should be regularly scrutinized and checked for blood flow in the flap by temperature and laser Doppler.[37] An acoustic evaluation of vessel patency using an 8 MHz transcutaneous Doppler is done percutaneously with the probe on the overlying the perforator blood vessel on the flap. This spot is demarcated by the surgeons. The Doppler signal is examined periodically to detect any decrease in flow.

If arterial flow is compromised, the flap is cold, has pallor, with prolonged capillary refill time, lack of bleed on puncture, and silence of arterial (triphasic) Doppler signal. On the contrary, if the venous outflow is blocked, the flap has warmth, is swollen, has a dusky discoloration, has brisk capillary refill time, prompt bleed of dark blood on puncture, and absolutely no venous Doppler signal (usually a continuous signal).

STEPS TO SAVE AN ISCHEMIC FREE FLAP

If it is detected early at the onset and managed instantly (within 6 hours), 75% of flaps with a partial anastomotic failure can be saved. The categorical step to save a compromised flap is surgical intervention and emergency re-exploration to scrutinize the vasculature for distortions and constrictions, reassess flow and stability of suture site, probe for any clot formation, execute embolectomy if needed, or perform intra-arterial thrombolysis.

Similar anesthetic principles used intraoperatively for flap harvesting and anastomosis should be carried on in the adverse circumstances of jeopardized flap perfusion, to provide an ideal condition that encourages finest flap flow.[3]

RECENT ADVANCES

Nowadays, a lot of advances have been made with 3D imaging platform to plan the reconstruction. The imaging and planning platform used is—iPlan 3.0 (Brainlab®, Feldkirchen, Germany). This platform allows for planning preoperatively with 3D tools about the alignment, autosegmentation, etc. with atlas function and a three-dimensional modification with a tool named SmartShaper. This helps not only with preoperative data analysis but also with postoperative quality control. In addition, this platform helps in intraoperative navigation of the virtual plan which is crucial for face and skull base surgeries.[38]

CONCLUSION

Free flap surgery provides aesthetic reconstruction after major tissue loss. But, the surgery carries high risk of failure after long painstaking hours of hard work by the entire team. Hence, meticulous care should be taken to make the surgery successful.

REFERENCES

1. Quinan J. Anesthesia for Reconstructive Free Flap Surgery. Anaesth Intens Care Med. 2009;10(1):26-31.
2. McCauley P, Moore M, Duggan E. Anaesthesia for reconstructive free flap surgery for head and neck cancer. Br J Hosp Med. 2022;83(5):1-9.
3. Nimalan N. Anaesthesia for free flap breast reconstruction. Br J Anaesth. 2015;16(5):162-6.
4. Ishimaru M, Ono S, Suzuki S, Matsui H, Fushimi K, Yasunaga H. Risk factors for free flap failure in 2,846 patients with head and neck cancer: A national database study in Japan. J Oral Maxillofac Surg. 2016;74:1265-70.

5. Haughey BH, Wilson E, Kluwe L, Piccirillo J, Fredrickson J, Sessions D, et al. Free flap reconstruction of the head and neck: Analysis of 241 cases. Otolaryngol Head Neck Surg. 2001;125:10-7.
6. Lese P, Biedermann R, Constantinescu M, Grobbelaa AO, Olariu R. Predicting risk factors that lead to free flap failure and vascular compromise: A single unit experience with 565 free tissue transfers. J Plast Reconstruct Aesthetic Surg. 2021;74(3):512-22.
7. Khan MTA, Rajesh A, Montorfano L, Lue M, Wong Won B, Wang HT, et al. Evaluation of modified frailty index for predicting post-operative outcomes after lower-extremity free-flap reconstruction. Microsurgery. 2023;43(7):657-64.
8. Dhatariya K. How to prepare people with diabetes for surgery. Diab Prim Care. 2018;20:53-4.
9. de Vries FE, Gans SL, Solomkin JS, Allegranzi B, Egger M, Dellinger EP, et al. Meta-analysis of lower perioperative blood glucose target levels for reduction of surgical-site infection. Br J Surg. 2017;104:e95-e105.
10. Rosado P, Cheng HT, Wu CM, Wei FC. Influence of diabetes mellitus on postoperative complications and failure in head and neck free flap reconstruction: a systematic review and meta-analysis. Head Neck. 2015;37(4):615-8.
11. Tasch C, Pattiss A, Maier S, Lanthaler M, Pierer G. Free Flap Outcome in Irradiated Recipient Sites: A Systematic Review and Meta-analysis. Plast Reconstr Surg Glob Open. 2022;10(3):e4216.
12. Kroll SS, Robb GL, Reece GP, Miller MJ, Evans GR, Baldwin BJ, et al. Does prior irradiation increase the risk of total or partial free-flap loss? J Reconstr Microsurg. 1998;14(4):263-8.
13. Jayaram K, Rao P, Gurajala I, Ramachandran G. Evaluation of the Effect of Regional Anaesthesia on Microvascular Free Flaps. Turk J Anaesthesiol Reanim. 2018;46(6):441-6.
14. O'Neill AC, Haykal S, Bagher S, Zhong T, Hofer S. Predictors and consequences of intraoperative microvascular problems in autologous breast reconstruction. J Plast Reconstruct Aesthet Surg. 2016;69(10):1349-55.
15. Sumer BD, Myers LL, Leach J, Truelson JM. Correlation between intraoperative hypothermia and perioperative morbidity in patients with head and neck cancer. Arch Otolaryngol Head Neck Surg. 2009;135:682-6.
16. Cook TM, Andrade J, Bogod DG, Hitchman JM, Jonker WR, Lucas N, et al. The 5th National Audit Project (NAP5) on accidental awareness during general anaesthesia: patient experiences, human factors, sedation, consent and medicolegal issues. Anaesthesia. 2014;69:1102-16.
17. Cláudia M, Maria EL, Rita C, Dora C, José Pedro A. Anaesthesia and Surgical Microvascular Flaps. Rev Bras Anestesiol. 2012;62:563-79.
18. Jackson TD, Wannares JJ, Lancaster RT, Rattner DW, Hutter MM. Does speed matter? The impact of operative time on outcome in laparoscopic surgery. Surg Endosc. 2011;25:2288-95.
19. Chang YT, Wu CC, Tang TY, Lu CT, Lai CS, Shen CH. Differences between total intravenous anesthesia and inhalation anesthesia in free flap surgery of head and neck cancer. PLoS One. 2016;11:e0147713.
20. Rajan S, Moorthy S, Paul J, Kumar L. Effect of dexmedetomidine on postoperative hemodynamics and outcome of free flaps in head and neck reconstructive surgeries. Open Anesthesiol J. 2016;10:12-8.
21. Yang X, Li Z, Gao C, Liu R. Effect of dexmedetomidine on preventing agitation and delirium after microvascular free flap surgery: A randomized, double-blind, control study. J Oral Maxillofac Surg. 2015;73:1065-72.
22. Aps C, Cox RG, Mayou BJ, Sengupta P. The role of anaesthetic management in enhancing peripheral blood flow in patients undergoing free flap transfer. Ann R Coll Surg Engl. 1985;67:177-9.
23. Funk D, Bohn J, Mutch WA, Hayakawa T, Buchel F. Goal-directed fluid therapy for microvascular free flap reconstruction following mastectomy: A pilot study. Plast Surg. 2015;23:231-4.
24. Motakef S, Mountziaris PM, Ismail IK, Agag RL, Patel A. Perioperative management for microsurgical free tissue transfer: Survey of current practices with a comparison to the literature. J Reconstr Microsurg. 2015;3:355-63.
25. Rose L, Prado N, Mulvey D, Laugharne D, Jones K, Stenhouse J. Vasoactive agents do not adversely influence the success of maxillofacial microvascular free-flap surgery: A retrospective analysis. Int J Anesth Res. 2016;4:327-30.
26. Chen C, Nguyen MD, Bar-Meir E, Hess PA, Lin S, Tobias AM, et al. Effects of vasopressor administration on the outcomes of microsurgical breast reconstruction. Ann Plast Surg. 2010;65:28-31.
27. Inglis MS, Edwards JM, Robbie DS, Breach NM. The anaesthetic management of patients undergoing free flap reconstructive surgery following resection of head and neck neoplasms: A review of 64 patients. Ann Royal Coll Surg Eng. 1988;70:235-8.
28. Pršić A, Kiwanuka E, Caterson SA, Caterson EJ. Anticoagulants and statins as pharmacological agents in free flap surgery: Current rationale. Eplasty. 2015;15:e51.
29. Sun TB, Chien SH, Lee JT, Cheng LF, Hsu LP, Chen PR. Is dextran infusion as an antithrombotic agent necessary in microvascular reconstruction of the upper aerodigestive tract? J Reconstr Microsurg. 2003;19:463-6.
30. Ferri A, Varazzani A, Valente A, Pedrazzi G, Bianchi B, Ferrari S, et al. Perioperative pain management after fibular free flap harvesting for head-and-neck reconstruction using mini-catheters to inject local anesthetic: A pilot study. Microsurgery. 2018;38:295-9.
31. Giordano S, Veräjänkorva E, Koskivuo I, Suominen E. Effectiveness of local anaesthetic pain catheters for abdominal donor site analgesia in patients undergoing free lower abdominal flap breast reconstruction: A meta-analysis of comparative studies. J Plastic Surg Hand Surg. 2013;47:428-33.

32. Erni D, Banic A, Signer C, Sigurdsson GH. Effects of epidural anaesthesia on microcirculatory blood flow in free flaps in patients under general anaesthesia. Eur J Anaesthesiol. 1999;16:692-8.
33. Habib AM, Zanaty OM, Anwer HF, Abo Alia D. The effect of paravertebral block on maxillofacial free flap survival. Int J Oral Maxillofac Surg. 2017;46:706-11.
34. Zhong T, Wong KW, Cheng H, Ojha M, Srinivas C, McCluskey SA, et al. Transverse abdominis plane (TAP) catheters inserted under direct vision in the donor site following free DIEP and MS-TRAM breast reconstruction: a prospective cohort study of 45 patients. J Plast Reconstr Aesthet Surg. 2013;66:329-36.
35. Gillan C, God A. Anaesthetic considerations for major cancer resection and free flap reconstruction in oral cancer: a review. J Oral Maxillofac Anesth. 2023;2:18.
36. Hanasono MM, Butler CE. Prevention and Treatment of Thrombosis in Microvascular Surgery. J Reconstr Microsurg. 2008;24(5):305-14.
37. Adams J, Charlton P. Anesthesia for microvascular free tissue transfer. Br J Anaesth. 2003;3:33-7.
38. Weitz J, Grabenhorst A, Singer H, Niu M, Grill FD, Kamreh D, et al. Mandibular reconstructions with free fibula flap using standardized partially adjustable cutting guides or CAD/CAM technique: a three- and two-dimensional comparison. Front Oncol. 2023;13:1167071.

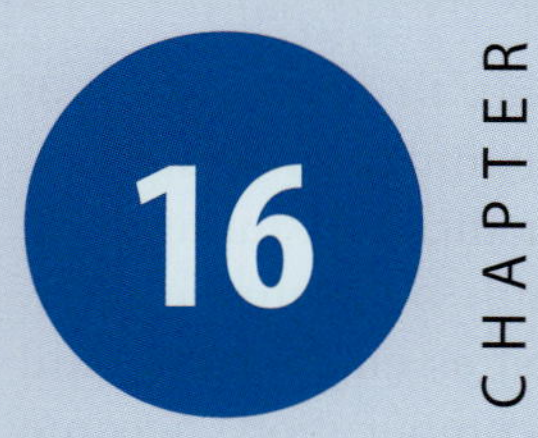

CHAPTER

Postoperative Issues in the Management of Head and Neck Cancer Surgery

NK Vinod, S Ramkiran

INTRODUCTION

Head and neck cancer surgeries are associated with significant perioperative challenges and associated morbidity attributable to its intrinsic procedural-related complexities. Radical composite resections, microvascular osseomyocutaneous flap reconstruction involving nerve-sparing techniques along with its regenerative reconstruction, speech-swallowing and airway-related challenges, vascular repair and reconstruction, complex skull base surgeries, functional endocrine surgeries, meningeal and lymphatic leak reinforcement procedures, ophthalmic structural and functional preservation techniques, and prosthetic cranial along with dental implant reconstruction and postirradiation cochlear implant surgeries pose extreme competitive decision-making challenges and efforts need to be directed in order to prevent complications arising due to complex head and neck cancer surgeries.

Radiation therapy, neoadjuvant chemotherapy, and targeted immunotherapy add up to the complications after surgery resulting in mucositis, delayed wound healing, fistula formation, stomal dehiscence, and chronic pain syndromes. Cosmetic, nutritional, and psychological impacts of major resection further complicate the quality of outcomes after head and neck cancer surgery. Astute prehabilitation of patients becomes necessary before undertaking major head and neck cancer surgeries which are followed by vocational, functional, and occupational rehabilitation (along with cosmetic reinforcements) which add to the quality of life (QOL) and recovery after surgery.

COMPLICATIONS OF HEAD AND NECK SURGERIES

The complications arising as a sequel after surgery may be classified into patient related, tumor related, and treatment related. Further, the complications could be subdivided as major and minor. Clavien Dindo proposed a five-grade classification which correlated well with length of hospital stay. Prediction of surgical risk within 30 days after surgery was proposed by American College of Surgeons National Surgical Quality Improvement Program (ACS NSQIP) but could not demonstrate efficacy involving microvascular free flap reconstruction. Similarly, the complications associated with concomitant chemoradiation associated with head and neck cancer surgery have not been well represented, although isolated Delphi techniques exist.[1-6]

Patient-related Complications

Patient Comorbidities

Functional and physical status limitation, age-related functional decline, cognitive decline, frailty, and sarcopenia are common manifestations associated with advanced head and neck malignancy. They attribute to crippling complications in the form of dysphagia, drooling, xerostomia, mucositis, and trismus.

Cardiopulmonary Compromise

Postoperative myocardial infarction, unstable angina, congestive heart failure, and ventricular arrhythmias occur in 2–5% of head and neck cancer surgery (bearing up to 20% mortality implication).[7] Preoperative revised cardiac risk index fairly predicts postoperative major adverse cardiac events, but may not represent subsequent intervening care pathways. Cardiac biomarkers in the form of troponins and pro-B-type natriuretic peptide provide prognostication in patients at risk for adverse cardiac events perioperatively. Patients who are immobilized beyond 24 hours pose an additional risk for development of thromboembolism. Prophylactic anticoagulation along with mechanical pneumatic compression devices and early ambulation constitute medical management.

Pulmonary prehabilitation in the form of deep breathing exercises, incentive spirometry, smoking cessation along with brief nicotine supplementation in nonhabilitated subset, secretion clearance and high frequency oscillatory chest compression devices in the form of compression vests, and positive expiratory pressure device and acapella is routinely employed. Poor functional status and Assess Respiratory Risk in Surgical Patients in Catalonia risk index (ARISCAT) score predict postoperative pulmonary complications and widely utilized as predictive surgical score. Elderly patients with underlying pneumonia may present with delirium and possess functional limitation in performing daily activities. Nebulization, inhaled steroids, secretion thinners, and antibiotics may be needed in select patients. Patients with preexisting tracheostomy pose increased risk for postoperative pneumonia.[7,8]

Obesity and Obstructive Sleep Apnea

Morbid obesity has been associated with obstructive sleep apnea and pulmonary hypertension in extreme cases leading to respiratory-related adverse events in immediate postoperative period needing assistance in ventilation with either noninvasive continuous/intermittent bi-level positive airway pressure or invasive ventilator support in critical care unit. Preoperative sleep study would guide postoperative airway management.

Preexisting Neurologic and Psychological Disorders

Most common postoperative complication in head and neck cancer subset has been delirium which occurs in 30% of patient population. This may be directly attributable to nutritional deficiency (thiamine), co-addiction to tobacco, alcohol, opioid, and psychotropic substances of abuse which often may occur irrespectively in elderly patients with preexisting lacunar microinfarcts and white matter hypodensities. Preexisting neurocognitive disorders, diabetes mellitus, metabolic disorders, drug interactions, infections, and dementia need to be evaluated prior to surgery. Psychologic counseling as part of prehabilitation often brings out subtle history of dementia and helps identify patients at risk for delirium.

Often, the stress mediators, surgical pain, and unacclimatized intensive care unit environment could predispose to development of postoperative delirium. Early ambulation after surgery becomes extremely vital in preventing delirium by allowing the patient to return to their familiar environment. Hyponatremia and hypoalbuminemia predispose further to development of delirium postoperatively. Early recognition of symptoms, avoidance of benzodiazepine premedication, minimizing opioids, use of dexmedetomidine in intensive care, maintaining normothermia as well as euglycemia, and prevention of hypoxia and cardiac complications become primordial in management of delirium.[7,9]

Substance Addiction

Tobacco use, alcohol withdrawal, psychotropic substance dependence, and opioid addiction due to preexisting opioid use are commonly encountered in patients presenting for head and neck cancer surgeries, most often getting detected only in early postoperative period.

Endocrine Disorders

Thyroid disorders need to be evaluated with a holistic approach including baseline cardiopulmonary assessment with astute follow-up, secondary to thyroid hormonal fluctuations, multiple endocrine neoplasia (MEN) syndromes involving secreting adrenal tumors, coexisting radiation-induced parathyroid adenoma, and hypercalcemia with associated renal damage. Retrosternal extension may pose extreme challenges perioperatively needing sternotomy and extracorporeal life support **(Fig. 1)**. Elderly patients may manifest with extreme lethargy, drowsiness, and depression in the postoperative intensive care unit which may be associated with sick euthyroid syndrome, subclinical hypothyroidism, and myxedema coma on one hand and apathetic thyrotoxicosis lacking any sympathetic manifestations on the other side of the spectrum. To further complicate decision making, Grave's disease, inflammatory thyroiditis, and autoimmune thyroiditis may need differentiation in reaching a clinical diagnosis.

Parathyroid adenoma may be associated with MEN syndrome which need to be evaluated with vigilance and to further rule out pheochromocytoma **(Fig. 2)**. Pituitary adenoma involving posterior pituitary usually manifests with central diabetes insipidus, high serum osmolality, and hypernatremia. Pancreatic adenoma associated with MEN presents with insulinoma leading to persistent hypoglycemia, whereas VIPoma manifests with watery diarrhea leading to significant dyselectrolytemia. Diabetes mellitus may manifest with autonomic disturbances, ketoacidosis, and hyperosmolar metabolic disturbances leading to insulin resistance.

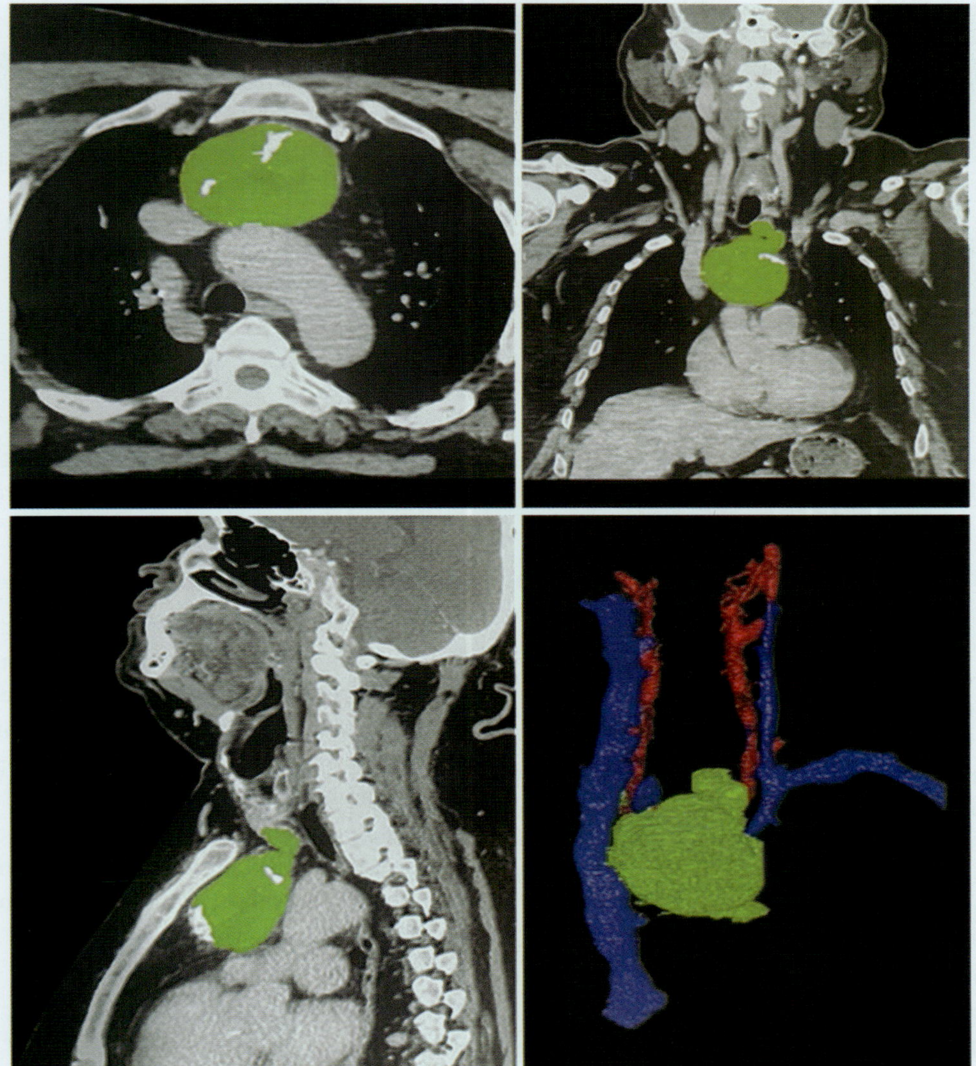

Fig. 1: Retrosternal extension of thyroid.

Anemia and Hypoalbuminemia

Anemia manifesting as hematocrit <25% has been associated with increased risk of postoperative complications, whereas in the cardiovascular subset patients, a hematocrit <30% has been associated with increased risk of developing postoperative cardiac complications, morbidity, and mortality. Nutritional deficiency anemia, bleeding from tumor, metastatic liver and kidney disease, hemolytic anemia, chemotherapy-related bone marrow suppression, and immune-mediated myeloid reactions are commonly associated with perioperative anemia.[7]

Nutrition-related Disorders

Cancer-associated cachexia has widely become recognized with tumor-related anorexia, oral mucositis, painful deglutition, and inability to chew contributing to about 40% incidence in head and neck cancer patients.[7] Protein–calorie malnutrition seen in both acute and chronic forms further worsens anorexia attributable to tumor metabolic byproducts and glucose drain by cytokines, as well as phagocytes involved in tumor metabolism. Micronutrients, vitamins, minerals, and trace elements directly influence cellular immune response with broader implications toward cancer therapy.

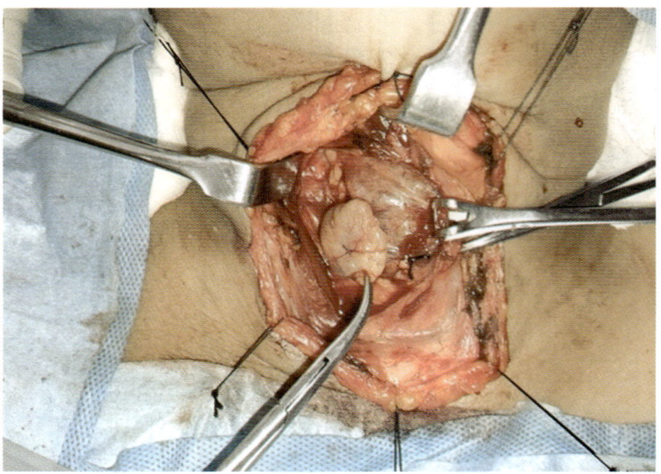

Fig. 2: Parathyroid adenoma.

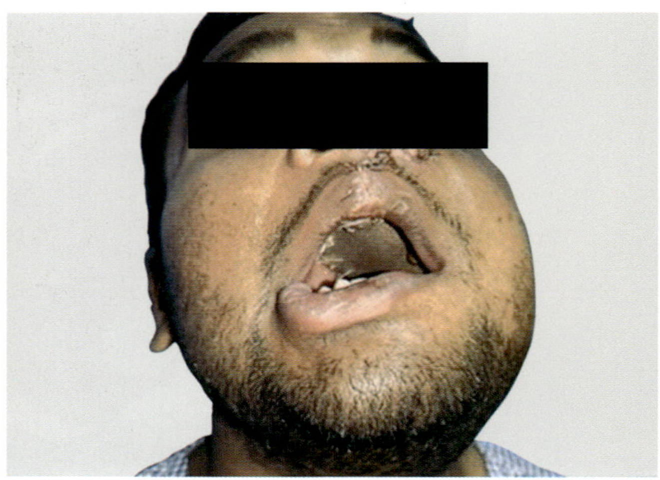

Fig. 3: Airway compromise after intraoral free flap.

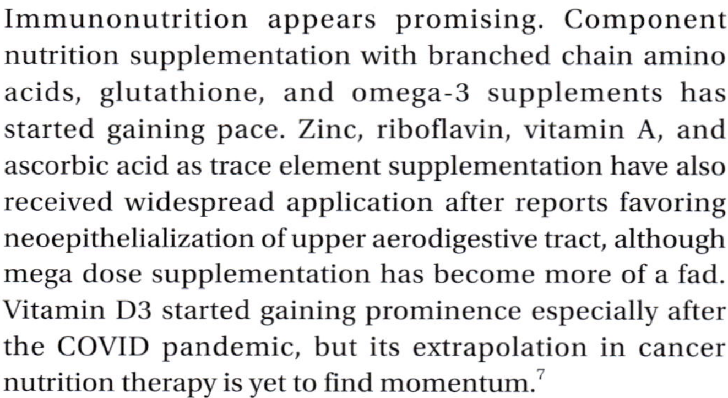

Immunonutrition appears promising. Component nutrition supplementation with branched chain amino acids, glutathione, and omega-3 supplements has started gaining pace. Zinc, riboflavin, vitamin A, and ascorbic acid as trace element supplementation have also received widespread application after reports favoring neoepithelialization of upper aerodigestive tract, although mega dose supplementation has become more of a fad. Vitamin D3 started gaining prominence especially after the COVID pandemic, but its extrapolation in cancer nutrition therapy is yet to find momentum.[7]

Though a lot of research on clinical nutrition-related cancer prevention and immunomodulation has been trending, most have unfortunately been based on animal, tissue culture, epidemiological, or retrospective studies. The postsurgical cancer patients are a unique subset; wherein, most immunonutrition principles may not be replicable in an environment of superadded stress-induced catabolism. Enteral and parenteral nutritional formulae often do not live up to the expectation carried by in vitro studies. It remains still unclear the overall impact of improved nutritional support upon the prognosis and QOL among head neck cancer surgical patients, who are further subjected to chemo-immuno-radiation. There exists, in future, a tremendous potential for nutrition-based research in improving QOL, which needs to be explored among head and neck cancer patients.[7,10,11]

Metabolic Disorders and Dyselectrolytemia

Hyperglycemia, hyponatremia, and hypomagnesemia may be associated with underlying renal and liver dysfunction.

Coagulopathy and Thromboembolism

Routine prophylaxis with low-molecular-weight heparin may not be indicated in all head and neck cancer patients presenting for surgery. Graded compression stockings, intermittent pneumatic compression devices, and early ambulation often provide prophylaxis against thromboembolism. Coagulopathy in head and neck cancer patients needs referral to hematologist, as such patients may present in varying clinical manifestations from minor bleeding diathesis attributable to factor deficiency to major hematologic syndromes.[7]

Procedure-related Complications

Oral Surgery-related Complications

Primary goals of patients undergoing oral surgery are to preserve function of speech, swallowing, mastication, and aesthetic facial contour. Airway complications although rare could be fatal in cases of hemorrhage, foreign body (retained throat pack), postoperative trismus, and mucosal obstruction may necessitate tracheostomy **(Fig. 3)**. Vascular catastrophes after associated neck dissection may result due to carotid dissection. Patients operated with marginal and segmental mandibulectomy surgeries are associated with reconstruction from external plating devices, fixation implants, three-dimensional reconstructive implant models, and autologous bone grafting. Lingual nerve, mental nerve, and marginal mandibular nerves may become entrapped in soft tissue fibrosis after reconstruction surgery leading to poor

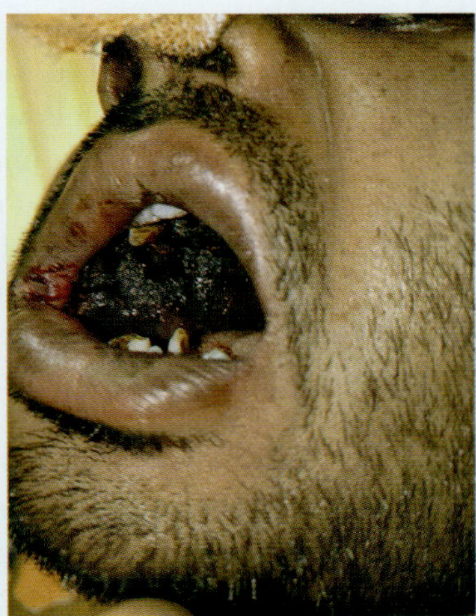
Fig. 4: Intraoral flap congestion.

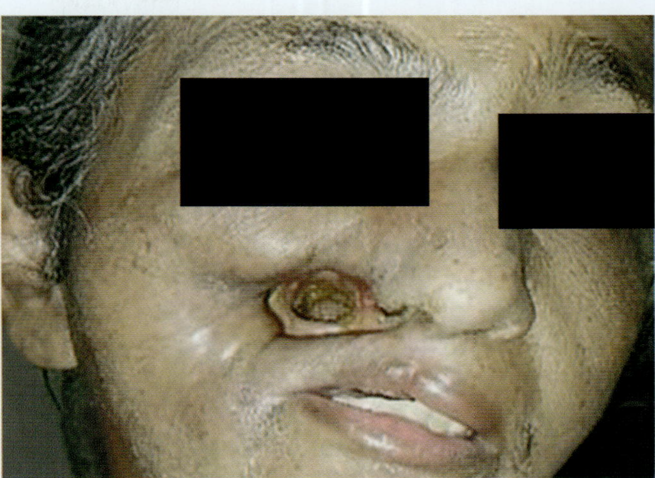
Fig. 5: Pharyngocutaneous fistula.

functional outcomes. Resurgeries may be required after initial free flap surgery due to flap failure wherein there may be venous congestion of the flap or poor arterial supply **(Fig. 4)**. This may necessitate subsequent soft tissue only reconstruction.[7]

Neck Surgery-related Complications

Injury to the cervical plexus, marginal mandibular branch of facial nerve, accessory nerve, brachial plexus, and sympathetic branches around the carotid sheath may be damaged. Vascular injury in the form of injury to jugular vein and carotid artery may lead to torrential hemorrhage. Chyle leak, air leak, and pulmonary complications may occur in the immediate postoperative period. Delayed complications include facial edema, fistula formation, wound infection flap loss, vascular rupture, and local recurrence of tumor **(Figs. 5 to 7)**. Quality of recovery depends upon the shoulder function and prevention of neck contracture.[7]

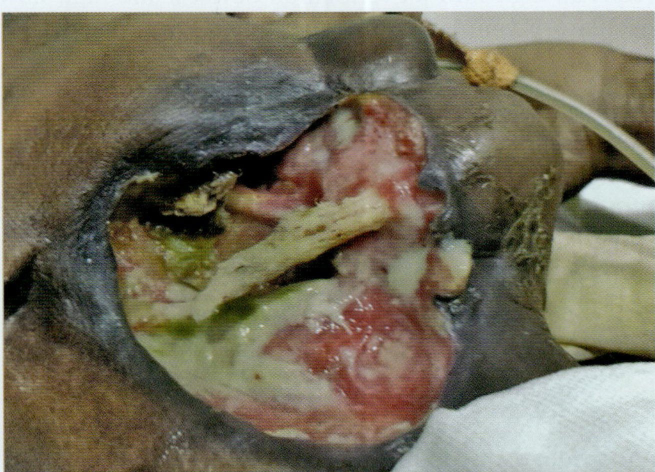
Fig. 6: Flap failure and dehiscence with infection.

Endoscopic Neck Surgery Complications

Endoscopic neck surgery includes endoscopic thyroidectomy and video-assisted thyroidectomy. Video-assisted neck surgery has evolved simultaneously along with conventional neck surgery, wherein insufflation of carbon dioxide under low pressure facilitates surgical dissection. The incidence of subcutaneous emphysema, pneumomediastinum, compression of major vessels, hypercarbia, and acidosis are considered high due to an associated autonomic sympathetic stimulation response.

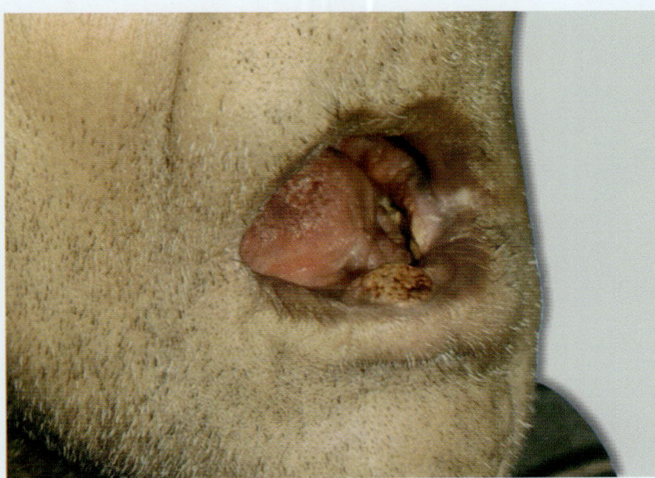
Fig. 7: Tumor recurrence after partial glossectomy.

Microlaryngeal Surgery and Related Complications

Microlaryngeal surgery has grown beyond the conventional operating microscope to include 3D operating exoscope, yet the devastating complications have found significant reduction owing to utility of laser safety.

Laser-related airway and surgical fires are the most devastating complications of head and neck laser surgeries, with associated disability and disfigurement affecting patient outcome. The "Fire triad" is composed of oxygen-enriched atmosphere, flammable skin preparation agents/drapes, and laser (electrosurgical) ignition source **(Fig. 8)**.[7]

The utility of high-flow oxygen delivery devices in the form of transnasal humidified rapid insufflation ventilator exchange (THRIVE) delivered by high-flow nasal cannula (HFNC), high-flow jet ventilation devices, and high-flow oscillatory ventilation (HFOV) needs to be used with extreme caution in laser surgery.

Endocrine Surgery Complications

Endocrine surgeries involve thyroid, parathyroid, and pituitary surgeries in relation to head and neck cancer surgeries.

Thyroid and Parathyroid Surgery Complications

Thyroid and parathyroid surgeries are associated with inherent complications due to involvement of recurrent laryngeal nerve leading to hoarseness of voice, dyspnea, and stridor based upon the extent of injury, being unilateral or bilateral, partial or complete transection, permanent or temporary, needing laryngoplasty or thyroplasty or neurorrhaphy. Intraoperative nerve monitoring of recurrent laryngeal nerve is routinely followed to reduce risk of nerve injury by utilizing less invasive and continuous monitoring through an electrode-embedded endotracheal tube **(Figs. 9 and 10)**. Airway ultrasound performed at the end of procedure may help identify the vocal cord palsy. Video-stroboscope is utilized to diagnose laryngeal nerve injury, as routine flexible fiberoptic laryngoscopy may not detect vocal cord palsy.

Hypocalcemia may occur with hypoparathyroidism which may be transient or permanent, owing to underlying ischemic insult. A rapid immunoradiometric parathyroid hormone assay may be needed for detecting parathyroid disorder. Single-photon emitting computed tomography, utilizing technetium 99 isotope—Sestamibi scan (99m Tc-sestamibi SPECT/CT) is used for rapid diagnosis of ischemic insult to the parathyroid **(Fig. 11)**. Bleeding and hematoma formation need to be identified early during postoperative period. Airway complications in the form of tracheomalacia secondary to retrosternal extension may pose difficult extubation in the postoperative period necessitating tracheal splinting, stenting, or tracheostomy.[7]

Pituitary Adenoma Surgical Complications

Pituitary adenoma excision by performance of a functional endoscopic sinus surgery (FESS) exposure serves as a minimally invasive approach to the anterior skull base. The associated fluid and electrolyte imbalance in the form of diabetes insipidus, central secretion inhibition leading to syndrome of inappropriate adrenocorticotropic

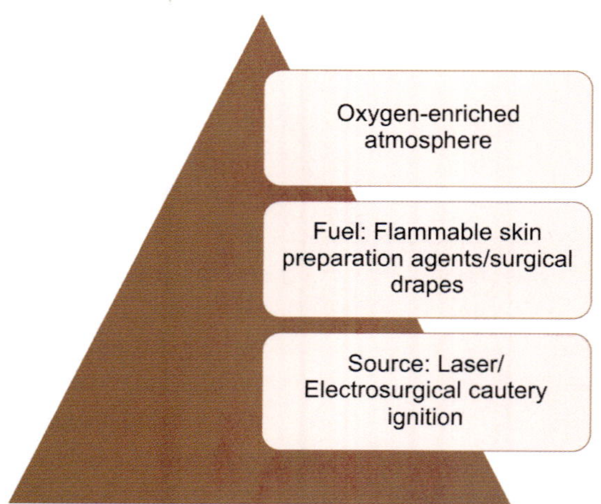

Fig. 8: Fire triad in laser surgery.

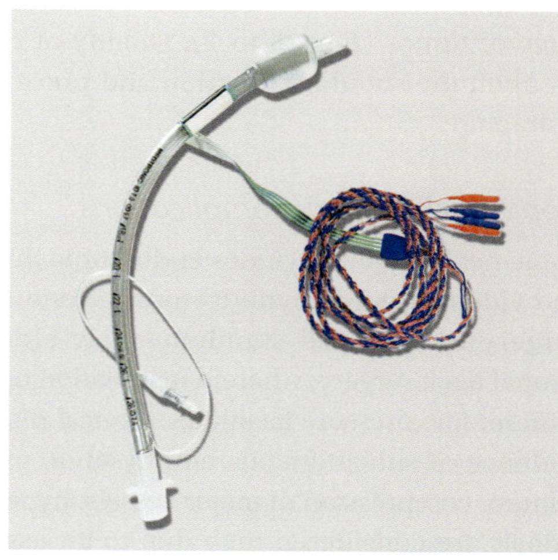

Fig. 9: Nerve monitoring embedded endotracheal tube.

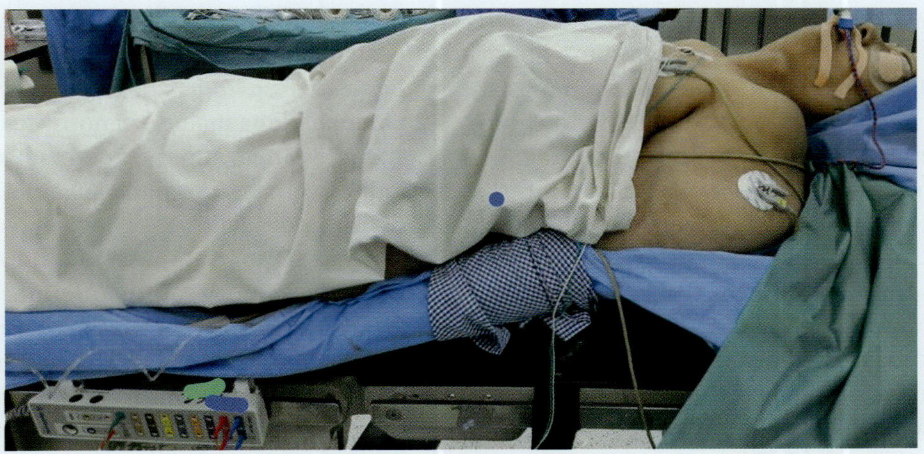

Fig. 10: Intraoperative nerve monitoring.

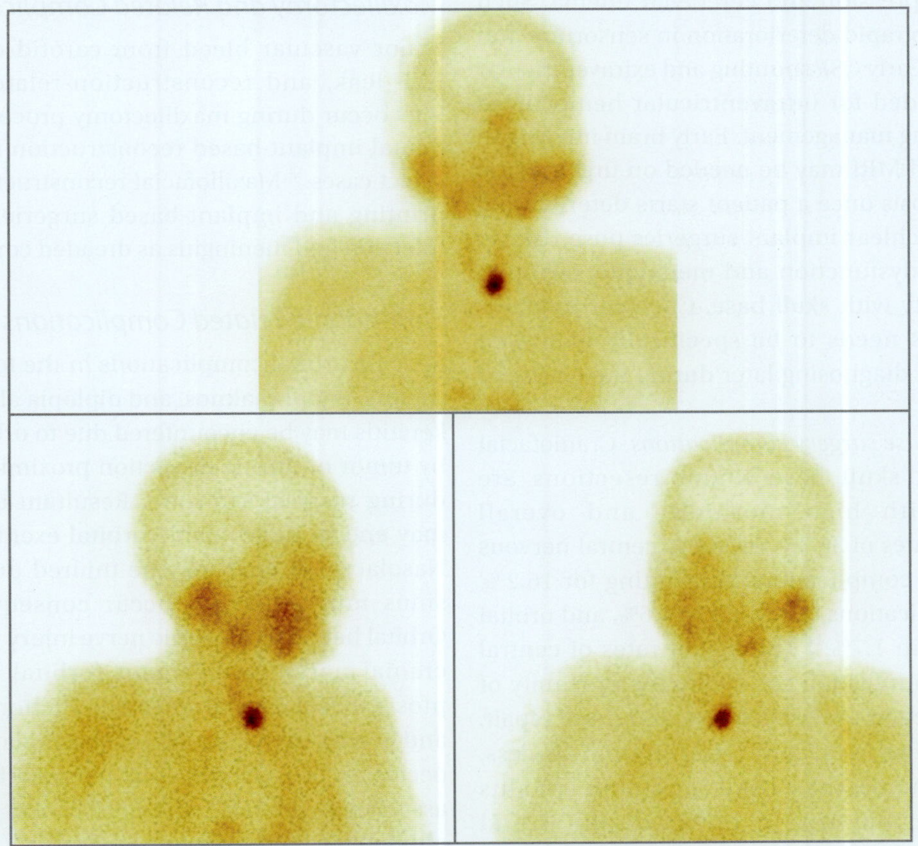

Fig. 11: Sestamibi SPECT scan of left lower parathyroid with increased focal uptake.

anti-diuretic hormone (SIADH), and pituitary apoplexy are major complications seen in the postoperative period necessitating hormonal supplementation and swift fluid-electrolyte correction.

Skull Base and Intracranial Neurosurgery-related Complications

Skull base surgery includes anterior skull base, lateral skull base, and posterior skull base (neuro-otology).

Acoustic neuroma constitutes most of the posterior and lateral skull base surgeries, whereas pituitary tumor excision via nasal endoscopy constitutes the majority of anterior skull base approach. Cerebrospinal fluid (CSF) leak, pneumocephalus, vascular injury, ischemic complications, stroke, seizures, cranial nerve injury, meningeal infection, and brain abscess are the most common complications associated with neurosurgical procedures. CSF drainage procedures in the form of lumbar drain and endoscopy-related leak containment repair procedures may be indicated in a few patients. Frontal lobe syndrome, involving memory and behavioral changes, may occur in patients operated upon the cribriform plate and anterior skull base. Acoustic neuroma patients may present with cerebellar hematoma leading to brainstem compression and cerebellar edema. Such patients proceed to rapid deterioration in sensorium and progressive coma. Early CSF shunting and extraventricular drain may be needed for intraventricular hemorrhage subsequently during management. Early brain imaging in the form of CT and MRI may be needed on urgent basis to establish diagnosis once a patient starts deteriorating neurologically. Cochlear implant surgeries pose risk for vestibular system dysfunction and meningitis owing to inner ear proximity with skull base. Cochlear implant-related meningitis needs to be specifically identified earlier, rather than diagnosing later during the course of hospital stay.[7]

- *Anterior skull base surgery complications:* Craniofacial resection and skull base tumor resections are associated with high morbidity and overall complication rates of 36.3%, owing to central nervous system-related complications accounting for 16.2%, systemic complications occurring in 4.6%, and orbital complications in 1.7%.[12] The higher rates of central nervous system infection are due to the proximity of the CSF, ventricular drain insertion, and dural repair. CSF leak, meningitis, seizures, intracranial abscess, intracranial hematoma, and pneumocephalus constitute the majority of both intradural and extradural central nervous system complications.
- *Lateral base surgery complications:* Proximity to the cranial nerves III to XII closely bounded by sphenoid and petrous ridge poses a risk for complications arising due to hemorrhage from the inaccessible internal carotid artery. Ischemic brain injury, cerebrovascular complications, CSF leak, and labyrinthine injury (leading to hearing loss and vestibular dysfunction) need to be anticipated.
- *Posterior fossa surgery complications:* Acoustic neuroma complications include venous hemorrhage from the sigmoid sinus, superior petrosal sinus, and jugular bulb which need immediate hemostasis with collagen or oxidized cellulose packing, bipolar cauterization, or bone wax application. Venous air embolism, venous infarction, injury to the anterior inferior cerebellar artery, increased intracranial pressure, seizures, CSF leak, meningitis, and lower cranial nerve palsy are major complications. Cerebrovascular accident, autonomic dysfunction, and brainstem infarct may pose significant life-threatening mortality.

Maxillectomy and Related Complications

Major vascular bleed from carotid-cavernous fistula, CSF leak, and reconstruction-related complications may occur during maxillectomy procedures. Palatal and dental implant-based reconstruction may be needed in select cases.[13] Maxillofacial reconstruction surgery by 3D printing and implant-based surgeries involve implant infection and meningitis as dreaded complications.

Ophthalmic-related Complications

Specific orbital complications in the form of optic nerve trauma, enophthalmos, and diplopia along with exposure keratitis may be encountered due to orbital floor invasion by tumor or during dissection proximity to orbital cavity during surgical exposure. Resultant nonfunctional eye may end in unavoidable orbital exenteration **(Fig. 12)**. Nasolacrimal duct may be injured during surgery and sinus mucocele may occur consequently **(Fig. 13)**. Orbital hemorrhage, optic nerve injury with simultaneous cranial nerve involvement (orbital apex syndrome), ptosis, nasolacrimal duct obstruction, globe invasion, and postoperative visual loss (secondary to retinal artery occlusion or ischemic optic neuropathy) are commonly associated with head and neck cancer surgeries needing ophthalmic cross-referral.

Minimally Invasive Transoral Robotic Surgery Complications

Transoral robotic surgery (TORS) is associated with complications which may be TORS related or non-TORS related **(Fig. 14)**. TORS-related complications could be

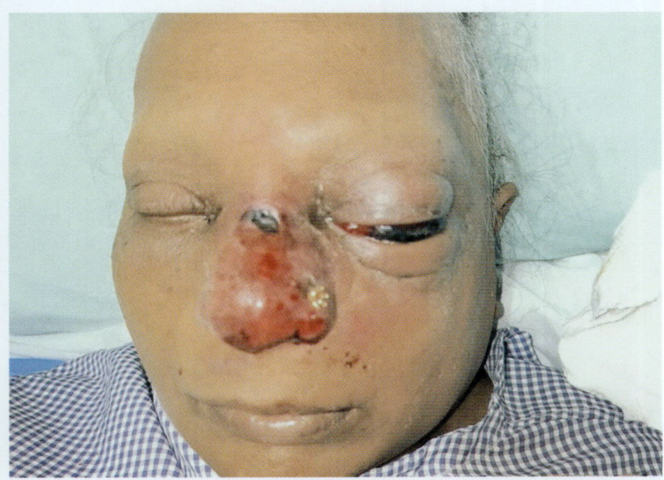

Fig. 12: Orbital encroachment leading to nonfunctional eye.

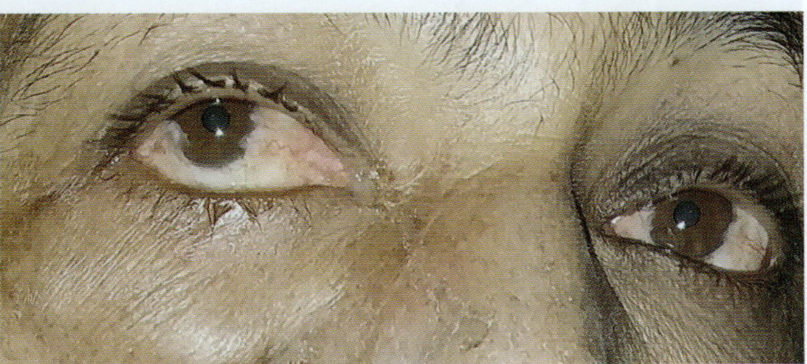

Fig. 13: Nasolacrimal duct involvement leading to constant teary right eye.

subdivided into major and minor complications. The most common being bleeding, dysphagia, oropharyngeal trauma, dental injury, hypoglossal/lingual nerve injury, localized pain in surgical area, ophthalmic injury, and aspiration pneumonia. Infections arising outside the oropharynx and neck complications account for non-TORS-related complications. Bleeding tonsillar fauces after TORS may need external carotid ligation performed as an emergency procedure **(Figs. 15 and 16)**.

Reconstructive Surgery and Its Complications

Free tissue transfer, microvascular free flap reconstruction, pedicle myocutaneous flap, and autologous bone graft-related complications are considered.

Reconstruction procedure complications:

- *Reconstruction by free grafts:* Includes avascular skin (split skin and full thickness skin graft), cartilage grafts, bone grafts, and fat grafts which require a

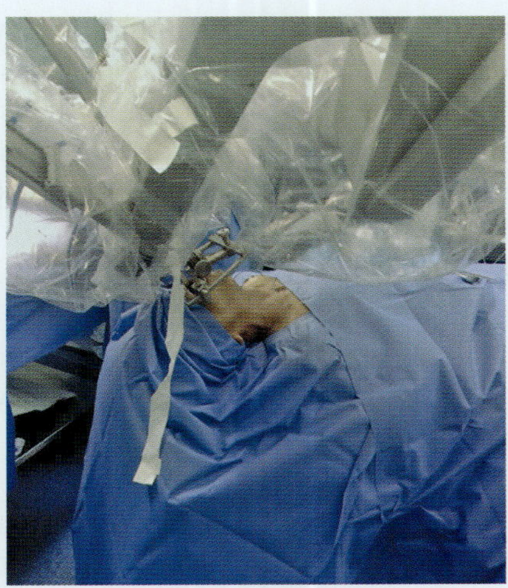

Fig. 14: Transoral robotic surgery imposing challenges.

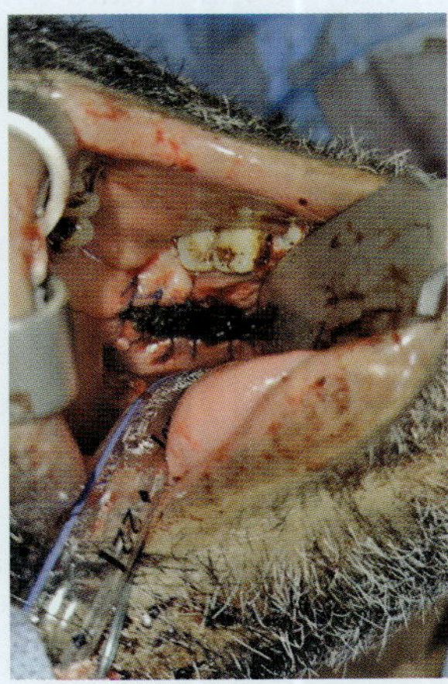

Fig. 15: Bleeding tonsillar fauces after TORS needing hemostat control. (TORS: transoral robotic surgery)

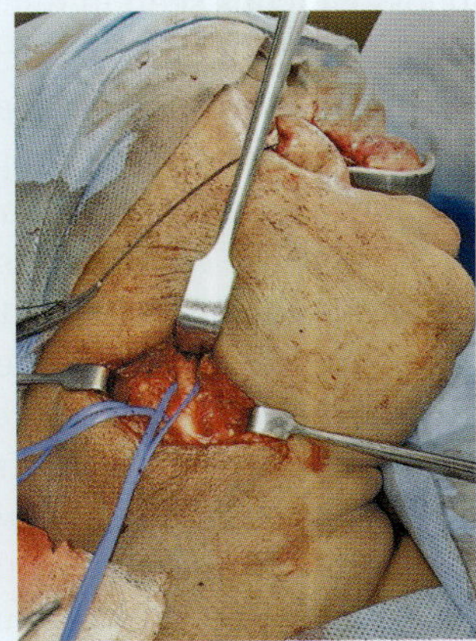

Fig. 16: External carotid artery ligation as salvage for uncontrolled bleeding.

well-vascularized recipient bed for survival with neovascularization and fibrin deposition, occurring by 48–72 hours. Proper care of donor site is of utmost importance. Hematoma, infection, and necrosis at the recipient site may lead to graft failure which needs to be addressed on a priority basis.

- *Local facial flap reconstructions:* Provide soft tissue coverage along with cosmetic benefit. The flap survival depends upon multiple factors and failure is predominantly due to impaired tissue oxygenation. Bleeding from the flap tissue margin, although clinically reliable, may not always predict the actual graft survival. Doppler flow, laser Doppler elastometry, dermato fluorometry, oximetry, and infrared flow cameras tagged with indocyanine green have been utilized as a surrogate for flow determination across the flap, which may be inaccurate when extrapolated clinically. Complications of local facial flaps are ischemia, infection, hemorrhage, and hematoma formation.
- *Pedicle myocutaneous flaps:* Viability of such flaps depends upon the native blood supply from the flap pedicle and by the muscle perforators. These flaps are robust in view of preserved vascular supply from the pedicle and considered as reliable flaps. Pectoralis major myocutaneous flap, trapezius, latissimus dorsi, platysma, temporalis, and nasolabial myocutaneous flaps are commonly performed when resource constraints exist for microvascular free flap reconstruction. Common complications of pedicle-based flaps include flap necrosis, infections, and hematoma formation. Partial flap loss is seen more commonly in pedicle-based flaps as against a complete flap loss which is seen in microvascular free flap reconstruction.
- *Free tissue transfers by microvascular free tissue transfer:* Cover large complex defect areas of composite resection with better functional and cosmetic outcomes from distant donor sites. Most common osseocutaneous flaps include free fibula and scapular flaps; whereas, soft tissue bulk yielding flaps include anterolateral thigh, lateral arm, radial forearm, and rectus abdominis flaps. Most free tissue transfer grafts suffer from ischemia time with ensuing revascularization as well as neovascularization. Numerous local and systemic factors play a role in flap failure including vessel morphology, endothelial response, and thrombus generation upon the microcirculation. Reperfusion injury and coagulation cascade factors along with the endothelial response guided by platelet dynamics dictate the time-sensitive flap survival[14] **(Fig. 17)**.

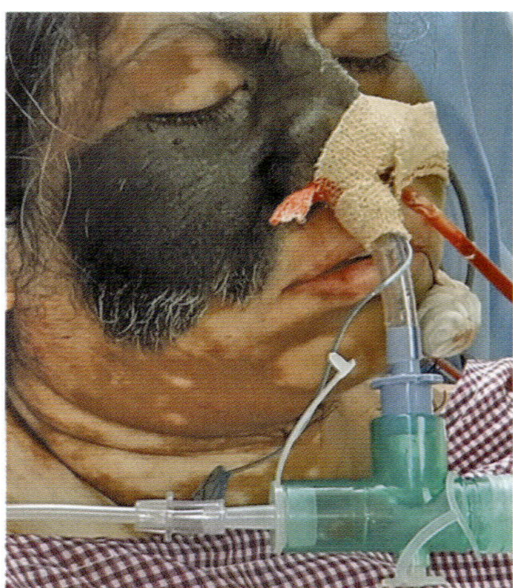

Fig. 17: Hairy nevus on the face resembling flap failure.

Dental-related Complications

Chewing and swallowing need to be facilitated after head and neck surgery, for which efficient dental rehabilitation needs to be incorporated. Preradiation dental evaluation is an essential prerequisite necessitating extraction of septic teeth foci. Osteoradionecrosis (ORN) after mandibular surgery typically may occur after dental extraction especially after an adjuvant radiation therapy, which needs to be recognized early as a nonhealing ulcer at surgical site with an exposed underlying bone and multiple fistulae **(Fig. 18)**. The term ORN needs to be differentiated from osteonecrosis, which in turn occurs after dental extraction following bisphosphonate therapy, provided for management of metastatic bone tumors in order to prevent osteoporosis **(Fig. 19)**. The indication for bisphosphonates has narrowed down to management of moderate to severe hypercalcemia secondary to breast malignancy, multiple myeloma, and metastatic osteolytic lesions (prostate malignancy).[7]

Salivary Gland Surgery-related Complications

Glandular surgery—parotid, submandibular, and cervical lymph node dissection—may lead to salivation and swallowing-related problems which is considered debilitating. Salivary fistulae, nerve injury (facial/greater auricular/auriculotemporal/hypoglossal), and Frey syndrome are complications commonly encountered.

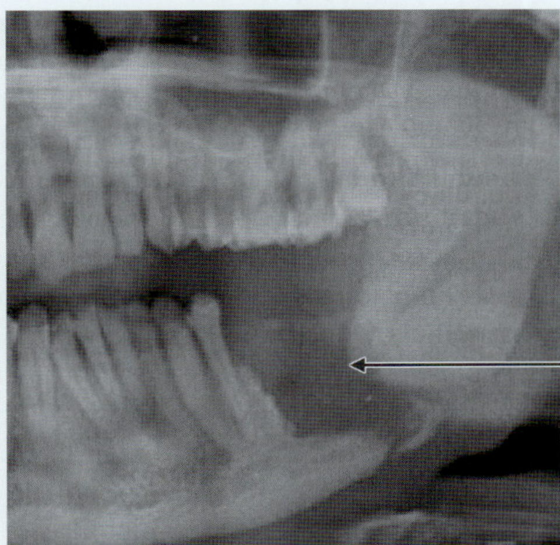

Fig. 18: Osteoradionecrosis mandible (pointer indicates destroyed bone at lower molar).

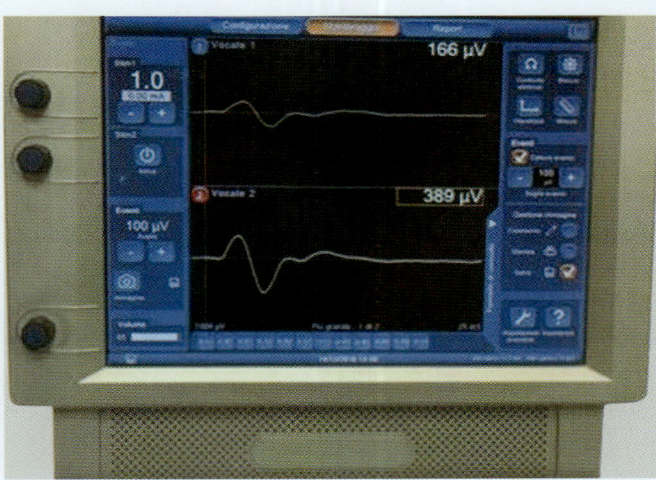

Fig. 20: Electromyography-based neuromonitoring.

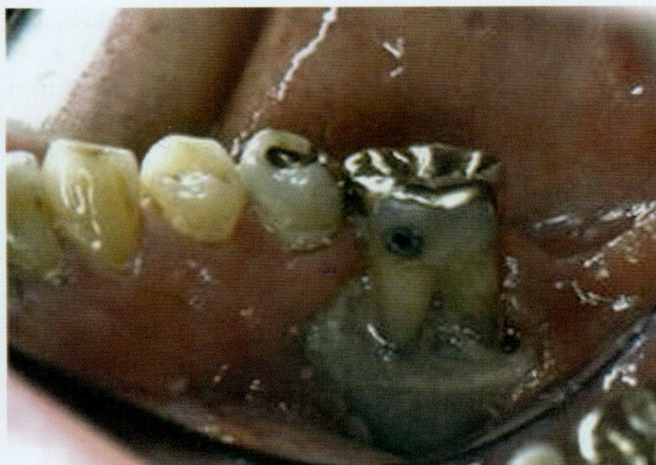

Fig. 19: Osteonecrosis mandible (post-dental extraction implant).

Intraoperative nonpulsed nerve stimulator and electromyography-based nerve monitoring, utilized judiciously, could detect and prevent facial nerve injury **(Fig. 20)**.

Interventional Radiology-related Complications

Complications related to interventional radiological procedures could be subdivided into local and systemic complications. Local complications constitute 0.6–23.2% of all complications ranging from allergic reactions to local anesthetic or contrast, wound infection, hematoma, pseudoaneurysm due to dissecting vessel, arteriovenous fistula formation, and thromboembolism.[7] Systemic complications occur in 0.5–9.4% patients ranging from idiosyncratic reactions to contrast-related anaphylactoid reactions, needing supportive therapy in an intensive care unit.[7] Complications related to interventional radiology also range from minor to major complications; the most devastating ones being visual loss, thromboembolic stroke, carotid blowout, cranial nerve palsy, and intraparenchymal hemorrhage. Interventional radiology procedures in cath lab may be needed to carryout emergency control of hemorrhage as well as achieve endovascular control **(Fig. 21)**.

Treatment-related Complications

Airway-related, drug-related, and surgery-related functional debility have been frequently encountered due to iatrogenic causes.

Airway-related Complications

Establishing airway control during surgery may need awake intubation which may result in turbinate injury, septal injury, adenotonsillar injury, vocal cord injury, arytenoid avulsion, and unidentified subglottic injury. Hoarseness of voice may lead to poor quality of speech. Trismus occurring in the postoperative period may affect the QOL in head and neck cancer patients **(Fig. 22)**. Neck contractures, shoulder movement restriction, and vocal cord palsy lead to overall poor QOL.

Radiation-induced osteonecrosis and dental caries may lead to poor oral hygiene and infection. Salivary gland-related complications may result in drooling and sialorrhea. Silent microaspirations may occur due

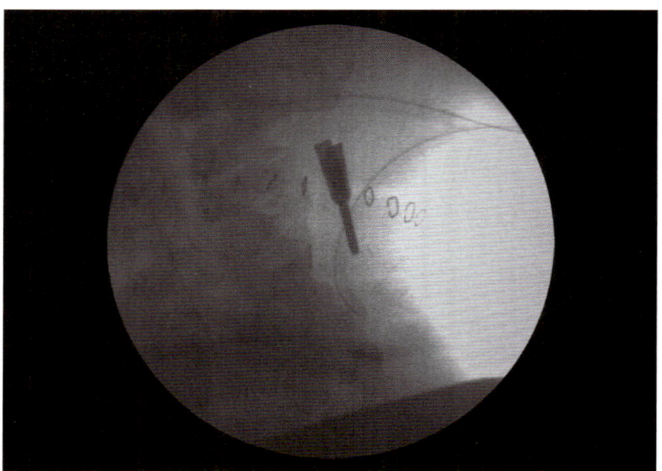

Fig. 21: Interventional radiology-guided vascular intervention.

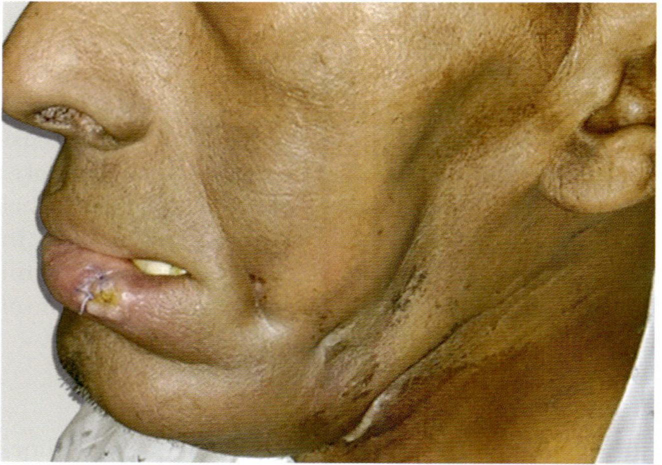

Fig. 22: Postoperative trismus.

to incoordinated swallowing. Mandibulectomy affects laryngeal suspension which may result in risk of aspiration during swallowing. Tumors involving tongue base and floor of mouth are associated with adverse airway-related events, and such patients should not be considered for immediate extubation after surgery.

Prophylactic tracheostomy is usually advocated in segmental mandibulectomy crossing the midline which is an independent risk factor for adverse airway events. Extubation guidelines have been defined by different airway societies (Difficult Airway Society, All India Difficult Airway Association). Failed extubation may occur in head and neck cancer surgery and no time should be lost in resecuring definitive airway in such a scenario. Failed intubation and unanticipated reintubation increase the morbidity and length of stay in hospital. Patient may be taken inside the operating room for reintubation, with facility for backup tracheostomy available in the crisis. Tracheostomy and tracheostoma-related complications may occur, leading to stricture formation over a period of time, needing serial dilatation procedures eventually culminating in tracheal stenting. Other complications associated with tracheostomy include dysphonia, hemorrhage, stenosis, fistula, mucous plug, or clot leading to aspiration pneumonia. Complete airway obstruction may occur if tracheostomy care bundles are not strictly adhered with policy.[15-19]

Radiation Therapy-related Complications

Complications of radiation therapy are predominantly related to mucositis, exposure dermatitis, dry mouth, salivary gland dysfunction (xerostomia), dysphagia, laryngeal edema, hypothyroidism, ORN, hearing loss, and myelitis.

The evolution of intensity-modulated radiation therapy (IMRT) has dramatically reduced toxicity rates associated with conventional radiation exposure by better dose distribution. The improvements have gained pace with betterment of quality-of-life outcomes, with respect to preservation of salivary function, swallowing, and ORN. The combination of IMRT along with free radical scavenger-based radioprotectants like amifostine has significantly reduced incidence of xerostomia.[7]

Chemotherapy, Chemoprevention, and Immunotherapy-related Complications

The emergence of novel neoadjuvant chemotherapeutic agents combined with immunotherapy has revolutionized traditional palliative intent patients to a new horizon of curative intent in head and neck cancer treatment. Added on to these established agents, chemoprevention by biological therapy has taken long strides, though with cautious interpretation of results, in the form of α-tocopherol, β-carotene, and cis-retinoic acid. Cytoreduction achieved by the above combination therapy, along with locoregional radiosensitization, has emerged to have better functional preservation and minimal toxicities while simultaneously benefiting patients from tumor recurrence.[7]

Transfusion-related Complications

Immunomodulation associated with perioperative blood and product transfusion (TRIM—transfusion-related immunomodulation) has been gaining a lot of momentum, and transfusion-sparing strategies have become evolved. Acute lung injury (TRALI—transfusion-related acute lung injury), transfusion-associated circulatory overload (TACO), transfusion-associated graft-versus-host disease (TA-GVHD), risk of infections, inflammatory cytokine cascade, febrile nonhemolytic transfusion reaction (FNHTR), and hemolytic transfusion reactions are complications gaining more research interest.

Wound and Infection-related Complications

Wound healing involves a complex interaction between cellular signaling and cellular mediators, toward an effort in unison to heal the injured tissues. Many interactions modulate healing processes, including preexisting diabetes with its glycation end products and superimposed infection. Aging, poor nutrition, hypothermia, irradiation, smoking, prolonged steroid exposure, improper tissue handling resulting in tissue edema, and impaired cellular oxygenation–perfusion pose definitive threat toward the healing–remodeling process. Contamination by aerodigestive–respiratory tract microorganisms due to spillage, aspiration, and fistula formation facilitates accelerated wound infection requiring prolonged systemic antibiotic therapy. Impaired/failed wound healing results in fistula formation, whereas its other extreme spectrum of overactive healing resulting in hypertrophic scars with ensuing contractures, limit functional and cosmetic outcomes.[7,20,21]

Functional Debility-related Complications

Neuralgia, Neurapraxia, and Intraoperative Nerve Injury

Neuromonitoring and nerve-sparing surgeries have taken precedence toward achieving functional recovery. Early neck–shoulder functional exercises are initiated in early postoperative period. The role of physiotherapist and occupational therapist becomes crucial in achieving functional outcomes after head and neck cancer surgery.

Speech and Dysphagia

Speech and swallowing restoration to normalcy and as close to preoperative functional state has been the cornerstone target for head and neck surgeries in view of its associated functional morbidity. Regional pedicled flaps, local free tissue transfer, nerve transfer, cervicofacial advancement, and microvascular reconstruction aid in adding the cosmetic value along with functional rehabilitation.[7]

QUALITY OF LIFE INDICATORS

Health-related quality of life (HRQOL), frailty, and instrumental activities of daily living have taken precedence as a parameter to evaluate postoperative surgical success. Numerous tools provide preoperative decision-making ability among patients before undergoing surgery, by incorporating a composite predictive surgical scoring involving mini mental state examination (MMSE), Eastern Cooperative Oncology Group performance status (ECOG), American Society of Anesthesia (ASA) physical status, Portsmouth Physiological Operative Severity Score for enumeration of Mortality and morbidity (P-POSSUM), American College of Surgeons National Surgical Quality Improvement Program (ACS-NSQIP), and Acute Physiology Chronic Health Evaluation (APACHE IV) score postoperatively for predicting length of stay in ICU as well as outcome prediction after surgery and associated mortality.[7] Similarly, disease-specific QOL indicator tools such as European Organization for research into treatment of cancer QOL questionnaire for head and neck cancer, functional assessment of cancer therapy head and neck (FACT-H and N), and University of Washington QOL questionnaires are specifically designed and validated for head and neck cancer functional outcomes. Symptom-specific qualitative tools such as the MD Anderson dysphagia inventory and voice-related quality of life (VRQOL) are gaining importance.[7]

Achieving complete tumor resection (R0 resection) associated with its draining lymphatic channels along with cosmetic preservation alone does not stand ground in today's cancer care. Today's requirements are much more demanding with goals toward preservation of QOL, activities of daily living, and functional preservation. Nerve-sparing surgeries to preserve functionality are attaining significance. Mastication, speech, and swallowing functional preservation are gradually gaining importance much more than cosmetic recovery. Xerostomia, dysgeusia, dysphagia, drooling, and dysphonia are considered crippling after head and neck surgery, and every effort needs to be put in to prevent these complications. Similarly, orocutaneous fistula, pharyngocutaneous fistula, Chyle leak, and postoperative trismus could be disgruntling to the postoperative patients. Strictures involving pharyngo-laryngeal-tracheoesophageal conduits, soft tissue fibrosis, neck contractures, edema, and trismus lead to both cosmetic and functional poor outcomes after surgery; whereas, xerostomia, mucositis, strictures, caries, and ORN lead to debilitating outcomes after chemoradiation along with its associated toxicities. Reflux, regurgitation, and pharyngo-esophageal dysfunction due to swallowing disorder could progress to fatal aspiration culminating in airway catastrophe.

Stomal stenosis leading to postoperative stridor and dysphagia after laryngectomy can lead significant impact on QOL. Tracheoesophageal puncture-related complication while instilling tracheoesophageal voice prosthesis (TEP) impairs VRQOL significantly. Tumor recurrence in a postoperative patient could devastate the patient completely. Inoperability of advanced proliferating tumors could essentially shatter the patient and hope of the family.[7]

Multimodal interdisciplinary rehabilitation of patient takes precedence, with speech-swallowing therapist, physical therapist, occupational therapist, psychological therapist, and dietician pitching in along with the patient's family, to ensure smooth recovery. Functional recovery and cosmetic recovery are targeted simultaneously to ensure patient to be back to activities of routine. Prevention of stiffness, rigidity, and contractures assumes importance during functional recovery. Stomal care providers, speech and swallowing experts, and dental implant/prosthetic rehabilitation become the cornerstone for early patient recovery and preserved QOL.

ROLE OF PAIN AND PALLIATIVE CARE

The principles of pain management after head and neck cancer surgeries include restoration of physical, occupational, and emotional functionality, by pharmacological, nonpharmacological, occupational, and interventional management techniques. Chronic pain and pain syndromes are associated with select head and neck cancer surgeries leading to debility. Recognition of the neuropathic pain component early limits the opioid usage in this nonresponsive subset leading to prevention of chronic opioid use. Opioid-sparing techniques followed by opioid de-escalation and opioid substitution by agonist-antagonist combination have bettered pain practice.

Bisphosphonates and calcitonin have been utilized in metastatic bony pain and bone infiltrating tumors, though the practical risk of osteonecrosis still exists. Methadone, naloxone-buprenorphine, and cannabinoids have recently emerged to fill pain treatment gaps after head and neck cancer surgery along with select neuroablation procedures. Cryo/radiofrequency ablation of select ganglia and radiosurgical gamma-knife has revolutionized interventional pain management in head and neck cancer.

RISK REDUCTION STRATEGIES

Strategies for risk reduction to prevent complications have incorporated predictive prognostic surgical scoring systems [American Society of Anesthesiologist (ASA), National Surgical Quality Improvement Program (NSQIP), and Physiological and Operative Severity Score for enumeration of mortality and Morbidity (POSSUM)], comorbidity indices (Charlson, Klabunde, Washington University, head and neck cancer index), prehabilitation (nutritional, psychological, and physiotherapy), anemia, electrolyte, and hypoalbuminemia correction, frailty assessment and frailty indices (modified five-point frailty index—mFI-5), obesity, diabetes, obstructive sleep apnea, and cardiorespiratory adverse events management, addiction cessation toward tobacco, psychotropic drugs, and alcohol, preoperative opioid weaning strategies, enhanced recovery protocols (ERAS), surgical safety checklist incorporation, transfusion-related risk and its threshold reduction, reexploration and its effect on QOL, functional outcomes rather than isolated survival outcomes in quality evaluation, airway intervention in the form of tracheostomy, stoma-related complication reduction, incorporation of endotracheal intubation, and extubation bundles, perioperative nerve-sparing techniques, prevention and early management of inadvertent nerve injury, and regular conduct of morbidity-mortality audits, quality of care along with patient safety audits.[1,7]

CONCLUSION

The management of head and neck cancer surgeries presents a complex array of complications, ranging from postoperative infections and wound healing issues to long-term functional impairments such as dysphagia, speech difficulties, and facial disfigurement. While advances in surgical techniques and multidisciplinary care have significantly improved patient outcomes, the risks inherent in these procedures remain substantial. Early identification and proactive management of these complications are crucial for minimizing morbidity and improving QOL. Therefore, it is essential for healthcare professionals to adopt a holistic approach that integrates vigilant postoperative care, prehabilitation, and ongoing patient education. A patient-centered model of care that emphasizes both physical and psychological recovery will be key to achieving optimal outcomes in head and neck cancer surgery.

REFERENCES

1. Ronen O, Robbins KT, Shaha AR, Kowalski LP, Makitie AA, Florek E, et al. Emerging concepts impacting head and neck cancer surgery morbidity. Oncol Ther. 2023;11:1-13.
2. Vosler PS, Orsini M, Enepekides DJ, Higgins KM. Predicting complications of major head and neck oncological surgery: an evaluation of the ACS NSQIP surgical risk calculator. J Otolaryngol Head Neck Surg. 2018;47:21.
3. Tierney W, Shah J, Clancy K, Lee MY, Ciolek PJ, Fritz MA, et al. Predictive value of the ACS NSQIP calculator for head and neck reconstruction free tissue transfer. Laryngoscope. 2020;130:679-84.
4. Dindo D, Demartines N, Clavien PA. Classification of surgical complications: a new proposal with evaluation in a cohort of 6336 patients and results of a survey. Ann Surg. 2004;240:205-13.
5. Monteiro E, Sklar MC, Eskander A, de Almeida JR, Shrime M, Gullane P, et al. Assessment of the Clavien-Dindo classification system for complications in head and neck surgery. Laryngoscope. 2014;124:2726-31.
6. Vallur S, Dutta A, Arjun AP. Use of Clavien-Dindo classification system in assessing head and neck surgery complications. Indian J Otolaryngol Head Neck Surg. 2020;72:24-9.
7. Eisele David W, Smith Richard V. Complications in head and neck surgery, 2nd edition. Philadelphia (PA): Mosby; 2009.
8. Buitelaar DR, Balm AJM, Antonini N. Cardiorespiratory complications after major head and neck surgery. Head Neck. 2006;28:595-602.
9. Vaurio LE, Sands LP, Wang Y, Mullen EA, Leung JM. Postoperative delirium: the importance of pain and pain management. Anesth Analg. 2006;102(4):1267-73.
10. Rabinovitch R, Grant B, Berkey BA. Impact of nutritional support on treatment outcome in patients with locally advanced head and neck squamous cell cancer treated with definitive radiotherapy: A secondary analysis of RTOG trial 90-03. Head Neck. 2006;28:287-96.
11. Yuvzsen T, Davis MP, Walsh D. Systematic review of the treatment of cancer associated anorexia and weight loss. J Clin Oncol. 2005;23:8500-11.
12. Ganly I, Patel SG, Singh B. Complications of craniofacial resection for malignant tumors of skull base: Report of an international collaborative study. Head Neck. 2005;27:445-51.
13. Unlu HH, Goktan C, Asian A. Injury to lacrimal apparatus after endoscopic sinus surgery; surgical implications from active transport dacryocystography. Otolaryngol Head Neck Surg. 2001;124:308-12.
14. McMahon JD, MacIver C, Smith M, Stathopoulos P, Wales C, McNulty R, et al. Postoperative complications after major head and neck surgery with free flap repair—prevalence, patterns, and determinants: a prospective cohort study. Br J Oral Maxillofac Surg. 2013;51(8):689-95.
15. Tsai CH, Liu YC, Chen PR, Loh CY, Kao HK. Risk factors for postoperative adverse airway events in patients with primary oral cancer undergoing reconstruction without prophylactic tracheostomy. Asian J Surg. 2024;47:1763-8.
16. Gupta K, Mandlik D, Patel D, Patel P, Shah B, Vijay DG, et al. Clinical assessment scoring system for tracheostomy (CASST) criterion: objective criteria to predict preoperatively the need for a tracheostomy in head and neck malignancies. J Craniomaxillofac Surg. 2016;44(9):1310-3.
17. Lapis PN, DeLacure MD, Givi B. Factors in successful elimination of elective tracheotomy in mandibular reconstruction with microvascular tissue. JAMA Otolaryngol Head Neck Surg. 2016;142(1):46-51.
18. Ledderhof NJ, Carlson ER, Heidel RE, Winstead ML, Fahmy MD, Johnston DT. Are tracheotomies required for patients undergoing composite mandibular resections for oral cancer? J Oral Maxillofac Surg. 2020;78(8):1427-35.
19. Meier J, Wunschel M, Angermann A, Ettl T, Metterlein T, Klingelhöffer C, et al. Influence of early elective tracheostomy on the incidence of postoperative complications in patients undergoing head and neck surgery. BMC Anesthesiol. 2019;19(1):43.
20. Broughton G, Janis JE, Attinger CE. The basic science of wound healing. Plast Reconstr Surg. 2006;117(7):12S-34S.
21. Paydarfar JA, Birkmeyer NJ. Complications in head and neck surgery: a meta-analysis of postlaryngectomy pharyngocutaneous fistula. Arch Otolaryngol Head Neck Surg. 2006;132(1):67-72.

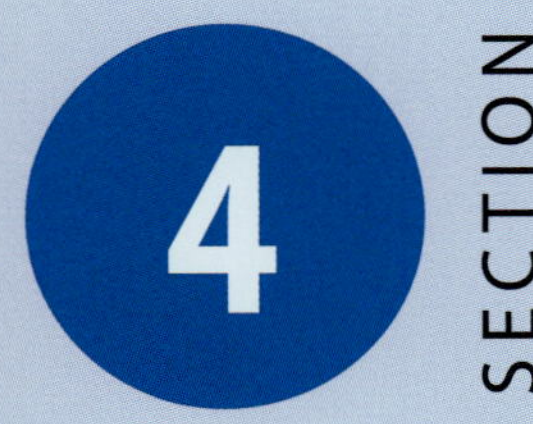

Section 4: Breast Onco-Surgeries

17 CHAPTER

Anesthesia for Breast Onco-Surgeries

Massimo Lamperti, Jesto Kurian, Amit Jain

INTRODUCTION

Breast cancer is one of the most common cancers worldwide.[1] Female gender is the most substantial breast cancer risk factor.[2] Approximately 99% of breast cancer patients are female, and only 0.5–1% of breast cancers occur in men. As per 2022 estimates, breast cancer accounts for 670,000 deaths globally.[3] Also, with time, the prevalence of breast cancer is on the rise.[2] As almost 80% of all breast cancer patients require oncosurgery as a part of their treatment, the number of breast surgeries performed every year is increasing.[4] Most of these surgeries are performed under general anesthesia (GA) combined with various types of regional anesthesia (RA) techniques for adequate pain relief in the postoperative period.[2] Less common is the practice of awake breast surgeries utilizing sole RA techniques.[5] In this chapter, the authors will first provide brief information about breast cancer classification and knowledge about the chemotherapy agents, hormonal and immunological adjuvants, or neoadjuvants commonly used in managing breast cancer patients. Subsequently, the types of breast cancer surgery commonly performed as treatment options will be discussed along with the anesthetic management of a patient for breast cancer surgery. Lastly, we will shed light on the current evidence on the impact of perioperative anesthesia techniques on breast cancer recurrence rates.

BREAST CANCER CLASSIFICATION

Breast cancer is a highly heterogeneous neoplasm with distinct histopathological characteristics that can often be grouped into four different molecular subtypes based on the immunohistochemical expression of hormone receptors: estrogen receptor positive (ER+), progesterone receptor positive (PR+), human epidermal growth factor receptor positive (HER2+), and triple-negative breast cancer (TNBC), which is characterized by the lack of expression of any of the above receptors.[1] The molecular subtyping carries prognostic and treatment significance (**Box 1**).[1]

NONSURGICAL TREATMENT IN BREAST CANCER

While most women with breast cancer will have some surgery to remove the tumor, depending on the type of breast cancer and how advanced it is, the patient may need other types of treatment as well, either before (neoadjuvant) or after surgery (adjuvant), or sometimes both.[4] Typically, treatment is based on the type of breast cancer and its stage. Other factors, including comorbidities, menopause status, and personal preferences, are also considered.

BOX 1: Classification of breast cancer.

Classification based on histological subtypes:
- Preinvasive cancer (25%)
- Ductal carcinoma in situ (80%)
- Lobular carcinoma in situ (20%)
- Invasive cancer (75%)
- Invasive ductal carcinoma (80%)
- Invasive lobular carcinoma (10%)
- Other (10%)

Classification based on molecular subtypes:
- Luminal A (40%): ER +, PR+, HER2 –
  - Prognosis: Good
  - Treatment: Hormonal therapy
- Luminal B (20%): ER +, PR ±, HER2 –
  - Prognosis: Intermediate
  - Treatment: Hormonal/chemotherapy
- HER2 positive (10–15%): ER ±, PR ±, HER 2 –
  - Prognosis: Intermediate to bad
  - Treatment: Hormonal/chemotherapy/Herceptin
- Triple negative (15–20%): ER –, PR –, HER 2 +
  - Prognosis: Bad
  - Treatment: Chemotherapy

(ER: estrogen receptor; PR: progesterone receptor; HER2: human epidermal growth factor receptor 2)

BOX 2: Nonsurgical treatment in breast cancer.

Radiotherapy:
- External beam radiation for breast cancer:
  - Whole breast radiation
  - Accelerated partial breast irradiation:
    - Intraoperative radiation therapy (IORT)
    - 3D-conformal radiotherapy (3D-CRT)
    - Intensity-modulated radiotherapy (IMRT)
    - Brachytherapy
  - Chest wall radiation
  - Lymph node radiation
- Brachytherapy:
  - Intracavitary brachytherapy
  - Interstitial brachytherapy

Adjuvant and neoadjuvant chemo drugs:
- Anthracyclines, such as doxorubicin (Adriamycin) and epirubicin (Ellence)
- Taxanes, such as paclitaxel (Taxol) and docetaxel (Taxotere)
- 5-fluorouracil (5-FU) or capecitabine (Xeloda)
- Cyclophosphamide (Cytoxan)
- Carboplatin (Paraplatin)

Hormone therapy:
- Drugs that block estrogen receptors:
  - Selective estrogen receptor modulators (SERMs): Tamoxifen, Toremifene
  - Selective estrogen receptor degraders (SERDs): Fulvestrant, Elacestrant
- Drugs that lower estrogen levels:
  - Aromatase inhibitors (AIs): Letrozole, Anastrozole, Exemestane
  - Luteinizing hormone-releasing hormone (LHRH) agonists: Goserelin, Leuprolide

A nonsurgical treatment plan may involve radiotherapy or drug therapy. The detailed description of this topic is out of the scope of the current chapter, but **Box 2** provides a list of nonsurgical treatment options used in the management of breast cancer.

BREAST SURGERY TYPES IN BREAST CANCER PATIENTS

Patients with breast cancer have some surgery as part of their treatment. The type of breast surgery may vary from removal of cancerous tissue to restoration of the breast's shape after the cancer is removed or to relieve the symptoms of advanced cancer.

Radical mastectomy, also known as Halsted radical mastectomy, once a common approach to removing breast cancer, is now rarely indicated. Radical mastectomy involves removing the whole breast, all the lymph nodes under the arm (axillary lymph node dissection), and the chest wall muscles under the breast. Now, it may be indicated only when breast cancer has spread to the chest wall muscles. The surgery is extensive, with more disfiguration and more significant postoperative complications.

Modified radical mastectomy: It involves removing the entire breast, including the nipple and most of the lymph nodes underlying the arm (axillary lymph node dissection), with or without the underlying skin. However, the underlying chest muscles will be left in place, unlike a traditional radical mastectomy. It is less extensive and disfiguring but is equally effective as radical mastectomy in the early stage of breast cancer.

Simple or total mastectomy: In this surgery, the entire breasts will be removed. However, the underlying chest wall muscles and sometimes armpit lymph nodes are secured. Approximately 30% of patients require total mastectomy because of personal choice or their unsuitability for some form of breast conservation surgery. Some patients wish to have prophylactic mastectomies for risk reduction surgery, which can be simple, skin-sparing, or nipple-sparing mastectomy.

Nipple-sparing mastectomy: In this surgery, the entire breast tissue is removed, but the nipples are kept intact.

Breast conservation surgery such as lumpectomies or partial mastectomy: Lumpectomy is the removal of the cancerous part of the breast tissue and some normal tissue around it. Wide local excision of the tumor with a histological confirmation that a minimum margin (typically 5 mm) of normal tissue has been excised around the tumor along with adjuvant or neoadjuvant radiotherapy or chemotherapy is equally effective compared to total mastectomy alone.

If a mammogram or ultrasound has detected the cancer and is not palpable, either of the two types of a localization procedure is required to assist the surgeon in removing the tumor.

Wire localization: The radiologist inserts a localizing wire on the morning of surgery, and hours may elapse before the operation begins. The wire sticks out from the breast and must be carefully secured with a bandage, so it does not become dislodged during this waiting period.

Seed insertion: This new technique involves placing a radioactive pellet, or "seed," in the breast next to the tumor. The seed method holds several advantages over wire localization. The seed can be implanted up to 5 days before surgery. Patients do not need to take any special precautions, as the amount of radioactivity in the seed is very low, and they can arrive at the hospital closer to their scheduled surgery time. Because the seed is nestled entirely within the breast, it does not shift around the way a localizing wire can. During the operation, the surgeon uses a small Geiger counter to locate the seed and remove the tumor and a rim of surrounding tissue, including the seed.

Multifocal disease, inflammatory breast cancer, and prior radiation to the breast are some of the contraindications for breast conservation strategies.

AXILLARY LYMPH NODE DISSECTION

Axillary lymph node dissection (ALND), axillary lymphadenectomy, or axillary dissection involves dissecting the lymph nodes within the axilla en bloc. Three levels of axillary lymph nodes are defined anatomically. Typically, level one and level two lymph nodes are taken during ALND dissection and level three nodes are not sought after.

In recent years, sentinel lymph node biopsy (SLNB) has replaced ALND in clinically node-negative patients. However, ALND may still be indicated in clinically positive axillary lymph nodes that have been proven with biopsy in a patient who is not planning on undergoing neoadjuvant chemotherapy or persistently positive lymph nodes after neoadjuvant therapy, in patients with inflammatory breast cancer, patients with three or more axillary sentinel nodes that are positive for cancer, in axillae with failed radiotracer and isosulfan blue dye (also known as lymphazurin/methylene blue) during SLNB, and following axillary lymph node recurrence after prior breast cancer treatment.

Axillary lymph node dissection is associated with a higher risk of lymphedema of the ipsilateral upper limb, upper limb sensory loss, increased length of hospital stay, and prolonged time to recovery from normal activities than the minimally invasive technique of SLNB.

SENTINEL LYMPH NODE BIOPSY

The sentinel lymph node is usually located by intraparenchymal injection of blue dye alone or in combination with intradermal administration of a radiolabeled colloid near the tumor site.[4] In breast cancer, the combination of blue dye and radiotracer has markedly increased the sensitivity of SLNB.[2,6-8] Approximately 50% of the dye is weakly bound to serum albumin to form an albumin-blue dye complex.[9] The albumin-blue dye complex is selectively picked up by regional afferent lymphatics, which causes lymphatic vessels and nodes to be identifiable by their bright blue color. The lymph nodes (typically one to four) with the highest radioactive signals are identified as sentinel lymph nodes. As the sentinel lymph node is the first node or group of lymph nodes that drains from the primary cancer, it is most likely to contain metastatic disease. Removal of the sentinel lymph node, commonly known as SLNB, is equally effective at predicting the status of axillary lymph nodes with far fewer adverse effects than ALND.[4,10] Women with positive SLNB may require subsequent ALND and/or further adjuvant treatment.

The use of dyes for SLNB is not without concerns. Isosulfan blue (lymphazurin 1%), the most used blue dye for SLNB in the United States, is associated with severe allergic reactions and anaphylaxis in 1–3% of patients.[9,11,12] The severity of allergic reactions can range from a mild allergic reaction (urticaria and erythema) to anaphylaxis that is characterized by hypotension, pulmonary edema, and cardiovascular collapse. Patent Blue V is another dye used for SLNB.[2] The National Audit Project 6 identified Patent Blue V dye as the fourth most common cause of perioperative anaphylaxis.[13] A safer option in terms of risk of anaphylaxis is methylene blue.[7] However, small doses of methylene blue can absorb significant light in the red (660 nm) range to produce spurious desaturation on pulse oximetry. Also, discoloration of skin and body fluids may occur, confusing the postoperative setting.[2]

The development of the one-step nucleic acid amplification assay may allow for the rapid detection of micrometastasis and could provide an alternative to pathology for examining SLNB.[8]

RECONSTRUCTION

Breast reconstruction surgery is often performed after primary tumor excision to restore the size and shape of the breast to near-normal status.[2,3,14] Such a surgery can either be performed immediately following the initial surgery for breast tumor excision or delayed until a later date. Immediate reconstruction is usually considered in noninvasive cancers and risk reduction surgery. Breast reconstruction can be performed using artificial implants (prostheses) or autologous grafts.

- Prosthetic reconstruction is usually referred to as breast augmentation, and it involves either one- or two-stage procedures. In a two-stage procedure, a tissue expander, a flat "water balloon," is placed under the pectoralis muscles. It will be gradually filled (expanded) during office visits to create space for a future prosthesis. The second surgery replaces the tissue expander with a breast implant, which is generally silicone in nature.
- Either of the two techniques can perform autologous graft reconstruction of breast:
    1. *Pedicled (rotational) flaps of tissue:* A flap of skin, fat, and muscle with accompanying vessels obtained from the adjacent tissue. The transverse rectus abdominis myocutaneous (TRAM) flap is the most utilized pedicle graft for breast reconstruction. An ellipse of lower abdominal tissue is reflected along with perforating vessels into the defect of the breast. In patients at higher risk of flap failure, such as in the presence of diabetes and smoking, TRAM flaps are not suitable, and latissimus dorsi (LD) flaps can be used. Pedicled flaps can involve long surgical times, increased operative blood loss, mainly if performed as immediate reconstruction, and severe acute postoperative pain.[2,14]
    2. Free flaps, such as the deep inferior epigastric perforator (DIEP) flap, are harvested from the donor site and transferred to the breast for reconstruction. The DIEP spares the rectus abdominis muscle and solely uses skin and fat. This minimizes the abdominal complications associated with the TRAM flap. However, as the free flap requires microsurgical anastomosis, there exists a higher risk of flap failure due to microvascular thrombosis.[2,14] Additionally, these are lengthy procedures (>8 h) and, like pedicled flaps, are associated with severe postoperative pain.

CONDUCT OF ANESTHESIA

Preoperative Assessment

Most patients with breast cancer are middle-aged and older females. About 50% of these patients are 62 or younger.[3] Many of these patients have ASA I or ASA II physical status with no or minimal significant systemic illness. Preoperative anxiety is widespread in patients awaiting breast cancer surgery.[2] A prior visit at preanesthesia testing and assessment by an anesthetist before surgery may help in the psychological preparation of these patients and ease anxiety. It allows for perioperative risk stratification, optimization of their comorbidities, determining the suitability for ambulatory surgery, and planning for conducting anesthesia, including RA and postoperative analgesia.

Most of the patients scheduled for breast cancer surgery might have received neoadjuvant hormonal, chemo-, or radiotherapy, and adverse effects from such a treatment should be considered along with other premorbid medical conditions.

Neoadjuvant and adjuvant chemotherapy is often given every 2 or 3 weeks for 4, 6, or 8 cycles (repeats) for up to 3–6 months in total.[4] The optimal timing for surgery is between 4 and 8 weeks following completion of neoadjuvant chemotherapy. Adjuvant chemotherapy is best timed within 90 days of surgery to improve outcomes.[15] These patients usually receive monitored anesthesia care for port insertion for chemotherapy.

Anesthesiologists must have a thorough understanding of the adverse effects of chemotherapeutic agents used in breast cancer treatment.[4] Doxorubicin, epirubicin, and other chemo drugs can cause cardiomyopathy and prolong the QT interval. The risk is highest if the drug is used for a long time or in high doses or when these drugs are used with other medications that can cause heart damage (such as those that target HER2).[4] The presence of other cardiac risk factors, such as family history of heart problems, high blood pressure, and diabetes, can further increase the risk of chemotherapy-induced cardiac toxicity.[2] These events can occur at any stage after treatment, even years after the initial chemotherapy regimen.[16] The patient should be assessed for symptoms of cardiac dysfunction before surgery, and investigations, such as ECG or echocardiography, may be required.

Neoadjuvant therapy can cause myelosuppression that may manifest as pancytopenia (anemia, thrombocytopenia, and neutropenia) in the perioperative period.[17] This may predispose these patients to increased bleeding risk, need for blood transfusion, and risk of infection and sepsis in the perioperative period. Myelosuppression usually reverses within 4–8 weeks after completion of chemotherapy.[2,4,17] Issues should be identified and managed before surgery. Prevalence of anemia in breast cancer patients may range from 41 to 82%.[18] Coexisting iron deficiency can be diagnosed using serum ferritin and transferrin saturation assay. Preoperative intravenous iron therapy in breast cancer patients with iron deficiency may reduce the need for intraoperative and postoperative blood transfusion. In case of expected blood loss, some patients may require blood cross-matching for transfusion.

Hormonal agents (e.g., tamoxifen or aromatase inhibitors) used in neoadjuvant treatment may be continued in the perioperative period.[2] These include agents, such as the monoclonal antibody trastuzumab (Herceptin), for human epidermal growth factor receptor 2-positive tumors. These agents can also be cardiotoxic and may increase the risk of perioperative venous thromboembolism (VTE).

Intraoperative Anesthetic Management

Despite counseling, patients with breast cancer may be anxious on the day of surgery. Despite an empathetic approach, pharmacological anxiolysis may be necessary in some of these patients.

Standard ASA monitoring during the perioperative period is appropriate for most cases. Monitoring should be applied in a way that allows adequate exposure for surgery and should be secured appropriately to avoid any disconnections and displacements during patient positioning and surgery. Usually, no monitoring is applied on the upper limb ipsilateral to the surgical site if the axilla needs to be explored. Electrocardiogram (ECG) electrodes should be placed on the back and may need to be secured with tapes to prevent dislodgment. In the case of bilateral breast surgery, occasionally, a blood pressure cuff may need to be applied on the lower limb. Invasive arterial pressure monitoring can be considered based on the patient's comorbidities and surgical complexity, especially for those with cardiac issues from neoadjuvant therapy and in free flap surgeries to assess the hemodynamic fluctuations. Invasive arterial monitoring allows early detection of hemodynamic variations after reperfusion instantly. Temperature monitoring is essential for procedures over 30 minutes. Breast reconstruction surgeries involving rotational pedicles or free-flaps can be very lengthy, and the torso remains largely exposed, resulting in a higher risk of intraoperative hypothermia. Using forced air warming devices, hot mattresses, and warmed intravenous fluids apart from maintaining ambient room temperature around 22°C can be considered to maintain normothermia.[19]

Intravenous access should preferably be obtained in the arm opposite the surgical site. This is especially important if axillary procedures are considered to reduce the risk of lymphedema.[20,21] The use of large-bore intravenous access for fluid and blood administration is recommended during lengthy surgeries, especially free flap surgeries. Consider central venous catheters (peripherally or centrally inserted) if intravenous cannulation is difficult, e.g., in patients after multiple cycles of chemotherapy.

Breast surgeries are usually performed under GA, which is often supplemented by RA for postoperative analgesia.[2] Both intravenous and inhalational induction techniques can be used to induce GA. With their related benefits and side effects, anesthesia can then be maintained effectively with total intravenous anesthesia (TIVA) or inhalational anesthetics.

The airway can be secured with supraglottic airway devices for short breast surgeries, but lengthy procedures, especially those involving breast reconstructions, require frequent changes of positions during the procedure and securing the trachea with tracheal intubation should be preferred.

A supine position with the arm on the operative side abducted is the usual position for single breast surgery. For bilateral breast surgeries, both arms can be abducted in a "crucifix" position. Overabduction of the arm should be avoided to prevent brachial plexus injury. Continuous observation is also essential to prevent brachial plexus injuries due to overstretching or misalignment of the neck and shoulders. For long breast surgeries, especially free flap and reconstructive surgeries, the head is supported and fixed on the table so that the head and neck are stable when given a steep head-up position.[22]

Specific Considerations in Flap Surgery

In LD flap surgery, patients may need to be positioned laterally during the procedure, necessitating careful monitoring of airway devices and intravenous access. To prevent pressure sores, jelly cushions and pressure-relieving mattresses should be utilized for long surgeries.

Minimize hypothermia and hypotension, as these can increase the risk for vasoconstriction, impairing the flap perfusion. Maintaining normothermia and euvolemia with adequate mean arterial pressures can flap perfusion and overall reconstruction outcome. Similarly, adequate lung ventilation, avoiding hypocapnia and hypoxia, is essential to ensure good graft perfusion and oxygen delivery.[21,22]

While excess fluid administration can worsen tissue edema, impairing graft microcirculation, it is equally important to avoid hypovolemia, which can reduce cardiac output and graft perfusion. Euvolemia should be considered in most scenarios. At the end of the procedure, a sitting position may be requested to assess symmetry.

Blood pooling and reduced venous return can lead to hemodynamic instability. Be prepared to administer vasopressors and fluid boluses to maintain hemodynamic stability.

Foley's catheter should be inserted ideally in long surgeries, especially flap surgeries, to assess the urine output perioperatively. Maintaining euvolemia is a crucial component for flap survival, so intraoperative urine output is an indicator of the patient's euvolemic status perioperatively.[21]

Given the increased risk of thromboembolism in cancer patients undergoing surgery, preventive measures against VTE should be considered in the perioperative period. Apply compression stockings for shorter procedures and sequential calf compression devices for longer ones to reduce the risk of VTE. Early pharmacological VTE prophylaxis should be initiated postoperatively once the surgical hemostasis is achieved following major breast cancer surgeries. Some institutes follow preprocedural subcutaneous heparin as thromboprophylaxis.[22]

Special Consideration during Sentinel Lymph Node Biopsy

As the American Society of Breast Surgery mentioned, ALND has been replaced by SLNB and it is required when patients are in the early stage of "cN0". The surgery can be performed under GA or deep sedation with local anesthesia (LA). There are two motor nerves of concern in axillary surgery: the long thoracic that supplies serratus anterior (SA) and the thoracodorsal nerve that supplies LD. Long-acting muscle relaxants are avoided during axillary dissection and recovery from neuromuscular blockade is ensured during SLNB, allowing surgeons to identify these motor nerves.

Intraoperative implications of blue dye use during SLNB are discussed in the above sections.[2,7,13]

Postoperative Anesthetic Management

Patients undergoing free-flap procedures will need general and flap monitoring in a high-dependency unit for at least 24 hours. Flap monitoring should continue for several postoperative days.[22]

Key considerations for postoperative care include:

- *Intraoperative principles:* Maintaining the same principles used during surgery to manage the flap in the postoperative period is important.
- *Temperature control:* Depending on individual institutional practices, patients may require a warm room to enhance flap perfusion.
- *Pain management:* Regular use of simple analgesics, such as paracetamol and nonsteroidal anti-inflammatory drugs (NSAIDs), can be beneficial alongside RA. Multimodal analgesia is the key to perioperative analgesia management in breast surgeries. The PROSPECT guideline recommends the use of evidence-based perioperative multimodal pain management techniques in breast surgery **(Table 1)**.[23]

TABLE 1: Prospect guidelines on perioperative analgesia management for breast surgeries.

Recommendations	*Minor breast surgery*	*Major breast surgery*
Preoperative and intraoperative interventions	• Paracetamol (Grade B) and conventional NSAIDs (Grade A) or COX-2-selective inhibitors (Grade B) • Gabapentin (Grade A) • Dexamethasone (Grade B) • Local anesthetic wound infiltration (Grade A)	• Paracetamol (Grade B) and conventional NSAIDs (Grade A) or COX-2-selective inhibitors (Grade B) • Gabapentin (Grade A) • Dexamethasone (Grade B) • PVB (Grade A) • PECS blocks if no axillary node dissection or PVB is contraindicated (Grade A) • Local anesthetic wound infiltration may be added to regional analgesia techniques (Grade A)
Postoperative interventions	• Paracetamol (Grade B) and conventional NSAIDs (Grade A) or COX-2-selective inhibitors (Grade B) • Opioids as rescue (Grade B)	• Paracetamol (Grade B) and conventional NSAIDs (Grade A) or COX-2-selective inhibitors (Grade B) • Opioids as rescue (Grade B) • Continuous PVB if catheter in place (Grade B)

(NSAIDs: nonsteroidal anti-inflammatory drugs; COX: cyclooxygenase; PVB: paravertebral block; PECS: pectoral nerve)

- *Postoperative nausea and vomiting (PONV) prevention:* Antiemetics prophylaxis is generally provided during the intraoperative phase, and rescue antiemetics should be prescribed to treat PONV.[22]

Regional Anesthesia Options for Breast Surgery

Regional anesthesia techniques, often used in conjunction with GA, have become increasingly popular in the perioperative management of patients undergoing breast cancer surgery. Multiple methods have been adopted in clinical literature with variable success rates and risks:

- Thoracic paravertebral block (TPVB)
- Pectoral nerve block (PECS) I and II
- Serratus anterior plane block
- Erector spinae block (ESB)
- Transversus thoracic plane block (TTPB)
- Local anesthetic infusion analgesia
- Thoracic epidural anesthesia (TEA)

These RA techniques offer adequate postoperative analgesia, reduce the need for opioids, and help minimize PONV and have occasionally been used as the sole anesthesia technique for "awake breast surgery" in patients with high perioperative risk with GA.

Thoracic Paravertebral Block

The thoracic paravertebral block is a well-established technique that allows for the injection of LA into the paravertebral space, which connects with both the epidural and intercostal spaces.[24]

Technique overview:

- *Injection methods:*
    - *Single shot:* For procedures like mastectomy and axillary node dissection, a single-level block between T2–T4 can be performed **(Fig. 1)**. A single injection of 15 mL of LA generally provides somatic coverage across three dermatomes.
    - *Multiple-level injections:* Multiple injections can be administered for broader coverage. If the plan is to conduct surgery under a sole regional anesthetic technique, two-level injections unilateral (for single breast surgery) or bilaterally (bilateral breast surgery) at T2–T3, T5–T6 with bupivacaine 0.375% with epinephrine 1:400,000, with 10–12 mL at each site (total of 40–48 mL) can be performed. If visualization is complex, attempt a more oblique ultrasound probe position or consider a sagittal paramedian approach. As analgesia may be incomplete for the axillary dissection, one may consider the addition of a pectoral nerve blocks (PECS) II block [i.e., ultrasound-guided PECS I, II, serratus plane (SP) block using either bupivacaine 0.25% or 0.375% with 60–70 mL volume].[25,26]

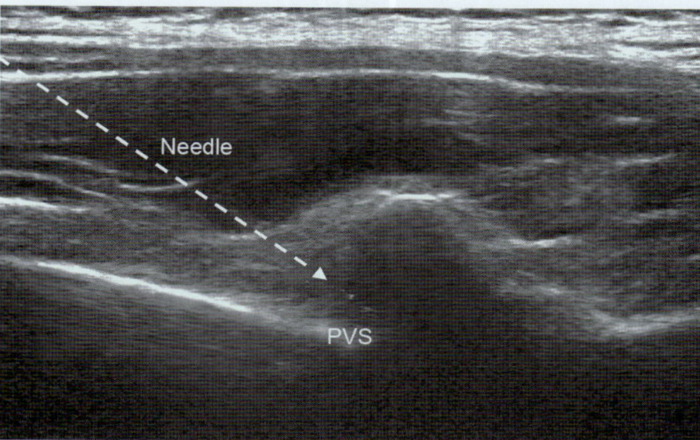

Fig. 1: Paravertebral block. The local anesthetic is deposited in the paravertebral space. (PVS: paravertebral space; LA: local anesthetic)

    - *Indwelling catheter:* Placement of a catheter in the paravertebral space for continuous analgesia may be an option.

Complications:

- *Frequency:* Complications are infrequent but can occur.
- *Potential issues:*
    - *Hypotension:* Intra- and postoperative hypotension may arise due to epidural spread of LA, usually manageable with small doses of vasopressors.
    - *Horner's syndrome:* Can occur in approximately 2% of cases
    - *Intravascular injection:* This may happen in about 0.5% of cases.
    - *Pneumothorax*
- *Technique failure:* The most common complication is technique failure, occurring in 10–15% of procedures, regardless of whether ultrasound or landmark techniques are used.

A recent review indicated that patients receiving either single-shot injections or paravertebral catheters experienced less acute pain in the first 72 hours post-surgery despite little impact on intra- and postoperative opioid consumption and PONV. There is evidence suggesting that

TPVB may help prevent chronic postsurgical pain after breast surgery at the 6-month mark.[24]

Thoracic Epidural Anesthesia

Thoracic epidural anesthesia at the level between T2–T5 can be used for analgesia during and after breast surgery. Due to its technical complexity and a 20% failure rate, TEA has largely been replaced by other techniques but is still relevant for prolonged reconstruction surgeries (e.g., TRAM, LD, and DIEP) and major bilateral operations. TEA poses a higher risk of hypotension and is not suitable for day-case procedures. Patients receiving TEA typically require monitoring in a high-dependency unit.

Pectoral Nerve Block (PECS I and II)

The PECS I and II are interfascial plane blocks introduced in 2012. PECS I blocks the medial and lateral pectoral nerves. PECS II targets the lateral branch of the intercostal nerve, including the intercostobrachial and long thoracic nerves, allowing for broader surgical coverage.[26]

- *Technique:*
  - Performed under ultrasound guidance, with the probe positioned below the lateral third of the clavicle
  - The needle is advanced to the space between the pectoralis major and minor (PEC 1) muscles at the third rib **(Fig. 2)** and then redirected to the deeper plane between the pectoralis minor and SA (PEC II) **(Fig. 3)**.
- *Dosage:*
  - *PECS I:* 0.2 mL/kg of dilute local anesthetic (e.g., 0.25–0.375% levobupivacaine, bupivacaine, 0.2–0.5% ropivacaine)
  - *PECS II:* 0.4 mL/kg
- *Benefits:* Fast-acting does not cause a sympathetic block and has been shown to reduce postoperative pain and opioid requirements compared to GA alone.

Serratus Anterior Plane Block

The SA plane block was first described for breast anesthesia in 2013. SA plane block aims to anesthetize the lateral cutaneous branches of thoracic intercostal nerves (T2–T12) for analgesia of the anterolateral chest wall.[27]

- *Technique:*
  - Conducted under ultrasound guidance using an in-plane approach
  - Local anesthetic is deposited deep to the LD muscle and superficial to the SA muscle in the mid-axillary area at the fourth or fifth rib **(Fig. 4)**.
- *Dosage:* The suggested dose is 0.2 mL/kg of long-acting local anesthetic.

The PECS and SA plane blocks are alternatives to TTPBs and thoracic epidurals. Due to the absence of neuraxial block risks, they are particularly suitable for day-case procedures. These blocks can be performed safely after the induction of GA, unlike TPVB or thoracic epidurals, which are typically administered. At the same time, the patient is awake to reduce nerve injury risk. PECS and SA

Fig. 2: PEC 1 block. The local anesthetic is deposited in the plane between pectoralis major muscle and pectoralis minor muscle at the level of third rib. (PM: pectoralis major; PMi: pectoralis minor; R3: third rib)

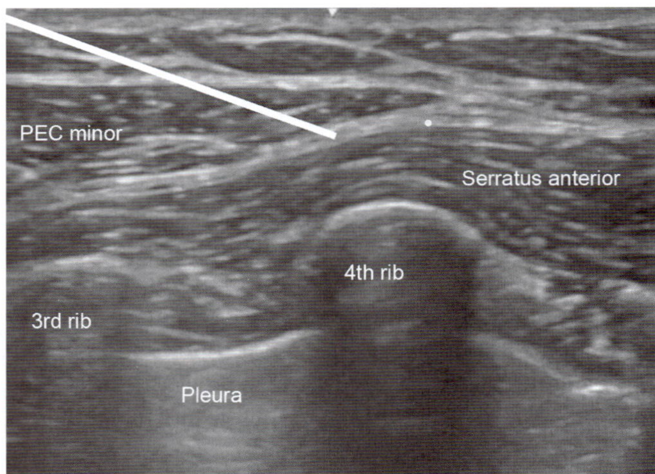

Fig. 3: PEC 2 block. The white line shows the direction of needle with tip in the plane between pectoralis minor and serratus anterior muscle at the level of fourth rib.

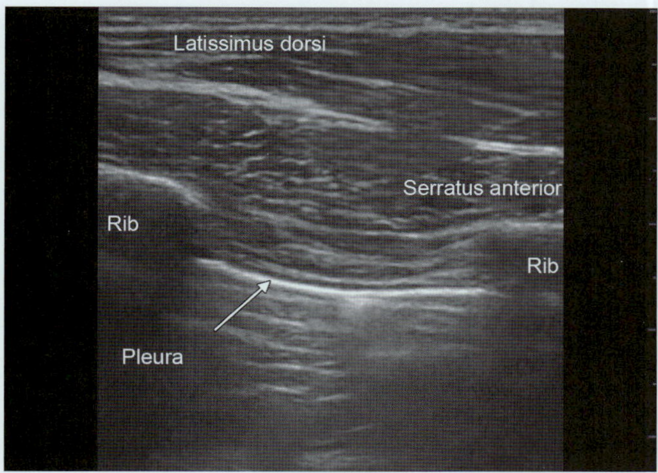

Fig. 4: Serratus anterior plane (SAP) block. The local anesthetic is deposited between the plane of serratus anterior muscle and latissimus dorsi muscle.

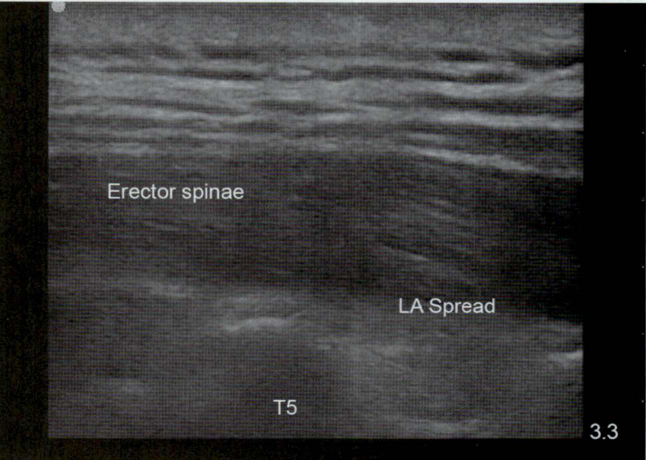

Fig. 5: Erector spinae block (ESB). The local anesthetic is deposited in the plane between erector spinae muscle and tip of traverse process of thoracic vertebrae. (T5: transverse process of fifth thoracic vertebra)

blocks are safe and easily performed under ultrasound guidance.

Erector Spinae Block

Erector spinae block is an emerging regional anesthetic technique that can be effectively utilized for analgesia in breast surgeries.[28]

Technique overview: The block targets the erector spinae muscle group, which runs along the spine. The injection is typically performed at the desired vertebral level to affect the dorsal rami of the spinal nerves.

- *Procedure:*
  - *Positioning:* The patient is usually in a sitting or lateral position.
  - *Ultrasound guidance:* An ultrasound probe is placed over the desired vertebrae, typically around T2 to T5.
  - *Injection:* A local anesthetic (e.g., 0.2% levobupivacaine) is injected in the plane between erector spinae muscle and tip of transverse process **(Fig. 5)**, allowing it to spread laterally to block the adjacent intercostal nerves.
- *Benefits:*
  - *Analgesia:* Provides effective postoperative pain relief, reducing the need for opioids.
  - *Safety:* Lower risk of complications compared to neuraxial blocks (e.g., no risk of spinal cord injury or neuraxial complications)
  - *Suitability:* Can be performed on awake patients, although it is also safe after induction of GA.
  - *Sympathetic block:* Unlike some traditional regional blocks, ESB typically does not cause significant sympathetic blockade, which is beneficial for maintaining hemodynamic stability.

Studies have shown that the ESB can provide comparable or superior analgesia compared to other regional techniques like TPVB and PECS blocks in patients undergoing breast surgery. Patients receiving the ESB report lower opioid consumption in the postoperative period.

Transversus Thoracic Plane Block

The TTPB involves injecting a local anesthetic bolus between the transversus thoracic muscle and the internal intercostal muscle at the fourth and fifth ribs near the costosternal junction. This block targets the anterior branches of the intercostal nerves (T2–T6) to provide analgesia for the internal mammary region. It is ideally used in conjunction with PECS I and II blocks for enhanced medial analgesia during breast surgery. A suggested injection volume is 15 mL of 0.15% levobupivacaine.

Local Anesthetic Infusion Analgesia

This method involves placing a catheter in the surgical wound to infuse a local anesthetic solution at a rate of 4–10 mL/hour using an active pumping mechanism.

It has been shown to provide better analgesia than a placebo, although comparative data against regional block techniques are limited. Recent studies indicate that combining local anesthetic infusion with PECS I and II blocks offers superior analgesia during the first 24 hours post-surgery compared to either technique used alone.

These regional anesthetic techniques provide effective pain relief and reduce the need for opioids, enhancing postoperative outcomes.

ANESTHESIA AND BREAST CANCER RECURRENCE

The debate about whether the anesthetic technique during cancer resection surgery affects the oncological outcomes in general and breast cancer, in particular, has been ongoing for more than a decade. Although the initial published retrospective studies indicated an association between the choice of anesthetic technique and long-term survival following breast cancer, a recent randomized controlled trial (RCT) of RA combined with propofol sedation in comparison to inhaled volatile GA combined with opioid analgesia for breast cancer surgery did not demonstrate a difference in cancer recurrence.[29]

- *Total intravenous anesthesia versus inhalational anesthesia and breast cancer recurrence:* The impact of anesthesia techniques and medications on long-term outcomes in early stage breast cancer has long intrigued both oncologists and anesthetists. Research suggests that propofol may offer advantages over volatile anesthetics like sevoflurane during breast cancer surgeries, as evidenced by biomarker studies showing propofol's superior inhibition of VEGF-C and TGF-β, increased activation of natural killer cells, and enhanced cancer cell apoptosis. However, the overall differences in long-term outcomes between propofol and volatile anesthetics remain less pronounced.

  A recent meta-analysis showed that propofol-based anesthesia can significantly enhance overall survival (OS) and locoregional recurrence-free survival (LRRFS) in nonmetastatic breast cancer patients compared to inhalational anesthesia. However, additional prospective RCTs are necessary to define the ideal patient population for propofol-based anesthesia and optimize its use in clinical settings.[30]
- *Role of RA and breast cancer recurrence:* The impact of anesthesia methods, especially RA, on cancer recurrence and metastasis after oncological surgery, is an area of increasing focus. Research indicates that RA can not only minimize opioid use but also hinder tumor recurrence by blocking sodium channels in cancer cells, reducing inflammation, and enhancing immune function. Additionally, opioids may promote tumor growth by causing immune suppression and stimulating cancer metastasis. Another way RA helps lower postoperative cancer recurrence is by decreasing growth factors that promote proliferation and angiogenesis.[31]

  There have been studies on various cancers and recurrence on the impact of RA. Still, there are only very few trials and hardly any meta-analysis on the effects of RA and breast cancer recurrence. Further meta-analysis and prospective studies are required to prove whether RA can prevent cancer recurrence.
- *Role of opioids and breast cancer recurrence:* Opioids remain the most used analgesics in managing cancer pain and are a crucial choice during surgery. Their benefits for cancer patients include improved quality of life, reduced neuroendocrine stress responses, and lower emotional stress, all of which contribute to better adherence to cancer treatments and positively impact survival. However, the existing evidence on whether opioids influence cancer outcomes is heterogeneous and unclear. While numerous preclinical, in vitro, and in vivo studies suggest a potential link between opioid use and cancer progression or metastasis, these findings have not been corroborated by clinical studies. Thus, there is insufficient evidence to justify avoiding these vital medications in breast cancer management. Recent randomized trials indicate that opioids should continue to be administered during surgery as analgesics in conjunction with anesthetic agents and used postoperatively for effective pain management related to cancer. Nevertheless, well-designed prospective studies are essential to further investigate the relationship between opioid use and OS in breast cancer patients.[32]

Overall, RCTs have not yet provided sufficient evidence that the anesthetic technique is associated with the recurrence rate or long-term outcomes in patients undergoing breast cancer surgery.

CONCLUSION

Breast cancer is one of the leading cause of cancer death in women. Most of the breast cancer patients require surgery as a part of the treatment.

The role of anesthesiologist in the peri operative period plays a crucial role in the overall outcome of the surgeries. Regional anesthesia technique and multimodal analgesia greatly helps in reducing postoperative pain and opioid consumption which is a key element in the postoperative outcome of breast onco-surgeries. Further studies are required to prove a direct relation between the anesthetic techniques including regional anesthesia techniques with overall outcome of the patient.

REFERENCES

1. Orrantia-Borunda E, Anchondo-Nuñez P, Acuña-Aguilar LE, Gómez-Valles FO, Ramírez-Valdespino CA. Subtypes of Breast Cancer. In: Mayrovitz HN (Ed). Breast Cancer. Brisbane (AU): Exon Publications; 2022. Chapter 3.
2. Sherwin A, Buggy DJ. Anaesthesia for breast surgery. BJA Educ. 2018;18(11):342-8.
3. World Health Organization. (2024). Breast cancer. [online] Available from https://www.who.int/news-room/fact-sheets/detail/breast-cancer. [Last accessed February, 2025]
4. National Cancer Institute. Breast Cancer Treatment (PDQ®)–Health Professional Version. [online] Available from https://www.cancer.gov/types/breast/hp/breast-treatment-pdq. [Last accessed February, 2025]
5. Vanni G, Costanzo G, Pellicciaro M, Materazzo M, Buonomo C, Federico T, et al. Awake Breast Surgery: A Systematic Review. In Vivo. 2023;37(4):1412-22.
6. White V, Harvey JR, Griffith CD, Youssef M, Carr M. Sentinel lymph node biopsy in early breast cancer surgery—working with the risks of vital blue dye to reap the benefits. Eur J Surg Oncol. 2011;37:101-8.
7. Ramin S, Azar FP, Malihe H. Methylene blue as the safest blue dye for sentinel node mapping: emphasis on anaphylaxis reaction. Acta Oncol. 2011;50:729-31.
8. Tamaki Y. One-step nucleic acid amplification assay (OSNA) for sentinel lymph node biopsy. Breast Cancer. 2015;22:230-4.
9. Liang MI, Carson WE 3rd. Biphasic anaphylactic reaction to blue dye during sentinel lymph node biopsy. World J Surg Oncol. 2008;6:79.
10. Cox CE, Salud CJ, Harrington MA. The role of selective sentinel lymph node dissection in breast cancer. Surg Clin North Am. 2000;80:1759-77.
11. Albo D, Wayne JD, Hunt KK, Rahlfs TF, Singletary SE, Ames FC, et al. Anaphylactic reactions to isosulfan blue dye during sentinel lymph node biopsy for breast cancer. Am J Surg. 2001;182:393-8.
12. Laurie SA, Khan DA, Gruchalla RS, Peters G. Anaphylaxis to isosulfan blue. Ann Allergy Asthma Immunol. 2002; 88:64-6.
13. Farooq S. (2018). Anaesthesia, surgery and life-threatening allergic reactions. [online] Available from http://www.nationalauditprojects.org.uk/NAP6Report#pt. [Last accessed February, 2025]
14. Petit JY, Rietjens M, Lohsiriwat V, Rey P, Garusi C, De Lorenzi F, et al. Update on breast reconstruction techniques and indications. World J Surg. 2012;36: 1486-97.
15. Chavez-MacGregor M, Clarke CA, Lichtensztajn DY, Giordano SH. Delayed initiation of adjuvant chemotherapy among patients with breast cancer. JAMA Oncol. 2016;2:322-9.
16. Shakir DK, Rasul KI. Chemotherapy induced cardiomyopathy: pathogenesis, monitoring and management. J Clin Med Res. 2009;1:8-12.
17. Allan N, Siller C, Breen A. Anaesthetic implications of chemotherapy. Contin Educ Anaesth Crit Care Pain. 2011;12:52-6.
18. Knight K, Wade S, Balducci L. Prevalence and outcomes of anemia in cancer: a systematic review of the literature. Am J Med. 2004;116 Suppl 7A:11S-26S.
19. National Institute for Health and Care Excellence. (2008) Hypothermia: prevention and management in adults having surgery. [online] Available from https://www.nice.org.uk/guidance/cg65/resources/hypothermia-prevention-andmanagement-in-adults-having-surgery-pdf-975569636293. [Last accessed February, 2025]
20. Cemal Y, Pusic A, Mehrara BJ. Preventative measures for lymphedema: separating fact from fiction. J Am Coll Surg. 2011;213:543-51.
21. Bodenham A. Vascular access after axillary lymph node surgery - a reply. Anaesthesia. 2017;72(1):128-9.
22. Nimalan N, Branford OA, Stocks G. Anaesthesia for free flap breast reconstruction. BJA Educ. 2016;16:162-6.
23. Jacobs A, Lemoine A, Joshi GP, Van de Velde M, Bonnet F; PROSPECT Working Group Collaborators. PROSPECT guideline for oncological breast surgery: a systematic review and procedure-specific postoperative pain management recommendations. Anaesthesia. 2020;75(5):664-73.
24. Terkawi AS, Tsang S, Sessler DI, Terkawi RS, Nunemaker MS, Durieux ME, et al. Improving Analgesic Efficacy and Safety of Thoracic Paravertebral Block for Breast Surgery: A Mixed-Effects Meta-Analysis. Pain Physician 2015;18(5):E757-80.
25. Kulhari S, Bharti N, Bala I, Arora S, Singh G. Efficacy of pectoral nerve block versus thoracic paravertebral block for postoperative analgesia after radical mastectomy: a randomized controlled trial. Br J Anaesth. 2016; 117(3):382-6.
26. Bashandy GM, Abbas DN. Pectoral nerves I and II blocks in multimodal analgesia for breast cancer surgery: a randomized clinical trial. Reg Anesth Pain Med. 2015;40(1):68-74.
27. Blanco R, Parras T, McDonnell JG, Prats-Galino A. Serratus plane block: a novel ultrasound-guided thoracic wall nerve block. Anaesthesia. 2013;68(11):1107-13.

28. Gürkan Y, Açıkalın EY. SP28 Erector spinae plane block (ESPB) for breast surgery. Reg Anesth Pain Med. 2022;47:A31.
29. Heaney A, Buggy DJ. Can anaesthetic and analgesic techniques affect cancer recurrence or metastasis? Br J Anaesth. 2012;109 Suppl 1:i17-i28.
30. Kim R, Kawai A, Wakisaka M, Kin T. Current Status and Prospects of Anesthesia and Breast Cancer: Does Anesthetic Technique Affect Recurrence and Survival Rates in Breast Cancer Surgery? Front Oncol. 2022;12:795864.
31. Sessler DI, Pei L, Huang Y, Fleischmann E, Marhofer P, Kurz A, et al. Breast Cancer Recurrence Collaboration. Recurrence of breast cancer after regional or general anaesthesia: a randomised controlled trial. Lancet. 2019; 394(10211):1807-15.
32. Thomas TE, Bowers K, Gomez D, Morgan O, Borowsky PA, Dutta R, et al. The association between perioperative opioids and breast cancer recurrence: a narrative review of the literature. Transl Breast Cancer Res. 2023;4:12.

Section 5: Thoracic Onco-Anesthesia

18 CHAPTER

One-Lung Ventilation

Jyotsna Goswami, Viplab Patro, Neha Desai

INTRODUCTION

The lungs, located on either side of the thoracic cavity, are anatomically distinct organs but function together as a single unit, inflating and deflating together to maintain normal oxygen and carbon dioxide levels in the blood. However, certain clinical situations require separation of the two lungs to facilitate the surgical exposure for thoracic surgeries, or to isolate the healthy lung from a diseased lung to prevent soiling or to allow differential ventilation. This process, known as lung isolation, allows each lung to operate independently by carefully preparing the airway through appropriate techniques and instrumentation. Despite its advantages, one-lung ventilation (OLV) poses significant challenges, such as airway manipulation-related trauma and significant physiological changes, in terms of ventilation-perfusion mismatch and the early onset of hypoxia.

This review will discuss the techniques of lung isolation techniques both in adults and pediatric patients, the general principles and physiology of OLV, its management, and complications, devices used for OLV and their placement.[1]

INDICATIONS FOR ONE-LUNG VENTILATION

The OLV is employed either for the surgical exposure or to protect the healthy lung from the diseased one.[2]

Thoracic Surgeries

- *Respiratory system:*
  - Lung resection procedures
    - Bullectomy
    - Pneumonectomy
    - Lobectomy
    - Wedge resection
  - Video-assisted thoracoscopic surgery (VATS)
  - Decortication
  - Diaphragmatic hernia repair (thoracic approach)
  - Single-lung transplant (management of postoperative complications)
- *Cardiovascular system:*
  - Minimally invasive cardiac surgeries
    - Valve repairs/replacements
  - Aortic arch surgeries
    - Dissecting aneurysm repair
  - Pericardial procedures
    - Repair of pericardial window
    - Pericardiectomy
- *Esophagus:*
  - Minimally invasive thoraco-laparoscopic esophagectomy

Nonthoracic Surgeries

- Anterior fixation of the thoracic spine

CONTRAINDICATIONS OF ONE-LUNG VENTILATION

- Dependence on bilateral mechanical ventilation.
- Patients with severe pulmonary disease or past history of (h/o) pulmonary resection may not tolerate OLV, when selective lobar blockade may be an option.
- Placement of a double-lumen endotracheal tube may not be technically possible in a patient with an intraluminal airway mass restricting access to the tracheobronchial tree.

ANATOMICAL CONSIDERATIONS

A thorough understanding of the anatomy of the tracheobronchial tree is essential to perform OLV safely. The use of fiberoptic bronchoscope or flexible intubating

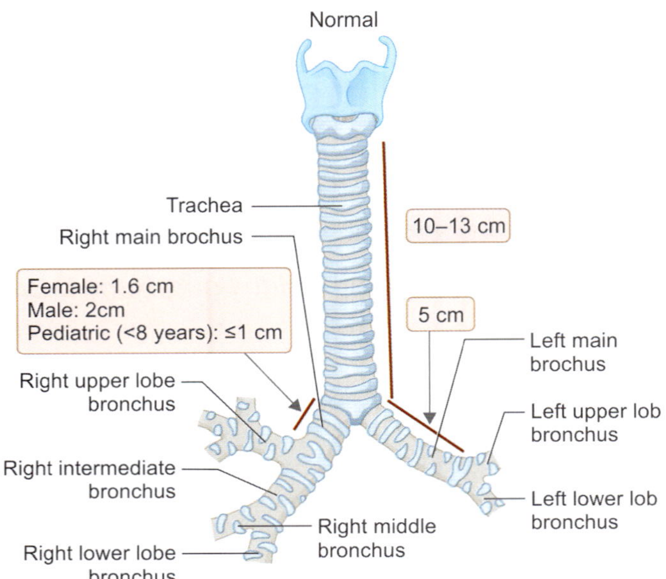

Fig. 1: Anatomy of tracheobronchial tree.[3]

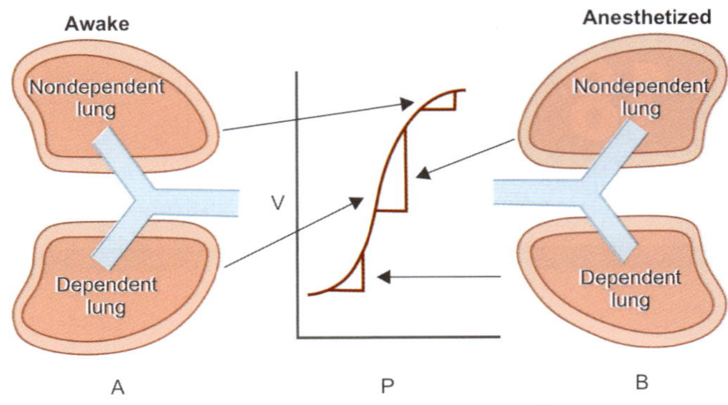

Fig. 2: Lung compliance curve.[4]

video-endoscope (FIVE) enables us to have a good visualization of the airway anatomy.

The trachea is about 10–13 cm long and has 12 concentric cartilaginous rings, which are deficient in their posterior aspect. The trachea divides into two mainstem bronchi, the left and right main bronchus (RMB) at the carina that is at the level of the sternal angle **(Fig. 1)**.

The left main bronchus (LMB) continues for about 5 cm, then it branches into the left lower lobe bronchus (LLLB) and left upper lobe bronchus (LULB). The RMB is shorter, wider, and more vertical than the left side. The RMB gives off the right upper lobe (RUB) bronchus and continues further as the bronchus intermedius. The take-off of the RUB bronchus is about 2.0 cm in adult men and about 1.6 cm in adult females **(Fig. 1)**.[3] A knowledge of tracheal anatomy helps the anesthesiologist to position the double-lumen tube for selectively isolating one lung for ventilation.

PHYSIOLOGICAL CONSIDERATIONS

It is very important to understand the changes in physiology caused by differential ventilation of the two lungs. In an awake patient, the dependent part of a lung receives more blood supply than the nondependent part due to gravity. The dependent part also gets preferentially more ventilation as it is slightly more compressed than the nondependent lung and therefore has a greater compliance once the atelectatic airways at the base have been opened. Ventilation (V) and perfusion (Q) are relatively well matched and shunt (lung that is perfused but not ventilated) is only 1–2% in a healthy person.

After anesthesia, the diaphragm and chest muscles are paralyzed resulting into decrease in the functional residual capacity (FRC) and also the mediastinal weight becomes unsupported as the surrounding structures become relaxed. So in an anesthetized patient, the upper nondependent lung becomes more compliant and moves to the position where the lower lung sits on the curve in the awake patient. The lower lung moves down the curve past the inflection point **(Fig. 2)**.[4] When the chest is opened, the upper lung becomes even easier to ventilate as there is no restriction by the chest wall. Blood supply is still determined by gravity, which now results into V/Q mismatch. This is even worse when the top lung is collapsed as there is then no ventilation to that lung, but there is still perfusion.

The initiation of OLV stops ventilation to one lung, which should create a 50% right-to-left shunt and relative hypoxemia if perfusion remain unchanged. However, the actual shunt fraction is usually only 20–30% for the following reasons:[5]

- Surgical manipulation of the atelectatic lung obstructs vascular flow to the nonventilated lung.
- Due to lateral positioning during thoracic surgery, the dependent lung gets a gravitational increase in perfusion, which is also ventilated. As the dependent ventilated lung is within the closed side of the chest and is exposed to the weight of the contralateral hemithorax contents, there is increase in lung elastance.[6]
- Mechanical collapse of the nondependent lung diverts the blood flow toward the dependent ventilated lung.

Lack of ventilation and therefore hypoxia in the collapsed lung causes a phenomenon called hypoxic pulmonary vasoconstriction (HPV), which modulates the blood flow to hypoxic regions of the lungs.[7] During OLV, HPV reduces shunt flow through the nonventilated lung by 40–50% and thus decreases the degree of hypoxemia.[8] By causing pulmonary vasoconstriction, alveolar hypoxia diverts blood away from poorly/nonventilated areas to better ventilated areas and thereby improves V/Q mismatch. Clinically, HPV is proportional to the degree of local hypoxia, and is initiated primarily in response to an alveolar oxygen partial pressure (PaO_2) <100 mm Hg.[9] The onset is usually two-phase such as initial rapid onset phase in minutes and a delayed phase in hours. After oxygenation and ventilation are re-established, the attenuation of HPV follows a reverse two-phase pattern and may not completely return to normal for several hours.[8] This is an important consideration in the case of bilateral sequential thoracic procedures, such as bilateral wedge resections for lung metastases, in which patients tend to desaturate more during the OLV of the second lung.

A number of anesthetic factors may influence HPV, some of which may be controlled by the management of the anesthetic.

The factors potentiating HPV, which causes less shunt and improves oxygenation are:[9]

- Metabolic and respiratory acidosis
- Hypercapnia
- Mild decreased mixed venous oxygenation
- Hyperthermia

The factors decreasing HPV, which causes increased shunt and worsening of oxygenation, are:

- Metabolic and respiratory alkalosis
- Hypocapnia
- Hypothermia
- Increased left atrial pressure
- Administration of a volatile inhalation anesthetic at a dose >1 minimum alveolar concentration (MAC)
- Hemodilution

EQUIPMENT

Double-lumen tubes (DLTs) and bronchial blockers (BBs) are special airway devices to achieve OLV. They are used to collapse one lung selectively to facilitate surgical exposure and direct the airflow to the other lung. The choice of device to achieve lung separation depends on the patient's anatomy, the procedure, availability, and the operator's preference.[2]

Double-Lumen Tubes

The design of the DLT used in the current practice of thoracic anesthesia is the Robertshaw design or disposable polyvinyl chloride (PVC). DLTs are two tubes of different lengths fused side by side to form a single unit. Their design enables independent ventilation of each lung through separate breathing circuits or a shared circuit using a Y-connector. The two tubes separate at the proximal end to allow independent connections. On the distal end, the shorter tube ends in the mid-trachea and the longer tube extends into the main-stem bronchus of the targeted lung (left or right). The tracheal portion curves anteriorly, while the bronchial portion curves at a right angle, with the concavity directed toward the targeted bronchus. Left-sided DLTs are commonly used due to the anatomical alignment of the LMB. Right-sided DLTs have an extra opening for the RUL bronchus. Position of the RUL opening varies depending on the design of the tube. It may be incorporated within the oblique cuff (e.g., Broncho-Cath®) or may be situated between two smaller cuffs (e.g., Rusch® tubes). Most DLTs are made of disposable plastic with color-coded components such as white for tracheal component and blue for bronchial component. DLTs are available in varying sizes from 26 to 41 Fr for adult and 26 to 28 Fr (left-sided only) for children. The size indicates the external diameter (ED) of the tube in cm.[10]

Tracheal cuff, when inflated, enables positive pressure ventilation for both lungs and isolates them from the external environment. Bronchial cuff, when inflated, separates the two lungs, allowing isolation or selective ventilation. Cross-sectional design features a D-shaped lumen for enhanced stability and functionality. Advantages include reliable lung separation, independent or selective lung ventilation, and easily adapted to surgical requirements.

Endobronchial Blockers

Endobronchial blockers (EBBs) are balloon-tipped devices designed to isolate and collapse specific lung segments. When inserted into the desired bronchus, the inflatable balloon occludes the airway, preventing aeration of the targeted lung segment, which leads to its collapse distal to the blockage.

Key Features

- Stylet-like design with an low-pressure high-volume cuff at the tip.
- Provides selective and precise lung segment isolation.
- Useful in patients where DLTs may not be suitable, such as in pediatric cases or those with challenging airway anatomy.

The EBBs are versatile tools in achieving lung isolation for various surgical and nonsurgical indications.[11]

Various types of EBBs are available now. They have different characteristics as described below:

	Arndt	*Cohen*	*Fuji Uniblocker*	*E-Z blocker*	*Univent*
Size (Fr)	5, 7, 9	9	5 F, 9F	7	7.5–12 mm (tube size)
Guidance feature	Wire loop to snare FOB	Deflecting tip with wheel device	None, preshaped	Double-lumen bifurcated tip	Preshaped integrated (within the tube) torque control
Smallest recommended TT size	• 9 Fr-8 mm • 7 Fr-7 mm • 5 Fr-4.5 mm	8 mm	9 Fr-8 mm 5 Fr-4.5 mm	8 mm	
Central lumen	1.8 mm	1.8 mm	2 mm	1.4 mm	2 mm
Murphy eye	Present in 9 Fr	Present	None	None	None
Disadvantages	Not visualized during insertion	Expensive		Lumen too small	Size too big

Techniques of Double-Lumen Tubes Insertion

As the left-sided DLT placement is less challenging than the right-sided one, the most commonly used DLT is the left-sided DLT, irrespective of which side requires the isolation.

After induction, the following steps are taken to place a left-sided DLT:

- A direct laryngoscopy using a Macintosh blade is used for laryngoscopy as the DLT is a large tube, and this technique provides the maximum space for its insertion.
- The DLT is introduced with a rigid stylet with the endobronchial curvature facing anteriorly.
- After the DLT passes through the vocal cords, the stylet is removed and the tube is then rotated by a 90° angle anticlockwise to the left until the blue bronchial lumen faces left and the tracheal lumen faces right.
- The tube is advanced until resistance is met. The tracheal cuff may be inflated at this moment, and the connector is attached to start ventilation.
- The DLT position should be confirmed with a fiberoptic bronchoscope (pediatric size 3.5) to ensure the tracheal lumen opening is above the carina and bronchial lumen is in the left bronchus.
- The bronchial cuff can now be inflated with 1–2 mL of air.
- Bilateral ventilation confirmation is by auscultation. Air entry should be audible in bilateral lungs at this point.
- Next, lung isolation is confirmed with selective tracheal and bronchial lumens clamping.
- Only the left lung should be inflated when ventilation through the bronchial lumen completes.
- Only the right lung should inflate when clamping the bronchial lumen and ventilating through the tracheal lumen.

The inability to perform a direct laryngoscopy is a contraindication to using a DLT. In such a situation, a BB may be a suitable alternative.[12]

How to Give Proper Deflation of the Nonventilated Lung

Complete collapse of the nonventilated lung will facilitate surgical exposure. Following measures help to improve collapse:

- Denitrogenate both lungs by ventilating with either 100% oxygen (O_2) or a nitrous oxide (N_2O)/O_2 mixture for several minutes prior to initiating OLV.[13] Replacing the poorly absorbed nitrogen in the nonventilated lung with more soluble O_2 or N_2O will facilitate collapse.[14]
- Apply low suction (20 cmH_2O) until the nonventilated lung has collapsed well.[15]

- When a BB is used, disconnect the anesthetic circuit and allow a prolonged expiration for 20–30 seconds, or until the end-tidal carbon dioxide ($ETCO_2$) falls to zero. Then begin OLV after inflating the cuff of the BB under direct vision with the flexible intubating scope.[14]
- Use pressure-controlled ventilation during OLV to avoid the peaks in airway pressure that may occur during volume-controlled ventilation (e.g., due to surgical manipulation in the chest or patient coughing). This decreases the chance of inadvertent reinflation of the nonventilated lung due to gas being forced past the inflated cuff of the DLT or BB device.

VENTILATION STRATEGY

The OLV can result in a spectrum of lung injury such as barotrauma, volutrauma, atelectrauma, biotrauma, etc., and ultimately severe lung injury.[16] The incidence of acute lung injury (ALI) is around 2–4% following lung resection[17-19] and 8–12% after pneumonectomy.[18,20] Mortality from ALI is around 40%.[21] Investigators have used inflammatory bio markers (such as cytokines) to detect ALI and to predict future multiorgan dysfunction and death.[16]

To prevent these ALI, lung protective ventilation strategy has been adapted, which is as follows:[22]

- *Low tidal volume (TV) ventilation:* 4–6 mL/kg (6–8 mL/kg during two-lung ventilation)—low TV has been shown to decrease inflammatory markers.[23]
- Adjustment of respiratory rate to maintain $ETCO_2$ and arterial carbon dioxide tension ($PaCO_2$) near the patient's baseline.
- *Positive end-expiratory pressure (PEEP):* 5–10 cmH_2O if TV is low [0–5 cmH_2O in patients with chronic obstructive pulmonary disease (COPD)].
- *Limited airway pressures:* Plateau inspiratory pressures <30 cmH_2O
- *Minimum fraction of inspired oxygen (FiO_2):* Minimum level to maintain arterial oxygen saturation (SpO_2) >90%.
- *Permissive hypercapnia:* Low TV results into hypercapnia, which may be beneficial during OLV, as it potentiates HPV.[24] It leads to a rightward shift of the oxyhemoglobin dissociation curve, which increases oxygen delivery to tissues leading to improved wound healing and less infectious complications.[25] However, the risk of increased intracranial pressure, pulmonary hypertension, myocardial depression, and decreased renal perfusion should be balanced with this beneficial effect.
- *PEEP level:* Application of PEEP prevents atelectasis and thus reduce injury from the mechanical stress of repetitive inflation and deflation cycles in the alveoli.[26] It is not clear how much PEEP should be applied to get the beneficial effect. Some study showed that PEEP of 10 cmH_2O is required with low TV to maintain adequate lung function in abdominal surgery[27] and other study showed that PEEP of 5 cmH_2O decreased inflammatory markers.[28] Whereas some authors showed that low TV (5 mL/kg-1) accompanied by 5 cmH_2O PEEP provides comparable arterial oxygenation and intrapulmonary shunt fraction during OLV as higher TV (10 mL/kg-1) without PEEP. Recently a multicenter randomized controlled trial used individualized one lung approach (iOLA) which included an alveolar recruitment maneuver to 40 cmH_2O of end-inspiratory pressure followed by individualized PEEP titrated to best respiratory system compliance, and individualized postoperative respiratory support with high-flow oxygen therapy. They found that during OLV, iOLA was associated with a reduced risk of severe postoperative pulmonary complications when compared with conventional lung-protective ventilation.[29]

HYPOXEMIA DURING ONE-LUNG VENTILATION

Hypoxia during OLV occurs in approximately 5% of patients, with SpO_2 falling below 90%.[5] The primary pathophysiological mechanism is impaired ventilation-perfusion (V/Q) matching within the lungs. The nonventilated lung continues to receive blood flow, which does not participate in gas exchange leading to the development of regions with low V/Q ratio or intrapulmonary shunt. Besides OLV itself, V/Q ratio is also influenced by patient position, anesthesia, cardiac output, mode of ventilation, the presence of preexisting lung disease, and factors that affect HPV.[30]

Management of Hypoxia During One-Lung Ventilation

Effective management involves predicting, preventing, and treating hypoxia in stepwise manner.

Predicting Hypoxia during One-Lung Ventilation

No single factor can fully predict hypoxia. Several factors may increase the risk and predict the likelihood of hypoxia during OLV.

- Preexisting low PaO_2
- *Left-sided ventilation:* Due to smaller size left lung.
- Higher forced expiratory volume in 1 second (FEV1)
- Supine as compared to lateral position

Preventing Hypoxia during One-Lung Ventilation

- *Preoxygenation:* Before initiating OLV, preoxygenation with 100% oxygen for 3–5 minutes can improve oxygen reserves and prolong the time before hypoxia occurs.
- *Positioning:* Proper patient positioning, such as ensuring the dependent lung is adequately ventilated, can improve oxygenation during OLV.
- *Application of PEEP:* Applying PEEP to the ventilated lung can prevent atelectasis and maintain lung volume, thus reducing the risk of hypoxia.
- *Alveolar recruitment maneuvers:* Implementing alveolar recruitment maneuvers in the ventilated lung (e.g., intermittent sustained inflation) can help improve gas exchange.
- *Minimize surgical compression:* Ensuring that the nonventilated lung is not excessively compressed by surgical retraction or the mediastinum can reduce V/Q mismatch.

Treating Hypoxia during One-Lung Ventilation

If hypoxia develops during OLV, it can be treated using the following interventions:[31]

- *Initial treatment is to increase FiO_2:* Administering 100% oxygen to the patient can enhance oxygenation, but it may not be sufficient in severe cases of hypoxia.
- To check the position of the lung isolation device using flexible intubating scope and reposition as needed.
- Suction to clear secretions or blood, which may block the airway.
- Cardiac output should be optimized with the use of vasopressors or inotropes, to optimize blood flow to the ventilated lung.

If still hypoxia persists, the ventilatory settings should be revisited as follows:

- *Alveolar recruitment:* A recruitment maneuver such as a sustained inflation of the ventilated lung can help reopen collapsed alveoli and improve oxygenation.
- Increasing PEEP up to 10 cmH_2O to the ventilated lung can help minimize atelectasis and improve oxygenation.[32]
- Continuous positive airway pressure (CPAP) 5–10 cmH_2O to the nonventilated lung reduces shunt fraction.[33] But it should be used only when hypoxemia does not subside with other measures, as any small flow to the operative lung causes partial inflation, which will affect surgical exposure.
- Insufflation of a low flow of oxygen (3 L/min) via a suction catheter in the lumen of the DLT to the nonventilated lung at the start of OLV has been shown to decrease the incidence of subsequent hypoxemia.[34]
- High frequency jet ventilation to the nonventilated lung can be used as an alternative to CPAP to improve oxygenation and decrease shunt.[35]
- The nonventilated lung may be intermittently inflated and ventilated, although this often requires interruption of the surgical procedure.
- If the patients do not tolerate collapse of an entire lung, then the collapse of only the operative lobe can be achieved with a BB placed in the bronchus of this lobe.[36]
- The surgeon can decrease shunt by mechanically restricting pulmonary blood flow to the operative lung.[37]
- Inhaled nitric oxide (NO) as a pulmonary vasodilator[38] and the use of nebulized prostacyclin to the ventilated lung can be useful during OLV.[39]

Reexpansion of Nonventilated Lung

At the end of resection, the upper nonventilated lung should be reexpanded to reinflate all atelectatic areas, except in case of pneumonectomy. A sustained inflation at low levels of positive airway pressure (20–30 cmH_2O for 10–15 seconds) helps this reexpansion, which should be repeated for optimal recruitment of lung tissue. The expansion should be applied under direct observation of the lung either in an open chest, or on the monitor during VATS. This ensures gradual but complete recruitment of residual lung tissue with application of the minimum sustained positive pressure that is necessary.

After pulmonary resection, the sustained inflation helps to detect bronchial air leaks. Higher pressures over >30 cmH_2O can exacerbate ALI or result into new air leaks after pulmonary resection.

Subsequently, two-lung ventilation is restarted with a protective ventilation strategy and the minimum FiO_2 that maintains oxygen saturation >93%.

Choice of Anesthesia

Type of anesthesia (inhalation versus intravenous) does not affect oxygenation during OLV, or incidence of lung injury and therefore should be based on standard considerations unrelated to OLV.[5]

PEDIATRIC ONE-LUNG VENTILATION

Advances in thoracic surgery have seen a paradigm shift in pediatric thoracic surgery with more procedures being done thoracoscopically in the last 20 years than before. Pediatric patients can present for a wide range of thoracic procedures in varying ages from neonates/preterms to teenagers. A thorough understanding of pediatric physiology, anatomical, and developmental changes, techniques of lung isolation, and OLV are essential for a pediatric anesthesiologist.

ANATOMICAL IMPLICATIONS FOR ONE-LUNG VENTILATION

The understanding of the pediatric airway has substantially improved during the last several decades based on multiple studies on autopsy specimens and various computed tomography guided evaluations of the airway.[40-42] Anatomic differences relevant for OLV in children are:

- The width of the left mainstem bronchus is smaller than the right mainstem bronchus and requires an endotracheal tube (ETT) half size smaller for endobronchial intubation. In neonates up to 3 months old, even a 3.0 uncuffed ETT may be difficult to insert, and a 2.5 size tube may be needed.[43]
- The distance from the carina to the take-off of the RUB is <1 cm in most children up to 8 years of age, thus increasing the chances of the ETT being distal to the upper lobe and exacerbating hypoxemia and hypercarbia in these patients. However, the take-off for the left upper lobe is usually 3 times greater giving the anesthesiologist a larger margin of safety for placing an ETT or BB.[44]
- The neonatal trachea has an average anteroposterior (AP) diameter of about 4.3 mm in both male and female, which grows uniformly for both until the age of 14 years, when the female trachea stops growing. However, the male trachea continues to grow till 19 years of age up to 16–18 mm. The trachea is elliptical in shape with the AP diameter less than the transverse diameter, hence sizing of devices should take this into consideration.[45]

PHYSIOLOGICAL CONSIDERATIONS FOR ONE-LUNG VENTILATION

In the awake subject in the upright position, ventilation is preferentially distributed to the dependent regions of the lung with an increasing gradient from the upper segments to the most dependent segments of the lung. Perfusion follows a similar pattern due to gravitational forces resulting in well matched V/Q ratio with maximum oxygenation.

Several factors lead to a mismatch in V/Q ratios during thoracic surgery. GA, neuromuscular blockade, mechanical ventilation, lateral position, all reduce FRC of both lungs. Surgical retraction and single-lung ventilation lead to collapse of the operative lung, favoring ventilation in the dependent lung. Hypoxia in the nondependent lung initiates HPV which directs blood away to better ventilated areas of the lung. HPV begins within seconds, peaking at 15–20 minutes, with a second peak at around 2 hours. All these compensatory mechanisms help to optimize the V/Q ratio with adequate oxygenation.[44,46] HPV is maximal with partial pressure of oxygen in venous blood (PvO_2) is normal. Inhalational agents and other vasodilating agents with high or low inspired oxygen fraction (FiO_2) can impair HPV. The effects of the lateral decubitus position however differ in infants compared to older children and adults.[46] In adults and older children, placing the healthy lung dependent leads to optimal oxygenation with better V/Q matching due to favorable ventilation and perfusion of the dependent lung due to gravitational forces, thus facilitating surgery in the diseased nondependent lung. Whereas, in infants, oxygenation is better with the healthy lung in the nondependent or "up" position. The main reasons for these differences are:[47,48]

- The mostly cartilaginous, compressible rib-cage of infants cannot fully support the dependent lung. Hence, the FRC is close to residual volume predisposing them to airway closure at tidal breathing.
- Due to their small size, the hydrostatic pressure gradient between the dependent and nondependent lungs is much lesser than in adults, thus diminishing the effect on ventilation and perfusion.
- The abdominal pressure gradient acting on the dependent diaphragm is significantly decreased in infants, thus reducing the advantage of the dependent diaphragm.

All these factors along with a higher metabolic rate make infants more prone to hypoxemia during OLV.

TECHNIQUES FOR LUNG ISOLATION IN INFANTS AND CHILDREN

One-lung ventilation in infants and children can be achieved via single lumen ETT, balloon tipped BBs, DLT, or a univent tube.

Single Lumen Endotracheal Tube

Selective endobronchial insertion of a conventional single lumen ETT remains the simplest means of lung isolation. It is generally the best option for neonates and very young infants. Right sided endobronchial intubation can be easily accomplished by simply advancing the ETT until the breath sounds on the left disappear. Care must be taken to avoid advancing the tube too distally to prevent occlusion of the RUB. For left endobronchial intubation, the recommended technique is to turn the bevel of the tube 180°, rotate the head to the right, and then advance the tube until breath sounds on the right side disappear. However, it is recommended to use a flexible bronchoscope for correct placement of the ETT.[49] It is vital to note that the distance between the tip of the tube and the proximal end of the cuff should be less than the length of the mainstem bronchus to ensure that the cuff is within the bronchus.[50] The advantage of this technique is that it is simple, and isolation can be quickly achieved in emergency situations such as pulmonary hemorrhage or pneumothorax. Paquet et al. have reported the successful isolation of whole lung for lavage with two single lumen ETTs, one endobronchial, and one in the trachea for ventilation.[51]

Disadvantages of endobronchial intubation are:[44,46]

- *Failure to provide adequate seal in the bronchus:* Operative lung may not collapse fully, contamination of the nonoperative lung.
- Inability to suction and provide CPAP to the operative lung.
- Potential for obstruction of the RUB bronchus, if the take-off is short.
- ETT may be occluded by secretions/debris.

Double Lumen Tubes

As described in the earlier sections, DLTs are essentially two tubes of unequal length moulded together to facilitate lung isolation and OLV. DLTs remain the gold standard of lung isolation in adults. The technique of insertion in adolescents remains the same as in adults. The smallest size of DLT available is 26 Fr (Rusch, Duluth, GA), which is approximately equivalent to a 6.5 ETT making it suitable for use in children above 8 years of age. Up to the age of 16 years, the size needed can be estimated by the equation "Size = Age* 1.5 + 14." After the age of 16 years, the male and female trachea vary in size, and the size required may be estimated based on sex and height as in adults.[45] Placement of a DLT must preferably be confirmed with a bronchoscope to ensure correct side and depth of insertion. As in adults, left-sided DLTs are preferred due to ease of insertion and avoidance of occlusion of the RUB.

Advantages of DLTs include ease of insertion, high quality of lung isolation, ability to suction, and apply CPAP to the operative lung and to quickly alternate between one-lung and two-lung ventilation, and reduced chances of contamination.[44,45] Disadvantages include size limitation, unsuitability for patients with difficult airways or upper airway abnormalities or those requiring postoperative ventilation and higher incidence of upper airway and tracheal injuries.[45,50]

Marraro has described the "Marraro Paediatric Endobronchial Bilumen Tube®" (mPEBT) which consists of two uncuffed medical grade PVC tubes attached laterally to each other. Different sizes of the mPEBT are suitable for use in neonates, infants, and children up to 4–5 years old. Absence of cuff and lateral attachment of the tubes allows a size larger than would be required to be used in these patients. However, the tube is currently available only as a special product.[52]

Bronchial Blockers

Balloon tipped BBs are the technique of choice for OLV in pediatric patients under the age of 6 years. These can be placed intraluminal or extraluminally. Presently, the devices available for use in pediatric patients are the Fogarty embolization catheters (Edwards Life Sciences, Irvine, CA), Arndt BB (Cook Medical, Bloomington, IN), 5F Fuji Uniblocker (Ambu, Columbia, MD), and the EZ-Blocker (Teleflex, Wayne, PA).

Fogarty embolectomy catheters were the devices first described for achieving OLV in children, with the earliest description in 1969.[53] Except the 2 and 3 Fr catheters, they all have a guidewire which allows the tip to be flexed at 20° and directed into the desired bronchus. The catheter may be placed within or outside the ETT lumen. Inflation of the low volume, high pressure cuff must be done under bronchoscopic visualization to prevent injury to the mucosa and dislodgement due to overinflation. Absence of a central channel makes deflation of the lung slow via absorption atelectasis and inability to apply suction to the operative lung.[45]

The *Arndt BB* is the most commonly used and most well documented of all BBs in children. It has a 4-way adapter, a high-volume low-pressure cuff and a removable guidewire with a loop at the distal end which slides over the bronchoscope to facilitate its insertion into the desired bronchus.[44] After insertion, the guidewire may be removed to use the central lumen for suction and CPAP. The blocker is available in three sizes (5, 7, and 9 Fr) and can be used with in patients with 5.0 ETT. Size 9 Fr can be used with ETTs of size 7.5 mm and above, 7 Fr with sizes 6.0 and 7.0 mm, and 5 Fr with .5–5.5 mm. For younger patients, the blocker may be placed extraluminal under visual guidance.[50]

The *5 Fr Fuji Uniblocker* is suitable for children up to 8 years old. It has a stiff shaft and a preformed angled tip, which can be rotated to insert into the desired bronchus. It has a 3 mL high-volume low-pressure cuff which should be inflated under bronchoscopic visualization. However, there is no central lumen for suctioning or CPAP.[45]

The *EZ-Blocker* is a "Y-shaped" BB with a two 4 cm distal ends connected to the shaft. It is designed to sit on the carina making insertion easier and dislodgement less likely. Though approved for use in adults, there are reports of extraluminal use of this blocker in children above 6 years of age. The blocker is placed extraluminally using a 5.5 uncuffed ETT as a conduit under direct laryngoscopy. Once through the glottic opening, the ETT is removed and another appropriate size tube for the patient is inserted with repeat laryngoscopy for ventilation. Placement of the BB is confirmed with bronchoscopy.[54,55]

Univent Tube

The Univent tube is a basically an ETT with a movable BB incorporated in an additional lumen. The tube comes in 3 sizes, 3.5, .5, and 5.5 mm. The size indicates the internal diameter (ID) of the ventilating lumen. The ED of 3.5 mm tube is 8 mm, making it suitable only for children 6 years and above. The tube is inserted in the conventional way followed by rotating it 90° to the operative side and advancing the blocker under bronchoscopy guidance. The main disadvantage of the Univent tube is the small ID increasing airway resistance and limiting the size of the bronchoscope that can be used. Also, due to the size limitations, there is only narrow age range (6–8 years), where the tube can be safely used.[45,56]

MANAGEMENT OF ONE-LUNG VENTILATION IN CHILDREN

Presently, there are no evidence-based recommendations for ventilation strategies during OLV in pediatric patients. There are very few studies evaluating effect of lung protective ventilation in children, those that are reported did not use PEEP in control groups, thus confounding the results.[44] The following measures may be followed for safely conducting OLV in children:[44,50]

Confirm correct placement of the isolation device after positioning for surgery with a bronchoscope.

- Begin with 100% oxygen to increase margin of safety, especially in endobronchial intubation, to promote absorption atelectasis of the operative lung and to promote redistribution of the blood flow to the dependent lung.
- The FiO_2 can then be gradually reduced to maintain saturation above 92%. Continue ventilation with TV at 4–6 mL/kg body weight, 5–10 cmH_2O PEEP to the dependent lung.
- Inspired concentration of the inhaled anesthetic should be kept <1 MAC to avoid excessive inhibition of HPV and to maintain cardiac output.
- CPAP as low as 1–2 cmH_2O may be applied to the operative lung to improve oxygenation. More than 10 cmH_2O CPAP must be avoided to avoid interference with the surgery.
- Adequate cardiac output must be maintained to prevent excessive fall in mixed venous oxygen content.
- On completion of surgery, the nonventilated lung should be gradually reexpanded with positive airway pressure of 20–30 cmH_2O sustained over 10–15 seconds. Overinflation should be avoided to prevent volutrauma.
- Some degree of hypercarbia is expected, but it usually resolves with resumption of two-lung ventilation.

MANAGEMENT OF HYPOXEMIA DURING ONE-LUNG VENTILATION

In most instances, SpO_2 >90% is acceptable in children. The actual incidence of hypoxemia in this group of patients remains unknown. If the saturation falls below 90% for >2 minutes, the following steps can be applied:[44]

Inform the surgeon about drop in saturation.

- Increase FiO_2 to 100%.
- Recruitment maneuver to the dependent lung.

- Increase PEEP up to 10 cmH_2O, while monitoring hemodynamic parameters.
- CPAP to the operative lung, if not already applied.
- Confirm position of the isolation device (BB/DLT/ETT) with a bronchoscope.
- If saturation does not improve with these measures, convert to two-lung ventilation and continue surgery with intermittent OLV and manual retraction of the operative lung.

CONCLUSION

Indications for OLV—OLV is ventilation of one lung while allowing the other to collapse. Indications include:

- Surgical exposure during thoracic surgery.
- Isolation of one lung from the other for the treatment of pulmonary pathology.

Contraindications for OLV—dependence on bilateral mechanical ventilation, and intraluminal airway masses.

Physiology of OLV—differential ventilation of both the lungs include ventilation/perfusion mismatch and HPV.

Lung-protective ventilation strategies—during OLV, protective ventilation strategy minimizes lung injury, which is as follows:

- Low TV ventilation (4–6 mL/kg).
- Respiratory rate adjusted to maintain $ETCO_2$ and $PaCO_2$ near the patient's baseline.
- PEEP 5–10 cmH_2O, except in patients with severe obstructive disease.
- Limited airway pressures (plateau inspiratory pressures <30 cmH_2O), or pressure-controlled ventilation.
- FiO_2 should be titrated to maintain oxygen saturation >90%.

Management of hypoxemia during OLV—we initially increase oxygen to 100%. If this is not effective, we temporarily return to two-lung ventilation to bring the oxygen saturation above 90%, and then perform the following maneuvers

- Increase FiO_2 to 100%.
- Check lung isolation device position using the flexible intubating scope (FIS), and reposition as indicated.
- Suction to remove blood or secretions, if any, from major bronchi.
- Optimize cardiac output.
- Perform recruitment maneuvers on the ventilated lung.
- Add 5 cmH_2O PEEP to ventilated side, use with caution in patients with obstructive pulmonary disease.
- Add CPAP 5–10 cmH_2O to the nonventilated lung.
- The nonventilated lung may be intermittently reinflated and ventilated.
- The surgeon may consider clamping flow to the operative lung.

Reexpanding the nonventilated lung—reexpansion with a sustained inflation at low levels of positive airway pressure (e.g., 20–30 cmH_2O for 10–15 seconds), reinflates all atelectatic areas of the nonventilated lung and detect bronchial air leaks. This maneuver may be repeated for optimal recruitment of lung tissue.

REFERENCES

1. Miller RD, Eriksson LI, Fleisher LA, Wiener-Kronish JP, Young WL. Anesthesia for Thoracic Surgery. In: Slinger P, Javier HT (Eds). Miller's Anesthesia, 7th edition. Philadelphia: Elsevier; 2006.
2. Cohen E. Current Practice Issues in Thoracic Anesthesia. Anesth Analg. 2021;133(6):1520-31.
3. Wooten C, Patel S, Cassidy L, Watanabe K, Matusz P, Tubbs RS, et al. Variations of the tracheobronchial tree: Anatomical and clinical significance. Clin Anat. 2014; 27(8):1223-33.
4. Strachan L. WFSA Resource Library. One-lung Ventilation. [online] Available from https://resources.wfsahq.org/atotw/one-lung-ventilation/ [Last accessed February, 2025]
5. Karzai W, Schwarzkopf K. Hypoxemia during one-lung ventilation: prediction, prevention, and treatment. Anesthesiology. 2009;110(6):1402-11.
6. Chiumello D, Formenti P, Bolgiaghi L, Mistraletti G, Gotti M, Vetrone F, et al. Body position alters mechanical power and respiratory mechanics during thoracic surgery. Anesth Analg. 2020;130(2):391-401.
7. Lagier D, Zeng C, Fernandez-Bustamante A, Vidal Melo MF. Perioperative Pulmonary Atelectasis: Part II. Clinical Implications. Anesthesiology. 2022;136(1):206-36.
8. Sylvester JT, Shimoda LA, Aaronson PI, Ward JPT. Hypoxic pulmonary vasoconstriction. Physiol Rev. 2012; 92(1):367-520.
9. Lohser J. Managing hypoxemia during minimally invasive thoracic surgery. Anesthesiol Clin. 2012;30(4):683-97.
10. Hao D, Saddawi-Konefka D, Low S, Alfille P, Baker K. Placement of a double-lumen endotracheal tube. N Engl J Med. 2021;385(16):e52.
11. Amjad MA, Khan A, Khan AR. Use of an endobronchial blocker where a double-lumen tube failed to ventilate: A case report of a distorted tracheobronchial anatomy. Cureus. 2022;14(11):e32047.
12. Mehrotra M, Jain A. Single-lung ventilation. In: StatPearls. Treasure Island (FL): StatPearls Publishing; 2024.
13. Ko R, McRae K, Darling G, Waddell TK, McGlade D, Cheung K, et al. The use of air in the inspired gas mixture

during two-lung ventilation delays lung collapse during one-lung ventilation. Anesth Analg. 2009;108(4):1092-6.

14. Yoshimura T, Ueda K, Kakinuma A, Sawai J, Nakata Y. Bronchial blocker lung collapse technique: nitrous oxide for facilitating lung collapse during one-lung ventilation with a bronchial blocker. Anesth Analg. 2014;118(3):666-70.
15. Narayanaswamy M, McRae K, Slinger P, Dugas G, Kanellakos GW, Roscoe A, et al. Choosing a lung isolation device for thoracic surgery: a randomized trial of three bronchial blockers versus double-lumen tubes. Anesth Analg. 2009;108(4):1097-101.
16. Lohser J, Slinger P. Lung injury after one-lung ventilation: A review of the pathophysiologic mechanisms affecting the ventilated and the collapsed lung. Anesth Analg. 2015;121(2):302-18.
17. Licker M, de Perrot M, Spiliopoulos A, Robert J, Diaper J, Chevalley C, et al. Risk factors for acute lung injury after thoracic surgery for lung cancer. Anesth Analg. 2003;97(6):1558-65.
18. Dulu A, Pastores SM, Park B, Riedel E, Rusch V, Halpern NA. Prevalence and mortality of acute lung injury and ARDS after lung resection. Chest. 2006;130(1):73-8.
19. Alam N, Park BJ, Wilton A, Seshan VE, Bains MS, Downey RJ, et al. Incidence and risk factors for lung injury after lung cancer resection. Ann Thorac Surg. 2007;84(4):1085-91; discussion 1091.
20. Jeon K, Yoon JW, Suh GY, Kim J, Kim K, Yang M, et al. Risk factors for post-pneumonectomy acute lung injury/acute respiratory distress syndrome in primary lung cancer patients. Anaesth Intensive Care. 2009;37(1):14-9.
21. Lohser J. Evidence-based management of one-lung ventilation. Anesthesiol Clin. 2008;26(2):241-72, v.
22. Boisen ML, Schisler T, Kolarczyk L, Melnyk V, Rolleri N, Bottiger B, et al. The year in thoracic anesthesia: Selected highlights from 2019. J Cardiothorac Vasc Anesth. 2020;34(7):1733-44.
23. Colquhoun DA, Leis AM, Shanks AM, Mathis MR, Naik BI, Durieux ME, et al. A lower tidal volume regimen during one-lung ventilation for lung resection surgery is not associated with reduced postoperative pulmonary complications. Anesthesiology. 2021;134(4):562-76.
24. Balanos GM, Talbot NP, Dorrington KL, Robbins PA. Human pulmonary vascular response to 4 h of hypercapnia and hypocapnia measured using Doppler echocardiography. J Appl Physiol Bethesda Md (1985). 2003;94(4):1543-51.
25. Lytle FT, Brown DR. Appropriate ventilatory settings for thoracic surgery: intraoperative and postoperative. Semin Cardiothorac Vasc Anesth. 2008;12(2):97-108.
26. Grichnik KP, Shaw A. Update on one-lung ventilation: the use of continuous positive airway pressure ventilation and positive end-expiratory pressure ventilation-clinical application. Curr Opin Anaesthesiol. 2009;22(1):23-30.
27. Satoh D, Kurosawa S, Kirino W, Wagatsuma T, Ejima Y, Yoshida A, et al. Impact of changes of positive end-expiratory pressure on functional residual capacity at low tidal volume ventilation during general anesthesia. J Anesth. 2012;26(5):664-9.
28. Michelet P, D'Journo XB, Roch A, Doddoli C, Marin V, Papazian L, et al. Protective ventilation influences systemic inflammation after esophagectomy: a randomized controlled study. Anesthesiology. 2006;105(5):911-9.
29. Ferrando C, Carramiñana A, Piñeiro P, Mirabella L, Spadaro S, Librero J, et al. Individualised, perioperative open-lung ventilation strategy during one-lung ventilation (iPROVE-OLV): a multicentre, randomised, controlled clinical trial. Lancet Respir Med. 2024;12(3):195-206.
30. Shum S, Huang A, Slinger P. Hypoxaemia during one lung ventilation. BJA Educ. 2023;23(9):328-36.
31. Cowan J, Hutton M, Owen A, Lam D, Bracco D, Hurdle H, et al. Cognitive aids for the management of thoracic anesthesia emergencies: Consensus guidelines on Behalf of a Canadian Thoracic Taskforce. J Cardiothorac Vasc Anesth. 2022;36(8 Pt A):2719-26.
32. iPROVE Network investigators, Belda J, Ferrando C, Garutti I. The effects of an open-lung approach during one-lung ventilation on postoperative pulmonary complications and driving pressure: A descriptive, multicenter national study. J Cardiothorac Vasc Anesth. 2018;32(6):2665-72.
33. Fujiwara M, Abe K, Mashimo T. The effect of positive end-expiratory pressure and continuous positive airway pressure on the oxygenation and shunt fraction during one-lung ventilation with propofol anesthesia. J Clin Anesth. 2001;13(7):473-7.
34. Jung DM, Ahn HJ, Jung SH, Yang M, Kim JA, Shin SM, et al. Apneic oxygen insufflation decreases the incidence of hypoxemia during one-lung ventilation in open and thoracoscopic pulmonary lobectomy: A randomized controlled trial. J Thorac Cardiovasc Surg. 2017;154(1):360-6.
35. Abe K, Oka J, Takahashi H, Funatsu T, Fukuda H, Miyamoto Y. Effect of high-frequency jet ventilation on oxygenation during one-lung ventilation in patients undergoing thoracic aneurysm surgery. J Anesth. 2006;20(1):1-5.
36. Campos JH. Update on selective lobar blockade during pulmonary resections. Curr Opin Anaesthesiol. 2009;22(1):18-22.
37. Ishikawa S, Nakazawa K, Makita K. Progressive changes in arterial oxygenation during one-lung anaesthesia are related to the response to compression of the non-dependent lung. Br J Anaesth. 2003;90(1):21-6.
38. Rocca GD, Passariello M, Coccia C, Costa MG, Di Marco P, Venuta F, et al. Inhaled nitric oxide administration during one-lung ventilation in patients undergoing thoracic surgery. J Cardiothorac Vasc Anesth. 2001;15(2):218-23.
39. Kim N, Lee SH, Joe Y, Kim T, Shin H, Oh YJ. Effects of inhaled iloprost on lung mechanics and myocardial function during one-lung ventilation in chronic obstructive pulmonary

disease patients combined with poor lung oxygenation. Anesth Analg. 2020;130(5):1407-14.
40. Hammer GB, Fitzmaurice BG, Brodsky JB. Methods for single-lung ventilation in pediatric patients. Anesth Analg. 1999;89(6):1426-9.
41. Szelloe P, Weiss M, Schraner T, Dave MH. Lower airway dimensions in pediatric patients-A computed tomography study. Paediatr Anaesth. 2017;27(10):1043-9.
42. Wani TM, Rafiq M, Terkawi R, Moore-Clingenpeel M, AlSohaibani M, Tobias JD. Cricoid and left bronchial diameter in the pediatric population. Paediatr Anaesth. 2016;26(6):608-12.
43. Downard MG, Lee AJ, Heald CJ, Anthony EY, Singh J, Templeton TW. A retrospective evaluation of airway anatomy in young children and implications for one-lung ventilation. J Cardiothorac Vasc Anesth. 2021;35(5):1381-7.
44. Templeton TW, Piccioni F, Chatterjee D. An Update on one-lung ventilation in children. Anesth Analg. 2021; 132(5):1389-99.
45. Letal M, Theam M. Paediatric lung isolation. BJA Educ. 2017;17(2):57-62.
46. Hammer GB. Single-lung ventilation in infants and children. Paediatr Anaesth. 2004;14(1):98-102.
47. Heaf DP, Helms P, Gordon I, Turner HM. Postural effects on gas exchange in infants. N Engl J Med. 1983;308(25):1505-8.
48. Mansell A, Bryan C, Levison H. Airway closure in children. J Appl Physiol. 1972;33(6):711-4.
49. Kubota H, Kubota Y, Toyoda Y, Ishida H, Asada A, Matsuura H. Selective blind endobronchial intubation in children and adults. Anesthesiology. 1987;67(4):587-9.
50. Choudhry DK. Single-lung ventilation in pediatric anesthesia. Anesthesiol Clin N Am. 2005;23(4):693-708, ix.
51. Paquet C, Karsli C. Technique of lung isolation for whole lung lavage in a child with pulmonary alveolar proteinosis. Anesthesiology. 2009;110(1):190-2.
52. CoLab. Selective endobronchial intubation in paediatrics: the Marraro Paediatric Bilumen Tube. [online] Available from https://colab.ws/articles/10.1111%2Fj.1460-9592.1994.tb00174.x [Last accessed February, 2025].
53. Vale R. Selective bronchial blocking in a small child. Case report. Br J Anaesth. 1969;41(5):453-4.
54. Piccioni F, Vecchi I, Spinelli E, Previtali P, Langer M. Extraluminal EZ-blocker placement for one-lung ventilation in pediatric thoracic surgery. J Cardiothorac Vasc Anesth. 2015;29(6):e71-3.
55. Templeton TW, Templeton LB, Lawrence AE, Sieren LM, Downard MG, Ririe DG. An initial experience with an Extraluminal EZ-Blocker®: A new alternative for 1-lung ventilation in pediatric patients. Paediatr Anaesth. 2018;28(4):347-51.
56. Fabila TS, Menghraj SJ. One lung ventilation strategies for infants and children undergoing video assisted thoracoscopic surgery. Indian J Anaesth. 2013;57(4):339-44.

19

CHAPTER

Anesthesia for Lung Resection for Cancer

Priya Ranganathan

INTRODUCTION

Surgery remains the key curative treatment for operable lung cancer. The spectrum of surgical resections include both nonanatomical wedge resections and anatomical excisions such as segmentectomy, lobectomy, bilobectomy, and pneumonectomy. Lung resection is considered a high-risk surgery associated with substantial perioperative morbidity, and therefore it is important to ensure that postoperative cardiopulmonary function is maintained. The goal of surgical planning is to exclude patients who would be at unacceptable risk while including those who are likely to benefit from surgery.

PREOPERATIVE CONCERNS

Patients presenting for resection for lung cancer are often elderly and chronic smokers (though the incidence of lung cancer among nonsmokers is also on the rise). The impact of increased age and smoking on various organ systems needs to be kept in mind. Many of them may have received preoperative chemotherapy with or without radiation therapy, with resultant short- and long-term toxicity. It is important to assess the 4M's associated with lung cancer—mass effect such as obstructive pneumonia, superior vena cava syndrome or chest wall involvement, effects of medications (chemotherapy or radiation therapy), metabolic effects such as electrolyte abnormalities or Eaton–Lambert syndrome, and whether there are metastases (bone, liver, adrenal, or brain).[1]

Preoperative work-up focuses on assessment of cardiopulmonary function to ensure that the patient will have adequate ability to meet his oxygen requirements after resection and will not end up as a respiratory cripple. This includes assessment of lung mechanics (which affects the ability to cough, clear secretions, and increase minute ventilation based on activity), the diffusion capacity (which determines alveolar gas exchange) and overall cardiopulmonary interaction which determines the functional status. This approach has been described as the "three legged stool" approach to assessment **(Flowchart 1)**.[1] It is important to remember that intra-operative handling, postoperative atelectasis or infection can hamper the function of the remaining lung, decreasing postoperative lung function below predicted levels.

Assessment of Lung Mechanics

The most commonly used measure of lung mechanical function is the forced expiratory volume in the first second

Flowchart 1: Three-legged stool approach for assessment for lung resection.

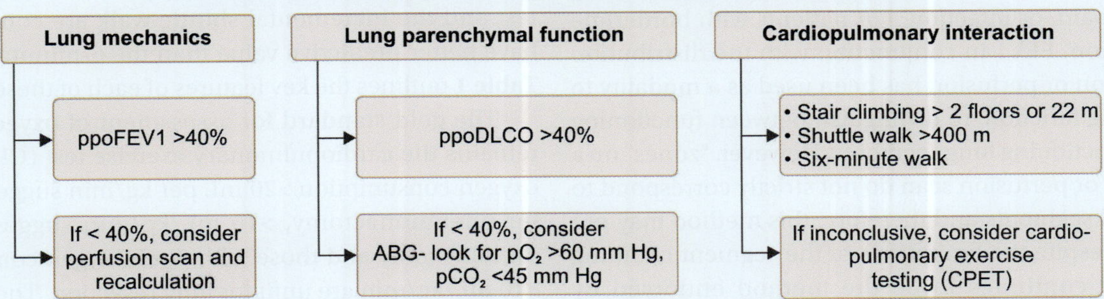

(DLCO: diffusion capacity for carbon monoxide; ppoFEV1: predicted postoperative forced expiratory volume in the first second)

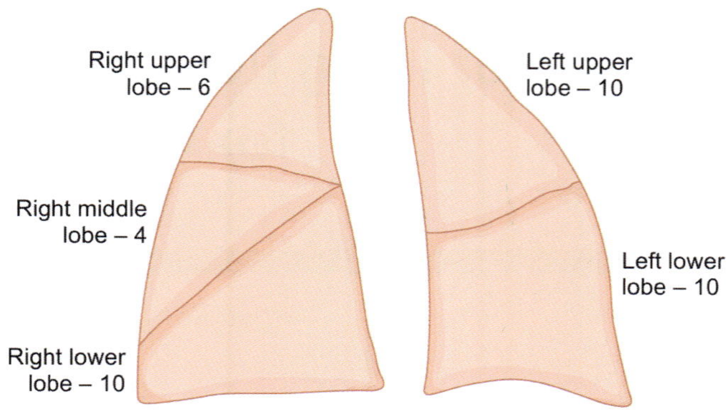

Fig. 1: Schematic representation of the number of segments in each lung.

(FEV1). Earlier, patients with absolute values of FEV1 of 1.5 liters for a lobectomy and 2 liters for a pneumonectomy were considered fit for surgery.[2] However, recent guidelines focus on calculation of predicted postoperative FEV1 (ppoFEV1) based on the number of segments to be resected.[3,4] **Figure 1** is a schematic representation of the number of segments in each lung.

ppoFEV1% is calculated as preoperative FEV1% × [1–(number of segments resected/19)]. Traditionally, ppoFEV1 >40% has been considered adequate for lung resection, with lower values predictive of increased morbidity and mortality. More recent guidelines suggest that ppoFEV1 as low as 30% may be considered in specific cases.[3,4] One of the fallacies of calculating ppoFEV1 using the segment-counting method is that it assumes that the lung to be resected is functioning and therefore, underestimates the true postoperative FEV1. If the resected lung is chronically collapsed or hyperinflated, then resection may actually allow the remaining healthy lung segments to expand with paradoxical improvement in lung function. Another important point to note is that whereas ppoFEV1 reflects lung function 3–6 months after surgery, it is possible that FEV1 may drop much lower in the immediate postoperative period due to lung handling, pain, or infection. For patients with borderline lung function, FEV1 in conjunction with the distribution of ventilation or perfusion has been used as a modality to predict lung function, to distinguish between functioning and nonfunctioning lung segments. However, "zones" on a ventilation or perfusion scan do not strictly correspond to anatomical segments and therefore, this method may not be valid. Despite the limitations of the segment counting method, it continues to be the method endorsed by most guidelines.[3,4] A systematic review identified several other methods of predicting postoperative lung function, including single photon emission computed tomography (SPECT), computed tomography volume and density (CT-VD), vibration response imaging (VRI), perfusion magnetic resonance imaging (MRI), ventilation CT, and CT volumetry and partial densitometry; however, none of these techniques have gained wide acceptance.[5]

Assessment of Lung Parenchymal Function

A separate but equally important measure of lung function is the ability to exchange gases, and this is measured by the diffusion capacity for carbon monoxide (DLCO). Predicted postoperative DLCO (ppoDLCO) can be calculated by methods similar to those described for FEV1. ppoDLCO <40% (and <30% according to more recent guidelines) is an independent risk factor for postoperative morbidity.[3,4]

Do We Need to Measure both Forced Expiratory Volume in the First Second and Diffusion Capacity for Carbon Monoxide?

Since FEV1 and DLCO measure different aspects of lung function, it is important to measure both, and there may be poor correlation between the two measures. A significant proportion of patients may have normal FEV1 and reduced DLCO. It has been suggested that the predicted postoperative product (product of ppoFEV1 and ppoDLCO) is a useful measure of morbidity with cutoff values <1,650 associated with increased complications.[6,7]

Assessment of Cardiopulmonary Interaction

Oxygen flux and the ability to increase oxygen supply to meet physiological demands (the oxygen reserve) depends on cardiopulmonary interaction. In its simplest form, this is measured using low technology submaximal tests such as stair climbing test, incremental shuttle walk test, and the 6-minute walk test. Of these, the stair-climbing test and the incremental shuttle walk are considered to have better predictive value than the 6-minute walk test. **Table 1** outlines the key features of each of these tests.

The gold standard for assessment of oxygen reserve remains the cardiopulmonary exercise test (CPET). Peak oxygen consumption >20 mL per kg/min suggests fitness for pneumonectomy, >15 mL/kg/min suggests fitness for lobectomy and those with peak oxygen consumption <10 mL/kg/min are unfit for lung resection. The cutoff for anaerobic threshold varies between 10 and 11 mL/kg/min.

CARDIAC RISK ASSESSMENT

Since smoking is a risk factor for lung cancer as well as ischemic heart disease, patients should be carefully evaluated to rule out active cardiac conditions that may increase perioperative risk. Smoking is also a risk factor for chronic obstructive pulmonary disease, which predisposes to right heart dysfunction. Lung resection further places a strain on the right heart due to the increased pulmonary vascular resistance. Initial cardiac evaluation includes a detailed history, examination, and 12 lead electrocardiography (ECG). A resting 2D ECHO may be helpful to evaluate left and right ventricular contractility. The thoracic revised cardiac risk index (Thoracic RCRI) consisting of cerebrovascular disease (1.5 points), cardiac ischemia (1.5 points), renal disease (1 point), and pneumonectomy (1.5 points) is used to predict risk category and subsequent risk-stratified evaluation including cardiac stress testing and coronary angiography.[8] **Flowchart 2** shows the algorithm for assessment of cardiac risk, and subsequent evaluation in patients presenting for lung resection.[3] **Flowchart 3** summarizes the overall strategy for assessment of cardiopulmonary function in patients presenting for lung resection.[3]

RISK SCORING SYSTEMS

Several risk scoring systems have been used to predict adverse postoperative outcomes in lung resection. Some of these are generic scores such as the Charlson comorbidity index, the POSSUM (Physiologic and Operative Severity Score for the enUmeration of Mortality and morbidity) score, the Portsmouth-POSSUM (P-POSSUM) score, and the ARISCAT (Assess Respiratory Risk in Surgical Patients in Catalonia) score.[9-11] There are also other scores which are specific to thoracic surgery or lung resection. Examples of these include the thoracic revised cardiac risk index (ThRCRI) (described in an earlier section) with a ThRCRI

TABLE 1: Submaximal tests of cardiopulmonary interaction.

Stair climbing • 20 steps of 6 inches each	• *5 flights:* Excellent • *3 flights:* Good • *2 flights or less:* High risk • *<22 meters:* High risk
Incremental shuttle walk test (10 meters distance)	<400 meters or <25 shuttles or desaturation >4% considered high risk
6-minute walk test (Less reliable than the other tests)	• Benchmark for distance unclear • Desaturation >4% considered high risk

Flowchart 2: Algorithm for assessment of cardiac risk, and subsequent evaluation in patients presenting for lung resection.

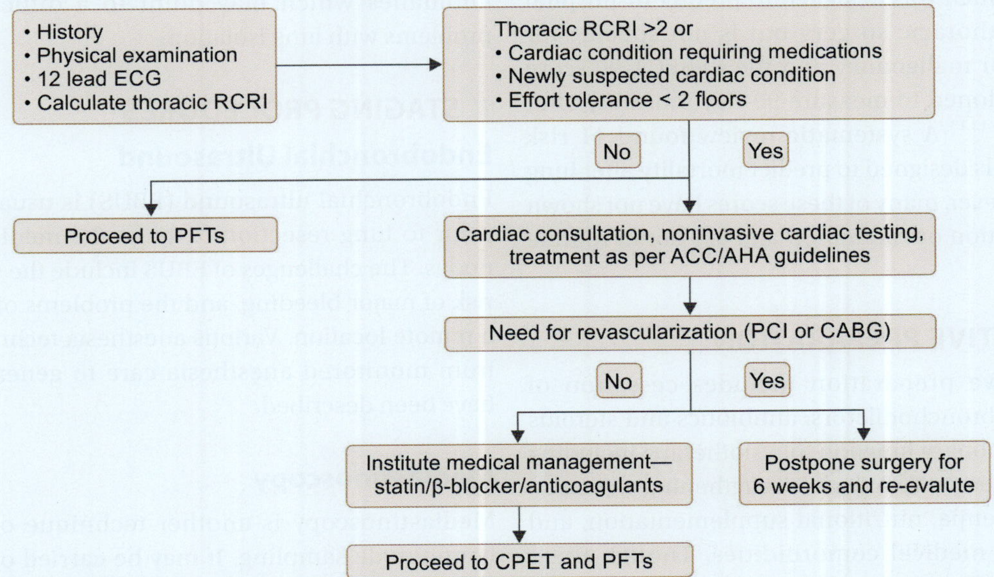

(CPET: cardiopulmonary exercise testing; PFT: pulmonary function testing)

Source: Adapted from Brunelli A, Kim AW, Berger KI, Addrizzo-Harris DJ. American College of Chest Physicians evidence-based clinical practice guidelines. Chest. 2013;143(5 Suppl):e166S-e190S.

Flowchart 3: Combined algorithm for cardiopulmonary testing for assessment for lung resection.

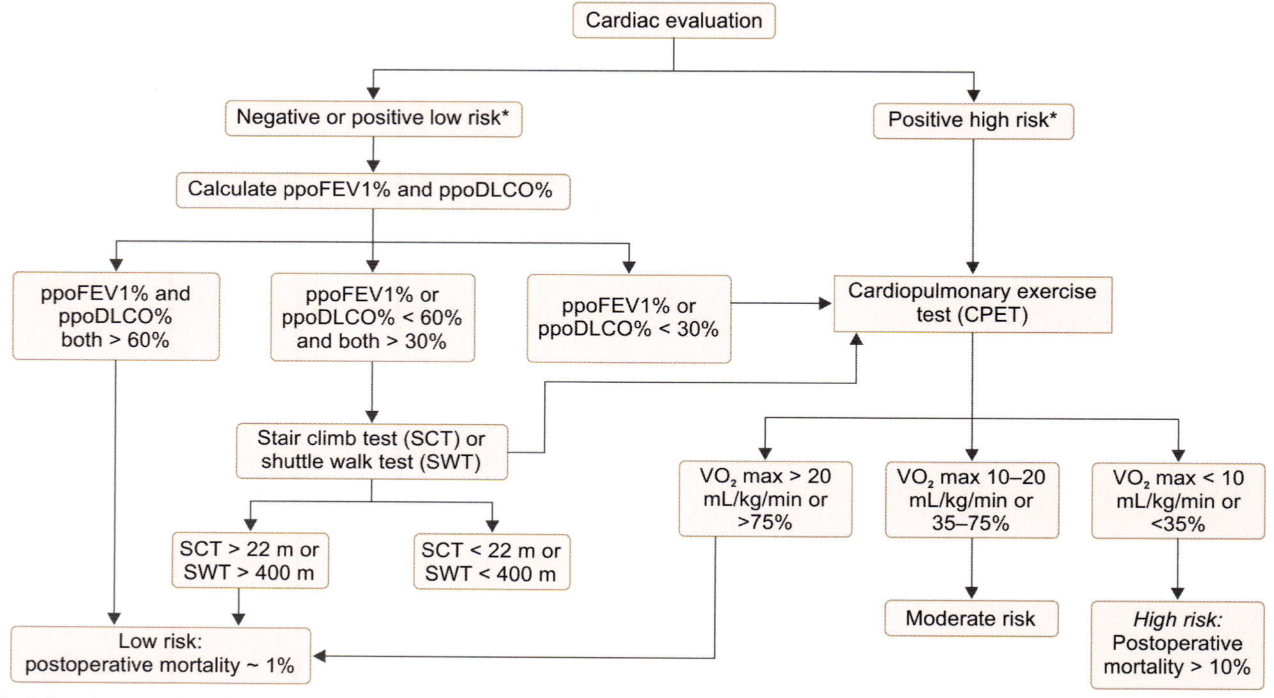

*Risk defined as per Flowchart 2

Source: Adapted from Brunelli A, Kim AW, Berger KI, Addrizzo-Harris DJ. American College of Chest Physicians evidence-based clinical practice guidelines. Chest. 2013;143(5 Suppl):e166S-e190S.

greater than 2.5 associated with significantly higher postoperative cardiac morbidity after thoracic surgery, the Thoracoscore which was designed to predict in-hospital mortality after thoracic surgery but is not specific for lung resection or malignancy and the RESECT-90 score which was developed to measure 90-day mortality after lung resection.[8,12,13] A systematic review found 11 risk prediction models designed to predict mortality after lung resection.[14] However, many of these scores have not shown good discrimination or calibration and are not in routine use.[15]

PREOPERATIVE PREPARATION

The preoperative preparation includes cessation of smoking, use of bronchodilators, antibiotics and steroids to optimize pulmonary function, physiotherapy including incentive spirometry and muscle strengthening exercises, correction of anemia, nutritional supplementation, and optimization of medical comorbidities. Though there is inadequate evidence regarding the impact of many of these interventions, they are integral to the enhanced recovery guidelines.

The anesthesiologist needs to review the patient's imaging and bronchoscopy to identify any airway anomalies which may point to a difficult airway or problems with lung isolation.

STAGING PROCEDURES

Endobronchial Ultrasound

Endobronchial ultrasound (EBUS) is usually performed prior to lung resection to stage the mediastinal lymph nodes. The challenges of EBUS include the shared airway, risk of major bleeding, and the problems of anesthesia in a remote location. Various anesthesia techniques ranging from monitored anesthesia care to general anesthesia have been described.

Mediastinoscopy

Mediastinoscopy is another technique of mediastinal lymph node sampling. It may be carried out as a stand-alone procedure but is usually performed in the same setting just prior to the planned resection. The complications of mediastinoscopy include airway and vascular compression, arrhythmias, risk of major bleeding, and pneumothorax. Anesthesiologists should consider lower limb vascular access, monitoring of saturation on the right upper limb, and the use of invasive blood pressure monitoring.

Anesthesia Management for Lung Resection

The key requirements for a good surgical exposure and favorable outcomes are safe and effective lung isolation, protective lung ventilation, judicious fluid management, appropriate monitoring, good pain relief, and adherence to enhanced recovery principles.

Lung Isolation Techniques

Three techniques can be used for lung isolation during surgery: Double lumen tubes, bronchial blockers, and endobronchial intubation with a single lumen tube. Of these, the first two are the preferred techniques. **Table 2** offers a comparison of some key features of double lumen tubes and bronchial blockers.

Protective Lung Ventilation during One-Lung Ventilation

One-lung ventilation (OLV) is an independent risk factor for postoperative pulmonary complications attributed to atelectasis-reexpansion and ischemia reperfusion in the nonventilated lung, and high volumes and pressures in the ventilated lung. Whereas traditional OLV of the dependent lung aimed to prevent hypoxemia and hypercarbia through large tidal volumes, avoidance of positive end-expiratory pressure (PEEP), high oxygen fractions, and high respiratory rates to maintain normocapnia, the focus is now on prevention of lung injury through lung protective strategies such as low tidal volumes, lower inspiratory pressures, inspired oxygen fraction titrated to acceptable saturation, titrated PEEP to optimize oxygenation, and respiratory rates to allow permissive hypercapnia.[16] The use of volume controlled ventilation (VCV) versus pressure controlled ventilation (PCV) during OLV has been debated but there is inadequate evidence to support one of the two techniques. **Table 3** outlines the key features of protective OLV.

Hypoxemia during One-Lung Ventilation

The OLV creates an obligatory shunt where the nonventilated operative lung receives perfusion but no

TABLE 3: Protective one-lung ventilation.

Key features of protective one-lung ventilation	
Tidal volume	4–6 mL per kg
FiO_2	Decreased to maintain acceptable saturation (88–92%)
Positive end-expiratory pressure (PEEP)	5–10 cmH_2O (titrated as per driving pressure, watch for intrinsic PEEP)
Peak pressure	<35 cmH_2O
Plateau pressure	<25 cmH_2O
Permissive hypercapnia	
Recruitment maneuvers to the ventilated lung	
Continuous positive airway pressure (CPAP) to the nonventilated lung	

TABLE 2: Comparison of key features of double lumen tubes and bronchial blockers.

	Double lumen tubes	***Bronchial blockers***
Time to collapse	Faster	Slower
Intraoperative malposition	Less frequent	More frequent
Application of continuous positive airway pressure (CPAP) to nonventilated lung	Possible and effective	Not possible
Quality of suction	Better	Poor
Alternate lung isolation	Possible	Possible only with EZ blocker
Trauma during insertion	More	Less
Use in difficult airway	Not possible	Preferred
Size determination	More difficult	Easier
Selective lobar blockade	Not possible	Possible
Postoperative mechanical ventilation	Needs tube change	No tube change needed

Flowchart 4: Management of hypoxemia during one-lung ventilation (OLV).

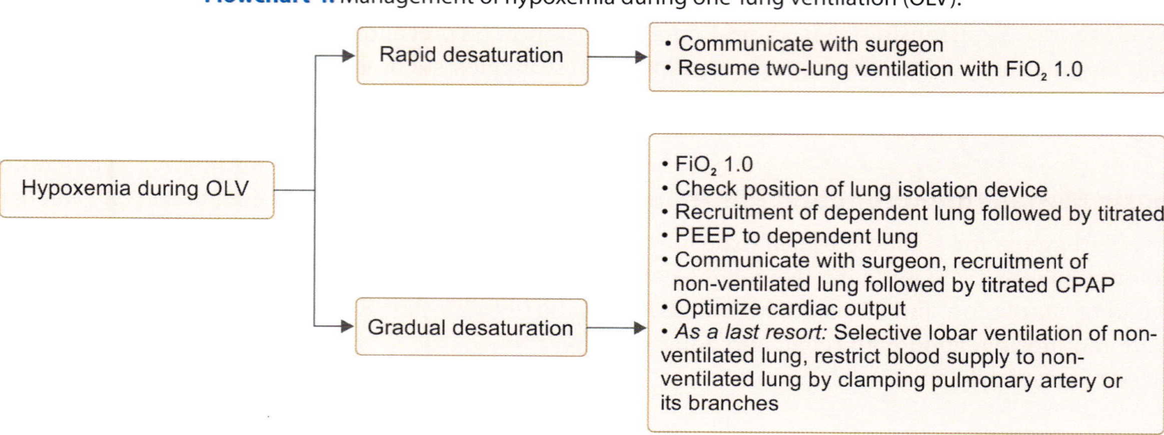

(CPAP: continuous positive airway pressure; PEEP: positive end-expiratory pressure)

ventilation. This could lead to hypoxemia during OLV. In addition, the dependent ventilated lung may also have areas of atelectasis and shunting due to positioning. The use of continuous positive airway pressure (CPAP) to the operative lung can be considered in cases of refractory hypoxemia. Shunting in the nonventilated lung is decreased by the effects of gravity (in the lateral decubitus position) and hypoxic pulmonary vasoconstriction (HPV), and can be further minimized by proper positioning, recruitment maneuvers, and the use of titrated levels of PEEP. **Flowchart 4** outlines the management of hypoxemia during OLV.

Choice of Anesthetic Agent

Total intravenous anesthesia with propofol decreases intraoperative shunt and results in better intraoperative oxygenation parameters than inhalational agents. However, the use of inhalational anesthesia during OLV results in decreased alveolar inflammation. A narrative review concluded that there is inadequate evidence to support the use of either one of these techniques.[17]

Fluid Management

Fluid overload can exacerbate lung injury and contribute to right ventricular dysfunction. At the same time, restrictive fluid therapy and hypovolemia are risk factors for renal injury. Judicious fluid management using a goal directed approach is the best approach. A systematic review found that goal-directed fluid therapy was superior to restricted fluid therapy in preventing pulmonary complications after lung resection.[18] However, as discussed in the section in the following text, choosing the appropriate goal in the context of OLV can be a challenge since the predictive value of dynamic indices such as stroke volume variation or pulse pressure variation remains debatable. The Enhanced Recovery after Surgery guidelines for lung resection recommend intraoperative and postoperative fluid infusion rate of 1–2 mL/kg/h with the use of balanced crystalloids, aiming for a perioperative positive fluid balance < 1,500 mL.[19] The judicious use of vasopressors to counter anesthetic-induced vasodilatation along with early return to enteral feeds helps to avoid fluid overload.

Appropriate Monitoring

Standard monitors include electrocardiogram, pulse oximetry, capnography, noninvasive blood pressure, temperature, and depth of neuromuscular monitoring. If total intravenous anesthesia (TIVA) techniques are used, it is recommended to use depth of anesthesia monitors. All major lung resections require invasive arterial monitoring to allow beat to beat pressure monitoring as well as frequent sampling. The use of central venous pressure as a static parameter has limited value; however, it may be helpful in cases of difficult peripheral venous access, for vasopressor infusions and sampling. Cardiac output monitoring has some limitations—the reliability of stroke volume variation during open thorax and low tidal volume ventilation is questionable; however in certain cases, absolute values of stroke volume may be useful to plan fluid therapy and the use of inotropes or vasopressors.

Flowchart 5: Plan for extubation after lung resection.

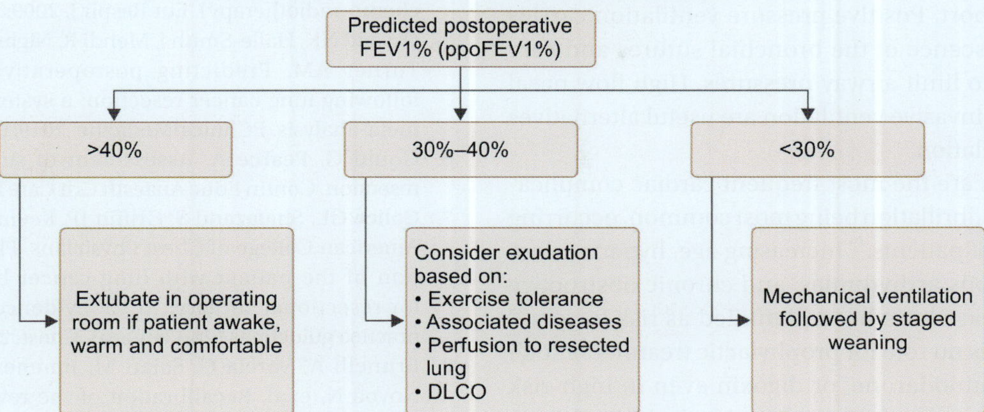

(DLCO: diffusion capacity for carbon monoxide; ppoFEV1: predicted postoperative forced expiratory volume in the first second)
Source: Adapted from Slinger P, Darling G. Preanesthetic Assessment for Thoracic Surgery. Slinger P (Ed). Principles and Practice of Anesthesia for Thoracic Surgery. Springer Science; 2011.

Analgesia Techniques

Thoracotomy is considered one of the most painful incisions with substantial acute and chronic pain. Thoracoscopy is believed to be less painful but can also be associated with moderate-to-severe acute and chronic pain. The PROSPECT guidelines recommend thoracic epidural or paravertebral block with continuous LA infusion as first line therapy in thoracotomy.[20] For minimally invasive surgery, thoracic epidural is not recommended; however paravertebral block or erector spinae block may be used.[21] Multimodal analgesia including paracetamol and nonsteroidal anti-inflammatory agents allow optimal pain management.

Extubation after Lung Resection

The decision to extubate in the operating room depends on the preoperative lung functions and the expected incidence of postoperative respiratory failure and complications. **Flowchart 5** depicts an algorithm for extubation of patients after lung resection.

Enhanced Recovery after Surgery in Lung Resection

Guidelines for enhanced recovery after lung surgery were published in 2019 and include recommendations for 45 items related to perioperative care.[19] Key recommendations include preoperative counseling, nutritional screening, smoking cessation, prehabilitation for high-risk patients, avoidance of fasting, carbohydrate loading, avoidance of preoperative sedatives, venous thromboembolism prophylaxis, prevention of hypothermia, short-acting anesthetics to facilitate early emergence, regional anesthesia, nausea and vomiting control, opioid-sparing analgesia, euvolemic fluid management, minimally invasive surgery, early chest drain removal, avoidance of urinary catheters, and early mobilization after surgery.

EMERGING TECHNIQUES

Minimally invasive lung resection (video-assisted thoracoscopic or robotic surgery) allows smaller incisions, three-dimensional visualization, better access, potentially less pain, and faster recovery after lung resection. The key anesthetic concerns include challenges with patient positioning in extreme positions, inability to access the patient during the surgery, and management of CO_2 elimination due to the combined effect of capnothorax and one-lung ventilation. Tubeless (nonintubated) video-assisted thoracoscopic surgery (niVATS) involves the avoidance of paralysis and lung isolation devices, and is performed in a spontaneously breathing patient, usually with a supraglottic airway device under locoregional anesthesia.[22,23] It is postulated to have fewer pulmonary complications and faster recovery, and shown to be safe.[24] Challenges include prevention of hypoventilation due to open thorax and effects of anesthesia.

COMPLICATIONS AFTER LUNG RESECTION

Pulmonary complications after lung resection include atelectasis, pneumonia, and respiratory failure. The management includes physiotherapy, antibiotics, and ventilatory support. Positive pressure ventilation carries the risk of dehiscence of the bronchial sutures and care must be taken to limit airway pressures. High flow nasal oxygen and noninvasive ventilation are useful alternatives to invasive ventilation.

Arrhythmias are the most frequent cardiac complications, with atrial fibrillation being most common, occurring in around 12% of patients.[19] Increasing age, hypertension, male sex, previous arrhythmias, and chronic obstructive pulmonary disease have been identified as risk factors.[19] However, there is no role for prophylactic treatments such as β-blockers, amiodarone, or digoxin even in high-risk patients. Right ventricular strain and right heart failure may occur especially after right-sided pneumonectomies, in patients with preexisting right heart strain and in fluid overload.

Surgical complications include persistent air leak and bronchopleural fistula. Pneumonectomies carry the risk of mediastinal shift, cardiac herniation, or cardiac torsion which may present as sudden hemodynamic collapse.

CONCLUSION

Pulmonary resection for lung cancer is associated with substantial morbidity and mortality. Advances in surgical and anesthesia techniques have resulted in an increased number of high-risk patients presenting for complex procedures. A stepwise approach to preoperative evaluation can help in risk-stratification and optimization, to improve perioperative outcomes.

REFERENCES

1. Slinger P, Campos JH. Anesthesia for Thoracic Surgery, in Miller's Anesthesia. Philadelphia: Elsevier Inc.; 2011. pp. 1648-716.e8.
2. British Thoracic Society; Society of Cardiothoracic Surgeons of Great Britain and Ireland Working Party. BTS guidelines: guidelines on the selection of patients with lung cancer for surgery. Thorax. 2001;56:89-108.
3. Brunelli A, Kim AW, Berger KI, Addrizzo-Harris DJ. Physiologic evaluation of the patient with lung cancer being considered for resectional surgery: Diagnosis and management of lung cancer, 3rd edition. American College of Chest Physicians evidence-based clinical practice guidelines. Chest. 2013;143:e166S-e190S.
4. Brunelli A, Charloux A, Bolliger CT, Rocco G, Sculier JP, Varela G, et al.; European Respiratory Society and European Society of Thoracic Surgeons joint task force on fitness for radical therapy. ERS/ESTS clinical guidelines on fitness for radical therapy in lung cancer patients (surgery and chemo-radiotherapy). Eur Respir J. 2009;34(1):17-41.
5. Oswald NK, Halle-Smith J, Mehdi R, Nightingale P, Naidu B, Turner AM. Predicting postoperative lung function following lung cancer resection: a systematic review and meta-analysis. EClinicalMedicine. 2019;15:7-13.
6. Gould G, Pearce A. Assessment of suitability for lung resection. Contin Educ Anaesth Crit Care Pain. 2006:97-100.
7. Colice GL, Shafazand S, Griffin JP, Keenan R, Bolliger CT; American College of Chest Physicians. Physiologic evaluation of the patient with lung cancer being considered for resectional surgery: ACCP evidenced-based clinical practice guidelines (2nd edition). Chest. 2007;132:161S-77S.
8. Brunelli A, Varela G, Salati M, Jimenez MF, Pompili C, Novoa N, et al. Recalibration of the revised cardiac risk index in lung resection candidates. Ann Thorac Surg. 2010;90(1):199-203.
9. Copeland GP, Jones D, Walters M. POSSUM: a scoring system for surgical audit. Br J Surg. 1991;78(3):355-60.
10. Prytherch DR, Whiteley MS, Higgins B, Weaver PC, Prout WG, Powell SJ. POSSUM and Portsmouth POSSUM for predicting mortality. Physiological and Operative Severity Score for the enUmeration of Mortality and morbidity. Br J Surg. 1998;85:1217-20.
11. Canet J, Gallart L, Gomar C, Paluzie G, Vallès J, Castillo J, et al.; ARISCAT Group. Prediction of postoperative pulmonary complications in a population-based surgical cohort. Anesthesiology. 2010;113(6):1338-50.
12. Falcoz PE, Conti M, Brouchet L, Chocron S, Puyraveau M, Mercier M, et al. The Thoracic Surgery Scoring System (Thoracoscore): risk model for in-hospital death in 15,183 patients requiring thoracic surgery. J Thorac Cardiovasc Surg. 2007;133(2):325-32.
13. Taylor M, Martin GP, Abah U, Sperrin M, Smith M, Bhullar D, et al.; North West Thoracic Surgery Collaborative (NWTSC). Development and internal validation of a clinical prediction model for 90-day mortality after lung resection: the RESECT-90 score. Interact Cardiovasc Thorac Surg. 2021;33(6):921-7.
14. Taylor M, Hashmi SF, Martin GP, Shackcloth M. A systematic review of risk prediction models for perioperative mortality after thoracic surgery. Interact Cardiovasc Thorac Surg. 2021;32(3):333-42.
15. Zorrilla-Vaca A, Grant MC, Rehman M, Sarin P, Mendez-Pino L, Urman RD, et al. Performance comparison of pulmonary risk scoring systems in lung resection. J Cardiothorac Vasc Anesth. 2023;37(9):1734-43.
16. Kozian A, Schilling T. Protective Ventilatory Approaches to One-Lung Ventilation: More than Reduction of Tidal Volume. Curr Anesthesiol Rep. 2014;4:150-9.
17. Parab S, Gaikwad S, Majeti S. Inhalational versus intravenous anesthetics during one lung ventilation in elective thoracic surgeries: A narrative review. Saudi J Anaesth. 2021;15(3):312-23.

18. Li X, Zhang Q, Zhu Y, Yang Y, Xu W, Zhao Y, et al. Effect of perioperative goal-directed fluid therapy on postoperative complications after thoracic surgery with one-lung ventilation: a systematic review and meta-analysis. World J Surg Oncol. 2023;21:297.
19. Batchelor TJP, Rasburn NJ, Abdelnour-Berchtold E, Brunelli A, Cerfolio RJ, Gonzalez M, et al. Guidelines for enhanced recovery after lung surgery: recommendations of the Enhanced Recovery After Surgery (ERAS®) Society and the European Society of Thoracic Surgeons (ESTS). Eur J Cardiothorac Surg. 2019;55(1):91-115.
20. Joshi GP, Bonnet F, Shah R, Wilkinson RC, Camu F, Fischer B, et al. A systematic review of randomized trials evaluating regional techniques for post-thoracotomy analgesia. Anesth Analg. 2008;107(3):1026-40.
21. Feray S, Lubach J, Joshi GP, Bonnet F, Van de Velde M; PROSPECT Working Group *of the European Society of Regional Anaesthesia and Pain Therapy. PROSPECT guidelines for video-assisted thoracoscopic surgery: a systematic review and procedure-specific postoperative pain management recommendations. Anaesthesia. 2022;77(3):311-25.
22. Anile M, Vannucci J, Ferrante F, Bruno K, De Paolo D, Bassi M, et al.; NIVATS Interest Group. Non-Intubated Thoracic Surgery: Standpoints and Perspectives. Front Surg. 2022;9:937633.
23. Starke H, Zinne N, Leffler A, Zardo P, Karsten J. Developing a minimally-invasive anaesthesiological approach to non-intubated uniportal video-assisted thoracoscopic surgery in minor and major thoracic surgery. J Thorac Dis. 2020;12(12):7202-17.
24. Wang L, Wang D, Zhang Y. Comparison of postoperative pulmonary complications and intraoperative safety in thoracoscopic surgery under non-intubated versus intubated anesthesia: a randomized, controlled, double-blind non-inferiority trial. Updates Surg. 2024;76(8): 2863-73.

CHAPTER 20

Anesthesia for Esophagectomy

Shagun Bhatia Shah, Uma Hariharan, Rajiv Chawla

INTRODUCTION AND HISTORICAL BACKGROUND

Esophagectomy for esophageal cancer entails substantial mortality and morbidity, with a 5-year survival rate below 50%,[1] and complication rate ranging from 33 to 50%, subject to whether the surgery is conducted in low-volume or high-volume centers.[2,3] Anesthesia for esophagectomy requires a multidisciplinary approach, involving anesthesiologists, surgeons, pulmonologists, and critical care specialists to ensure the best outcomes for the patient. More than a century ago, in 1913, Dr Franz Torek, a pioneering thoracic surgeon, performed the first thoracic esophagectomy employing the left transpleural approach. The anesthetic technique utilized was the Meltzer–Auer method of intratracheal insufflation of air and ether. The surgery lasted 2 hours, 43 minutes, and the patient survived 13 years before dying of unrelated causes.[4]

EPIDEMIOLOGY

Esophageal cancer is the eighth most common cancer worldwide, the fifth most common in India, and the third most common in Indian males. As per latest GLOBOCAN data (2022), there were 511,054 new cases (eleventh most common incidence) and 445,391 annual deaths (seventh most common cancer mortality) worldwide, with 70,637 new cases and 66,410 deaths (fifth most common incidence and mortality) in India alone.[5,6] Both incidence and mortality of carcinoma esophagus are projected to nearly double by 2050 **(Fig. 1)**.[7] There are significant geographical variations in the incidence of esophageal cancer, Malawi in Eastern Africa being the hotspot. East Asia (Bangladesh, China), eastern and southern Africa, and Iran, have the highest prevalence. Esophageal cancer is more common in men, the male-to-female ratio being 3:1.[7] The incidence rises with age, peaking above 60 years.

TYPES OF ESOPHAGEAL CANCER AND THEIR PATHOPHYSIOLOGY

Squamous cell carcinoma (SCC) is predominantly found in the upper and middle thirds of the esophagus and is more common in the developing world.[8] Adenocarcinoma usually afflicts the terminal one-third of the esophagus, occurs more frequently in developed nations, where it exhibits a rising incidence. Chronic gastroesophageal reflux results in metaplasia, followed by low grade dysplasia, high grade dysplasia, and eventually adenocarcinoma esophagus.[9] Midesophageal SCC is currently far more common than adenocarcinoma in India. Although the rates of gastroesophageal junctional adenocarcinoma are increasing, no evidence of an increase in the lower esophageal cancer in last 20 years has been observed in India.[10]

RISK FACTORS

Lower socioeconomic status is associated with a higher risk of esophageal cancer, attributable to lifestyle factors (diet, smoking, and alcoholism), and limited access to quality healthcare. Consumption of tobacco and alcohol in conjunction with low intake of fruits and vegetables and excessive ingestion of smoked/pickled food are powerfully associated with SCC. Environmental exposure to certain chemicals and pollutants, preexisting achalasia, tylosis, and prior caustic injury to the esophagus are other risk factors for SCC.[11] Chronic gastroesophageal reflux disease (GERD) may lead to Barrett's esophagus, a precursor to adenocarcinoma. Obesity is strongly associated with an increased risk of adenocarcinoma. Smoking is less strongly associated with adenocarcinoma compared to SCC. High dietary intake of fatty foods and low intake of fruits and vegetables are other risk factors.[11]

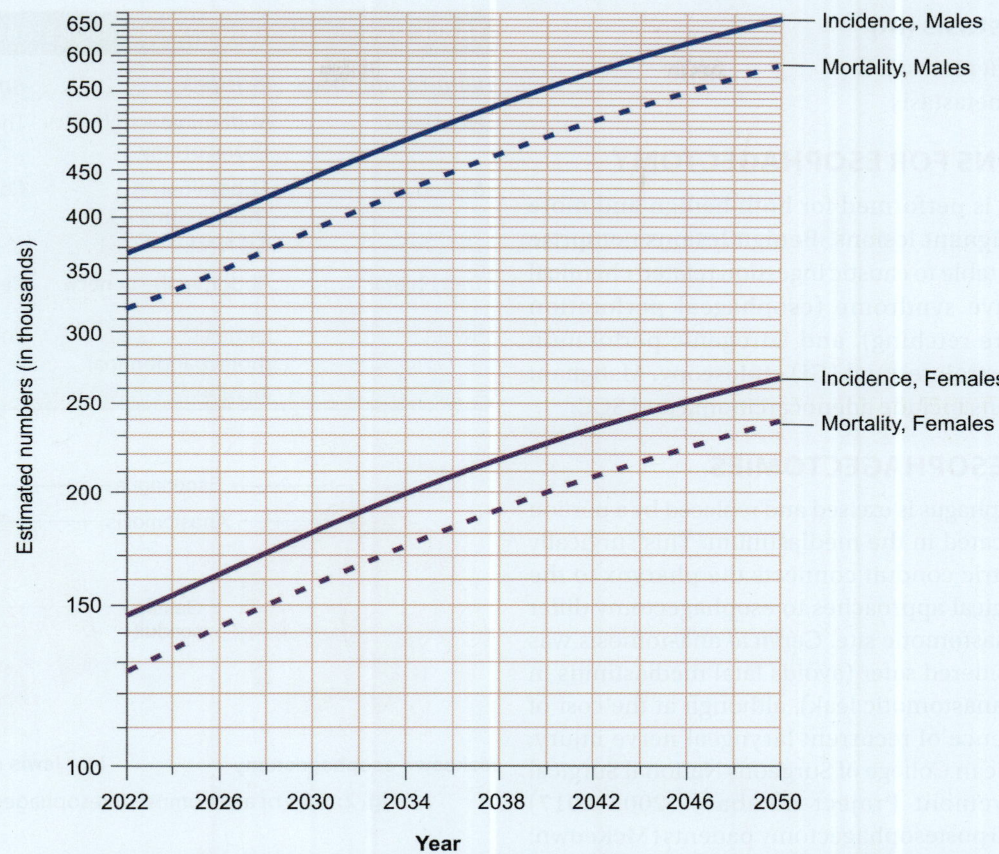

Fig. 1: Current incidence and mortality from esophageal cancer and projection till 2050.
Source: Adapted from GLOBOCAN statistics.

PREVENTION AND SCREENING

Lifestyle modifications such as cessation of tobacco and alcohol abuse, maintaining a healthy weight, and a fruit and vegetable rich diet can lower the risk. Regular endoscopic surveillance in patients with Barrett's esophagus for detecting early changes can reduce the risk of progression to adenocarcinoma.

TUMOR, NODES, METASTASIS STAGING

Tumor, nodes, metastasis (TNM) staging for esophageal cancer summarized in the following text is the most commonly used classification. The 7th UICC-AJCC staging system provides a better prognostic stratification of overall survival postesophagectomy especially for adenocarcinomas.[12]

- T_X: Primary tumor cannot be assessed
- T_0: No evidence of primary tumor
- T_{is}: High-grade dysplasia (malignant cells confined by the basement membrane)
- T_1: Invasion of lamina propria/muscularis mucosae/ submucosa by tumor
- T_{1a}: Tumor invades lamina propria/muscularis mucosae
- T_{1b}: Tumor invades submucosa
- T_2: Tumor invades muscularis propria
- T_3: Tumor invades adventitia
- T_4: Tumor invades adjacent structures
- T_{4a}: Tumor resectable and invades pleura/pericardium/ azygos vein/diaphragm/peritoneum
- T_{4b}: Unresectable tumor that invades adjacent structures (aorta, vertebral body, and trachea)

Regional Lymph Nodes (N)

- N_X: Regional lymph nodes cannot be assessed
- N_0: No regional lymph node metastasis
- N_1: Metastasis in 1–2 regional lymph nodes
- N_2: Metastasis in 3–6 regional lymph nodes
- N_3: Metastasis in ≥7 regional lymph nodes

Distant Metastasis (M)

- M_0: No distant metastasis
- M_1: Distant metastasis

INDICATIONS FOR ESOPHAGECTOMY

Esophagectomy is performed for both benign and more commonly, malignant lesions. Benign lesions comprise strictures attributable to caustic ingestion related chemical burns, Boerhaave syndrome (esophageal perforation caused by severe retching), and iatrogenic perforation during upper gastrointestinal (GI) endoscopy. Malignant esophageal lesions include adenocarcinoma and SCC.

TYPES OF ESOPHAGECTOMIES

The diseased esophagus is excised and replaced by a portion of stomach relocated in the mediastinum. This surgically constructed gastric conduit connects the pharynx to the duodenum. Surgical approaches to esophagectomy differ mainly in the anastomotic site. Cervical anastomosis was historically considered safer (avoids fatal mediastinitis in the event of an anastomotic leak), although at the cost of increased incidence of recurrent laryngeal nerve injury. As per the American College of Surgeons National Surgical Quality Improvement Project database (2005–2017) comprising 6,136 postesophagectomy patients (McKeown: 1,676; Ivor Lewis: 4,.0460), McKeown esophagectomy was associated with higher rates of superficial surgical site infections (8.02% vs. 3.67%), anastomotic leaks (9.12% vs. 7.71%), prolonged intubation (15.06% vs. 10.10%), reintubation (15.30% vs. 10.34%), and return to the operating room (16.46% vs. 11.32%).[13] Another recent meta-analysis, places the overall mortality after intrathoracic anastomotic leakage at 11% (21/200 patients) versus 14% (10/73 patients) after cervical anastomotic leakage.[14] Overall incidence of postesophagectomy anastomotic leak is 7.2% and 13.6% with a high mortality of 6–50%.[15] The incision and anastomotic sites for various types of esophagectomies are depicted in **Table 1** and **Figure 2**.

- *Ivor Lewis esophagectomy:* This is ideal for lesions of the lower end of esophagus and unsuitable for lesions superior to the carinal level.
- *McKeown esophagectomy:* This is the preferred approach for lesions above the gastroesophageal junction right upto the clavicle.
- *Trans-hiatal esophagectomy:* Notably, one-lung ventilation (OLV) is not required for this approach.
- *Sweet esophagectomy:* Obsolete technique involving a left sided thoracotomy.

TABLE 1: Comparison of surgical approaches to esophagectomy.

Surgical approach	*Incisions*	*Anastomotic site*
Ivor Lewis	Abdominal + right (Rt) Thoracotomy	Thoracic
McKeown	Abdominal + Rt Thoracotomy + left (Lt) Neck	Cervical
Trans-hiatal	Abdominal + Lt neck	Cervical
Sweet	Large Lt thoracoabdominal incision	Thoracic

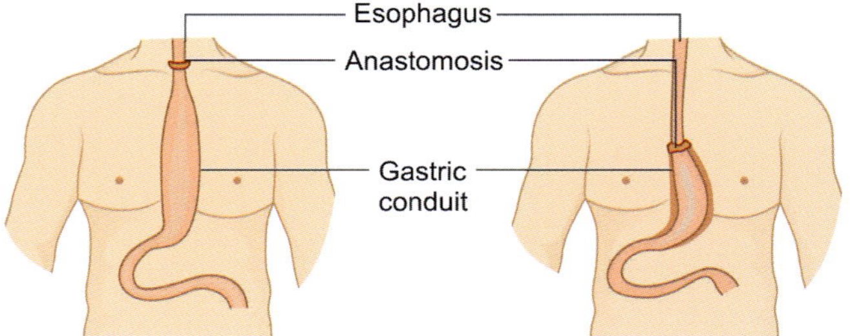

Fig. 2: Sites of anastomosis in esophagectomy.

All the above esophagectomies[14-16] are amenable to either an open, hybrid, totally minimally invasive, or robotic-assisted approach.

ANESTHETIC CONSIDERATIONS

Preanesthetic Checkup

A thorough preoperative evaluation (PAC) with risk stratification and planning for perioperative course is vital for a successful outcome. History, signs, and symptoms of esophageal cancer should be meticulously elicited. Dysphagia, initially for solids, eventually progressing to include liquids (esophageal lumen <13 mm) is the most common symptom.[17,18] Weight loss due to tumor-related anorexia and dysphagia is the second most common symptom. Bleeding (iron deficiency anemia), epigastric or retrosternal pain, bone pain (metastatic disease), hoarseness (recurrent laryngeal nerve involvement), and intractable coughing or frequent pneumonia (tracheobronchial fistulas caused by direct invasion of tumor through the esophageal wall and into the mainstem bronchus) comprise other symptoms. On physical examination, typically, no signs (except for malnutrition) can be elicited unless the cancer has undergone metastasis. Hepatomegaly and lymphadenopathy (laterocervical or supraclavicular nodes) reflect metastasis. During cardiopulmonary exercise testing, an inability to deliver 800 mL/min/m^2 oxygen and a low anaerobic threshold (AT) [observed in postneoadjuvant chemotherapy (NACT) patients] correlates with perioperative risk.[17]

A detailed preanesthetic checkup is a basic prerequisite for thoracic surgery. It begins with counseling, nutritional risk assessment, and prehabilitation. The patients should be advised to discontinue smoking. Malnutrition is a mismatch between requirement and intake of nutrients. If intake is higher than requirement, obesity results which is associated with adenocarcinoma esophagus. If requirement is higher than intake we have an undernourished patient more prone to SCC. Preoperative malnutrition is common (prevalence of 65% in onco-surgeries). It negatively impacts surgery by leading to poor treatment tolerance, increased morbidity, length of stay (LOS), 30-day readmission rate, and hence, mounting cost to healthcare systems. Malnutrition is an independent prognostic factor in onco-surgical patients. Nutritional risk assessment is crucial since malnutrition is a modifiable risk factor amenable to prehabilitation. Inadequate oral intake has a multifactorial causation. Anorexia, tumor-derived cytokines [interleukin (IL)-1, IL-6, and tumor necrosis factor (TNF)-α], oral ulcers caused by multivitamin deficiency or chemotherapy, low socioeconomic status (poor access to fruits, vegetables, healthcare/screening facilities, and lack of awareness), malabsorption syndromes, metabolic abnormality, esophageal cancer per se (progressive dysphagia for energy-dense solids followed by liquids), surgical stress response, cancer cachexia, muscle protein depletion, and systemic inflammation are the main causes of malnutrition. Preoperative nutritional screening (PONS) is a modified version of malnutrition universal screening tool (MUST) which is based on height and weight and assigns risk for body mass index (BMI) <18.5, unintentional weight loss, and decreased oral intake. PONS changed the BMI cutoff for age to >65 years and added low albumin levels as a biochemical marker of malnutrition.[19] Prehabilitation with oral nutritional supplements is recommended for patients who fail to consume 75% of their daily goal calories, while nasogastric (NG) tube feeding is indicated for patients consuming <50%.[17] Immunonutrition (arginine, omega-3 unsaturated fatty acids such as eicosapentaenoic acid, nucleotides) merits further evidence.

Physiotherapy and bronchodilators for chronic obstructive pulmonary disease (COPD) patients should be provided. Plan of postoperative analgesia should be explained to the patient including familiarity with patient controlled intravenous and epidural devices.

Investigations

Blood investigations include complete blood count, hepatorenal function tests, fasting blood sugar, thyroid function tests, coagulation profile (prothrombin time including International normalized ratio, partial thromboplastin time). Miscellaneous tests include chest radiograph, ventilation-perfusion scintigraphy, computed tomography (CT)-scan, and an electrocardiogram. Airway assessment to rule out any tracheal compression by the esophageal tumor or mediastinal lymph nodes is imperative. Tests to assess lung function include arterial blood gas (ABG), pulmonary function tests (PFT), predicted postoperative forced expiratory volume in one second (PPO FEV_1) or diffusing capacity of lungs for carbon monoxide (DLCO) <60% on exercise testing. These are further elaborated in the three-legged stool[20] as shown in **Figure 3**.

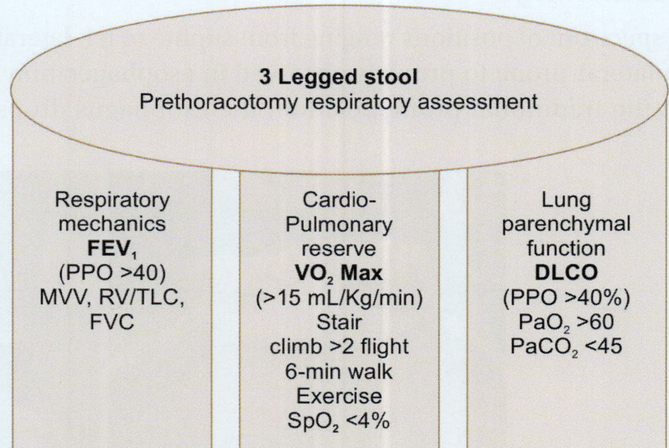

Fig. 3: Three legged stool for prethoracotomy respiratory assessment. (DLCO: Diffusing capacity of the lungs for carbon monoxide; FEV_1: Forced expiratory volume in first second; FVC: Forced vital capacity; MVV: Maximum voluntary ventilation; PPO: Predicted postoperative; $PaCO_2$: Partial pressure of carbon di oxide in arterial blood; PaO_2: Partial pressure of oxygen in arterial blood; RV: Residual Volume; TLC: Total lung capacity; VO_2: Maximum oxygen consumption during aerobic activity)

International guidelines on noncardiac surgery place esophagectomy under the high-risk surgery category (expected 30-day cardiovascular death or myocardial infarction risk >5%).[21] Thorough premature atrial complexes (PAC) workup, streamlined perioperative course, and surgical expertise in high volume centers diminish the mortality rate.[22]

Review PAC is performed a day prior to scheduled surgery. The anesthesiologist reviews the initial assessment and test results, assesses difficulty of lung isolation by examining the chest radiograph and CT scan, and assesses the risk of hypoxemia during OLV. The airway anatomy serves as a guide to choosing the optimal lung isolation device [double lumen tube (DLT) versus bronchial blocker (BB)] and the tracheal/left bronchial diameter predicts the optimal DLT size.

Intraoperative Management

Two large bore intravenous cannulas should be secured in the operation theater (OT). The NG tube is introduced postanesthetic induction, before positioning the patient. NG tube is partially withdrawn and repositioned with surgical guidance during gastric conduit formation. NG decompression of the gastric conduit is a standard practice to protect the anastomosis, identify any GI bleeding, and to monitor gastric secretion volume.[23]

Positioning

A spectrum of positions ranging from supine to left lateral to lateral-prone to prone is observed in esophagectomy. In the traditional prone position, the esophagus drops anteriorly out of its normal position and simplifies dissection. Disadvantages include raised central venous pressure (CVP), elevated mean pulmonary arterial and intraocular pressures, and reduced lung compliance.[24,25]

The abdominal phase is a common factor in all three techniques of esophagectomy (*Transhiatal:* **Fig. 5**, Ivor Lewis, McKeown). The reverse Trendelenburg position is optimal for this phase.

Thoracoscopic phase is encountered in both Ivor Lewis and McKeown esophagectomies. The left lateral decubitus/45° semiprone position facilitate this phase **(Fig. 4)**. The DLT position is fiberoptically verified once the patient is turned lateral, and OLV employed for this phase.

Neck anastomosis is practiced in Mc Keown esophagectomy. Supine position with head turned to the right side is employed during this phase.

Monitoring

Besides standard monitors, an arterial line (invasive blood pressure, ABG analysis), and a CVP line are secured, although CVP has doubtful value in presence of

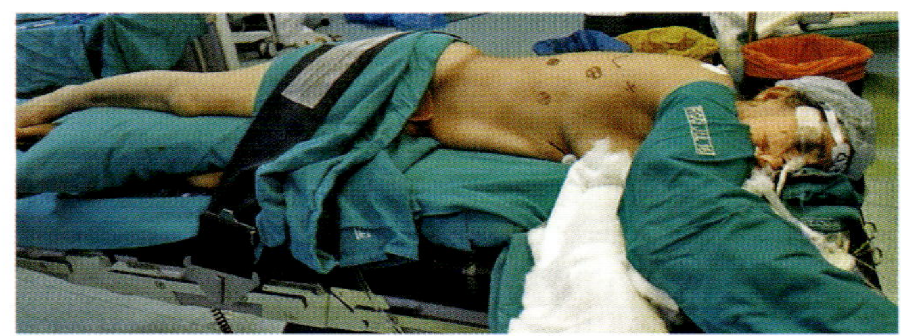

Fig. 4: Lateral positioning for esophagectomy.

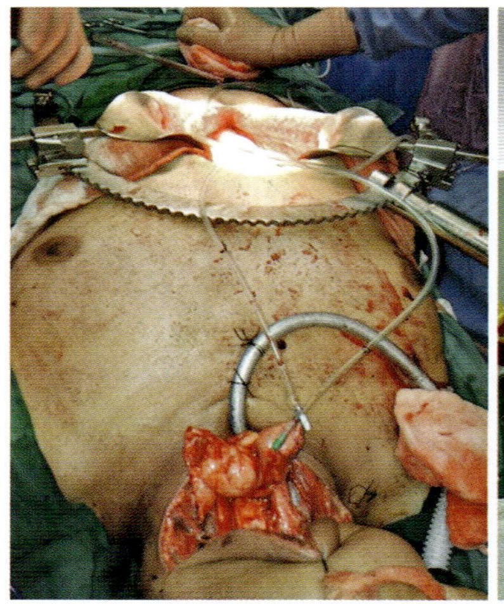

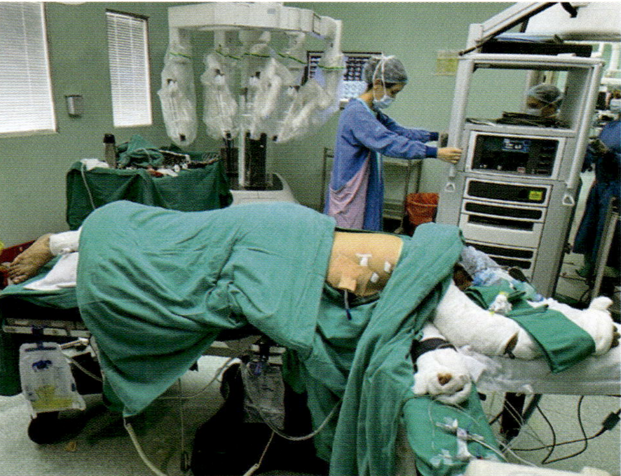

Fig. 5: Transhiatal esophagectomy (left side) and McKeown esophagectomy (right side).

pneumoperitoneum or capnothorax. Peripheral nerve stimulator (PNS) guided deep neuromuscular block and bispectral index (BIS) guided propofol or dexmedetomidine infusion, transesophageal echocardiography (TEE) (hemodynamic monitoring, assessing myocardial function), and continuous spirometry constitute additional important monitoring tools.

Aspiration prophylaxis: H_2-receptor antagonist [intravenous (IV) ranitidine 50 mg], prokinetics (IV metoclopramide 10 mg; 1 hour preoperatively), and an antacid (per oral sodium citrate 30 mL 10 minutes preoperatively), coupled with rapid sequence intubation are recommended for aspiration prophylaxis.

ANALGESIA

Both neuraxial and IV routes are employed for intraoperative analgesia and seamlessly blend with postoperative patient controlled IV and epidural analgesia.

Thoracic Epidural Catheter and Paravertebral Blocks

A thoracic epidural catheter placed in the T_6–T_7 dermatome level provides catheter incision congruence and suffices both, for the transthoracic and transabdominal incisions. A thoracic epidural is considered the gold standard for esophagectomies owing to myriad benefits such as preemptive analgesia, better postoperative pain relief, opioid-sparing effect, augmented blood flow to the anastomosis, early extubation, reduced venous thromboembolism risk, and reduced length of hospital stay due to adequate pain relief.[17,18,23] Paravertebral blocks are equally efficacious for thoracotomies, have fewer side effects including pulmonary complications and are a useful alternative when encountered with difficult epidurals.[26]

Opioids and Other Intravenous Analgesics

Cervical incision pain, shoulder pain from lateral positioning, or pain from very large incisions not covered by epidurals, necessitate IV opioid administration (morphine 0.1 mg/kg, fentanyl 2–3 μg/kg). Dexmedetomidine infusion during OLV is opioid sparing and simultaneously reduces volatile anesthetic requirement. IV paracetamol infusion 1 g may also be used preemptively before the surgical incision. Benefit with IV lignocaine, IV magnesium, and IV ketamine infusions have also been reported.[17,18]

CLINICAL PEARLS IN ONE-LUNG VENTILATION

Lung Isolation Devices

Double lumen tubes (DLTs) remain the gold-standard lung isolation devices during esophagectomies. A left sided DLT is preferred over a right sided DLT, due to the higher margin of safety (right upper bronchus may get blocked by a malpositioned slot on the right DLT). Difficulty in DLT placement may be encountered at four levels: difficulty in navigating the tip of DLT to the glottis, DLT impaction at glottic aperture, DLT impaction beyond glottis (cricoid cartilage/ primary bronchial opening), and DLT negotiating the wrong bronchus.

Bronchial blockers constitute a valuable alternative when distorted upper airway anatomy precludes optimal DLT placement. Single-cuff BB usually need to be placed through a single lumen (SLT) endotracheal tube (Coopdech BB), but some BB possess a designated SLT (Univent BB). Lung isolation techniques utilizing a combination of both BB and DLT have also been reported.[27] Some of the commonly used lung isolation devices are tabulated here for ready reference **(Table 2)**.[27-30]

Lung Protective Ventilatory Parameters During One-Lung Ventilation

During OLV the nonventilated lung is susceptible to atelectotrauma and ischemia-reperfusion injury. The ventilated lung is vulnerable to volutrauma and barotrauma, oxygen toxicity due to high FiO_2, and cardiovascular issues attributable to shunts and elevated pulmonary artery pressure. The historical use of high tidal volumes Sans positive end expiratory pressure (PEEP) to prevent atelectasis and minimize shunt has now been abandoned, and replaced by, low tidal volume, lung-protective strategies and permissive hypercarbia.

Volume controlled ventilation (VCV) mode is usually utilized to ensure a fixed tidal volume. Pressure controlled ventilation (PCV) is switched on in special scenarios such as emphysematous bullae, postpneumonectomy status, or in lung transplant recipients. Ventilatory parameters during OLV for esophagectomy include maintaining an FiO_2 of 1, tidal volume 5–6 mL/kg (keeping peak and plateau airway pressures lower than 35 cmH_2O and 25 cmH_2O, respectively), and respiratory rate >12 breaths/min (to maintain $PaCO_2$ 35–40 mmHg).

TABLE 2: Lung isolation devices.

Lung isolation device	*Color coding of cuffs*	*Bronchus entered*	*Guiding mechanism*
• Robertshaw DLT (Bronchocath • Sheridan, Shiley)	• Tracheal (White) • Bronchial (Blue)	*Opposite* to side of Sx	Two preformed concavities
Ambu VivaSight DLT	• Tracheal (White) • Bronchial (Blue)	*Opposite* to side of Sx	Integrated camera at distal end of tracheal lumen
Ankor DLT	• Tracheal (White) • Carinal (Green) • Bronchial (Blue)	*Opposite* to side of Sx	Carinal cuff is inflated and this third cuff blocks the right bronchial opening, so that the bronchial DLT lumen is directed to the left main bronchus
Coopdech BB	• Bronchial (White)	*Same* as side of Sx	Angulated tip
Arndt BB	• Bronchial (White)	*Same* as side of Sx	Wire loop
Univent BB	• Tracheal (Blue, on designated SLT) • Bronchial (White)	*Same* as side of Sx	Designated tube with channel for BB in concavity
EZ BB	• Rt Bronchial (Blue) • Lt Bronchial (Yellow)	*Both* bronchi entered	Two distal cuffed branches spring open, bifurcation resting on carina

(BB: bronchial blocker; DLT: double lumen tube; SLT: single lumen tube; Sx: surgery)

A PEEP of 5 cmH_2O to the ventilated lung is utilized except in COPD patients. Optimal DLT/BB positioning is reaffirmed after lateral positioning. If the peak airway pressure exceeds 40 cmH_2O during OLV, then DLT/BB malposition can be expected.[17,18,23]

During OLV, restrictive intravenous fluid therapy using balanced crystalloids is recommended. Total intravenous anesthesia using propofol/dexmedetomidine is preferable to volatile anesthetics.

Hypoxemia in One-Lung Ventilation

The first reaction to hypoxemia in OLV should be to increase FiO_2 to 1, and then review possible explanations such as a malpositioned DLT, secretions blocking the DLT, and administration of vasodilators. After rectifying these if hypoxemia persists then the standard management comprises continuous positive airway pressure (CPAP) (5–10 cmH_2O, 5 L/min) to nondependent lung, which is the most effective measure, and PEEP (5–10 cmH_2O) to dependent lung which remains the least effective measure. Intermittent two-lung ventilation and frequent recruiting maneuvers can be employed. Clamping the pulmonary artery is a last resort. McKesson CPAP System is a commercially available device attachable to the nonventilated lung lumen of the DLT. It incorporates an adjustable valve that supplies pressures (1–10 cmH_2O).

Anatomy of tracheobronchial tree, bronchoscopy using a fiberscope, and chest imaging constitute the ABCs to be mastered for adequate lung isolation.

A mental image of the tracheobronchial tree anatomy allows you to detect and rectify optimal DLT positioning/malpositioning in the airway. The right lung comprises three lobes (upper, middle, and lower), whereas the left lung contains only two lobes (upper and middle). On fiberoptic visualization through the tracheal lumen of DLT, the primary carina appears sharp and the rim of the blue cuff of the left DLT should be visible as the bronchial lumen disappears into the left bronchus. The right main bronchus is then negotiated, to identify the right upper lobe. In case the carina is not visualized fiberoptically, it usually means that the bronchial lumen is wrongly placed into the right bronchus. If the carina is blunt and broad, with further bifurcations visible within both the supposedly main bronchial lumens, then it is secondary carina and lobar bronchi that are being mistaken for the main carina. A grossly distorted tracheobronchial tree as evidenced on a computerized tomography (CT) scan advocates the use of BBs as lung isolation devices. DLT size is conventionally determined by the height/stature and gender of the patient. As a thumb rule a 35F left-sided DLT for female patients and a 37F left-sided DLT for most Indian male patients suffice for esophagectomy. Tracheal diameter and left bronchial diameter on CT scan, chest radiograph or point of care ultrasound correlate well with the DLT size. Cricoid cartilage diameter has generated considerable research interest recently for gauging the optimal DLT size.

Goal Directed Fluid Therapy

Without entering into the controversy of liberal versus restrictive fluid therapy, goal directed fluid therapy (GDFT) using pleth variability index (PVI) of 10 (co-oximeter reading) or stroke volume variation (SVV) of 10 using an advanced hemodynamic monitor as a goal, should be used. A point to be emphasized is that with the thorax open, the dynamic indices [systolic pressure variation (SPV), pulse pressure variation (PPV), and SVV] become inaccurate.[31] Eternal vigilance for ongoing fluid losses (intake/output fluid balance) and the maintenance of normal vital signs are more reliable. Does not have much prognostic value while a pulmonary artery catheter is too invasive for routine use. Avoid hypotension and use the hypotension prediction index, if available on your advanced hemodynamic monitor. Avoid norepinephrine and phenylephrine in the setting of hypovolemia (PVI >13). Norepinehrine and phenyleprhine are acceptable in normovolemic states (PVI <13). A physiological balanced crystalloid (Ringer lactate, sterofundin, and plasmalyte) is the intravenous fluid of choice.

Blood Products Transfusion

Minimally invasive techniques have reduced intraoperative blood loss. Moreover, perioperative red blood cell (RBC) transfusions are associated with increased postoperative complications and a higher mortality risk postesophagectomy.[32,33] Hence, hemoglobin 7 g/dL should be the transfusion trigger in the absence of cardiac disease and with adequate organ perfusion (serum lactate below 2 mmol/L, urine output above 0.5 mL/kg/h, $ScVO_2$ >70%, and hemodynamic stability). A higher transfusion trigger [hemoglobin (Hb) <8–9 g/dL] is advisable in presence of inadequate organ perfusion and with associated cardiac comorbidity.

Miscellaneous Empirical Drugs

Methylprednisolone administered at the induction of anesthesia reportedly reduces pulmonary inflammation. Contrarily, chronic steroid is a known risk factor for adverse outcome postesophagectomy. Sivelestat, a neutrophil elastase inhibitor is prescribed in Japan and South Korea for acute respiratory distress syndrome (ARDS) prophylaxis and therapy.[34] Multicentric robust randomized controlled trials are required to prove/refute these claims.

Postoperative Care

Tracheal extubation on the OT table itself is a safe option after uneventful surgery with vital signs stable, oxygen saturation optimal, hemodynamic stability, normothermia, adequate pain control, and neuromuscular block reversal.[18,23]

Postoperative nausea vomiting: Multimodal drug therapy with ondansetron and dexamethasone included is promising. Aprepitant could be a second line drug.

Postoperative pain relief: Multimodal postoperative pain relief applied in a step-down fashion is recommended postesophagectomy **(Table 3)**. Regional techniques overlapping with IV medication and lastly IV medication supplemented with oral adjuncts (once oral intake is permitted) like gabapentinoids to prevent chronic pain. Patient controlled intravenous and epidural anesthesia techniques for delivering opioids are fast gaining favor.[17,35,36]

Postoperative Complications

Respiratory complications (pneumonia, ARDS) are the most common (17–51%).[37] Other complications of esophagectomy include chylothorax, hemothorax, atrial fibrillation, phrenic nerve injury, brachial plexus injury, recurrent laryngeal nerve palsy, and anastomotic leak. Intraoperative lung-protective ventilation, GDFT, postoperative chest physiotherapy, and early mobilization

TABLE 3: Postoperative pain relief application.

***Regional*→→**	***Systemic*→→**	***Oral***
Thoracic epidural	Opioids	Gabapentin
Paravertebral block	NSAIDs	Pregabalin
Erector spinae plane block	Acetaminophen	Low dose tricyclic antidepressants
Intercostal nerve block	Ketamine	Ketorolac
Transversus abdominis plane (AP) block	Lignocaine	Tramadol
Intrapleural	Magnesium	Morphine
Intrathecal	Dexamethasone	Caffeine

(NSAIDs: nonsteroidal anti-inflammatory drugs)

after esophagectomy reduce postoperative pulmonary complications. Causes of atrial arrhythmia include direct contact during thoracic dissection, pericardial irritation, sepsis, anastomotic leak, preexisting cardiac comorbidity, age, or raised right atrial pressure after OLV.[23] Recurrent laryngeal nerve palsy (4–67% patients) may produce inadequate cough, reflux, and aspiration, but is usually partial and transient.[37,38] The presenting symptom of hoarseness maybe delayed since narrowing of glottic chink due to vocal cord edema occurs in the immediate postoperative period and paradoxically aids adduction of vocal cords.

SPECIAL CONSIDERATIONS

Neoadjuvant Chemotherapy

This is typically used in T_3 or N_1 disease after a staging laparotomy for biopsy and peritoneal lavage fluid. Chemotherapeutic drug combinations include cisplatin/5-fluorouracil, paclitaxel/carboplatin, cisplatin/fluoropyrimidine, and oxaliplatin/5-fluorouracil. Cisplatin is cardiotoxic, hepatotoxic, and nephrotoxic while 5-fluorouracil is cardiotoxic and hepatotoxic. Leukopenia (risk of infection), and thrombocytopenia (risk of hemorrhage) may persist in some of these post-NACT patients posted for esophagectomy.[17] There is paucity of Indian randomized, prospective studies on chemoradiation, induction chemotherapy, and palliative chemotherapy in esophageal cancers as per the Indian Council of Medical Research consensus document for management of esophageal cancer.[39]

Bleomycin Chemotherapy

Traditionally, bleomycin was administered as a chemotherapeutic agent for esophageal cancer both intravenously and by the intra-arterial route, but has now been discontinued.[40] Pulmonary fibrosis is a known adverse effect of bleomycin. High-dose oxygen exposure is one of the risk factors for pulmonary toxicity. In bleomycin-induced pulmonary toxicity, supplemental oxygen therapy becomes a synergistic toxin with bleomycin, especially in patients under general anesthesia. In the event patients giving a history of bleomycin exposure, require oxygen administration, inspired oxygen concentration is recommended to be kept at the lowest level (FiO_2 of 0.22–0.25), that provides adequate tissue oxygenation.[41] This creates a catch-22 situation and may result in hypoxemia during OLV where FiO_2 approximating 1 is desirable.

Enhanced Recovery after Surgery Protocol

The enhanced recovery after surgery (ERAS) protocol requires coordinated, multidisciplinary efforts **(Fig. 6)**.[42,43] Adherence to all the following ERAS elements has been shown to reduce length of hospital and surgical intensive care unit (SICU) stays and promote return to intended oncologic treatment (RIOT). An audit of degree of compliance and outcomes completes the feedback loop.[43]

Preoperative Optimization

- Patient counseling
- Tumor board
- Prehabilitation; Nutrition (80% malnourished)
- Preoperative complex carbohydrate (maltodextrin) drink
- Reduce fasting
- Antibiotic prophylaxis
- Thromboprophylaxis
- No bowel preparation
- No premedication

Intraoperative Stress Reduction

- *Timing:* 3–6 weeks following NACT; 6–10 weeks following NACRT
- Thoracic epidural
- Short-acting anesthetics
- *GDFT:* Balanced crystalloids
- Optimize OLV
- Opioid-sparing multimodal analgesia
- Normothermia and active warming
- Mutimodal antiemetics

Postoperative Protocolized Normalization

- Opioid-sparing analgesia [thoracic epidural analgesia (TEA), nonsteroidal anti-inflammatory drugs (NSAIDs), celecoxib, paracetamol (PCM), gabapentin, and ketorolac]
- No NG tubes
- No chest tubes
- Early oral nutrition
- Early removal of urinary catheters
- Avoid postoperative nausea and vomiting (PONV)
- Stimulation of gut motility (chewing gum)
- Avoid salt-water overload
- Early mobilization

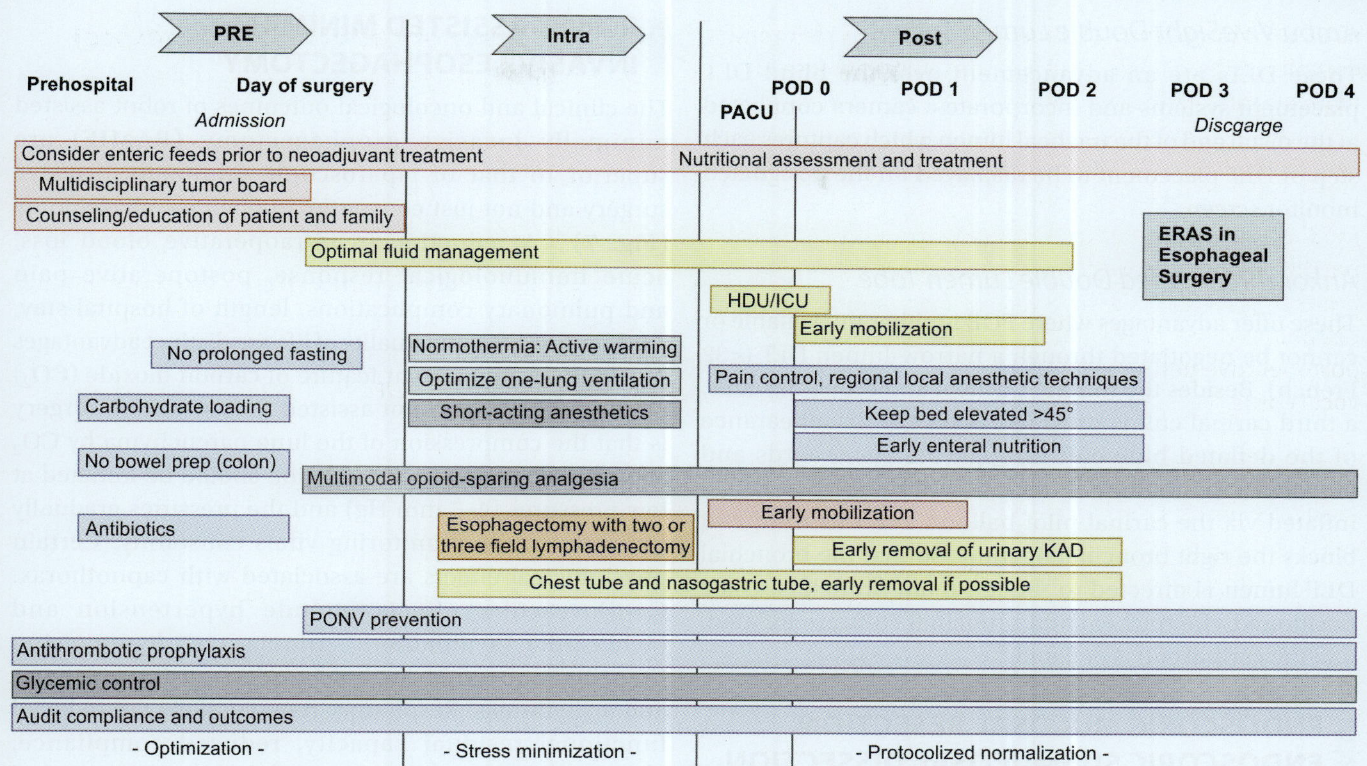

Fig. 6: The enhanced recovery after surgery (ERAS) protocol for esophagectomy. (PONV: postoperative nausea and vomiting)

Nontechnical Skills and Team Work

A successful thoracic anesthesiologist must master the nontechnical skills of communication, task management, situational awareness, teamwork, and decision making.[44,45]

He must communicate with the surgeon to confirm positioning for surgery, ensure that the urinary bladder is catheterized by the surgeon before the patient is turned lateral and confirm the plan for surgery. If the surgeon plans to operate the abdomen first, the anesthesiologist should intubate with a single lumen tube (SLT) first, followed by a DLT if the lesion is found resectable. If the surgical plan involves opening the thorax first, a DLT first followed by change to SLT for abdomen and neck is the ideal course of airway management. Intraoperative communication by loudspeaker is desirable.

Anesthesiologist must communicate with the OT technician so that DLT of the correct size and side, correct BB type, tooth guard, a videolaryngoscope (for anticipated difficult DLT placement), and fiberoptic bronchoscope (FOB) for confirmation of DLT placement are readily available in the OT. The biochemistry and transfusion department must be informed about the requirement of blood and blood products and intraoperative ABG. The SICU staff must be told beforehand about any anticipated postoperative ventilatory support requirement so that they may cater to the availability of a ventilator-bed, transport ventilator, and transport monitors.

Recent Advances

C-Mac D-blade Guided Double Lumen Tube Placement

The D-blade is known to improve glottic visualization, improving the Cormack–Lehane grade by at least one grade compared to a normal blade. The distal concavity of the DLT is shaped as per the D-blade concavity, and the DLT blue/bronchial cuff can be visualized on the monitor as it disappears through the vocal cords. While the remaining procedure commencing with counterclockwise rotation of the DLT still remains blind, this technique has the additional advantage of less cuff rupture. The frequency of wrong-sided DLT placement is marginally higher but is easily corrected under FOB guidance.[46]

Ambu VivaSight Double Lumen Tube

These DLTs are an advancement over the blind DLT placement systems and incorporate a camera connected at the distal end of the tracheal lumen which captures each step of DLT placement to be displayed on the designated monitor screen.[28]

Ankor three-cuffed Double Lumen Tube

These offer advantages where FOB is either unavailable or cannot be negotiated through a narrow-lumen DLT (<32 French). Besides the routine tracheal and bronchial cuffs, a third carinal cuff is provided. After the disappearance of the deflated blue cuff through the vocal cords and anticlockwise rotation of the left DLT, the carinal cuff is inflated via the carinal pilot balloon and this third cuff blocks the right bronchial opening, so that the bronchial DLT lumen is directed to the left main bronchus. Once positioned, the tracheal and bronchial cuffs are inflated, and the carinal cuff is deflated.[29]

ENDOSCOPIC MUCOSAL RESECTION, ENDOSCOPIC SUBMUCOSAL DISSECTION

Endoscopic management of early esophageal cancer confined to the mucosa (T1a) employing endoscopic mucosal resection (EMR), endoscopic submucosal dissection (ESD) is a recent advancement attributable to the low risk of lymph node involvement at this stage. Radiofrequency ablation (RFA), cryotherapy, and free-hand mucosal resection are other modalities of treatment.[39]

ROBOT ASSISTED MINIMALLY INVASIVE ESOPHAGECTOMY

The clinical and oncological outcomes of robot assisted minimally invasive esophagectomy (RAMIE) are superior to that of laparoscopic minimally invasive surgery and not just conventional open esophagectomy **(Fig. 7)**.[47] A reduction in intraoperative blood loss, acute immunological response, postoperative pain and pulmonary complications, length of hospital stay, readmission rate, and quality of life are distinct advantages of RAMIE. An important feature of carbon dioxide (CO_2) pneumothorax for robot assisted thoracoscopic surgery is that the compression of the lung parenchyma by CO_2 acts as a retractor. CO_2 insufflation should be initiated at low pressures (4–5 mm Hg) and the pressures gradually increased while monitoring vitals constantly. Certain physiological effects are associated with capnothorax. Cardiovascular effects include hypertension and tachycardia (sympathetic stimulation), hypotension (impaired venous return), bradycardia (vagal stimulation), and arrhythmias. Respiratory repercussions are reduced functional residual capacity, reduced compliance, increased ventilatory pressures (peak, plateau, and mean airway pressures), and barotrauma including pneumothorax, and atelectasis.[48,49] Rise in CVP, pulmonary artery pressure (PAP), and pulmonary capillary wedge pressure (PCWP) also occur. Insufflation of CO_2 at 8–10 mm Hg for 30–40 minutes in the right hemithorax (not left) results in a reduced mean arterial pressure, and cardiac index. Renal/metabolic effects include reduced

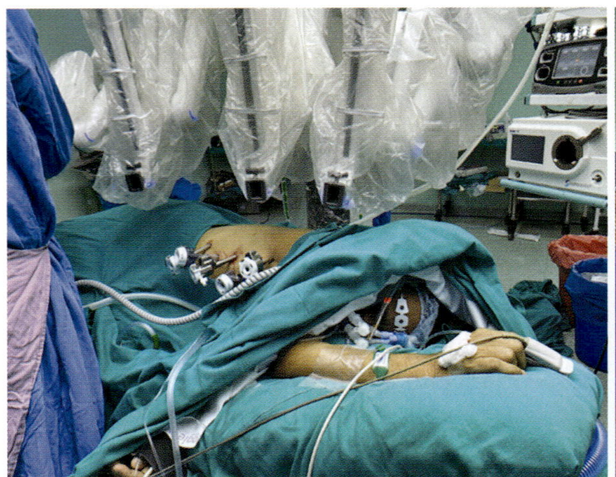

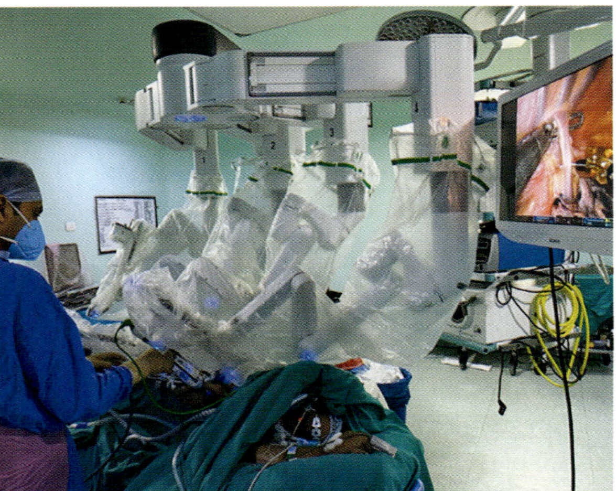

Fig. 7: Robot assisted minimally invasive esophagectomy in progress.

renal perfusion, activation of the renal–angiotensin–aldosterone system, and increased antidiuretic hormone. GI effects comprise raised intra-abdominal pressure with attendant increased risk of gastric regurgitation and splanchnic ischemia.

Complications such as carbon dioxide gas embolism, sudden cardiac arrest, and extra-peritoneal spread of CO_2 may occur.[47-49] Subcutaneous emphysema, also known as surgical emphysema, are usually heralded by a steadily increasing $EtCO_2$ level despite increasing minute ventilation. This is an indication to meticulously palpate the chest and neck of the patient for any crepitations and obtain PCO_2 levels from an ABG analysis. Damage to the contralateral pleura may result in CO_2 flow to contralateral chest, difficult ventilation, and hemodynamic compromise.

Potential impaired intraoperative coagulation and tumor cell proliferation, metastasis, and invasion directly associated with high insufflation pressure and prolonged insufflation time are other concerns.

MINIMALLY INVASIVE ANESTHESIA (MIA) FOR MINIMALLY INVASIVE SURGERY (MIS)

The first reported use of two-lung ventilation (TLV) in minimally invasive esophagectomy (MIE) was by Palanivelu et al. in 2006 in 130 patients being operated in prone position. A very low rate of postoperative pneumonia, without complications such as tracheal or lung injury was encouraging.[50]

Is TLV a possible good alternative to OLV in MIE?

Double lumen tubes exhibit several disadvantages. These include a complicated preoperative intubation and a complicated intraoperative management. Intraoperative hypoxemia is more common during OLV. Pulmonary oxidative stress due to lung reexpansion and postoperative atelectasis are more frequently encountered with a DLT. The larger external diameter of the DLT may have consequences such as vocal cord injury, postoperative sore throat/hoarseness, injury to posterior bronchial wall, hemorrhage, and tracheal rupture.[51] Surgical issues too exist, like reduced mobility of the trachea and bronchus caused by DLT, hampering subcarinal lymph node dissection. Another disadvantage of DLTs is the need to change the DLT to a single-lumen ETT if mechanical ventilation is required after surgery.

An SLT has several advantages over a DLT. Faster and easier placement, reduced risk of intraoperative displacement, and better oxygenation constitute a few of them. Exposure of the operative field, although inferior to that with DLT, is also adequate, especially in robotic esophagectomy.[51,52] However, if conversion to open esophagectomy is required, TLV should be changed to OLV. An SLT-BB combination (introducing a BB through the SLT in situ) is a good option in this scenario, since it is more convenient, faster, and safer than removing the SLT, followed by placing a DLT.

TELEROBOTIC SURGERY

In principle, telerobotic surgery is a milestone technology that could potentially bring the expertise of distinguished surgeons to remote locations (Tier 2/3 cities, war arenas, outbreaks, and outer space). In telerobotic surgery, surgeon's console houses the operating surgeon or the "master", who is several miles away from the "slave" robotic arms docked onto the patient. The surgeon's commands are communicated to the slave manipulator via fiberoptic cables. Currently, the major limitations of telerobotic surgery are high cost of fiberoptic cables and network, time latency of data transmission and communication.[53] Artificial intelligence and 6G network infrastructure, can aid in securing minimal-latency, high-bandwidth, secure and private connections to guarantee surgical precision without compromising patient safety. Roundtrip latency, or time lag between the surgeon's action and his perception of the robot response on his console, lower than 200 ms is critical for telerobotic surgery.[54] Globally, the first telerobotic cancer surgery was conducted in June 2024 in a prostatic cancer patient in Beijing, while the master surgeon console was 8,000 miles away in Rome. A round-trip latency of 135 ms could be attained.[55] The first telerobotic cancer surgery in India was a cystoprostatectomy performed in the same month (June 2024) by the distinguished robotic surgeon, Dr SK Rawal **(Fig. 8)**. He was stationed in a surgeon's console in Gurugram while the patient was operated by slave robotic arms of the indigenous robotic system SSI Mantra, in an OT in Rajiv Gandhi Cancer Institute Rohini, 35 km away.[56,57] This has paved the way for a telerobotic esophagectomy in the near future.

CONCLUSION

We have witnessed a paradigm shift from open posterolateral thoracotomy to robot-assisted minimally invasive esophagectomy as a clinically and oncologically safe technique. In tandem with this rapid advancement in

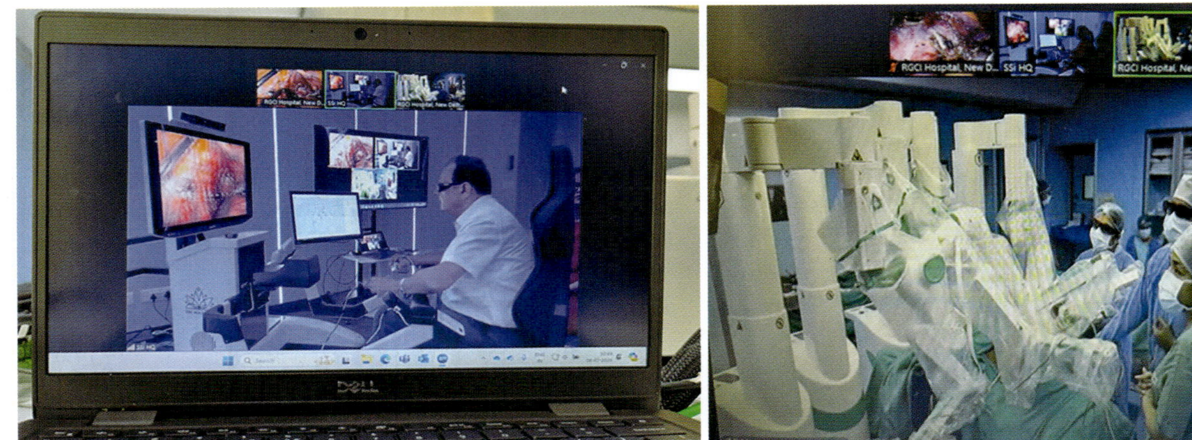

Fig. 8: The first telerobotic oncosurgery in India in progress.

surgical techniques, anesthetic techniques too have become less invasive with an acceptance of two-lung ventilation via a SLT for robotic esophagectomy. However, OLV is an art and science which every anesthesiologist must master, since this is the standard technique in open esophagectomy as well as a fallback technique for complicated robotic esophagectomy patients. Centralization of care to high-volume ERAS protocol compliant centers has reduced the morbidity and mortality.

REFERENCES

1. van Hagen P, Hulshof MC, van Lanschot JJ, Steyerberg EW, van Berge Henegouwen MI, Wijnhoven BP, et al. Preoperative chemoradiotherapy for esophageal or junctional cancer. N Engl J Med. 2012;366(22):2074-84.
2. Zheng R, Tham EJH, Rios-Diaz AJ, Grenda TR, Evans NR 3rd, Rosato EL, et al. A 10-year ACS-NSQIP analysis of trends in esophagectomy practices. J Surg Res. 2020;256:103-11.
3. Abdelsattar ZM, Habermann E, Borah BJ, Moriarty JP, Rojas RL, Blackmon SH. Understanding failure to rescue after esophagectomy in the United States. Ann Thorac Surg. 2020;109(3):865-71.
4. Tovell RM. Intratracheal Anesthesia. Anesth Analg. 1931; 10(3):97-103.
5. WHO. (2024). Cancer factsheets. [online] Available from https://gco.iarc.who.int/today/en/fact-sheets-cancers [Last accessed February, 2025].
6. WHO. (2024). Global cancer observatory. [online] Available from https://gco.iarc.who.int/media/globocan/factsheets/populations/356-india-fact-sheet [Last accessed February, 2025].
7. WHO. (2024). Cancer tomorrow. [online] Available from https://gco.iarc.who.int/tomorrow/en/dataviz/trends?multiple_populations=1&cancers=6 [Last accessed February, 2025].
8. Abnet CC, Arnold M, Wei WQ. Epidemiology of esophageal squamous cell carcinoma. Gastroenterol. 2018; 154(2):360-73.
9. Domper Arnal MJ, Ferrández Arenas Á, Lanas Arbeloa Á. Esophageal cancer: Risk factors, screening and endoscopic treatment in Western and Eastern countries. World J Gastroenterol. 2015;21(26):7933-43.
10. Choksi D, Kolhe KM, Ingle M, Rathi C, Khairnar H, Chauhan SG, et al. Esophageal carcinoma: An epidemiological analysis and study of the time trends over the last 20 years from a single center in India. J Fam Med Primary Care. 2020;9(3):1695-9.
11. Napier K, Scheerer M, Misra S. Esophageal cancer: a review of epidemiology, pathogenesis, staging workup and treatment modalities. World J Gastrointest Oncol. 2014;6(5):112-20.
12. Talsma K, van Hagen P, Grotenhuis BA, Steyerberg EW, Tilanus HW, van Lanschot JJ, et al. Comparison of the 6th and 7th Editions of the UICC-AJCC TNM Classification for Esophageal Cancer. Ann Surgical Oncol. 2012;19(7):2142-8.
13. Sabra MJ, Alwatari YA, Wolfe LG, Xu A, Kaplan BJ, Cassano AD, et al. Ivor Lewis vs Mckeown esophagectomy: analysis of operative outcomes from the ACS NSQIP database. General thoracic and cardiovascular surgery. 2020;68(4):370-9.
14. Verstegen MH, Bouwense SA, van Workum F, Ten Broek R, Siersema PD, Rovers M, et al. Management of intrathoracic and cervical anastomotic leakage after esophagectomy for esophageal cancer: a systematic review. World J Emerg Surg. 2019;14:1-12.
15. Pace M, Minervini A, Goglia M, Cinquepalmi M, Moschetta G, Antolino L, et al. Overall survival following anastomotic leakage after surgery for Carcinoma of the

Esophagus and Gastroesophageal Junction: a systematic review. In Vivo. 2023;37(4):1423-31.
16. Verstegen MH, Slaman AE, Klarenbeek BR, van Berge Henegouwen MI, Gisbertz SS, Rosman C, et al. Outcomes of patients with anastomotic leakage after transhiatal, McKeown or Ivor Lewis esophagectomy: a nationwide cohort study. World J Surg. 2021;45(11):3341-9.
17. Howells P, Bieker M, Yeung J. Oesophageal cancer and the anaesthetist. BJA Education. 2017;17(2):68-73.
18. Deana C, Vetrugno L, Bignami E, Bassi F. Peri-operative approach to esophagectomy: a narrative review from the anesthesiological standpoint. J Thor Dis. 2021;13(10):6037.
19. West MA, Wischmeyer PE, Grocott MP. Prehabilitation and nutritional support to improve perioperative outcomes. Curr Anesthesiol Rep. 2017;7(4):340-9.
20. Slinger P, Darling G. Preanesthetic assessment for thoracic surgery. In: Slinger P (Ed). Principles and practice of anesthesia for thoracic surgery. Switzerland AG: Springer Nature; 2019. pp. 13-41.
21. Kristensen SD, Knuuti J, Saraste A. 2014 ESC/ESA Guidelines on non-cardiac surgery: cardiovascular assessment and management: The Joint Task Force on non-cardiac surgery: cardiovascular assessment and management of the European Society of Cardiology (ESC) and the European Society of Anaesthesiology (ESA). Eur Heart J. 2014;35(35):2383-431.
22. Low DE, Kuppusamy MK, Alderson D, Cecconello I, Chang AC, Darling G, et al. Benchmarking Complications Associated with Esophagectomy. Ann Surg. 2019; 269(2):291-8.
23. Carney A, Dickinson M. Anesthesia for esophagectomy. Anesthesiol Clin. 2015;33(1):143-63.
24. Yatabe T, Kitagawa H, Yamashita K, Hanazaki K, Yokoyama M. Comparison of the perioperative outcome of esophagectomy by thoracoscopy in the prone position with that of thoracotomy in the lateral decubitus position. Surgery today. 2013;43(4):386-91.
25. Kikuchi H, Hiramatsu Y, Matsumoto T, Soneda W, Kawata S, Hirotsu A, et al. The hybrid position is superior to the prone position for thoracoscopic esophagectomy with upper mediastinal lymphadenectomy. Ann Lap Endosc Surg. 2020;5:1-9.
26. Ding X, Jin S, Niu X. A comparison of the analgesia efficacy and side effects of paravertebral compared with epidural blockade for thoracotomy: an updated meta-analysis. PLOS One. 2014;9(5):e96233.
27. Shah SB, Chawla R, Hariharan U, Shukla S. An algorithm for difficult double lumen tube placement and troubleshooting a malpositioned double lumen tube harnessing A, B, Cs of lung isolation. Indian J Anaesth. 2022;66(6):328-32.
28. Schuepbach R, Grande B, Camen G, Schmidt AR, Fischer H, Sessler DI, et al. Intubation with VivaSight or conventional left-sided double-lumen tubes: A randomized trial. Can J Anaesth. 2015;62(7):762-9.
29. Kim N, Byon HJ, Kim GE, Park C, Joe YE, Suh SM, et al. A randomized controlled trial comparing novel triple-cuffed double-lumen endobronchial tubes with conventional double-lumen endobronchial tubes for lung isolation. J Clin Med. 2020;9(4):977-81.
30. Hariharan U, Shah SB, Mittal A, Bhargava AK. C-Mac guided bronchial blocker (COOPDECH™) insertion for one lung ventilation in an adolescent with difficult airway. J Anaesthesiol Clin Pharmacol. 2014;30:591-2.
31. Marik PE, Lemson J. Fluid responsiveness: an evolution of our understanding. Br J Anaesth. 2014;112(4):617-20.
32. Lee J, Chin JH, Kim JI, Lee EH, Choi IE. Association between red blood cell transfusion and long-term mortality in patients with cancer of the esophagus after esophagectomy. Dis Esophagus. 2018;31(2).
33. Kaufmann KB, Baar W, Glatz T, Hoeppner J, Buerkle H, Goebel U, et al. Epidural analgesia and avoidance of blood transfusion are associated with reduced mortality in patients with postoperative pulmonary complications following thoracotomic esophagectomy: a retrospective cohort study of 335 patients. BMC Anesthesiol. 2019;19(1):162.
34. Pan T, Tuoerxun T, Chen X, Yang CJ, Jiang CY, Zhu YF, et al. The neutrophil elastase inhibitor, sivelestat, attenuates acute lung injury in patients with cardiopulmonary bypass. Front Immunol. 2023;14:1082830.
35. Fiorellia A, Mazzella A, Passavanti B, Sansone P, Chiodini P, Iannotti M, et al. Is pre-emptive administration of ketamine a significant adjunction to intravenous morphine analgesia for controlling postoperative pain? A randomized, double-blind, placebo-controlled clinical trial. Interact Cardiovasc Thorac Surg. 2015;21(3):1-7.
36. Visser E, Marsman M, van Rossum PS, Cheong E, Al-Naimi K, van Klei WA, et al. Postoperative pain management after esophagectomy: a systematic review and meta-analysis. Dis Esophagus 2017;30(10):1-11.
37. Sharma S. Management of complications of radical esophagectomy. Indian J Surg Oncol. 2013;4(2):105-11.
38. Paul S, Altorki N. Outcomes in the management of esophageal cancer. J Surg Oncol. 2014;110(5):599-610.
39. ICMR. Esophagus. Available from https://www.icmr.nic.in/sites/default/files/guidelines/Esophagus%20final%20ICMR2014_0.pdf [Last accessed February, 2025].
40. Maruta K, Sato E, Nishi M. Effect of arterial infusion of bleomycin on esophageal carcinoma-an evaluation by nuclear cytophotometry. Jpn J Clin Oncol. 1983;13:683-91.
41. Verma R. Supplemental oxygen therapy in bleomycin-induced pulmonary toxicity. Medical Journal, Armed Forces India. 2011;67(2):194.
42. Rubinkiewicz M, Witowski J, Su M, Major P, Pędziwiatr M. Enhanced recovery after surgery (ERAS) programs for esophagectomy. J Thorac Dis. 2019;11(5):S685-S691.
43. Low DE, Allum W, De Manzoni G, Ferri L, Immanuel A, Kuppusamy M, et al. Guidelines for perioperative care in

esophagectomy: Enhanced recovery after surgery (ERAS®) society recommendations. World J Surg. 2019;43(2):299-330.
44. Chawla R, Shah SB, Kumar M. Chapter 5; Soft Skills (Non-Technical Skills) and Anaesthesiologist; In: Kulkarni AP editor. Treatise on Clinical Anesthesia. 1st ed. New Delhi: Jaypee Brothers 2022.
45. Radhakrishnan B, Katikar MD, Myatra SN, Gautam PL, Vinayagam S, Saroa R. Importance of non-technical skills in anaesthesia education. Indian J Anaesth. 2022;66(1):64-9.
46. Shah SB, Bhargava AK, Hariharan U, Mittal AK, Goel N, Choudhary M. A randomized clinical trial comparing the standard Mcintosh laryngoscope and the C-Mac D blade videolaryngoscope™for double lumen tube insertion for one lung ventilation in onco surgical patients. Indian J Anaesth. 2016;60(5):312-8.
47. Biere SS, van Berge Henegouwen MI, Maas KW, Biere SS, van Berge Henegouwen MI, Maas KW, et al. Minimally invasive versus open oesophagectomy for patients with oesophageal cancer: a multicentre, open-label, randomised controlled trial. Lancet. 2012;379(9829):1887-92.
48. Minimally invasive versus open oesophagectomy for patients with oesophageal cancer: a multicentre, open-label, randomised controlled trial. Lancet. 2012;379:1887-92.
49. Xue M, Liu J, Lu M, Zhang H, Liu W, Tian H. Robotic assisted minimally invasive esophagectomy versus minimally invasive esophagectomy. Front Oncol. 2024;13:1293645.
50. Kingma BF, de Maat MFG, van der Horst S, van der Sluis PC, Ruurda JP, van Hillegersberg R. Robot-assisted minimally invasive esophagectomy (RAMIE) improves perioperative outcomes: a review. J Thorac Dis. 2019;11(5):S735-S742.
51. Palanivelu C, Prakash A, Senthilkumar R, Senthilnathan P, Parthasarathi R, Rajan PS, et al. Minimally invasive esophagectomy: thoracoscopic mobilization of the esophagus and mediastinal lymphadenectomy in prone position-experience of 130 patients. J Am Coll Surg. 2006;203(1):7-16.
52. Lin M, Shen Y, Feng M, Tan L. Is two lung ventilation with artificial pneumothorax a better choice than one lung ventilation in minimally invasive esophagectomy? J Thorac Dis. 2019;11(5):S707-12.
53. Patel M, Wilson A, Ong C. Double-lumen tubes and bronchial blockers. BJA education. 2023;23(11):416-24.
54. Rocco B, Moschovas MC, Saikali S, Gaia G, Patel V, Sighinolfi MC. Insights from telesurgery expert conference on recent clinical experience and current status of remote surgery. J Robotic Surg. 2024;18(1):240.
55. Mohan A, Wara UU, Arshad Shaikh MT, Rahman RM, Zaidi ZA. Telesurgery and robotics: An improved and efficient era. Cureus. 2021;13(3):e14124.
56. CGTN. 2024. Chinese team perform world-first robotic surgery from Rome in Beijing Available from https://newseu.cgtn.com/news/2024-06-12/Chinese-team-perform-world-first-robotic-surgery-from-Rome-in-Beijing-1um4yx45Ixq/p.html [Last accessed February, 2025].
57. Healthworld.com. 2024. RGCIRC undertakes telesurgery for cancer care. [online] Available from https://health.economictimes.indiatimes.com/news/hospitals/rgcirc-undertakes-telesurgery-for-cancer-care/111113966 [Last accessed February, 2025].

21 CHAPTER

Anesthesia for Mediastinal Mass

Anjali Pingle, Aishwarya Ramkrishnan

INTRODUCTION

Mediastinum (medieval Latin—mediastinus, meaning midway) is the central compartment of the thoracic cavity located between the two pleural sacs. The mediastinum contains major airways, major vessels, and crucial nerves in close proximity to each other in a confined space. The presence of any space-occupying lesion in this vicinity **(Fig 1.)**—whether encountered in the operation theater, intensive care unit, or emergency room—poses a challenge to the anesthesiologist. Three factors are crucial to successful management of the effects of mediastinal masses on the airway and vasculature: (1) A thorough understanding of the anatomy and physiology of the thorax, (2) complete clinical and radiological evaluation, and (3) a comprehensive strategy for the conduct of perioperative care.

ANATOMY OF THE MEDIASTINUM AND THE TUMORS INVOLVING MEDIASTINUM

The mediastinum contains several vital organs and acts as a conduit for structures traversing the thorax to the abdomen. It is divided into superior and inferior mediastinum. The inferior mediastinum is further divided into anterior, middle, and posterior sections **(Table 1)**.

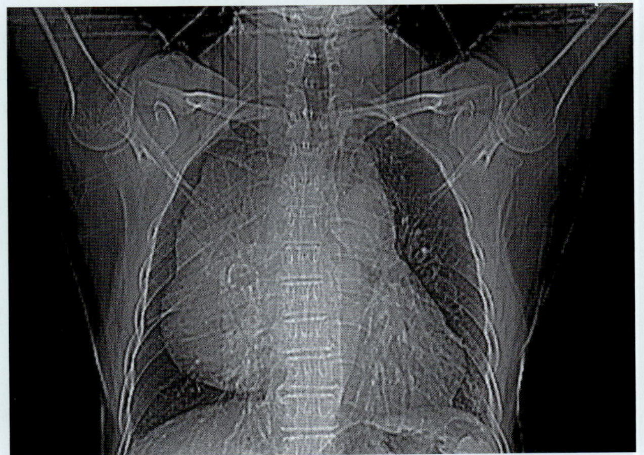

Fig. 1: X-ray showing mediastinal mass.

COMMON MEDIASTINAL TUMORS AND THE CURRENT TREATMENT REGIMENS FOR EACH TYPE

The most common hematological diseases of the mediastinum are represented by Hodgkin lymphoma (HL), diffuse large B-cell lymphoma (DLBCL), and primary mediastinal large B-cell lymphoma (PMBCL).

Hodgkin lymphoma is treated with ABVD (Doxorubicin, Bleomycin, Vinblastine, and Dacarbazine) as the first line of treatment. The other treatment options include novel antibody-drug conjugate—brentuximab and auto/allogenic hematopoietic stem cell transplantation. DLBCL is the most common type of non-Hodgkin lymphoma. It is an aggressive tumor, typically presenting with rapidly enlarging lymphadenopathy. The chemotherapy regimen includes upfront chemoimmunotherapy with R-CHOP regimen (Rituximab, Cyclophosphamide, Doxorubicin, Vincristine, and Prednisone), combined with biological agents, including ibrutinib, bortezomib, or lenalidomide, which give variable results.[2]

Pediatric patients with T-lymphoblastic lymphoma (T-LBL) and classical Hodgkin's lymphoma (CHL) have excellent prognosis with cure rates >90%, in contrast to adult patients, who present with complex subtypes.

Mediastinal germ cell tumors (GCTs) show a typical bimodal age distribution, with the first peak in infancy and the first few years of childhood, i.e., up to 4–5 years of age (mainly teratoma and yolk sac tumors), and thereafter in adolescence and young adulthood, i.e., starting at 12–13 years of age (seminoma). Thymomas are the most frequently occurring mediastinal tumor in adults.[3]

TABLE 1: Mediastinal boundary and content.[1,2]

	Boundaries	*Contents*	*Pathology involved*	*Pediatric*
Superior	Extend superiorly by thoracic inlet, inferiorly by transverse thoracic plane, laterally by pleura, anteriorly by the posterior surface of manubrium sterni, and posteriorly by T1–T4 thoracic vertebrae	Thymus, trachea, esophagus Arteries: Aortic arch, brachiocephalic trunk, left common carotid artery, left subclavian artery, superior vena cava, brachiocephalic veins, the arch of the azygos, thoracic duct	Retrosternal and intrathoracic goiter	Lymphoma
Anterior	From the posterior surface of the lower sternum to the anterior surface of pericardium and great vessels, lies between pleural cavities, extends from thoracic inlet to the diaphragm	Thymus, trachea, esophagus, large veins, large arteries, thoracic duct, sympathetic trunk, lymph nodes, ectopic thyroid gland, and parathyroid tissues	Thymic carcinoma, thymoma, germ cell tumor, teratoma, lymphoma	Lymphoma (most common), thymoma (rare) germ cell tumor
Middle	Between the anterior mediastinum and the anterior border of the vertebral bodies	Heart and pericardium, great vessels, vagus and phrenic nerves	Parathyroid adenoma	Lymphoma, lymph node from abdominopelvic tumors
Posterior	Posterior to the middle mediastinum	Intercostal nerves, thoracic spinal ganglion, and sympathetic chain	Neurogenic tumors, schwannoma	Sympathetic ganglion tumor (early years of age)

Surgical resection is the first line of treatment for thymomas: Nonresectable tumors are managed with CAP (Doxorubicin, Cisplatin, and Cyclophosphamide) regimen.

Thoracic neuroblastomas occur in the posterior mediastinum and may not cause any symptoms and are usually diagnosed by imaging studies incidentally. Presenting symptoms may range from chronic cough to acute breathlessness. Thoracic neuroblastomas can present with Horner's syndrome and can cause neurologic symptoms, including weakness, limping, paralysis, and even bladder and bowel dysfunction.

Huge mediastinal masses which are chemosensitive should undergo appropriate chemotherapy preoperatively. Steroids and preoperative radiotherapy can be considered in some cases. Steroids are known to cause shrinkage of tumor size, especially in lymphomas, but have limited role in tumors of thymic origin. Steroids in lymphoma patients are to be used with caution, as they can trigger tumor lysis syndrome[4] and can also cause diagnostic confusion (up to 22% inaccuracy in diagnosis of lymphoma, if prebiopsy steroids are administered).[5] The administration of preoperative steroids can distort cellular morphology, compromise the accuracy and timeliness of a histological diagnosis, and thereby alter the choice of and response to therapy. This risk-benefit ratio of prebiopsy steroid should be considered in the high-risk patient. As an anesthesiologist, understanding the pathophysiology of the various mediastinal tumors and the effects of their treatment regimen is crucial for anticipating potential complications during the perioperative period.

PREOPERATIVE EVALUATION

The focus should be to elicit both local and systemic effects of the tumor.

Local Effects of a Mediastinal Mass

1. *Dyspnea in the supine position*: This symptom helps gauge the tumor's mass effect on the airway. Dyspnea severity in the supine position can be categorized as follows:
   - *Asymptomatic*: No symptoms are present.
   - *Mild*: The patient can lie supine but may experience a mild cough or pressure symptoms due to the mediastinal mass.
   - *Moderate*: The patient can lie supine only briefly before symptoms worsen.
   - *Severe*: The patient cannot lie supine at all.[1]

   For symptomatic patients, inquire about the most comfortable position that alleviates dyspnea (e.g., sitting or lateral). This information helps understand the mass effect and potential relieving factors, which can guide positioning during anesthesia induction and a rescue position in the event of airway compromise or hemodynamic collapse intraoperatively.

2. *Mass effect on blood vessels*: Superior and anterior mediastinal masses can compress the great vessels, potentially causing superior vena cava syndrome. Clinical signs include headache, neck and facial swelling, venous distention in the neck, and the Pemberton sign (Hugh Pemberton 1946) (positive Pemberton's sign—the patient raises both arms until the forearms touches the sides of the face, if facial congestion and cyanosis, respiratory distress develop after approximately one minute) demonstrates the presence of latent pressure in the thoracic inlet.
3. Other symptoms may include chest pain, back pain, dysphagia, and syncope.

Systemic Effects

Mediastinal tumors can be associated with paraneoplastic syndromes. For example, thymoma may be associated with myasthenia gravis in about 30% cases (detected through antiacetylcholine receptor antibody testing). A thorough history and clinical examination for any signs of muscle weakness should be conducted. Acetylcholine antibody levels should be determined.

Other paraneoplastic syndromes such as pure red cell aplasia and hypogammaglobulinemia are commonly seen with thymic tumors. Thyroid evaluation is important in patients with suspected retrosternal extension of goiter.

PREOPERATIVE INVESTIGATION

Imaging

Chest X-ray is used for initial screening, while CT chest provides detailed information, including the exact location, size, extent, airway caliber, and proximity of vessels **(Figs. 2A and B)**. A CT chest is particularly valuable for identifying airway compression, determining its location (whether it affects the trachea, carina, or main bronchi), and assessing the extent and percentage of luminal compression and luminal wall invasion. If the airway diameter is narrowed by 50% or more at any level due to extraluminal compression (measured at the narrowest cross-sectional area on the CT slice), it can complicate airway management for the anesthesiologist. This information helps in planning the management strategy, but CT alone cannot fully predict respiratory complications. Another important factor for perioperative planning is the size of the mediastinal mass. Masses occupying more than 50% of the thoracic cavity—measured by the mediastinal mass ratio (the ratio of the transverse diameter of the mediastinal mass to the maximum transverse diameter of the chest)—are significant. The incidence of respiratory collapse increases with the size of the mass, the incidence being 2.1% for masses <31% of the chest diameter, 10.5% for masses between 32% and 44%, and 33.3% for masses >45%.[6] If the patient is unable to tolerate supine position, the patient can be positioned lateral or even prone for imaging. With modern fast CT scanners, scan times are under 20 seconds and if needed,

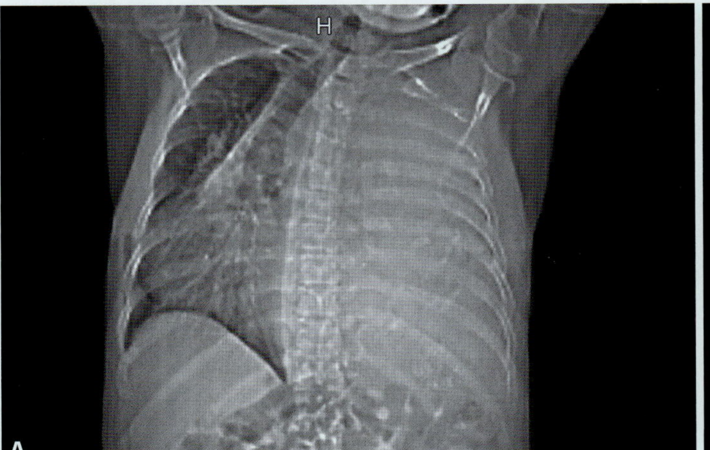

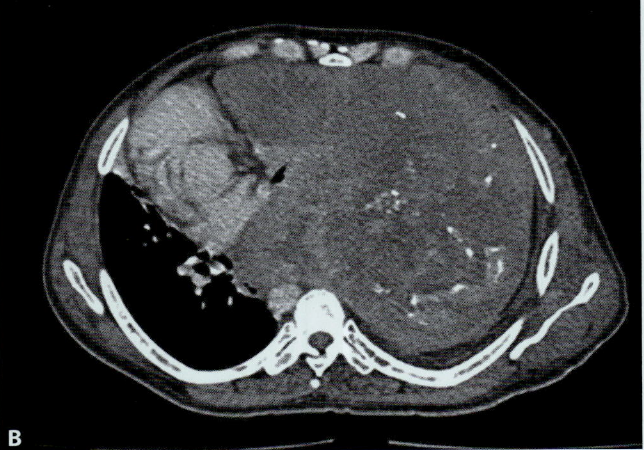

Figs. 2A and B: (A) X-ray showing huge homogenous opacity involving the hemithorax with mediastinal and tracheal shift; (B) CT scan reveals a huge mass arising from the mediastinum involving the whole of the left hemithorax with severe tracheal compression.

the patient's head and chest can be elevated to 30° without affecting scan quality.

The most important information to be derived from the CT plates is the location and extent of the lesion and especially the presence of a landing zone for the ETT. The exact length where the tube tip should be placed to the incisors should be measured in advance, either with the help of the radiologist or prior to induction, with a pediatric fiberoptic scope.

Pulmonary Function Tests

Performed in an upright position, pulmonary function tests (PFTs) offer an objective assessment of airway obstruction. Among these tests, the peak expiratory flow rate (PEFR) is the most useful for risk assessment. According to Schamberger's criteria, a tracheal area <50% combined with a PEFR <50% indicates a high risk for airway collapsibility with anesthesia induction.[6]

Flow–Volume Loops

Obtaining flow–volume loops requires patient cooperation and effort. There is poor correlation with patient symptoms and degree of tracheal deviation and stenosis.[7] Their utility in identifying the level of obstruction is limited and does not provide significant clinical benefits

They were of value in the era when imaging was not available but have been rendered obsolete due to the availability of three-dimensional pictures with CT scans. Increased mid-expiratory plateau when changing the position from upright to supine was said to be pathognomonic of variable intrathoracic airway obstruction and an indicator of high risk for airway collapse during induction of anesthesia. They are usually performed in the sitting position and measure maximal inspiratory and expiratory volumes and may be useful in quantifying the dynamic change in the airway which cannot be obtained in CT scans which is a static image done in the supine position **(Fig. 3)**.[8]

Virtual Bronchoscopy

Virtual bronchoscopic imaging is the 3D reconstruction from a multislice CT, can help in the preoperative evaluation and planning of the management of mediastinal mass, and evaluate the status of tracheal or bronchial compression. It gives precise idea of length and diameter of the compressed tracheal segment. It also allows us to determine the tracheal tube size, which can be passed safely. The advantage of this technique is that it is noninvasive and helps to see beyond compressed trachea which may be difficult to pass with a real bronchoscope.[9]

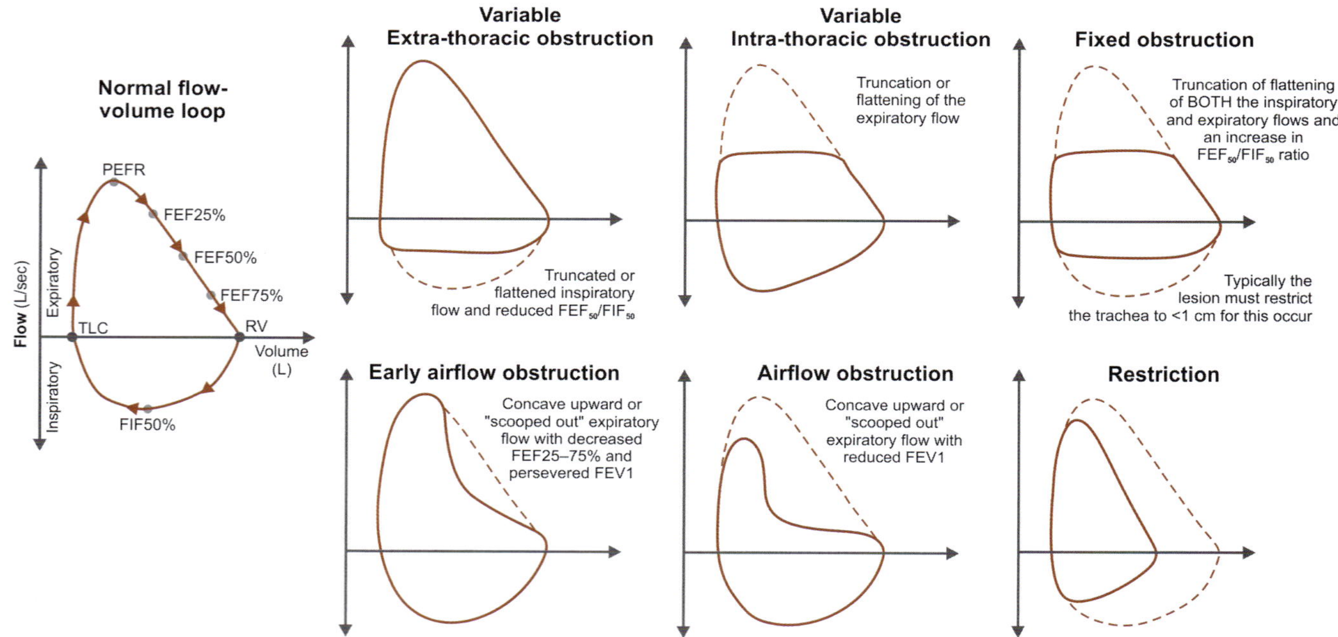

Fig. 3: Pulmonary function: Flow–volume loops.

Bronchoscopy

All patients should undergo bronchoscopy just prior to induction of anesthesia. This procedure provides a dynamic, real-time assessment of the airway, aiding in the planning of anesthetic management. It helps identify the exact location of luminal narrowing, the segments involved, and any intraluminal extensions.

Cardiac evaluation

Cardiac evaluation is crucial for functional evaluation and optimization of these patients as they may be associated with pericardial effusion, which should be quantified using echocardiography. The presence of pericardial effusion is a strong predictor of intraoperative cardiovascular collapse. Preoperative pericardiocentesis is advisable prior to a planned biopsy or procedure.[10]

Comprehensive cardiac functional assessment, including ECG and echocardiography, is essential for managing these major surgeries. In patients with cardiovascular symptoms, or in those patients who are unable to give an adequate history, echocardiography helps to assess compression of the heart, and systemic or pulmonary vasculature. If compromise is suspected, echo should be done in the sitting position and the patient made to lie supine and repeated to know the dynamic changes. Inferior vena cava volume and collapsibility should be assessed in the preoperative period, to assess the volume status of the patient. It also helps to identify the patients who are at risk of intraoperative cardiovascular collapse.

POSTERIOR MEDIASTINAL MASSES

The posterior mediastinal masses are less likely to cause any airway compromise or vascular compression, but if they are large and involve the left hemithorax they can compress the heart chambers, especially the atrial chambers. Detailed history and imaging help to rule out these features and if any compression of cardiac chambers is suspected, extracorporeal membrane oxygenation (ECMO) should be instituted prior to anesthesia induction.[11]

DIFFERENCE BETWEEN PEDIATRIC AND ADULT MEDIASTINAL MASS

The commonest mediastinal tumors in children are lymphomas, which respond well to chemotherapy. These children may present to the anesthetist for diagnostic procedures which are mandatory for initiation of treatment but carry the risk of airway compression.

Low-risk patients are defined as those who are asymptomatic and have no postural or radiological compression findings. Moderate-risk patients are those who have moderate postural symptoms and whose tracheal compression is below 50%. Patients with a cross-sectional area of 50% or mediastinal mass ratio above 45% are defined as those at high risk for airway compression.

Respiratory complications are more common in pediatric patients than adults as the cartilaginous structures in the airway are more compressible than in adults, and eliciting a detailed history of the symptoms is also difficult in children which may lead to an underestimation of symptoms. Children with severe respiratory compromise for whom a needle biopsy is not feasible without sedation or general anesthesia should be treated with steroids, empirical chemotherapy, and radiotherapy as life-saving measures and biopsy should be planned after the airway is safe to be handled.[12]

PROCEDURES PERFORMED FOR DIAGNOSIS AND TREATMENT OF MEDIASTINAL MASS

Patients may present for anesthesia for various diagnostic or therapeutic interventions. This requires meticulous planning and care, especially in nonoperating room (NORA) locations.

- *Image-guided biopsy:* Various options are available for biopsy of mediastinal masses such as image guided (CT/USG), mediastinotomy, video-assisted thoracoscopic surgery (VATS), and open surgical biopsy. Each of the techniques has its pros and cons. The choice of technique depends on tumor size, location, age, and performance status. Image-guided transthoracic biopsy is most commonly used.
- *Mediastinoscopy:* A mediastinoscope is inserted beneath the manubrium to take the biopsy for histological diagnosis.[13]
- *Mediastinal mass excision:* Various surgical approaches are used. Sternotomy is the most common approach used but anterolateral thoracotomy is also used if the mass involves one hemithorax. VATS may be used if space is available but not suitable for masses >10 cm.[14]

EFFECT OF ANESTHESIA ON AIRWAY CALIBER IN MEDIASTINAL MASS

The mass effect on the airway may not always be apparent in the awake state. However, under anesthesia, smooth muscle tone is reduced and diaphragmatic excursions are minimized with cephalad displacement of the diaphragm. It was hypothesized that both these factors reduce the transpleural pressure gradient that keeps the airway dilated, thus leading to collapse of the tracheobronchial tree and airway compromise under anesthesia. A recent study by Hartigan et al. has failed to prove these assumptions. The study was designed to observe the airway diameter in patients ($n = 17$) with large mediastinal masses with moderate-to-severe airway obstruction (more than 50%) under various stages of anesthesia.

The bronchoscopy images of the airway of various patients were captured during spontaneous ventilation, induction of anesthesia, initiation of positive-pressure ventilation, and after administration of muscle relaxant. These images were evaluated by experienced, independent bronchoscopists. The changes in the anterior–posterior diameter of the airway were marked as mean airway patency score and classified as positive or negative, depending on whether they were between 25% and 50%, above, or below the baseline. It was found that there was no significant change in the mean airway patency score after anesthesia induction. Positive-pressure ventilation was effective in maintaining airway patency even after administration of muscle relaxants. They demonstrated that maintaining spontaneous ventilation and assisting with positive-pressure ventilation helps to avoid major airway compromise in patients with large mediastinal masses.[15]

The recent data shows that positive-pressure ventilation with muscle paralysis does not alter the airway caliber and also maintains the peak inspiratory flow and expiratory flow rates. Any reduction in expiratory flow can be compensated by increasing the expiratory time, by changing the I:E ratio to 1:1.[16] However, this new observation should not impact our risk stratification or our planning of the airway management in patients with mediastinal masses. The most successful strategy is staged inductions rather than conventional inductions in this patient group, with a flexibility to back off at any stage.

TABLE 2: Factors influencing surgical and anesthesia management in airway-related procedures.

Patient factors	Specific airway problem, comorbidities, body habitus, elective or emergency(stridor) procedure
Surgical factors	Planned surgical intervention and surgical urgency
Anesthesia factors	Training, skill set, experience of high volume of similar cases, recent case familiarity, frequency of exposure to the clinical scenario
Organizational factors	Environment, high-volume center, rapport of team members, communication, available assistance, equipment including backup, local policies and protocols

TABLE 3: Monitoring, equipment, and personnel requirements for airway management in surgical procedures.

Standard monitoring	ECG, plethysmography, capnography
Depth of anesthesia monitoring	Agent gas monitor, BIS (bi-spectral index), or entropy-based monitoring
Additional monitoring	Airway pressures, neuromuscular monitoring, temperature, urine output
Blood pressure monitoring	• Noninvasive BP for low-risk patients • Invasive arterial BP for high-risk patients (preinduction)
Equipment in operation theater	• Syringe pumps, forced air warmers, fluid warmers, rapid infuser systems, intermittent pneumatic compression devices • Rigid bronchoscope (RB) ready in the OR/NORA site • Cardiopulmonary bypass setup if planned
Personnel requirements	• Personnel skilled in the use of RB present throughout the case • Adequate staff for patient position changes (lateral/prone) in case of respiratory compromise (ideally four) • Cardiovascular team if required

ANESTHETIC MANAGEMENT

The aim of preoperative assessment is to identify high-risk patients and avoid major complications. Preoperative optimization and multidisciplinary planning is crucial for all high risk patient. Disease progression from the day of preoperative assessment to the day of surgery, can change the risk profile. Hence, it is mandatory to look at all the images taken recently along with the bronchoscopy findings in the immediate preoperative period. Many factors influence a clinician's decisions in a patient at risk of airway compromise or hemodynamic collapse as enumerated in **Table 2**.[17]

Anesthesia induction should always be done in propped-up position or sitting position is optimal in symptomatic patients. Induction of anesthesia should be titrated and slow, maintaining spontaneous ventilation as far as possible. Dexmedetomidine has been found to be safe and useful for procedural sedation for biopsy and also for awake fiberoptic bronchoscope (FOB) guided intubation.[18]Airway should be secured and either awake or spontaneous ventilation preserved if possible. Muscle relaxants can be used if adequate ventilation can be achieved with face mask after induction. It should be confirmed by capnography and adequate time for expiration should be set.

Awake fiberoptic-guided intubation becomes the standard technique of airway management in cooperative patients with tracheal compression >50%. Care should be taken to position the distal end of the tube distal to the level of obstruction. Armored/flexometallic tubes are used in these patients to prevent intraoperative airway collapse.

ROLE OF CARDIOPULMONARY BYPASS FOR OXYGENATION IN ANTERIOR MEDIASTINAL MASS

Earlier reports have suggested that cardiopulmonary bypass (CPB) should be kept standby as a rescue method but femoral cannulation takes 5–20 minutes. This delay may be fatal in an emergency.[14] In high-risk individuals, with severe positional symptoms due to airway or cardiovascular compression, femoral cannulation should be done under local anesthesia, prior to induction of general anesthesia, so that bypass can be initiated without delay in an emergency.[7] CPB/extracorporeal membrane oxygenation (ECMO) pump and circuit should be primed and ready. Partial bypass can be instituted via femoral vessels (2.5 L/min flow). It is now possible to introduce a cannula into the superior vena cava via the femoral route which can achieve total bypass (5 L/min flow) with the use of suction, in patients where it is deemed necessary.[19] It should be considered an integral part of airway management (assuring oxygenation) in low-lying mediastinal masses with bronchial or carinal compression.[6] This decision is to be taken with the knowledge that institution of ECMO/CPB involves anticoagulation, most commonly heparinization.[3]

HEMODYNAMIC COLLAPSE IN MEDIASTINAL MASS

There are various reasons for hypotension in patients with mediastinal masses, which include obstruction of the great vessels by the mass or massive hemorrhage.[10]

The mass may compress the heart leading to mechanical obstruction and reduction in cardiac output due to decreased venous return. Immediate rescue involves sternotomy and lifting of the tumor to manage the hemodynamic compromise. These patients will need CPB initiated to maintain the circulation and tissue perfusion.

Tracheal compression leading to reduction in expiratory flow may cause progressive air trapping and result in tension pneumothorax and hemodynamic collapse. Intercostal drain placement is required.

Intraoperative blood loss is anticipated in these patients, and wide bore peripheral or central IV access (Swan–Ganz introducer) should be secured. Central venous access is mandatory for inotropic support. Femoral vessels are preferred in cases where internal jugular vein (IJV) or superior vena cava (SVC) cannulation may interfere with the surgical field. Venous access should be secured in the lower limb in patients with SVC obstruction and where a possibility of breaching the major thoracic vessels exists. Availability of blood and blood products should be confirmed prior to induction. Massive blood transfusion protocol should be activated in case of any injury to major vessels. Hypothermia should be avoided by using warming blankets and fluid warmers. The use of cardiac output monitoring is beneficial in individualizing fluid management for major resections. Liberal fluid administration should be avoided to prevent postoperative pulmonary complications.[20]

EXTUBATION AND POSTOPERATIVE CARE

Patients without any preoperative airway compromise can be extubated on table. Phrenic nerve involvement and intactness should be discussed with surgeons prior to extubation. Suspected tracheomalacia, long-standing goiter, suspected recurrent laryngeal nerve (RLN) or phrenic nerve injury, hemodynamic instability, massive blood transfusion, and associated lung resections are common indications for elective postoperative ventilation (EPOV). EPOV is also indicated in large mediastinal masses associated with prolonged surgical resection times.

POSTOPERATIVE PAIN MANAGEMENT

Modality of pain management used depends on the surgical approach. Multimodal analgesia is preferred. Epidural analgesia is the gold standard for sternotomy and thoracotomy pain. However, epidural is not advisable in patients with vascular involvement or in cases with the possibility of requiring CPB, in view of the use of anticoagulants. Opioid-based patient-controlled analgesia can be used in such patients. According to some authors, a new modality, parasternal intercostal blocks, can be used and has been shown to provide superior pain relief and reduce postoperative pulmonary complications.[21]

CONCLUSION

As always, effective preoperative assessment and planning determine success. To summarize, in these high-risk cases, favorable outcomes are likely in the hands of proficient clinicians working in high-volume centers, with systems in place and where the team functions cohesively as a single unit. At all times, communication is the key.

REFERENCES

1. Garg R, Bhatnagar S. Textbook of Onco-Anesthesiology. Singapore: Springer; 2021.
2. Conci N, Grilli G, Dall'Olio FG. Principles of medical and oncological management of giant masses of the mediastinum: a narrative review. Mediastinum. 2022;6:35.
3. Ramanathan K, Leow L, Mithiran H. ECMO and adult mediastinal masses. Indian J Thoracic Cardiovasc Surg. 202137:338-43.
4. Belay Y, Yirdaw K, Enawgaw B. Tumor lysis syndrome in patients with hematological malignancies. J Oncol. 2017:2017:9684909.
5. Borenstein SH, Gerstle T, Malkin D, Thorner P, Filler RM. The effects of prebiopsy corticosteroid treatment on the diagnosis of mediastinal lymphoma. J Pediatr Surg. 2000;35(6):973-6
6. Shamberger RC, Holzman RS, Griscom NT, Tarbell N, Weinstein HJ, Wohl ME. Prospective evaluation by computed tomography and pulmonary function of children with mediastinal masses tests. Surgery. 1995;118(3):468-71.
7. Slinger P, Karsli C, St E. Management of the patient with a large anterior mediastinal mass: recurring myths. Curr Opin Anaesthesiol. 2007;20(1):1-3
8. Wong P, Liew G, Kothandan H. Anaesthesia for goitre surgery: A review. Proc Singapore Healthcare. 201524:165-70.
9. De Wever W, Vandecaveye V, Lanciotti S, Verschakelen JA. Multidetector CT-generated virtual bronchoscopy: An illustrated review of the potential clinical indications. Eur Respir J. 200423:776-82.
10. Béchard P, Létourneau L, Lacasse Y, Côté D, Bussières JS. Perioperative Cardiorespiratory Complications in Adults with Mediastinal Mass Incidence and Risk Factors. Anesthesiology. 2004;100(4):826-34; discussion 5A.
11. Anderson DM, Dimitrova GT, Awad H. Patient with Posterior Mediastinal Mass Requiring Urgent Cardiopulmonary Bypass [Internet]. Anesthesiology. 2011;114(6):1488-93,
12. Azizkhan RG, Dudgeon DL, Buck JR, Colombani PM, Yaster M, Nichols D, et al. Life-Threatening Airway Obstruction as a Complication to the Management of Mediastinal Masses in Children. J Pediatr Surg. 1985; 20(6):816-22.
13. Ku CM, Slinger P. Anesthesia for Patients with Mediastinal Masses. Principles and Practice of Anesthesia for Thoracic Surgery. DOI 10.1007/978-1-4419-0184-2_14, © Springer Science+Business Media, LLC 2011.
14. Li WWL, Van Boven WJP, Annema JT, Eberl S, Klomp HM, de Mol BAJM. Management of large mediastinal masses: Surgical and anesthesiological considerations. J Thorac Dis. 2016;8(3):E175-84.
15. Hartigan PM, Karamnov S, Gill RR, Ng JM, Yacoubian S, Tsukada H, et al. Mediastinal Masses, Anesthetic Interventions, and Airway Compression in Adults: A Prospective Observational Study. Anesthesiology. 2022; 136(1):104-14.
16. Sarkiss M, Jimenez CA. The evolution of anesthesia management of patients with anterior mediastinal mass. Mediastinum. 2023:7:16.
17. Cook TM, Morgan PJ, Hersch PE. Equal and opposite expert opinion. Airway obstruction caused by a retrosternal thyroid mass: Management and prospective international expert opinion. Anaesthesia. 2011;66:828-36.
18. Olix DJ, Carollo DS, Ural KG. Dexmedetomidine Used to Maintain Spontaneous Ventilation in a Patient With Anterior Mediastinal Mass and Superior Vena Cava Syndrome. Ochsner J. 2023;23(4):363-6.
19. Parker LP, Marcial AS, Brismar TB, Broman LM, Prahl Wittberg L. Cannulation configuration and recirculation in venovenous extracorporeal membrane oxygenation. Sci Rep. 2022;12(1):16379.
20. Li X, Zhang Q, Zhu Y, Yang Y, Xu W, Zhao Y, et al. Effect of perioperative goal-directed fluid therapy on postoperative complications after thoracic surgery with one-lung ventilation: a systematic review and meta-analysis. World J Surg Oncol. 2023;21(1):297
21. Chen H, Song W, Wang W, Peng Y, Zhai C, Yao L, et al. Ultrasound-guided parasternal intercostal nerve block for postoperative analgesia in mediastinal mass resection by median sternotomy: a randomized, double-blind, placebo-controlled trial. BMC Anesthesiol. 2021;21(1):98.

CHAPTER

Anesthesia for Tracheal Resection

Swapnil Parab

INTRODUCTION

Tracheal resection is a complex surgery that presents unique challenges for an anesthesiologist. Sharing an airway with the surgeon presents challenges in intraoperative ventilation of the lungs. This chapter will discuss the indications, preoperative evaluation, airway and ventilation management during the surgery, and postoperative care required in patients with tracheal resection surgery.

INDICATIONS OF TRACHEAL RESECTION

Tracheobronchial pathologies that need tracheal resection are listed in **Box 1**.

Pathophysiology of Critically Obstructive Tracheal Lesion

The nature and degree of airway obstruction depend on the narrowest diameter of the trachea and the location of the lesion. Lesions around the upper trachea are usually extrathoracic lesions, while intrathoracic pathologies compress the middle and lower tracheal segments. Airway obstruction caused by extrathoracic mass is usually fixed and affects both inspiratory and expiratory flows. As a result, stridor appears during inspiration and exhalation.

On the other hand, intrathoracic masses usually produce dynamic airway obstruction, as pleural pressure plays a role in the movement of the mass. During spontaneous breathing, the pleural pressure becomes negative. Also, the inflow of air in the trachea increases the intratracheal pressure. Thus, the mass is pulled away from the airway, relieving the degree of the obstruction. During exhalation, the mass is no longer pulled away from the airway, thus obstructing the expiratory flow. Hence, the patient has relatively smooth inspiration but an effortful and prolonged exhalation during spontaneous breathing. The nature of stridor is usually expiratory.

During positive-pressure ventilation, the dynamic airway obstruction worsens the inspiratory flows, as the pleural pressure becomes positive during inspiration and pushes the mass toward the airway. Hence, positive-pressure ventilation becomes difficult for the patient, who breathes well spontaneously. This is the reason for maintaining spontaneous breathing during the induction of patients who have dynamic airway obstruction. Spontaneous breathing drive is maintained in inhalational induction, whereas intravenous induction abolishes it. This is why inhalational induction is chosen in patients with critical airway obstruction. However, recent evidence from a prospective observational study of 17 patients with large mediastinal masses showed no significant change in airway patency following the induction of anesthesia and administration of muscle relaxants. Although it is performed in a small sample size, this study questions the conventional ideology of central airway obstruction and its management.[1]

BOX 1: Indications of tracheal resection.

Pathologies that require tracheal resection:
- *Tracheal stenosis*:
  - Postintubation
  - Post-traumatic
  - Postinfectious (e.g., tuberculosis)
  - Post-chronic granulomatous inflammation (e.g., sarcoidosis)
- *Tracheal tumors*:
  - Adenoid cystic carcinoma
  - Squamous cell carcinoma
  - Carcinoid
  - Tracheal papilloma
  - Metastasis from thyroid, renal, breast, and lung cancers
- Congenital anomalies (tracheal agenesis/tracheomalacia)
- Trachea-esophageal fistula
- Traumatic tracheal injury

Secondly, another difference between intrathoracic and extrathoracic obstruction is that external pressure of neck mass on the airway can be relieved by mechanical lifting of the mass postinduction of the patient. For example, a large thyroid mass compressing the trachea in the neck can be lifted off the trachea by mechanical efforts or by changing the patient's position from supine to lateral. However, intrathoracic obstruction cannot be relieved by this method. Hence, the intrathoracic obstruction should always be managed carefully, and a rigid bronchoscope to splint open the airway should always be kept ready.

PREOPERATIVE EVALUATION

Preoperative evaluation of the patient planned for tracheal resection should include a detailed history taking and general examination to ensure fitness for general anesthesia. It would include an assessment of comorbidities and their control, history of medications and addictions, previous medical and surgical treatments, recording the vitals, and examination of cardiorespiratory systems. Also, recent blood investigations, namely hemogram, renal and liver function tests, electrocardiogram, and chest radiograph, should be assessed.

- As far as trachea-bronchial pathology is concerned, certain additional points should be assessed in history taking. The inability to lie supine indicates a significant obstruction involving the trachea's lower end. A history of hemoptysis indicates a vascular lesion. Audible breathing or stridor usually appears when the lumen is compromised to less than 50% of its original size.
- Tracheal lesions are often asymptomatic in the early phase. Symptoms are insidious in onset and are often misdiagnosed for tuberculosis or exacerbation of bronchial asthma. Hence, it is not uncommon to find patients receiving antituberculosis treatment, bronchodilators, and steroids. The side effects of these medications should be assessed carefully during preoperative evaluation.
- The two most helpful investigations are computed tomography (CT) scan and bronchoscopy. The location of the lesion in the trachea-bronchial tree and the narrowing of the lumen of the airway must be assessed using a CT scan. Minimal tracheal/bronchial diameter available for passage of the endotracheal tube should be measured. It would help to plan airway management. Three-dimensional reconstruction of the CT scan provides a virtual bronchoscopic vision of the airway. However, real-time bronchoscopy is necessary to assess the histology, consistency, vascularity, and extent of the lesion. Anesthesiologists and surgeons must see the bronchoscopy video preoperatively to plan airway management and the extent of resection.
- Pulmonary function tests and flow–volume loops were used to assess the dynamic nature and location of airway obstruction. However, they need not be done as precise information can be easily obtained using CT scans and bronchoscopy.
- Total or partial obstruction of the bronchus results in the collapse of the lung distal to the obstruction. Infection and consolidation may occur in the lung parenchyma. During bronchoscopy, attempts should be made to obtain the secretions distal to the obstructed area, and antibiotics should be administered based on the culture-sensitivity report.

PREPARATION OF THE OPERATION THEATER

In addition to the standard monitors and devices required for general anesthesia, additional equipment that should be kept ready in the operation theater (OT) are mentioned in **Box 2**.

INTRAOPERATIVE MONITORING

In addition to standard monitoring during general anesthesia (namely electrocardiogram, pulse oximeter, end-tidal carbon dioxide monitor, temperature monitor), the following monitoring should be instituted in case of tracheal resection:

- Bispectral index (BIS) to monitor the depth of anesthesia during the "open airway" phase
- Nerve monitoring for recurrent laryngeal nerves (either a special endotracheal tube with vocal cord movement sensors or thyroid cartilage electrodes)
- Neuromuscular monitoring
- Invasive blood pressure monitoring, in case of patients with critically obstructed airways or severe/poorly controlled comorbidities
- Central line insertion is usually not required unless the patient carries severe or poorly controlled cardiac comorbidities. Either subclavian or femoral veins are cannulated.
- In case of a critically obstructed airway, preparation for venovenous cardiopulmonary bypass (CPB) is done electively.

BOX 2: Preparation of the operation theater.

For cross-field ventilation:
- Adequate size endotracheal tubes, sufficient to pass by the side of the lesion into distal airway (4.0 mm × 6.5 mm)
- Microlaryngeal tubes for delivering ventilation distal to the obstructive lesion (5F, 5.5F, and 6.0F)
- Small-sized flexometallic tubes for endobronchial placement during cross-field ventilation (in carinal resection) (28F, 30F, 32F, 34F, and 36F)
- A sterile breathing circuit with appropriate connectors such as catheter mount/angle piece
- A sterile camera cover sheath to cover the breathing circuit in surgical field
- An infusion pump for total intravenous anesthesia delivery

For apneic oxygenation/jet ventilation:
- A sterile bougie/endobronchial blocker tube/suction catheter
- Auxiliary flow meter with oxygen flow tubing
- High-flow oxygen delivery circuit
- Manual jet ventilator
- HFJ ventilator
- Narrow-caliber catheter or bougie
- Hunsaker's tube

For nonintubated oxygenation technique:
- Adequate size second-generation laryngeal mask airway
- An infusion pump for total intravenous anesthesia delivery
- BIS monitor
- Neuromuscular monitor
- Additionally, all preparation for emergency cross-field ventilation

Additional equipment:
- Rigid bronchoscope (in case of intrathoracic obstructive lesions)
- Adult and pediatric bronchoscope (5.2 mm ED and 3.8 mm ED)

(BIS: bispectral index; HFJ: high-frequency jet)

INDUCTION OF ANESTHESIA AND AIRWAY MANAGEMENT PLAN

It is crucial to carefully decide on the plan for anesthesia induction and airway management. Findings from a recent bronchoscopy help in this decision. Depending on the nature of the airway obstruction and the location of the lesion, the strategy for anesthesia induction and airway management can be planned.

The schematic algorithm for anesthesia induction and airway management is shown in **Flowchart 1**.

Awake versus Asleep Airway Management

Awake airway management is performed in critically obstructive lesions in the lower trachea. Dynamic intrathoracic obstructions get worse on positive-pressure ventilation. Hence, awake airway management prevents the collapse of the intrathoracic airway by maintaining spontaneous breathing throughout the airway management. The risk involved in this approach is sudden airway obstruction when the bronchoscope is passed through the narrow lumen of the airway beside the lesion ("a cork-in-the-bottle" effect). The patient can become hypoxic, and the operator can lose the cooperation of the patient. Also, during awake airway management, excellent topical anesthesia of the oropharyngeal and tracheal mucosa is essential. The "spray as you go" (SAYGO) technique can be employed during bronchoscopy. Also, the airway can be managed in a sitting position in patients who cannot lie supine.

In nonobstructive lesions, the airway can be managed following the anesthesia induction with intravenous agents and muscle relaxants.

Keeping the Tube above the Lesion or Passing Beyond it

The endotracheal tube is passed beyond the lesion for upper tracheal lesions, and it is kept above the lesion for lower tracheal lesions.

Passage of the tube beyond the lesion must always be done using a fiberoptic bronchoscope. Vascular lesions bleed at times, leading to the passage of blood clots into the distal airway. In such cases, care should be taken to use a small endotracheal tube to avoid abrasion with the lesion. In case of airway bleed, the endotracheal tube should be quickly passed beyond the lesion, and the cuff should be inflated to avoid aspiration of blood clots. Trendelenburg position should be given to allow gravitational drainage of blood into the proximal trachea. A cryoprobe or electrocautery and adrenaline–saline washes are used to control the bleeding in the airway.

When the endotracheal tube is positioned above the lesion, ventilation settings should be adjusted to allow high peak airway pressure, low tidal volume, and low ratio of inspiration to expiration. It allows exhalation to complete and prevents auto-PEEP generation.

When the endotracheal tube is positioned beyond the lesion, care should be taken to avoid endobronchial intubation. Also, the endotracheal tube needs to be withdrawn when the surgeon cuts open the trachea.

Flowchart 1: Plan for anesthesia induction and airway management in tracheal resection.

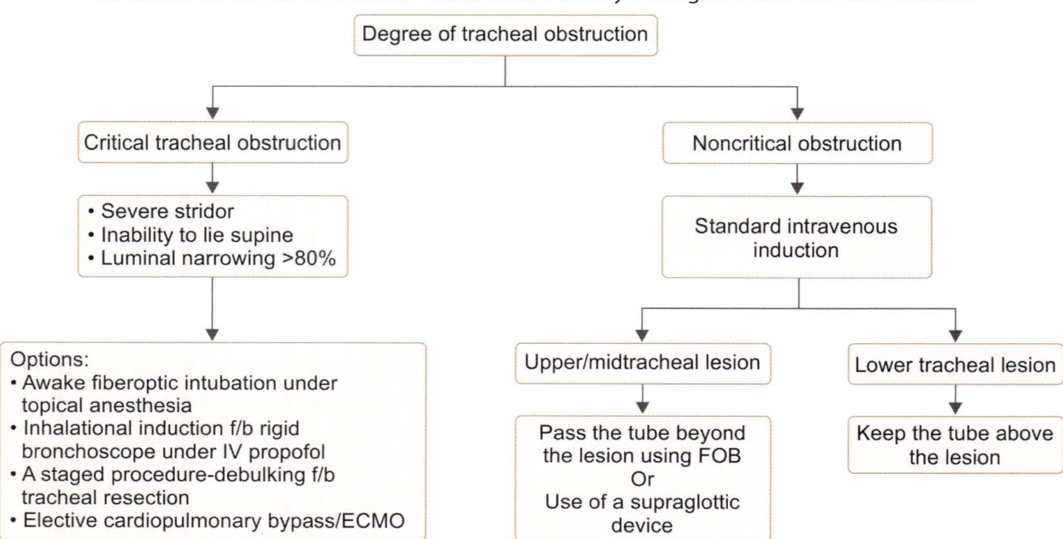

(ECMO: extracorporeal membrane oxygenation; FOB: fiberoptic bronchoscope; f/b: followed by)

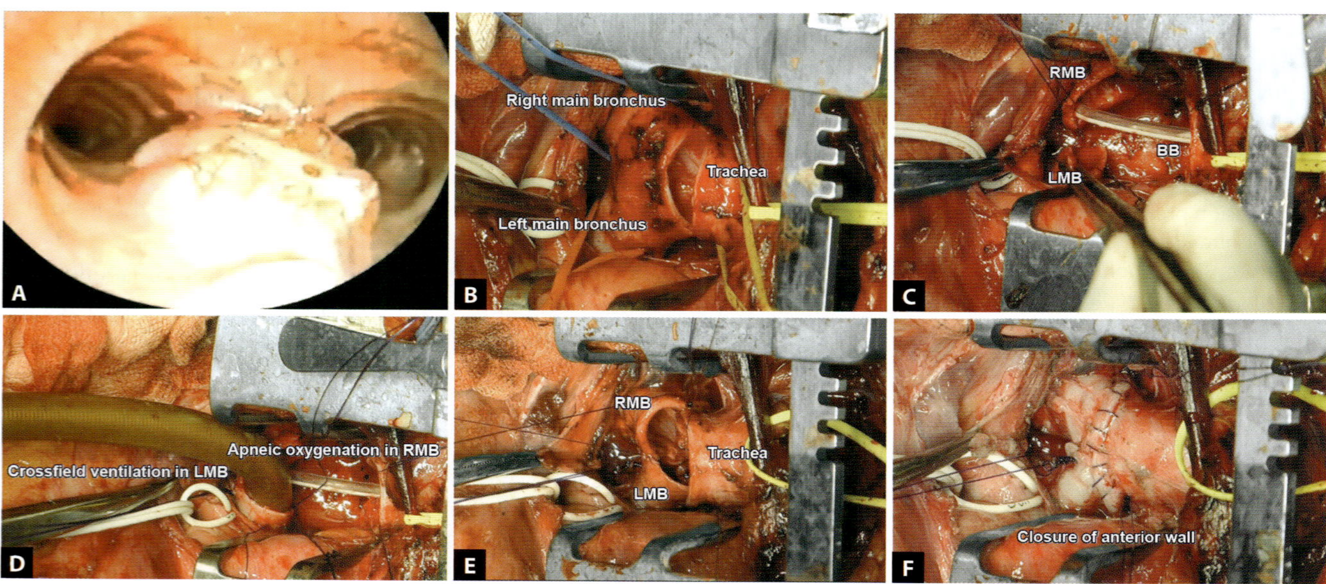

Figs. 1A to F: Steps in carinal resection. (A) Tracheal tumor at the lower end of the trachea; (B) Opening of the trachea; (C) Apneic oxygenation through a bronchial blocker inserted in the right main bronchus; (D) Cross-field ventilation using an armored tube in the left main bronchus. Also note that the apneic oxygenation of the right lung is continued through a bronchial blocker; (E) Closure of the posterior tracheal wall; (F) After complete closure of trachea and bronchi.

SURGICAL STEPS IN TRACHEAL RESECTION AND ANESTHESIA IMPLICATIONS (SEE FIGS. 1A TO F)

The surgical approach to tracheal resection depends on the location of the lesion and the extent of the resection. For the upper tracheal lesions, the cervical approach is employed. A laryngectomy with upper tracheal resection may be required for malignant lesions in the subglottic region. For mid-tracheal lesions, the cervical approach may require additional partial median sternotomy to access the anterior carina and tracheobronchial junctions. Laryngeal drop is an additional procedure to avoid the stress at the anastomosis. For isolated lower tracheal or carinal resection, median sternotomy is performed. However, for carinal resection, which involves additional resection of pulmonary parenchyma, posterolateral thoracotomy or a clamshell incision is preferred.

The information about how much trachea can be resected without tension at the anastomotic site varies in the literature. Grillo et al. showed in the cadaveric studies that up to 4.5 cm of the trachea, i.e., approximately seven tracheal rings, can be resected and anastomosed without compromising blood supply and the tension across the suture line. Adult patients can have up to 50% of the trachea resected. However, it must be remembered that postoperative anastomotic complications increase significantly when resections exceed 4 cm in length.[2] In pediatric patients, approximately 30% of tracheal length can be resected.[3]

Tracheal resection surgery has three phases: Dissection, mobilization and resection, and anastomosis. The first phase involves dissecting important mediastinal structures such as the superior vena cava, pericardium, and vagus and phrenic nerves. Arrhythmias and hemodynamic instability are likely during this phase of the surgery. Invasive arterial blood pressure monitoring and adequate vascular access (especially on the lower limb, considering the risk of injury to the superior vena cava) are essential during this phase. Blood supply to the trachea is segmental, with blood vessels entering from the lateral wall. Hence, anteroposterior dissection avoids vascular compromise.

Tracheal cuts are always taken under bronchoscopic guidance. Before the tracheal cuts, inhalational anesthetic is turned off, and the lungs are ventilated with 100% oxygen to increase oxygen reserve. It helps to increase the apnea time after the trachea is open. The depth of anesthesia is maintained by intravenous infusion of injection propofol and is monitored using the BIS. The endotracheal tube cuff is deflated, and the tracheal tube is withdrawn proximally under direct vision through the open trachea. Cross-field ventilation or apneic oxygenation is instituted to maintain the oxygenation. Thorough suction in the surgical field prevents the aspiration of blood clots into the distal airway. The resected segment is sent to the histopathology laboratory to ensure the disease-free margins.

The two ends of the trachea are mobilized adequately to achieve tension-free anastomosis. Anastomosis of the trachea's posterior walls requires removal of the endotracheal tube. Oxygen saturation is carefully monitored during the apneic period, and cross-field ventilation is resumed when it drops to 90%. The purpose of ventilation is not only to regain oxygenation but also to achieve decarboxylation. During the carinal resection, the lungs are ventilated by passing two small-sized endotracheal tubes into each bronchus. Care should be taken to avoid volutrauma and barotrauma to the lungs. Good communication between the surgical and anesthesia teams is essential during this period.

Once the posterior and lateral walls are anastomosed, ventilation is resumed using the endotracheal tube in the proximal trachea and the anterior wall is closed. Water-tight anastomosis is ensured. The position of the endotracheal tube is adjusted to avoid the presence of a cuff at the anastomotic line.

INTRAOPERATIVE VENTILATION STRATEGIES DURING TRACHEAL RESECTION

During the surgery, conventional positive-pressure ventilation continues till the time the trachea is cut open by the surgeon. After tracheotomy, ventilation into the distal airway is carried out by one of the following different methods, namely:

- Crossfield ventilation
- Apneic oxygenation
- Jet ventilation
- Spontaneous breathing
- Extracorporeal membrane oxygenation (ECMO)/ cardiopulmonary bypass (CPB)

A schematic representation of some of these methods is shown in **Figure 2**. It is important to note the benefits and disadvantages of each method and then choose a method or combination of two methods to achieve the desired outcomes. **Figure 2** combines a few photographs showing the intraoperative ventilation strategies used in a case of carinal resection. The choice of intraoperative ventilation strategy depends on the operator's expertise, the lesion's anatomy, the patient's physiology, and equipment availability.

Crossfield Ventilation

Crossfield ventilation is the most employed technique for intraoperative ventilation. The surgeon inserts a sterile tube into the distal end of the trachea and connects it to the

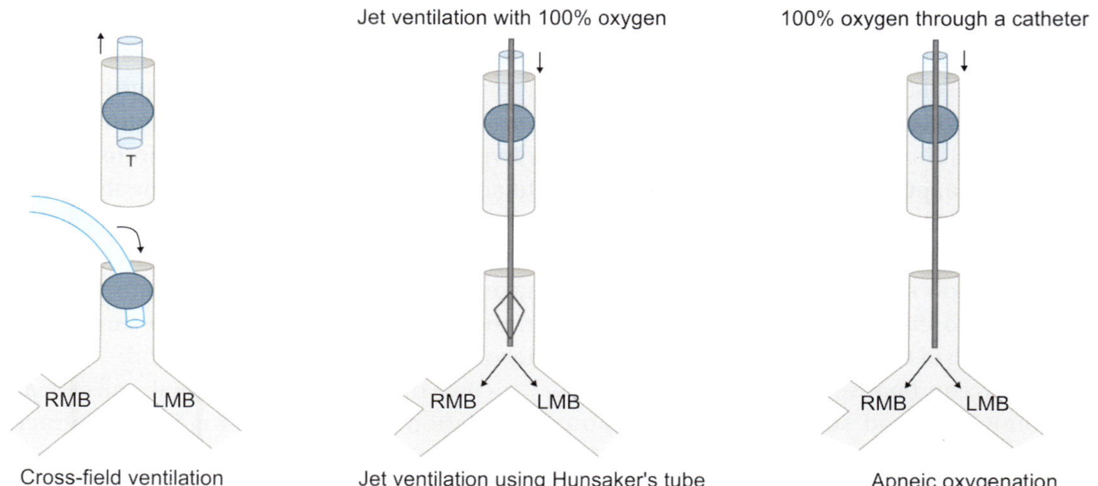

Fig. 2: A schematic representation of intraoperative ventilation and oxygenation strategies during tracheal resection.

breathing circuit to resume positive-pressure ventilation. During carinal resection, two small-sized endotracheal tubes are inserted into two bronchi. Ventilation is alternated with intermittent apnea, during which the tube is removed to facilitate the closure of the posterior and anterior walls of the tracheal ends. Oxygen saturation is closely monitored, and ventilation is resumed as soon as the oxygen saturation drops below a critical level of 90%. The advantage of this technique is that oxygenation and decarboxylation are taken care of by intermittent ventilation. The disadvantages of this technique are multiple interruptions in the surgical work and the possibility of a breach of sterility of the surgical field.

Apneic Oxygenation

This technique involves the continuous flow of oxygen into the lungs so that oxygenation is maintained during the period of apnea. The flow of oxygen is facilitated through a small catheter connected to an oxygen flowmeter. High flow rates (15–30 L/min) help in gas exchange and provide continuous positive pressure to prevent the collapse of the lung, thus prolonging the period of apnea. Also, a small caliber of the catheter helps the surgeon to work around the catheter and minimize interruptions in the surgical work. The disadvantages of this technique are hypercarbia and interference with the use of the cautery due to high oxygen concentration in the surgical field.

Jet Ventilation

In-flow of oxygen can also be achieved using a manual or automated jet ventilator device. Intermittent jets of pressurized gas (100–250 kPa) are administered at a low (10/min) or high frequency (75–400/min) using a manual or automated jet ventilator. During high-frequency jet ventilation (HFJV), inspiration time, frequency and driving pressure are adjusted on the ventilator to deliver low tidal volumes (2 mL/kg) at 75–400 breaths per minute. Gas transfer is achieved through various mechanisms such as Taylor's dispersion or pendelluft phenomenon. Exhalation is passive. Jet ventilation is delivered through a sturdy catheter or a specialized tube-like Hunsaker's tube to prevent the "whiplash" effect of the distal tip of the catheter. Jet ventilation provides a stable surgical field, achieves oxygenation, and requires minimal interruptions in the surgical procedure. However, it may lead to splashing of blood and secretions in the surgical field. Also, there is a possibility of barotrauma and hypercarbia during jet ventilation.[4]

Nonintubated Spontaneous Breathing

In this technique, the patient is either conscious or sedated, but spontaneous breathing is maintained throughout the surgery. It is a relatively new technique employed in patients with cervical tracheal resection. Various regional analgesic techniques, like a cervical epidural or superficial cervical plexus block, are performed to provide analgesia at the surgical site. Additionally, surgeons perform vagal nerve block or topical anesthesia at the trachea-bronchial mucosa to prevent coughing and bucking. Neuromuscular blockers are avoided. As the patient breathes spontaneously, ambient air is sucked into the distal end of the open airway, which helps in oxygenation and decarboxylation. The flow of oxygen in the surgical field can enrich the oxygen content of inspired air. Depth of anesthesia is maintained by intravenous infusion of anesthetic agents like propofol. Respiratory depression due to the use of an anesthetic agent may lead to alveolar hypoventilation, resulting in desaturation and hypercarbia. Careful monitoring of oxygen saturation, respiratory rate, depth of anesthesia (by the BIS monitor), and hemodynamic parameters is required to ensure the safety of the patient. All the preparation for the conversion to general anesthesia with controlled ventilation should be ready as it may be necessary to manage critical desaturation. The advantage of this technique is that surgical work is not interrupted. Also, the lack of neuromuscular blockers allows intraoperative recurrent laryngeal nerve monitoring. Airway instrumentation is avoided. Spontaneous breathing rules out ventilation-induced lung injury, helping in reducing postoperative pulmonary complications and hospital stay. Periods of apnea are minimized, which reduces the re-expansion and reperfusion injury to the lungs and pulmonary vasculature. Disadvantages of the technique are the possibility of critical desaturation, hypercarbia, bucking, and coughing. Also, the positive-pressure leak test cannot be performed at the end of the anastomosis. Contraindications for this approach include ASA 3 patients, reactive airway disease, obesity, poorly compliant lungs, and difficult upper airway. This technique is still new and requires more evidence for its application. There have been many case reports and case series where nonintubated tracheal resections have been performed in spontaneously breathing patients.[5-7]

Cardiopulmonary Bypass or Extracorporeal Membrane Oxygenation

Cardiopulmonary bypass or ECMO is applied in critically obstructed airways (where a rigid bronchoscope cannot be negotiated beyond the lesion) and in conditions where the pathology is closely related to cardiac structures. Additional indications include tracheal surgeries in infants and major tracheobronchial injuries. It is always an elective option where vascular catheters are inserted before anesthesia induction. Veno-venous or veno-arterial catheters are employed in this option. ECMO is preferred over CPB as it requires less heparinization [activated clotting time (ACT) 150–180 seconds] than CPB (ACT450–480 seconds). Additionally, ECMO can be performed using peripheral cannulas as well. Disadvantages of ECMO include systemic heparinization and cost.[8]

EXTUBATION AND POSTOPERATIVE CARE

It is the best practice to extubate the trachea following the resection anastomosis if the patient is warm and awake. Continuing postoperative ventilation carries many disadvantages, such as the requirement of sedation in the postoperative period, the possibility of migration of the endotracheal tube across the anastomosis, endobronchial intubation and resultant desaturation, and anastomotic dehiscence due to positive-pressure ventilation. It is important to avoid excessive movement of the neck at the time of recovery from anesthesia. Adequate analgesia and reversal of neuromuscular blockade facilitate smooth emergence from anesthesia. Many surgeons use a "mental stitch" to maintain the flexion attitude of the neck and prevent neck extension. The patient is encouraged to start enteral nutrition if there are no concerns about recurrent laryngeal nerve injury. In case of concerns about vocal cord dysfunction, feeding is resumed through Ryle's tube. There is no need to continue the postoperative antibiotics. Multimodal analgesia is offered using a combination of paracetamol, nonsteroidal anti-inflammatory drugs (NSAIDs), and regional blocks such as superficial cervical plexus block.

POSTOPERATIVE COMPLICATIONS

Tracheal resection is a complex surgery that requires careful patient selection and meticulous surgical skills. Despite the improvements in the surgical skills, morbidity of the surgical procedure remains between 9 and 45% and mortality between 0 and 5%.[9-16]

Postoperative complications following tracheal resection surgeries are described in the following text.

Anastomotic Leak

Anastomotic leak is a dangerous and life-threatening complication following the tracheal resection. Post-operative mortality has been reported to be significantly high after anastomotic complications as compared to other complications following tracheal surgery. Risk factors for anastomotic leak include comorbidities of patient (e.g., long-standing and poorly controlled diabetes mellitus), infection, previous tracheobronchial irradiation, resection of the longer tracheal segment resulting in tension at the suture line, and laryngotracheal resection. It usually occurs in within days to the first 2 weeks after the surgery. The presenting symptoms and signs include cough, hemoptysis, subcutaneous emphysema, air leak in the intercostal drain, and stridor. Surgical re-exploration and stabilization of the airway should be the priority in such situations. Small defects can be buttressed with vascularized tissue grafts. Other management includes antibiotics, control of blood sugar, drainage of infectious collections, and neck flexion. Hyperbaric oxygen treatment may improve surgical healing.

Tracheal Stenosis

Tracheal strictures and restenosis occur weeks and months after the tracheal resection and have an insidious onset. Patients present with stridor or difficulty in breathing. Postoperative infection, subclinical leak at the suture line, and tension across the suture line are usually the causes of the inflammation at the suture line that results in scar tissue formation. Tracheal strictures are treated with balloon dilatation, insertion of tracheal stents, or re-surgery.

Tracheal Fistula

Trachea-innominate fistula is a devastating complication that carries precipitous mortality. The patient presents with massive hemoptysis and hemodynamic instability. It is often preceded by "sentinel bleed" in the form of minor hemoptysis. Infection and inflammation at the anterior suture line may erode into the innominate artery to create a fistula. Immediate surgical re-exploration with control of the airway is essential.

Trachea-esophageal fistula is relatively rare and is the cause of inflammation at the posterior suture line. Infection and collection of secretions are often the causes, and systemic antibiotics and drainage of collections are required. Surgical exploration to close the fistula may require additional resection of the tracheal segment involved in the fistula.

Recurrent Laryngeal Nerve Palsy

Recurrent laryngeal nerve palsy is a rare surgical complication resulting in unilateral or bilateral vocal cord palsy. The patient presents with a hoarse voice and a weak cough. Bilateral palsy may cause stridor and require a surgical airway. Unilateral palsy improves with time, and any intervention is rarely required.

CONCLUSION

Tracheal resection is challenging for surgical and anesthesia teams as they share and operate upon the airway. Careful airway management and flexible and accommodative ventilation strategies are as essential as meticulous surgical skills during the surgery. Cooperative communication between the two teams is the way to success.

REFERENCES

1. Hartigan PM, Karamnov S, Gill RR, Ng JM, Yacoubian S, Tsukada H, et al. Mediastinal Masses, Anesthetic Interventions, and Airway Compression in Adults: A Prospective Observational Study. Anesthesiology. 2022;136(1):104-14.
2. Wright CD, Grillo HC, Wain JC, Wong DR, Donahue DM, Gaissert HA, et al. Anastomotic complications after tracheal resection: prognostic factors and management. J Thorac Cardiovasc Surg. 2004;128:731-9.
3. Wright CD, Graham BB, Grillo HC, Wain JC, Mathisen DJ. Pediatric tracheal surgery. Ann Thorac Surg 2002;74:308-13; discussion 314.
4. Musil P, Harsanyi S, Torok P, Paulikova M, Moens D, Kalas L, et al. Application and Technical Principles of Catheter High-Frequency Jet Ventilation. Adv Respir Med. 2023;91(4):278-87.
5. Li S, Liu J, He J, Dong Q, Liang L, Cui F, et al. Video-assisted transthoracic surgery resection of a tracheal mass and reconstruction of trachea under non-intubated anesthesia with spontaneous breathing. J Thorac Dis. 2016;8(3):575-85.
6. Jiang L, Liu J, Gonzalez-Rivas D, Shargall Y, Kolb M, Shao W, et al. Thoracoscopic surgery for tracheal and carinal resection and reconstruction under spontaneous ventilation. J Thorac Cardiovasc Surg. 2018;155(6):2746-54.
7. Parab SY, Humane S, Pai P, Karimundackal G. Anaesthesia management of 'tubeless' tracheal resection. Indian J Anaesth. 2022;66(6):471-2.
8. He B, Zhang S, Ren L, Zhou Y, Chen Q, Tang J, et al. Case report: Thyroid carcinoma invading trachea: Multidisciplinary resection and reconstruction assisted by extracorporeal membrane oxygenation. Front Oncol. 2023;12:990600.
9. Amorós JM, Ramos R, Villalonga R, Morera R, Ferrer G, Díaz P. Tracheal and cricotracheal resection for laryngotracheal stenosis: experience in 54 consecutive cases. Eur J Cardiothorac Surg. 2006;29:35-9.
10. Marulli G, Rizzardi G, Bortolotti L, Loy M, Breda C, Hamad AM, et al. Single-staged laryngotracheal resection and reconstruction for benign strictures in adults. Interact Cardiovasc Thorac Surg. 2008;7:227-30; discussion 230.
11. Cordos I, Bolca C, Paleru C, Posea R, Stoica R. Sixty tracheal resections—single center experience. Interact Cardiovasc Thorac Surg. 2009;8:62-5; discussion 65.
12. Krajc T, Janik M, Benej R, Lucenic M, Majer I, Demian J, et al. Urgent segmental resection as the primary strategy in management of benign tracheal stenosis. A single center

experience in 164 consecutive cases. Interact Cardiovasc Thorac Surg. 2009;9:983-9.

13. Mutrie CJ, Eldaif SM, Rutledge CW, Force SD, Grist WJ, Mansour KA, et al. Cervical tracheal resection: New lessons learned. Ann Thorac Surg. 2011;91:1101-6.
14. Bibas BJ, Terra RM, Oliveira AL Jr, Tamagno FL, Minamoto H, Cardoso PFG, et al. Predictors for postoperative complications after tracheal resection. Ann Thorac Surg. 2014; 98:277-82.
15. Piazza C, Del Bon F, Paderno A, Grazioli P, Mangili S, Lombardi D, et al. Complications after tracheal and cricotracheal resection and anastomosis for inflammatory and neoplastic stenoses. Ann Otol Rhinol Laryngol. 2014;123:798-804.
16. D'Andrilli A, Maurizi G, Andreetti C, Ciccone AM, Ibrahim I, Poggi C, et al. Long-term results of laryngotracheal resection for benign stenosis from a series of 109 consecutive patients. Eur J Cardiothorac Surg. 2016;50:105-9.

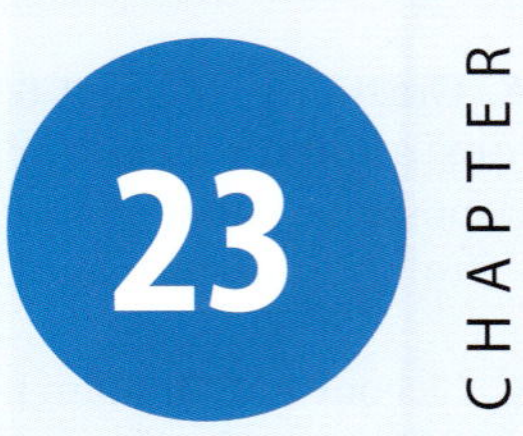

Anesthesia for Interventional Pulmonary Procedures

Bindiya G Salunke

INTRODUCTION

Interventional pulmonology (IP) is a budding subspecialty in pulmonary medicine that is taking the limelight rapidly. The first bronchoscopy was performed by Gustav Killian in the year 1897, for right main stem foreign body retrieval, and in 1968 Ikeda and colleagues introduced the flexible bronchoscope, which has undergone significant advancements since then.[1,2] IP involves minimally invasive procedures and has made the diagnosis and management of complex airway, lung, and pleural diseases possible. The range of procedures has expanded significantly, with interventional pulmonologists now utilizing advanced techniques for both diagnostic and therapeutic purposes, particularly in the management of thoracic malignancies and complex noncancerous conditions, such as chronic obstructive pulmonary disease (COPD) and interstitial lung disease. The significant shift in IP procedure from traditional diagnostic approaches to complex therapeutic interventions such as bronchial thermoplasty, endobronchial stenting, and ablation techniques for airway tumors is made possible with the advancements in technology.[3-5]

Anesthesia is an integral part of these procedures, ensuring patient safety, comfort, and procedural success. Hence, these procedures demand skilled and trained anesthetists due to the complexity of cases, shared airways, and underlying comorbidities of patients, and most of the time these procedures are done in non-operating room (NORA) settings or in intervention radiology suits. Depending on the complexity of the procedure the anesthesia management will change ranging from sedation or monitored anesthesia care (MAC) for simple bronchoscopy procedures to the need for specialized ventilation strategies such as jet ventilation for advanced procedures. Maintaining the oxygenation of a patient along with the adequate depth of anesthesia may become challenging at times in certain situations, such as central airway procedures. Effective collaboration between the anesthesiology and IP teams is vital to navigating shared airway challenges, minimizing risks, and optimizing outcomes.

With advancements in IP, a need for every anesthesiologist to keep updated regarding the planned approach to such patients to optimize patient outcomes and procedural success. This chapter explores the principles, techniques, and innovations in anesthesia for IP procedures, emphasizing patient safety and procedural success.

COMMON INTERVENTIONAL PULMONOLOGY PROCEDURES

Interventional pulmonology procedures can be categorized into diagnostic and therapeutic procedures. Diagnostic procedures are further divided into basic and advanced.[6]

Basic Diagnostic Procedures

These are minimally invasive and can typically be performed under MAC or mild sedation.

- Flexible bronchoscope
- Endobronchial biopsy
- Bronchoalveolar lavage (BAL) or brushing
- Transbronchial biopsy
- Conventional transbronchial needle aspiration (TBNA)

Advanced Diagnostic Procedures

These generally require general anesthesia or deep sedation due to their complexity. Examples include:

- Endobronchial ultrasound (EBUS)
- Cryobiopsy
- Bronchoscopic transparenchymal nodule biopsy

Advanced Therapeutic Procedures

These procedures predominantly involve the use of rigid bronchoscopy and require general anesthesia. Examples include:

- Tracheal stent placement
- Central airway debulking procedures
- Bronchial thermoplasty
- Intrabronchial valve or coil placement
- Bronchoscopic steam ablation

An alternative method to classify anesthesia management is to categorize procedures based on the type of bronchoscopy procedures involved:

- *Rigid bronchoscopy procedures:* These typically require general anesthesia with muscle relaxation to ensure optimal airway control.
- *Flexible bronchoscopy procedures:* These are usually performed under MAC or mild sedation, but some may necessitate deep sedation or general anesthesia based on the complexity of the procedure and the patient's comorbidities.

PREOPERATIVE ASSESSMENT

A comprehensive preoperative evaluation is crucial to minimize risks and ensure the success of interventional pulmonary procedures. These patients often present with significant respiratory and systemic comorbidities, such as COPD, interstitial lung disease, diabetes, and cardiovascular conditions, which add complexity to anesthetic management.

Patient History and Physical Examination

Patient assessment starts from a detailed history and physical examination. History of respiratory symptoms such as dyspnea, stridor, and wheezing, which indicates airway obstruction. A history suggestive of difficult airway for procedure access such as prior surgeries, radiation therapy, and trauma can also affect airway anatomy. Documenting comorbidities such as COPD, interstitial lung disease, or cardiovascular disease is essential, as these conditions often coexist and share common risk factors, particularly smoking. Recognizing these comorbidities is essential, as patients may require additional evaluations and specific investigations to optimize their preoperative condition.

On physical examination, airway examination is an important assessment along with systemic examination. An anesthetist shares the airway of the patient with the pulmonologist during these procedures, and preparing strategies for managing a difficult airway or handling complications is a key aspect of preoperative planning.

Diagnostic Evaluation

In certain situations, may need to evaluate pulmonary function through baseline tests such as forced expiratory volume (FEV1) and forced vital capacity (FVC). These values help assess respiratory reserve and predict the risk of perioperative complications, such as hypoventilation and desaturation.[1] Additionally, imaging studies, including chest X-rays and computed tomography (CT), are very important for identifying location, the extent of airway abnormalities, and proximity and invasion of surrounding structures, especially major vessels and the heart.[7,8] These investigations guide the planning of the procedure, particularly in patients with significant central airway obstruction. Routine blood investigations and cardiovascular assessments, such as electrocardiogram (ECG) and echocardiography, should be performed based on the patient's history to evaluate cardiac function and identify any additional risks.

To assess cardiorespiratory function and identify any additional risks, simple tests like the 6-minute walk test can provide a general understanding of the patient's condition. If the results are unusually low, further evaluation may be needed using stress tests such as dobutamine stress echocardiography, cardiopulmonary exercise testing (CPET), or the Bruce protocol stress test.

PREOPERATIVE OPTIMIZATION

After a preoperative evaluation, optimization is essential to reduce perioperative complications. For patients with obstructive airway disease, bronchodilator therapy can help improve pulmonary function. Additionally, physiotherapy (particularly chest physiotherapy) plays a crucial role in enhancing respiratory mechanics. In specific conditions such as hyperactive airway and repeated airway instrumentation steroid therapy or antibiotic therapy may be indicated.[9] All these interventions help to minimize perioperative complications and reduction of postoperative pulmonary complications.

COLLABORATIVE PLANNING

Finally, effective preoperative preparation depends on close collaboration between the anesthesiology, IP team and also, technical staff, and nursing teams. To ensure smooth execution, a briefing and debriefing session should be conducted for every procedure. This session should include all involved personnel in the procedure room. Detailed discussions should cover the anesthetic plan, the required level of sedation, and strategies for airway and complication management. These discussions ensure that everyone involved is well-informed about the procedure steps and adequately prepared to manage emergencies, such as complete airway obstruction, hypoxia, or severe bleeding. Also, the risk stratification of high-risk patients needs to be done in collaboration as well.

A thorough preoperative evaluation and effective risk management by the anesthesia team can significantly improve patient safety and the success of IP procedures. However, in urgent situations, such as patients with an obstructed airway needing urgent tracheal debulking or cases of foreign body aspiration, there may not be enough time for a full evaluation and an anesthetist may have to proceed with a brief history, physical examination, and available investigations. Similarly, for diagnostic procedures critical to deciding treatment such as in cancer patients and extensive preoperative evaluations, including advanced tests such as stress tests and sleep study may not always be necessary.

ANESTHETIC TECHNIQUES

A comprehensive overview of anesthesia management for interventional pulmonary procedures, emphasizing the importance of patient safety, airway management, sedation techniques, and the management of potential complications. Depending on the complexity of the procedure and patient comorbidities the anesthesia technique will vary, ranging from moderate sedation for diagnostic bronchoscopy to general anesthesia for complex therapeutic interventions, such as rigid bronchoscopy and airway stenting. For further ease let us divide it into flexible fiberoptic bronchoscopy procedures and rigid bronchoscopy procedures. **Table 1** enumerates common IP procedures and anesthesia techniques.

TABLE 1: Common interventional pulmonology procedures and anesthesia techniques.

Interventional pulmonology procedure	*Description of procedure*	*Indications*	*Anesthesia management*	*Special considerations*
FOB	Visualization of an airway with a flexible bronchoscope	• For examination of the airway • Aids in diagnostic evaluation such as BAL, bronchial washing, and TBNA	• Mild to moderate sedation • Topical anesthesia for airway • Oxygen supplementation • Bite block to avoid injury to the bronchoscope	Watch for complications such as apnea, hypopnea, and airway spasms
BAL	FOB-guided saline washing of the lung	Infection, interstitial lung disease, or malignancy	Same as for FOB	Same as above
TBNA	FOB-guided needle biopsy of mediastinal or hilar lymph nodes	For diagnosis or staging of lung cancer or mediastinal lymph node metastasis	• Deep sedation or general anesthesia • TIVA • Airways generally secured via ETT or SGA	In addition to FOB complications, risk of bleeding and pneumothorax
EBUS	Ultrasound guidance for TBNA or biopsy	For diagnosis or staging of lung cancer or mediastinal lymph node biopsy	• Deep sedation or general anesthesia • TIVA • Airways generally secured via ETT or SGA	USG guidance helps in identifying the lymph nodes (better yield) and surrounding major vessels (injury to major vessels can be avoided)
Airway dilation (balloon dilation)	Stenotic areas in the airway are dilated using balloon dilatation	Benign or malignant airway stenosis	General anesthesia, intubation, or SGA	• Compromised airway preprocedure • Rigid bronchoscopy should be available as a standby

Contd...

Contd...

Interventional pulmonology procedure	***Description of procedure***	***Indications***	***Anesthesia management***	***Special considerations***
Tracheobronchial stenting	Insertion of stents into the trachea or bronchi to maintain airway patency	Malignant or benign airway obstruction	General anesthesia, intubation.	• Procedure can be performed using both rigid or flexible bronchoscopes • Compromised airway preprocedure • Risk of stent migration, and bleeding
Bronchial thermoplasty	Application of thermal energy to reduce airway smooth muscle in asthma	Severe, persistent asthma not responsive to medications	General anesthesia, intubation	• Invasive procedure • Risk of airway spasms is high
Thermal ablation techniques (e.g., laser, cryotherapy, electrocautery, or APC)	All these modalities to treat obstructive airway lesions or tumors	Malignant airway obstruction	General anesthesia, intubation, or via rigid bronchoscope	• Risk of airway fire • Risk of hypoxia and bleeding
Rigid broncho-scopy	Use of a rigid bronchoscope for airway intervention	Removal of foreign bodies, massive hemoptysis, stenting, or central airway debulking	• General anesthesia • Muscle relaxation (frequently utilized)	Airway protection and ventilation are critical
Endobronchial valve/coil placement	Insertion of valves or coils to treat severe emphysema or airway collapse	Severe emphysema and atelectasis	General anesthesia, intubation	High-risk procedure requiring close monitoring of ventilation and oxygenation

(APC: argon plasma coagulation; BAL: bronchoalveolar lavage; EBUS: endobronchial ultrasound; ETT: endotracheal tube; FOB: flexible bronchoscopy; SGA: supraglottic airway; TBNA: transbronchial needle aspiration; TIVA: total intravenous anesthesia)

Common anesthetic management in both rigid and flexible bronchoscopy are:

- All the routine American Society of Anesthesiologists (ASA) standard monitors should be attached to patients, sometimes we may need more invasive monitoring such as invasive blood pressure monitoring and cardiac output monitoring in certain high-risk situations (both procedure-wise or patient comorbidity-wise) for both cardiovascular monitoring and for arterial blood gas analysis to evaluate oxygenation and ventilation. When we utilize general anesthesia, especially with muscle relaxants, bispectral index (BIS) monitoring should be used to monitor the depth of anesthesia.[10,11] Capnography is one of the important monitors for early diagnosis of hypoventilation or apnea, however continuous monitoring of chest movement with respiration will always be the best monitoring for spontaneously breathing patients. Transcutaneous carbon dioxide ($PtCO_2$) monitoring helps to assess ventilation in a noninvasive way.
- Follow the routine fasting guidelines as the risk of aspiration is very high during these procedures due to unprotective airway, majority of times.
- *Use of antisialogog:* The American College of Chest Physicians (ACCP) advises against routine use of anticholinergics but its use decreases secretions and makes visualization of the airway easy as well as helps to increase the efficacy of topical anesthesia. However, one should keep in mind that it may result in undesirable side effects, including prolonged dry mouth, tachycardia, and arrhythmia. For better efficacy, it should be administered 30 minutes prior to the procedure.[12]

- Oxygenation preoperatively as well as perioperatively via different modalities ranging from nasal prongs, high-flow nasal cannula (HFNC), jet ventilation, or controlled ventilation.
- Should always avoid using volatile anesthetic agents as these procedures involve frequent airway suctioning and disconnection of anesthesia circuits to allow the introduction of a bronchoscope and this can lead to operating theater (OT) contamination as well as the risk of inadequate depth of anesthesia (not possible to determine the concentration of volatile anesthetic agent administered to the patient).[13,14]

ANESTHESIA FOR FLEXIBLE BRONCHOSCOPY PROCEDURES

Basically, fiberoptic flexible bronchoscopy is utilized for noninvasive procedures such as BAL, bronchial brushing, and dynamic airway examination or for invasive procedures, such as EBUS or TBNA. For both invasive and noninvasive procedures, a topical local anesthetic should be used for airway preparation. For noninvasive procedures, good topical airway anesthesia alone may be sufficient, with mild sedation if needed. However, for invasive procedures, general anesthesia is typically used to minimize complications, ensure patient comfort, and facilitate the pulmonologist's work. Many noninvasive procedures are done without an anesthesiologist unless the patient has some high-risk comorbidities. However, all the ASA-recommended monitors should be attached to a patient while performing these procedures.

Like awake intubation, even while performing flexible bronchoscopy we need to utilize the STOP[15] strategy (sedation, topicalization, oxygenation, and performance) for better results.

If the procedure is planned via a nasal route, a topical nasal vasoconstrictor before nasotracheal intubation is recommended as it reduces the incidence of epistaxis.

Topical Anesthesia

Effective topicalization of the airway with local anesthetics is essential for successful performance and is recommended by the ACCP as it reduces the dose of sedative agents required for patient cooperation and also decreases cough.[16] Lignocaine is the most commonly used local anesthetic. Systemic absorption of the drug is variable when administered by different techniques/delivery systems; however, the maximum dose of topical lignocaine should never exceed 9 mg/kg lean body weight to avoid local anesthetic toxicity. Different techniques utilized for airway topical anesthesia employ the use of lignocaine spray (10% lignocaine), nebulization, transtracheal injection of 4% or 2% lignocaine, or spray as you go (SAYGO) with topical lignocaine. Invasive nerve blocks to block the glossopharyngeal nerve and superior laryngeal nerve are rarely used presently as these blocks give similar results as a topical local anesthetic with lesser complication rates.[17,18]

Sedation Techniques

For flexible bronchoscopy procedures, good patient counseling and reassurance, and some degree of sedation are required for better patient cooperation and satisfaction. Sedation should not affect spontaneous respiration and the cardiovascular system and should be administered with great caution.

Drugs which can be used are:

- Dexmedetomidine is an excellent agent for sedation as it causes anterograde amnesia, anxiolysis, and analgesia with minimal effects on respiration.
- Remifentanyl has a rapid onset and offset of action, anti-tussive action as well as analgesic properties.
- Propofol is also employed for the same purpose by many anesthesiologists but it is best used as a target-controlled infusion as monotherapy or in combination with remifentanil.[19] Even propofol boluses can be employed in short bronchoscopy procedures. Propofol has multiple advantages such as rapid onset and shorter recovery times and decreased reports of postoperative pain, nausea, and breathlessness, however, it has a narrow therapeutic window resulting in respiratory depression, apnea, and cardiovascular compromise. This is the main reason that propofol should always be administered by a certified anesthesia provider and not by a proceduralist. Short-acting benzodiazepines such as midazolam alone and in combination with an opioid is also one of the commonly used modalities.
- Ketamine in combination with midazolam or propofol is also an effective alternative.

A good balance with diligent titration of these sedation agents ensures adequate sedation and anxiolysis as well as maintaining spontaneous ventilation. Noninvasive FOBs are generally performed under mild sedation with good topical airway preparation. For dynamic flexible bronchoscopy, where forced inspiration and expiration are needed to be performed by the patient, minimal sedation with midazolam or fentanyl just adequate to minimize the patient's anxiety is advisable. Similarly, for BAL and bronchial lavage minimal sedation with anxiolysis is advisable.

However, for invasive bronchoscopy procedures such as EBUS and TBNA generally require moderate to deep sedation or general anesthesia. The method of sedation should be individualized depending on the operator's experience, patient comorbidities, and duration of the procedure. Infusion of propofol along with additional boluses of short-acting opioids is used as common practice.[20,14]

Ventilation and Oxygenation

As mentioned above selected procedures can be done under minimal sedation in spontaneously breathing patients without securing the airway. Oxygenation with nasal prongs or humidified high-flow nasal oxygen (HFNO) (40–60 L/min) and bite block to avoid damage to the bronchoscopy is mostly sufficient in such short procedures. The advantage of HFNO is that along with maintaining the oxygenation of patients, it also prevents hypercapnia. Sometimes when bronchoscopy is required in patients with respiratory failure, especially for BAL or bronchial lavage, positive pressure ventilation is provided via resuscitation face mask or special mask called the *Janus mask* (Biomedical Srl, Florence, Italy) while bronchoscopy is performed.[21]

For invasive bronchoscopy procedures where deep sedation or general anesthesia is desired, it is always advisable to secure the airway with either supraglottic devices or an endotracheal tube. A laryngeal mask airway, especially an I-gel of size 4 is preferred over an endotracheal tube due to multiple advantages over endotracheal tube (ETT) like the ease of placement without much stimulation, it is incorporated with bite block (I-gel) and allows evaluation of high tracheal lesions like sampling of high-level, i.e., station 2 of mediastinal lymph nodes. The I-gel size 4 allows easy passage of the bronchoscope (external diameter = 5.9 mm) as well as EBUS scope (external diameter = 6.9 mm) and also ETT (external diameter = up to 7 mm) as it has an internal diameter of 12.3 mm.[14] ETT placement is recommended in certain situations like the placement of SGA is difficult, patient has severe gastroesophageal reflux or in the anticipated difficult airway. The appropriate size of ETT should be selected according to the size of a bronchoscope.

A patient can be kept on spontaneous ventilation or positive pressure ventilation depending on the need of the procedure. Only in certain situations such as apnea, desaturation, hypercapnia, and hypoxia, does a patient need positive pressure ventilation.

ANESTHESIA FOR RIGID BRONCHOSCOPY

The rigid bronchoscope is made up of a hollow metal tube with a distal beveled fenestrated end and a proximal end with three openings for an optical device, a port for ventilation, and a working channel. Its size can vary from a diameter of 3–14 mm and length of usually 43 cm for bronchoscope and 33 cm for tracheoscope. Rigid bronchoscopy is an advanced and invasive procedure that presents challenges to anesthesiologists to facilitate airway intervention while maintaining ventilation and oxygenation.[22]

Rigid bronchoscopy is employed to bypass an obstruction in situations of anterior mediastinal mass or in procedures that require a large working channel, such as foreign body removal, mechanical dilatation of the central airway, airway stent placement, and central airway lesion debulking.

Pharmacological Anesthesia Management

General anesthesia with muscle relaxants is typically required for these procedures. Here the introduction of the rigid scope requires good muscle relaxation for less airway trauma and to avoid patient movement as well as for a better field for the pulmonologist. It is advisable to use BIS in these patients to ensure adequate depth of anesthesia while utilizing TIVA. Another important aspect with the use of muscle relaxants is that it should be administered only after confirming that the ventilation is possible and visible chest rise is seen. Additional boluses of propofol may be needed during placement of scope and during airway manipulation. The use of opioids to decrease postprocedure pain, decreases the cardiovascular responses to the procedure as well as decreases the requirement of propofol. Confirmation of adequate muscle relaxation reversal at the end of the procedure with neuromuscular monitoring is advisable as patients who undergo rigid bronchoscopy have decreased pulmonary reserve and they cannot tolerate residual paralysis.[23]

Ventilation and Oxygenation

It is a difficult task to ventilate and maintain oxygenation for a patient needing rigid bronchoscopy. Here a hollow metal tube is inserted in the central airway of a patient which acts as a sole conduit for oxygenation as well as a working channel for pulmonologists. Also, a rigid bronchoscope cannot give a perfect seal with the trachea and there is a huge air leakage around the scope. Ideally, the breathing circuit is connected to the port provided at the proximal end of the bronchoscope, and the patient is ventilated by packing the oropharynx with gauze and external manipulation on the trachea to minimize the leak around the scope. There are different ventilation strategies employed with rigid bronchoscopes including apneic oxygenation, spontaneous-assisted ventilation, controlled mechanical ventilation, and jet ventilation.[24]

- Apneic ventilation is a very commonly employed approach that includes ventilating patients with 100% FiO_2 by occluding the working channel, followed by stopping ventilation to allow pulmonologist to perform their procedure via the working channel. While monitoring the oxygen saturation of the patient. As soon as the patient's oxygen saturation drops to a certain predecided level (around 92%), the procedure is halted, and the patient is ventilated with 100% oxygen till the patient's oxygen saturation is 100% and end-tidal carbon dioxide ($ETCO_2$) is within normal range. Once the oxygenation improves, again the procedure is restarted till further desaturation and this cycle will repeat till the procedure is completed.[24] The disadvantages of this strategy of ventilation are that it leads to cardiovascular instability, acid–base disturbances as well as increased procedure duration due to multiple breaks for ventilation intermittently.
- Another ventilation strategy is spontaneous-assisted ventilation. Here the patient is maintained on spontaneous ventilation with 100% oxygen via a breathing circuit being connected to the rigid bronchoscope and respiratory support is provided as needed. However, this strategy of ventilation is associated with increased incidences of coughing, laryngospasm, higher incidence of desaturation, awareness as well as airway trauma in comparison to controlled ventilation.[25]
- Another ventilation strategy is controlled ventilation, here the patient is given positive pressure ventilation via the rigid bronchoscope throughout the procedure. To achieve this Silastic caps are used on the ports of the rigid scope and oropharyngeal packing with a throat pack around the rigid bronchoscope is done to minimize air leaks. The major disadvantages of this strategy are circuit leaks and hypoxia.
- Jet ventilation is the most commonly utilized strategy of ventilation in rigid bronchoscopy procedures. Here a high-pressure gas is applied in short bursts to an open airway which helps to achieve high FiO_2 via the Venturi principle. The greatest advantage of this strategy is that it delivers oxygen in rapid, low-tidal-volume bursts, ensuring adequate ventilation with minimal interruptions in procedure and good technical access.[26] There are two modes of jet ventilation available are manual jet ventilation and mechanical jet ventilation as high-frequency jet ventilation (HFJV) (120–600 respirations/min) or low-frequency jet ventilation (LFJV) (10–30 respirations/min).[26] The manual jet ventilation utilizes a handheld valve connected to 100% oxygen with a pressure limiting device which allows gas to be delivered to a patient at 50 psi or less. However, despite of all the advantages, a patient on jet ventilation needs to be monitored closely to avoid complications, such as barotrauma, air trapping, and hypercapnia. Respiratory rate, duration of breath, and driving pressure are decided by the anesthetist which usually is 10–14 breaths/min of respiratory rate with 30–40% of inspiration duration. This ventilation setting with a limitation of driving pressure of around 20 PSI is recommended for prevention of barotrauma and auto-positive end-expiratory pressure (auto-PEEP).[27] Continuous monitoring of chest rise and oxygen saturation will guide the adequacy of ventilation and oxygenation. PCO_2 monitoring either with repeated arterial blood gas measurements during the procedure or by transcutaneous capnographic monitoring can also guide the adequacy of ventilation.
- *Extracorporeal membrane oxygenation (ECMO):* ECMO is another alternative used in critically obstructed central airway management when the risk of cardiorespiratory arrest is very high. However, the establishment of vascular assessment and setting of an ECMO machine requires significant time. Hence, patients who are likely to require ECMO should be identified as preprocedure, and cannulation should be performed before proceeding with the airway intervention.[28,29]
  - Once the procedure is completed, the patient's respiration is supported till complete recovery from neuromuscular blocking agents and sedation. This can be achieved by face mask ventilation or the use of a supraglottic airway device, especially laryngeal mask airway (LMA). LMA is preferred as along with

providing respiratory support, it also allows airway and vocal cord inspection with FOB if needed. In the recovery phase, the head-up position with supplemental oxygen, especially with HFNO is commonly utilized to decrease respiratory distress and coughing.

SPECIAL SITUATIONS

- *Thermal ablation techniques (e.g., laser, cryotherapy, electrocautery, or argon plasma coagulation):* The use of laser or electrocautery or argon plasma coagulation (APC) needs to consider certain specific interventions to avoid catastrophic complications, which is airway fire. However, the use of APC is less likely to cause airway fire as argon displaces oxygen away during use. As well known, a combination of three components is required for fire to occur and that is an ignitor (a heat-based surgical device such as a laser or electrocautery), an oxidizer (oxygen or nitrous oxide), and fuel (tissue, mesh, or plastic devices).[30] Therefore, it is recommended to keep low FiO_2 with end-tidal O_2 be below 40% and avoid the use of nitrous oxide whenever laser, electrocautery, or APC systems are activated.[31] Another maneuver is to keep an adequate distance of these probes from the tip of the bronchoscope (minimum 1 cm) and the tip of ETT (minimum 4 cm), this will help to decrease exposure to oxygen. Also, the use of gauze or cotton as a throat pack should be avoided as well as the clearing of charred tissue must be done frequently as it can act as fuel for fire.[30] **Figures 1A to C** display the airway patency post-debulking procedure.
- Argon gas embolization is another life-threatening complication associated with APC use and prevention of this with the use of low flow of argon gas as well as avoiding direct contact with vessels is recommended as a preventive measure.[32]
- The use of cryotherapy is very abundant similar to the use of electrocautery and laser in debulking of airway tumors. This method does not pause a risk for airway fire but is associated with pneumothorax and hypoxia due to the rapid conversion of liquid nitrous oxide to gaseous form. Hence, preoxygenation with 100% oxygen, holding ventilation during its use, and allowing free expiration can act as preventive measures.[33] It is also known to cause airway bleeding during the debulking of the airway as it tears the tissue, so the use of cold saline, adrenaline saline, or using a Fogarty catheter or bronchial blocker to cause tamponade effect are few measures to overcome this situation.
- *Balloon bronchoplasty:* This technique utilizes navigation of a silicone balloon using FOB or rigid

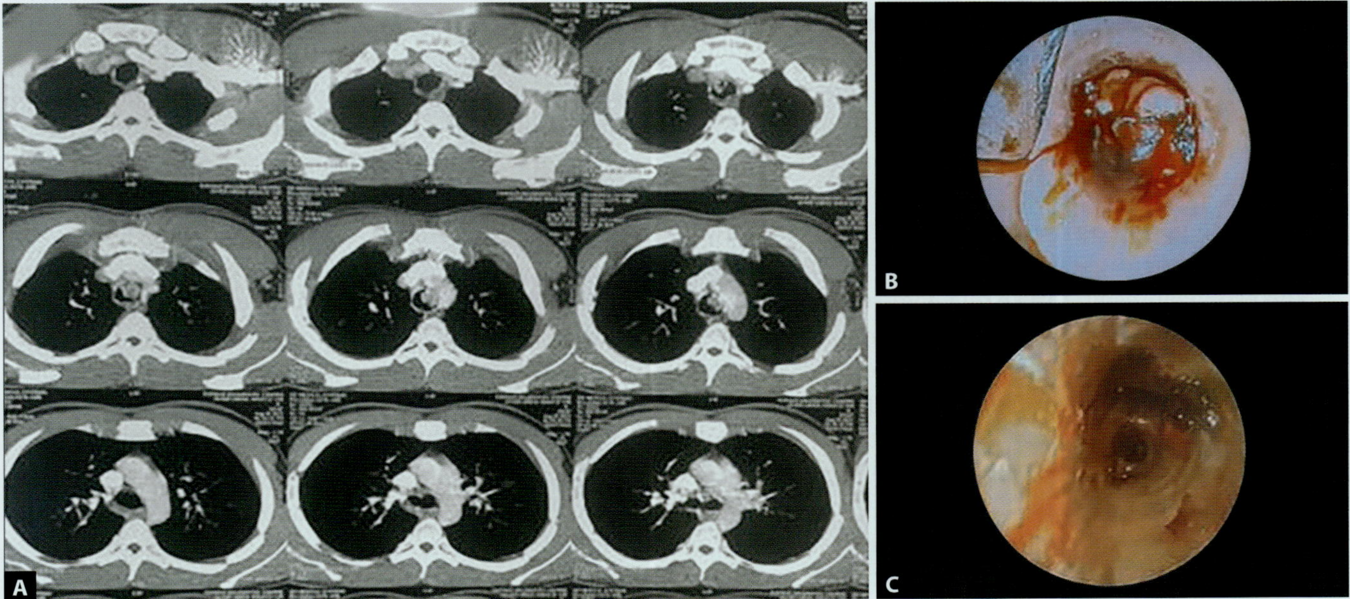

Figs. 1A to C: A patient scheduled for tracheal debulking. (A) Computed tomography (CT) scan showing an intratracheal lesion; (B) Preprocedure bronchoscopic view of the lesion; and (C) Postdebulking bronchoscopic view showing a clear distal view of the carina and main bronchi.

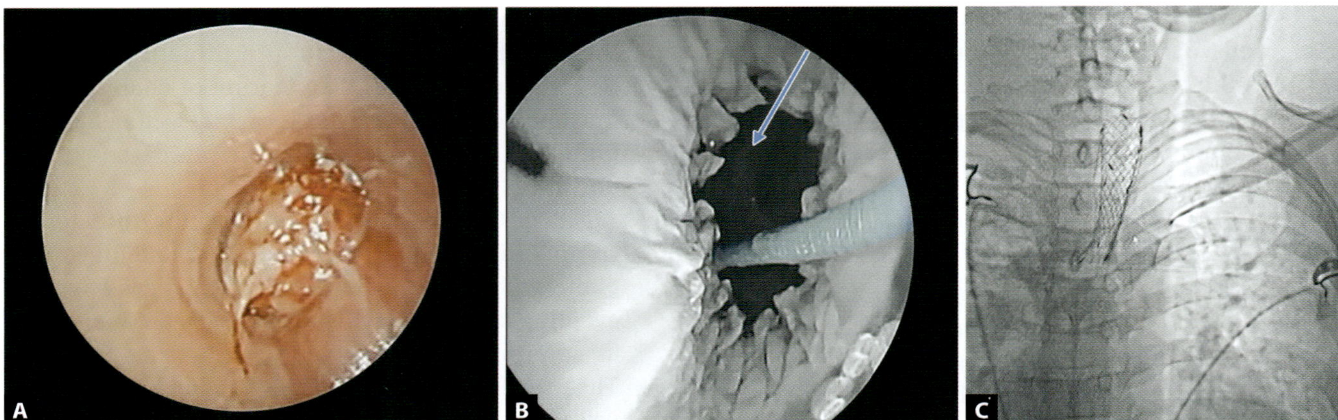

Figs. 2A to C: Near-complete obstruction of the trachea scheduled for tracheal stenting. (A) Presenting bronchoscopic view of the lesion; (B) Poststenting bronchoscopic view showing the stent in place, with the arrow pointing towards the patent primary carina; and (C) Postprocedure X-ray showing the stent in situ.

bronchoscopy into a stenotic region, followed by incremental and pressurized inflation to treat tracheal stenosis. Airway rupture, bleeding airway spasm, tracheitis, and pneumomediastinum are complications seen with this technique.[34]

- *Airway stent:* Stenting of a central airway with metal or silicon stents is another option especially with malignancy and palliative patients to relieve airway obstruction. Placement of silicon stent requires rigid bronchoscopy, whereas metal stent can be deployed FOB guided under fluoroscopy. The patient warrants general anesthesia for the precision of stent placement and to avoid coughing and displacement of a stent. Stent migration, stent obstruction, pneumothorax, and dissemination of postobstructive pneumonia are a few specific complications with airway stents. Chronically placed stents can present with fistula formation with adjacent structures, such as broncho vascular fistula and esophagorespiratory fistula. **Figures 2A to C** show the airway before and after airway stenting.
- *Bronchial thermoplasty* is a technique utilized in the treatment for difficult-to-treat asthma. Here, controlled radiofrequency energy is applied to the airway wall, leading to a reduction in airway smooth muscle mass and eventually increasing airflow.[35]
- *Endobronchial valves:* This technique is used in the treatment of severe emphysema and asthma as an alternative to lung volume reduction surgery. Here, a one-way valve is placed bronchoscopically in segmental or subsegmental bronchi thereby restricting flow during inspiration and allowing passive exhalation and secretion clearance. The endobronchial valves have also been used in the management of persistent postoperative leaks. This procedure is associated with complications, such as bronchospasm, COPD exacerbation, pneumothorax, and valve migration.[36,37]

COMPLICATIONS AND MANAGEMENT

Diagnostic interventional pulmonary procedures are generally safe with very low complication rates whereas certain therapeutic procedures and anesthetic techniques may cause certain complications which are listed further. To ensure patient safety, early recognition and management of these complications are very important to avoid severe morbidity and mortality. **Table 2** enumerates the common complications during interventional pulmonology procedures.

Airway Complications

Trauma to the patient's airway such as injury to dentures, vocal cord trauma, and tracheal or bronchial perforation can be seen in rigid bronchoscopy and is more likely in inexperienced pulmonologists or if patient movement or coughing occurs during the procedure.

Airway compromise like complete airway obstruction can occur in patients with central airway lesions after administration of sedation and anesthesia. Adequate preoxygenation of patients and employing apneic oxygenation strategies, especially jet ventilation are very effective in overcoming this complication.

TABLE 2: Complications and risk management in interventional pulmonology procedures.

Complication	*Interventional pulmonology procedure*	*Risk factors*	*Prevention strategies*	*Management*
Airway obstruction	All procedures	Obesity, difficult anatomy, deeper depth of sedation	Ensure titrated sedation, Identify difficult airway preprocedure, monitor airway patency	Reposition the airway device, assist in ventilation
Hypoxia	All procedures	Preexisting lung disease, poor ventilation	• Preoxygenation • Supplemental oxygen periprocedural continuous monitoring of SpO_2	Increase FiO_2, use positive pressure ventilation, consider intubation
Laryngospasm	All procedures	Light sedation, irritant exposure, hyperactive airway	Ensure deep sedation and adequate topical anesthesia	• Apply positive pressure, administer Increased depth of anesthesia • Use muscle relaxant
Arrhythmias	All procedures	Underlying heart disease, hypoxia, hypercapnia	Continuous ECG monitoring ensures stable oxygenation and ventilation	Administer antiarrhythmic drugs, treat underlying causes
Pneumothorax	EBUS, airway dilation (balloon dilation), rigid bronchoscope, and endobronchial valves	• Mechanical ventilation, needle biopsy procedures • High airway pressures	• Careful insertion and gentle aspiration of a biopsy needle • Use appropriate pressure-controlled ventilation, monitor ventilation pressures	Chest X-ray postprocedure, 100% FiO_2, intercostal drainage
Bleeding	EBUS, TBNA, and thermal ablation techniques	Antiplatelet therapy, anticoagulation, injury to major vessels	• Assess coagulation profile, discontinue antiplatelet/anticoagulation • Careful examination for major vessels via EBUS probe before needle insertion. Gentle procedure without trauma	Convert to rigid bronchoscopy for control, tamponade or cautery for bleeding control
Airway perforation	Airway dilation, rigid bronchoscopy	High balloon pressure, anatomical deformity	Gradually inflate a balloon, monitor airway pressures, limit inflation time	Ventilate via a secure airway, chest X-ray postprocedure
Airway fire	Thermal ablation techniques	High oxygen concentration, use of electrocautery or laser	Maintain low FiO_2, use laser or electrocautery cautiously	Extinguish fire immediately, secure the airway, and administer ventilatory support
Cardiovascular instability	All procedures especially with rigid bronchoscopy	High-risk cardiovascular disease, sedation	Monitor ECG, maintain adequate fluid status, and provide oxygen supplementation	Administer vasoactive drugs as needed, optimize fluid balance, and ensure airway protection

(EBUS: endobronchial ultrasound ; ECG: electrocardiogram; SpO2: peripheral capillary oxygen saturation)

In patients with a tracheal or bronchial stent, their migration in the distal airway can cause airway obstruction requiring immediate reintervention.

Airway spasm is another common complication and maintaining adequate depth of sedation and generous topical airway anesthesia can help in decreasing the incidents.

Hypoxemia

The majority of patients posted for these procedures have compromised respiratory reserve and a definitive airway is always not possible to establish. Also, a shared airway between the pulmonologist and anesthetist posed these patients more at risk of hypoxia. Also, these procedures are more prone to different ventilation strategies like apneic ventilation and spontaneous ventilation which may lead to hypoventilation and desaturation. Hypoxia is also a major complication faced due to difficulty in ventilation in central airway debulking cases. As mentioned above use of liquid nitrogen in cryotherapy can also lead to hypoxia. Prevention with adequate preoxygenation and periprocedure oxygenation via different modalities such as jet ventilation and HFNO are employed. In cases of central airway debulking or severely compromised lung, an option of ECMO should be considered.

Hemodynamic Instability

Hemodynamic instability during these procedures is not uncommon. Deeper sedation requires high doses of agents like propofol and this can commonly lead to hypotension. More hemodynamic changes are seen in elderly patients or patients with preexisting cardiovascular compromise. This complication can be managed by titration of anesthetic agents or the use of vasoactive agents. Arrhythmias are commonly seen in these procedures and are commonly related to hypercapnia.

Hemorrhage

Procedures such as a transbronchial biopsy, ablative therapies, and debulking of central airway procedures can present with a rare but life-threatening complication and that is bleeding. In such situations protecting the airway from a collection of blood is the primary aim along with control of bleeding. Securing a definitive airway, positioning a patient in head low position to avoid soiling of distal airway, and trying to stop bleeding with either cold saline or adrenaline irrigation or tamponade with bronchial blocker or Fogarty blocker are necessary measures should be activated immediately. If all these measures fail, emergency surgical intervention needs to be performed.

With the use of EBUS, the sampling of mediastinal nodes in close proximity to major vessels has also become very convenient, as color Doppler and ultrasonography help in identifying the exact location of these vascular structures.

It is recommended to withhold antiplatelets (except low-dose aspirin) and anticoagulants before these procedures to minimize the risk of bleeding, however, it should be individualized considering the risk-benefit ratio for each patient.

Pneumothorax

Pneumothorax is also very rare, however, all bronchoscopy patients especially biopsy patients and tracheal balloon dilation patients should be evaluated after 30–60 minutes and imaging is considered in patients with any positive signs. Barotrauma with jet ventilation if not used properly can also lead to this catastrophic complication.

Airway Fire

As described in special consideration in the above text.

ENHANCED RECOVERY PATHWAYS

In addition to preoperative optimization, emphasizing enhanced recovery protocols in IP procedures plays a crucial role in early recovery and minimizing post-procedure pulmonary complications. Strategies such as shorter anesthesia duration, use of short-acting anesthesia agents, multimodal analgesia, early mobilization and resumption of feeding, and early establishment of post-procedure chest physiotherapy are the key elements of an enhanced recovery pathway.

CONCLUSION

Anesthesia for interventional pulmonary procedures is a dynamic and challenging field. Anesthesiologists play a crucial role in from preoperative evaluation, and intraoperative management to postoperative care. These procedures are complex and necessitate a deeper understanding of anesthesia techniques. Collaborative decision-making and pre-procedure discussion with the whole team involved in the procedure are necessary to plan the depth of sedation, mode of ventilation, and preparedness for complication mitigation.

REFERENCES

1. Finlayson GN, Shaipanich T, Durkin C. Bronchoscopic Procedures. In: Slinger P (Ed). Principles and Practice of Anesthesia for Thoracic Surgery. Germany: Springer, Cham; 2019. pp. 197-217.
2. Ikeda S, Yanai N, Ishikawa S. Flexible bronchofiberscope. Keio J Med. 1968;17(1):1-16.
3. Arias S, Lee HJ. The future of interventional pulmonology. Semin Respir Crit Care Med. 2014;35(6):763-8.
4. Beaudoin EL, Chee A, Stather DR. Interventional pulmonology: an update for internal medicine physicians. Minerva Med. 2014;105(3):197-209.
5. In: Ernst A, Herth FJF (Eds). Principles and practice of interventional pulmonology. New York: Springer-Verlag; 2013.

6. de Lima A, Kheir F, Majid A, Pawlowski J. Anesthesia for interventional pulmonology procedures: a review of advanced diagnostic and therapeutic bronchoscopy. Can J Anaesth. 2018;65(7):822-36.
7. Lee KS, Lunn W, Feller-Kopman D, Ernst A, Hatabu H, Boiselle PM. Multislice CT evaluation of airway stents. J Thorac Imaging. 2005;20(2):81-8.
8. Baroni RH, Ashiku S, Boiselle PM. Dynamic CT evaluation of the central airways in patients undergoing tracheoplasty for tracheobronchomalacia. Am J Roentgenol. 2005; 184(5):1444-9.
9. Wood D. Airway stenting. Chest Surg Clin N Am. 2003; 13(2):211-29.
10. Bould MD, Mahtani DG, Davies R, Roughton M, Hunter DN, Kelleher A. Bispectral index values during elective rigid bronchoscopy: a prospective observational pilot study. Anaesthesia. 2007;62(5):438-45.
11. Myles PS, Leslie K, McNeil J, Forbes A, Chan MT. Bispectral index monitoring to prevent awareness during anaesthesia: the B-Aware randomised controlled trial. Lancet Lond Engl. 2004;363(9423):1757-63.
12. Wahidi MM, Jain P, Jantz M, Lee P, Mackensen GB, Barbour SY, et al. American College of Chest Physicians consensus statement on the use of topical anesthesia, analgesia, and sedation during flexible bronchoscopy in adult patients. Chest. 2011;140(5):1342-50.
13. Pawlowski J. Anesthetic considerations for interventional pulmonary procedures. Curr Opin Anaesthesiol. 2013; 26(1):6-12.
14. Sarkiss M, Kennedy M, Riedel B, Norman P, Morice R, Jimenez C, et al. Anesthesia technique for endobronchial ultrasound-guided fine needle aspiration of mediastinal lymph node. J Cardiothorac Vasc Anesth. 2007;21(6):892-6.
15. Ahmad I, El-Boghdadly K, Bhagrath R, Hodzovic I, McNarry AF, Mir F, et al. Difficult Airway Society guidelines for awake tracheal intubation (ATI) in adults. Anaesthesia. 2020;75(4):509-28.
16. Majid A, Gaurav K, Sanchez JM, Berger RL, Folch E, Fernandez-Bussy S, et al. Evaluation of tracheobronchomalacia by dynamic flexible bronchoscopy. A pilot study. Ann Am Thorac Soc. 2014;11(6):951-5.
17. Xue FS, Liu HP, He N, Xu YC, Yang QY, Liao X, et al. Spray-as-you-go airway topical anesthesia in patients with a difficult airway: a randomized, double-blind comparison of 2% and 4% lidocaine. Anesth Analg. 2009;108(2):536-43.
18. Kostyk P, Francois K, Salik I. Airway Anesthesia for Awake Tracheal Intubation: A Review of the Literature. Cureus. 2021;13(7):e16315.
19. Johnston KD, Rai MR. Conscious sedation for awake fibreoptic intubation: a review of the literature. Can J Anaesth. 2013;60(6):584-99.
20. Yarmus L, Akulian J, Gilbert C, Mathai SC, Sathiyamoorthy S, Sahetya S, et al. Comparison of moderate versus deep sedation for endobronchial ultrasound transbronchial needle aspiration. Ann Am Thorac Soc. 2013;10(2):121-6.
21. Cabrini L, Landoni G. A novel non-invasive ventilation mask to prevent and manage respiratory failure during fiberoptic bronchoscopy, gastroscopy and transesophageal echocardiography. Heart Lung Vessels. 2015;7(4):297-303.
22. José RJ, Shaefi S, Navani N. Anesthesia for bronchoscopy. Curr Opin Anaesthesiol. 2014;27(4):453-7.
23. Murphy GS, Brull SJ. Residual neuromuscular block: lessons unlearned. Part I: definitions, incidence, and adverse physiologic effects of residual neuromuscular block. Anesth Analg. 2010;111(1):120-8.
24. Pathak V, Welsby I, Mahmood K, Wahidi M, MacIntyre N, Shofer S. Ventilation and anesthetic approaches for rigid bronchoscopy. Ann Am Thorac Soc. 2014;11(4):628-34.
25. Liu Y, Chen L, Li S. Controlled ventilation or spontaneous respiration in anesthesia for tracheobronchial foreign body removal: a meta-analysis. Paediatr Anaesth. 2014; 24(10):1023-30.
26. Evans E, Biro P, Bedforth N. Jet ventilation. Contin Educ Anaesth Crit Care Pain. 2007;7:2-5.
27. Putz L, Mayné A, Dincq AS. Jet Ventilation during rigid bronchoscopy in adults: a focused review. BioMed Res Int. 2016;2016: 4234861.
28. Kim CW, Kim DH, Son BS, Cho JS, Kim YD, Hoseok I, et al. The feasibility of extracorporeal membrane oxygenation in the variant airway problems. Ann Thorac Cardiovasc Surg. 2015;21(6):517-22.
29. McLenon M, Bittle GJ, Jones K, Menaker J, Pham SM, Iacono AT, et al. Extracorporeal lung support as a bridge to airway stenting and radiotherapy for airway-obstructing pancoast tumor. Ann Thorac Surg. 2016;102(1):e7-9.
30. Smith LP, Roy S. Operating room fires in otolaryngology: risk factors and prevention. Am J Otolaryngol. 2011; 32(2):109-14.
31. Remz M, Luria I, Gravenstein M, Rice SD, Morey TE, Gravenstein N, et al. Prevention of airway fires: do not overlook the expired oxygen concentration. Anesth Analg. 2013;117(5):1172-6.
32. Reddy C, Majid A, Michaud G, Feller-Kopman D, Eberhardt R, Herth F, et al. Gas embolism following bronchoscopic argon plasma coagulation: a case series. Chest. 2008;134(5): 1066-9.
33. Moore RF, Lile DJ, Abbas AE. Current status of spray cryotherapy for airway disease. J Thorac Dis. 2017; 9(Suppl 2):S122-9.
34. McArdle JR, Gildea TR, Mehta AC. Balloon bronchoplasty: its indications, benefits, and complications. J Bronchol Interv Pulmonol. 2005;12(2):123-7.
35. Cox G. New interventions in asthma including bronchial thermoplasty. Curr Opin Pulm Med. 2008;14(1):77-81.
36. McKenna RJ. Endobronchial valves for the treatment of emphysema. Semin Thorac Cardiovasc Surg. 2008; 20(4):285-9.
37. Klooster K, ten Hacken NH, Hartman JE, Kerstjens HA, van Rikxoort EM, Slebos D-J. Endobronchial valves for emphysema without interlobar collateral ventilation. N Engl J Med. 2015;373(24):2325-35.

SECTION

Hepato-Pancreato-Biliary and Gastrointestinal Onco-Anesthesia

24 CHAPTER

Anesthesia for Nontransplant Major Liver Resections

Lakshmi Kumar, Kshama Balakrishna, Sudhindran Surendran

INTRODUCTION

Liver cancers are the fifth most common cancers and feature as the third common cause of deaths due to cancers. Nearly 90% of primary hepatic malignancies are due to hepatocellular carcinomas (HCCs) and the 5-year survival can improve between 50 and 70% if they present early for ablation or resection.[1] Cholangiocarcinoma is less common form of hepatic malignancy and many of them are advanced at the time of presentation and less than a fifth are amenable for resection.[2] Hepatic metastasis from colorectal cancers occurs in nearly 25–50% patients with colorectal malignancies and hepatectomy is the best form of treatment.[3]

Knowledge of the hepatic anatomy and improved techniques of resection have contributed to improved outcomes after surgery. This chapter will cover resections for malignancies and anesthetic management and postoperative care.

IMPLICATIONS OF HEPATECTOMY FOR THE ANESTHESIOLOGIST

The liver is the largest internal organ and is unique in its segmental break down of its architecture into independent functional units, centered on portal triads, constituted by terminal branches of vein, hepatic artery, and the bile duct. The liver has a dual blood supply from the hepatic artery and the portal vein. The portal vein, which provides 80% liver's blood supply, is formed by the confluence of the superior mesenteric and the splenic veins. The arterial supply is from the hepatic artery that is a branch of the celiac axis which in turn divides into the right and left hepatic artery. The hepatic veins, the right, middle, and left hepatic veins, drain into the inferior vena cava (IVC).

Hepatocytes can exhibit an altered cell division process whereby mitosis occurs without the completion of cytokinesis, leading to the formation of binuclear polyploid cells.[4] It is unique in that the hepatocytes are capable of regeneration that has allowed resection of nearly 70% of the liver with regrowth of the remnant liver.

The hepatic lobule is a hexagonal structural unit of the liver **(Fig. 1A)**. At each of the vertices is the portal triad with the hepatic artery, portal vein, and branches of the bile duct. The blood flow to the cells is arranged centripetally from the portal triad such that the areas around the central vein receive the least supply and are vulnerable to ischemic damages during perioperative hypotension. The liver acinus is a functional unit of the liver and has the hepatocytes lined by a layer of endothelial cells **(Fig. 1B)**.

PREOPERATIVE TESTS FOR EVALUATION

A complete blood count, renal function evaluation, blood sugar, and electrolytes must be performed prior to major surgery. A chest X-ray and 12-lead ECG must always be performed.

The presence of comorbidities such as hypertension, diabetes, ischemic heart disease (IHD) and dyslipidemia, cerebrovascular accident (CVA), and underlying prothrombotic states needs assessment. Hypertensive patients can continue their antihypertensive medications in usual doses until surgery except for angiotensin receptor blockers (ARB) and angiotensin-converting enzyme inhibitors (ACE I) that should be discontinued if doses are on the night before or the morning of surgery. This is required as their continued use can result in intractable hypotension perioperatively in major surgeries. Diabetic patients can be risk profiled by the duration of diabetes, need for insulin, and the presence of microvascular complications.

Indications for preoperative echocardiogram include patients with IHD, valvular HD, and those with poor effort tolerance. Patients with a previous history of IHD will need a transthoracic echocardiogram for left ventricular (LV) dysfunction and wall motion

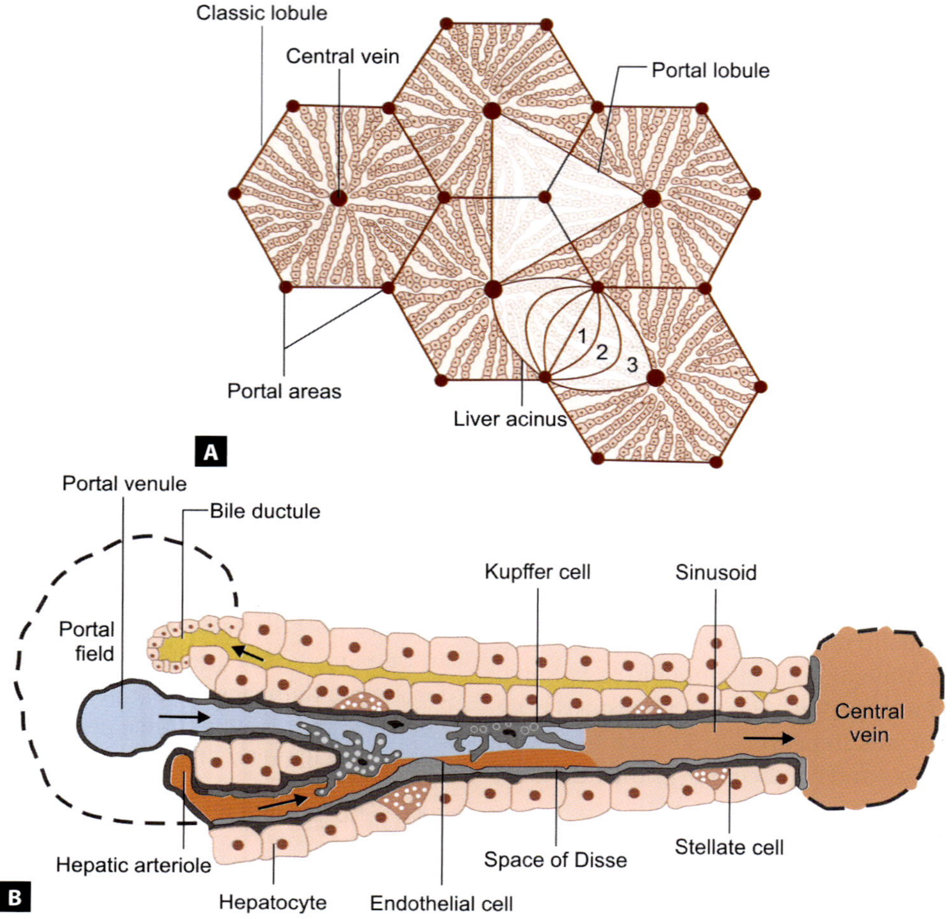

Fig. 1A and B: (A) Hepatic lobule; (B) Hepatic acinus.

abnormalities. Rarely, aneurysmal LV or an organized clot or valve abnormalities may be incidental pick-ups on echocardiography. Advanced tests such as a treadmill test (TMT) or coronary angiogram need to be individualized. Risk is stratified with Lee's revised cardiac risk index (high-risk surgery, diabetic on insulin, creatinine >2.0 mg/dL, CVA, and history of pulmonary edema).

Patients who are on dual antiplatelet therapy for coronary stents >12 months can have clopidogrel withheld and low-dose aspirin with low-molecular-weight heparin (LMWH) continued perioperatively.

Smokers and patients with history suggestive of chronic obstructive pulmonary disease (COPD) can be tested for lung signs, chest X-ray, and a 6-minute walk test or two flight stair climb in the pre-anesthesia clinic (PAC) for evaluation of cardiorespiratory reserve. Significant COPD, Gold class 3 and above, can pose significant risks for postoperative pulmonary complications and should be considered for surgery weighing risks versus benefits.

Evaluation of liver function tests:

- *Hepatocellular function:* Aspartate and alanine aminotransferases (AST and ALT). ALT is more specific for hepatocyte inflammatory injury. Elevated levels can be seen with chemotherapy, metabolic-associated steatohepatitis, or alcoholic hepatitis.
- *Markers of obstruction/cholestasis:* Alkaline phosphatase, 5'-nucleotidase, and gamma-glutamyl transferase
- *Synthetic function:* Serum albumin, coagulation factors: Prothrombin time/international normalized ratio (INR), activated partial thromboplastin time (aPTT), and fibrinogen

- *Bilirubin:* Conjugated hyperbilirubinemia typically indicates liver pathology, whereas elevated levels of unconjugated bilirubin are often associated with hemolysis or congenital deficiencies in conjugating enzymes, such as Gilbert's syndrome.

Patients older than 70 years, with higher levels of bilirubin (>11 mg/dL), hypoproteinemia (serum albumin <3.0 mg/dL), renal dysfunction, and malignant etiology, are noted to have poorer outcomes. In patients with obstructive jaundice, concerns on perioperative hydration and correction of coagulation with administration of vitamin K need attention.

CIRRHOSIS

Cirrhosis is a pathological dysfunction of the liver consequent to hepatocyte injury that results from a variety of insults. Injury to the sinusoidal endothelial cells leads to the creation of dense extracellular matrix in the subendothelial space of Disse. With the progression of injury, the stellate cells transform to fibrogenic cells called myofibroblasts. This results in the loss of hepatic architecture, fibrosis, and development of portal hypertension (PHT).

Table 1 outlines the modified Child–Pugh–Turcotte grading system, which is used to assess liver function and prognosis.

In conditions with excessive rise in bilirubin such as primary biliary cirrhosis and sclerosing cholangitis, 1 point is allotted for bilirubin <4 mg/dL, 2 points for 4–10 mg/dL, and 3 points for bilirubin >10 mg/dL. Child A represents 5–6 points, Child B 7–9 points, and Child C 10 points and above.

The MELD scoring or Model for End-Stage Liver Disease is superior to the Child score and is the inclusion of creatinine and elimination of subjective factor assessment such as ascites and encephalopathy. MELD incorporates the natural logarithm of INR, creatinine, and bilirubin as given by the formula below:

$$\text{MELD} = 11.2 \times \ln \text{INR} + 9.57 \times \ln \text{Creatinine (mg/dL)} + 3.78 \times \ln \text{Bilirubin (mg/dL)} + 6.43$$

$$\text{MELD-Na} = \text{MELD} + 1.32 \times (137 - \text{Na}) - [0.033 \times \text{MELD} \times (137 - \text{Na})]$$

These formulas are cumbersome to remember and values can be obtained by an online calculator www.mdcalc.com.

Child A or MELD <8 is considered safe for hepatectomy and worse grades carry a high mortality after hepatectomy.

TABLE 1: Modified Child–Pugh–Turcotte grading.

Parameters	*1 point*	*2 points*	*3 points*
Albumin (g/dL)	>3.5	2.8–3.5	<2.8
PT prolongation	<4 seconds	4–6 seconds	>6 seconds
INR	<1.7	1.7–2.3	>2.3
Ascites	Absent	Slight/moderate	Tense
Encephalopathy	None	Grade I–II	Grade III–IV
Bilirubin (mg/dL)	<2	2–3	>3

(INR: international normalized ratio; PT: prothrombin time)

PREOPERATIVE OPTIMIZATION

Radical hepatic resection although deemed urgent can be delayed for better optimization of the patient to improve outcomes. A series of recommendations have been proposed as a part of Enhanced Recovery After Surgery (ERAS) guidelines.[5] They include preoperative counseling and scope for nutritional improvement if the patients appears to be malnourished (>10–15% weight loss in 6 months or if serum albumin is <3.0 mg/dL).

While allowing clear fluids until 2 hours prior to procedure is supported by moderate level of evidence in those without contraindications, carbohydrate (CHO) loading the night before and 2 hours prior has a lower recommendation. Even though diabetics are excluded from preoperative CHO loading, diabetics given CHO drink did not manifest a glycemic response and contrarily showed improved blood glucose levels in comparison to water among a study in patients undergoing colorectal surgery.[6]

Premedication should avoid a long-acting anxiolytic particularly in patients with underlying cirrhosis or obstruction to the biliary system. Proton pump inhibitors and a prokinetic can be considered on the night before surgery.

Thromboprophylaxis with LMWH (enoxaparin 20 mg subcutaneously 12 hours prior to surgery) and use of deterrent stockings are recommended.

Outcomes after hepatectomy can be improved by optimization of associated comorbidities. Diabetes is often associated with poorer outcomes after hepatectomy due to altered immune functions and liver steatosis. Correction and optimization of blood sugars may improve outcomes. Medications used for diabetes can confound measurements of lactates and can contribute to lactic acidosis (metformin). Short-acting insulin should be instituted preoperatively. Newer medications such as sodium-glucose cotransporter-II (SGLT-II) inhibitors are associated with euglycemic ketoacidosis (eKA) and should be discontinued a few days before surgery.[7] Renal dysfunction is an independent predictor of poor outcomes following hepatectomy.

Anemia is also predictive of a poorer outcome following hepatectomy. Correction of anemia, if possible, preoperatively with parenteral iron therapy can improve outcomes.

Neoadjuvant chemotherapy is often used to reduce the tumor size in patients with metastatic colonic cancer; however, chemotherapy can damage the liver parenchyma. For example, irinotecan can cause chemotherapy-associated steatohepatitis (CASH), while oxaliplatin may lead to sinusoidal obstruction. Both of these effects can impair the function of the residual liver and result in postoperative liver dysfunction. 5-fluorouracil, doxorubicin, cyclophosphamide, and trastuzumab can result in cardiomyopathy and myocardial dysfunction. A mandated time period of 4–6 weeks is needed after chemotherapy to allow recovery and an echocardiogram is needed at the completion of chemotherapy.[8]

Hepatocellular carcinoma can develop in patients with a background of cirrhosis and/or viral infections and a cirrhotic liver can increase the risks of posthepatectomy liver failure (PHLF) that is defined as INR over 1.7 and bilirubin over 3 mg/dL (50-50 criteria) after the 5th postoperative day (POD).[9] Factors that predispose to the occurrence of PHLF include advancing age, diabetes, sepsis, renal insufficiency, cardiopulmonary compromise, and thrombocytopenia.[10] Fatty livers with steatosis >30% are more prone to PHLF that manifests as increased ischemia reperfusion (IR) injury due to altered sinusoidal circulation. At least 50% future liver remnant (FLR) is needed for hepatectomy in steatotic livers compared to the 30% in normal healthy livers.

Among surgical factors, blood losses of >1.2 L, IVC repair, and resection of tissues around the porta and duodenum can predispose to PHLF. The quality and volume of remnant liver contribute to small for size syndrome (SFSS). In patients with cirrhosis, hepatectomy can be safely performed in Child A and is considered unsafe in Child B and above.

SEGMENTS AND DIVISIONS OF THE LIVER IN THE CONTEXT OF HEPATECTOMY[11]

Although the pathway of the ligamentum teres divides the liver into right and left lobes, the functional division of the liver is by the middle hepatic vein. The portal vein branches divide the left lobe of the liver into lateral segment (II) and an inferior segment (III) while the medial segment divides into superior IVa and inferior IVb by the portal vein branches. The right lobe liver is divided into anterior segments (V and VIII) and posterior segments (VI and VII) by the right hepatic vein and into superior and inferior segments by the right portal vein. Segment I, the caudate lobe, lies over the IVC and receives the portal blood flow from both the right and left branches of the portal vein.

A classical right hepatectomy involves resection of segments V–VIII and left hepatectomy involves resection of segments II–IV. Extended right hepatectomy involves resection of all segments to the right of umbilical fissure (IV–VIII and sometimes I) and extended left hepatectomy entails resection of segments II, III, IV, V, and VIII **(Fig. 2)**.

VASCULAR CONTROL DURING LIVER RESECTION

The techniques available for vascular control to decrease blood losses during hepatic resection vary and are relevant to the anesthesiologist by virtue of the hemodynamic impact. Pringle's maneuver (PM) or clamping of the portal triad is most commonly used and period of 10-minute occlusion is followed by at least 5 minutes recovery **(Fig. 3)**. The process can allow up to 1 hour of portal triad clamping during resections.

Studies have shown that during PM, the central venous pressure (CVP) decreases and splanchnic flow is reduced accompanied by a decrease in cardiac output (CO) and an activation of the sympathoadrenal responses with a fall in CO. The release is accompanied by a vasodilation-related fall in blood pressure and the anesthesiologist needs to be equipped to handle this.[12]

The PM is generally well tolerated although it is associated with up to 40% increase in systemic vascular resistance and 10% decreases in CO. PM is not recommended for >1 hour in normal livers and 30 minutes in pathologic livers due to its impact with IR injuries. Concerns on the PM in hepatic malignancies exist due to possible implications in tumor recurrence.[13]

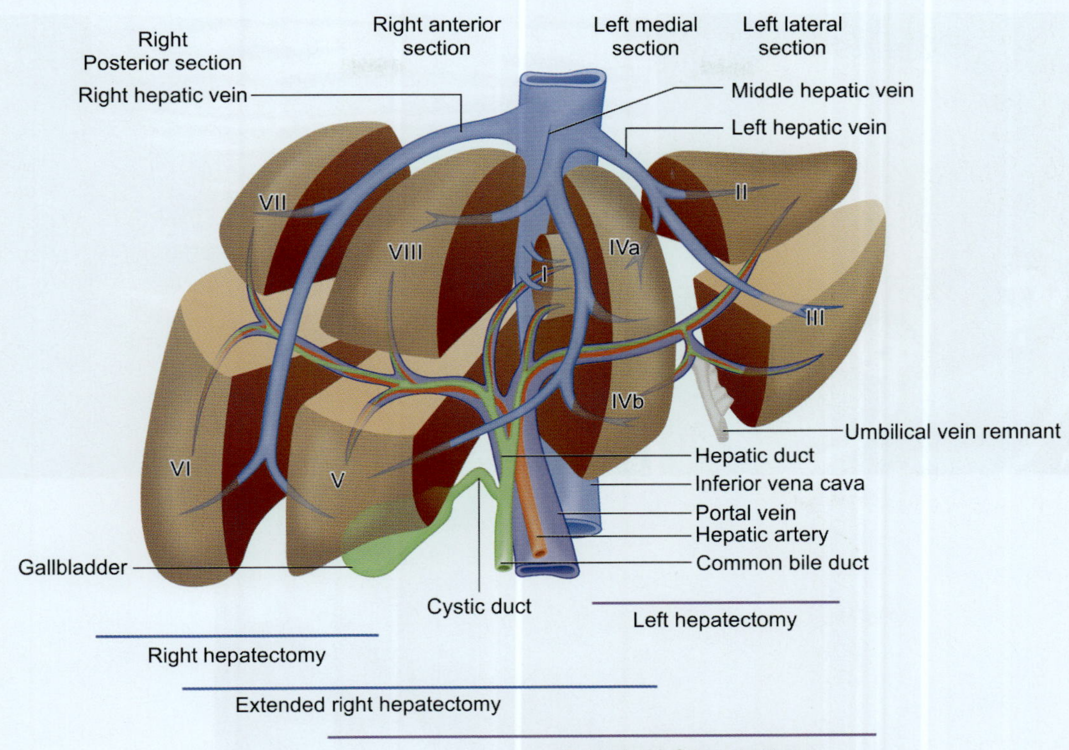

Fig. 2: Anatomical divisions of the liver.

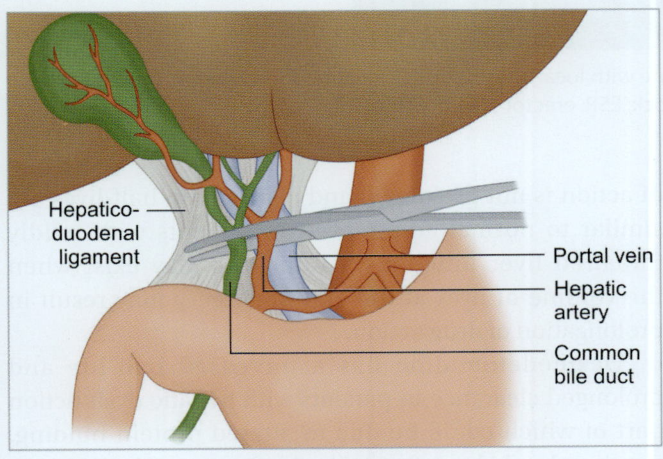

Fig. 3: Pringle's maneuver.

Inflow occlusion by clamping of the hepatic pedicle can reduce blood losses during resection but while it can reduce the bleed from the hepatic artery and portal vein, it does not address back bleeding from the hepatic veins. Ischemic preconditioning is another technique described wherein the short period of ischemia prepares the liver hepatocytes for subsequent ischemic periods.

CONDUCT OF ANESTHESIA

In an open surgery, epidural analgesia is the analgesic technique of choice. Postoperative coagulopathy seen following surgery raises concerns on the safety of epidural, but several studies have endorsed the safety in patients with normal livers and normal preoperative platelets and prothrombin times.[14] Measurements of dynamic tests of coagulation have shown hyperfibrinogenemia as an acute phase reactant that restores the coagulation to a normal profile. This probably explains the safety and the nonoccurrence of epidural hematomas in this patient group.

In minimally invasive surgery, the port holes are along a transverse line along the umbilicus and the retrieval is through a Pfannenstiel incision **(Fig. 4A)**. An epidural is considered too invasive for this group of patients.

Bilateral erector spinae blocks, paravertebral blocks, and transverse abdominal plane (TAP) blocks are available

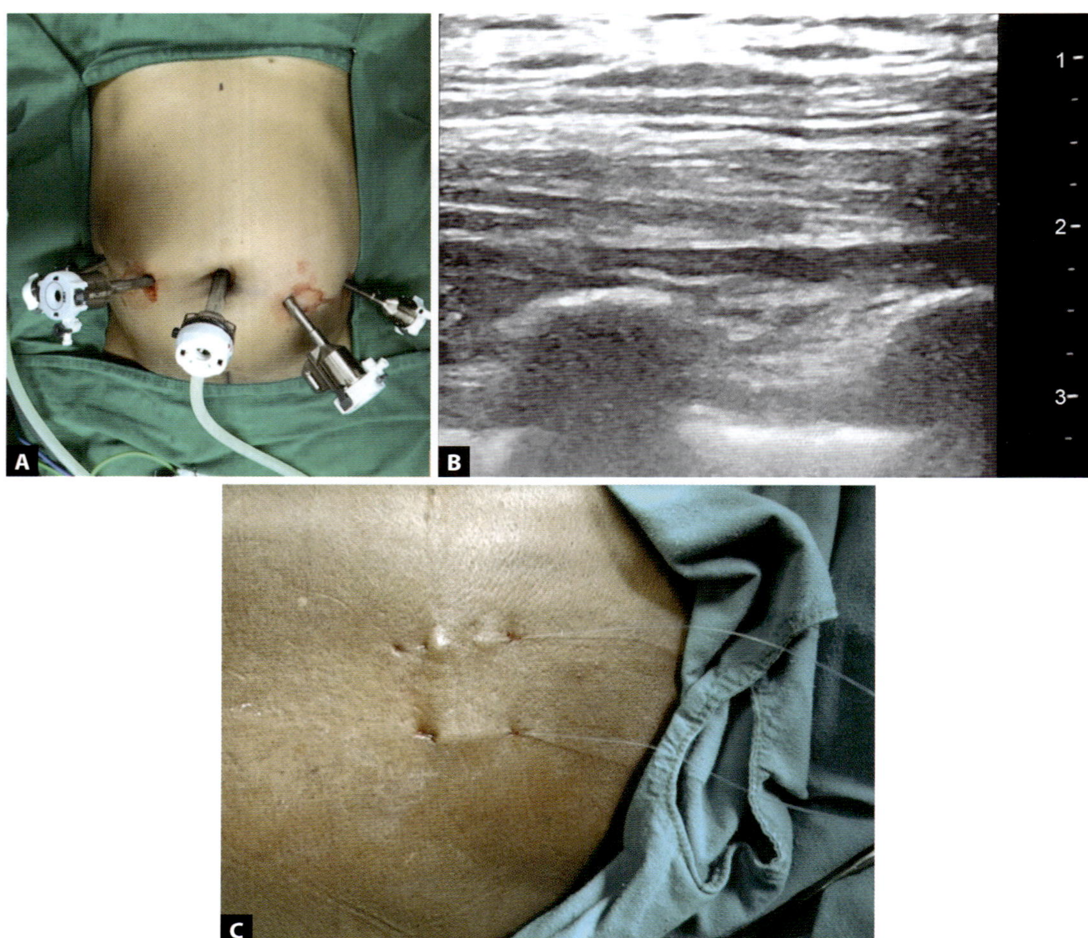

Fig. 4A to C: (A) Port placement in robotic hepatectomy; (B) ESB plane with local anesthetic. (C) Bilateral ESP catheters for continuous analgesia. (ESB: erector spinae block; ESP: erector spinae plane)

alternatives. Introduction of catheters in the erector spinae plane (ESP) allows a continuous administration of anesthetic drugs for pain relief **(Figs. 4B and C)**. Care should be taken for assessment of the volume of local anesthetic and potential local anesthetic-induced systemic toxicity (LAST) with the use of large volumes of local anesthetics and availability of 20% Intralipid as an antidote should be confirmed while practicing blocks.

Induction of anesthesia can be performed with fentanyl 2 μg/kg, midazolam 1–2 mg, and propofol titrated to loss of verbal response. Elevated bilirubin levels are seen in cholangiocarcinomas and anesthesia may need adjustments for drug metabolism. Bilirubin is bound to albumin and free fraction of administered drugs can increase. Propofol, etomidate, and ketamine are lipid soluble with a high hepatic extraction ratio. Their duration of action is not prolonged and elimination half-lives are similar to normal adults even in patients with mildly impaired liver functions.[15] Concerns may exist when the volume of liver at the end of surgery may result in prolongation of drug action.

Dexmedetomidine has a increased half-life and prolonged clearance in patients with hepatic dysfunction part of which could be due to altered protein binding. Caution should be exercised in the dosage as the duration could be prolonged. Sevoflurane or isoflurane can be used as inhalational agents. Fentanyl remains the best analgesic available, caution must be paid to the fact that it can accumulate in lipid storage sites contributing to redistribution.

Remifentanil (Ultiva) is a short-acting opioid with onset of 90 seconds and a context sensitivity half-life of

4 minutes even while used as an infusion. It is metabolized by nonspecific esterases and may have a role in patients with cirrhosis with limited volume following hepatic resection.

Rapid sequence induction may be restricted to liver tumors that rarely causes duodenal obstruction and full stomach and is not routinely practiced. Succinylcholine can be used as pseudocholinesterase levels are normal until the liver is affected as in end-stage liver disease (ESLD). Rocuronium is an alternative bearing in mind that hepatic metabolism may be slowed. Atracurium and cisatracurium are relaxants of choice as they have a nonorgan-related elimination.

Epidural opioid is useful analgesic option during surgery. This avoids vasodilation and hypotension relating to the use of an epidural local anesthetic. Preservative-free morphine 2–3 mg in 10 mL saline through the epidural at the start of surgery provides adequate analgesia.

FLUID MANAGEMENT IN HEPATIC SURGERY

Can a liver rendered intermittently ischemic through vascular management strategies like PM handle the metabolism of lactate in intravenous (IV) fluids? Lactate is the buffer or base present in the most commonly used crystalloid Ringer's lactate in surgery. The lactate in the IV fluid is converted to bicarbonate by liver metabolism; however, a diseased liver or when the volume of liver remnant is less than adequate, lactate metabolism is interrupted. This and the fact that lactate serves as a marker for tissue perfusion and assessment of liver function[16] have led to the use of an acetated balanced salt solution Plasmalyte[17] in liver surgeries.

Plasmalyte has a biochemical composition most physiologic with that of human plasma, notably, chloride of 98 mmol/L, and contains bases of acetate 27 mmol/L and gluconate 23 mmol/L. It contains no calcium and hence compatible with blood and the second base does not add to alkalosis but is filtered at the kidney. In comparison to lactate metabolism, acetate is advantageous, in that it does not stimulate gluconeogenesis, faster conversion to bicarbonate, metabolism by nonhepatic sites, and most importantly does not interfere with the measurement of lactate levels.[18] Several studies have looked at metabolic profiles of acetated solutions in living donor hepatectomy. Bicarbonate and base excess were better with Ringer's acetate,[19] while studies using Plasmalyte showed lesser lactate and also lesser bilirubin and prothrombin time and increased albumin in comparison to lactated Ringer's solution.[20] Normal saline is not preferred as it is not considered a balanced solution because it does not contain a buffer (lactate or acetate). A study on healthy volunteers showed a decrease in renal blood flow velocity and hyperchloremia with the use of normal saline in comparison with Plasmalyte[21] and a retrospective analysis showed an increased incidence of complications in abdominal surgery with normal saline.[22,23] Subsequent studies failed to demonstrate any impact on renal function with either normal saline or Ringer's lactate.[24,25]

The practice is to use Ringer's lactate initially and switch to Plasmalyte if an elevation in lactate is noted. If hepatic resection is accompanied by a decrease in urine output or hyperkalemia, then ½ NS with added soda bicarbonate (37.5 mL of 8.4% solution to 460 mL ½ NS) is preferred.

Synthetic colloids, hetastarch, and gelatins may be used as per preferences of the centers. While there are no studies directly establishing a correlation between hetastarch and renal dysfunctions, there is no evidence to support the use in major surgery or in patients at risk for developing postoperative renal dysfunction.[26,27] Gelatins (Haemaccel/Gelaspan) are used in some centers as a colloid to minimize fluid administration. It carries a small risk of associated anaphylaxis and may also affect coagulation by affecting the von Willebrand factor (vWF) in the vascular endothelium **(Table 2)**.

Albumin is the natural colloid and is increasingly being used on account of its safety in comparison with synthetic colloids. It is fairly expensive and being prepared from human plasma carries risks of antigenicity and anaphylaxis. In liver resection surgery with large volume losses, albumin is used as a supplement to volume and reduction of extravascular fluid accumulation. Lower preoperative albumin levels correlate with increased postoperative complications in liver surgery.[28] The recommendations for use are limited even in cirrhotics and are mainly for correcting ascitic losses and treating hepatorenal syndrome.[29]

Guidelines for blood and product transfusions are comparable to that of major surgeries. A massive transfusion protocol can be activated in the context of sudden major hemorrhages that will involve transfusions of packed red blood cell (PRBC):fresh frozen plasma (FFP):platelets as 1:1:1 along with fibrinogen as cryoprecipitate, more slow

TABLE 2: Constituents of IV fluids used in practice.

Strength (mmol/L)	*Plasmalyte*	*Ringer's lactate*	*Normal saline*	*Hydroxyethyl starch (130/0.4)*	*Gelaspan 4%*
Osmolarity	294	278	308	286.5	284
Sodium (Na^+)	140	131	154	137	151
Potassium (K^+)	5	5	–	4	4
Chloride (Cl^-)	98	111	154	110	103
Calcium (Ca^{2+})	–	2	–	–	1
Magnesium (Mg^{2+})	1.5	–	–	1.5	1
Lactate (bicarbonate)	–	29	–	–	–
Acetate	27	–	–	34	24
Gluconate	23	–	–	–	–

(IV: intravenous)

ongoing losses can be addressed with PRBCs largely and plasma when larger volumes of blood are lost or when there is evidence of ongoing coagulopathy.

Point-of-care tests (POCTs) of coagulation help in transfusion of appropriate products. A meta-analysis of transfusions in major oncological hepatic surgeries suggests that there may be evidence for increased complications and tumor recurrence with overtransfusions and suggests adoption of restrictive transfusion practices in hepatic surgery.[30]

Point-of-care Testing of Coagulation

Thromboelastography (TEG) and rotational thromboelastometry (ROTEM) are viscoelastic tests that can be performed and provide an assessment of clotting from a dynamic state, i.e., combination of procoagulant and anticoagulant factors **(Fig. 5)**. A sample of blood is placed in a cuvette and is rotated through an arc. The formation of a clot slows the movement of the pin and the trace of the changes in pin movement is displayed as a graph. The time for the formation of the clot, rate of fibrin link-up, the clot strength, and any lysis of the clot can be obtained from the graph. The advantage of this is that transfusions are specific to the factor deficiencies and can reduce volume in transfusions.[31]

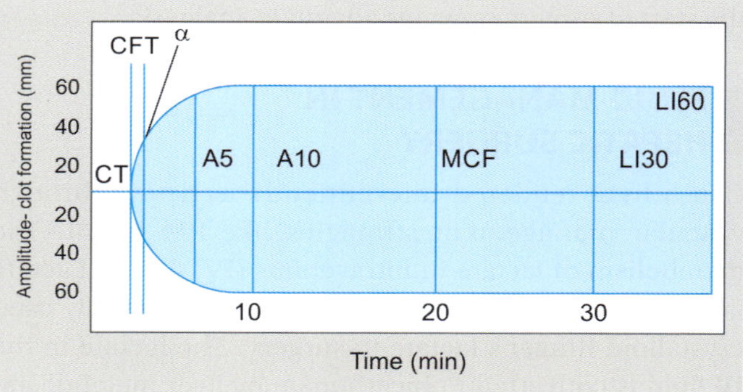

Fig. 5: Rotational thromboelastometry (ROTEM). (CT: clotting time; CFT: clot formation time; A5: amplitude at 5 minutes; A10: amplitude at 10 minutes; MCF: maximum clot firmness)

Hemodynamic Monitoring and Central Venous Pressure

Central venous pressure monitoring measurement reflects the right atrial pressure and preload. Although CVP may not be an accurate monitor of volume assessment owing to various factors affecting it such as position of the liver, clamping of vascular structures, position of the patient, and variation in intra-abdominal pressure, especially in laparoscopic and robotic liver resection surgeries, CVP measurements still have a role in these surgeries. Preferred sites of CVP monitoring include internal jugular vein and subclavian vein. A low CVP strategy decreases hydrostatic pressure in the IVC at the level of hepatic veins, thereby allowing better surgical dissection of the portal structures, IVC, and hepatic veins with minimal bleeding.[32] In minimally invasive surgeries, due to increases in intra-abdominal pressures, the reading of the CVP can be unreliable. The anesthesiologist needs to collaborate with the surgeon's assessment of IVC filling for an accurate volume status. The thumb rule is a visualized distensibility of the IVC with respiratory variations which implies a low volume status similar to the IVC collapsibility measured by abdominal ultrasound.

Hemodynamic monitoring is fundamental as surgery involves rapid blood loss, handling of liver and hilar structures, vascular clamping, and risk of vascular injury, which can lead to significant hemodynamic changes under anesthesia.[33] The preferred site of IBP monitoring is the radial artery; however, the femoral artery may be desired in cases with extensive vascular involvement. Studies comparing the radial versus the femoral pressures during liver transplant state although the systolic pressures can vary, the mean arterial pressures are comparable and can be used interchangeably.[34] High vasopressor supports can result in peripheral vasoconstriction and make a radial trace unreliable.

Most new workstations use pulse pressure variation (PPV) derived from the IBP automatically. This is based upon the cardiorespiratory changes and derives the volume responsiveness based upon blood pressure variations with respiration.

In high-risk hepatic resections, such as cholangiocarcinomas with extensive vascular involvement, additional monitoring modalities such as CO measurement may be beneficial in management. These include the FloTrac/Vigileo (Edwards Life Sciences, Irvine, CA, USA) or ProAQT (Getinge) that requires no calibration.

Both provide a real-time monitoring when connected to radial arterial catheter through a unique sensor. When the central venous line is connected, the systemic vascular resistance is derived. Hemodynamic information such as stroke volume variation (SVV), stroke volume index (SVI), cardiac index (CI), and systemic vascular resistance index (SVRI) can be obtained, which can be used in early goal-directed management.[35]

A newer innovation for CO has been introduced using artificial intelligence. Capstesia™ (GalenicApp, Vitoria, Spain) smartphone application for Android™/iOS™ systems is a software downloaded into a smartphone.[36] This allows the calculation of a patients CO by analyzing the pulse contour of a snapshot of the arterial trace after the inputs of heart rate, systolic and diastolic pressures, and a recent study has found this to be comparable with the readings from the FloTrac-Vigileo.

Cardiac output monitoring by PiCCO (Getinge-Pulsioflex) using transpulmonary thermodilution requires a central IBP. This can provide additional information on intrathoracic blood volume indices, global end diastolic volumes and extravascular lung water indices may be obtained, which can refine and guide optimal fluid management.

Pulmonary artery catheters and transesophageal echocardiography (TEE) are also available options in high-risk cases. The small but significant complications associated with PAC have eliminated their use in the OR. The direct visualization of the heart in real time in TEE allows for instantaneous assessment of changes in global and regional contractility, rapid diagnosis of ventricular dilatation and failure, rapid optimization of hypovolemia, and intraoperative diagnosis and management of air embolism and thromboembolism.[37]

Ischemia Reperfusion Injury

Any surgery for cancer is associated with a risk of cancer recurrence that can be linked to tumor handling and IR injury. When the liver cells are rendered ischemic during clamping for resection, the ATP supply to the mitochondria is depleted. This opens the calcium channels that increase mitochondrial permeability and result in cell death. When the blood supply is reestablished, the high succinic acid in hypoxic tissue results in the formation of reactive oxygen species. Apoptosis, endothelial dysfunction, and inflammation are mechanisms of manifestations of IR injury.[38]

In order to reduce cancer recurrence, an anterior surgical approach is recommended over the conventional approach that requires liver mobilization as the first step. Anterior approach involves inflow control, parenchymal transection, and outflow control prior to mobilization of the right lobe. This technique is shown to increase the disease-free period post-surgery.

Other measures to reduce recurrence are maintenance of normothermia, use of opioid-sparing anesthetic techniques, and avoiding excessive transfusion that can produce immunosuppression.

ASSOCIATING LIVER PARTITION AND PORTAL VEIN LIGATION FOR STAGED HEPATECTOMY (ALPPS)

Associating liver partition with portal vein ligation is a technique to improve resectability in patients with poor functional reserve of liver. In this procedure, the first stage involves portal vein ligation without dissection of the pedicle combined with in situ splitting of the liver. After allowing a week for the nontumor-containing lobe to hypertrophy, a completion second stage is done to remove the malignancy.[39,40] A systematic review of this procedure has stated that hypertrophy of 61–93% occurs over a median of 9–14 days, 95–100% cases progress to second stage completion and that there is high likelihood of R0 resection (86–100%).[41]

Anesthesia management can be tailored to maintain the mean arterial pressures that can maintain hepatic perfusion. An epidural is included and invasive lines are mandated. Local anesthetic infusions through epidural are avoided to reduce hypotension but opioids can be safely used at lower doses. Induction drugs, opioids, inhalational agents, and relaxants are selected to have shortest duration of action.

Patients are often extubated at the end of the procedure and monitored in high-dependency units for a week before they can be scheduled for the second stage. Institutional policies for the management of invasive lines for this period can be followed.

POSTOPERATIVE CARE

The postoperative care ensures an early recovery following hepatectomy. Patients are usually extubated and shifted to the ICU. They are nursed in a 30° head-up position to reduce aspiration risks. ERAS guidelines recommend an early removal of Ryle's tube and drains when possible. Fluids (balanced salt solutions) with acetate as base are used for the 1st POD, dextrose may be added if the patient is not taking adequately orally. The target is to maintain an even balance, if associated renal or electrolyte issues are not present.

FAST HUG BID is the mnemonic used to follow the care of the patient: F—feeding, A—analgesia, S—sedation, T—thromboprophylaxis, H—head elevation, U—ulcer prophylaxis, G—glycemic control, B—bowel, I—indwelling lines, and D—de-escalation of antibiotics.

Analgesia in open surgery is most common with epidural analgesia. Contrary to the belief that epidurals in hepatectomy can be associated with epidural hematomas, its safety has been established in many studies.[42] The postsurgical state may actually be prothrombotic and has been seen in TEGs in donor hepatectomy who demonstrates a hyperfibrinogenemia. In minimally invasive surgery, a multimodal strategy involving injection paracetamol 1 G TID and local anesthetic infusions through ESP catheters or IV opioids can be used.

Intravenous phosphate supplementation is needed to provide phosphate for new regenerating hepatocytes and 6–20 mmol/day is needed for patients. N-acetyl cysteine is a glutathione precursor and free radical scavenger and although there are no proven benefits, an infusion of 350–500 mg/h is given for a few days.

Thromboprophylaxis is recommended but the deranged coagulation (INR) will not allow use of heparins. Thromboembolic stockings can be used and early ambulation encouraged.

Branched-chain amino acids when administered were associated with an improved subjective well-being in patients post hepatic resection.[43]

CONCLUSION

Anesthesia for hepatic resections requires an understanding of the pathophysiological state and effects of anesthetics on residual liver functions that can be temporarily deranged. Availability of newer and advanced monitoring equipment and drugs that are easily metabolized has improved outcomes. Multidisciplinary ICU support and care enhances patient care and outcomes in major hepatectomies.

REFERENCES

1. Allaire M, Goumard C, Lim C, Le Cleach A, Wagner M, Scatton O. New frontiers in liver resection for hepatocellular carcinoma. JHEP Rep. 2020;2(4):100134.
2. Cillo U, Fondevila C, Donadon M, Gringeri E, Mocchegiani F, Schlitt HJ, et al. Surgery for cholangiocarcinoma. Liver Int. 2019;39 Suppl 1:143-55.
3. Martin J, Petrillo A, Smyth EC, Shaida N, Khwaja S, Cheow HK, et al. Colorectal liver metastases: Current management and future perspectives. World J Clin Oncol. 2020;11:761-808.
4. Dewhurst MR, Ow JR, Zafer G, van Hul NKM, Wollmann H, Bisteau X, et al. Loss of hepatocyte cell division leads to liver inflammation and fibrosis. PLoS Genet. 2020;16:e1009084.
5. Bayramov N, Mammadova SH. A review of the current ERAS guidelines for liver resection, liver transplantation and pancreatoduodenectomy. Ann Med Surg. 2022;82:104596.
6. Kumar L, Ashok A, Sudhakar A, Sreekumar G. Preoperative maltodextrin in minimally invasive colorectal surgery: Is it safe for diabetics? A randomised controlled trial. Indian J Anaesth. 2023;67:1084-9.
7. Kartha AP, Irimpan J, Thomas DE, Kumar L. Euglycaemic ketoacidosis after abdominal surgery: Implications of SGLT2 inhibitors for anaesthesiologists – A case study. Indian J Anaesth. 2023;67:840-1.

8. Patel J, Jones CN, Amoako D. Perioperative management for hepatic resection surgery. BJA Educ. 2022;22:357-63.
9. Balzan S, Belghiti J, Farges O, Ogata S, Sauvanet A, Delefosse D, et al. The "50-50 criteria" on postoperative day 5: an accurate predictor of liver failure and death after hepatectomy. Ann Surg. 2005;242:824-8.
10. Ray S, Mehta NN, Golhar A, Nundy S. Post hepatectomy liver failure - A comprehensive review of current concepts and controversies. Ann Med Surg (Lond). 2018;34:4-10.
11. Aragon RJ, Solomon NL. Review Article. Techniques of hepatic resection. J Gastrointest Oncol. 2012;3:28-40.
12. Guest RV. The principles of liver resection. Surgery (Oxford). 2023;41:350-8.
13. Snowden C, Prentis J. Anesthesia for Hepatobiliary Surgery. Anesthesiol Clin. 2015;33:125-41.
14. Jacquenod P, Wallon G, Gazon M, Darnis B, Pradat P, Virlogeux V, et al. Incidence and Risk Factors of Coagulation Profile Derangement After Liver Surgery. Anesth Analg. 2018;126:1142-7.
15. Rothenberg DM, O'Connor CJ, Tuman KJ. Anaesthesia and the hepatobiliary system. In: Miller RD (Ed). Miller's Anaesthesia, 8th edition. Philadelphia: Elsevier Saunders; 2014. Chapter 73. pp. 2244-65.
16. Watanabe I, Mayumi T, Arishima T, Takahashi H, Shikano T, Nakao A, et al. Hyperlactemia can predict the prognosis of liver resection. Shock. 2007;28:35-8.
17. Weinberg L, Collins N, Van Mourik K, Tan C, Bellomo R. Plasma-Lyte 148: A clinical review. World J Crit Care Med. 2016;5:235-50.
18. Zander R. (2019). Fluid Management. [online] Available from https://www.physioklin.de/fileadmin/user_upload/literatur/z/Zander_Fluid_Management_032020v.pdf. [Last accessed February, 2025]
19. Kumar L, Seetharaman M, Rajmohan N, Ramamurthi P, Rajan S, Varghese R. Metabolic profile in right lobe living donor hepatectomy: Comparison of lactated Ringer's solution and normal saline versus acetate based balanced salt solution—a pilot study. Indian J Anaesth. 2016;60:719-25.
20. Shin WJ, Kim YK, Bang JY, Cho SK, Han SM, Hwang GS. Lactate and liver function tests after living donor right hepatectomy: A comparison of solutions with and without lactate. Acta Anaesthesiol Scand. 2011;55:558-64.
21. Chowdhury AH, Cox EF, Francis ST, Lobo DN. A randomized, controlled, double-blind crossover study on the effects of 2-L infusions of 0.9% saline and plasma-lyte® 148 on renal blood flow velocity and renal cortical tissue perfusion in healthy volunteers. Ann Surg. 2012;256:18-24.
22. Shaw AD, Bagshaw SM, Goldstein SL, Scherer LA, Duan M, Schermer CR, et al. Major complications, mortality, and resource utilization after open abdominal surgery: 0.9% saline compared to Plasma-Lyte. Ann Surg. 2012;255:821-9.
23. Krajewski ML, Raghunathan K, Paluszkiewicz SM, Schermer CR, Shaw AD. Meta-analysis of high-versus low-chloride content in perioperative and critical care fluid resuscitation. Br J Surg. 2015;102:24-36.
24. Weinberg L, Li MH-G, Churilov L, Macgregor C, Garrett K, Eyles J, et al. The effects of 0.9% saline versus Plasma-Lyte 148 on renal function as assessed by creatinine concentration in patients undergoing major surgery: A single-centre double-blinded cluster crossover trial. PLoS One. 2021;16(5):e0251718.
25. Maheshwari K, Turan A, Makarova N, Ma C, Esa WAS, Ruetzler K, et al. Saline versus Lactated Ringer's Solution: The Saline or Lactated Ringer's (SOLAR) Trial. Anesthesiology. 2020;132:614-24.
26. Futier E, Garot M, Godet T, Biais M, Verzilli D, Quattara A, et al. Effect of Hydroxyethyl Starch vs Saline for Volume Replacement Therapy on Death or Postoperative Complications Among High-Risk Patients Undergoing Major Abdominal Surgery: The FLASH Randomized Clinical Trial. JAMA. 2020;323:225-36.
27. Xu Y, Wang S, He L, Yu H, Yu H. Hydroxyethyl starch 130/0.4 for volume replacement therapy in surgical patients: a systematic review and meta-analysis of randomized controlled trials. Perioper Med. 2021;10(1):16.
28. Kuhlmann AD, Spies C, Schulte E, Jara M, von Haefen C, Mertens M, et al. Preoperative hypoalbuminemia in liver surgery: an observational study at a university medical centre. BMJ Open. 2023;13:e068405.
29. Callum J, Skubas NJ, Bathla A, Keshavarz H, Clark EG, Rachwerg B, et al. Use of Intravenous Albumin: A Guideline From the International Collaboration for Transfusion Medicine Guidelines. Chest. 2024;166(2):321-38.
30. Bennett S, Baker LK, Martel G, Shorr R, Pawlik TM, Tinmouth A, et al. The impact of perioperative red blood cell transfusions in patients undergoing liver resection: a systematic review. HPB (Oxford). 2017;19:321-30.
31. Abeysundara L, Mallett S, Clevenger B. Point-of-Care Testing in Liver Disease and Liver Surgery. Semin Thromb Hemost. 2017;43:407-15.
32. Wilks JA, Hancher-Hodges S, Gottumukkala VNR. Contemporary perioperative anaesthetic management of hepatic resection. Adv Anesth. 2016;34:85-103.
33. Blasi A, Biancofore G, Green D. Haemodynamic monitoring during liver transplant surgery. In: Milan Z, Goonasekera C (Eds). Anesthesia for Hepatico-Pancreatic-Biliary Surgery and Transplantation. Switzerland AG: Springer Nature; 2021. pp. 195-208.
34. Thomas M, Kumar L, Jain P, Sarma C, Paul S, Surendran S. Correlation between radial and femoral arterial blood pressure during reperfusion in living donor liver transplantation. Indian J Anaesth. 2021;65:302-8.
35. Manecke GR Jr, Auger WR. Cardiac output determination from the arterial pressure wave: clinical testing of a novel algorithm that does not require calibration. J Cardiothoracic Vasc Anesth. 2007;21:3-7.
36. Shah SB, Bhargava AK, Hariharan U, Vishvakarma G, Jain CR, Kansal A. Cardiac output monitoring:

A comparative prospective observational study of the conventional cardiac output monitor Vigileo™ and the new smartphone-based application Capstesia™. Indian J Anaesth. 2018;62:584-91.

37. De Pietri L, Mocchegiani F, Leuzzi C, Montalti R, Vivarelli M, Agnoletti V. Transoesophageal echocardiography during liver transplantation. World J Hepatol. 2015;7:2432-48.
38. Maspero M, Yilmaz S, Cazzaniga B, Raj R, Ali K, Mazzaferro V, et al. The role of ischaemia-reperfusion injury and liver regeneration in hepatic tumour recurrence. JHEP Rep. 2023;5:100846.
39. Ciria R, Briceño J. The ALPPS procedure—As limited procedures as possible, leads to improved survival. Hepatobiliary Surg Nutr. 2022;11:636-9.
40. Popescu GA, Alexandrescu ST, Grigorie RT, Stoica L, Apavaloaie CA, Hrehoreţ D. GOOD TO KNOW: The ALPPS Procedure—Embracing a New Technique. Chirurgia (Bucur). 2017;112:332-41.
41. Bertens KA, Hawel J, Lung K, Buac S, Pineda-Solis K, Hernandez-Alejandro R. ALPPS: challenging the concept of unresectability—a systematic review. Int J Surg. 2015; 13:280-7.
42. Koul A, Pant D, Rudravaram S, Sood J. Thoracic epidural analgesia in donor hepatectomy: An analysis. Liver Transpl. 2018;24:214-21.
43. Wrighton LJ, O'Bosky KR, Namm JP, Senthil M. Postoperative management after hepatic resection. J Gastrointest Oncol. 2012;3:41-7.

25 CHAPTER

Anesthesia for Pancreatic Cancer Surgeries

Arun Muthukumar, Juan Jose Guerra-Londono, Carlos Eduardo Guerra-Londono

INTRODUCTION

In 2020, there were approximately 510,566 new cases and 467,005 deaths attributed to pancreatic cancer, constituting approximately 5% of all cancer deaths worldwide.[1] Despite its relatively low incidence (12th in incidence worldwide), pancreatic cancer has surpassed breast cancer as the third-leading cause of cancer death in North America and Europe and the sixth globally.[2] High-income countries in these regions are responsible for the majority of pancreatic cancer cases, presumably due to the aging population and lifestyle choices that increase their exposure to risk factors such as smoking, obesity, and diabetes.[3] Worldwide, pancreatic cancer duplicated its incidence, deaths, and disability-adjusted life-years between 1990 and 2017.[3] In addition to risk factors, the improvements in diagnostic imaging since the 1990s have been central to an improved diagnosis and staging of this condition.[4] Pancreatic cancer is generally regarded as a disease with poor survival, with surgery remaining the most important means to improve it.

Neoplasms from the pancreas can be histologically categorized into epithelial and nonepithelial neoplasms.[5] The epithelial component of the organ is composed of endocrine and exocrine glands. Roughly 80% of the malignant tumors of the pancreas arise from exocrine glands, specifically the ducts, which are known as pancreatic ductal adenocarcinomas (PDAC).[6] Due to this histologic dominance, the terms pancreatic cancer and PDAC are often used interchangeably.[5] Tumors of endocrine origin are categorized and managed differently.[7]

Patients undergoing pancreatic surgery can present multiple challenges for the anesthesiologist. First, the disease often coexists with significant comorbidity and the presence of systemic disease-related conditions, including those related to neoadjuvant therapy. Second, surgical techniques can result in major changes in the anesthetic plan, such as the need for goal-directed hemodynamic therapy (GDHT), neuraxial anesthesia, endocrine management, and perioperative anticoagulation. As a result, various anesthesia techniques, including general anesthesia (GA), total intravenous anesthesia (TIVA), and regional anesthesia have been thoroughly investigated in the context of pancreatic surgeries. In this chapter, we will discuss anesthetic management for adults undergoing pancreatic cancer surgery. We will present preoperative, intraoperative, and postoperative considerations, highlighting important aspects of the surgical technique and the implications for hemodynamic management. The authors acknowledge that the impact of anesthesia technique on cancer progression or recurrence remains largely controversial and is not central to the scope of this chapter. At the time of writing, the authors cannot recommend a particular anesthetic technique or medication to be administered with the sole purpose of reducing the risk of cancer progression.

PREOPERATIVE ASSESSMENT

Comorbid Conditions

The most common modifiable risk factors for pancreatic cancer include obesity, diabetes, and alcohol consumption.[8] These should be identified and addressed promptly in the preoperative period. Because pancreatic cancer tends to occur with increasing frequency in older individuals, cardiovascular, liver, and metabolic diseases frequently coexist. Diabetes management requires optimal glycemic control to minimize perioperative complications such as infection and delayed wound healing.[9] The loss of functional pancreatic tissue from cancer can indeed result in worsening or new-onset diabetes mellitus. When patients are amenable to upfront surgery, time to address these factors may be limited. However, in those undergoing neoadjuvant or induction treatments, these conditions must be optimized.

Ductal Occlusion, Malabsorption, Body Composition, and Deconditioning

Pancreatic head cancer may present with signs and symptoms of ductal occlusion.[10] Evidence shows that patients with ductal occlusion have worse overall and recurrence-free survival at 3 years postoperatively.[10] These patients are known to have organ damage, which increases the duct-to-parenchyma ratio, leading to pancreatic exocrine insufficiency and malabsorption. This is evidenced clinically by reduced nutritional and anthropometric indices regardless of neoadjuvant treatment.[10] Preoperative biliary drainage is generally avoided as it increases the risk of postoperative complications. Nonetheless, it may be necessary in patients with significant hyperbilirubinemia (>15 mg/dL), cholangitis, or undergoing neoadjuvant therapy.[11]

Preoperative sarcopenia is an independent risk factor for the development of clinically relevant postoperative pancreatic fistula.[12] Recent meta-analyses also suggest that it negatively impacts both the overall and progression-free survivals of patients undergoing curative treatment.[13,14] Excess visceral fat and sarcopenia can further predict poor outcomes after pancreatic surgery.[15] The Malnutrition Universal Screening Tool (MUST) or the Patient-Generated Subjective Global Assessment (PG-SGA) can screen cancer patients for malnourishment. Serum albumin, prealbumin, and transferrin levels provide insight into the nutritional status of these patients.[16] A multidisciplinary team should assess the nutritional and physical status of the patients and identify those patients that may require pancreatic enzyme replacement therapy in the preoperative period to improve their nutritional status.[10]

Deconditioning in patients with cancer refers to the physical decline resulting from prolonged inactivity or chronic illness, characterized by reduced muscle strength, endurance, and overall functional capacity. Recent evidence suggests that prehabilitation programs can improve physical function and quality of life in the preoperative period and reduce the length of stay (LOS).[17] Prehabilitation programs may improve muscle strength, body composition, and cardiopulmonary fitness in preparation for surgery. In major abdominal surgery, a 4-week in-hospital supervised multimodal prehabilitation program reduced the risk and severity of postoperative complications.[18]

Nonsurgical Therapies

Current evidence recommends all patients undergoing surgical resection of PDAC receive adjuvant chemotherapy (after surgery).[19] The evidence is conflicting about the potential of neoadjuvant therapies to maximize total resection or effect in overall survival.[19] Nonetheless, patients with borderline or unresectable tumors are the main candidates for neoadjuvant or induction therapies (chemotherapy and radiation) to reduce the tumor size, which may allow a complete resection.[6,7,19] Recent evidence found that patients who received neoadjuvant therapy for pancreatic cancer had a significant increase in muscle mass, which can be a result of reduced tumor burden and cancer-induced inflammation.[20]

Recommended regimens such as gemcitabine, nab-paclitaxel, and FOLFIRINOX (i.e., combination of fluorouracil, leucovorin, irinotecan, and oxaliplatin) can lead to side effects such as neutropenia, thrombocytopenia, and anemia, and demand careful management to ensure patients are in the best possible condition for surgery.[7] Hematologic abnormalities increase the risk of infections, bleeding, and poor wound healing, making thorough preoperative assessment and optimization crucial. Preoperative anemia is an independent predictor of postoperative complications after pancreatic surgery.[21] Overall, the management of anemia (red blood cell transfusions or erythropoiesis-stimulating agents), neutropenia (growth factors), and thrombocytopenia (stimulators or platelet transfusion) should be performed as otherwise clinically indicated.

DAY OF SURGERY

Cancer survivors have a significant psychological burden, both from cancer as well as its treatment. Addressing individual patients' needs, including the management of anxiety, options for regional analgesia, and expectations of the perioperative environment [e.g., postoperative intensive care unit (ICU) admission, transfusion] is paramount. However, the routine use of anxiolytics, antiacids, or antisialagogues on the day of surgery is not recommended. In addition, signs or symptoms of gastric outlet obstruction should alert the need for rapid sequence induction. Finally, the high prevalence of gastrointestinal symptoms in these patients highlights the need to address postoperative nausea and vomiting (PONV) (e.g., scopolamine, aprepitant).

Approximately 50% of patients with pancreatic cancer experience pain. During the disease course, the pain of pancreatic cancer may radiate from the abdomen to the back. In one study, a higher stage and involvement of the pancreatic body were associated with a higher prevalence of pain. Overall, employing a multimodal pain regimen can reduce the opioid burden on this population.[22]

Despite the invasiveness and at times prolonged postoperative stay, patients undergoing pancreatic cancer surgery benefit from an enhanced recovery after surgery (ERAS) protocol.[11] While the ERAS society guidelines for pancreatoduodenectomy (PD) recommend preoperative gabapentinoids, recent evidence has challenged its benefit on acute postoperative pain.[23] Some key points relevant to anesthesiologists include:

- *Preoperative care:* Patient education, nutritional assessment, limited preoperative fasting, carbohydrate loading, and selective biliary stenting.
- *Prehabilitation:* Encouraging physical activity and respiratory exercises.
- *Anesthetic management:* Multimodal analgesia and maintenance of normothermia via active body surface warming.
- *Surgical techniques:* Laparoscopic PD should be performed in highly experienced, high-volume centers. Clinicians can expect a longer procedural time and reduced blood loss.
- *Intraoperative care:* GDHT and antibiotic prophylaxis.
- *Postoperative care:* Early mobilization, early oral intake [i.e., protocol signifies the importance of early oral intake from postoperative day (POD 1)], and glycemic control.
- *Monitoring and assessment:* Regular assessment of pain, gastrointestinal function, and recovery progress.
- *Discharge planning:* Criteria for discharge readiness and postdischarge follow-up.

INTRAOPERATIVE CONSIDERATIONS

Surgical Planning

Upon diagnosis of a pancreatic mass, the differential diagnosis includes adenocarcinomas, acinar and mucinous tumors, as well as tumors of neuroendocrine origin. Each has a different biological behavior and necessitates a distinct surgical approach.[24] Typically, PDAC without distant metastatic disease may be classified into three surgical stages: resectable, borderline-resectable, and unresectable (locally advanced or the presence of metastasis).[6,7] This classification is defined based on the degree of vessel involvement, which includes the celiac trunk, superior mesenteric artery (SMA), portal vein (PV), or superior mesenteric vein (SMV).[6,7]

Tumors of the body and tail of the pancreas typically require distal pancreatectomy (DP) with en-bloc splenectomy.[7] In contrast, those involving the head will typically undergo a PD or Whipple procedure, which will remove the head of the pancreas, part of the duodenum, and common bile duct, the gallbladder, and possibly part of the stomach.

In general, resectable tumors do not have any radiographic evidence of SMV or PV distortion, and computed tomography shows clear fat planes around the celiac trunk, hepatic artery, and SMA. Borderline resectable tumors can have venous involvement of SMV and PV, so long as there is the ability to perform a safe resection and reconstruction. In the arterial system, borderline resectable tumors can show encasement of the gastroduodenal artery up to the hepatic artery or its abutment but without compromising the celiac trunk significantly. Finally, tumor contact with the SMA (head tumor) or celiac trunk (body or tail) should not exceed 180° of the vessel's wall. Naturally, these recommendations rely on the surgeon's experience and ability to reconstruct the vascular supply.[7] Other less common surgical procedures include the total pancreatectomy, minimally invasive surgeries (laparoscopic or robotic-assisted), and the Appleby procedure.[25] A recent meta-analysis of randomized controlled trials (RCTs) demonstrated that minimally invasive pancreatic surgery reduces LOS and intraoperative blood loss, at the expense of a lengthier procedure.[26] It is possible that minimally invasive surgery also reduces the rate of surgical site infections.[26] A summary of the different surgical approaches, indications, and techniques is available in **Table 1**. The anesthesia team should be aware of the staging and surgical approach, as these will determine the extent of surgery, vascular reconstruction, and potential intraoperative events. For instance, Whipple procedures often require manual pressure from the surgeon on the PV and inferior vena cava during tumor dissection, reducing venous return, and cardiac preload, and ultimately causing hypotension even in the absence of surgical bleeding. Active communication with the surgeon is strongly advised to determine the most appropriate management.

Monitoring

Aside from the basic American Society of Anesthesiologists (ASA) monitoring standards, the recommendations

TABLE 1: Summarizes the different surgical techniques, indications, and considerations.

Distal pancreatectomy	Body/tail tumor	*Total (en bloc):* • Pancreas tail • Spleen *Possible:* Pancreas body (partial or total)	*Possible:* Vascular supply (rare)	• Less invasive. MIS more feasible • May not require invasive monitoring, unless significant bleeding is expected
Pancreaticoduodenectomy (*Whipple* procedure)	Head/neck tumor	*Total:* • Pancreas head • Common bile duct • Gallbladder *Partial or total:* Duodenum *Possible:* • Pancreas neck or body (partial) • Pylorus • Stomach (partial)	*Mandatory*:* • Gastrojejunostomy • Hepaticojejunostomy • Pancreatojejunostomy *Possible:* Vascular supply	• Major vessel compression • Higher risk of bleeding and transfusion • Fluid shifts • Extent of vessel dissection affects potential blood loss
Distal pancreatectomy with celiac artery resection (*Appleby* procedure)	Neck/body tumor or tumor affecting the celiac trunk or roots of common hepatic or splenic arteries. *The tumor cannot extend to the pancreas head*	*Total:* • Pancreas neck, body, and tail • Celiac artery • Spleen *Possible:* Stomach (partial)	*Possible:* Vascular supply in case collateral flow to the liver is impaired	Rarely indicated. Complex vascular resection of the celiac artery warrants invasive monitoring, careful fluid management and preparation for massive transfusion
Total pancreatectomy	• Multifocal tumors • Locally advanced tumors	*Total:* • Pancreas • Duodenum • Common bile duct • Gallbladder *Possible:* Stomach (partial)	*Mandatory*:* • Gastrojejunostomy • Hepaticojejunostomy *Possible:* Vascular supply	Rarely indicated

*Reconstruction technique will largely depend on patient anatomy. Options include Roux-en-Y reconstruction and conventional loop reconstruction.[27] Obesity is a risk factor for pancreatic ductal adenocarcinomas (PDAC), and some patients may have prior history of gastric bypass. This will likely result in a more challenging PD.[28]
(PD: pancreaticoduodenectomy; MIS: minimally invasive surgery)

for intraoperative monitoring follow the surgical considerations explained in **Table 1**. Pancreatic cancer surgeries are typically considered major abdominal surgeries. Thus, surgery-specific considerations revolve around the monitoring of circulation, the need for invasive hemodynamic monitoring, and the plans for intraoperative and postoperative pain management. In adults undergoing noncardiac surgery, older age, female gender, and higher ASA physical status independently predict the risk of intraoperative hypotension.[29]

- *Open surgical approaches:* Open surgical approaches require large-bore intravenous access. As studies continue to support the safety of temporary vasopressor use via peripheral intravenous lines, central venous lines are rarely indicated. In addition, the hemodynamic shifts imply intra-arterial catheter blood pressure monitoring, blood gases, and electrolytes. In these cases, using minimally invasive hemodynamic monitoring (e.g., LIdCO, FloTrac) can help identify and treat the cause of hypotension. Total pancreatectomies require frequent arterial blood samples for close metabolic monitoring and titration of the insulin infusion, which in this case is essential to prevent a state of diabetic ketoacidosis. An exception to the hemodynamic monitoring in open surgical approaches may be a DP with clear surgical planes and easy exposure in patients with few risk factors for intraoperative hypotension.

- *Minimally invasive approaches (i.e., laparoscopic and robotic-assisted):* These procedures have less risk of bleeding, albeit with the need for reverse Trendelenburg and pneumoperitoneum, which can lead to reduced preload and hypotension. Positioning will typically allow access to the extremities if invasive hemodynamic monitoring is not placed before or immediately after anesthetic induction. Unless there are surgical concerns, a robotic DP will typically not require invasive hemodynamic monitoring.

Core body temperature monitoring is commonly done with an esophageal probe. Bladder, rectal, and axillary sites do not accurately represent the core body temperature. If intraoperative hyperthermic intraperitoneal chemotherapy is indicated, additional temperature monitoring includes bladder and intra-abdominal tissue temperatures. Active warming is encouraged via forced-air convection warming of the upper and/or lower body.

Blood gas and metabolic monitoring are reserved for cases in which an arterial line is obtained, such as those with extensive resections (e.g., Whipple, Appleby), fluid shifts, severe preoperative anemia, or total pancreatectomy. The frequency of blood drawn should be determined on an individual basis and as clinically indicated. In cases of total pancreatectomy, blood draws may be necessary every 30 minutes or every hour.

Anesthetic Management

Induction of Anesthesia

Induction of anesthesia is most commonly intravenous, including a hypnotic (e.g., propofol), a muscle relaxant (e.g., rocuronium), and an analgesic (e.g., fentanyl). Etomidate can be useful in patients with significant cardiovascular comorbidity (e.g., decreased ejection fraction) due to a better hemodynamic profile when compared to propofol. Patients with pancreatic cancer are often malnourished and frail and have increased susceptibility to hemodynamic instability following induction. Slow titration of the hypnotic agent can significantly reduce the induction dose and decrease the risk of hypotension postinduction. Vasopressors should be immediately available.

Maintenance of Anesthesia

Both balanced inhalational volatile anesthesia (INVA) and TIVA have been used in patients undergoing pancreatectomy. Propofol-based TIVA has the primary advantage of reducing the risk of PONV. Some literature suggests that TIVA may offer greater oncologic benefits and increased recurrence-free survival than INVA.[30] Makito et al. evaluated the Japanese Diagnosis Procedure Combination database (n = 196,303) and found no significant difference in overall survival (OS) and recurrence-free survival (RFS) between TIVA and INVA for patients undergoing gastrointestinal surgeries, including pancreatic surgeries.[31] This large-scale study suggested that the choice of anesthesia may not significantly impact long-term cancer prognosis. While some studies have shown better outcomes following propofol-based TIVA in gastrointestinal tumor patients, a multicenter trial evaluated the effects of TIVA and INVA in pancreatic adenocarcinoma patients undergoing surgery by measuring circulating tumor cells on days 0, 3, 7, and at 6 and 12 months. The trial found no significant difference between the types of anesthesia in reducing the time to recurrence ($p = 0.589$) and in reducing the levels of circulating tumor cells between the two groups [hazard ratio (HR) 2.7, 95% confidence interval (CI) 0.35–1.67].[32]

General Anesthesia versus Combined General-Epidural Anesthesia

While GA is the standard of practice in patients with pancreatic carcinoma undergoing major surgeries, combining GA with thoracic epidural analgesia (TEA) in pancreatic cancer surgeries can provide superior analgesia, reduced opioid consumption, and with similar or better oncologic outcomes compared to GA alone.[33,34] Notably, epidural anesthesia carries a higher risk of intraoperative hypotension. Nonetheless, TEA promotes the return of gastrointestinal function, which could improve recovery and LOS. Mixed evidence exists on the effect of TEA on postoperative outcomes. For instance, Kim et al. noted that epidural analgesia increases the hospital stay anywhere from 6 to 7 days following postpancreaticoduodenectomy to DP.[35] In contrast, a meta-analysis by Pöpping et al. found that TEA significantly reduced postoperative pain scores and opioid consumption compared to systemic analgesia alone. There were no significant differences between groups (TEA or patient-controlled intravenous analgesia) in the clinical, surgical, or postoperative characteristics, including LOS.[36] In the postoperative period, TEA is continued with lower concentrations of local anesthetics (e.g., 0.125% or 0.0625% bupivacaine, 0.1% ropivacaine) with or without epidural opioids (e.g., fentanyl, hydromorphone).

Regarding anticoagulation, TEA can be considered in all patients receiving prophylaxis. Readers are referred to the current regional anesthesia guidelines.[37] For patients requiring therapeutic anticoagulation, such as during vascular reconstruction, TEA can still be considered when anticoagulation is limited to the intraoperative period. Communication with the surgeon is strongly advised to confirm any plans for vascular reconstruction and the need for postoperative anticoagulation, as therapeutic anticoagulation contraindicates TEA.

Anesthetic Adjuvants

Ketamine has advantages as an opioid-sparing alternative, particularly in patients with chronic opioid use. Furthermore, one study demonstrated the expression of the N-methyl-D-aspartate (NMDA) receptor type R2a in pancreatic cancer cells, where ketamine and esketamine inhibited cell proliferation and cell death in pancreatic cancer cells.[38] The clinical impact of this is yet to be determined.

Dexmedetomidine is also a useful opioid-sparing adjuvant, with a beneficial hemodynamic profile. A recent randomized controlled trial showed that intraoperative dexmedetomidine reduced the early postoperative inflammatory response in patients undergoing laparoscopic pancreaticoduodenectomy, as explained by the reduced neutrophil to lymphocyte ratio ($p < 0.032$).[39]

Intravenous lidocaine infusions (e.g., 2 mg/kg/h after a 1.5 mg/kg bolus) constitute another opioid-sparing alternative. In a recent randomized controlled trial of adults undergoing pancreatectomy, the group assigned to lidocaine had a lower mean intraoperative sufentanil dose, without any difference in postoperative complications or LOS. Differences in oncologic outcomes were mixed.[40]

Hemodynamic Management

Pancreatic surgeries can result in significant hemodynamic changes due to extensive dissection near major blood vessels and the potential for substantial blood loss. A long-standing debate still exists about the optimal hemodynamic management strategy. Three fluid management strategies can be identified: liberal, restrictive, and GDHT. Because the definition of each strategy varies widely in the literature, caution is advised when interpreting the results of clinical studies, particularly when the control group is not clearly defined ("standard of care") or when data is retrospective. Regardless of the strategy, the main priority is to avoid intraoperative hypotension (i.e., mean arterial pressure <65 mm Hg).

Liberal fluid management: Liberal strategies generally favor fluid administration over vasopressor use by ensuring a minimum volume of fluids per hour of surgery. When using this strategy, an overall positive fluid balance is expected. In the RELIEF (Restrictive versus Liberal Fluid Therapy for Major Abdominal Surgery) trial, a liberal strategy consisted of an initial bolus of 10 mL/kg of body weight followed by an infusion of 8 mL/kg/h until the end of surgery.[41] Fluid infusion rates could be decreased after the first 4 hours if clinically indicated. The main benefits of a liberal strategy are a reduced vasopressor requirement and decreased risk of acute kidney injury. Nonetheless, liberal strategies carry a risk of fluid overload, which can raise concerns such as postoperative ileus due to interstitial and bowel edema.

Restrictive fluid management: Limits fluid administration to a net zero fluid balance, preventing fluid overload, edema, and complications. Mixed evidence exists on the benefit of restrictive strategies in major abdominal surgery. Retrospective data suggests an increased risk of complications when >4,400 mL of fluids are administered during the first 24 hours.[42] Furthermore, hospitals with more restrictive fluid strategies (<10 mL/kg/h) have reduced rates of pancreatic fistula.[43] In the RELIEF trial, which randomized some 1,490 participants to restrictive (net zero) or liberal strategies, patients undergoing a restrictive strategy were more likely to require vasopressor support. No differences in the rates of major postoperative complications or disability-free survival were noted between groups, except for a higher risk of acute kidney injury in those assigned to a restrictive strategy.[41] While avoidance of excessive fluid administration can be beneficial, restrictive strategies carry a risk of vasopressor use and acute kidney injury.

Goal-directed hemodynamic therapy: Consists of a management algorithm that maintains hemodynamic variables within predefined goals. GDHT relies on monitoring of parameters such as stroke volume variation (SVV), pulse pressure variation, systemic vascular resistance, and cardiac output. As such, GDHT aims to optimize cardiac output and tissue perfusion, presumably balancing the benefits of both restrictive and liberal approaches. Lopes et al. randomized 100 high-risk surgical patients and found a lower complication rate (34% vs. 57%, $p = 0.04$) and shorter hospital stay (mean difference of 1.16 days) in the GDHT group.[44] Furthermore, a meta-analysis of RCTs showed that the GDHT group had significantly fewer gastrointestinal complications (23.5% vs. 50%, $p = 0.036$) and shorter ICU stays (2.3 vs. 4.1 days, $p = 0.021$).[45] Moreover, Sultzer et al. suggested that incorporating GDHT before the reconstructive phase of pancreaticoduodenectomy may contribute to lower postoperative rates of pancreatic leak and delayed gastric emptying. The authors also stressed that the optimal threshold of SVV <12 resulted in a significant 15.4% reduction in postpancreaticoduodenectomy complications compared to patients with SVV >12.[46] These findings strongly support GDHT over other fluid administration techniques for pancreatic cancer patients undergoing major surgeries, offering improved outcomes, reduced complications, and shorter hospital stays.

Glucose Control

Impaired glucose tolerance is present in most patients diagnosed with pancreatic adenocarcinoma and up to half of the patients can have preexisting diabetes. Hyperglycemia is known to increase the risk of infections, prolonged hospital stays, and mortality. Avoiding blood glucose levels above 180 mg/dL with standard-of-care perioperative guidelines is sufficient in most patients. However, patients undergoing total pancreatectomy should be treated similarly to patients with type 1 diabetes.

POSTOPERATIVE CONSIDERATIONS

Multimodal Analgesia

- *Regional analgesia:* Aside from TEA, fascial plane blocks [e.g., transversus abdominis plane (TAP) block] are acceptable alternatives to TEA for patients undergoing pancreatic cancer surgery. Fascial plane blocks are most commonly a single-injection procedure and are not expected to provide analgesia beyond 24 hours. In 2019, Solis-Velasco et al. showed that pancreatic cancer patients who received a TAP block with bupivacaine had fewer morphine requirements than patients who did not receive them, without any difference in postoperative morbidity and LOS.[47] There is still controversy between TAP blocks and TEA in major abdominal surgeries. Overall, one can expect higher postoperative opioid requirements in those undergoing TAP blocks (as opposed to TEA),[48] without major differences in the quality of recovery. The TAP block offers a few advantages over TEA, such as promoting early ambulation, reducing the need for intensive monitoring, and minimizing episodes of hypotension. As of now, we are not aware of major trials of TEA versus TAP (or other fascial plane alternatives) in adults undergoing pancreatic cancer surgery.
- *Nonsteroidal anti-inflammatory drugs (NSAIDs) and acetaminophen:* Perioperative NSAIDs are an important opioid-sparing modality in multimodal analgesia. Due to the gastrointestinal and renal side effects associated with them, the ERAS guidelines issue caution when starting NSAIDs postoperatively. In contrast, acetaminophen has a better safety profile and can routinely be started in the preoperative period, with or without other NSAIDs.
- *Intravenous Patient-controlled analgesia (PCA):* PCA is useful during the first 2–3 postoperative days. Once bowel function has resumed, transition to oral opioids is encouraged.

Postoperative Morbidity and Mortality

Improvements in perioperative surgical and anesthetic management have contributed to decreased mortality rates for pancreatic cancer. Overall, mortality from pancreatic surgery ranges from 2 to 5% and can result from cardiovascular, infectious, respiratory, or hemorrhagic complications.[49] In contrast, complications are frequent, with 30–60% of patients experiencing them.[49] The most common complications after pancreatic cancer surgery include pancreatic fistula (~20%), delayed gastric emptying (8–45%), intra-abdominal infections (1–12%), and hemorrhage (3–13%). Postoperative complications are important because they increase the risk of death and disability and prolong hospital LOS. As a result, it is not uncommon for perioperative pathways to include immediate admission to the ICU. With the advent of minimally invasive techniques, reduced blood loss, and patient optimization, the need for ICU admission continues to decrease.

Pancreas Transplant after Pancreatic Cancer Surgery

The evolution of pancreatic transplantation (i.e., either islet or partial organ transplantation) for patients with end-stage malignancy following pancreatic resection has progressed in recent years.[50] Although still an emerging field with ongoing research questions, pancreatic transplant patients can become increasingly common in the perioperative setting. The management of these patients can be particularly complex during the preoperative and postoperative periods due to challenges such as graft rejection and the administration of immunosuppressants. Pancreatic islet autotransplantation may improve glucose control and reduce insulin requirements. In addition, it avoids immunosuppression when compared with allograft pancreatic transplantation.

CONCLUSION

Pancreatic cancer is a leading cause of cancer death worldwide. Adults with pancreatic cancer present for surgical intervention with significant comorbidity and the presence of consequences of cancer or cancer treatment. Surgical techniques can vary from open approaches, with or without vascular reconstruction, to minimally invasive robotic approaches. This results in major changes in the anesthetic plan, such as the need for goal-directed hemodynamic therapy, neuraxial anesthesia, endocrine management, and perioperative anticoagulation. As such, we strongly recommend open communication with the surgeon to understand the surgical plan and devise an anesthetic management that aligns the surgical concerns. The use of ERAS pathways is encouraged, with careful review of updated evidence to modify pre-existing recommendations. The anesthetic technique should be tailored to concerns regarding hemodynamic management, multimodal analgesia, and postoperative care to improve postoperative outcomes. Currently, the evidence does not support an anesthetic technique solely to reduce the risk of cancer progression.

REFERENCES

1. Bray F, Laversanne M, Sung H, Ferlay J, Siegel RL, Soerjomataram I, et al. Global cancer statistics 2022: GLOBOCAN estimates of incidence and mortality worldwide for 36 cancers in 185 countries. CA Cancer J Clin. 2024;74(3):229-63.
2. Siegel RL, Giaquinto AN, Jemal A. Cancer statistics, 2024. CA Cancer J Clin. 2024;74(1):12-49.
3. Collaborators GBDPC. The global, regional, and national burden of pancreatic cancer and its attributable risk factors in 195 countries and territories, 1990-2017: a systematic analysis for the Global Burden of Disease Study 2017. Lancet Gastroenterol Hepatol. 2019;4(12):934-47.
4. Yu J, Yang X, He W, Ye W. Burden of pancreatic cancer along with attributable risk factors in Europe between 1990 and 2019, and projections until 2039. Int J Cancer. 2021;149(5):993-1001.
5. Haeberle L, Esposito I. Pathology of pancreatic cancer. Transl Gastroenterol Hepatol. 2019;4:50.
6. Conroy T, Pfeiffer P, Vilgrain V, Lamarca A, Seufferlein T, O'Reilly EM, et al. Pancreatic cancer: ESMO clinical practice guideline for diagnosis, treatment and follow-up. Ann Oncol. 2023;34(11):987-1002.
7. Network NCC. (2024). Pancreatic Adenocarcinoma. [online] Available from https://www.nccn.org/professionals/physician_gls/pdf/pancreatic.pdf [Last accessed February, 2025].
8. Sung H, Ferlay J, Siegel RL, Laversanne M, Soerjomataram I, Jemal A, et al. Global Cancer Statistics 2020: GLOBOCAN Estimates of Incidence and Mortality Worldwide for 36 Cancers in 185 Countries. CA Cancer J Clin. 2021; 71(3):209-49.
9. Ata A, Lee J, Bestle SL, Desemone J, Stain SC. Postoperative hyperglycemia and surgical site infection in general surgery patients. Arch Surg. 2010;145(9):858-64.
10. Hidaka Y, Tanoue S, Ayukawa T, Takumi K, Noguchi H, Higashi M, et al. Impact of pancreatic ductal occlusion on postoperative outcomes in pancreatic head cancer patients undergoing neoadjuvant therapy. J Gastroenterol. 2004;59(9):858-68.
11. Melloul E, Lassen K, Roulin D, Grass F, Perinel J, Adham M, et al. Guidelines for Perioperative care for pancreatoduodenectomy: enhanced recovery after surgery (ERAS) Recommendations 2019. World J Surg. 2020;44(7):2056-84.
12. Nishida Y, Kato Y, Kudo M, Aizawa H, Okubo S, Takahashi D, et al. Preoperative sarcopenia strongly influences the risk of postoperative pancreatic fistula formation after pancreaticoduodenectomy. J Gastrointest Surg. 2016; 20(9):1586-94.
13. Thormann M, Hinnerichs M, Barajas Ordonez F, Saalfeld S, Perrakis A, Croner R, et al. Sarcopenia is an independent prognostic factor in patients with pancreatic cancer—a Meta-analysis. Acad Radiol. 2023;30(8):1552-61.
14. Zhong L, Liu J, Xia M, Zhang Y, Liu S, Tan G. Effect of sarcopenia on survival in patients after pancreatic surgery: a systematic review and meta-analysis. Front Nutr. 2023;10:1315097.
15. Pecorelli N, Carrara G, De Cobelli F, Cristel G, Damascelli A, Balzano G, et al. Effect of sarcopenia and visceral obesity on mortality and pancreatic fistula following pancreatic cancer surgery. Br J Surg. 2016;103(4):434-42.

16. Wigmore SJ, Plester CE, Richardson RA, Fearon KC. Changes in nutritional status associated with unresectable pancreatic cancer. Br J Cancer. 1997;75(1):106-9.
17. Bundred JR, Kamarajah SK, Hammond JS, Wilson CH, Prentis J, Pandanaboyana S. Prehabilitation prior to surgery for pancreatic cancer: A systematic review. Pancreatology. 2020;20(6):1243-50.
18. Molenaar CJL, Minnella EM, Coca-Martinez M, Ten Cate DWG, Regis M, Awasthi R, et al. Effect of multimodal prehabilitation on reducing postoperative complications and enhancing functional capacity following colorectal cancer surgery: The PREHAB Randomized Clinical Trial. JAMA Surg. 2023;158(6):572-81.
19. Springfeld C, Ferrone CR, Katz MHG, Philip PA, Hong TS, Hackert T, et al. Neoadjuvant therapy for pancreatic cancer. Nat Rev Clin Oncol. 2023;20(5):318-37.
20. Sandini M, Patino M, Ferrone CR, Alvarez-Perez CA, Honselmann KC, Paiella S, et al. Association between changes in body composition and neoadjuvant treatment for pancreatic cancer. JAMA Surg. 2018;153(9):809-15.
21. Xu JY, Tian XD, Yang YM, Song JH, Wei JM. Preoperative Anemia Is a Predictor of Worse Postoperative Outcomes Following Open Pancreatoduodenectomy: A Propensity Score-Based Analysis. Front Med (Lausanne). 2022; 9:818805.
22. D'Haese JG, Hartel M, Demir IE, Hinz U, Bergmann F, Buchler MW, et al. Pain sensation in pancreatic diseases is not uniform: the different facets of pancreatic pain. World J Gastroenterol. 2014;20(27):9154-61.
23. Verret M, Lauzier F, Zarychanski R, Perron C, Savard X, Pinard AM, et al. Perioperative use of gabapentinoids for the management of postoperative acute pain: A systematic review and meta-analysis. Anesthesiology. 2020;133(2):265-79.
24. Yeo CJ, Cameron JL, Lillemoe KD, Sitzmann JV, Hruban RH, Goodman SN, et al. Pancreaticoduodenectomy for cancer of the head of the pancreas. 201 patients. Ann Surg. 1995;221(6):721-31; discussion 31-3.
25. Cannella R, Borhani AA, Zureikat AH, Tublin ME. Appleby Procedure (Distal Pancreatectomy With Celiac Artery Resection) for locally advanced pancreatic carcinoma: indications, outcomes, and imaging. Am J Roentgenol. 2019;213(1):35-44.
26. Pfister M, Probst P, Muller PC, Antony P, Klotz R, Kalkum E, et al. Minimally invasive versus open pancreatic surgery: meta-analysis of randomized clinical trials. BJS Open. 2023;7(2):zrad007.
27. Grobmyer SR, Hollenbeck ST, Jaques DP, Jarnagin WR, DeMatteo R, Coit DG, et al. Roux-en-Y reconstruction after pancreaticoduodenectomy. Arch Surg. 2008;143(12): 1184-8.
28. Peng JS, Corcelles R, Choong K, Poturalski M, Gandhi N, Walsh RM, et al. Pancreatoduodenectomy after Roux-en-Y gastric bypass: technical considerations and outcomes. HPB (Oxford). 2018;20(1):34-40.
29. Schnetz MP, Danks DJ, Mahajan A. Preoperative identification of patient-dependent blood pressure targets associated with low risk of intraoperative hypotension during noncardiac surgery. Anesth Analg. 2023;136(2): 194-203.
30. Zhang Y, Wang F, Zhang H, Wei Y, Deng Y, Wang D. Volatile anesthesia versus propofol-based total intravenous anesthesia: A retrospective analysis of charts of patients who underwent elective digestive tract cancer curative surgeries. Medicine (Baltimore). 2022;101(29):e29169.
31. Makito K, Matsui H, Fushimi K, Yasunaga H. Volatile versus total intravenous anesthesia for cancer prognosis in patients having digestive cancer surgery. Anesthesiology. 2020;133(4):764-73.
32. Lahoud MJ, Kourie HR, Antoun J, El Osta L, Ghosn M. Road map for pain management in pancreatic cancer: A review. World J Gastrointest Oncol. 2016;8(8):599-606.
33. Call TR, Pace NL, Thorup DB, Maxfield D, Chortkoff B, Christensen J, et al. Factors associated with improved survival after resection of pancreatic adenocarcinoma: a multivariable model. Anesthesiology. 2015;122(2):317-24.
34. Lin KJ, Hsu FK, Shyr YM, Ni YW, Tsou MY, Chang KY. Effect of epidural analgesia on long-term outcomes after curative surgery for pancreatic cancer: A single-center cohort study in Taiwan. J Chin Med Assoc. 2022;85(1):124-8.
35. Kim SS, Niu X, Elliott IA, Jiang JP, Dann AM, Damato LM, et al. Epidural analgesia improves postoperative pain control but impedes early discharge in patients undergoing pancreatic surgery. Pancreas. 2019;48(5):719-25.
36. Popping DM, Elia N, Marret E, Remy C, Tramer MR. Protective effects of epidural analgesia on pulmonary complications after abdominal and thoracic surgery: a meta-analysis. Arch Surg. 2008;143(10):990-9; discussion 1000.
37. Narouze S, Benzon HT, Provenzano D, Buvanendran A, De Andres J, Deer T, et al. Interventional Spine and Pain Procedures in Patients on Antiplatelet and Anticoagulant Medications (Second Edition): Guidelines From the American Society of Regional Anesthesia and Pain Medicine, the European Society of Regional Anaesthesia and Pain Therapy, the American Academy of Pain Medicine, the International Neuromodulation Society, the North American Neuromodulation Society, and the World Institute of Pain. Reg Anesth Pain Med. 2018;43(3):225-62.
38. Malsy M, Gebhardt K, Gruber M, Wiese C, Graf B, Bundscherer A. Effects of ketamine, s-ketamine, and MK 801 on proliferation, apoptosis, and necrosis in pancreatic cancer cells. BMC Anesthesiol. 2015;15:111.
39. Chen YX, Du L, Wang LN, Shi YY, Liao M, Zhong M, et al. Effects of dexmedetomidine on systemic inflammation and postoperative complications in laparoscopic

pancreaticoduodenectomy: A double-blind randomized controlled trial. World J Surg. 2023;47(2):500-9.
40. Zhang H, Qu M, Guo K, Wang Y, Gu J, Wu H, et al. Intraoperative lidocaine infusion in patients undergoing pancreatectomy for pancreatic cancer: a mechanistic, multicentre randomised clinical trial. Br J Anaesth. 2022;129(2):244-53.
41. Myles PS, Bellomo R, Corcoran T, Forbes A, Peyton P, Story D, et al. Restrictive versus liberal fluid therapy for major abdominal surgery. N Engl J Med. 2018;378(24):2263-74.
42. Gilgien J, Hubner M, Halkic N, Demartines N, Roulin D. Perioperative fluids and complications after pancreatoduodenectomy within an enhanced recovery pathway. Sci Rep. 2020;10(1):17898.
43. Healy MA, McCahill LE, Chung M, Berri R, Ito H, Obi SH, et al. Intraoperative fluid resuscitation strategies in pancreatectomy: Results from 38 Hospitals in Michigan. Annals of Surgical Oncology. 2016;23(9):3047-55.
44. Lopes MR, Oliveira MA, Pereira VO, Lemos IP, Auler JO, Jr Michard F. Goal-directed fluid management based on pulse pressure variation monitoring during high-risk surgery: a pilot randomized controlled trial. Crit Care. 2007;11(5):R100.
45. Giglio MT, Marucci M, Testini M, Brienza N. Goal-directed haemodynamic therapy and gastrointestinal complications in major surgery: a meta-analysis of randomized controlled trials. Br J Anaesth. 2009;103(5):637-46.
46. Sulzer JK, Sastry AV, Meyer LM, Cochran A, Buhrman WC, Baker EH, et al. The impact of intraoperative goal-directed fluid therapy on complications after pancreaticoduodenectomy. Ann Med Surg (Lond). 2018;36:23-8.
47. Solis-Velasco MA, Ore Carranza AS, Stackhouse KA, Verkoulen K, Watkins AA, Akhouri V, et al. Transversus abdominis plane block reduces pain and narcotic consumption after robot-assisted distal pancreatectomy. HPB (Oxford). 2019;21(8):1039-45.
48. Wu Y, Liu F, Tang H, Wang Q, Chen L, Wu H, et al. The analgesic efficacy of subcostal transversus abdominis plane block compared with thoracic epidural analgesia and intravenous opioid analgesia after radical gastrectomy. Anesth Analg. 2013;117(2):507-13.
49. Ho CK, Kleeff J, Friess H, Büchler MW. Complications of pancreatic surgery. HPB (Oxford). 2005;7(2):99-108.
50. Aref A, Zayan T, Pararajasingam R, Sharma A, Halawa A. Pancreatic transplantation: Brief review of the current evidence. World J Transplant. 2019;9(4):81-93.

CHAPTER 26

Anesthesia for Stomach and Gallbladder Cancer Surgeries

Punitha Chockalingam, Nairita Das, Pritha Raj

INTRODUCTION

Anesthesia plays a vital role in the management of patients undergoing stomach and gallbladder cancer surgeries, significantly impacting the perioperative phase and overall outcomes. In this chapter, we will explore the detailed anesthetic considerations focusing on the unique challenges posed by these patients as most of them are malnourished, anemic, and defunctionalized with multiple comorbidities. We will give an overview of various effective management strategies that can be adapted.

GASTRIC CANCER

Gastric cancer (GC) is the fifth most common cancer and cause of death due to cancer in the world with nearly a million new cases[1] reported every year. It is expected to increase by >70% worldwide by 2045.[2] In India it is the seventh most common cause of cancer with male preponderance.

SURGICAL ANATOMY AND PHYSIOLOGY OF THE STOMACH

The stomach is a hollow organ located in the epigastric region of the abdomen and its primary functions are digestion to form chyme, microbial defenses, and synthesis of intrinsic factor to aid in absorption of vitamin B_{12} and peristalsis. The stomach can be anatomically divided into four parts—fundus, cardia, body, and pylorus **(Fig. 1)**. Histologically, the gastric glands in the epithelial layer have four specialized cells: surface mucus cells, parietal cells, chief cells, and neuroendocrine cells. Parietal cells secrete gastric hydrochloric acid whereas chief cells are responsible for the production of the proteolytic enzyme,

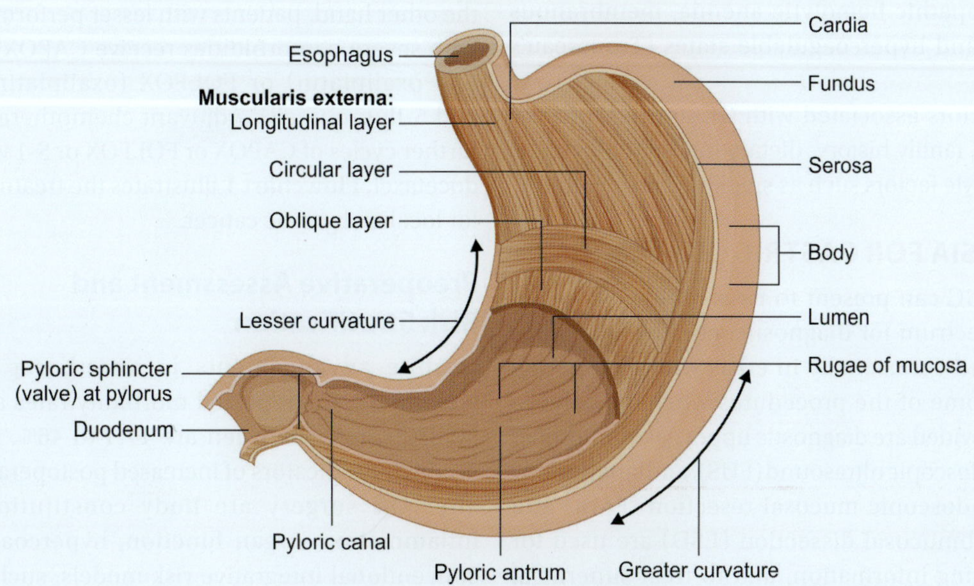

Fig. 1: Parts and layers of the stomach.

pepsinogen. The arterial supply is from the branches of the celiac trunk and the venous drainage is into the portal vein. The lymphatic drainage varies depending on the region of the stomach but ultimately drains into the celiac lymph node. Parasympathetic nerve supply is by the vagus and sympathetic is from the celiac plexus.

CLASSIFICATION OF GASTRIC CANCER

Ninety percentage of GCs are adenocarcinomas further classified by Lauren into intestinal, diffuse and mixed types.[3] The other rare gastric malignancies are gastrointestinal stromal tumors, lymphomas, and neuroendocrine tumors. The intestinal-type, the more common variant appears to follow a multistep progression that is usually initiated by *Helicobacter pylori* infection.[4] The 8th edition of the tumor, node, metastasis (TNM) staging by the American Joint Committee on Cancer (AJCC) is widely used for prognosticating and management of GC.[5]

CLINICAL PRESENTATION

Patients present with weight loss, persistent abdominal pain, history of gastric ulcer, dysphagia, early satiety, occult gastrointestinal bleeding, anemia, and abdominal mass. The common sites of metastasis are liver, peritoneum, and lymph nodes which present as jaundice, liver mass, Krukenberg tumor of the ovary, ascites, and left supraclavicular lymphadenopathy. Other sites of metastasis include central nervous system, bone, and intrathoracic or soft tissue. The paraneoplastic features are microangiopathic hemolytic anemia, membranous nephropathy, and hypercoagulable states (Trousseau's syndrome).

The risk factors associated with GC are *Helicobacter pylori* infection, family history, dietary intake of processed meat, and lifestyle factors such as smoking and alcohol.

ANESTHESIA FOR GASTRIC CANCER

Patients with GC can present to us at various stages of the disease spectrum for diagnostic, curative, palliative procedures, and occasionally in crisis with obstruction or bleeding. Some of the procedures where anesthesia services are provided are diagnostic upper gastrointestinal endoscopy, endoscopic ultrasound (EUS), and laparoscopy for staging. Endoscopic mucosal resection (EMR) and endoscopic submucosal dissection (ESD) are used for diagnosis, staging information, and to treat superficial lesions such as dysplasia or intramucosal carcinoma.[6] Upfront gastrectomy with D1 resection implies removal of the perigastric lymph nodes and those along the left gastric artery. D1+ and D2 implies removal of additional lymph nodes along the proper or common hepatic artery, splenic artery, or celiac axis with superior outcomes compared with D1 resection.[7] Presence of advanced stage (≥T2 or ≥N1) warrants completion of neoadjuvant chemotherapy (NACT) followed by definitive surgery. The extent of gastric resection (subtotal/total/proximal) depends on the location of the tumor in the stomach.

Laparoscopic approach has resulted in fewer complications, faster recovery, and oncological equivalence except total gastrectomy. Minimally invasive approaches are adopted in high volume centers with adequate expertise however patient selection is of prime importance.

With technical advances, future GC surgery will most likely become increasingly minimally invasive and will probably take advantage of the rapidly developing robotic technologies with faster recovery and similar cancer outcomes.[8] Heated intraperitoneal chemotherapy (HIIPEC) and pressurized intraperitoneal aerosol chemotherapy (PIPAC) are options available for the treatment of peritoneal spread of GC and are becoming part of the treatment protocol.[9]

Chemotherapy for GC includes drugs such as 5-fluorouracil, cisplatin, oxaliplatin, capecitabine, paclitaxel, leucovorin, docetaxel, irinotecan, trastuzumab, and ramucirumab. Patients with good functional status usually receive NACT with FLOT regimen consisting of 5-fluorouracil, leucovorin, oxaliplatin, and docetaxel. On the other hand, patients with lesser performance status or with severe comorbidities receive CAPOX (capecitabine and oxaliplatin) or FOLFOX (oxaliplatin, leucovorin, and 5-fluorouracil). Adjuvant chemotherapy consists of further cycles of CAPOX or FOLFOX or S-1 with or without docetaxel. **Flowchart 1** illustrates the treatment algorithm for localized gastric cancer.

Preoperative Assessment and Risk Stratification

Despite advancements in anesthesia and surgical techniques, the reported morbidity rates after resection for GC ranges between are 17.4 to 46%.[11] Some of the predictive indicators of increased postoperative morbidity after GC surgery are body constitution, nutrition, inflammation, organ function, hypercoagulation, and conventional integrative risk models, such as American Society of Anesthesiologists (ASA) classification, POSSUM,

Flowchart 1: Treatment algorithm for localized gastric cancer.

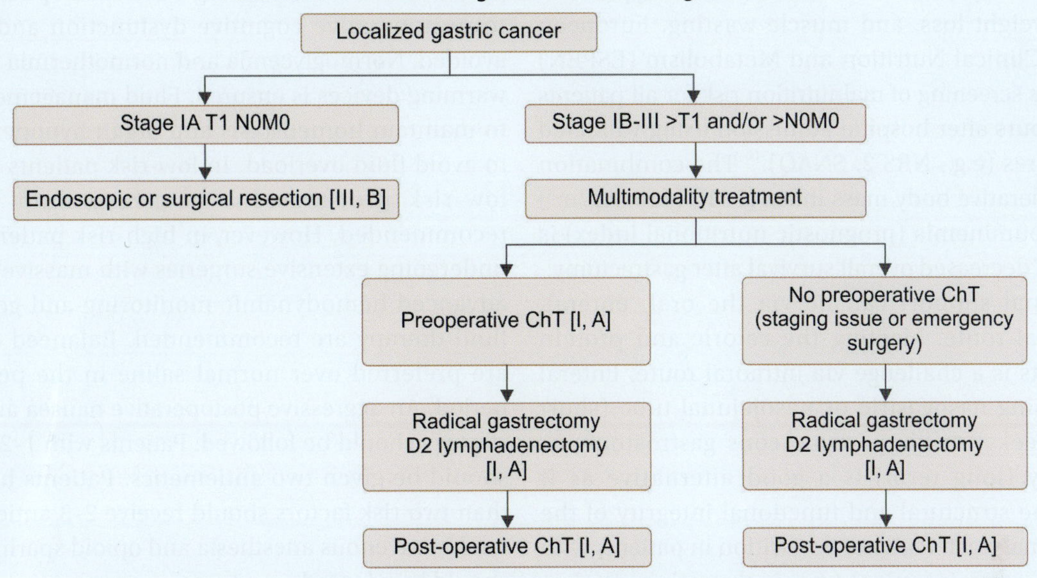

Source: Reproduced from ESMO clinical practice guideline for diagnosis, treatment, and follow-up.[10]

and APACHE II.[12] Patients with GC are smokers with comorbidities such as hypertension, chronic obstructive pulmonary disease, and coronary artery disease and they come to the preanesthetic clinic in a malnourished, anemic, and defunctionalized state. Patients with compromised functional status and significant comorbidities need special investigations such as exercise electrocardiogram (ECG), cardiopulmonary testing, pulmonary function tests, etc., for risk stratification. Patients with distal GC having features of gastric outlet obstruction (GOO) such as vomiting, dehydration, and electrolyte abnormalities need preoperative optimization of fluid and electrolyte abnormalities and correction of acidosis.

Smoking and alcohol cessation should be advised at least 4 weeks prior to surgery and the patient must receive adequate pharmacological and psychological support in doing so.

Chemotherapy related side effects must be recognized, documented, and addressed. Cisplatin, oxaliplatin, docetaxel, and paclitaxel may cause peripheral neuropathy and preoperative neurological deficits must be recorded before regional anesthesia. 5-fluorouracil can cause severe mucositis and lead to a traumatic airway management. Epirubicin can cause cardiotoxicity and hence functional cardiac assessment is mandatory. The increased incidence of thrombosis and infection due to presence of totally implantable long term vascular access for chemotherapy affects the morbidity in GC patients considerably.

Preoperative Optimization

Prehabilitation in Gastric Cancer

Multimodal programs which include nutrition, supervised physical activity, and psychological counseling show improved postoperative physical performance, muscle strength, and quality of life in patients with esophagogastric cancers.[13] The impact of prehabilitation is maximum in patients with low grade tumors undergoing minimally invasive surgery when applied for at least 2 weeks prior to surgery.

Anemia has been shown to be a poor prognostic factor in GC, affecting overall survival and disease-free survival.[14] Due to the poor oral tolerance and time constraint, intravenous iron therapy is recommended. Blood transfusions must be restricted to severely anemic patients as they have immune modulating effects and have been proven to increase cancer recurrence.

Endurance training, respiratory muscle, and resistance training must be encouraged as a part of home-based exercise program as they are found to enhance recovery.

Nutrition

Nutritional prehabilitation is the most important pillar in patients with GC[15] as preoperative nutritional condition directly affects postoperative prognosis, overall survival, and disease-specific survival. A large proportion of GC patients develop the anorexia-cachexia syndrome characterized by decreased food intake, hypoalbuminemia, weight loss, and muscle wasting. European Society for Clinical Nutrition and Metabolism (ESPEN) recommends screening of malnutrition risk for all patients within 48 hours after hospital admission using validated questionnaires (e.g., NRS 2, SNAQ).[16] The combination of low preoperative body mass index (BMI) (<18.5kg/m^2) and hypoalbuminemia (prognostic nutritional index) is predictive of decreased overall survival after gastrectomy.

Nutritional support can be via the oral, enteral, or parenteral route. Meeting the caloric and protein requirements is a challenge via intraoral route. Enteral nutrition using nasogastric or nasojejunal tube (short term 2–3 weeks) or via percutaneous gastrostomy or jejunostomy (long term) is a good alternative as it preserves the structural and functional integrity of the gastrointestinal tract. Parenteral nutrition in patients with inaccessible gastrointestinal tract is through central or peripheral veins but they are prone for catheter related blood stream infections. Immunonutrition with arginine, omega 3 fatty acids, and nucleotides in the perioperative phase have been shown to reduce overall complications and length of hospital stay but not mortality in patients undergoing major gastrointestinal surgery.[17]

INTRAOPERATIVE MANAGEMENT

Premedication

In the absence of GOO and gastroparesis, clear fluids or carbohydrate containing drink is recommended as it improves insulin sensitivity, reduces perioperative stress response, and increases patient comfort apart from decreasing postoperative nausea and vomiting.

A standard anesthetic protocol[18] consists of general anesthesia with regional analgesia. Patients with GOO need a rapid sequence induction. Induction of anesthesia may be associated with profound hypotension and needs optimal fluid resuscitation and vasopressor support. Depth of anesthesia should be monitored and a minimum alveolar concentration of 0.7–1.3 or bispectral index (BIS) between 40 and 60 is recommended. Avoiding excessive depth of anesthesia helps in reducing side effects and facilitates early awakening. Long-acting neuromuscular blockers should be avoided. It is advisable to use neuromuscular monitoring and to wait for a train of four ratio >0.9 to avoid residual paralysis and micro aspiration. Long-acting opioids and sedatives must be avoided as they delay time to recovery and discharge. In elderly patients even short-acting benzodiazepines may lead to postoperative cognitive dysfunction and should be avoided. Normoglycemia and normothermia using active warming devices is ensured. Fluid management is aimed to maintain homeostasis and organ hypoperfusion and to avoid fluid overload. In low-risk patients undergoing low-risk procedures a near-zero fluid balance is recommended. However, in high-risk patients or those undergoing extensive surgeries with massive fluid shifts, advanced hemodynamic monitoring and goal directed fluid therapy are recommended. Balanced crystalloids are preferred over normal saline in the perioperative period. An aggressive postoperative nausea and vomiting strategy should be followed. Patients with 1–2 risk factors should be given two antiemetics. Patients having more than two risk factors should receive 2–3 antiemetics and total intravenous anesthesia and opioid sparing strategies should be adopted.

Pain Management

Aggressive pain management is mandatory for gastrectomy to avoid postoperative pulmonary complications. A multimodal and opioid sparing approach should be adopted.[19] For open surgeries thoracic epidural has been traditionally considered the gold standard as it reduces the dynamic pain scores, time to return of bowel function, time to mobilization, and pulmonary complications. Although there is no difference in overall morbidity or length of hospital stay, epidural combined with general anesthesia has shown lower rates of metastasis and recurrence due to anti-inflammatory effects.[20] Epidural opioids such as morphine and hydromorphone reduce the postoperative systemic opioid consumption. Other alternatives to neuraxial blockade are abdominal plane blocks such as transversus abdominis plane (TAP), Quadratus lumborum block, and external oblique intercostal block. Intravenous lignocaine infusion maybe a good adjunct however because of safety issues and unproven benefits its widespread use cannot be recommended. The pain in minimally invasive surgeries is maximum in the initial 24 hours after which it reduces remarkably. Hence, intrathecal opioid is useful and is widely in practice. Patient-controlled analgesia using intravenous opioid is an effective option. Procedure specific postoperative pain management—(PROSPECT) guidelines available for the laparoscopic sleeve gastrectomy can be extrapolated for all minimally invasive gastrectomy **(Box 1)**.

However, it has not recommended TAP block, α-2 adrenergic agonists, magnesium sulfate, and intraperitoneal local anesthetic infiltration.

Enhanced Recovery after Gastrectomy

Perioperative care protocols have been developed by the Enhanced Recovery after Surgery (ERAS) study group with the overall aim of reducing complications, improving outcomes, reducing length of hospital stay, and optimizing resources. Several gastrectomy specific recommendations[22] exist and have been elaborated in **Table 1**.

BOX 1: PROSPECT guidelines 21 for perioperative pain management of laparoscopic gastrectomy

Preoperative and intraoperative period:

- Paracetamol (Grade A)
- Nonsteroidal anti-inflammatory drug (NSAID) or cyclooxygenase-2 (COX-2) selective inhibitor (Grade A)
- Single, low dose of intravenous (IV) dexamethasone (Grade A)
- Gabapentinoids, when paracetamol and/or NSAID/COX-2 selective inhibitor are not possible (Grade A)

Postoperative period:

- Paracetamol (Grade A)
- NSAID or COX-2 selective inhibitor (Grade A)
- Rescue opioid (Grade A)

TABLE 1: Enhanced recovery after surgery recommendations for gastrectomy.

Intervention	*Level of evidence*	*Grade of recommendation*
Preoperative nutrition	Very low	Strong
Preoperative oral pharmaco-nutrition	Moderate	Weak
Minimally invasive techniques	High	Strong
Wound catheters and TAP block	Low	Weak
Nasogastric/nasojejunal decompression	High	Strong
Avoid abdominal drains	High	Strong
Early postoperative diet and artificial nutrition	Moderate	Weak
Audit	Low	Strong

(TAP: transversus abdominis plane)

POSTOPERATIVE MANAGEMENT

Postoperative delirium can be reduced by avoidance of prolonged fasting, disturbance in sleep cycle or medications such as benzodiazepines and atropine. Strategies aimed at enabling early return of bowel function such as reducing systemic opioids, early mobilization, early oral intake, and optimal fluid strategy should be adopted. Enteral nutrition via a feeding jejunostomy should be resumed as early as 6 hours after gastrectomy as this preserves the integrity of the gastrointestinal tract.

Postoperative Complications after Gastrectomy

Postgastrectomy patients can develop early complications such as anastomotic leaks, strictures, gastrointestinal obstruction, and gastric stasis. Many patients develop a typical postgastrectomy "Dumping syndrome" caused by the destruction or bypass of the pyloric sphincter. Dumping symptoms include gastrointestinal discomfort (e.g., nausea, vomiting, cramps, and diarrhea) as well as vasomotor symptoms (e.g., diaphoresis, palpitations, and flushing). Dietary (carbohydrate avoidance) therapies work well for dumping syndrome. Long-term complications in the remnant stomach include peptic ulcer disease and remnant cancer. Postgastrectomy patients also develop several nutritional deficiencies. Anemia develops in 50% patients postgastrectomy. The main cause of anemia is iron deficiency which is due to the reduction in gastric acid secretion and bypassing of the duodenum. Vitamin B_{12} deficiency develops within 1 year postgastrectomy due to lack of intrinsic factor secreted by the parietal cells of the gastric glands. Older age, high neutrophil-lymphocyte ratio (NLR), and major postoperative complications are independent risk factors causing delay in return to indented oncological therapy.[23]

PALLIATIVE ISSUES IN ADVANCED GASTRIC CANCER

Approximately 35% of GC are detected in stage IV with a median overall survival of 9–10 months.[24] They may present with obstruction, bleeding, ascites, or pain. Early introduction of systematic palliative care in these patients improves their quality of life[25] and reduces the need for aggressive end of life care in these patients.[26,27] The anesthetic concerns are an extremely malnourished, dehydrated patient with electrolyte abnormalities needing a rapid sequence induction along with aggressive volume resuscitation. Anesthetic should be tailored to reduce morbidity and facilitate early discharge from the hospital. Endoscopic intervention is the first line of management for bleeding GCs followed by transcatheter arterial embolization (TAE) or palliative gastrectomy. Patients who have GOO may need palliative surgical bypass or self-expanding stent placement or EUS guided gastrojejunostomy.[28]

Malignant ascites is another debilitating problem, and these patients require repeated paracentesis for symptom relief. A novel therapy has been developed in Japan called KM-CART which filters the malignant cell rich ascites and reinfuses cell free ascites. This reinfusion can cause disseminated intravascular coagulation and these patients need vigilant monitoring.[29] Pain in advanced GC is severe and often associated with obstructive symptoms.[30] Opioids are the mainstay of treatment, but adjuvants help in reducing their dose and side effects. Celiac plexus neurolysis is a good option and has been shown to benefit these patients.[31] Neuromodulation and intrathecal drug delivery systems are other promising modalities for patients with advanced disease.

GALLBLADDER CANCER

Gallbladder cancer (GBC) and bile duct cancer are collectively termed biliary tract cancers. While they share common risk factors and symptoms, their incidence and treatment differ.

Incidence

The GBC is the most common primary biliary tumor and the 6th most common gastrointestinal tumor.[32] The incidence is one in 100,000 per year in western countries, but it is significantly higher in less developed countries such as India, China, and Chile where near epidemic rates are reported. Cholangiocarcinoma (CCA) is an epithelial malignancy arising from the biliary ducts accounting for 3% of gastrointestinal malignancies. It is the second most common primary hepatic malignancies responsible for 20% of the deaths from hepatobiliary cancers and 13% of the total cancer mortality.[33,34] The incidence of CCA is rising due to their silent clinical course, lack of reliable biomarkers, difficult anatomical location, and highly desmoplastic nature. Prognosis is poor with a dismal 5-year survival rate of 5–13%. Currently, cholelithiasis diagnosis followed by cholecystectomy are the only prevention strategy in high risk populations.[35]

Surgical Anatomy

The gallbladder (GB) is a pear shaped organ located beneath the liver, **(Fig. 2)** between the segments IV (left) and segment V (right). It consists of the fundus, body, infundibulum, and neck. The cystic duct joins the common hepatic duct (CHD) to form the common bile duct (CBD). It lies in close proximity to multiple vital structures which includes the liver, porta hepatis (hepatic hilum), hepatoduodenal ligament (holds the CBD, proper hepatic artery, and main portal vein), pancreas, and colon. Therefore, resection of these vital structures is necessary to achieve surgical clearance in advanced GBC.[36]

Intrahepatic bile ducts drain the right and left liver parenchyma, forms the right and left hepatic ducts, and unites to form the CHD. It becomes CBD after the cystic duct joins the CHD. This then descends on the right of the proper hepatic artery and lies anterior to the portal vein. The CBD is joined by the pancreatic duct to form a common channel, the ampulla of Vater. This runs in the duodenal wall and opens into the second part of the duodenum.

Based on the origin of the disease, CCA is classified into intrahepatic (iCCA) and extrahepatic (eCCA) **(Fig. 3)**. eCCA is further divided into perihilar (pCCA) and distal (dCCA). iCCA arises from the second order bile ducts, within the liver parenchyma, while pCCA or Klatskin tumor arises from the extrahepatic second order bile ducts and extends up to the insertion of the cystic duct. dCCA is confined to the CBD below the cystic duct.[37] pCCA accounts for nearly 60–70% of all CCA. Identifying

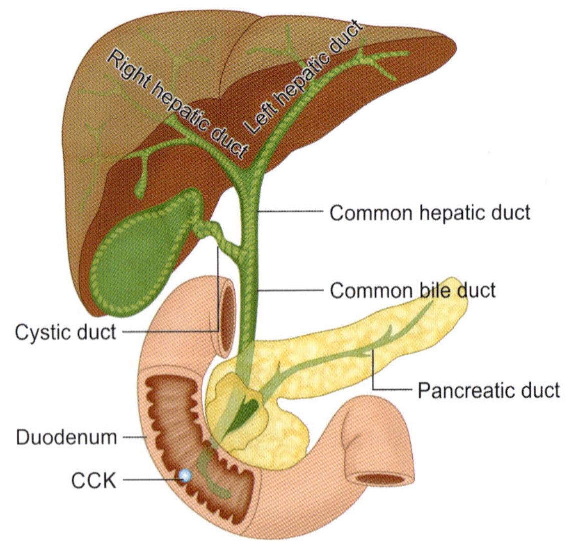

Fig. 2: Gallbladder anatomy.

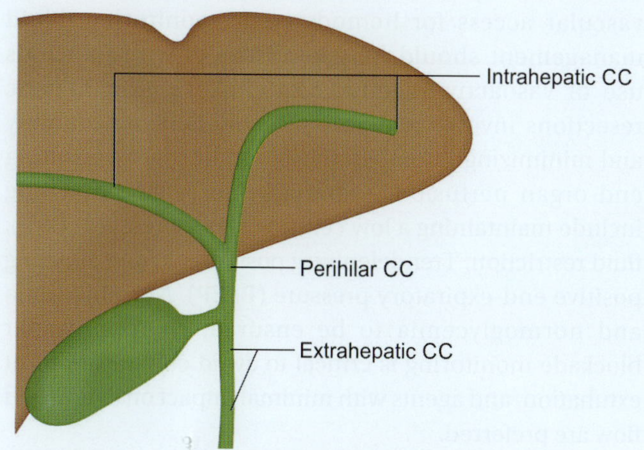

Fig. 3: Biliary duct system anatomy.

the exact anatomical location of these tumors is crucial in distinguishing their molecular and biological patterns and in determining the choices for systemic therapy.[38]

CLINICAL PRESENTATION

The GBC and CCA present with icterus, abdominal pain, weight loss, and nausea. GBC is usually asymptomatic and shows vague symptoms such as dyspepsia which may mimic glycogen storage disease. Abdominal pain occurs at later stages. A hard nontender lump maybe palpable in the right hypochondrium with hepatomegaly due to cholestasis or ascites develops due to peritoneal spread or hypoalbuminemia. The common sites of metastasis are the liver, lungs, bone, and brain.

The iCCA typically presents with dull right quadrant abdominal pain, weight loss, and raised alkaline phosphatase levels, mild icterus, and often incidentally diagnosed during cirrhosis evaluation. eCCA has features of obstructive jaundice with abdominal pain, weight loss, and fever, and may rarely present with cholangitis or paraneoplastic syndromes such as porphyria cutanea tarda.[39] Metastasis from iCCA commonly spreads to other intrahepatic locations, peritoneum, lungs, and pleura. The pCCA metastasizes mainly in the liver while the dCCA, metastasize later in the course of disease, to liver, lungs, and peritoneum.

The common risk factors of GBC and CCA are chronic cholecystitis, cholelithiasis, chemical dye exposure, obesity, primary sclerosing cholangitis, and inflammatory bowel disease. Familial adenomatous polyps and diabetes are found to cause GBC. Cirrhosis and hormonal use are linked with CCA.

ANESTHESIA FOR GALLBLADDER CANCER AND CHOLANGIOCARCINOMA

Patients may present for diagnostic procedures such as EUS for lymph node sampling or staging laparoscopy requiring monitored anesthesia care or conscious sedation. Laparoscopic evaluation precedes the surgery to assess disease burden and resectability which depends on location of the tumor, its relation to the intrahepatic and vascular structures, the future liver remnant (FLR) and the function of the FLR postresection.[40] Patients with incidental GBC after cholecystectomy, reresection, and portal lymphadenectomy is done to ensure microscopic negative margins.[35] Surgical procedures entail extended/radical cholecystectomy which includes the GB, a wedge of the liver based on infiltration, an extended hepatectomy, or biliary reconstruction with lymphadenectomy. It may include pancreaticoduodenectomy, combined resection of adjacent organs (stomach, duodenum, jejunum, and colon), vascular resection with reconstruction or even hepato-pancreatic-duodenectomy.[36] Patients with early iCCA disease (<2 cm) might be candidates for liver transplantation. Though hepatectomy with regional lymphadenectomy is the treatment of choice. For pCCA surgical resection includes extended hepatectomy with en-bloc resection of the extrahepatic biliary system and regional lymphadenectomy. However for the dCCA—surgical resection includes pancreaticoduodenectomy or Whipple's procedure with removal of the GB and bile duct, head of pancreas, and the 1st part of the duodenum.

As per the National Comprehensive Cancer Network (NCCN) guidelines, in locoregionally advanced CCA with liver/nodal spread neoadjuvant therapy using gemcitabine/cisplatin, gemcitabine/capecitabine, capecitabine/cisplatin, capecitabine/oxaliplatin, and 5 fluorouracil/cisplatin are tried. Systemic chemotherapy for GBC revolves around gemcitabine and cisplatin. The efficacy of these trials are conflicting. It is imperative to know the implications of these emerging options such as targeted therapy via fibroblast growth factor receptor (FGFR) inhibitors (pemigatinib) and immunotherapy on the principle of immune checkpoint blockade.

Preoperative Evaluation and Risk Assessment

These patients present to the preanesthesia clinic with malnutrition, cachexia, anemia, deranged liver functions, and obstructive jaundice. A detailed evaluation of the patient's general condition including the nutritional status, and systemic evaluation along with laboratory and radiological evaluation helps in predicting the morbidity of the procedure and aids in meticulous planning. Neoadjuvant therapy induced toxicities such as hepatotoxicity and cardiotoxicity must be thoroughly assessed. Predictors of postoperative complications are ASA grade, age, extent of resection, perioperative blood transfusion, and preexisting cirrhosis.

Preexisting liver disease mandates the use the Child-Turcotte-Pugh score (CTP) or MELD score based stratification to evaluate liver function. A MELD score of 10–15 denotes increased risk.[41] Other comorbidities must be optimized such as hyperglycemia as they may cause higher operative mortality.

Future Liver Remnant Assessment

Volumetric assessment of the FLR is done using computed tomography (CT) and magnetic resonance imaging (MRI). The FLR volume correlates well with the function of FLR and predicts the risk of posthepatectomy-liver failure (PHLF). In patients with well-preserved liver function, a FLR of 20% may be sufficient. But in patients with steatohepatitis/NAFLD/posthepatotoxic chemotherapy, an FLR of 30–40% is needed.[42] Indocyanine green (ICG) dye can be used to gauge dynamic function of the liver.[43] In patients undergoing significant liver resections as part of CCA/GBC may need preoperative augmentation of the FLR. Different techniques adopted include:

- Portal vein embolization (PVE)
- Portal vein ligation (PVL)
- Liver venous deprivation (LVD)
- Associating liver partition and PVL for staged hepatectomy (ALPPS)

These procedures are often done in patients with low FLR, or when tumor is adjacent to vital structures.

Prehabilitation

Prehabilitation includes anemia correction with blood transfusion, addressing coagulation abnormalities with vitamin K or fresh frozen plasma, and managing electrolyte imbalances. Smoking and alcohol cessation are advised for at least 4 weeks preoperatively. Preoperative biliary drainage may be necessary for some patients. Respiratory exercises, including incentive spirometry, and adherence to ERAS guidelines where applicable, are recommended.

INTRAOPERATIVE CONSIDERATIONS

Standard anesthesia techniques include general anesthesia with controlled ventilation, along with invasive vascular access for hemodynamic monitoring. Fluid management should be goal-directed, with judicious use of vasoactive agents. Key challenges in hepatic resections involve maintaining hemodynamic stability and minimizing intraoperative blood loss while ensuring end-organ perfusion.[44] Strategies to reduce bleeding include maintaining a low central venous pressure (CVP), fluid restriction, Trendelenburg positioning, and avoiding positive end-expiratory pressure (PEEP). Normothermia and normoglycemia to be ensured. Neuromuscular blockade monitoring is critical to avoid complications at extubation, and agents with minimal impact on liver blood flow are preferred.

ANALGESIC MANAGEMENT

A multimodal, opioid-sparing analgesic regimen is preferred, including continuous wound infusions and regional blocks such as the TAP and erector spinae blocks. IV paracetamol is generally safe, with dose adjustments for patients with compromised liver function. A maximum dosage of 3 g/day may be used safely.[45] NSAIDs may be used cautiously depending on renal function and other comorbidities.

Effective analgesia is crucial for faster recovery and reducing complications. Thoracic epidural analgesia (TEA), once a standard approach, is now less favored due to technical challenges, risk of complications, and hemodynamic instability. Intrathecal morphine (ITM) is a more reliable option with fewer side effects and quicker recovery.[44]

ENHANCED RECOVERY AFTER SURGERY AS PART OF BILIARY TRACT AND GALLBLADDER MALIGNANCY SURGERIES

Specific ERAS guidelines for bile duct and GB surgeries are lacking.[46] However, the protocols adapted from pancreaticoduodenectomy are applicable. The components include:[47]

- *Preoperative biliary drainage:* This should be avoided unless necessary, as it may increase postoperative complications without improving mortality.
- *Analgesia:* Emphasizing a multimodal, opioid-sparing approach.
- *Goal-directed fluid management:* Essential for maintaining hemodynamic stability.
- *Antibiotic prophylaxis:* Single-dose prophylaxis should be administered preincision with repeat dosing as necessary.

- *Thromboprophylaxis:* Includes both pharmacological and mechanical measures.
- *Diet and nutrition:* A tailored approach with early return to normal diet where applicable.

ANESTHESIA FOR ENDOSCOPIC PROCEDURES

Endoscopic procedures such as percutaneous transhepatic biliary drainage (PTBD) and endoscopic biliary drainage (EBD) are used for preoperative preparation or for palliative management in unresectable tumors.[40] These procedures pose challenges due to compromised liver function and positional challenges. General anesthesia with careful selection of short-acting agents is vital, considering the potential impact on liver function.[48] Correction of coagulopathies, electrolyte imbalances, and hydration is critical in these cases.

PALLIATIVE PROCEDURES

Advanced GBC often presents with biliary stasis or with GOO. EBD for malignant jaundice and surgical/EUS guided gastrojejunostomy are the treatment options available. Surgical options are least preferred due to their morbidity. Endoscopic radiofrequency ablation (RFA), intraluminal brachytherapy (IBT), and endoscopic photodynamic therapy (PDT) have been studied for the management of biliary malignancies.[49]

POSTOPERATIVE CARE AND COMPLICATIONS

Postoperative care requires ICU monitoring with a focus on liver function and following ERAS protocols to expedite recovery. Complications include cardiac events, respiratory infections, renal dysfunction, and sepsis.

Common postsurgical complications after biliary tract tumors are given in the **Table 2**.

Less common complications are intra-abdominal sepsis, portal vein and hepatic artery thrombosis, and venous thromboembolism.

- *Postoperative hemorrhage:* Hemodynamic instability with an ongoing intra-abdominal bleed which exceeds 1L, needs exploratory laparotomy. Early radiological imaging and correction of coagulopathy are the key interventions.
- *Bile leak:* It is defined by the International study group of liver surgery (ISGLS) as bilirubin level three times higher in drains than the serum concentration.

TABLE 2: Timeline of complications after biliary duct cancer surgeries.

Complication	*Incidence*	*Onset*	*Presentation*
Surgical site infection	30%	<7 days of surgery	Swelling, induration, tenderness, discharge at site
Bile leak	4–17%	Days after surgery	General condition is poor
Biliary fistulae	4–27%	Days to weeks postsurgery	Abdominal pain, tenderness, bile leak through wound
Hepatic failure	8–12%	On or after POD 5	Elevated INR and bilirubin on or after POD 5
Hemorrhage	<3%	Immediate or delayed	Increased drain output, drop in Hb, hemodynamic instability

(Hb: hemoglobin; INR: international normalized ratio)

Prompt diagnosis and immediate drainage of biliary collection or biliary peritonitis is essential.

- Venous thromboembolism (VTE): Routine chemoprophylaxis is recommended, even if hepatectomy is part of the surgical plan.
- *Postsurgical hepatic failure (PHLF):* ISGLS defines PHLF as "A postoperatively acquired deterioration in the ability of the liver (in patients with normal and abnormal liver function) to maintain its synthetic, excretory and detoxifying function, characterized by increase in the INR and hyperbilirubinemia on or after postoperative day 5."[43] PHLF is graded into severity (A, B, and C) denoting perioperative mortality of 0% for grade A to 54% for grade C, with grade B requiring noninvasive intensive care management. Risk factors for PHLF in patients undergoing resection of primary bile duct tumors or GBC along with hepatectomy are:
- Prolonged surgical time
- Excessive intraoperative blood loss
- Small FLR/extensive resection
- Ischemia/reperfusion
- Sepsis

Hence, patient selection with adequate optimization of comorbidities for the proposed extent of surgery helps in prevention of PHLF. Careful monitoring of postoperative liver function, liver enzymes, coagulation, mentation, and supportive therapy with fresh frozen plasma (FFP), vitamin K, albumin and diuretics, rarely mechanical ventilation, and dialysis hasten the hepatic recovery.

- *Hepatic artery thrombosis (HAT) and portal vein thrombosis*[50] *(PVT):* This rare complication occurs when extensive vascular reconstruction has been done. Acute PVT thrombosis may lead to portal hypertension with development of varices and subsequent hemorrhage and ascites. Chronic PVT may present as abdominal pain due to involvement of superior mesenteric vessels leading to bowel ischemia. HAT is managed with anticoagulants and fluids occasionally may need an angioplasty or surgical thrombectomy. PVT managed with anticoagulants, thrombolysis, or surgical thrombectomy. Laparotomy maybe needed to redo the anastomosis.

CONCLUSION

The perioperative management of stomach cancer requires a multidisciplinary approach. CCA and GB carcinoma are aggressive tumors, often presenting at an advanced stage. We as Onco anesthesiologists have an indispensable role throughout these patient's cancer journey starting from diagnosis till the end-of-life care. Therefore, understanding the disease pathology, various treatment options, and close communication with the surgical team and patient are the relevant factors that will help to improve patient satisfaction and their outcome.

REFERENCES

1. Bray F, Laversanne M, Sung H, Ferlay J, Siegel RL, Soerjomataram I, et al. Global cancer statistics 2022: GLOBOCAN estimates of incidence and mortality worldwide for 36 cancers in 185 countries. CA Cancer J Clin. 2024;74(3):229-63.
2. WHO. Cancer Tomorrow. [online] Available from whttps://gco.iarc.who.int/tomorrow/en/dataviz/tables?cancers=7&populations=935_900 [Last accessed February, 2025].
3. Lauren P. The two histological main types of gastric carcinoma: diffuse and so-called intestinal-type carcinoma. An attempt at a histo-clinical classification. Acta Pathol Microbiol Scand. 1965;64:31-49.
4. Ferreira RM, Machado JC, Figueiredo C. Clinical relevance of Helicobacter pylori vacA and cagA genotypes in gastric carcinoma. Best Pract Res Clin Gastroenterol. 2014;28(6):1003-15.
5. Edge SB, American Joint Committee on Cancer AC. AJCC cancer staging handbook: from the AJCC cancer staging manual. New York: Springer; 2010.
6. Ono H, Yao K, Fujishiro M, Oda I, Uedo N, Nimura S, et al. Guidelines for endoscopic submucosal dissection and endoscopic mucosal resection for early gastric cancer (second edition). Digestive Endoscopy. 2021;33(1):4-20.
7. Japanese gastric cancer association. Japanese gastric cancer treatment guidelines 2018 (5th edition). Gastric Cancer. 2021;24(1):1-21.
8. Smyth EC, Nilsson M, Grabsch HI, van Grieken NC, Lordick F. Gastric cancer. Lancet. 2020;396(10251):635-48.
9. Khan H, Johnston FM. Current role for cytoreduction and HIPEC for gastric cancer with peritoneal disease. J Surg Oncol. 2022;125(7):1176-82.
10. Lordick F, Carneiro F, Cascinu S, Fleitas T, Haustermans K, Piessen G, et al. Gastric cancer: ESMO Clinical Practice Guideline for diagnosis, treatment and follow-up. Ann Oncol. 2022;33(10):1005-20.
11. Kurita N, Miyata H, Gotoh M, Shimada M, Imura S, Kimura W, et al. Risk Model for Distal Gastrectomy When Treating Gastric Cancer on the Basis of Data From 33,917 Japanese Patients Collected Using a Nationwide Web-based Data Entry System. Ann Surg. 2015;262(2):295-303.
12. Kanda M. Correction to: Preoperative predictors of postoperative complications after gastric cancer resection. Surg Today. 2020;50(3):321.
13. Mareschal J, Hemmer A, Douissard J, Dupertuis YM, Collet TH, Koessler T, et al. Surgical Prehabilitation in Patients with Gastrointestinal Cancers: Impact of Unimodal and Multimodal Programs on Postoperative Outcomes and Prospects for New Therapeutic Strategies—A Systematic Review. Cancers (Basel). 2023;15(6):1881.
14. Huang XZ, Yang YC, Chen Y, Wu CC, Lin RF, Wang ZN, et al. Preoperative anemia or low hemoglobin predicts poor prognosis in gastric cancer patients: A meta-analysis. Dis Markers. 2019;2019:7606128.
15. Bennett H, Harris R. To feed or not to feed - review of post-operative feeding strategies after gastric cancer surgery and impact on outcomes. Clin Nutr ESPEN. 2022;48:83.
16. Muscaritoli M, Arends J, Bachmann P, Baracos V, Barthelemy N, Bertz H, et al. ESPEN practical guideline: Clinical Nutrition in cancer. Clin Nutr. 2021;40(5):2898-913.
17. Shen J, Dai S, Li Z, Dai W, Hong J, Huang J, et al. Effect of Enteral Immunonutrition in Patients Undergoing Surgery for Gastrointestinal Cancer: An Updated Systematic Review and Meta-Analysis. Front Nutr. 2022;9:941975.
18. Feldheiser A, Aziz O, Baldini G, Cox BPBW, Fearon KCH, Feldman LS, et al. Enhanced Recovery After Surgery (ERAS) for gastrointestinal surgery, part 2: Consensus statement for anaesthesia practice. Acta Anaesthesiol Scand. 2016;60(3):289-334.
19. Pirie K, Traer E, Finniss D, Myles PS, Riedel B. Current approaches to acute postoperative pain management after major abdominal surgery: a narrative review and future directions. Br J Anaesth. 2022;129(3):378-93.
20. Pei JP, Zhang CD, Liang Y, Zhang C, Wu KZ, Zhao ZM, et al. Effects of epidural combined with general anesthesia versus general anesthesia alone in gastric cancer surgery:

a propensity score matching analysis. Ann Transl Med. 2020;8(7):798435.

21. ESRA. Laparoscopic sleeve gastrectomy 2018. [online] Available from https://esraeurope.org/prospect/procedures/laparoscopic-sleeve-gastrectomy-2018/summary-recommendations-11/ [Last accessed February, 2025].
22. Desiderio J, Trastulli S, D'Andrea V, Parisi A. Enhanced recovery after surgery for gastric cancer (ERAS-GC): Optimizing patient outcome. Transl Gastroenterol Hepatol. 2020;5:11.
23. Ramos MFKP, de Castria TB, Pereira MA, Dias AR, Antonacio FF, Zilberstein B, et al. Return to Intended Oncologic Treatment (RIOT) in Resected Gastric Cancer Patients. J Gastroint Surg. 2020;24(1):19-27.
24. Howlader N, AM N, M K, D M, A B, M Y, et al. SEER Cancer Statistics Review. J Natl Cancer Inst. 2019.
25. Scarpi E, Dall'Agata M, Zagonel V, Gamucci T, Bertè R, Sansoni E, et al. Systematic vs. on-demand early palliative care in gastric cancer patients: a randomized clinical trial assessing patient and healthcare service outcomes. Supportive Care Cancer. 2019;27(7):2425-34.
26. Merchant SJ, Brogly SB, Goldie C, Booth CM, Nanji S, Patel S V., et al. Palliative Care is Associated with Reduced Aggressive End-of-Life Care in Patients with Gastrointestinal Cancer. Ann Surg Oncol. 2018;25(6):2336-45.
27. Harada K, Zhao M, Shanbhag N, Baba H, Ajani J a. Palliative care for advanced gastric cancer. Expert Rev Anticancer Ther. 2020;20(7):575-80.
28. Kim BS, Yang SY, Lee WD, Song JS, Yang MA, Jung GM, et al. Endoscopic Ultrasonography-guided Gastrojejunostomy for Patients with Gastric Outlet Obstruction and Pyloric Metal Stent Dysfunction. Korean J Gastroenterol. 2022;79(6):260-4.
29. Matsusaki K, Ohta K, Yoshizawa A, Gyoda Y. Novel cell-free and concentrated ascites reinfusion therapy (KM-CART) for refractory ascites associated with cancerous peritonitis: Its effect and future perspectives. Int J Clin Oncol. 2011;16(4):395-400.
30. Hamada H. Interventional Management of Chronic Visceral Pain Syndrome. Anesth Analg. 2021;132(6):e98.
31. Ambai VT, Singh V, Boorman DW, Neufeld NJ. Celiac plexus neurolysis for abdominal cancers: going beyond pancreatic cancer pain. Pain Rep. 2021;6(1):e930.
32. Halaseh SA, Halaseh S, Shakman R. A Review of the Etiology and Epidemiology of Gallbladder Cancer: What You Need to Know. Cureus. 2022;14(8):e28260.
33. Kirstein MM, Vogel A. Epidemiology and Risk Factors of Cholangiocarcinoma. Visc Med. 2016;32(6):395-400.
34. Saha SK, Zhu AX, Fuchs CS, Brooks GA. Forty-Year Trends in Cholangiocarcinoma Incidence in the U.S.: Intrahepatic Disease on the Rise. Oncologist. 2016;21(5):594-9.
35. Gamboa AC, Maithel SK. The Landmark Series: Gallbladder Cancer. Ann Surg Oncol. 2020;27(8):2846-58.
36. Cha C, Brandt WS. Surgical anatomy of the hepatobiliary system. In: Surgical and Perioperative Management of Patients with Anatomic Anomalies. Springer International Publishing. 2020. pp. 205-34.
37. Valle JW, Borbath I, Khan SA, Huguet F, Gruenberger T, Arnold D, et al. Biliary cancer: ESMO clinical practice guidelines for diagnosis, treatment and follow-up. Ann Oncol. 2016;27(suppl 5):v28-v37.
38. Banales JM, Marin JJG, Lamarca A, Rodrigues PM, Khan SA, Roberts LR, et al. Cholangiocarcinoma 2020: the next horizon in mechanisms and management. Nat Rev Gastroenterol Hepatol. 2020;17(9):557-88.
39. Sökmen M, Demirsoy H, Ersoy Ö, Gökdemir G, Akbayir N, Karaca Ç, et al. Paraneoplastic porphyria cutanea tarda associated with cholangiocarcinoma: Case report. Turkish J Gastroenterol. 2007;18(3):897-907.
40. Zori AG, Yang D, Draganov PV, Cabrera R. Advances in the management of cholangiocarcinoma. World J Hepatol. 2021;13(9):1003-18.
41. Delis SG, Bakoyiannis A, Biliatis I, Athanassiou K, Tassopoulos N, Dervenis C. Model for end-stage liver disease (MELD) score, as a prognostic factor for post-operative morbidity and mortality in cirrhotic patients, undergoing hepatectomy for hepatocellular carcinoma. HPB. 2009;11(4):351-7.
42. Memeo R, Conticchio M, Deshayes E, Nadalin S, Herrero A, Guiu B, et al. Optimization of the future remnant liver: review of the current strategies in Europe. Hepatobiliary Surg Nutr. 2021;10(3):350-63.
43. Bekheit M, Grundy L, Salih AK, Bucur P, Vibert E, Ghazanfar M. Post-hepatectomy liver failure: A timeline centered review. Hepatobiliary Pancreat Dis Int. 2023;22(6):554-69.
44. Patel J, Jones CN, Amoako D. Perioperative management for hepatic resection surgery. BJA Educ. 2022;22(9):357-63.
45. Murphy V, Koea J, Srinivasa S. The efficacy and safety of acetaminophen use following liver resection: a systematic review. HPB. 2022;24(1):1-8.
46. Quinn LM, Mann K, Jones RP, Bathla S, Stremitzer S, Dunne DF, et al. Defining enhanced recovery after resection of peri-hilar cholangiocarcinoma. Eur J Surg Oncol. 2019;45(8):1439-45.
47. Melloul E, Lassen K, Roulin D, Grass F, Perinel J, Adham M, et al. Guidelines for Perioperative Care for Pancreatoduodenectomy: Enhanced Recovery After Surgery (ERAS) Recommendations 2019. World J Surg. 2020;44(7):2056-84.
48. Tetzlaff JE, Vargo JJ, Maurer W. Nonoperating room anesthesia for the gastrointestinal endoscopy suite. Anesthesiol Clin. 2014;32(2):387-94.
49. Schepis T, Boškoski I, Tringali A, Bove V, Costamagna G. Palliation in Gallbladder Cancer: The Role of Gastrointestinal Endoscopy. Cancers (Basel). 2022;14(7):1686.
50. Russell MC. Complications following hepatectomy. Surg Oncol Clin N Am. 2015;24(1):73-96.

27 CHAPTER

Anesthesia for Colorectal Surgeries

Aanchal Kakkar, Anupama Gill Sharma, Akhil Agarwal

INTRODUCTION

The incidence of colorectal (CR) surgeries has increased worldwide owing to an increase in the incidence of CR cancers.[1] CR surgery is associated with increased morbidity and mortality. There are ample anesthesia concerns for CR surgeries, be it for intestinal obstruction, perforation, diverticulitis, or high-risk CR malignancy.

A systematic preoperative assessment and optimization, predefined perioperative anesthesia goals, and preemptive strategies to avoid postoperative complications are a must to have a good outcome for CR surgeries. In 2005, the Enhanced Recovery After Surgery (ERAS) Society formulated ERAS guidelines to decrease the perioperative stress, standardize the anesthesia technique, maintain postoperative physiological function, and accelerate the recovery after CR surgery. These evidence-based guidelines were updated in 2018.[2] ERAS guidelines provide evidence of structured multimodal protocols with a multidisciplinary approach, which can be applied at every stage of the perioperative period.

PREOPERATIVE MANAGEMENT

Preoperative assessment helps us in the identification and optimization of high-risk patients.

Apart from counseling of the patient and taking written informed consent, the goals of preoperative assessments also include:

- Optimization of preexisting comorbidities
- Maintaining the hydration/euvolemic status of the patient
- Correction of any metabolic or electrolyte disorder

It is pertinent to understand the basic physiology of CR oxygenation and blood flow and the factors affecting them while optimizing the patient for CR surgery.

Perioperative smoking, low hematocrit, atherosclerosis, cardiac failure, and chronic obstructive pulmonary disease can lead to colonic tissue hypoxia. Other factors affecting the CR blood flow also include:

- Increased Intraluminal or intra-abdominal pressure
- Hypovolemic status of the patient
- Metabolic or electrolyte disorders
- Sepsis

Many of the above factors affecting the oxygenation and blood flow to the colonic tissue can be corrected in the preoperative period, especially for an elective surgery.

ERAS guidelines recommend the optimization of the patients' right from the preadmission time.

Preadmission Information, Education, and Counseling

All patients must be provided with adequate information regarding the disease and procedure to allay the fear and anxiety. The patient's and caregiver's counseling should be done in a dedicated area by the multidisciplinary team (including a surgeon, anesthesiologist, intensivist, nurse, or allied health professional)

Preoperative Optimization

A detailed history and clinical assessment should be done for the patients. Many of the patients presenting with CR diseases may have preexisting cardiac and/or pulmonary diseases. The patients should be optimized for their preexisting comorbidities and the medication should be continued in the preoperative period.

Prehabilitation

Enhanced Recovery After Surgery protocols recommend prehabilitation. It is a process in the continuum of care that occurs between the time of diagnosis and the beginning of acute treatment. Prehabilitation includes:

- Physiological, nutritional, and psychological assessments

- Identify the concerns and optimizations with required interventions

Prehabilitation promotes the physical and psychological health of the patients and thereby reduces the incidence of postoperative complications.

Preoperative nutritional screening and supplementation 7–10 days prior to surgery reduces perioperative infections, complications, and anastomotic leaks. There are many tools available to assess the malnutrition in these patients, such as the Malnutrition Universal Screening Tool (MUST), Subjective Global Assessment (SGA), and Patient-Generated Subjective Global Assessment (PG-SGA). Iron deficiency anemia due to blood loss or chronic inflammation should be managed. A preoperative Hb minimum of 8 gm/dL should be targeted for patients with cardiac, renal, and pulmonary diseases. Nutritional deficiencies, especially hypoalbuminemia, anemia, and dyselectrolytemia, should be recognized and corrected as all these are associated with poor outcomes of the CR surgeries. The hydration should be maintained for all the patients

Cessation of alcohol, smoking, and tobacco is advised at least 1 month prior to surgery. Based on the amount of consumption, alcoholism is associated with various complications such as intraoperative cardiomyopathy, arrhythmias, cardiac ischemia, and infection being the most common.

Smoking is also associated with various intraoperative and postoperative complications such as bronchospasm, atelectasis, hypoxia, wound infections, and thromboembolic phenomena.

Preoperative Preparation

The general fitness of a patient is a better predictor for outcome after surgery for CR cancer than chronological age.[3] Most of the patients for CR surgeries undergo mechanical bowel preparation (MBP) and insertion of a nasogastric tube. Both MBP and nasogastric tube insertion have been challenged in the literature. Hence, the practice may differ from institute to institute and surgeon to surgeon. As a general rule, all patients should be started on maintenance fluid preoperatively to maintain the hydration status, and serum electrolytes must be checked in the morning of surgery. In elective CR surgery, nondiabetic patients and without delayed gastric emptying, 6-hour fasting for solids and 2-hour for clear fluids including carbohydrate (CHO) drinks is recommended. Preoperative carbohydrate loading (Complex CHO—maltodextrin, 12.5%, 285 mOsm/kg, 800 mL in the evening before surgery and 400 mL 2–3 hours before induction of anesthesia) has shown to improve well-being, reduce complications, shortening time to recovery of the bowel along with a decrease in perioperative insulin resistance.[2]

TABLE 1: Preoperative recommendations and benefits.

Preoperative recommendations	***Benefits***
Preoperative patient counseling	To reduce patient stress and anxiety prior to surgery
Prehabilitation	To reduce the impact of surgical stress and increase functional capacity
Improving nutritional status	To prevent excessive protein breakdown and catabolism
Smoking/alcohol cessation	To avoid potential pulmonary and thromboembolic events and reduce the risks of wound infection, sepsis, and pneumonia
Thromboembolic prophylaxis	To reduce the risk of venous thromboembolisms during and after surgery
Antimicrobial Prophylaxis	To reduce the risk of postoperative infections

A written informed consent highlighting the high-risk factors should be taken. Preoperative anxiety should be allayed with effective and complete communication regarding the nature of surgery. Benzodiazepines may be used with caution whereas drugs such as melatonin and gabapentinoids may be used for this purpose.

Preoperative antibiotic prophylaxis can reduce surgical site infections from 39 to 13%. Oral or intravenous (IV) antibiotic cephalosporin in combination with metronidazole should be administered within 60 minutes prior to skin incision.

Thromboprophylaxis—prophylactically Low-molecular-weight heparin (LMWH) should be started in CR malignancies and bedridden patients in the preoperative period to be stopped 12 hours prior to surgery.

Medications—some patients with CR malignancies are on neoadjuvant chemotherapy and hence need preoperative investigation and optimization as per the medical oncologist.

Preoperative recommendations and benefits are mentioned in **Table 1**.

INTRAOPERATIVE MANAGEMENT

Anesthesia techniques can influence the time to discharge and bowel function. ERAS protocols in CR surgery represent a paradigm shift toward patient-centered care and also in fast-track surgery. A single dose of gabapentin or pregabalin, administered preoperatively, is associated with decreased postoperative pain and opioid consumption.

The combination of balanced general anesthesia (GA) and the regional block is increasingly recognized as an optimal approach for CR surgery. General anesthesia is preferred for complex, lengthy surgeries or when pneumoperitoneum is required. Regional anesthesia is best reserved for smaller localized procedures or as an adjunct to GA for analgesia as it reduces the reliance on systemic opioids and lowers the risk of ileus, sedation, nausea and vomiting postoperatively. The approach should be tailored as per patient comorbidities, surgical technique, and recovery goals. A minimallly invasive surgical technique is associated with reduced postoperative complications and hospital. Evidence-based anesthetic management focuses on maintaining hemodynamic stability, optimizing ventilation, providing effective analgesia, and minimizing postoperative complications. Standard monitoring as per American Society of Anaesthesiologists (ASA) guidelines (ECG, NIBP, pulse oximetry , end tidal carbon dioxide) along with temperature and urinary output monitoring should be done. Invasive monitoring such as intra-arterial blood pressure (IABP), central venous pressure (CVP) along with monitoring of depth of anesthesia and neuromuscular monitoring, may be required in high-risk surgery. As most of the CR surgeries are of prolonged duration, pneumatic compression devices as a means of thromboprophylaxis should be applied wherever feasible.

Goals for an intraoperative period:

- Adequate depth of anesthesia
- Hemodynamic stability
- Maintain euvolemia
- Adequate oxygenation and ventilation
- Avoid hypothermia
- Adequate analgesia

Anesthetic Agents and Technique

Rapid sequence induction (RSI) or modified RSI should be done for patients with bowel obstruction or having significant aspiration risk. Standard induction with short-acting anesthetics including propofol, fentanyl (remifentanil/sufentanil), and sevoflurane and a short-acting neuromuscular blockade should be done. Total intravenous anesthesia (TIVA) reduces postoperative nausea and vomiting (PONV) and may be preferred in ERAS protocols. Some studies suggest that exposure to inhalational anesthesia is associated with an increased risk of cancer recurrence after CR surgery compared to TIVA.[4] It is suggested that the immune-modulating effects of inhalation anesthesia may create a favorable environment for metastasis formation in curative cancer surgery. The effect of the type of anesthesia may not be as substantial in a low-surgical stress setting. Since inhalational anesthetics are primarily given to the weakest of patients, a more rapid discharge and return of bowel function is found in patients receiving TIVA compared to inhalational anesthesia.[5]

Fluid Management

Goal-directed fluid therapy (GDFT) using dynamic indices such as stroke volume variation (SVV) and pulse pressure variation (PVV) may be used. The aim of fluid therapy is to maintain intravascular volume, cardiac output, and tissue perfusion without causing fluid overload. Crystalloid use may be minimized to prevent interstitial edema and ileus. Colloids or blood products may be given as per hemodynamic parameters and laboratory values. Evidence favors restrictive or individualized fluid strategies to reduce postoperative complications such as anastomotic leaks.[6] There is no standard definition of restrictive fluid therapy. ERAS guidelines recommend aiming for a zero-fluid balance and euvolemic during the intraoperative period and first postoperative day in elective CR surgeries.[2,7]

Arterial hypotension should be treated with vasopressors when administering intravenous fluid boluses fails to improve the stroke volume significantly (stroke volume >10%). Inotropes should be considered in patients with reduced myocardial contractility (cardiac index <2.5 L/min) to achieve adequate oxygen delivery.[8,9]

Analgesia

There is an increased emphasis on multimodal opioid-sparing techniques for analgesia. Hence, GA along with regional is the preferred choice of anesthesia in these patients. Opioids can cause postoperative delirium, delayed return of bowel function, and PONV, leading to delayed recovery.

The choice of analgesia with thoracic epidural has several benefits, and there is strong evidence for its recommendation.[10] Apart from providing excellent analgesia, it has the advantage of improved intestinal blood flow, oxygenation and motility, reduced incidence of postoperative ileus, and better GI recovery. It is most suitable for enhanced recovery after open surgery.

Intraoperative opioids along with postoperative patient-controlled analgesia (PCA) with fentanyl may provide excellent analgesia although it has the disadvantage of reduced GI motility, increased duration of postoperative ileus, constipation, and PONV.

Wound infiltration with local anesthetic can decrease pain scores and opioid consumption.

Local perianal anesthetic infiltration with a posterior perineal block with 0.125% bupivacaine and 0.5% lignocaine has been shown to be a safe and effective method for intraoperative analgesia in anorectal surgeries which also minimizes the incidence of urinary retention and other associated complications.[11]

Transversus abdominis plane (TAP) block and quadratus lumborum (QL) block can provide good quality pain relief with early resumption of diet and reduce opioid consumption. TAP block has consistently shown to decrease the pain intensity at rest within 24 hours of both laparoscopic and open surgeries; however, the effect is more profound in open surgeries.[12]

Systemic lignocaine infusion in a dose of 1.5–3 mg/kg/h can reduce the incidence of PONV and time to first flatus and bowel movement, but it may carry the risk of hypotension.[13,14]

Acetaminophen 1 gm and nonsteroidal anti-inflammatory drugs (NSAIDs) such as ketorolac give a good pain control with less opioid consumption and reduced ileus.[15]

Temperature Regulation

The importance of prevention of intraoperative hypothermia is well established. General anesthesia as well as neuraxial anesthesia affects the thermoregulation. Because of peripheral vasodilation heat loss from the body leads to redistribution of heat from the core to the periphery. The temperature of the operating room further adds to the stress of intraoperative hypothermia. Even minimal intraoperative hypothermia can lead to impaired immune function, making patients more prone to postoperative wound infections. In the postoperative period, hypothermic patients may have shivering which in turn increases the oxygen demand exponentially. Other adverse effects of hypothermia include arrhythmias, cardiac ischemia, coagulopathy, and vasoconstriction, leading to reduced colonic blood flow.[2]

Thus, maintaining normothermia is a must to do, especially in high-risk patients having long extensive CR surgeries. Temperature monitoring can be done using skin temperature probes or oropharyngeal temperature probes, later being more accurate. Warm fluids should be used for intravenous as well as irrigation purposes. Forced air-warming devices or warm blankets should be used to maintain normothermia.[2]

Antiemetic Prophylaxis

A multimodal regimen for PONV prophylaxis should be employed. Injection of ondansetron (4 mg) or a combination of dexamethasone (4–8 mg) and ondansetron 4 mg is commonly used for high-risk patients. TIVA has been shown to reduce the risk of PONV markedly.[5] It has been found that postoperative supplemental oxygen at 80% fraction of inspired oxygen (FiO_2) in comparison to 30% reduces the incidence of PONV two- to fivefold after CR surgery, possibly due to decreased serotonin levels in plasma.[16] Liberal use of opioids has also been shown to increase the risk of PONV.[17] Some studies suggest that preoperative carbohydrate loading may decrease PONV.[18] Several scoring systems have been described for the prediction of PONV, with simpler ones appearing to provide better discrimination (The most commonly used are Koivuranta score and Apfel's simplification of this score).[19] Patients having 1–2 risk factors should receive a two-drug combination prophylaxis using first-line antiemetics. Patients with more than 2 risk factors should receive 2–3 antiemetics. For persistent PONV, salvage therapy may be provided using a multimodal approach with different classes of drugs from those used for prophylaxis.[20] There are several classes of first-line antiemetic drugs, including dopamine (D2) antagonists (e.g., droperidol), serotonin (5HT3) antagonists (e.g., ondansetron), and corticosteroids (e.g., dexamethasone).

Surgical Access

Minimally invasive surgery (MIS) for both colonic and rectal resection is well established and, in many countries, it has become the standard of care. Laparoscopic technique is preferred over open laparotomy because of various complications associated with the latter, such as increased postoperative pain, nausea vomiting, lung atelectasis, hypoxia, and delayed recovery. Technological advancements in the last two decades have gained speed in the field of robotic CR surgery, a procedure that limits excessive blood loss via 3D pinpoint precision capability resulting in finer marginal resections, a greater number of lymph node resections, and earlier bowel recovery.[21] Smaller surgical incisions, less discomfort, and a shorter hospital stay are some of the significant benefits. The patient should be safely strapped to the table to prevent sliding down after positioning. Two anesthesiologists along with surgeons, circulating and scrub nurses, and technicians should always be available in the operation theater (OT). The chief surgeon is docked onto the robotic station. A clear and close communication between the team members is the key to a successful uneventful surgery. Laparoscopic and robotic surgeries need insufflation of the peritoneum to create space for operating. High intra-abdominal pressure can impair cardiac function, ventilation, and renal blood flow (RBF).[22] Reducing the intra-abdominal pressure <10–12 mm Hg minimizes the changes in the physiological effects of pneumoperitoneum **(Fig. 1)**.

Considerations for Robotic Surgery

Docking is defined as attaching patient cart instrument arms to the patient after positioning of patient and insertion of ports. After docking, adjustments of the operating table or patient become difficult. Anesthesia workstations should be positioned in a way that allows patients' monitors to be accessible and visible. Glaucoma patients should be identified and handled with extra precaution as the patient position is associated with increased intraocular pressure and cerebral blood flow.[24] All ASA standard monitoring, hourly urinary output, neuromuscular monitoring (TOF), bispectral (BIS) index, and respiratory gas monitoring are essential as even slightly inadequate depth of anesthesia can have deleterious effects. ABP and CVP may be monitored in high-risk cases. Balanced GA with cuffed ETT should be provided. Three-point ETT cuff palpation technique is a simple, reliable, and effective way to prevent endobronchial tube migration during robotic pelvis surgery.[25] Lung protective ventilation with positive end-expiratory pressure (PEEP) decreases the likelihood of atelectasis, improves respiratory mechanics, and restores functional residual capacity (FRC). The degree of limb extension, stirrup position, padding of bony prominences, and eyes should be frequently assessed to avoid any nerve injuries. Intravenous balanced salt solutions are preferred targeting near-zero fluid balance and euvolemia.

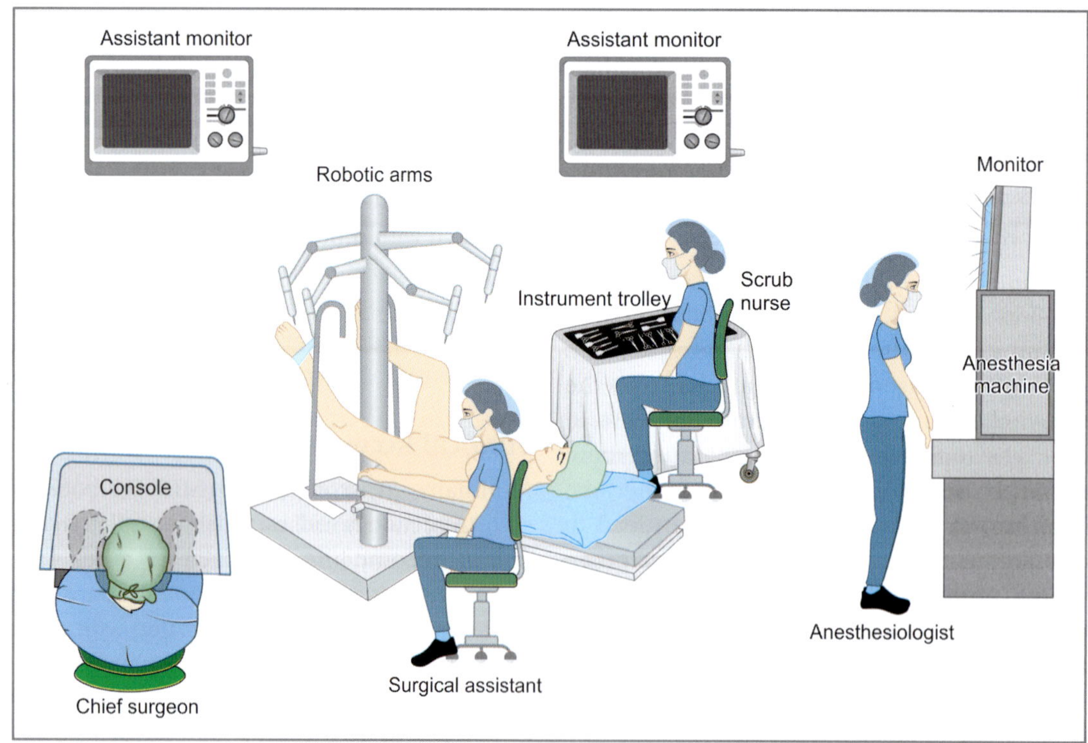

Fig. 1: A typical operating room setup.[23]

TABLE 2: Intraoperative recommendations and their benefits.

Intraoperative recommendations	*Benefits*
Opioid-sparing or minimal opioid administration	Early recovery of bowel function and decreased postoperative nausea and vomiting
Normothermia	Better wound healing and fewer wound infections
Euvolemia/zero-fluid balance	Less bowel edema, early recovery
Antiemetic prophylaxis	Prevents postoperative nausea and vomiting
Minimally invasive approach	To reduce the risk of complications and postoperative pain

Pneumoperitoneum and patient position can increase chances of airway edema, leading to unsuccessful extubation. An airway leak test may be performed prior to extubation.[26]

Intraoperative recommendations and their benefits are mentioned in **Table 2**.

POSTOPERATIVE MANAGEMENT

Extubation

Neuromuscular monitoring should be a standard of care with objective monitoring being more accurate than basic peripheral nerve stimulators. Reversal of neuromuscular blocking agent (NMBA) to a TOF ratio of 90% is important to avoid residual paralysis and risk of postpulmonary complications.[27] Injection of neostigmine with injection glycopyrrolate or injection atropine is commonly used for reversing the NMBA. Sugammadex can also be used, if available.[28]

Recovery after open CR surgery can be hastened by adopting perioperative evidence-based enhanced or fast-tracked/accelerated recovery pathways.[29]

The postoperative period in CR surgeries (both open and laparoscopic) focuses on addressing pain, respiratory function, hemodynamic stability, gastrointestinal recovery, and potential complications. Postoperative nasogastric tubes should not be used routinely; if inserted during surgery, they should be removed before reversal of anesthesia.[30]

Postoperatively, patients should be kept propped up with oxygen supplementation and continuous monitoring of vital parameters should be continued. One must evaluate for existing comorbidities, procedure-associated risks, and possible intraoperative complications such as subcutaneous emphysema, delayed hypercarbia, and capnothorax. The key emphasis should be on adequate analgesia and early ambulation.[31]

Opioid-sparing technique is associated with early mobilization and fewer complications.[32] Acetaminophen is an integral part of it and can be administered easily. NSAIDs and COX 2 drugs are also vital parts of a multimodal strategy. Lignocaine and dexmedetomidine infusions do reduce postoperative pain although there are limited studies that have assessed the combination of these systemic additives.[33,34] Dose of lignocaine ranges from 1.5 to 3 mg/kg/h depending on the bolus given (0–1.5 mg/kg).[13,14]

Thoracic epidural analgesia (TEA) (T7-T10) with a mixture of a low dose of LA and lipophilic opioids remains the gold standard in patients undergoing open CR surgery and reduces the metabolic and neuroendocrine stress response.[35,36] The same analgesic benefits are not demonstrated in laparoscopic CR surgery.[37] Regional abdominal wall blocks such as TAP given at 2 points or 4 points under USG guidance provide analgesic coverage to the ant abdominal wall from T10 to L1 in minimally invasive laparoscopic surgeries.[38]

Antiemetic (injection of ondansetron) should be continued for PONV prophylaxis. Deep vein thrombosis (DVT) prophylaxis (mechanical or pharmaceutical) along with good chest physiotherapy is of prime importance in postoperative period.[29]

Recent reviews of risk factors for DVT include ulcerative colitis, advanced malignancy, hypercoagulable state, steroid use, advanced age, and obesity.[39] Patients undergoing major CR surgery should have dual prevention from DVT with mechanical thromboprophylaxis by well-fitting compression stockings and/or intermittent pneumatic compression until discharge and by receiving pharmacological prophylaxis with LMWH once daily for 28 days after surgery.[2]

Surgical stress can cause an acute depletion of arginine, which both impairs T-cell function and wound healing.[40] Hence, patients should be offered a normal oral diet with around 1,200–1,500 kcal as early as possible to reduce infectious complications and decrease morbidity.[41] Perioperative immunonutrition in malnourished patients is beneficial in CR cancer surgery.[42] Hyperglycemia is a risk

TABLE 3: Postoperative recommendations and their benefits.

Postoperative recommendations	*Benefits*
Early resumption of oral feeding	To reduce the risk of insulin resistance
Early mobilization	To support quick return to normal function, reduction of risk of pneumonia and deep vein thrombosis (DVT)
Avoidance of NG tubes, catheters, and drains	To reduce pain, discomfort, and the risk of pneumonia, while promoting the resumption of oral feeding
Multimodal analgesia	To control pain while sparing excessive opioid usage

factor for complications and should be avoided by using insulin if needed.

A near-zero fluid and electrolyte balance should be maintained by using balance salt solutions for replacement losses, and hypotonic crystalloid for pure maintenance needs to prevent loading with high concentrations of sodium and cations.[2,43]

Postoperative recommendations and their benefits are described in **Table 3**.

Emergency Surgery

Nearly about 30% of CR surgeries are emergent in nature such as perforated colonic diverticulitis, fulminant colitis, massive gastrointestinal (GI) hemorrhage, and traumatic injuries to the colon and rectum with higher morbidity, mortality, and longer hospital stay.[44] The goals should be to optimize hemodynamic stability with fluid resuscitation and vasopressors, ensure RSI to prevent aspiration, use lung-protective ventilation strategies, maintain normothermia and effective pain control, vigilantly monitor for complications such as sepsis, ileus, and anastomotic leak. The ERAS protocol adherence in emergency CR surgery has shown a lower overall rate of complication, lesser readmission rates, and mortality.[45]

CONCLUSION

Efficient anesthesia for colorectal surgeries involve a combination of general anesthesia, regional anesthesia and tailored pain management strategies. The anesthetic plan must be individualized based on patient factors such as age, comorbidities and the complexity of the surgery. Postoperative pain management approach should focus on reducing opioid consumption,with options like epidural analgesia, patient control analgesia (PCA), and non-opioid analgesics. Adhering to Enhanced recovery after surgery (ERAS) protocols can further improve patient outcomes and speed recovery.

REFERENCES

1. Fitzmaurice C, Akinyemiju TF, Al Lami FH, Alam T, Alizadeh-Navaei R, Allen C, et al.; Global Burden of Disease Cancer Collaboration. Global, regional, and national cancer incidence, mortality, years of life lost, years lived with disability, and disability adjusted life-years for 29 cancer groups, 1990 to 2016: a systematic analysis for the global burden of disease study, Global Burden of Disease Study. JAMA Oncol. 2018;4:1553-68.
2. Gustafsson UO, Scott MJ, Hubner M, Nygren J, Demartines N, Francis N, et al. Guidelines for Perioperative Care in Elective Colorectal Surgery: Enhanced Recovery After Surgery (ERAS®) Society Recommendations: 2018. World J Surg. 2019;43:659-95.
3. Oruç Z, Kaplan MA. Effect of exercise on colorectal cancer prevention and treatment. World J Gastrointest Oncol. 2019;11(5):348-66.
4. Hasselager RP, Hallas J, Gögenur I. Inhalation or total intravenous anaesthesia and recurrence after colorectal cancer surgery: a propensity score matched Danish registry-based study. Br J Anaesth. 2021;126(5):921-30.
5. Crone V, Hasselager RP, Fransgaard T, Gögenur I. Anaesthetic technique and outcomes after colorectal cancer surgery. Dan Med J. 2020;67(4):A04190255.
6. Deslarzes P, Jurt J, Larson DW, Blanc C, Hübner M, Grass F. Perioperative Fluid Management in Colorectal Surgery: Institutional Approach to Standardized Practice. J Clin Med. 2024;13(3):801.
7. Thiele RH, Raghunathan K, Brudney CS, Lobo DN, Martin D, Senagore A, et al. American Society for Enhanced Recovery (ASER) and Perioperative Quality Initiative (POQI) joint consensus statement on perioperative fluid management within an enhanced recovery pathway for colorectal surgery. Perioper Med (Lond). 2016;5:24.
8. Schwegler I, von Holzen A, Gutzwiller JP, Schlumpf R, Mühlebach S, Stanga Z. Nutritional risk is a clinical predictor of postoperative mortality and morbidity in surgery for colorectal cancer. Br J Surg. 2010;97(1):92-7.
9. Gibbs J, Cull W, Henderson W, Daley J, Hur K, Khuri SF. Preoperative serum albumin level as a predictor of operative mortality and morbidity: results from the National VA Surgical Risk Study. Arch Surg. 1999;134(1):36-42.
10. Patel S, Lutz JM, Panchagnula U, Bansal S. Anesthesia and perioperative management of colorectal surgical patients - A clinical review (Part 1). J Anaesthesiol Clin Pharmacol. 2012;28(2):162-71.

11. Poskus T, Jakubauskas M, Čekas K, Jakubauskiene L, Strupas K, Samalavičius NE. Local Perianal Anesthetic Infiltration Is Safe and Effective for Anorectal Surgery. Front Surg. 2021;8:730261.
12. Viderman D, Aubakirova M, Abdildin YG. Transversus Abdominis Plane Block in Colorectal Surgery: A Meta-Analysis. Front Med (Lausanne). 2022;8:802039.
13. Dunn LK, Durieux ME. Perioperative Use of Intravenous Lidocaine. Anesthesiology. 2017;126(4):729-37.
14. Sun Y, Li T, Wang N, Yun Y, Gan TJ. Perioperative systemic lidocaine for postoperative analgesia and recovery after abdominal surgery: a meta-analysis of randomized controlled trials. Dis Colon Rectum. 2012;55(11):1183-94.
15. Chen JY, Ko TL, Wen YR, Wu SC, Chou YH, Yien HW, et al. Opioid-sparing effects of ketorolac and its correlation with the recovery of postoperative bowel function in colorectal surgery patients: a prospective randomized double-blinded study. Clin J Pain. 2009;25(6):485-9.
16. Greif R, Laciny S, Rapf B, Hickle RS, Sessler DI. Supplemental oxygen reduces the incidence of postoperative nausea and vomiting. Anesthesiology. 1999;91(5):1246-52.
17. Apfel CC, Philip BK, Cakmakkaya OS, Shilling A, Shi YY, Leslie JB, et al. Who is at risk for postdischarge nausea and vomiting after ambulatory surgery? Anesthesiology. 2012;117(3):475-86.
18. Singh BN, Dahiya D, Bagaria D, Saini V, Kaman L, Kaje V, et al. Effects of preoperative carbohydrates drinks on immediate postoperative outcome after day care laparoscopic cholecystectomy. Surg Endosc. 2015;29(11):3267-72.
19. Kappen TH, Moons KG, van Wolfswinkel L, Kalkman CJ, Vergouwe Y, van Klei WA. Impact of risk assessments on prophylactic antiemetic prescription and the incidence of postoperative nausea and vomiting: a cluster-randomized trial. Anesthesiology. 2014;120(2):343-54.
20. Eberhart LH, Mauch M, Morin AM, Wulf H, Geldner G. Impact of a multimodal anti-emetic prophylaxis on patient satisfaction in high-risk patients for postoperative nausea and vomiting. Anaesthesia. 2002;57(10):1022-7.
21. Shah MF, Nasir IUI, Parvaiz A. Robotic Surgery for Colorectal Cancer. Visc Med. 2019;35(4):247-50.
22. Demyttenaere S, Feldman LS, Fried GM. Effect of pneumoperitoneum on renal perfusion and function: a systematic review. Surg Endosc. 2007;21(2):152-60.
23. Khanna S, Das J, Kumar S, Mehta Y, Ahlawat R. Being intuitive: Starting a comprehensive multispecialty robotic surgery programme. OA Robot Surg. 2014;15:2-8.
24. Awad H, Santilli S, Ohr M, Roth A, Yan W, Fernandez S, et al. The effects of steep Trendelenburg positioning on intraocular pressure during robotic radical prostatectomy. Anesth Analg. 2009;109(2):473-8.
25. Mittal AK, Dubey J, Shukla S, Bhasin N, Dubey M, Jaipuria J. Efficacy of the three-point cuff palpation technique in preventing endobronchial tube migration during positioning in robotic pelvic surgeries. Indian J Anaesth. 2022;66(12):818-25.
26. Phong SV, Koh LK. Anaesthesia for robotic-assisted radical prostatectomy: considerations for laparoscopy in the Trendelenburg position. Anaesth Intensive Care. 2007;35(2):281-5.
27. Brull SJ, Prielipp RC. Neuromuscular monitoring and the cost of antagonism: when will we learn? Anaesthesia. 2017;72(12):1557-8.
28. Abad-Gurumeta A, Ripollés-Melchor J, Casans-Francés R, Espinosa A, Martínez-Hurtado E, Fernández-Pérez C, et al.; Evidence Anaesthesia Review Group. A systematic review of sugammadex vs neostigmine for reversal of neuromuscular blockade. Anaesthesia. 2015;70(12):1441-52.
29. Suryawanshi CM, Shah B, Khanna S, Ghodki P, Bhati K, Ashok KV. Anaesthetic management of robot-assisted laparoscopic surgery. Indian J Anaesth. 2023;67(1):117-22.
30. Nelson R, Edwards S, Tse B. Prophylactic nasogastric decompression after abdominal surgery. Cochrane Database Syst Rev. 2007;2007(3):CD004929.
31. Batley SE, Prasad V, Vasdev N, Mohan SG. Post-operative Pain Management in Patients Undergoing Robotic Urological Surgery. Curr Urol. 2016;9(1):5-11.
32. Ljungqvist O, Scott M, Fearon KC. Enhanced Recovery After Surgery: A Review. JAMA Surg. 2017;152(3):292-8.
33. Kranke P, Jokinen J, Pace NL, Schnabel A, Hollmann MW, Hahnenkamp K, et al. Continuous intravenous perioperative lidocaine infusion for postoperative pain and recovery. Cochrane Database Syst Rev. 2015;(7):CD009642.
34. Ge DJ, Qi B, Tang G, Li JY. Intraoperative Dexmedetomidine Promotes Postoperative Analgesia and Recovery in Patients after Abdominal Hysterectomy: A Double-Blind, Randomized Clinical Trial. Sci Rep. 2016;6:21514.
35. Block BM, Liu SS, Rowlingson AJ, Cowan AR, Cowan JA Jr, Wu CL. Efficacy of postoperative epidural analgesia: a meta-analysis. JAMA. 2003;290(18):2455-63.
36. Werawatganon T, Charuluxanun S. Patient controlled intravenous opioid analgesia versus continuous epidural analgesia for pain after intra-abdominal surgery. Cochrane Database Syst Rev. 2005;(1):CD004088.
37. Hübner M, Blanc C, Roulin D, Winiker M, Gander S, Demartines N. Randomized clinical trial on epidural versus patient-controlled analgesia for laparoscopic colorectal surgery within an enhanced recovery pathway. Ann Surg. 2015;261(4):648-53.
38. Keller DS, Ermlich BO, Delaney CP. Demonstrating the benefits of transversus abdominis plane blocks on patient outcomes in laparoscopic colorectal surgery: review of 200 consecutive cases. J Am Coll Surg. 2014;219(6):1143-8.
39. Iannuzzi JC, Aquina CT, Rickles AS, Hensley BJ, Probst CP, Noyes K, et al. Risk Factors for Post discharge Venothromboembolism After Colorectal Resection. Dis Colon Rectum. 2016;59(3):224-9.

40. Mauskopf JA, Candrilli SD, Chevrou-Séverac H, Ochoa JB. Immunonutrition for patients undergoing elective surgery for gastrointestinal cancer: impact on hospital costs. World J Surg Oncol. 2012;10:136.
41. Andersen HK, Lewis SJ, Thomas S. Early enteral nutrition within 24h of colorectal surgery versus later commencement of feeding for postoperative complications. Cochrane Database Syst Rev. 2006;(4):CD004080.
42. Weimann A, Braga M, Carli F, Higashiguchi T, Hübner M, Klek S, et al. ESPEN guideline: Clinical nutrition in surgery. Clin Nutr. 2017;36(3):623-50.
43. Prowle JR, Kirwan CJ, Bellomo R. Fluid management for the prevention and attenuation of acute kidney injury. Nat Rev Nephrol. 2014;10(1):37-47.
44. Bayar B, Yılmaz KB, Akıncı M, Şahin A, Kulaçoğlu H. An evaluation of treatment results of emergency versus elective surgery in colorectal cancer patients. Ulus Cerrahi Derg. 2015;32(1):11-7.
45. Lohsiriwat V, Jitmungngan R. Enhanced recovery after surgery in emergency colorectal surgery: Review of literature and current practices. World J Gastrointest Surg. 2019;11(2):41-52.

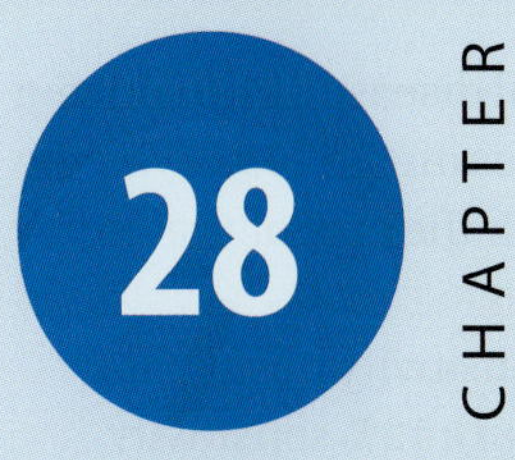

Anesthesia for Cytoreductive Surgery and Hyperthermic Intraperitoneal Chemotherapy

Sohan Lal Solanki

INTRODUCTION

Cytoreductive surgery (CRS) combined with hyperthermic intraperitoneal chemotherapy (HIPEC) offers a potentially effective treatment option for carefully selected patients with peritoneal carcinomatosis, originating either from primary peritoneal malignancies or secondary from gastrointestinal or gynecological cancers. This approach has significantly enhanced both survival rates and quality of life in these patients. Historically, before CRS and HIPEC were introduced, peritoneal malignancies were considered incurable, and palliative chemotherapy was the only available option.[1]

Dr Paul Sugarbaker pioneered this technique, initially applying it to treat pseudomyxoma peritonei (PMP) arising from the appendix. His work demonstrated that CRS and HIPEC could improve survival and quality of life.[2] Later, Verwaal et al. conducted a randomized trial comparing systemic chemotherapy to CRS combined with HIPEC. The results, with an 8-year follow-up, revealed a nearly twofold survival benefit (13 months vs. 22 months) in the HIPEC arm, and patients who achieved complete cytoreduction showed a median survival of 43 months.[3]

The global incidence of peritoneal cancers or carcinomatosis is increasing, resulting in substantial morbidity and mortality. Primary peritoneal surface malignancies include malignant peritoneal mesothelioma (MPM) and PMP, while secondary peritoneal malignancies arise from metastases of cancers such as colorectal, ovarian, and gastric tumors. Over recent years, the treatment landscape for peritoneal carcinomatosis has evolved significantly, with CRS, often combined with HIPEC, becoming the standard of care due to its proven effectiveness in improving outcomes.[1]

Cytoreductive surgery and HIPEC consist of three distinct phases. The first phase involves CRS, which entails the removal of all visible metastatic disease in the abdomen and pelvis through peritonectomy. This extensive surgical procedure removes both the peritoneal deposits and the primary tumor. The second phase, HIPEC, involves administering heated chemotherapy at temperatures between 41 and 43°C directly into the peritoneal cavity for 60–120 minutes. The final phase includes the removal of the chemotherapy solution, bowel reconstruction (if not performed before HIPEC), ensuring hemostasis, and closing the abdominal incision[4] **(Fig. 1)**.

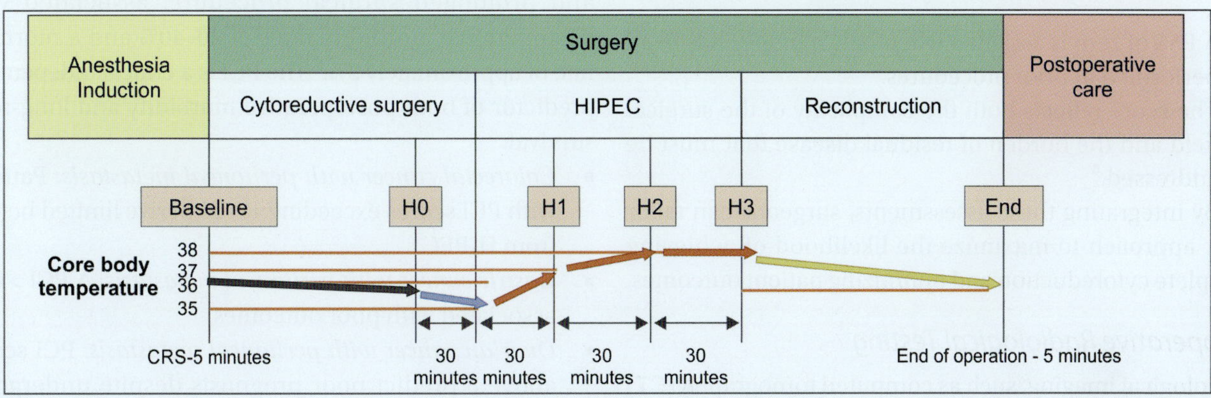

Fig. 1: The time course and phases of CRS-HIPEC. (CRS: cytoreductive surgery; HIPEC: hyperthermic intraperitoneal chemotherapy)

CYTOREDUCTIVE SURGERY

Cytoreductive surgery is a surgical strategy aimed at reducing tumor burden by resecting the primary tumor and/or metastatic deposits. This may involve complete or partial resection, with the goals of achieving disease cure, alleviating symptoms, preventing complications, and enhancing the patient's quality of life.

For most cancers, the primary objective of surgical management, whether through primary cytoreductive surgery (PCS) or interval cytoreductive surgery (ICS), is to achieve complete resection. PCS is performed upfront and may be followed by systemic chemotherapy, whereas ICS is undertaken after neoadjuvant chemotherapy, with or without subsequent systemic chemotherapy. Regardless of timing, the ultimate aim of CRS is to achieve total clearance of the peritoneal cavity, as residual disease at the end of surgery is a critical prognostic factor influencing survival outcomes.[5]

Disease Assessment

Prognostic indicators such as histopathology, the prior surgical score (PSS), the peritoneal cancer index (PCI), and the completeness of cytoreduction score (CC score) play a pivotal role in assessing peritoneal metastases from gastrointestinal and gynecological malignancies. These indicators provide valuable insights into the extent of disease and guide surgical planning.

Preoperative Assessment

Prior surgical score: The PSS is a quantitative measure used to evaluate the extent of previous surgical interventions in patients scheduled for CRS due to peritoneal metastases. It provides an estimate of the adhesions surgeons may encounter during definitive surgery and assesses the degree of tumor cell entrapment needing resection during CRS.

- A PSS of zero is assigned when only a biopsy has been performed in prior procedures.
- The score reflects both the complexity of the surgical field and the burden of residual disease that must be addressed.[6]

By integrating these assessments, surgeons can tailor their approach to maximize the likelihood of achieving complete cytoreduction and optimizing patient outcomes.

Preoperative Radiological Testing

Radiological imaging, such as computed tomography (CT) or magnetic resonance imaging (MRI), plays a critical role in evaluating the extent of peritoneal disease and assessing involvement of other organs preoperatively. However, the sensitivity of CT imaging varies with the size of the tumor nodules:

- *Small nodules (<0.5 cm):* 28% sensitivity
- *Moderate-sized nodules (0.5–5 cm):* 72% sensitivity
- *Large nodules (>5 cm):* Approximately 90% sensitivity[7]

Despite its utility, CT-based determination of the peritoneal cancer index (CT-PCI) can sometimes be unreliable, leading to inaccuracies in disease assessment.[8]

Intraoperative Assessment

Peritoneal cancer index: The PCI, also known as the peritoneal carcinomatosis index, is the most precise and validated system for intraoperative assessment of peritoneal cancer prognosis. It evaluates the disease burden or metastatic spread within the peritoneal cavity.

- *Scoring system:* The peritoneal cavity is divided into 13 regions (labeled 0–12). In each region, the size of the largest tumor nodule is measured and scored:
  - *Score 0:* No visible tumor
  - *Score 1:* Tumor size <0.5 cm
  - *Score 2:* Tumor size between 0.5 and 5 cm
  - *Score 3:* Tumor size >5 cm or confluent layers of small nodules
- *PCI calculation:* The scores from all 13 regions are summed to produce a total PCI, with a maximum score of 39. A higher PCI indicates greater disease burden and poorer prognosis. This scoring system remains the gold standard for intraoperative evaluation of peritoneal cancers[1] **(Fig. 2)**.

Postoperative Outcomes and Prognostic Indicators

Cytoreductive surgery–HIPEC is a technically demanding and prolonged surgical procedure, associated with postoperative morbidity rates of 20–40% and a mortality rate of approximately 3%.[9] The PCI is a critical independent predictor of both postoperative morbidity and long-term survival.

- *Colorectal cancer with peritoneal metastasis:* Patients with PCI scores exceeding 17–20 derive limited benefit from HIPEC.
- *Gastric cancer with peritoneal metastasis:* A PCI >12 is associated with poor outcomes.
- *Ovarian cancer with peritoneal metastasis:* PCI scores above 8 predict poor prognosis despite undergoing HIPEC.

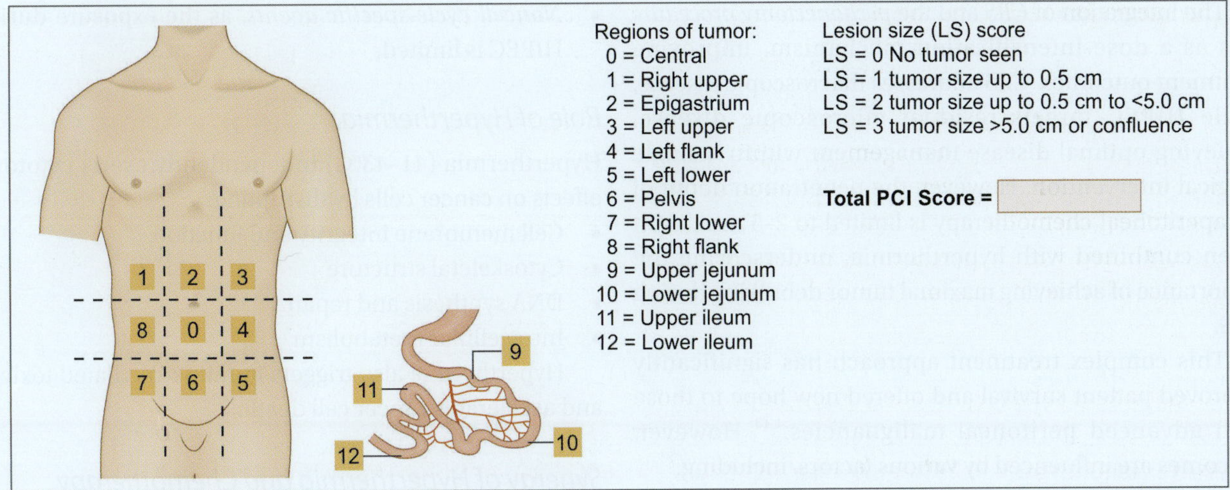

Fig. 2: Peritoneal cancer index (PCI).

- *MPM and PMP:* Unlike other cancers, there is no definitive PCI cutoff; however, higher PCI values generally correlate with worse long-term outcomes.[1]

Completeness of Cytoreduction

The primary goal of CRS is the thorough removal of all visible disease, with completeness evaluated using the *CC score*, as defined by Sugarbaker:

- *CC0:* No residual disease
- *CC1:* Residual nodules <2.5 mm
- *CC2:* Residual nodules between 2.5 mm and 2.5 cm
- *CC3:* Residual nodules >2.5 cm

A CC score of ≥2 denotes incomplete cytoreduction. Achieving *complete cytoreduction (CC0 or CC1)*is essential, as incomplete cytoreduction (CC ≥ 2) negates the therapeutic benefits of HIPEC.[10,11]

HYPERTHERMIC INTRAPERITONEAL CHEMOTHERAPY

Hyperthermic intraperitoneal chemotherapy involves delivering heated cytotoxic chemotherapy directly into the peritoneal cavity, targeting microscopic cancer cells that remain post-CRS and cannot be surgically removed. This approach aims to reduce cancer recurrence.

- *Procedure:* A single dose of chemotherapy—often oxaliplatin, mitomycin, doxorubicin, or cisplatin—is heated to 41–43°C and infused into the peritoneal cavity. The chemotherapeutic agents are mixed with a dialysate solution, heated in a specialized device (e.g., Belmont pump), and circulated through the abdominal cavity via an inlet channel. The fluid is then drained, reheated, and recirculated through an outlet channel.[1]
- *Advantages of HIPEC:*
  - Ensures optimal drug exposure by direct contact with microscopic residual cancer cells, avoiding barriers such as postoperative adhesions.
  - Utilizes a standardized technique to maximize chemotherapy distribution and dwell times.
  - Hyperthermia enhances the cytotoxicity of chemotherapeutic agents by increasing deoxyribonucleic acid (DNA) crosslinking and tumor penetration.
- *Toxicity of hyperthermia:* Hyperthermia induces cell damage through:
  - Membrane and nuclear alterations
  - Protein denaturation
  - *Disruptions in calcium permeability:* It is effects are more pronounced in hypoxic tumor cells due to the acidic environment, poor nutrition, and inadequate perfusion typically present in these tissues.[12]

The chemotherapy agents in HIPEC are designed to target microscopic metastatic cells within the peritoneal cavity. Hyperthermia itself has a cytotoxic effect, and its combination with chemotherapy creates a synergistic effect that enhances the destruction of cancer cells while reducing the risk of tumor recurrence. Additionally, the systemic absorption of intraperitoneal chemotherapy is minimal, allowing for the administration of higher doses compared to intravenous chemotherapy with fewer systemic side effects.[1]

The integration of *CRS* and the *peritonectomy procedure* acts as a dose-intensification mechanism, improving treatment outcomes. CRS addresses macroscopic disease, while HIPEC targets residual microscopic disease, achieving optimal disease management within a single surgical intervention. However, the penetration depth of intraperitoneal chemotherapy is limited to 2–5 mm, even when combined with hyperthermia, underscoring the importance of achieving maximal tumor debulking during CRS.[1]

This complex treatment approach has significantly improved patient survival and offered new hope to those with advanced peritoneal malignancies.[1,13] However, outcomes are influenced by various factors, including:

- Patient selection
- Primary cancer diagnosis
- Disease extent (e.g., PCI score)
- Surgical expertise
- Chemotherapeutic regimen
- Response to preoperative therapy

Numerous studies worldwide continue to refine the management strategies for CRS and HIPEC.

Multidisciplinary Approach

Cytoreductive surgery and HIPEC demand specialized surgical skills for the intricate resection of peritoneal tumors. Successful management involves a *multidisciplinary team* of healthcare professionals, including:

- Surgeons
- Anesthesiologists
- Critical care specialists
- Pulmonologists
- Allied healthcare workers, such as nurses, nutritionists, and physiotherapists

The teamwork among these professionals ensures the meticulous execution of the procedure, optimal perioperative care, and improved patient outcomes.

Chemotherapy Drugs in Hyperthermic Intraperitoneal Chemotherapy

The objective of HIPEC is to deliver high concentrations of chemotherapeutic agents directly to local tissues (20–1,000 times greater than plasma levels), minimizing systemic toxicity.[14] Ideal drugs for HIPEC are:

- *Large, high-molecular-weight, hydrophilic compounds* with slow peritoneal clearance, which enhance tumor cell penetration.
- *Noncell cycle-specific agents*, as the exposure during HIPEC is limited.

Role of Hyperthermia

Hyperthermia (41–43°C) independently exerts cytotoxic effects on cancer cells by disrupting:

- Cell membrane integrity and function
- Cytoskeletal structure
- DNA synthesis and repair
- Intracellular metabolism

Hyperthermia also triggers immune-mediated toxicity and accelerates cancer cell death.[15,16]

Synergy of Hyperthermia and Chemotherapy

The combination of hyperthermia and chemotherapy enhances drug efficacy through:

- Improved drug uptake
- Enhanced tumor penetration
- Altered pharmacokinetics and excretion[16]

Commonly Used Chemotherapeutic Agents

Commonly used chemotherapeutic agents are as follows:

- *Mitomycin-C (MMC):* A noncell cycle-specific agent synergistic with hyperthermia
- *Platinum-based drugs:*
    - Cisplatin, carboplatin, and oxaliplatin are commonly used due to their heat synergy.
- *Less commonly used agents:* Doxorubicin, docetaxel, paclitaxel, 5-fluorouracil (5-FU), and irinotecan[17]

Bidirectional Intraoperative Chemotherapy

Bidirectional intraoperative chemotherapy (BIC) combines intraoperative intravenous (IV) and intraperitoneal (IP) chemotherapy to create a bidirectional diffusion gradient across cancer cells.

- Common protocol:
    - *IV administration: 5-FU (400 mg/m^2)* and *leucovorin (20 mg/m^2)* in 250 mL of saline, administered rapidly 1 hour before initiating IP chemotherapy.
- BIC enhances chemotherapy delivery to peritoneal nodules, improving treatment efficacy.[18]

Systemic Toxicity of Intraperitoneal Chemotherapy

Systemic toxicity from IP chemotherapy is generally low **(Table 1)**, but some notable side effects include:

TABLE 1: Common chemotherapy agents used in HIPEC.

	Cytotoxic drugs commonly used for intraperitoneal (IP) administration				
Drug	***Heat synergy***	***Penetration depth, mm***	***Cell cycle-specific***	***AUC IP:IV ratio***	***Toxicities***
Carboplatin	Yes	0.5	No	2–10	Nephrotoxicity, neurotoxicity, GI bleeding, myelosuppression peripheral neuropathy
Cisplatin	Yes	1.0–3.0	No	8–21	
Oxaliplatin	Yes	1.0–2.0	No	3.5–16	
Mitomycin C	Yes	2.0	No	10–23.5	Nephrotoxicity, pulmonary toxicity, and myelosuppression
Paclitaxel	Minimal	0.5	Yes	1,000	Myelosuppression, and peripheral neuropathy
Fluorouracil	Minimal	0.2	Yes	250	Gastrointestinal, myelosuppression, and neurotoxicity

(AUC: area under the curve; IV: intravenous; GI: gastrointestinal; HIPEC: hyperthermic intraperitoneal chemotherapy)

- *Hematological toxicity:* Reported in 4–39% of patients.[19,20]
  - MMC-associated myelosuppression occurs in up to 28% of cases.[21]
- *Renal toxicity:*
  - *Renal insufficiency* is observed in 2–5% of patients, particularly with cisplatin.[19,20]
  - *Nephrotoxicity* is a known risk of cisplatin therapy.[22]
- *Intra-abdominal complications: Oxaliplatin* can cause intra-abdominal bleeding[23] and mild hepatotoxicity.

Carrier Solutions

The selection of the carrier solution for IP drug delivery plays a critical role in the pharmacokinetics of HIPEC. An optimal carrier solution enhances drug exposure to the peritoneal surface, ensures slower clearance from the peritoneal cavity, and maintains an adequate drug volume without causing adverse effects.[24] The two primary factors influencing drug delivery are the tonicity of the solution and the molecular weight of the solute. Higher molecular weight compounds and/or hypertonic solutions tend to result in slower clearance of the peritoneal fluid, thus prolonging the peritoneal exposure to the chemotherapy agents.[17] Currently, most centers recommend isotonic saline or dextrose-based peritoneal solutions, with 1.5% dextrose isotonic solutions being the most commonly used.[16]

Historically, oxaliplatin was administered in 5% dextrose-based solutions, as it was believed that chloride ions could degrade oxaliplatin into less cytotoxic metabolites. However, recent findings have shown that oxaliplatin can be safely used in chloride-containing solutions, which may even enhance its cytotoxicity.[1] Furthermore, using dextrose-based solutions can sometimes lead to perioperative complications such as hyperglycemia and hyponatremia.

Perfusion Techniques

Hyperthermic intraperitoneal chemotherapy can be administered using various techniques, including open and closed abdominal methods, with some variations such as semi-open, semi-closed, and laparoscopic approaches. However, no single method has been universally accepted as superior.

- *Closed abdominal technique:* This was the first technique developed and remains in use today. After cytoreductive surgery, Tenckhoff catheters, temperature probes, and drains are inserted through small incisions, and the skin edges are sutured tightly to create a closed circuit for the perfusion. The perfusate is distributed through continuous agitation of the abdomen externally.[24]
- *Open abdominal technique ("Coliseum technique"):* In this method, after cytoreduction, the same placement of catheters and probes is done, but the skin edges are suspended from a self-retaining retractor to allow the abdominal cavity to remain open. The surgeon manually stirs the perfusate within the cavity[24] **(Figs. 3 and 4)**.

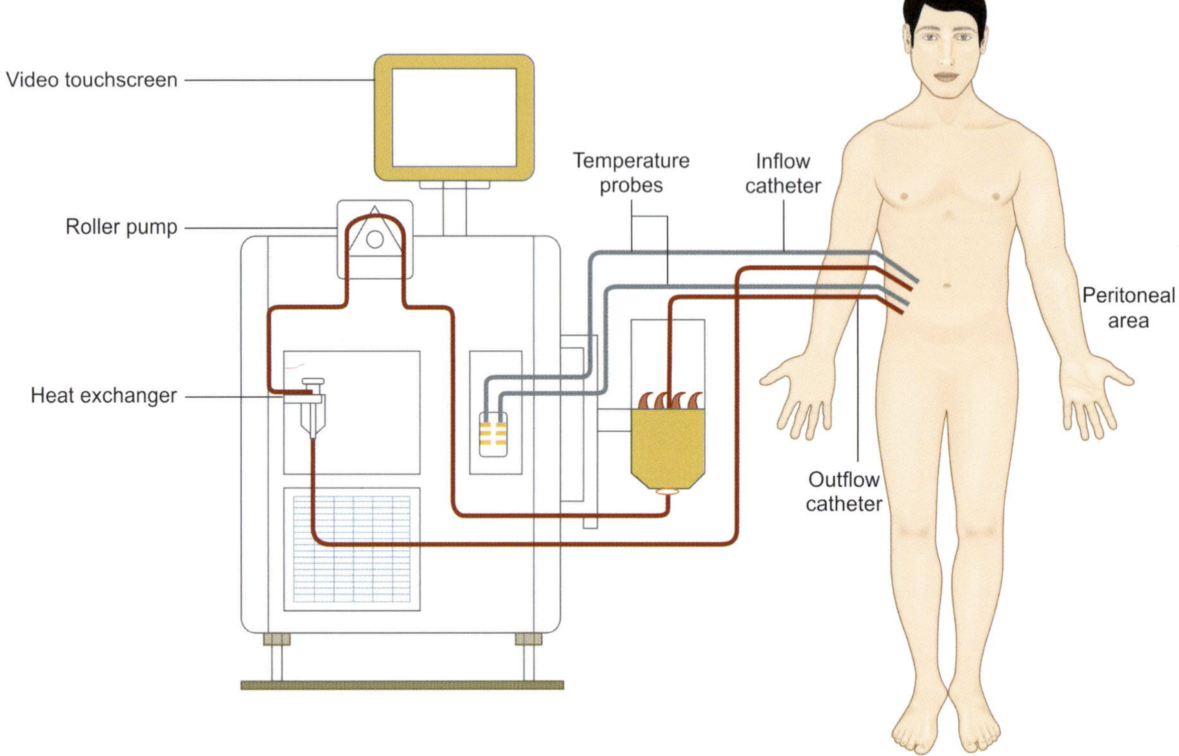

Fig. 3: The hyperthermic intraperitoneal chemotherapy (HIPEC) circuit.

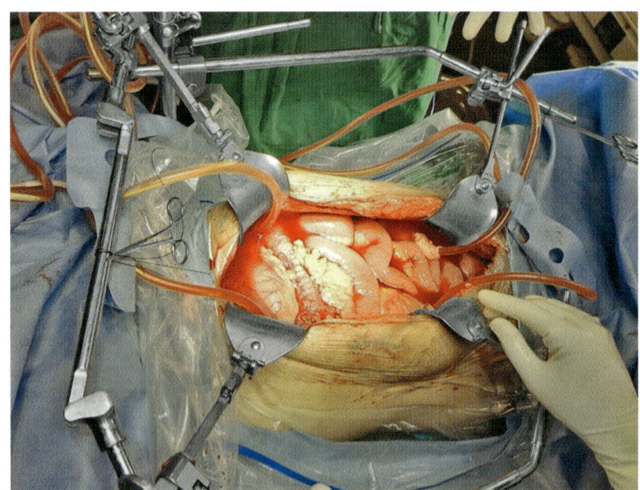

Fig. 4: The "Coliseum technique" of hyperthermic intraperitoneal chemotherapy (HIPEC).

A variety of automated hyperthermic perfusion pumps are now widely available, which typically include the following components:[25]

- A single-use circuit tubing with a reservoir
- A heat source
- A heat exchanger for heating the perfusate
- A roller pump to circulate the perfusate through the patient
- A return system (either a second roller pump or a vacuum source)
- Multiple temperature monitors

The amount of IP drug and the volume of the carrier solution are typically calculated based on the patient's body surface area (BSA). Common perfusate volumes are 1.5 L/m^2 or 2 L/m^2. During HIPEC, the perfusate circulates at a rate of 1 L/min with the aid of a roller pump. The heat exchanger maintains the perfusate temperature at 43–45°C, ensuring the intraperitoneal temperature stays within the desired range of 41–43°C. Once the perfusate circulates fully in and out of the abdomen, typically after reaching an intraperitoneal temperature of around 41.5°C, the chemotherapy drug is added, and the perfusion cycle is timed for 60–90 minutes, depending on the drug being used.[16,25]

ANESTHETIC MANAGEMENT

Cytoreductive surgery combined with HIPEC for peritoneal carcinomatosis is a complex and often prolonged procedure, depending on the extent of the disease in the abdomen. The complexity of this surgery can result in significant fluid shifts, blood loss, and associated hemodynamic, hematological, and metabolic disturbances. The lengthy CRS phase may lead to intraoperative anemia, hemodynamic instability, tissue hypoperfusion, and metabolic acidosis (e.g., lactic acidosis). Similarly, alterations in hemodynamics and metabolism can occur during the HIPEC phase and even in the early postoperative period, potentially leading to increased morbidity and mortality.[2,26,27]

During HIPEC, the transfusion of large volumes of cold intravenous fluids can significantly affect fluid status and cardiovascular dynamics, leading to an increase in heart rate, mean arterial pressure, and cardiac output. Although systemic absorption of chemotherapy drugs from the peritoneum is minimal compared to intravenous infusion, cardiotoxic chemotherapy agents such as doxorubicin (Adriamycin) may cause systemic effects. The chemotherapy agents can also induce systemic inflammatory responses, further destabilizing the cardiovascular system during the intraoperative and early postoperative periods, necessitating intensive care monitoring. Changes in tissue oxygenation, oxygen consumption, and electrolytes often require serial blood gas analyses throughout the procedure and recovery period. Therefore, continuous monitoring is critical during both the intraoperative and postoperative phases.

The morbidity and mortality rates following CRS and HIPEC can range from 12 to 65%. A well-coordinated team, including anesthesiologists, surgeons, intensivists, medical oncologists, and other healthcare providers such as clinical nutritionists and physiotherapists, is essential for optimal clinical outcomes.

Preoperative Workup and Prehabilitation

As with any major surgery, a thorough preoperative assessment is necessary. This includes a detailed medical history and evaluation of comorbid conditions and past treatments. Routine blood investigations should include complete blood count (CBC) with an absolute neutrophil count, liver and renal function tests, serum electrolytes, coagulation profiles, and a 12-lead electrocardiogram (ECG). Chest X-rays may not be necessary if the patient already has preoperative imaging such as chest and abdominal CT or MRI. A resting 2D echocardiogram is typically performed to assess heart function, as significant hemodynamic variations are expected during the perioperative period, with substantial IV fluid administration during the HIPEC phase. Cardiac stress tests may be indicated for patients with coronary artery disease or those with poor functional capacity. Pulmonary function tests should be considered for patients with chronic obstructive pulmonary disease (COPD), asthma, or other pulmonary diseases, especially those with large-volume peritoneal disease (e.g., PMP or MPM) who may require diaphragmatic stripping.[4]

Preoperative nutrition and physiotherapy are vital for reducing morbidity and mortality following CRS and HIPEC. Preoperative hypoalbuminemia is an independent predictor of major postoperative complications and can serve as a prognostic factor.[1,28] Malnourished patients may benefit from preoperative enteral nutrition (sip feed) or parenteral nutrition in cases where enteral nutrition is not feasible or adequate. Oral nutrition should be encouraged for all patients, even those with normal nutritional parameters.[29] The role of preoperative immunonutrition is still not well established. Anemia management should be initiated as soon as surgery is planned. Preoperative chest physiotherapy, incentive spirometry, and physical exercise should be implemented to support enhanced recovery. Pulmonary prehabilitation is particularly important in preventing postoperative pulmonary complications, especially in patients with large upper abdominal incisions or those undergoing diaphragmatic stripping.

The Society of OncoAnaesthesia and Perioperative Care recommends that patients be evaluated 1–4 weeks before the scheduled surgery for proper preoperative optimization. Alcohol and smoking cessation prior to surgery (as early as possible) should be encouraged to improve functional capacity and reduce postoperative complications.[30] These patients may be candidates for a locally adapted enhanced recovery after surgery (ERAS) pathway, although the implementation of ERAS for CRS-HIPEC surgeries is still under investigation.

Intraoperative Management

In the operating room, it is essential to adhere to a surgical safety checklist. Intraoperative monitoring should include basic American Society of Anesthesiologists (ASA) monitoring (electrocardiogram, end-tidal CO_2, noninvasive blood pressure, and pulse oximetry) along with invasive blood pressure monitoring. Cardiac output monitoring is advised for goal-directed fluid therapy, as patients may experience high cardiac output and stroke volume during and after HIPEC. Carrying over cardiac output monitoring into the postoperative period can aid in fluid management. A central venous catheter should be placed for monitoring central venous pressure, administering vasopressors, and delivering fluids. A large-bore IV line should be secured to facilitate the rapid infusion of fluids, blood, and blood products, with a rapid infuser available for sudden blood loss.

General anesthesia is the standard for this complex and prolonged procedure. A thoracic epidural catheter should be considered for intraoperative and postoperative pain management if not contraindicated. Epidural analgesia aids in early recovery and mobilization in the postoperative period, supporting the patient's ability to engage in chest physiotherapy and rehabilitation. Induction anesthesia typically involves opioids (e.g., fentanyl) along with a short-acting anesthetic (e.g., propofol or etomidate). A long-acting muscle relaxant such as vecuronium or rocuronium is used for intubation. Rapid sequence induction may be necessary in patients with large peritoneal deposits and ascites, as these conditions can increase intra-abdominal pressure and raise the risk of gastric aspiration.[1]

Endotracheal intubation is preferred over supraglottic airway devices since patients may require postoperative ventilation and are at higher risk of aspiration with supraglottic airways. Although there are no studies specifically investigating the safety of nitrous oxide in CRS-HIPEC procedures, it is generally considered safe. Total intravenous anesthesia (TIVA) or volatile anesthetics can be used for maintenance. Laboratory evidence suggests that volatile anesthesia combined with opioids may increase the malignant potential of tumors, promoting tumor invasion and proliferation.[31,32] However, a meta-analysis suggests that TIVA is associated with better overall and disease-free survival.[33] Interestingly, a large retrospective study on CRS-HIPEC showed that volatile anesthesia with opioids resulted in better 5-year survival and recurrence-free survival compared to TIVA.[34]

Hemodynamic Monitoring

Advanced hemodynamic monitoring is crucial as there are significant variations in hemodynamics during both the intraoperative and postoperative periods. The use of an arterial line along with arterial pressure-based cardiac output monitoring is invaluable for assessing the patient's hemodynamic status throughout surgery. This includes tracking parameters like stroke volume, stroke volume index, cardiac output, and cardiac index. Continuous monitoring of central venous pressure also provides insights into the patient's volume status.[1]

Serial monitoring of arterial and venous blood gases, lactate levels, and mixed central venous oxygen saturation ($ScVO_2$) can help evaluate the body's perfusion status. Regular blood gas analysis is necessary for tracking lactate levels, oxygenation, and base excess.

Electrolyte monitoring is equally critical, as both hyperkalemia and hypokalemia (particularly during or after the HIPEC phase) can lead to fatal arrhythmias. Blood glucose levels also tend to fluctuate during the surgery, and it is important to monitor them even in nondiabetic patients, as prolonged surgical stress and the infusion of heated chemotherapy can cause hyperglycemia.[35] Profound hyperglycemia and hyponatremia may arise if 5% dextrose is used as a perfusate for chemotherapy infusion.[36] Dilutional hypomagnesemia can also develop due to large fluid volumes and during platinum-based chemotherapy infusion.[37,38] Additionally, ionized calcium should be monitored, especially after significant blood loss and transfusions of blood products.

Temperature Management

Monitoring and managing body temperature is essential, as hypothermia can cause coagulopathy. Maintaining the patient's core body temperature within a normal range throughout the surgery is recommended. Hypothermia can occur during the prolonged cytoreduction phase of surgery, requiring the use of warming blankets and fluid warmers to maintain euthermia.

During HIPEC, body temperature typically rises above the normal range.[39] Temperature increases rapidly during the initial 30 minutes of HIPEC (H1 phase), gradually rising until the 60-minute mark (H2 phase), where it then plateaus (H3 phase). The maximum temperature is reached after 60 minutes of chemotherapy perfusion, reaching levels between 41–43°C.[40] To control the temperature, passive cooling (e.g., turning off warming devices) at least 30 minutes prior to the start of HIPEC (H0 phase) can be done if required but not essential.[1]

Higher perfusion temperatures correlate with more significant changes in serum glucose, sodium, and lactate levels.[41] Cooling measures, such as the infusion of cold crystalloid solutions, the use of cooling blankets, or placing cold saline bottles in the axilla and neck areas, can help. If the temperature continues to rise despite these measures and exceeds 39°C, the temperature of the chemotherapy perfusate may need to be reduced. Hyperthermia can be harmful, causing tachycardia, increasing metabolic demands, and potentially leading to convulsions and coagulation disturbances. Post-HIPEC hypothermia is also common, particularly after prolonged cytoreductive surgery, and can lead to severe complications when coupled with metabolic acidosis and hypokalemia.[42]

Fluid Management

Intraoperative fluid management is crucial as significant fluid shifts, blood loss, and electrolyte disturbances occur during surgery. Crystalloids are typically started at 2–4 mL/kg for maintenance, in addition to replacing any active losses. Goal-directed fluid therapy, guided by parameters like pulse pressure variation or stroke volume variation, is essential. Colantonio et al.[43] found that patients treated with goal-directed fluid therapy received less fluid overall, experienced lower morbidity, and had shorter postoperative hospital stays, without any increase in mortality.

Balanced solutions such as Ringer's lactate and acetate-containing solutions are typically used, and colloids like albumin may also be necessary. In patients with extensive disease and massive ascites, perioperative albumin administration is beneficial due to significant protein loss. Other starch-based colloids, such as hydroxyl ethyl starch (HES), are not recommended. Kajdi et al. reported that the use of HES solutions had negative effects on renal function[4] and caused increased bleeding tendencies as evidenced by thromboelastography (TEG).[44]

Allogeneic blood transfusions can lead to immunosuppression and increase morbidity and mortality in cancer surgery patients. It is recommended that the intraoperative goal be to maintain hemoglobin levels above 8 g/dL in CRS–HIPEC patients to optimize postoperative outcomes.[30] In cases of massive blood loss, a massive transfusion protocol should be followed.

Vasopressors, such as noradrenaline, are recommended to maintain adequate blood pressure and prevent fluid overload, which can lead to complications such as bowel edema, anastomotic leaks, and pulmonary edema.

Urine Output Monitoring

Monitoring urine output is a key indicator of renal and tissue perfusion. Ensuring adequate urine output is critical in preventing acute kidney injury (AKI), which is a common complication in CRS and HIPEC due to factors like hypotension and chemotherapy drugs. A minimum urine output of 0.5 mL/kg/hour should be maintained during the CRS phase, and it should be elevated to >2 mL/kg/hour during HIPEC and 1–2 mL/kg/hour during the reconstructive phase to promote the excretion of chemotherapy drugs.[1]

Use of cisplatin increases the risk of AKI, and patients receiving intraperitoneal cisplatin should have a higher urine output (2–4 mL/kg/hour). Diuretics are generally not recommended for increasing urine output; maintaining euvolemia is essential to ensure renal perfusion.[1]

Coagulation Monitoring

Coagulation abnormalities are common during CRS and HIPEC due to blood loss, hypothermia, hyperthermia, and chemotherapy agents. This can result in dilutional coagulopathy, which necessitates monitoring coagulation parameters closely. Routine prothrombin time (PT), international normalized ratio (INR), and activated partial thromboplastin time (aPTT) should be checked preoperatively and throughout the procedure, as well as in the postoperative period.[7] TEG or rotational thromboelastometry (ROTEM) can provide more detailed information about coagulation status compared to conventional tests.[1] Using TEG or ROTEM to guide transfusions of fresh frozen plasma (FFP) or cryoprecipitate can reduce unnecessary transfusions. Preemptive transfusions are not recommended unless specifically required.[30]

Extubation After Surgery

Extubation depends on several factors including the patient's preoperative health status, comorbidities, intraoperative blood loss, and the extent and duration of surgery.[1] Ideally, extubation should occur in the operating room to reduce postoperative complications, length of stay, and morbidity.[30]

However, if patients are unstable, with high vasopressor requirements, elevated lactate levels, or poor pulmonary function, extubation can be deferred, and the patient can be transferred to the intensive care unit (ICU) for elective postoperative ventilation.[1]

Extubation and Intensive Care Unit Management

Postponing extubation: In patients who experience significant intraoperative challenges such as unstable hemodynamics, high vasopressor requirements, significant blood loss, or compromised pulmonary function, the decision to extubate may be delayed. In such cases, patients are often transferred to the ICU for controlled postoperative ventilation.

Pain Management

- *CRS-HIPEC procedure:* Due to the extensive nature of the surgery, including large incisions and complex dissections, effective pain management is essential. The combination of thoracic epidural analgesia and IV paracetamol has been shown to significantly reduce the need for opioids after surgery.
- *Risks with epidural analgesia:* Epidural analgesia, while effective, carries risks such as hemodynamic instability and spinal hematoma, particularly in patients with coagulopathies or low platelet counts. For patients where epidural analgesia is contraindicated, patient-controlled analgesia (PCA) using opioids like fentanyl is an appropriate alternative.
- *Alternative techniques:* If epidural analgesia is not feasible, other regional techniques, such as the transverse abdominis plane block or rectus sheath catheter, can be employed for pain control.

Postoperative and Intensive Care Management

The postoperative and intensive care management is as follows:

- *Physiological responses:* After surgery, patients often exhibit tachycardia, hypotension, and metabolic disturbances, including acidosis and hyperlactatemia. Changes in respiratory function are common due to elevated intra-abdominal pressure and diaphragmatic splinting.
- *Coagulation and renal considerations:* Common postoperative issues include coagulation abnormalities such as low platelet count, alterations in INR, and kidney dysfunction due to reduced perfusion. These patients may also experience hyperglycemia as part of the stress response.
- *Postoperative care:* Immediate postoperative care involves fluid management, human albumin, and FFP, especially in the first few days. Nutritional support is also crucial, and many patients will need parenteral nutrition initially due to difficulties in tolerating enteral feeding.

Recovery and Complications

Recovery and complications include:

- *Recovery process:* Recovery after CRS-HIPEC involves regaining normal function across several domains, including physical, psychological, and social aspects. Protocolized mobilization has been shown to improve recovery, although patients with a high PCI tend to experience delayed recovery compared to those with a lower PCI.
- *Postoperative complications:* Common complications following surgery include anastomotic leaks, infections (e.g., intra-abdominal abscesses), pulmonary embolism, and gastrointestinal issues such as ileus or bowel perforation. The risk of early recurrence of the disease is associated with poorer survival outcomes, particularly in patients with extensive peritoneal disease.

Nutritional Considerations

Preoperative nutrition: The nutritional status of patients prior to surgery plays a critical role in their postoperative recovery and long-term survival. Most patients are unable to tolerate enteral feeding in the first few days post-surgery, making parenteral nutrition essential in the early recovery period.

Morbidity and Mortality

Newton et al. conducted a review to identify factors contributing to morbidity and mortality in patients undergoing CRS and HIPEC.[21] They found that for various types of cancer, the incidence of grade III–IV morbidity ranged from 22 to 34%, and mortality ranged from 0.8% to 4.1%. For colorectal cancer, PMP, and diffuse malignant peritoneal mesothelioma, mortality ranged from 2 to 4%. Gastric cancer showed a higher mortality rate (3.9 to 6.5% in two separate studies), while ovarian cancer had the lowest mortality rate at 0.8%. Age, hypoalbuminemia, and preoperative performance status were strongly linked to morbidity, while obesity showed a weaker correlation.

Operative factors, such as the PCI score, bowel resections, diaphragm involvement and stripping, distal pancreatectomy, and the surgeon's experience, were strongly associated with postoperative morbidity. In contrast, hepatobiliary procedures, urological interventions, and preoperative bevacizumab treatment were less strongly associated with postoperative complications. **Box 1** shows various surgical and non-surgical complications after CRS-HIPEC.

BOX 1: Postoperative complications after CRS–HIPEC.[45-56]

Surgical complications:
- Anastomotic leaks requiring reexploration
- Surgical bleeding
- Fistula formation
- Intra-abdominal abscess requiring drainage
- Bowel ischemia
- Deep wound infection
- Wound dehiscence
- Gastric or intestinal perforation
- Diaphragmatic hernia
- Postoperative ileus

Nonsurgical complications:
- Acute respiratory failure
- Postoperative hypovolemia
- Postoperative hypotension
- Septic shock
- Reintubation
- Acute blood loss anemia
- Pulmonary embolism
- Acute kidney injury
- Dilutional coagulopathy
- Hypoalbuminemia
- Cardiac arrhythmias
- Catheter-related bloodstream infections
- Prolonged mechanical ventilation
- ICU delirium
- Ventilator-associated pneumonia
- Hyperammonemia and hyperbilirubinemia

(CRS: cytoreductive surgery; HIPEC: hyperthermic intraperitoneal chemotherapy; ICU: intensive care unit)

PEDIATRIC CYTOREDUCTIVE SURGERY–HYPERTHERMIC INTRAPERITONEAL CHEMOTHERAPY

In children, CRS–HIPEC is typically performed for colorectal peritoneal tumors, desmoplastic round-cell tumors, and rhabdomyosarcoma.[57] Anesthesia is usually induced via inhalational or IV agents, combined with short-acting opioids. When there are no contraindications, a thoracic epidural catheter is often placed to provide perioperative analgesia and reduce opioid use. The anesthetic approach follows the same principles as other major abdominal surgeries in pediatric patients. Management in children is similar to that in adults, with the exception of age-related variations.

Central venous and arterial catheters are usually inserted for invasive monitoring. However, since many noninvasive cardiac output monitoring methods are not validated in pediatric patients, a cardiac output monitor is typically not used. Fluid management during CRS–HIPEC in children is crucial, and a fluid administration rate of 9 mL/kg/hour has been shown to maintain adequate urine output.[58,59] Hemoglobin levels should be maintained at or above 10 gm/dL.[59] The decision to extubate in the operating room or transfer the patient to the ICU for elective ventilation depends on the intraoperative course.

HYPERTHERMIC INTRATHORACIC THORACOABDOMINAL CHEMOTHERAPY

Pleural malignancies can originate from various cancers, such as malignant pleural mesothelioma, advanced thymoma with pleural spread, or peritoneal metastasis from PMP. Achieving local control over these tumors is challenging due to their diffuse and invasive nature. Pleural metastases from abdominal tumors, such as PMP, may occur due to diaphragmatic perforation during abdominal surgery or transdiaphragmatic lymphatic spread of the disease.[60]

The standard treatment approach for pleural malignancies remains controversial.[61] Many patients receive palliative chemotherapy, though multimodal therapy—comprising induction chemotherapy, surgical resection, adjuvant chemotherapy, and sometimes radiotherapy—can reduce local recurrence and improve patient outcomes.[62,63] Recently, CRS combined with intraoperative hyperthermic intrathoracic chemotherapy has been advocated to reduce local tumor spread and treat cancer.[64,65]

Cytoreductive surgery typically involves pleurectomy, decortication, or extrapleural pneumonectomy to remove macroscopic tumor deposits. Microscopic deposits, however, pose a significant risk for local recurrence, so local intracavitary chemotherapy is applied to provide a higher dose of the drug while minimizing systemic side effects. The regional hyperthermia enhances drug penetration. In cases of PMP, if diaphragmatic stripping is performed during CRS, it should not be closed during hyperthermic intraperitoneal chemotherapy to facilitate the flow of the chemotherapy agent into the thoracic cavity, enhancing its cytotoxic effects.[60] For pleural spread from peritoneal carcinomatosis, complete removal of peritoneal and pleural metastases is achieved by opening the diaphragm during abdominal surgery, followed by hyperthermic intraoperative thoracoabdominal chemotherapy infusion (HITAC).[66]

Complications associated with HITAC are similar to those of hyperthermic intraperitoneal chemotherapy (e.g., thrombocytopenia, bleeding, and systemic inflammation), with additional complications specific to HITAC, including pulmonary embolism, chest pain, dyspnea, bronchopleural fistula, pneumothorax, empyema, and air leaks.[66]

Before CRS and HITAC, patients must undergo thorough workups. They are prone to intraoperative bleeding, so adequate blood products must be available. Comprehensive evaluation of cardiorespiratory function is necessary, including a 12-lead ECG, 2D echocardiography, and stress tests. Pulmonary function can be assessed through tests of lung capacity, diffusion capacity, and effort tolerance. Both respiratory and cardiology specialists should be involved in the perioperative care alongside the surgeon and anesthesiologist. Preoperative chest physiotherapy and patient counseling on the surgery and pain management are essential.[1,66]

Anesthesia during the procedure is challenging due to blood and fluid loss, which varies depending on cancer load. Fluid administration should be guided by stroke volume and delta stroke volume to avoid pulmonary edema. Pulse pressure variation and stroke volume variation are unreliable during thoracotomy procedures. It is crucial to maintain normal temperature throughout the procedure. Chemotherapy in the intrathoracic cavity can increase fluid load, airway pressures, intrathoracic pressures, mediastinal shift, and reduce functional residual capacity.

Postoperative extubation following HITAC procedures has not been extensively studied. Extubation is usually preferred in the postanesthesia care unit due to significant fluid shifts and a reduction in pulmonary volumes postsurgery. Hemodynamic monitoring should continue until the patient is stable. Consideration should be given to the reduction in postoperative lung volume after lung resection. Temperature monitoring is also essential. Coagulopathy remains a significant concern postprocedure due to hyperthermia, blood loss, and inflammation. Adequate pain management is necessary to allow for spirometry and chest physiotherapy, which help reduce pulmonary complications.

PRESSURIZED INTRA-ABDOMINAL AEROSOLIZED CHEMOTHERAPY

Pressurized intra-abdominal aerosolized chemotherapy (PIPAC) is a novel method of delivering chemotherapy in the form of an aerosol under pressure within a closed abdominal cavity created using laparoscopy. This technique is typically used for patients with large-volume disease not suitable for surgery. The aerosol is generated using a nebulizer connected to a high-pressure IV injector. Various chemotherapeutic agents, such as doxorubicin (for ovarian and gastric cancers) and oxaliplatin (for colorectal and appendiceal cancers), are used in PIPAC. During the procedure, a therapeutic capnoperitoneum is maintained at 37°C for 30 minutes.[67]

The amount of chemotherapy administered during PIPAC is 5–20 times lower than the dose required for IV chemotherapy, but the concentration of the drug in the target tissue is double.[68] PIPAC can be repeated up to six times for patients with maximum PCI and those with symptoms like pain, ascites, diarrhea, or constipation. Over 60% of patients experience an improvement in PCI and symptom resolution. A 30-day mortality rate of 7% has been observed.[69]

Pressurized intra-abdominal aerosolized chemotherapy (PIPAC) is performed under general anesthesia and is a relatively short procedure. Standard ASA monitoring is used, and invasive blood pressure monitoring may be implemented.[70] After anesthesia induction, pneumoperitoneum is created laparoscopically. The chemotherapy agent is converted into an aerosol form by the nebulizer and injected under high pressure for 30 minutes. After the procedure, the aerosol is exsufflated with a special filter. Patients are usually extubated in the operating room and monitored in the postanesthesia recovery unit.

Since chemotherapy drugs are aerosolized during PIPAC, there is a risk of occupational exposure for operating room staff. These drugs can enter the body through inhalation, skin contact, or injection, and may cause adverse effects such as hair loss, headaches, irritation, hypersensitivity, congenital malformations, and an increased risk of other cancers.[71] Therefore, appropriate safety measures are required during the procedure.

All operating room personnel must wear an N-95 mask with a tight seal. The nebulizer and injector producing the aerosol must be remotely controlled, and no personnel should remain in the operating room during aerosol administration. The capnoperitoneum system must be airtight, and the aerosol must be exsufflated into a waste air system. During the procedure, there should be no CO_2 flow to avoid leaks and increased pressure. Laminar flow in the operating room is recommended, though studies have shown that PIPAC can be safely performed in nonlaminar flow environments with minimal occupational risk.[72-74]

CONCLUSION

CRS-HIPEC is an extensive and high-risk procedure requiring meticulous anesthetic management to optimize patient outcomes. Anesthesia for CRS-HIPEC involves a multimodal approach to address significant physiological challenges, including prolonged operative duration, extensive fluid shifts, massive blood loss, hypothermia, and chemotherapy-related systemic effects. General anesthesia with advanced hemodynamic monitoring, goal-directed fluid therapy, and multimodal analgesia—often incorporating regional techniques such as epidural or fascial plane blocks—are key components. Perioperative considerations include meticulous temperature management, prevention of coagulopathy, and vigilant renal protection due to nephrotoxic effects of chemotherapeutic agents. Additionally, ventilation strategies must be tailored to maintain adequate oxygenation and prevent respiratory complications, especially in patients with diaphragmatic stripping. Postoperatively, these patients often require intensive care monitoring due to the risk of complications such as systemic inflammatory response syndrome and multiorgan dysfunction.

REFERENCES

1. Solanki SL, Mukherjee S, Agarwal V, Thota RS, Balakrishnan K, Shah SB, et al. Society of Onco-Anaesthesia and Perioperative Care consensus guidelines for perioperative management of patients for cytoreductive surgery and hyperthermic intraperitoneal chemotherapy (CRS-HIPEC). Indian J Anaesth. 2019;63(12):972-87.
2. Sugarbaker PH, Ryan DP. Cytoreductive surgery plus hyperthermic perioperative chemotherapy to treat peritoneal metastases from colorectal cancer: Standard of care or an experimental approach? Lancet Oncol. 2012;13(8):e362-9.
3. Verwaal VJ, van Ruth S, de Bree E, van Sloothen GW, van Tinteren H, Boot H, et al. Randomized trial of cytoreduction and hyperthermic intraperitoneal chemotherapy versus systemic chemotherapy and palliative surgery in patients with peritoneal carcinomatosis of colorectal cancer. J Clin Oncol. 2003;21(20):3737-43.
4. Kajdi ME, Beck-Schimmer B, Held U, Kofmehl R, Lehmann K, Ganter MT. Anaesthesia in patients undergoing cytoreductive surgery with hyperthermic intraperitoneal chemotherapy: Retrospective analysis of a single centre three-year experience. World J Surg Oncol. 2014;12:136.
5. Revaux A, Rouzier R, Ballester M, Selle F, Daraï E, Chéreau E. Comparison of morbidity and survival between primary and interval cytoreductive surgery in patients after modified posterior pelvic exenteration for advanced ovarian cancer. Int J Gynecol Cancer. 2012;22(8):1349-54.
6. Jacquet P, Sugarbaker PH. Current methodology for clinical assessment of patients with peritoneal carcinomatosis. J Exp Clin Cancer Res. 1996;15:49-58.
7. Jacquet P, Jelinek JS, Sugarbaker PH, Steves MA. Evaluation of computer tomography in patients with peritoneal carcinomatosis. Cancer. 1993;72(5):1631-6.
8. Rivard JD, Temple WJ, McConnell YJ, Sultan H, Mack LA. Preoperative computed tomography does not predict resectability in peritoneal carcinomatosis. Am J Surg. 2014;207(5):760-5.
9. Chua TC, Yan TD, Saxena A, Morris DL. Should the treatment of peritoneal carcinomatosis by cytoreductive surgery and hyperthermic intraperitoneal chemotherapy still be regarded as a highly morbid procedure? A systematic review of morbidity and mortality. Ann Surg. 2009; 249(6):900-7.
10. Cotte E, Passot G, Gilly F-N, Glehen O. Selection of patients and staging of peritoneal surface malignancies. World J Gastrointest Oncol. 2010;2:31-5.
11. Coccolini F, Catena F, Glehen O, Yonemura Y, Sugarbaker PH, Piso P, et al. Complete versus incomplete cytoreduction in peritoneal carcinosis from gastric cancer, with consideration to PCI cut-off. Systematic review and meta-analysis. Eur J Surg Oncol. 2015;41(7):911-9.
12. Cowan RA, O'Cearbhaill RE, Zivanovic O, Chi DS. Current status and future prospects of hyperthermic intraoperative intraperitoneal chemotherapy (HIPEC) clinical trials in ovarian cancer. Int J Hyperthermia. 2017;33(5):548-53.
13. Glehen O, Mohamed F, Gilly FN. Peritoneal carcinomatosis from digestive tract cancer: New management by cytoreductive surgery and intraperitoneal chemohyperthermia. Lancet Oncol. 2004;5(4):219-28.
14. Webb CA, Weyker PD, Moitra VK, Raker RK. An overview of cytoreductive surgery and hyperthermic intraperitoneal chemoperfusion for the anesthesiologist. Anesth Analg. 2013;116(4):924-31.
15. Hildebrandt B, Wust P, Ahlers O, Dieing A, Sreenivasa G, Kerner T, et al. The cellular and molecular basis of hyperthermia. Crit Rev Oncol Hematol. 2002;43(1):33-56.
16. González-Moreno S, González-Bayón LA, Ortega-Pérez G. Hyperthermic intraperitoneal chemotherapy: Rationale and technique. World J Gastro Oncol. 2010;2(2):68-75.
17. Helderman RFCPA, Löke DR, Kok HP, Oei AL, Tanis PJ, Franken NAPK, et al. Variation in clinical application of hyperthermic intraperitoneal chemotherapy: A Review. Cancers (Basel). 2019;11(1):78.
18. Lemoine L, Sugarbaker P, Van der Speeten K. Drugs, doses, and durations of intraperitoneal chemotherapy: Standardising HIPEC and EPIC for colorectal, appendiceal, gastric, ovarian peritoneal surface malignancies and peritoneal mesothelioma. Int J Hyperthermia. 2017;33(5):582-92.

19. Mehta SS, Gelli M, Agarwal D, Goéré D. Complications of cytoreductive surgery and HIPEC in the treatment of peritoneal metastases. Indian J Surg Oncol. 2016;7(2):225-9.
20. Baratti D, Kusamura S, Laterza B, Balestra MR, Deraco M. Early and long-term postoperative management following cytoreductive surgery and hyperthermic intraperitoneal chemotherapy. World J Gastrointest Oncol. 2010;2(1):36-43.
21. Newton AD, Bartlett EK, Karakousis GC. Cytoreductive surgery and hyperthermic intraperitoneal chemotherapy: A review of factors contributing to morbidity and mortality. J Gastrointest Oncol. 2016;7(1):99-111.
22. Park BJ, Alexander HR, Libutti SK, Wu P, Royalty D, Kranda KC, et al. Treatment of primary peritoneal mesothelioma by continuous hyperthermic peritoneal perfusion (CHPP). Ann Surg Oncol. 1999;6(6):582-90.
23. Pomel C, Ferron G, Lorimier G, Rey A, Lhomme C, Classe JM, et al. Hyperthermic intra-peritoneal chemotherapy using oxaliplatin as consolidation therapy for advanced epithelial ovarian carcinoma. Results of a phase II prospective multicentre trial. CHIPOVAC study. Eur J Surg Oncol. 2010; 36:589-93.
24. Valle SJ, Alzahrani NA, Liauw W, Sugarbaker PH, Bhatt A, Morris DL. Hyperthermic intraperitoneal chemotherapy (HIPEC) methodology, drugs and bidirectional chemotherapy. Indian J Surg Oncol. 2016;7(2):152-9.
25. González-Moreno S, González-Bayón L, Ortega-Pérez G. Hyperthermic intraperitoneal chemotherapy: methodology and safety considerations. Surg Oncol Clin N Am. 2012;21(4):543-57.
26. Franko J, Ibrahim Z, Gusani NJ, Holtzman MP, Bartlett DL, Zeh HJ 3rd. Cytoreductive surgery and hyperthermic intraperitoneal chemoperfusion versus systemic chemotherapy alone for colorectal peritoneal carcinomatosis. Cancer. 2010;116(16):3756-62.
27. Schmidt C, Creutzenberg M, Piso P, Hobbhahn J, Bucher M. Peri-operative anaesthetic management of cytoreductive surgery with hyperthermic intraperitoneal chemotherapy. Anaesthesia. 2008;63(4):389-95.
28. Rothfield KP, Crowley K. Anesthesia considerations during cytoreductive surgery and hyperthermic intraperitoneal chemotherapy. Surg Oncol Clin N Am. 2012;21(4):533-41.
29. Burden S, Todd C, Hill J, Lal S. Pre-operative nutrition support in patients undergoing gastrointestinal surgery. Cochrane Database Syst Rev. 2012;11:CD008879.
30. Hübner M, Kusamura S, Villeneuve L, Al-Niaimi A, Alyami M, Balonov K, et al. Guidelines for perioperative care in cytoreductive surgery (CRS) with or without hyperthermic IntraPEritoneal chemotherapy (HIPEC): Enhanced recovery after surgery (ERAS®) Society Recommendations-Part I: Preoperative and intraoperative management. Eur J Surg Oncol. 2020;46(12):2292-310.
31. Byrne K, Levins KJ, Buggy DJ. Can anesthetic-analgesic technique during primary cancer surgery affect recurrence or metastasis? Can J Anesth. 2016;63(2):184-92.
32. Connolly C, Buggy DJ. Opioids and tumour metastasis: Does the choice of the anesthetic-analgesic technique influence outcome after cancer surgery? Curr Opin Anaesthesiol. 2016;29(4):468-74.
33. Yap A, Lopez-Olivo MA, Dubowitz J, Hiller J, Riedel B; Global Onco-Anesthesia Research Collaboration Group. Anesthetic technique and cancer outcomes: A meta-analysis of total intravenous versus volatile anesthesia. Can J Anaesth. 2019;66(5):546-61.
34. Zhou X, Zhang P, Luo W, Zhang L, Hu R, Sun Y, et al. Ketamine induces apoptosis in lung adenocarcinoma cells by regulating the expression of CD69. Cancer Med. 2018;7(3):788-95.
35. Stewart CL, Gleisner A, Halpern A, Ibrahim-Zada I, Luna RA, Pearlman N, et al. Implications of hyperthermic intraperitoneal chemotherapy perfusion-related hyperglycemia. Ann Surg Oncol. 2018;25(3):655-9.
36. Escobar B, Medina-Piedrahita P, Gómez-Henao P, Higuera-Palacio A, García-Mora M, Ruiz-Villa JO, et al. Cytoreductive surgery plus hyperthermic intraperitoneal chemotherapy: Main concepts for anaesthetists. Rev Col Anest. 2018;46(2):134-42.
37. Hakeam HA, Breakiet M, Azzam A, Nadeem A, Amin T. The incidence of cisplatin nephrotoxicity post hyperthermic intraperitoneal chemotherapy (HIPEC) and cytoreductive surgery. Ren Fail. 2014;36(10):1486-91.
38. Hayati F, Hossainzadeh M, Shayanpour S, Abedi-Gheshlaghi Z, Beladi Mousavi SS. Prevention of cisplatin nephrotoxicity. J Nephropharmacol. 2015;5(1):57-60.
39. Kamal JM, Elshaikh SM, Nabil D, Mohamad AM. The perioperative course and anesthetic challenge for cytoreductive surgery with hyperthermic intraperitoneal chemotherapy. Egypt J Anaesth. 2013;29(4):311-8.
40. Kanakoudis F, Petrou A, Michaloudis D, Chortaria G, Konstantinidou A. Anaesthesia for intra-peritoneal perfusion of hyperthermic chemotherapy. Hemodynamic changes, oxygen consumption and delivery. Anaesthesia. 1996;51(11):1033-6.
41. Ceelen W, De Somer F, Van Nieuwenhove Y, Vande Putte D, Pattyn P. Effect of perfusion temperature on glucose and electrolyte transport during hyperthermic intraperitoneal chemoperfusion (HIPEC) with oxaliplatin. Eur J Surg Oncol. 2013;39(7):754-9.
42. Solanki SL, Jhingan MAK, Saklani AP. Rebound hypothermia after cytoreductive surgery with hyperthermic intraperitoneal chemotherapy (CRS-HIPEC) and cardiac arrest in immediate postoperative period: a report of two cases and review of literature. Pleura Peritoneum. 2020;5(3):20200126.
43. Colantonio L, Claroni C, Fabrizi L, Marcelli ME, Sofra M, Giannarelli D, et al. A randomized trial of goal directed vs. standard fluid therapy in cytoreductive surgery with hyperthermic intraperitoneal chemotherapy. J Gastrointest Surg. 2015;19(4):722-9.

44. Rasmussen KC, Secher NH, Pedersen T. Effect of perioperative crystalloid or colloid fluid therapy on hemorrhage, coagulation competence, and outcome: A systematic review and stratified meta-analysis. Medicine (Baltimore). 2016;95(31):e4498.
45. Said ET, Sztain JF, Abramson WB, Meineke MN, Furnish TJ, Schmidt UH, et al. A dedicated acute pain service is associated with reduced postoperative opioid requirements in patients undergoing cytoreductive surgery with hyperthermic intraperitoneal chemotherapy. Anesth Analg. 2018;127(4):1044-50.
46. Osseis M, Weyrech J, Gayat E, Dagois S, Lo Dico R, Pocard M, et al. Epidural analgesia combined with a comprehensive physiotherapy program after cytoreductive surgery and HIPEC is associated with enhanced post-operative recovery and reduces intensive care unit stay: A retrospective study of 124 patients. Eur J Surg Oncol. 2016;42(12):1938-43.
47. McQuellon RP, Loggie BW, Lehman AB, Russell GB, Fleming RA, Shen P, et al. Long-term survivorship and quality of life after cytoreductive surgery plus intra-peritoneal hyperthermic chemotherapy for peritoneal carcinomatosis. Ann Surg Oncol. 2003;10(2):155-62.
48. Bouman EA, Theunissen M, Bons SA, van Mook WN, Gramke HF, van Kleef M, et al. Reduced incidence of chronic postsurgical pain after epidural analgesia for abdominal surgery. Pain Pract. 2014;14(2):E76-84.
49. Teoh DA, Hutton MJH, Else S, Walker A, Lee A, Mack LA. Epidural analgesia? A prospective analysis of perioperative coagulation in cytoreductive surgery and hyperthermic intraperitoneal chemotherapy. Am J Sur. 2019;217(5):887-92.
50. Van der Speeten K, Lemoine L, Sugarbaker P. Overview of the optimal perioperative intraperitoneal chemotherapy regimens used in current clinical practice. Pleura Peritoneum. 2017;2(2):63-72.
51. Owusu-Agyemang P, Soliz J, Hayes-Jordan A, Harun N, Gottumukkala V. Safety of epidural analgesia in the perioperative care of patients undergoing cytoreductive surgery with hyperthermic intraperitoneal chemotherapy. Ann Surg Oncol. 2014;21(5):1487-93.
52. Richardson J, Lönnqvist PA, Naja Z. Bilateral thoracic paravertebral block: Potential and practice. Br J Anaesth. 2011;106(2):164-71.
53. Padmakumar AV. Intensive care management of patient after cytoreductive surgery and HIPEC-A concise review. Indian J Surg Oncol. 2016;7(2):244-8.
54. Falcón Araña L, Fuentes-García D, Roca Calvo MJ, Hernández-Palazón J, Gil Martínez J, Cascales Campos PA, et al. Alterations in hemostasis during cytoreductive surgery and hyperthermic intraperitoneal chemotherapy in patients with peritoneal carcinomatosis. Cir Esp. 2015;93(8):496-501.
55. Arakelian E, Gunningberg L, Larsson J, Norlén K, Mahteme H. Factors influencing early postoperative recovery after cytoreductive surgery and hyperthermic intraperitoneal chemotherapy. Eur J Surg Oncol. 2011; 37(10):897-903.
56. Simkens GA, van Oudheusden TR, Luyer MD, Nienhuijs SW, Nieuwenhuijzen GA, Rutten HJ, et al. serious postoperative complications affect early recurrence after cytoreductive surgery and HIPEC for colorectal peritoneal carcinomatosis. Ann Surg Oncol. 2015;22(8):2656-62.
57. Zmora O, Hayes-Jordan A, Nissan A, Kventsel I, Newmann Y, Itskovsky K, et al. Cytoreductive surgery (CRS) and hyperthermic intraperitoneal chemotherapy (HIPEC) for disseminated intra-abdominal malignancies in children-a single-institution experience. J Pediatr Surg. 2018;53(7):1381-6.
58. Owusu-Agyemang P, Arunkumar R, Green H, Hurst D, Landoski K, Hayes-Jordan A. Anesthetic management and renal function in pediatric patients undergoing cytoreductive surgery with continuous hyperthermic intraperitoneal chemotherapy (HIPEC) with cisplatin. Ann Surg Oncol. 2012;19(8):2652-6.
59. Owusu-Agyemang P, Williams UU, Van Meter A, Zavala AM, Rebello E, Feng L, et al. Investigating the association between perioperative blood transfusions and outcomes in children undergoing cytoreductive surgery with hyperthermic intraperitoneal chemotherapy. Vox Sang. 2017;112(1):40-6.
60. Chua TC, Yan TD, Yap ZL, Horton MD, Fermanis GG, Morris DL. Thoracic cytoreductive surgery and intraoperative hyperthermic intrathoracic chemotherapy for pseudomyxoma peritonei. J Surg Oncol. 2009;99(5):292-5.
61. Ried M, Potzger T, Braune N, Diez C, Neu R, Sziklavari Z, et al. Local and systemic exposure of cisplatin during hyperthermic intrathoracic chemotherapy perfusion after pleurectomy and decortication for treatment of pleural malignancies. J Surg Oncol. 2013;107(7):735-40.
62. Zauderer MG, Krug LM. The evolution of multimodality therapy for malignant pleural mesothelioma. Curr Treat Options Oncol. 2011;12(2):163-72.
63. Rena O, Mineo O, Casadio C. Multimodal treatment for stage IVA thymoma: A proposable strategy. Lung Cancer. 2012;76(1):89-92.
64. Tilleman TR, Richards WG, Zellos L, Johnson BE, Jaklitsch MT, Mueller J, et al. Extrapleural pneumonectomy followed by intracavitary intraoperative hyperthermic cisplatin with pharmacologic cytoprotection for treatment of malignant pleural mesothelioma: A phase II prospective study. J Thorac Cardiovasc Surg. 2009;138(2):405-11.
65. Ried M, Potzger T, Braune N, Neu R, Zausig Y, Schalke B, et al. Cytoreductive surgery and hyperthermic intrathoracic chemotherapy perfusion for malignant pleural tumours: Perioperative management and clinical experience. Eur J Cardiothorac Surg. 2013;43(4):801-7.
66. Solanki SL, Bajaj JS, Rahman F, Saklani AP. Perioperative management of cytoreductive surgery and hyperthermic

intraoperative thoraco-abdominal chemotherapy (HITAC) for pseudomyxoma peritonei. Indian J Anaesth. 2019;63(2):134-7.

67. Horvath P, Yurttas C, Struller F, Bösmüller H, Lauer UM, Nadalin S, et al. Pressurized intraperitoneal aerosol chemotherapy (PIPAC) for peritoneal metastases in solid organ graft recipients: First experience. Ann Transplant. 2019;24:30-5.
68. Solass W, Kerb R, Mürdter T, Giger-Pabst U, Strumberg D, Tempfer C, et al. Intraperitoneal chemotherapy of peritoneal carcinomatosis using pressurized aerosol as an alternative to liquid solution: First evidence for efficacy. Ann Surg Oncol. 2014;21(2):553-9.
69. Alyami M, Mercier F, Siebert M, Bonnot PE, Laplace N, Villeneuve L, et al. Unresectable peritoneal metastasis treated by pressurized intraperitoneal aerosol chemotherapy (PIPAC) leading to cytoreductive surgery and hyperthermic intraperitoneal chemotherapy. Eur J Surg Oncol. 2019;47(1):128-33.
70. Solanki SL, Kumar PP, DeSouza A, Saklani AP. Perioperative concerns and management of pressurised intraperitoneal aerosolised chemotherapy: Report of two cases. Indian J Anaesth. 2018;62(3):225-8.
71. Solass W, Giger-Pabst U, Zieren J, Reymond MA. Pressurized intraperitoneal aerosol chemotherapy (PIPAC): Occupational health and safety aspects. Ann Surg Oncol. 2013;20(11):3504-11.
72. Graversen M, Detlefsen S, Bjerregaard JK, Fristrup CW, Pfeiffer P, Mortensen MB. Prospective, single-center implementation and response evaluation of pressurized intraperitoneal aerosol chemotherapy (PIPAC) for peritoneal metastasis. Ther Adv Med Oncol. 2018; 10:1758835918777036.
73. Delhorme JB, Klipfel A, D'Antonio F, Greget MC, Diemunsch P, Rohr S, et al. Occupational safety of pressurized intraperitoneal aerosol chemotherapy (PIPAC) in an operating room without laminar airflow. J Visc Surg. 2019;156(6):485-8.
74. Ametsbichler P, Böhlandt A, Nowak D, Schierl R. Occupational exposure to cisplatin/oxaliplatin during pressurized intraperitoneal aerosol chemotherapy (PIPAC)? Eur J Surg Oncol. 2018;44(11):1793-9.

29

CHAPTER

Anesthesia for Surgery of Retroperitoneal and Inferior Vena Cava Tumor

Sohan Lal Solanki, Aafreen Siddique

INTRODUCTION

Retroperitoneal tumors (RPTs) present unique challenges for anesthesiologists and surgeons alike. The complex anatomy of the retroperitoneal space, coupled with the potential for massive blood loss and hemodynamic instability, demands a thorough understanding of both basic principles and advanced techniques. The aim of this chapter is to present an in-depth overview of the anatomy of retroperitoneum, the physiological changes in hemodynamics associated with large RPTs, and anesthetic strategies for managing surgeries related to these tumors.

Literally, RPTs should refer to any neoplasms that occur in the retroperitoneal space. But practically it involves tumors arising from fat, loose connective tissue, muscle, fascia, blood vessels, nerves, or lymphatic tissue of the retroperitoneum, but it excludes tumors arising from retroperitoneal organs (such as the kidney, pancreas, suprarenal gland, and ureter).[1]

The retroperitoneal space is not a real compartment. However, in simple terminology, we can define retroperitoneum by its three-dimensional margins. Of course, the size and specific location of the mass in the retroperitoneum determine which of the many structures mentioned earlier constitute which specific margin.[2]

The retroperitoneum refers to an anatomical region situated posterior to the abdominal or peritoneal cavity. Organs that are not attached to the mesentery and are positioned between the abdominal wall and the parietal peritoneum are classified as being within the retroperitoneal space. This compartment has posterior parietal peritoneum as its anterior boundary and transversalis fascia as posterior boundary.[2]

It is further subdivided into three components: (1) The anterior pararenal, (2) the perirenal space, and (3) the posterior pararenal spaces.[3]

- The anterior pararenal space is bounded by the posterior parietal peritoneum anteriorly and the anterior renal fascia posteriorly. This space has ascending and descending colon, the duodenum, and the pancreas.
- The posterior pararenal space is bounded by the posterior renal fascia anteriorly, lateroconal fascia laterally, and the transversalis fascia posteriorly. This space primarily contains fat, small vessels, lymphatics, and no visceral organs. It is composed of fat, blood vessels, and lymphatics.[3]
- Located between the anterior and posterior renal fasciae, the perirenal space contains vital anatomical structures such as the adrenal gland, kidney, ureters, and renal vessels (**Fig. 1**).

Additionally, there exists a fourth, less clearly delineated area referred to as the great vessel space. This region is situated anterior to the vertebral bodies and psoas muscles, encompassing the aorta, inferior vena cava (IVC), and the surrounding adipose tissue.[3]

A diverse array of pathologies can be found within the retroperitoneum, including several rare benign tumors and malignant neoplasms that can manifest as either primary

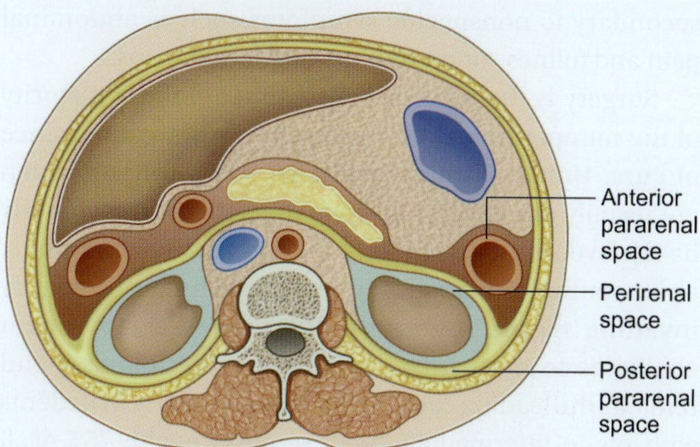

Fig. 1: Anatomy of retroperitoneal space.

or metastatic lesions. RPTs can cause a diagnostic dilemma and present several therapeutic challenges because of their rarity, relative late presentation, anatomical location, and also because these tumors are in close relationship with several vital structures in the retroperitoneal space.[4]

Primary retroperitoneal tumors are uncommon, accounting for 0.1–0.2% of all malignancies in the body; 80–90% of all primary RPTs are malignant. The most common secondary retroperitoneal neoplasms are lymph nodal masses. The solid neoplasms can be classified according to their tissue of origin into three main categories: (1) Mesodermal tumors, (2) neurogenic tumors, and (3) extragonadal germ cell tumors.[3]

Mesodermal tumors: These are the most prevalent type of RPTs and can originate from any tissue type found within the retroperitoneal spaces. They can be benign or malignant. Retroperitoneal sarcomas account for 90% of mesodermal primary retroperitoneal malignancies, with liposarcoma, leiomyosarcoma, and malignant fibrous histiocytoma (MFH) making up more than 80% of these tumors.

Neurogenic tumors: These constitute 10–20% of primary RPTs. In general, these conditions are more prevalent among younger patients, tend to be benign in nature, and are associated with a more favorable prognosis when compared to sarcomas. Neurogenic tumors can originate from ganglion cells, the paraganglionic system, or nerve sheaths. Abdominal neurogenic tumors usually follow the distribution of the sympathetic ganglia along the paraspinal region or arise from the adrenal medulla or the organ of Zuckerkandl.

Usually, RPTs are large at the time of presentation, as these tumors tend to grow without producing many symptoms. Therefore, most of the RPTs are diagnosed secondary to nonspecific symptoms such as abdominal pain and fullness or on routine health check-ups.[3]

Surgery is the mainstay of treatment for the majority of the retroperitoneal RPTs and offers a potential chance of cure. Unlike primary epithelial solid tumors, which are usually confined to a single organ and can generally be removed with resection of that organ, RPT commonly abuts multiple surrounding organs without necessarily invading them. Surgery of RPT poses a significant challenge to both surgeons and anesthesiologists and remains the leading cause of death, particularly in patients with low-to-intermediate-grade tumors [roughly 75% of all retroperitoneal sarcoma (RPS)].[5]

In the early stage, RPTs that are confined to relatively small areas with intact capsules can be removed by open, laparoscopic, or robotic techniques under general or epidural anesthesia. Smaller tumors may not need any specific anesthesia considerations.

However, most of the tumors are located more deeply into the abdomen with greater space for expansion and are generally asymptomatic in the early stage. When they grow over a period of time, tumors may fill the retroperitoneal space, abut, encase, or invade other structures, such as major vessels of the retroperitoneum. Symptoms do not appear until the boundary between the tumor and intestine or blood vessels becomes ill-defined. The deeper location and large size of the tumor pose challenges to both the surgical team and the anesthesia team.[6]

The main concerns while treating such bigger RPTs are:

- *Physiological changes:* Large RPTs, because of their size, cause alterations in normal physiologic parameters. Respiratory and hemodynamic compromise occur as a result of the tumor's intra-abdominal development and compression of organs. Large RPT leads to elevation of the bilateral diaphragm, decreased lung compliance, and high airway pressures.[7]

The phases of anesthesia can be categorized into two distinct periods: (1) Prior to and (2) following the excision of the tumor. In the preoperative phase, complications may arise related to respiratory function, hemodynamics, renal performance, and the gastrointestinal system **(Fig. 2)**. Conversely, in the postoperative phase, there is a swift reduction in intrathoracic pressure, which can lead to hemodynamic instability and the potential onset of reexpansion pulmonary edema (RPE). Hence, preoperative assessment, optimization, and careful planning of anesthesia management are mandatory for reducing perioperative complications.[7]

During general anesthesia for very large tumors, the administration of neuromuscular blocking drugs leads to the relaxation of the diaphragm. This relaxation, coupled with increased intra-abdominal pressure, results in decreased compliance of the lungs and thorax, thereby causing an increase in both peak and plateau airway pressures. One strategy to prevent this complication is to ensure spontaneous respiration with pressure support ventilation until abdominal decompression is accomplished, after which controlled ventilation can be initiated. It is essential to maintain the inspiratory pressure below 20 cmH_2O, the airway plateau pressure

Respiratory system

Mass that compress the diaphragm in a superior direction, causing

- Increase in pleural and thoracic pressure
- Increased dead space ventilation and a rise in PCO_2 levels
- Decrease in functional residual capacity
- High peak airway pressure and diminished lung and chest compliance
- Symptoms may include dyspnea, tachypnea, orthopnea, and decline in exercise tolerance

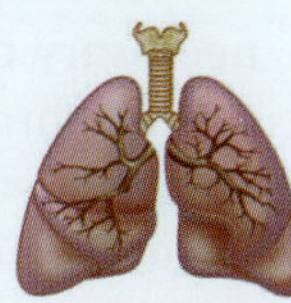

Cardiovascular system

Mass compression of the IVC and aorta

- Reduced right ventricular preload
- Increased left ventricular afterload
- Decreased cardiac output
- Increased systemic vascular resistance
- Increased jugular venous pressure
- Hypotension, tachycardia
- Compensatory vasoconstriction

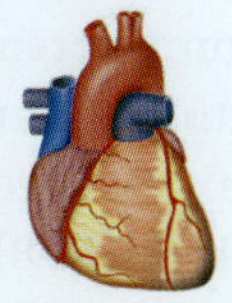

Gastrointestinal system

- Early satiety
- Stimulation of gastric acid secretion
- Abdominal distension
- Constipation
- Hiatus hernia

Renal system

- Mass compressing the ureter causing hydronephrosis and hydroureter
- Decreased urinary output
- Azotemia

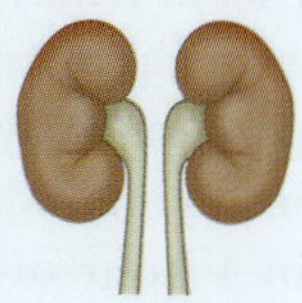

Fig. 2: Physiological effects of large retroperitoneal mass. (IVC: inferior vena cava)

under 30 cmH_2O, and the driving pressure below 15 cm H_2O. Anesthesiologists must remain vigilant to the possibility that spontaneous respiration may become inadequate, necessitating the eventual use of positive pressure ventilation and potentially, neuromuscular blocking agents. At this juncture, there is a risk of partial compromise to the hemodynamic system, so it is crucial to anticipate and prepare for this eventuality. The other strategy to prevent respiratory failure can be to perform surgery in a propped-up position when possible.

- Another concern during the management of this kind of tumor is excessive bleeding, which may be because of adhesions, infiltration of malignant tumor, compression of major vessels and collaterals, etc. Sometimes obtaining hemostasis is difficult because of a large tumor, a bigger raw area with continuous oozing, and the development of intravascular disseminated coagulation due to massive transfusion. As the incidence of bleeding in retroperitoneal surgeries is high, it is essential that blood-derived products are easily accessible, accompanied by rapid infusion devices.[8,9]
- Prolonged surgical times lead to the development of hypothermia due to the exposure of the peritoneal cavity and large fluid shifts. Blood loss can exacerbate hypothermia, as it necessitates volume replacement and the administration of blood products. Thus, passive and active warming techniques should be used.[10]
- *Risk of aspiration during intubation:* To rapidly secure the airway and avoid losing spontaneous respiration, video laryngoscopy should be preferred. Another option might be to utilize rapid sequence induction along with cricoid pressure, but this could result in difficulties with ventilation and oxygenation due to the cessation of spontaneous breathing. Furthermore, associated pneumonia can be a feature due to a poor ability to cough and the retention of secretions.[11]
- Acute kidney injury may occur due to obstruction and ischemia intraoperative or preoperative.
- Liver insufficiency may occur due to prolonged Pringle's maneuver in cases needing retrohepatic IVC resection.
- A large RPT can compress the IVC and may lead to reduced venous return, diminished cardiac output (CO), increased systemic vascular resistance, heightened cardiac workload, and the development of collateral circulation. The presence of intra-abdominal tumors can induce supine hypotension syndrome through aortocaval compression; therefore, positioning the patient in the left lateral decubitus can help mitigate this risk.[12]
- Additionally, during general and epidural anesthesia, there is a decrease in sympathetic activity, which can cause acute hypotension. When these factors are compounded by insufficient preoperative fluid status and the commencement of positive pressure ventilation, venous return can be severely compromised.[13]
- *Risk of RPE:* It is a noncardiogenic pulmonary edema that happens due to sudden reduction in thoracic pressure after removal of giant RPT, resulting in rapid expansion of lungs, which can lead to hemodynamic collapse.[14]

The mechanisms contributing to RPE are linked to the duration and intensity of lung collapse, surfactant depletion, increased permeability of the pulmonary vasculature, changes in pulmonary artery pressure, and the presence of inflammatory cytokines such as interleukin 8 (IL-8) and leukotriene B4. Sustained elevated intra-abdominal pressure can cause a bilaterally elevated diaphragm, leading to lung compression and subsequent collapse. RPE may develop swiftly after lung reexpansion following a prolonged collapse, especially if the lung has collapsed for 3 days or longer, or if over 2,000 mL of fluid has been removed, with symptoms potentially appearing within 1 hour of reexpansion. This condition shares characteristics with unilateral pulmonary edema that can occur after treatment for spontaneous pneumothorax. It is essential to implement a lung-protective ventilation strategy throughout the invasive mechanical ventilation process. Gradual reexpansion of the atelectatic lung is crucial to avoid RPE. Monitoring tidal volume during spontaneous breathing can assist in establishing a comparable tidal volume during controlled ventilation to mitigate the risk of RPE.[14]

- The use of epidural insertion remains a topic of debate. Increased intra-abdominal pressure can elevate the pressure within the epidural space, leading to engorgement of the Batson venous plexus. This, combined with potential technical challenges, raises the likelihood of developing an epidural hematoma. Additionally, the sympatholytic effects of local anesthetics introduced into the epidural space may further exacerbate hemodynamic instability. Current guidelines generally advise against the use of epidural anesthesia during surgery, although it may be appropriate for postoperative management. Given the infrequency of such large tumors, drawing definitive conclusions is challenging.[6]

ANESTHESIA MANAGEMENT

Preoperative Assessment

The evaluation must concentrate on gathering an extensive medical history, alongside assessing weight, height, body mass index, abdominal circumference, and nutritional status and conducting blood tests. Following this, further diagnostic evaluations, including an electrocardiogram (ECG), chest X-ray, and computed tomography (CT) scan, should be undertaken to evaluate the feasibility of surgery and to assist in anesthesia preparation. Additionally, venous Doppler ultrasonography of the lower limbs is necessary to investigate the potential presence of deep venous thrombosis resulting from chronic compression. Before advancing to surgery, it is imperative to confirm the ABO and Rh blood groups, as well as the availability of packed red blood cells (RBCs), fresh frozen plasma (FFP), and platelets. It is also advisable to have heating devices and compression stockings on hand.[6]

In individuals presenting with an adrenal mass, it is essential to evaluate their functional status and initiate endocrine treatment when necessary.[15] For patients scheduled to undergo retroperitoneal lymph node dissection (RPLND), a comprehensive history of prior chemotherapy treatments is crucial and beneficial.[16]

Prior to the surgery, a multidisciplinary approach is essential for careful preoperative evaluation. The surgical team—oncologist, along with the anesthesiologist, blood bank team, and intensive care team—should gather before surgery to discuss the overall strategies for the case. They should consider logistical issues, the type of tumor and its impact on physiological parameters, the surgical approach, the nature of the incision, the extent of resection, options, the time length of duration, potential interoperative risk, potential blood loss, the anesthetic plan, surgery and anesthesia-related complications, and postoperative management in intensive care facilities.[6]

Intraoperative Management

It is essential for the patient to undergo thorough preparation, which typically necessitates an extended preoperative period. Consideration should be given to the prophylaxis of aspiration pneumonia.

For most RPTs, general anesthesia is usually necessary because regional anesthesia alone cannot meet the operative requirements. Spinal anesthesia can disrupt the body's compensatory responses to blood loss by blocking sympathetic ganglia, which leads to vasodilation and hypovolemic shock. In contrast, general anesthesia not only alleviates patient discomfort but also supports respiratory and circulatory functions while allowing for effective monitoring of vital signs and hemodynamic changes. It is often the preferred option for patients with RPTs, who are at risk of significant intraoperative blood loss (IBL). When necessary, general anesthesia can be combined with epidural anesthesia to minimize the required dosage of medications **(Figs. 3A and B)**.

Standard American Society of Anesthesiologists (ASA) monitoring protocols must be implemented, accompanied

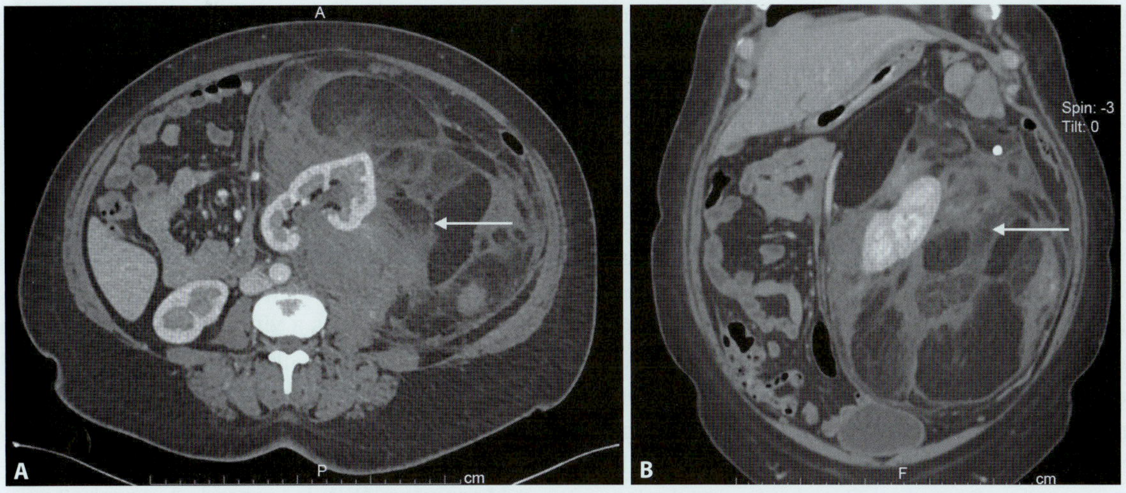

Figs. 3A and B: Giant primary leiomyosarcoma of retroperitoneum (white arrow).

by the placement of two large-bore intravenous peripheral catheters. Prior to the induction of anesthesia, it is crucial to obtain an invasive arterial pressure measurement, insert a central venous catheter, and place a urinary catheter.

Hemodynamic monitoring, which includes CO, pulse pressure variation (PPV), stroke volume variation (SVV), and continuous central venous pressure (CVP), can be conducted using a FloTracTM to evaluate fluid responsiveness during the surgical procedure. Whenever feasible, transesophageal echocardiography (TEE) may also assist in managing hemodynamics during anesthesia and is also important with respect to surgery in patients with IVC tumor thrombus. Entropy and the surgical plethysmographic index (SPI) are valuable tools for assessing the depth of anesthesia and the adequacy of analgesia, respectively.[17,18]

Awake intubation should be contemplated for airway management, or alternatively, rapid sequence induction with cricoid pressure may be performed. The McKenzie system can be utilized to effectively anesthetize the airway. Additionally, conscious sedation with target-controlled infusion (TCI) of remifentanil may be initiated. Following airway securement, either propofol or sevoflurane can be employed for the induction of anesthesia. To preserve spontaneous respiration with pressure support ventilation, the use of neuromuscular blocking agents should be avoided, as their administration could lead to ventilatory failure. Surgeons must be cognizant of the potential for decreased venous return and hypotension resulting from increased intrathoracic pressure when positive pressure ventilation is initiated. Anesthesia maintenance can be achieved with sevoflurane and remifentanil.[19]

Surgical procedures may be initiated in a semirecumbent position to mitigate the risk of supine hypotensive syndrome and respiratory distress. Following decompression, one can anticipate a decrease in airway pressure, enhanced lung compliance, and improved gas exchange. An increase in stroke volume and CO, along with a reduction in SVV, is expected due to the augmented venous return to the heart.

Maintaining appropriate temperature levels during surgery is associated with better clinical outcomes. Inadvertent perioperative hypothermia, which is defined as a core temperature dropping below 36°C, can result from disturbances in the body's natural temperature control mechanisms. Such disturbances may be caused by prolonged skin exposure, the use of anesthetic drugs, and the administration of significant quantities of intravenous and irrigation fluids. This hypothermic state can adversely influence both the surgical procedure and the patient's recovery trajectory.[19]

Surgical resection of RPTs often carries a substantial theoretical risk of considerable blood loss, estimated to exceed 500–1,000 mL. Significant intraoperative bleeding presents a considerable challenge for both surgeons and anesthesiologists. When IBL surpasses 2,000mL and is accompanied by massive blood transfusion (MBT), the risk of severe complications rises markedly. These complications may include coagulation disorders, secondary hemorrhages, renal dysfunction, thrombosis, cardiovascular incidents, and additional issues.[20]

Therefore, implementing patient blood management (PBM) should be prioritized in the perioperative care of these individuals. PBM involves the prompt application of evidence-based surgical practices aimed at reducing the need for allogeneic blood transfusions (ABT) and enhancing patient outcomes. This is achieved through three key strategies: (1) Optimizing RBC mass, minimizing blood loss and bleeding, and improving the body's physiological tolerance to anemia.[16]

In the context of reducing blood loss during surgery, intraoperative cell salvage and acute normovolemic hemodilution (ANH) are viable options. Research indicates that the implementation of cell salvage can lead to a 38% decrease in the need for allogeneic blood transfusions, translating to an average savings of approximately 0.68 units of RBCs per patient. While there have been apprehensions regarding the potential adverse effects of tumor cells being aspirated during surgery, a recent meta-analysis encompassing 34 observational studies found that the reinfusion of salvaged autologous blood in oncology procedures was linked to lower cancer recurrence rates and comparable mortality outcomes when contrasted with allogeneic blood transfusions. The preliminary safety of cell salvage has also been established in cases involving urologic cancers, hepatocellular carcinoma, and metastatic spinal tumors. Furthermore, the use of leukocyte depletion filters has proven effective in eliminating various tumor cells from salvaged blood, thereby encouraging a more widespread application of cell salvage techniques in cancer surgeries. Conversely, ANH presents a more cost-effective strategy for conserving blood intraoperatively, particularly in settings with limited resources. Its primary benefit is the enhancement of tissue oxygenation following surgical blood loss through the retransfusion of whole blood, which also mitigates the risks associated with dilutional coagulopathy and thrombocytopenia. Recent investigations have demonstrated the effectiveness of ANH in reducing the need for allogeneic blood transfusions across various surgical contexts, although its efficacy in minimizing bleeding has primarily been validated in cardiac surgery.[21]

The third and important strategy of PBM focuses on enhancing the patient's physiological capacity to tolerate anemia. Alongside evidence-based transfusion protocols, it is crucial to continuously optimize CO, ventilation, and oxygenation throughout the surgical procedure. Maintaining hemodynamic stability is important to ensure adequate organ perfusion. Furthermore, effective analgesia both during and after the operation to minimize oxygen consumption is important.[20]

Fluid management: Throughout the anesthesia process, it is highly recommended to utilize goal-directed fluid therapy, which can be effectively achieved through various hemodynamic monitoring techniques such as arterial pressure monitoring, CVP monitoring, pulse contour analysis, and TEE. Rather than relying solely on crystalloid resuscitation, damage control resuscitation employing a balanced approach in a 1:1:1 ratio (i.e., FFP, platelets, and RBCs) or the use of whole blood (WB) has been emphasized as a vital strategy in managing major hemorrhage. Transfusing FFP, platelets, and RBCs at a higher 1:1:1 ratio has been linked to a reduced incidence of complications and mortality among patients suffering from severe trauma.[22,23]

Moreover, WB is regarded as an optimal and advantageous choice for patients undergoing MBTs. Nonetheless, a significant challenge with WB transfusion is the time needed for safety testing, which can result in a considerable reduction of coagulation factors.[20]

In cases of substantial blood loss, the depletion of blood components occurs unevenly. The levels of coagulation factors may be inadequate to sufficiently elevate or sustain the already diminished plasma concentrations in patients experiencing bleeding. Research indicates that the median fibrinogen level decreases, with prothrombin time (PT) and activated partial thromboplastin time (APTT) significantly prolonged from the preoperative to postoperative periods. Studies involving surgical patients who received MBTs have demonstrated that higher fibrinogen levels at the conclusion of surgery correlate with improved survival rates. However, the administration of prothrombin complex concentrates (PCCs) and fibrinogen concentrates (FC) has been associated with an increased risk of thrombotic events in trauma patients in some studies and inversely associated with better outcomes in some studies.[20]

Pain Management and Postoperative Care

Pain relief in the postoperative period can be achieved using paracetamol, opioids, wound infiltration, or trunk blocks like the transversus abdominis plane (TAP) block. Analgesia can be effectively achieved by regional blocks, hence sparing the opioids and their side effects and enabling faster recovery. The patient requires intensive care unit (ICU) care for continuous monitoring of vital signs due to the risk of ongoing respiratory and hemodynamic issues, as well as potential blood loss, fluid shifts, or surgical complications. Given the relaxation of the abdominal and diaphragmatic muscles, it is sometimes advisable to delay extubation, which can be managed in the ICU.

Special Considerations

Retroperitoneal Lymph Node Dissection

The RPLND is an operation that is integral to the management of metastatic germ cell cancer. RPLND is most often performed in a postchemotherapy setting in patients with residual disease. Platinum-based chemotherapy may lead to considerable cardiovascular and respiratory complications, which may have implications in anesthesia for RPLND.[16]

Bleomycin is recognized for its potential to cause acute pulmonary toxicity, with documented incidences of bleomycin-induced pneumonitis ranging up to 42%. The association between bleomycin and acute respiratory distress syndrome (ARDS) after surgery was reported in 1978 shortly after the introduction of bleomycin as a chemotherapy agent.[16]

More recent papers have questioned the lifelong association of oxygen therapy and bleomycin exposure, particularly with the advent of restrictive fluid strategies and lung protective ventilation. Hence, during anesthesia, it is important to restrict fluids and to deliver as low a concentration of oxygen as is possible to maintain an $SPO_2 \geq 92\%$ and a $PaO_2 \geq 8$ kPa.[16]

A study with a 14-year follow-up indicates that among patients receiving cisplatin for the treatment of testicular cancer, there is a documented incidence of major cardiac events at 6%. Additionally, cisplatin is recognized for causing peripheral neuropathy, known as cisplatin-induced peripheral neuropathy (CIPN), which is another significant adverse effect. It has been observed that the neuropathy became more apparent in the postoperative period. The possible explanation may be related to patient and limb positioning.[16]

Pheochromocytoma or Other Secreting Tumors

All adrenal tumors must be evaluated for secretory function, and endocrine treatment must be initiated before planning surgery to avoid intraoperative catastrophes. Even so-called nonsecreting pheochromocytomas or paraganglioma may manifest catecholamine storm. Usually, catecholamine secretion from these tumors is triggered by direct pressure on the tumor, manipulation during surgery, or touching the mass through the abdominal wall. Serious complications can arise from a catecholamine storm, including severe hypertension, myocardial infarction, coronary spasm, arrhythmias, cardiomyopathy, stroke, and pulmonary edema. So, it is important that anesthesia team must anticipate such problems, remain vigilant throughout the procedure, and be ready with necessary drugs.[15]

Inferior Vena Cava Tumor

Leiomyosarcoma, while rare, represents one of the most frequently occurring primary tumors of the IVC. These tumors originate from smooth muscle cells of IVC. Surgical en bloc excision of the tumor is the mainstay of treatment. Depending upon the segment of IVC involved, nephrectomy or autotransplant of kidneys or liver may be needed **(Figs. 4A and B)**.

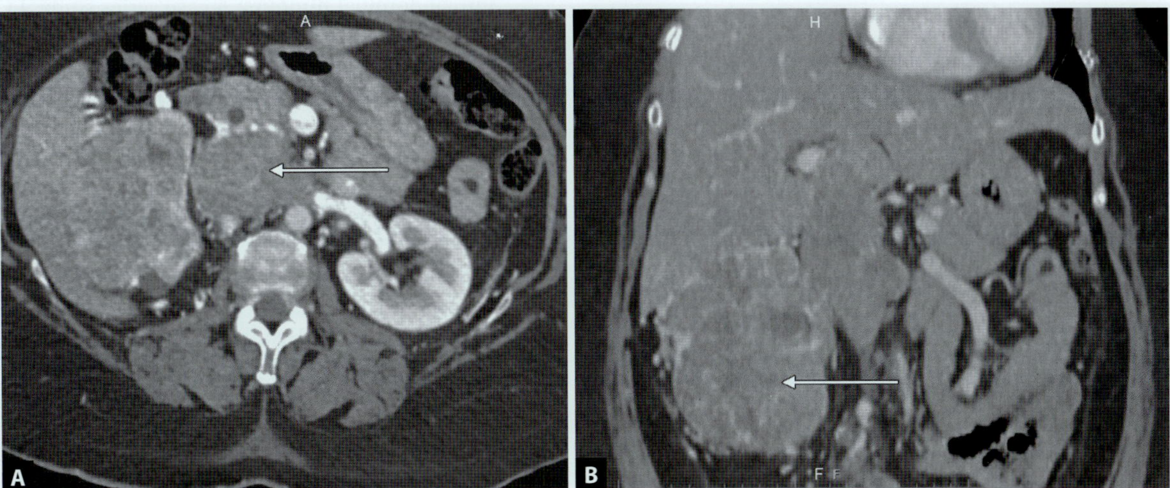

Figs. 4A and B: Right renal cell carcinoma with inferior vena cava (IVC) extension and IVC invasion.

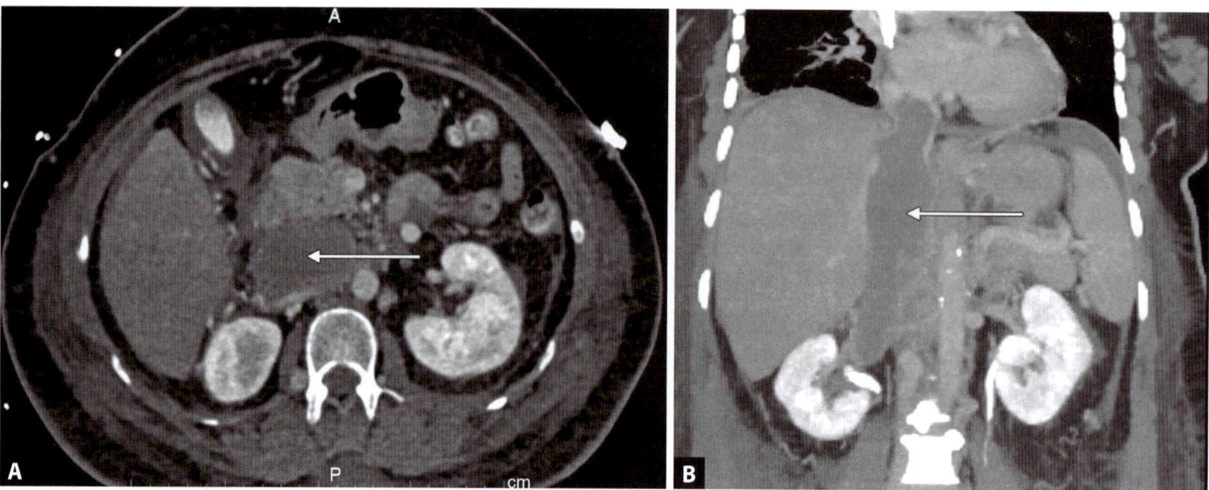

Figs. 5A and B: Primary leiomyosarcoma of inferior vena cava.

Renal cell carcinoma and adrenocortical carcinomas are the most common secondary tumors of IVC. In patients with IVC tumors with an intracardiac extension, cardiopulmonary bypass (CPB) may be needed **(Figs. 5A and B)**.

Intraoperatively, TEE evaluation is very important to properly assess extent of the tumor before cross-clamping the IVC and also to identify tumor embolization if any. Surgery for IVC tumors is associated with significant bleeding and requires liver mobilization, tumor embolization, IVC replacement, or cardiopulmonary bypass underlining the importance of multidisciplinary team approach involving liver surgeon, cardiovascular surgeon, anesthesia and intensive care team.

CONCLUSION

An effective perioperative management of large RPTs necessitates a multidisciplinary approach. Increasing awareness among physicians from different specialties about the systemic complications of these tumors can improve patient outcomes. Important factors to consider include targeted fluid management, slow expansion of lungs to avoid RPE, judicious use of blood and blood products, etc. Additional clinical research, particularly in the form of randomized clinical trials, is necessary to gain a better understanding of the perioperative complications associated with these tumors.

REFERENCES

1. Guan L, Li T, Zhu B, Yao L. Perioperative anesthetic management and preoperative precautions for retroperitoneal tumors. In: Luo CH (Ed). Retroperitoneal Tumors. Dordrecht, Netherlands: Springer; 2018. pp. 71-91.
2. Shi X, Luo CH. Surgical anatomy of the retroperitoneal and pelvic extraperitoneal space. In: Luo CH (Ed). Retroperitoneal Tumors. Dordrecht, Netherlands: Springer; 2018. pp. 1-16.
3. Osman S, Lehnert BE, Elojeimy S, Cruite I, Mannelli L, Bhargava P, et al. A comprehensive review of the retroperitoneal anatomy, neoplasms, and pattern of disease spread. Curr Probl Diagn Radiol. 2013;42(5):191-208.
4. Strauss DC, Hayes AJ, Thway K, Moskovic EC, Fisher C, Thomas JM. Surgical management of primary retroperitoneal sarcoma. Br J Surg. 2010;97(5):698-706.
5. Bonvalot S, Raut CP, Pollock RE, Rutkowski P, Strauss DC, Hayes AJ, et al. Technical considerations in surgery for retroperitoneal sarcomas: Position paper from E-Surge, a master class in sarcoma surgery, and EORTC-STBSG. Ann Surg Oncol. 2012;19(9):2981-91.
6. Grăjdieru O, Petrişor C, Bodolea C, Tomuleasa C, Constantinescu C. Anaesthesia management for giant intraabdominal tumours: A case series study. J Clin Med. 2024;13(5):1321.
7. Corp A, Thomas C, Adlam M. The cardiovascular effects of positive pressure ventilation. BJA Educ. 2021;21(6):202-9.
8. Madhu YC, Harish K, Gotam P. Complete resection of a giant ovarian tumour. Gynecol Oncol Case Rep. 2013;6:4-6.
9. Kb N, Pt P, Shivanna S, Cvr M. Anaesthetic implications and management of a giant ovarian cyst. J Clin Diagn Res. 2014;8(3):170-1.
10. Rauch S, Miller C, Bräuer A, Wallner B, Bock M, Paal P. Perioperative hypothermia—a narrative review. Int J Environ Res Public Health. 2021;18(16):8749.
11. Klucka J, Kosinova M, Zacharowski K, De Hert S, Kratochvil M, Toukalkova M, et al. Rapid sequence induction: An international survey. Eur J Anaesthesiol. 2020;37(6):435-42.
12. Bamba K, Watanabe T, Kohno T. Anesthetic management of a patient with a giant ovarian tumor containing 83 L of fluid. Springerplus. 2013;2(1):487.

13. Pierre SA, Jaeger MT, Siemens DR. Intra-operative inferior vena cava syndrome in a patient with autosomal dominant polycystic kidney disease. World J Urol. 2006;24(1):110-2.
14. Sohara Y. Reexpansion pulmonary edema. 2008;14(4): 205-9.
15. Kumar RA. Anesthetic management of a large retroperitoneal paraganglioma: A rare case report. J Clin Anesthesiol Res. 2020;1(1):1-6.
16. Stephens M, Murphy T, Hendry D. Anaesthesia for retroperitoneal lymph node dissection in the treatment of testicular cancer. BJA Educ. 2019;19(9):283-9.
17. Suehiro K, Tanaka K, Matsuura T, Funao T, Yamada T, Mori T, et al. The Vigileo-FloTracTM system: Arterial waveform analysis for measuring cardiac output and predicting fluid responsiveness: A clinical review. J Cardiothorac Vasc Anesth. 2014;28(5):1361-74.
18. Sánchez JIA, Ruiz JDC, Fernández JJD, Zuñiga WFA, Ospina-Tascón GA, Martínez LEC. Predictors of fluid responsiveness in critically ill patients mechanically ventilated at low tidal volumes: Systematic review and meta-analysis. Ann Intensive Care. 2021;11(1):28.
19. Feng D, Xu F, Wang M, Gu X, Ma Z. Anesthetic management of a patient with giant retroperitoneal liposarcoma: Case report with literature review. Int J Clin Exp Med. 2015;8(10):19530-4.
20. Wang J, Chen J, Liu K, Zhang H, Wei Y, Suo L, et al. Anesthetic management, morbidities and mortalities in retroperitoneal sarcoma patients experiencing perioperative massive blood transfusion. Front Oncol. 2024;14:1347248.
21. Droz NM, Lin J, Beach J, Vo C, Morrow K, Lyden SP, et al. Decreased transfusion requirements with use of acute normovolemic hemodilution in open aortic aneurysm repair. J Vasc Surg. 2021;74(6):1885-93.
22. Benes J, Giglio M, Brienza N, Michard F. The effects of goal-directed fluid therapy based on dynamic parameters on post-surgical outcome: A meta-analysis of randomized controlled trials. Crit Care. 2014;18(5):584.
23. Holcomb JB, Tilley BC, Baraniuk S, Fox EE, Wade CE, Podbielski JM, et al. Transfusion of plasma, platelets, and red blood cells in a 1:1:1 vs a 1:1:2 ratio and mortality in patients with severe trauma: The PROPPR randomized clinical trial. JAMA. 2015;313(5):471-82.

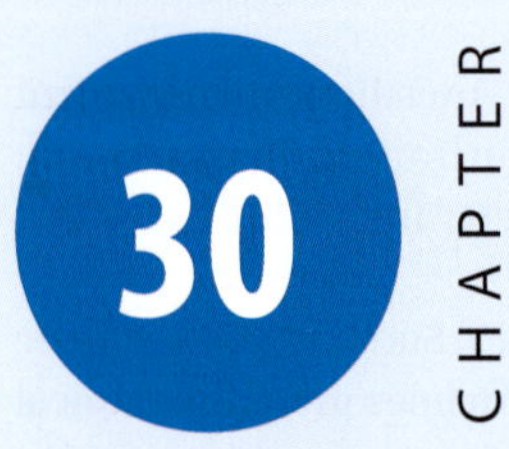

Hemodynamic and Fluid Management in Major Thoracic and Abdominal Cancer Surgeries

Rakesh Garg, Karthik AR, Prasanna Vani

INTRODUCTION

Fluid should be considered as a drug, and its excess or deficit can be detrimental to overall patient outcomes. Our understanding of perioperative fluid therapy and hemodynamic management has changed over the years based on continuously evolving evidence. Various strategies such as restrictive, liberal, goal-directed, moderate, and euvolemic have been described in the literature as regards the amount of fluid to be administered in the perioperative period. However, the definition of each strategy is vague and varies with each study group. On the whole, a well-accepted fact is that a balance should be achieved between organ perfusion and tissue edema. A lesser than required fluid with low perfusion causes end-organ damage, in particular acute kidney injury (AKI). A more than-required fluid will cause extravasation of excess fluid into the extravascular space, leading to tissue edema. This will lead to bowel edema, causing anastomotic dehiscence; pulmonary edema, causing acute lung injury; and limb edema. The amount of extravasation depends on the integrity of the capillary endothelium, plasma oncotic pressure, and the type and amount of fluid administered. The fluid and hemodynamic management goals in any surgery should be to optimize tissue perfusion and oxygen delivery.

ENDOTHELIAL GLYCOCALYX AND ENDOTHELIAL SURFACE LAYER

The vascular endothelium was regarded as the innermost layer of any blood vessel and the only layer of a capillary. It consists of a single layer of endothelial cells with tight junctions and a basal lamina. However, a fourth "jelly-like" layer was discovered in the late twentieth century using electron, confocal, and intravital microscopy. This layer was called the endothelial glycocalyx (Latin for "sweet husk").[1] It is present in the luminal side of the endothelium. It consists of negatively charged glycosaminoglycans anchored to proteoglycans.[2] The endothelial glycocalyx is a dynamic structure undergoing constant enzymatic and mechanical degradation and replenishment by the endothelial cells. It electrostatically interacts with circulating albumin and orosomucoid to form a physiologically active layer called the endothelial surface layer (ESL).[3] The ESL plays a vital role in regulating vascular permeability, coagulation, vascular rheology, and mediation of inflammation.[1] It also serves as a mechanosensor and mechanotransducer for the endothelial cells, activating endothelial nitric oxide synthase (eNOS) in response to blood-flow-related shear stress. This is responsible for the local flow-mediated vasodilatation.[4] Glycocalyx degradation and shedding is aggravated by various factors—sepsis, inflammation, hypervolemia, hyperglycemia, hemorrhagic shock, and ischemia-reperfusion. Thus, optimal perioperative fluid management should be targeted at maintaining the integrity of ESL.

REVISED STARLING MODEL OF FLUID EXCHANGE

Since 1896, when Starling first described the forces regulating fluid exchange across the capillaries, his work has been the mainstay in understanding pericapillary fluid physiology. He postulated that fluid movement across a capillary is the net of four parameters—capillary and interstitial hydrostatic pressures and capillary and interstitial colloid osmotic pressures (oncotic pressure). However, he could not measure the interstitial hydrostatic and interstitial oncotic pressure with the available technology. According to his theory, in a steady state, fluid is filtered from the arterial side of the capillaries and is reabsorbed from the venous side. However, with advancements in science in recent decades, measurement of interstitial hydrostatic and oncotic pressure became possible, and it was seen that fluid is not absorbed from the venous side, but the filtration rate reduces gradually down the capillary. The calculated initial capillary filtration rates were much higher than the observed rates. It was seen that lymphatic flow was the main channel of fluid reabsorption into the vascular system rather than the venular end of the capillaries. These observations required revising the conventional Starling's model of fluid exchange complemented by the pore-exit microgradients and glycocalyx-cleft model.[5]

Most fluid movement across the capillary occurs through the intercellular clefts in the endothelium. The endothelial glycocalyx on the luminal side covers the entrance to these clefts. The space beneath the intercellular cleft is called the subglycocalyx space **(Fig. 1)**. The communication pathway between the subglycocalyx space and the interstitial space is long and tortuous. Once considered the endothelium, the semipermeable membrane in the capillary is actually the glycocalyx layer. Thus, the interstitial oncotic pressure in the original Starling equation has to be substituted with the oncotic pressure of the subglycocalyx layer. The subglycocalyx oncotic pressure is very minimal compared to the interstitial oncotic pressure, and hence, the amount of fluid filtered in the arteriolar end of the capillary is lesser than what was estimated. Similarly, the significant amount of venular uptake of fluid once estimated does not happen in reality in most of the capillaries, the exceptions being kidneys and intestines. Thus, most tissues' lymphatic system forms the mainstay of interstitial fluid reabsorption.[5] A further description of capillary fluid dynamics is beyond the scope of this chapter, and the reader is encouraged to read about the evolving concepts in this intriguing field.

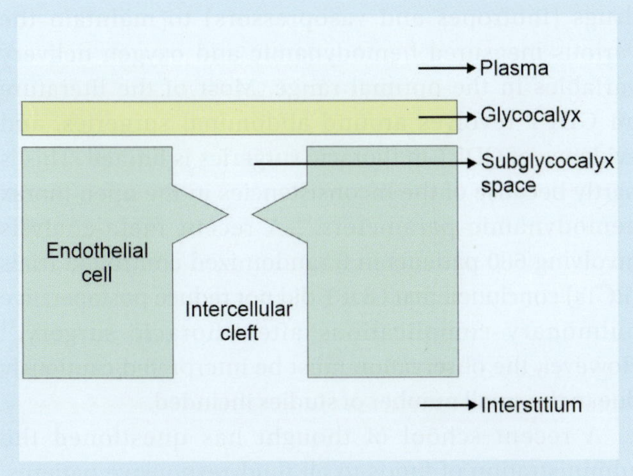

Fig. 1: Revised Starling model of fluid exchange.

DELETERIOUS EFFECT OF HYPERVOLEMIA

Hypervolemia is worthy of particular mention in capillary microregulation. It causes the dilution of plasma proteins and the release of atrial natriuretic peptide (ANP). Recent evidence shows that ANP causes glycocalyx shedding in a cyclic GMP-linked proteolytic pathway.[1] This causes increased vascular permeability and fluid extravasation, causing edema. Thus, a liberal perioperative fluid strategy is deleterious to patient outcomes.

HEART–LUNG INTERACTIONS

The cardiovascular system is primarily responsible for the perfusion of end organs with oxygenated blood. During positive-pressure mechanical ventilation, as in general anesthesia, the intrathoracic pressure and right atrial pressure increase, decreasing venous return to the right heart. Thus, the output of the right heart is reduced, which is reflected in the output of the left heart during expiration due to pulmonary transit time. The opposite happens during expiration, and the systemic cardiac output increases during inspiration.[6] Thus, there is a cyclical variation in the cardiac output with respiration. This variation is exacerbated during hypovolemia as the cardiac output becomes more preload-dependent. Hence, replacing fluids in such cases increases cardiac output.

Hypoperfusion could be due to many reasons, and hypovolemia is one of them. Not all patients with hypoperfusion would respond to fluid replacement. Those patients whose perfusion and cardiac output increase with fluid infusion are called fluid responders. If the cardiac output does not respond to fluid infusion, such patients are called fluid nonresponders. Whether a patient responds to fluid or not depends on which portion of the Frank–Starling curve the patient is. The Frank–Starling curve demonstrates that cardiac output increases with an increase in preload or venous return up to a certain extent, after which the increase is not appreciable. Thus, the curve plotted against venous return and cardiac output is curvilinear, with the first part being steep and later assuming a plateau. Identifying which portion of the curve a patient is at a given time would provide valuable information on whether the patient would be a fluid responder. This would prevent iatrogenic fluid overload in nonresponders. Several methods have been described to assess the clinical interaction between cardiac and pulmonary systems.[6]

METHODS TO EVALUATE CARDIOPULMONARY INTERACTIONS

Stroke volume variation (SVV) and pulse pressure variation (PPV) in the respiratory cycle derived from pulse wave analysis (PWA) are useful dynamic indicators of volume responsiveness. However, specific prerequisites need to be met for them to be valid. The lungs must be ventilated with at least 8 mL/kg tidal volume, more than what is routinely recommended in lung-protective ventilation. The heart should have a sinus rhythm, and PWA seems inconsistent in open thorax as in cardiac and thoracic surgeries. PWA is also inconsistent in spontaneous respiration, low lung compliance, increased intra-abdominal pressure, right heart failure, and high respiratory rate. Inferior vena cava diameter and its variations concerning the respiratory cycle have been used to predict fluid responsiveness. Transthoracic and transesophageal echocardiography (esophageal Doppler monitor) is used to visualize the heart directly, and measuring the aortic blood flow velocity during the respiratory cycle has been shown to predict fluid responsiveness.[6] Plethysmographic variability index derived from pulse oximetry, end-expiratory occlusion test, and dynamic arterial elastance derived from PPV and SVV have also been described in the literature to predict the need for vasopressors and fluids.[6] The noninvasive cardiac output monitor (NICOM) based on bioreactance is a sensitive and specific technique to assess fluid responsiveness. It is noninvasive and easily tolerated in conscious patients. It can be used in varied patient groups. Four surface electrodes are placed over the chest. Using bioreactance technology, the device tracks hemodynamic variables, including stroke volume (SV), SV variation, and CO. Passive leg raising and administration of a fluid challenge can be performed to study the response to fluids and the improvement in hemodynamic variables. It performs comparably to the esophageal Doppler monitor in guiding fluid therapy.[7]

THORACIC CANCER SURGERY

Perioperative fluid overload was seen to be an independent risk factor for postoperative pulmonary complications in lung resection surgeries.[8] Hence, the age-old teaching in thoracic anesthesia was to keep the patient dry. However, a very restrictive strategy can cause AKI and adversely affect overall patient outcomes. The most important parameter pointing toward good outcomes is to maintain euvolemia. This can be achieved by reducing the fasting time so the patient comes adequately hydrated to the operating room. The same principle is carried forward in the postoperative period, where the patient is allowed oral fluids as soon as possible after recovery from anesthesia. This, along with various other measures, encompasses the enhanced recovery after surgery (ERAS) perioperative care pathway, first popularized in colorectal surgery and now being adopted widely in most surgical specialties. The thoracic ERAS guidelines were jointly released by the ERAS Society and the European Society of Thoracic Surgeons (ESTS) in 2019.[9] Clear fluids are allowed until 2 hours before surgery, and recently, a more liberal strategy of "sip till send" allows about 150 mL/hr of fluids until the patient is shifted to the operating room for hip fracture surgeries without increasing the aspiration risk. Post-thoracic surgery, lung injury, and pulmonary edema are exacerbated by the usage of large intraoperative tidal volumes and various other factors. Thus, inappropriate fluid management is one of the factors of the multiple-hit theory in which systemic inflammatory response is the first hit.

GOAL-DIRECTED FLUID THERAPY

Although it is known that euvolemia is the ideal strategy to follow, achieving that in a heterogeneous group of patients is challenging. Customizing fluid therapy titrated to specific objective hemodynamic parameters is the essence of goal-directed fluid therapy (GDFT). GDFT includes the administration of fluids and vasoactive drugs (inotropes and vasopressors) to maintain the various measured hemodynamic and oxygen delivery variables in the optimal range. Most of the literature on GDFT revolves around abdominal surgeries, and evidence of GDFT in thoracic surgeries is limited. This is partly because of the inconsistencies in the open thorax hemodynamic parameters.[10] A recent meta-analysis involving 680 patients in 6 randomized controlled trials (RCTs) concluded that GDFT did not reduce postoperative pulmonary complications after thoracic surgery.[11] However, the observation must be interpreted cautiously due to the small number of studies included.

A recent school of thought has questioned the administration of fluids to all fluid-responsive patients. Fluid responsiveness might not necessarily equate to fluid necessity. Not all fluid-responsive patients require fluids. Being fluid-responsive is normal for some patients, and administering fluids until they become nonresponsive might cause a new pathologic state. Optimizing tissue perfusion is more important than optimizing cardiac output.[12] Recently, the efficacy of GDFT has been questioned in the context of ERAS pathways.[13] Studies comparing GDFT with and without ERAS protocols noted a wide variation in results. GDFT has significantly reduced morbidity and hospital and intensive care length of stay (LOS) in major abdominal surgeries. If participants were managed in the ERAS pathway, the benefit of GDFT was less pronounced and was observed only in intensive care LOS, not in morbidity or hospital LOS.[14] This might be because various factors of the multiple-hit hypothesis have been addressed in the ERAS protocol, and the contributory importance of one single factor reduces the overall picture. However, this cannot eliminate the importance of GDFT. A meta-analysis of 21 trials concluded that GDFT reduced postoperative complications irrespective of the amount of fluid administered perioperatively.[15] However, these benefits did not translate into reducing perioperative mortality. GDFT can be helpful in high-risk patients while guiding clinicians on the timing of fluid administration and appropriate usage of vasoactive drugs.[10]

ABDOMINAL SURGERY

A zero-balance fluid approach has been shown to reduce postoperative complications in elective abdominal surgery.[16] The fasting deficit is not extensive in a perioperative patient on clear liquids until 2 hours before surgery. Mechanical bowel preparation, which can induce functional hypovolemia, is not routinely recommended now. The concept of third space loss is also questioned. Surgical trauma, by itself, can cause edema and fluid accumulation. A positive balance with a weight gain of 3 kg in elective colonic resection has been shown to delay recovery of gastrointestinal function.[17] Interstitial edema with fluid infusion develops due to the fluids' osmotic gradient created and maintained by sodium and chloride. Excess sodium is eliminated slower than water, resulting in edema. Intravenous fluid does not remain in the intravascular compartment due to tissue injury during surgery. This results in tissue edema with excess fluid administration.

Considering the need for the delicate balancing of fluid, it is best to encourage oral liquids up to 2 hours before surgery and minimize the necessity for intravenous fluid replacement. Complex carbohydrate drink is recommended to improve insulin resistance and reduce postoperative vomiting.[18] Evidence shows that clear liquids up to 2 hours before surgery are not associated with increased gastric volume, have no increased risk of aspiration, and the residual volumes are less even in obese patients after 2 hours of clear liquids.[19] The fluid turnover in the perioperative period is 1–1.5 mL/kg/hr due to diuresis and insensible perspiration, evaporation from the wound, and retention in traumatized tissue, and these should be replaced by carbohydrate-containing hypotonic fluids. Sensible perspiration and gastrointestinal losses need replacement with balanced salt solutions. The timing of fluid replacement is also critical. Fluids should be administered early to correct hypovolemia before organ failure starts. Late optimization after organ failure can increase tissue edema due to increased vascular permeability.

VASOPRESSORS AND CHOICE OF FLUIDS

Goal-directed fluid therapy is often used in combination with vasopressors such as noradrenaline. Noradrenaline showed no adverse effects on microcirculatory blood flow or tissue oxygen tension in the intestinal tract.[20] In a meta-analysis of GDFT in combination with noradrenaline in abdominal surgeries, a reduced rate of complications, shortened LOS, and early resumption of solid feeds was noted.[21] There was no compromise on renal perfusion and microcirculatory blood flow at normal volume status using vasopressors. However, caution is needed in elderly patients and those with renal insufficiency.

Colloids do not have any advantages over crystalloids in terms of morbidity or tissue oxygenation despite the lower volumes of fluid infused in the colloid group.[22] Though the recent generation of hydroxy ethyl starches (HES) shows no higher risk of AKI, trial sequential analysis and confidence intervals of that meta-analysis do not exclude their harmful effects on renal function. The use of HES was also associated with higher RBC infusion rates. It is prudent to avoid HES in patients at risk of renal impairment.[23] Balanced crystalloids are a better choice of fluids in those cases.

OTHER FACTORS INFLUENCING OUTCOMES

Apart from fluid and hemodynamic parameters, a few other related parameters modify outcomes. So, these factors must be considered when assessing fluid-related outcomes. Duration of surgery is one of the determinants of fluid requirement. Bioimpedance data showed that the fluid ratio in interstitial space to infused volume is greater in surgeries lasting longer than 3 hours and more in injured tissues than uninjured tissue. The range of fluid infusion rate to maintain the critical plasma volume was narrower in long-duration surgery, especially in those extending more than 6 hours.[24]

Modes of ventilation have an interaction with fluid strategies. Patients in pressure support ventilation on liberal fluid therapy were found to be more prone to lung injury. Patients with liberal fluid with high positive end-expiratory pressures (PEEP) or sudden decrease in PEEP also had higher chances of lung injury. Positive-pressure ventilation can affect hemodynamics and precipitate organ damage in the context of restrictive fluid strategies. This gets exacerbated in the setting of high PEEP. Adjusting ventilatory parameters is recommended to gradually prevent adverse effects on hemodynamics.[25] The benefits of one fluid strategy over the other are negated if a lung-protective ventilation strategy is not employed.

In high-risk emergency surgeries such as colonic perforation and intestinal obstruction, the dynamics of fluid distribution are different. These patients had increased extracellular volume and positive fluid balance, leading to overhydration by the 5th postoperative day in half of them. This was accompanied by increased preload dependency in 12% in the immediate postoperative period and up to 58% by the 5th postoperative day. This progressive increase in extracellular water and preload dependency is due to vasoplegia and endothelial dysfunction. Understanding this in acute high-risk abdominal surgeries is important to avoid fluid overload. Invasive monitoring of cardiac output and correcting the primary cause are needed in such situations.[26]

PRACTICAL GUIDE

- Maintain good preoperative hydration with ERAS protocols: Drink carbohydrates 2 hours before surgery and avoid mechanical bowel preparation.
- Assess patient- and surgery-specific risk. When the risk is high on either parameter, follow goal-directed fluid management.
- In patients with low-to-moderate patient-specific and surgical risk, avoid crystalloid excess and use maintenance fluid at 2 mL/kg/hr, including the volume needed for drug infusions.
- Use isotonic balanced electrolyte solutions (e.g., Hartmann's) to avoid hyperchloremic acidosis.
- Replace blood loss with colloids or blood products.
- Correct hypovolemia early to prevent endothelial dysfunction.
- Encourage early resumption of oral fluids postoperatively.
- Review fluid orders daily and consider enteral before intravenous fluids.
- Goals of fluid management at the end of surgery are normothermia, normovolemia, no evidence of tissue hypoperfusion or hypoxia, no evidence of excess fluid ("zero balance"), hemoglobin >7 g/dL, no clinically significant coagulopathy, and minimal use of vasopressors.
- Factors that predict a poor outcome are greater age, higher ASA physical status, high blood loss, longer duration of surgery, evidence of hypovolemia or hypoperfusion (e.g., metabolic acidosis, blood lactate >2 mmol/L, central venous O_2 saturation <70%), use of high-dose vasopressors, intravenous fluids (>3.5 L total), and a positive fluid balance (>2 L on day of surgery).
- Indicators of central hypovolemia due to blood and fluid loss are tachycardia, hypotension, cold peripheries, low central venous pressure (CVP), low cardiac output, reduced SV, increased pulse pressure variation during positive-pressure ventilation, fluid responsiveness, low central venous O_2 saturation, and increased blood lactate. Central hypovolemia responds to volume therapy.
- In low- to moderate-risk surgery, there is no additional benefit of using GDFT in minimizing postoperative complications compared to mean arterial pressure-guided therapy.[27]
- The use of hemodynamic monitoring devices for GDFT strategy is recommended in the following situations: Major surgery with a 30-day mortality rate of >1%, major surgery with anticipated blood loss of >500 mL, major intra-abdominal surgery, intermediate-risk surgery (30-day mortality >0.5%) in high-risk patients (age >80 years, cardiovascular or cerebrovascular comorbidities, or peripheral arterial disease), and unexpectedly high blood loss and/or fluid loss requiring > 2 L of fluid replacement.
- Patients at high risk of complications, patients who are in poor physical status, hemodynamically unstable

patients, and those undergoing emergency surgeries benefit from invasive monitoring devices and require liberal fluid treatment, which can be tailored using goal-directed strategies.

CONCLUSION

Much of the evidence on fluid therapy emerges from various trials. Patients included in these trials might differ from those encountered in the clinical practice concerning race and ethnicity. Trials get outdated with changes in practice, such as ERAS, and with questionable reliability of monitoring techniques. Clinical judgement in the light of these evidences and periodic audit of the perioperative outcomes at each center should guide clinical practice. The goal should be on oxygen delivery and tissue oxygenation, rather than maintaining only blood pressure and volume status.

REFERENCES

1. Pillinger NL, Kam PCA. Endothelial Glycocalyx: Basic Science and Clinical Implications. Anaesth Intensive Care. 2017;45(3):295-307.
2. Alamilla-Sanchez ME, Alcala-Salgado MA, Cerezo Samperio B, Prado Lozano P, Diaz Garcia JD, Gonzalez Fuentes C, et al. Advances in the Physiology of Transvascular Exchange and A New Look At Rational Fluid Prescription. Int J Gen Med. 2023; 16:2753-70.
3. Pries AR, Secomb TW, Gaehtgens P. The endothelial surface layer. Pflüg Arch - Eur J Physiol. 2000;440(5):653-66.
4. Foote CA, Soares RN, Ramirez-Perez FI, Ghiarone T, Aroor A, Manrique-Acevedo C, et al. Endothelial Glycocalyx. In: Prakash YS (Ed). Comprehensive Physiology, 1st edition. New York: Wiley; 2022. pp. 3781-811.
5. Levick JR, Michel CC. Microvascular fluid exchange and the revised Starling principle. Cardiovasc Res. 2010;87(2):198-210.
6. Bennett VA, Aya HD, Cecconi M. Evaluation of cardiac function using heart-lung interactions. Ann Transl Med. 2018;6(18):356.
7. Waldron NH, Miller TE, Thacker JK, Manchester AK, White WD, Nardiello J, et al. A Prospective Comparison of a Noninvasive Cardiac Output Monitor Versus Esophageal Doppler Monitor for Goal-Directed Fluid Therapy in Colorectal Surgery Patients. Anesth Analg. 2014;118(5):966-75.
8. Arslantas MK, Kara HV, Tuncer BB, Yildizeli B, Yuksel M, Bostanci K, et al. Effect of the amount of intraoperative fluid administration on postoperative pulmonary complications following anatomic lung resections. J Thorac Cardiovasc Surg. 2015;149(1):314-21.e1.
9. Batchelor TJP, Rasburn NJ, Abdelnour-Berchtold E, Brunelli A, Cerfolio RJ, Gonzalez M, et al. Guidelines for enhanced recovery after lung surgery: recommendations of the Enhanced Recovery After Surgery (ERAS®) Society and the European Society of Thoracic Surgeons (ESTS). Eur J Cardiothorac Surg. 2019;55(1):91-115.
10. Şentürk M, Bingül ES, Turhan Ö. Should fluid management in thoracic surgery be goal directed? Curr Opin Anaesthesiol. 202235(1):89-95.
11. Han S, Wu X, Li P, He K, Li J. The impact of goal-directed fluid therapy on postoperative pulmonary complications in patients undergoing thoracic surgery: a systematic review and meta-analysis. J Cardiothorac Surg. 2024;19(1):60.
12. Takala J. Volume responsive, but does the patient need volume? Intensive Care Med. 2016;42(9):1461-3.
13. Batchelor TJP. Modern fluid management in thoracic surgery. Curr Opin Anaesthesiol. 2024;37(1):69-74.
14. Rollins KE, Lobo DN. Intraoperative Goal-directed Fluid Therapy in Elective Major Abdominal Surgery: A Meta-analysis of Randomized Controlled Trials. Ann Surg. 2016;263(3):465-76.
15. Messina A, Robba C, Calabrò L, Zambelli D, Iannuzzi F, Molinari E, et al. Association between perioperative fluid administration and postoperative outcomes: a 20-year systematic review and a meta-analysis of randomized goal-directed trials in major visceral/noncardiac surgery. Crit Care. 2021;25(1):43.
16. Voldby AW, Brandstrup B. Fluid therapy in the perioperative setting—a clinical review. J Intensive Care. 2016;4(1):27.
17. Lobo DN, Bostock KA, Neal KR, Perkins AC, Rowlands BJ, Allison SP. Effect of salt and water balance on recovery of gastrointestinal function after elective colonic resection: a randomised controlled trial. The Lancet. 2002;359(9320):1812-8.
18. Makaryus R, Miller TE, Gan TJ. Current concepts of fluid management in enhanced recovery pathways. Br J Anaesth. 2018;120(2):376-83.
19. Maltby JR, Pytka S, Watson NC, McTaggart Cowan RA, Fick GH. Drinking 300 mL of clear fluid two hours before surgery has no effect on gastric fluid volume and pH in fasting and non-fasting obese patients. Can J Anesth. 2004;51:111-5.
20. Hiltebrand LB, Koepfli E, Kimberger O, Sigurdsson GH, Brandt S. Hypotension during Fluid-restricted Abdominal Surgery. Anesthesiology. 2011;114(3):557-64.
21. Feng S, Yang S, Xiao W, Wang X, Yang K, Wang T. Effects of perioperative goal-directed fluid therapy combined with the application of alpha-1 adrenergic agonists on postoperative outcomes: a systematic review and meta-analysis. BMC Anesthesiol. 2018;18(1):113.
22. Reiterer C, Kabon B, Zotti O, Obradovic M, Kurz A, Fleischmann E. Effect of goal-directed crystalloid-versus colloid-based fluid strategy on tissue oxygen

tension: a randomised controlled trial. Br J Anaesth. 2019;123(6):768-76.

23. Pensier J, Deffontis L, Rollé A, Aarab Y, Capdevila M, Monet C, et al. Hydroxyethyl Starch for Fluid Management in Patients Undergoing Major Abdominal Surgery: A Systematic Review With Meta-analysis and Trial Sequential Analysis. Anesth Analg. 2022;134(4):686-95.
24. Tatara T, Nagao Y, Tashiro C. The Effect of Duration of Surgery on Fluid Balance During Abdominal Surgery: A Mathematical Model. Anesth Analg. 2009;109(1):211-6.
25. De Carvalho EB, Battaglini D, Robba C, Malbrain MLNG, Pelosi P, Rocco PRM, et al. Fluid management strategies and their interaction with mechanical ventilation: from experimental studies to clinical practice. Intensive Care Med Exp. 2023;11(1):44.
26. Cihoric M, Kehlet H, Højlund J, Lauritsen ML, Kanstrup K, Foss NB. Perioperative changes in fluid distribution and haemodynamics in acute high-risk abdominal surgery. Crit Care. 2023;27(1):20.
27. Stens J, Hering JP, Van Der Hoeven CWP, Boom A, Traast HS, Garmers LE, et al. The added value of cardiac index and pulse pressure variation monitoring to mean arterial pressure-guided volume therapy in moderate-risk abdominal surgery (COGUIDE): a pragmatic multicentre randomised controlled trial. Anaesthesia. 2017;72(9):1078-87.

SECTION 7

Gynecological Onco-Anesthesia

31 CHAPTER

Anesthesia for Major Gynecological Cancers

Yukti Sharma, Nishkarsh Gupta, Anju Gupta

INTRODUCTION AND OVERVIEW OF GYNECOLOGICAL CANCER

Malignant neoplasms are leading cause of premature death in most countries worldwide. Breast cancer and gynecological malignancies are common causes of death in the female population.[1]

An essential component of contemporary surgical care is anesthesia. The patient's result is influenced by the modern anesthesia used during perioperative treatment. If applicable, innovative regional anesthesia procedures may yield additional benefits for patients. Anesthesia is an inseparable element of modern surgical treatment. The modern anesthesia applied as a part of perioperative care influences the patient outcome **(Table 1)**.[8,9]

Some retrospective studies suggest different oncologic outcomes related to the anesthesia type used in surgical treatment.[10,11] Gynecologic oncology surgery is increasingly using robotic surgery, which necessitates changes in anesthetic management. Presenting current information on many facets of anesthetic treatment and associated topics in patients with gynecologic cancers is the goal of this chapter.

For ovarian cancer, midline laparotomy is recommended to surgically manage early ovarian cancers.

In early stage disease (stage 1a):

- Young woman → Unilateral oophorectomy or (fertility-sparing surgery) is done.
- Elderly woman → Hysterectomy and bilateral salpingo-oophorectomy
- In stage Ia, Grade 3 (ascites, rupture of capsule) diseases: Staging laparotomy → hysterectomy and bilateral salpingooophorectomy

Chemotherapy is considered for most patients:

- B. *In advanced stage disease*: Exploratory laparotomy → Cytoreductive or debulking surgery. This includes—total abdominal hysterectomy, bilateral salpingo-oophorectomy, complete omentectomy, retroperitoneal lymph node sampling, and resection of any metastatic tumor.
- C. Advanced stage disease

Chemotherapy: Chemotherapy is used widely following surgery to improve the result in terms of survival **(Table 2)**. Drugs are given for five or six cycles at 3–4 weekly interval.

- B. *Combined radiation and surgery*: Radiation (external and intracavitary) followed in 6 weeks by total abdominal hysterectomy and bilateral salpingo-oophorectomy
- *Contraindications of radiotherapy*: Presence of a pelvic mass, pelvic kidney, pyometra, pelvic abscess, previous laparotomies and/or adhesions with bowel and prior pelvic radiation.

ANESTHETIC CONSIDERATIONS

Preoperative Assessment and Optimization

Preoperative assessment is now routine practice in all patients undergoing major surgery. This makes it possible to conduct a comprehensive examination, determine the course of therapy, optimize the preoperative state, and allocate time for patient education and counseling, with special focus on measuring distant cancer spread and general risk factors such as smoking, obesity, and advanced age.

PREOPERATIVE CONSIDERATIONS

Disease-specific Considerations

89% of patients with advanced ovarian cancer suffer from ascites. Pleural effusions and malignant ascites are two specific signs of advanced ovarian cancer that are relevant to anesthesia. Perioperative ventilation may be hampered

TABLE 1: Gynecological cancers with incidence and staging.

Malignancy	*Presenting symptoms*	*Incidence*	*Staging*	*Diagnosis*
Cervical cancer	• Vaginal bleeding • Dyspareunia • Vaginal discharge (change in consistency, odor)	• In India, 2nd most common cause • Incidence rate of 18.3% and second leading cause of mortality rate of 9.1% as per GLOBOCAN 2020	• FIGO Classification • Stage IA is microinvasive (<3 mm) • Stages IB, IIA: Early invasive (>3 mm, <5 mm) • Stages IIB, III, and IVA: Advanced stages	• Inspection of vagina and cervix, colposcopy, hysteroscopy, biopsy, endocervical curettage, conization for assessment of extension and depth of tumor spread • FDG-PET and PET-CT for assessment of lymph node involvement and anatomic and metabolic spread of the disease[2]
Ovarian cancer	• Often asymptomatic in early stages • Pain in abdomen, pelvic region • Abdominal fullness • Ascites • Pleural effusion	In India, 3rd most common and lethal cancer type, accounting for 6.7% of observed cancer incidences[3] and has the worst prognosis[4]	• *Early stages:* Stage 1 when tumor is limited to one or both ovaries • In stage 2, there is pelvic spread of disease or primary peritoneal cancer • In stage 3, disease spreads beyond pelvis and/or to retroperitoneal lymph nodes • *Advance stage:* Stage 4 distant/ intraparenchymal spread	The diagnosis relies on imaging techniques, CA-125 blood tests, and surgical biopsies
Endometrial cancer	• 6th most common cancer among women all over the world • The incidence in 2020 was 16,413 in India[5]	• Abnormal vaginal bleed • Dyspareunia • Dysuria • Pelvic pain	• Stage 1 is when tumor is confined to uterus • Stage 2 invasion of cervical stroma • Stage 3 is local spread of tumor (serosal or adnexal invasion, vaginal or parametrial, pelvic lymph node involvement) • Stage 4 is when tumor extends to pelvic wall, lower 1/3rd vagina, hydronephrosis, nonfunctional kidney • Distant metastasis	• Physical examination • Endometrial biopsy • Dilatation and curettage • Hysteroscopy • CA-125 levels
Vaginal cancer	• Abnormal vaginal bleed • Mass in vagina • Dyspareunia • Dysuria	1–2% of all gynecologic cancers	• *Stage 1*: Tumor confined to vagina • *Stage 2*: Tumor invading paravaginal tissue • *Stage 3*: Tumor extending • to pelvic wall • *Stage 4*: Invasion of rectum or bladder mucosa or direct extension beyond true pelvis	• Colposcopy • Pap smear • Biopsy • Imaging

Contd...

Contd...

Malignancy	Presenting symptoms	Incidence	Staging	Diagnosis
Vulvar cancer	• Pruritus • Ulcer • Vaginal discharge • Pain[6]	GLOBOCAN 2018 data, vulvar cancer was placed at the 33rd rank among all new cases in India[7]	• *Stage 1:* Tumor confined to vulva or perineum • *Stage 2:* Tumor of any size with extension to lower third of vagina/ anus/ urethra with negative nodes • *Stage 3:* Tumor of any size with or without extension to adjacent perineal structure or nonfixed/nonulcerated genitofemoral nodes • *Stage 4:* Invasion of any of following upper urethra and/or vaginal mucosa, bladder mucosa, rectal mucosa, or fixed or ulcerated genitofemoral nodes	• Vulvoscopy • Biopsy (punch/ excisional) • Imaging

(CA: cancer antigen; CT: computed tomography; FDG: fluorodeoxyglucose; FIGO: International Federation of Gynecology and Obstetrics; PET: positron emission tomography)

TABLE 2: Common chemotherapy regimens for gynecological cancers.

Chemotherapeutic agent	Type	Common toxicities
Cisplatin	Alkylating agent	Nephrotoxicity
Cyclophosphamide	Apoptotic cell death[8-11]	Pulmonary toxicity, weight gain
Doxorubicin	Antitumor antibiotic	Cardiotoxicity, myelosuppression
Paclitaxel	Plant alkaloid	Myelosuppression, peripheral neuropathy
Docetaxel	Plant alkaloid	Pulmonary toxicity, myelosuppression
Carboplatin	Alkylating agent	Myelosuppression
Gemcitabine	Nucleic acid synthesis suppression	GI toxicity
5-FU	Antimetabolite	GI toxicity, myelosuppression, neurotoxicity
Irinotecan	Plant alkaloid	Myelotoxicity
Bleomycin	Breakage of single strand and double strand of DNA	Pulmonary inflammation and fibrosis
Epirubicin	Inhibition of nucleoside base triggering DNA cleavage	Hyperpigmentation of nail, myelosuppression

(GI: gastrointestinal)

by either. Ascites is usually managed by preoperative drainage.[12] Although pleural effusions are treated in a similar manner, precautions must be taken to prevent the pleural tap from causing tension pneumothorax during positive pressure ventilation in anesthesia.

Paraneoplastic syndrome: Gynecological cancers have been linked to the following paraneoplastic syndromes:

- *Ovarian cancer:* Cauda equina syndrome, retinopathy, nephritic syndrome, and cerebellar degeneration
- *Uterine:* Peripheral neuropathy, myelitis, retinopathy, encephalitis, dermatomyositis, and hypercalcemia

Anemia: More focus has been placed on managing anemia before surgery, a prevalent issue in advanced ovarian cancer. Anemia is linked to negative perioperative results such as requiring a blood transfusion and longer hospital stays,[13] as well as reduced survival in patients with ovarian cancer.[14]

Iron deficiency, either absolute due to poor nutritional intake or blood loss or the functional iron deficiency caused by impaired iron absorption in anemia of chronic disease, is the most common cause. Preoperative iron replacement has previously been advocated;[15] however, recent evidence[16] has failed to show a reduction in the frequency of intraoperative blood transfusion, postoperative complications, or mortality through the use of intravenous iron replacement in anemic patients prior to major elective abdominal surgery.

Neoadjuvant chemotherapy prior to surgical intervention is increasingly used in ovarian cancer,[17] and platinum-based agents such as cisplatin and carboplatin have a range of side effects of which the anesthetist should be aware. These include immunosuppression, and toxic effects on the pulmonary, cardiac, renal, and hepatic systems, that should be detected by the electrocardiogram (ECG), baseline echocardiography, and blood tests that are routine in the pre-assessment clinic.

Age-related Complications

Because of the later age group in which ovarian cancer usually presents, patients may have multiple unrelated comorbidities and advice regarding preoperative continuation and cessation of certain medications is important. Drugs generally continued include cardioactive, hypertensive, and psychiatric medications. Drugs generally omitted include oral contraceptive agents, antiplatelets, anticoagulants, and diabetic medications, each carrying specific advice as to how many doses to omit preoperatively.

Deep Vein Thrombosis Prophylaxis

There is 7–45% overall risk of deep vein thrombosis (DVT) and 1% risk of fatal embolisms. Release of tissue factor (TF) and procoagulant by tumor cells and gynecological malignancies raise the risk of thromboembolism. The interaction of tumor cells, platelets, monocytes, and macrophages, further procoagulant substances are released. Furthermore, patients are usually immobilized, in advance stage due to direct compression of major vessel causes venous stasis posing as risk factors for venous thromboembolism. As per local protocols, thromboprophylaxis should begin prior to surgery and continue following it.

Prehabilitation aims to aid the response to surgery and postoperative recovery by improving functional and metabolic reserves prior to the surgical procedure. It forms a cornerstone of enhanced recovery programs, which are increasingly recommended in the management of gynecological malignancy.[18] Although it may not be feasible to allow for prolonged prehabilitation in the perioperative interval, interventions such as nutritional counseling and support, exercise prescription,[19] and certain psychological interventions (e.g., counseling and stress reduction techniques) are achievable in the short term. Smoking cessation and reduction of alcohol intake should be encouraged and comorbidities such as diabetes and hypertension should be identified and treated. Enhanced recovery protocols are discussed further below.

The description of regional anesthesia (epidural or spinal injections) that are administered prior to induction of general anesthesia to the patient. Regional anesthesia promotes the recovery of bowel function and decreases the usage of opiates and their side effects, including nausea and vomiting.

INTRAOPERATIVE CONSIDERATIONS

Choice of Anesthesia Technique

Volatile anesthesia versus total intravenous anesthesia: Both volatile anesthesia (VA) and total intravenous anesthesia (TIVA) can be used for induction and maintenance of anesthesia along with opioid or nonopioid analgesic agents and sometimes various types of regional anesthesia.

Certain studies have indicated possible ways in which volatile anesthetics may increase the spread of cancer by altering the immune response, affecting the body's stress response to surgery, or impacting cancer cell signaling. Nevertheless, the molecular pathways responsible for these effects are not fully comprehended, and there are conflicting findings regarding the impact of volatile agents on various cancer cell types. Luo et al. discovered that in ovarian cancer cells, isoflurane enhances the cancerous properties by elevating levels of markers related to cell cycle, growth, and blood vessel formation: insulin-like growth factor (ILGF), vascular endothelial growth factor (VEGF), angiopoietin-1, and matrix metalloproteinases (MMPs).[20]

Amount of messenger ribonucleic acid (mRNA) for VEGF-A, MMP11, chemokine receptor CXCR2, and tumor growth factor-β (TGF-β) is significantly increased after exposure to volatile anesthetics, indicating the activation of cancer cell transformation, basement membrane degradation, and angiogenesis.[21]

Sevoflurane did not impact apoptosis, proliferation, or migration of cervical cancer cells, but it enhanced their chemosensitivity, indicating possible inhibitory effects on cervical cancer growth and spread.[22]

In contrast, propofol has anti-inflammatory, antioxidative, and antitumor effects by directly regulating key ribonucleic acid pathways and signaling in cancer cells.[23] Propofol regulates both microRNAs and long noncoding RNAs and regulates different signaling pathways. However, there are conflicting results about propofol's impact on migration and invasion of human breast cancer cell lines.[24,25]

Clinical studies on long-term outcomes after cancer surgery under VA and TIVA included outcomes were all-cause mortality, recurrence, and recurrence-free survival. TIVA was associated with slightly lower mortality after cancer surgery, while recurrence and recurrence-free survival were inconclusive. There was, however, considerable heterogeneity among the studies. The authors conducted a subgroup analysis for the other organs' involvement, but this did not demonstrate any significant difference between TIVA and VA [breast cancer: HR 1.14 (0.92–1.40), colorectal cancer: HR 0.57 (0.23 to 1.41)].[26]

Total intravenous anesthesia's beneficial effect in patients requiring significant surgical procedures that cause considerable tissue injury and provoke substantial neural and inflammatory responses.[27] The evidence provided in the research does not allow making definite conclusions. Nevertheless, numerous perioperative variables could impact the progression of cancer in gynecology patients.

Several ongoing prospective randomized controlled trials (RCTs) with oncological outcomes as primary endpoints may help us answer this question.[28,29]

Role of Anesthesia Drugs in Cancer Recurrence

Volatile anesthetics, opioids, and surgical stress response are the most frequently suggested factors that impair host defense against cancer recurrence metastasis in animal models reported that volatile agents might increase metastasis. However, there is no suggestion that local anesthetics are harmful to oncologic patients.[30]

Opioids: Opioids have been widely used in acute perioperative pain and for cancer-related pain. However, laboratory studies indicate some mechanisms which might influence tumor recurrence. For example, some opioids have been found to impair the function of natural killers, T-cells, or macrophages, promoting immunosuppression.[31] In addition, it has been shown that opioids can directly impact cancer growth via their action on μ-opioid receptors (MOR), which are overexpressed in some cancer cell lines.[32]

On the contrary, in a study, morphine decreases leukocyte transendothelial migration, thus reducing angiogenesis associated with tumor growth.[33] A systematic review aiming to validate the data about the link between opioids and tumor dissemination in colorectal cancer could not reveal the long-term impact on cancer-related outcomes due to the heterogeneity of the different studies.[34] Therefore, whether opioid use in surgery promotes cancer recurrence remains inconclusive. Surgical stress may cause many biologic changes, including activation of neural and inflammatory signaling pathways, suppression of cell-mediated immunity, and release of proangiogenic factors.[27]

The data in many studies underlines the significance of minimizing postoperative pain. Uncontrolled pain can be a mediator of the tumor-promoting effects.[35] The animal model study supports the hypothesis that the provision of pain relief attenuates surgery-induced metastatic susceptibility.[36] The best regimen for anesthetic management to improve long-term oncology prognosis should be volatile agents free anesthesia alongside regional techniques combined with an opioid-sparing strategy. There is insufficient evidence to promote specific anesthetic management, and more large-scale research is necessary to prove a link between anesthetic techniques and metastasis.

A related debate is the use of intravenous lidocaine infusion: Local anesthetic, both as regional anesthesia and intravenous infusion, has been suggested to reduce cancer recurrence.[37,38] Again, clinical trials are not supportive[39] and this potential advantage appears to have been outweighed by the serious, life-threatening risks posed by intravenous lidocaine therapy.[40]

Intraoperative Monitoring

Standard ASA II monitoring and whether invasive monitoring is required should be individualized depending upon the severity of tumor invasion, comorbidities, ASA grade, and in cases where large fluid shifts with the potential for hemodynamic instability are anticipated should be done.

Furthermore, if ascitic fluid is rapidly drained upon abdominal opening, patients with a substantial volume of ascites may have abrupt hemodynamic decompensation. Central venous cannulation is advised for patients who may require intraoperative vasopressor assistance in order to ensure adequate perfusion. Due to adhesions and fibrosis, patients who have previously undergone interval debulking or chemotherapy prior to surgery may lose more blood. Because blood loss may be diluted by ascites and irrigation fluid, estimating blood loss might be difficult. Blood products must be easily accessible and utilized in accordance with institute protocol. Urinary catheterization is required for surgical procedures as well as for monitoring hourly urine output.

In patients without preexisting renal disease, urine output of >0.5 mL/kg/h is expected.[41]

Arterial blood gas analysis should be performed at regular intervals for both gas exchange and glucose parameters. Metabolic derangements due to fluid shifts, blood product use, and preexisting conditions or medications are common and should be corrected.

Perioperative hyperglycemia is a separate indicator of negative surgical results such as slow wound healing, infection at the surgical site, cute kidney injury, longer hospital stays, and higher chances of death after surgery in both diabetic and nondiabetic groups.[42] The maintenance of intraoperative glucose levels between 110 and 180 mg% through the use of subcutaneous or intravenous insulin is recommended, with regular monitoring of glucose levels in order to minimize the risk of hypoglycemia.[43]

Intraoperative Fluid Management

Fluid management during major gynecologic oncology surgeries faces great challenges due to the distinctive characteristics of patients with gynecologic malignancies as well as features of the surgical. Goal-directed fluid therapy (GDFT) during surgery has been shown to be successful in decreasing postoperative issues in major colorectal and gynecological operations.[44]

Goal-directed fluid management (GDFM) includes the evaluation of fluid sensitivity and cardiac functions using dynamic and static parameters to measure cardiac output such as pulse pressure variation (PPV), systolic pressure variation (SPV), and pleth variability index (PVI) in order to optimize oxygen supply to tissues during surgery. Randomized controlled trials and meta-analyses have reported superior outcomes for GDFM in terms of organ damage, mortality, wound healing, length of hospital stay, and length of ICU stay compared to liberal fluid management (LFM).[45]

COMMON GYNECOLOGICAL SURGICAL PROCEDURES

The common types of surgery include salpingo-oophorectomy, hysterectomy, lymphadenectomy, peritonectomy, omentectomy, and surgical debulking of the tumor **(Figs. 1 and 2)**. The aim is to remove the bulk of the tumor, after which platinum-based chemotherapy is usually offered.[46]

Additionally, hyperthermic chemotherapy may be delivered to the peritoneal cavity directly after cytoreductive surgery. Radiotherapy is rarely used in the management of ovarian cancer, apart from the treatment of metastases. Radical surgery may also involve the need to operate on or near major arteries and veins (e.g., iliacs), bladder, and ureters, and rarely, liver or spleen where there are metastases. Some surgeons favor stripping the diaphragmatic surface of any metastatic deposits, which may include entering the thoracic cavity.

The entire surgery can now be performed laparoscopically, where access permits. Surgery duration is long, rarely less than 5 hours and often much longer.

Open versus Laparoscopic Surgery

The open and laparoscopic approaches present their own respective challenges for anesthesia. Open surgery

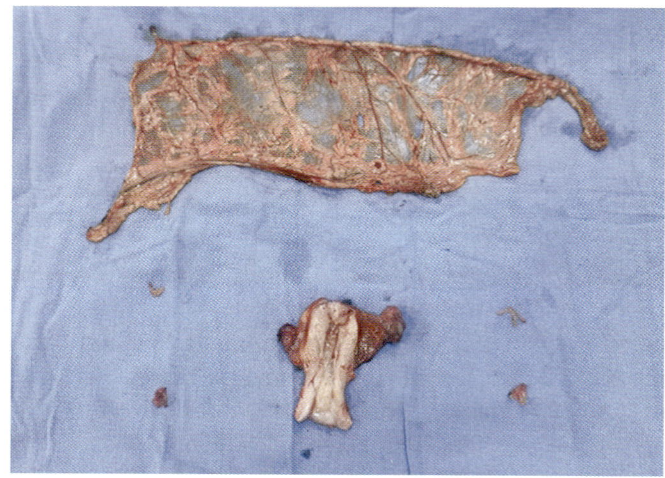

Fig. 1: Specimen of TAH + BSO with omentectomy. (BSO: bilateral salpingo-oophorectomy; TAH: total abdominal hysterectomy)

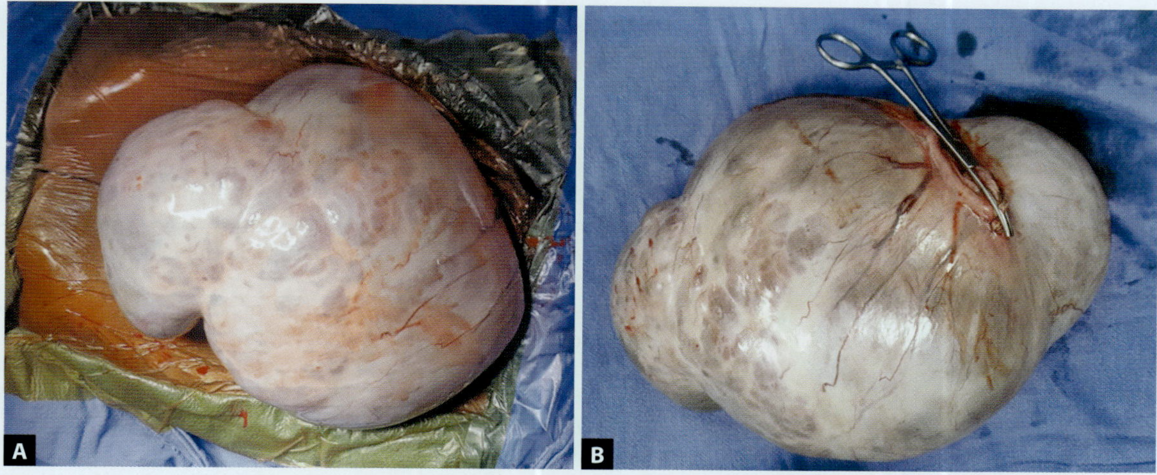

Figs. 2A and B: Large solid cystic adnexal mass in 71-year-old 45 kg BMI 15.7 kg/m^2 elderly female.

requires particular attention to postoperative analgesia and postoperative intravenous patient-controlled analgesia (opiate PCA) or patient-controlled epidural analgesia (PCEA) is commonplace.

The laparoscopic approach requires attention to intraoperative patient positioning, usually in the steep head-down, Trendelenburg position.

Positioning Concerns

Specific concerns for the anesthetist include impaired pulmonary function and potential for reduced ventilation (which can in turn require high inflation pressures), airway and facial edema, increased intraocular and intracranial pressure, and the risk of nerve injury.

Another aspect of the Trendelenburg position's ergonomics is that gynecologists frequently stand patient's head end while using a laparoscope to view down into the pelvis. As a result, the anesthetist must arrange the operating area and anesthesia machine appropriately. Because surgery takes a long time, it is crucial to pay close attention to positioning. In extended cases, repositioning may be necessary at different intervals, particularly for patients who are at high risk of pressure damage, such as those who are fragile or obese.[47]

Extubation

It is complex and multifactorial and is best tailored individually on a case-to-case basis. It begins with the resolution of respiratory failure and/or the disease that prompted initiation of mechanical ventilation. Overall criteria include, but are not limited to:

- The patient should be able to protect the airway, maintain airway patency, have a strong cough, and have minimal secretions.
- Fraction of inspired oxygen (FiO_2) requirement <50% with positive end-expiratory pressure (PEEP) <10 cm of water, and PFR >150
- The four most important things to remember are mental status, oxygenation, ventilation, and expectoration (acronym, *MOVE*).
- Devoid of significant cardiovascular instability/vasopressor requirement

POSTOPERATIVE CONSIDERATIONS

Immediate anesthetic issues include acute pain management, postoperative nausea and vomiting (PONV), delirium in geriatric patients, and surgical complications.

Postoperative analgesia should be a continuation of the intraoperative analgesia, along with a multimodal approach where possible.

Postoperative Analgesia

For gynecological oncological surgery, postoperative pain treatment options are mentioned in **Table 3**.

PROSPECT (procedure-specific postoperative pain management) guidelines:[52]

PROSPECT provides clinicians with supporting arguments for and against the use of various interventions in postoperative pain based on published evidence and expert opinion.

TABLE 3: Various modalities used for postoperative analgesia.

Site	Technique	Comment
Regional anesthesia		
Neuraxial	• *Intrathecal morphine* • Epidural anesthesia	• Morphine acts by binding to μ-opioid receptor via G-protein receptor • *Hydrophilic nature:* Slower uptake and greater bioavailability at the spinal cord's dorsal horn compared with other hydrophobic opioids (fentanyl and sufentanil) • *Dose:* 100–500 μg (effect a dose of less than 300 μg is recommended)[48,49] • Associated with a lower incidence of postoperative complications and improves cardiovascular, respiratory, and gastrointestinal morbidity, lower wound complications but more prolonged urinary catheter use, and higher postoperative hypotension endpoints compared to systemic analgesia[50] • Cornerstone of ERAS pathway
Peripheral nerve blocks	TAP block	• Local anesthetic (LA) is deposited into a plane between the transversus abdominis and internal oblique muscles during a TAP block • T10–T12 dermatomes are covered when LA deposited in lateral abdominal wall • T9–12 in posterior TAP block • Subcostal block covers T6–T12
	Quadratus lumborum block (QLB)	• LA deposition concerning quadratus lumborum muscle, lateral—QLB1, posterior—QLB2, anterior—QLB3, and intramuscular QLB injected directly into the quadratus lumborum muscle • LA spreads along thoracolumbar and endothoracic fascia blocking such structures as intercostal, subcostal, iliohypogastric, and ilioinguinal nerves and reaching the paravertebral spaces • Bilateral QLB provided better intra- and postoperative analgesia in patients undergoing total abdominal hysterectomy than bilateral TAP[51]
	Erector spinae plane block	• LA in the plane deep into erector spinae muscles and superficial transverse processes • Wide cephalocaudal distribution along with several levels and into paravertebral space anteriorly and laterally in the intercostal spaces
Systemic analgesia	Paracetamol, selective cyclooxygenase-2 (COX-2) inhibitors, or conventional nonsteroidal anti-inflammatory drugs (NSAIDs)	• As part of a balanced analgesia, regular administration of nonopioid analgesics to patients undergoing surgeries involving severe pain may help reduce opioid doses and adverse effects while also improving the quality of analgesia
Preemptive analgesia	Ketamine, dexmedetomidine, acetaminophen, NSAIDs, and dexamethasone	• Medication administered before surgery with the goal of minimizing or preventing pain afterward is known as preemptive analgesia • In MIGS (Minimal Invasive Gynecological Surgery), preemptive blocks with a good cost-benefit ratio, such as paracervical, triple antibiotic paste, or pudendal block, seem to have the most consistently positive impact on postoperative pain

(ERAS: enhanced recovery after surgery; TAP: transverse abdominis plane)

Various recommendations are:

- Epidural anesthesia combined with general anesthesia or combined spinal–epidural anesthesia, in high-risk patients (grade A)
- Strong opioids administered in enough time to secure sufficient analgesia when the patient wakes (grade A)
- Cyclooxygenase-2 (COX-2) selective inhibitors or conventional nonsteroidal anti-inflammatory drugs

(NSAIDs), in combination with strong opioids for high-intensity pain (VAS = 50) or with weak opioids for moderate- (VAS < 50 > 30) or low-intensity pain (VAS = 30) (grade A)

- Strong opioids by IV PCA or by fixed IV dosing titrated to pain intensity (grade A)
- Local anesthetic skin infiltration at the proposed site of incision (grade A) but intraoperative wound infiltration is recommended.
- Epidural single dose for postoperative analgesia is not recommended (grade A).

Enhanced Recovery after Surgery

Enhanced recovery after surgery (ERAS) protocols are multimodal perioperative care pathways designed to achieve early recovery after surgical procedures by maintaining preoperative organ function and reducing the profound stress response following surgery. The key elements of ERAS protocols include preoperative counseling, optimization of nutrition, standardized analgesic and anesthetic regimens, and early mobilization.[53]

- Key components routinely used in practice are
- Avoiding prolongation of fasting period, application of antibiotic prophylaxis
- Application of thromboprophylaxis
- Application of midthoracic, epidural anesthesia/ analgesia
- Goal-directed fluid therapy
- Maintenance of normothermia (heating the body, and use of warmed up intravenous fluids)
- Multimodal analgesia with application of midthoracic, epidural anesthesia/analgesia, regional anesthesia techniques, and use of nonopioid oral analgesics/ NSAIDs
- Prevention of nausea and vomiting
- Earlier removal of catheters
- Initiation of oral intake at an early period
- Early mobilization

Outcomes of Enhanced Recovery after Surgery in Gynecologic Oncology

Improvements in length of stay, complications, cost, opioid use, and patient satisfaction have been shown when ERAS is implemented in gynecologic oncology. Results have been found to improve more when ERAS rules are followed more closely. The median opioid consumption among gynecologic oncology patients decreased by 72%, according to Meyer and colleagues' analysis of opioid use with ERAS protocol implementation,[54] and the ERAS population demonstrated faster resolution of impairment in activities with earlier resolution of fatigue, and earlier return to unimpaired walking.[55] ERAS has been found to decrease the risk of gastrointestinal complications and is associated with shortened time to first flatus and lower rates of paralytic ileus.[55]

RECENT ADVANCES

Robotic Surgery

Robotic surgery nowadays plays a vital role in surgical procedures. This surgical method enhances ergonomics, improves visualization of the surgical area, and reduces tissue damage by stabilizing instruments, all done through a minimally invasive procedure. Yet, robotic surgery has its constraints. This method necessitates extra surgical education to enhance the tactile response between the patient and surgeon and results in higher expenses and longer operating room durations.

There are also new challenges for the anesthetic team. They include different patient's body positioning, risk of hemodynamic instability, changes in respiratory mechanics, and limited access to the patient during the procedure.

Body Positioning

The Trendelenburg position is necessary for most gynecological procedures **(Table 4)**. Nevertheless, it is advisable to avoid placing high-risk patients in a very steep Trendelenburg position (>30°) due to potential hemodynamic changes and effects on intracranial and intraocular pressure.

The main preventative measures in the operating area are careful patient securing and appropriate padding.[56] Gynecologic oncology patients do not represent the group of increased risk of position-related injury. Patients with gynecologic oncology are not at higher risk for position-related injuries.[57] During surgery, uncontrolled patient displacement is avoided by using anti-skid materials.[58]

During robotic surgery, multidisciplinary team members from the nursing, surgical, and anesthesia departments should be involved in patient care. Relative contraindications for robotic surgery may include patients with various risk factors, such as excessive obesity and preexisting neurological, ocular, or cardiovascular conditions.

TABLE 4: Effects of Trendelenburg position on various organ systems.

System	*Changes*
Cardiovascular system	• Increase in systemic vascular resistance, mean arterial pressure, myocardial oxygen consumption • Decrease in renal, portal, and splanchnic flow
Respiratory system	• Increase in ventilation-perfusion mismatch, peak airway pressure (P_{peak}) • Decrease in functional residual capacity, vital capacity, compliance • Pulmonary congestion and edema • Hypercarbia, respiratory acidosis
Central nervous system	Increase in intracranial pressure, cerebral blood flow and intraocular pressure
Endocrine	• Catecholamine release • Activation of renin–angiotensin system
Others	• Gastroesophageal regurgitation • Venous air embolism • Neuropraxia • Tracheal tube displacement • Facial and airway edema • Visceral/vascular injury • Ischemic optic neuropathy and corneal abrasion

Optimizing ventilation is made possible by the protective lung ventilation technique that was extrapolated from acute respiratory distress syndrome (ARDS) patients treated in critical care units. The international expert panel-based consensus recommendations suggest a PEEP of 5 cmH_2O and a low tidal volume (TV) of 6–8 mL/kg predicted body weight. Furthermore, when performing recruitment maneuvers, the lowest effective pressure and shortest sufficient time should be used.[59]

Obese patients may benefit from bridging respiratory support to decrease the risk of postoperative pulmonary complications. It includes noninvasive ventilation with continuous positive airway pressure (CPAP)/PEEP or high-flow nasal cannulas systems to improve the outcome in this population.

Robotic Surgery in Gynecological Cancers

Despite great expectations from minimal invasive robotic surgery, it is not preferred in all gynecological procedures in oncologic patients. For example, laparotomy is associated with better outcomes in early-stage cervical cancer than a minimally invasive approach.[60] Similar benefits can be observed for ovarian cancer.[61]

A recently published meta-analysis involving endometrial cancer patients found benefits from robotic-assisted surgery, allowing for a shorter hospital stay, lowering conversion rate to laparotomy, decreasing blood loss, and overall complications with a similar duration of surgery. However, robotic surgery was associated with higher costs.

CONCLUSION

Patients presenting for gynecologic oncology surgery have unique anesthetic challenges due to patient comorbidities, extensive surgical procedures, and the need for optimal perioperative pain management. One needs to follow a multimodal analgesia and enhanced recovery pathway. One also needs to follow a goal-directed fluid therapy and manage proactively for perioperative thromboembolism. A multidisciplinary approach involving anesthesiologists, surgeons, and oncologists is required for effective perioperative care.

REFERENCES

1. World Health Organization. (2020). WHO Report on Cancer: setting priorities, investing wisely and providing care for all. [online] Available from https://www.who.int/publications/i/item/who-report-on-cancer-setting-priorities-investingwisely-and-providing-care-for-all. [Last accessed February, 2025]
2. Dalal A. D C Dutta's Textbook of Gynaecology and Textbook of Obstetrics. J Obstet Gynaecol India. 2016;66(4):303-4.
3. Mhatre A, Koroth J, Manjunath M, Kumar SS, Gawari R, Choudhary B. Multi-omics analysis of the Indian ovarian cancer cohort revealed histotype-specific mutation and gene expression patterns. Front Genet. 2023;14:1102114.
4. Cabasag CJ, Fagan PJ, Ferlay J, Vignat J, Laversanne M, Liu L, et al. Ovarian cancer today and tomorrow: A global assessment by world region and human development index using GLOBOCAN 2020. Int J Cancer. 2022;151(9):1535-41.
5. International Agency for Research in Cancer. Cancer Today. [online] Available from https://gco.iarc.fr/today/factsheets-populations. [Last accessed February, 2025]
6. Beller U, Quinn MA, Benedet JL, Creasman WT, Ngan H, Maisonneuve P, et al. Carcinoma of the vulva. In: Devita Jr VT, Lawrence TS, Rosenberg SA (Eds). Cancer: Principles and Practice of Oncology, 11th edition. Philadelphia: Lippincott Williams &Wilkins; 2018. pp. 2133-58.
7. Bray F, Ferlay J, Soerjomataram I, Siegel RL, Torre LA, Jemal A. Global cancer statistics 2018: GLOBOCAN estimates of incidence and mortality worldwide for 36 cancers in 185 countries. CA Cancer J Clin. 2018;68:394-424.
8. Nelson G, Altman AD, Nick A, Meyer LA, Ramirez PT, Achtari C, et al. Guidelines for pre- and intra-operative

care in gynecologic/oncology surgery: Enhanced Recovery After Surgery (ERAS®) Society recommendations—Part I. Gynecol Oncol. 2016;140(2):313-22.

9. Hübner M, Kusamura S, Villeneuve L, Al-Niaimi A, Alyami M, Balonov K, et al. Guidelines for Perioperative Care in Cytoreductive Surgery (CRS) with or without hyperthermic intraperitoneal chemotherapy (HIPEC): Enhanced Recovery After Surgery (ERAS®) Society Recommendations—Part II: Postoperative management and special considerations. Eur J Surg Oncol. 2020; 46(12):2311-23.
10. Lee JH, Kang SH, Kim Y, Kim HA, Kim BS. Effects of propofol-based total intravenous anesthesia on recurrence and overall survival in patients after modified radical mastectomy: a retrospective study. Korean J Anesthesiol. 2016;69(2):126-32.
11. Enlund M, Berglund A, Ahlstrand R, Walldén J, Lundberg J, Wärnberg F, et al. Survival after primary breast cancer surgery following propofol or sevoflurane general anesthesia—A retrospective, multicenter, database analysis of 6305 Swedish patients. Acta Anaesthesiol Scand. 2020;64(8):1048-54.
12. Kietpeerakool C, Rattanakanokchai S, Jampathong N, Srisomboon J, Lumbiganon P. Management of drainage for malignant ascites in gynaecological cancer. Cochrane Database Syst Rev. 2019;(12):CD007794.
13. Musallam KM, Tamim HM, Richards T, Spahn DR, Rosendaal FR, Habbal A, et al. Preoperative anaemia and postoperative outcomes in non-cardiac surgery: a retrospective cohort study. Lancet. 2011;378:1396-407.
14. Caro JJ, Salas M, Ward A, Goss G. Anemia as an independent prognostic factor for survival in patients with cancer: a systemic, quantitative review. Cancer. 2001;91:2214-21.
15. Muñoz M, Acheson AG, Auerbach M, Besser M, Habler O, Kehlet H, et al. International consensus statement on the perioperative management of anaemia and iron deficiency. Anaesthesia. 2017;72:233-47.
16. Richards T, Baikady RR, Clevenger B, Butcher A, Abeysiri S, Chau M, et al. Preoperative intravenous iron to treat anaemia before major abdominal surgery (PREVENTT): a randomised, double-blind, controlled trial. Lancet. 2020;396(10259):1353-61.
17. Elies A, Rivière S, Pouget N, Becette V, Dubot C, Donnadieu A, et al. The role of neoadjuvant chemotherapy in ovarian cancer. Expert Rev Anticancer Ther. 2018;18:555-66.
18. Schneider S, Armbrust R, Spies C, du Bois A, Sehouli J. Prehabilitation programs and ERAS protocols in gynecological oncology: a comprehensive review. Arch Gynecol Obstet. 2020;301:315-26.
19. Steffens D, Young J, Beckenkamp PR, Ratcliffe J, Rubie F, Ansari N, et al. Feasibility and acceptability of pre-operative Physical Activity to improve patient outcomes After major cancer surgery: study protocol for a pilot randomised controlled trial (PEPA Trial). Trials. 2018;19:112.
20. Luo X, Zhao H, Hennah L, Ning J, Liu J, Tu H, et al. Impact of isoflurane on malignant capability of ovarian cancer in vitro. Br J Anaesth. 2015;114(5):831-9.
21. Iwasaki M, Zhao H, Jaffer T, Unwith S, Benzonana L, Lian Q, et al. Volatile anaesthetics enhance the metastasis related cellular signalling including CXCR2 of ovarian cancer cells. Oncotarget. 2016;7(18):26042-56.
22. Ding J, Zhang L, Zeng S, Feng T. Clinically relevant concentration of sevoflurane suppresses cervical cancer growth and migration through targeting multiple oncogenic pathways. Biochem Biophys Res Commun. 2019;514(4):1179-84.
23. Jiang S, Liu Y, Huang L, Zhang F, Kang R. Effects of propofol on cancer development and chemotherapy: Potential mechanisms. Eur J Pharmacol. 2018;831:46-51.
24. Li Q, Zhang L, Han Y, Jiang Z, Wang Q. Propofol reduces MMPs expression by inhibiting NF-κb activity in human MDAMB-231 cells. Biomed Pharmacother. 2012;66(1):52-6.
25. Ecimovic P, Murray D, Doran P, Buggy DJ. Propofol and bupivacaine in breast cancer cell function in vitro — role of the NET1 gene. Anticancer Res. 2014;34(3):1321-31.
26. Jin Z, Li R, Liu J, Lin J. Long-term prognosis after cancer surgery with inhalational anesthesia and total intravenous anesthesia: a systematic review and meta-analysis. Int J Physiol Pathophysiol Pharmacol. 2019;11(3):83-94.
27. Sessler DI, Riedel B. Anesthesia and Cancer Recurrence: Context for Divergent Study Outcomes. Anesthesiology. 2019;130(1):3-5.
28. National Library of Medicine. (2022). Cancer and Anesthesia: Survival After Radical Surgery — a Comparison Between Propofol or Sevoflurane Anesthesia (CAN). [online] Available from https://clinicaltrials.gov/ct2/show/NCT01975064. [Last accessed February, 2025].
29. National Library of Medicine. (2025). General Anesthetics in cancer resection Surgery (GA-CARES) Trial (GA-CARES). [online] Available from https://clinicaltrials.gov/ct2/show/NCT03034096. [Last accessed February, 2025]
30. National Library of Medicine. (2022). Volatile Anaesthesia and Perioperative Outcomes Related to Cancer Feasibility Study (VAPOR-C). [online] Available from https://clinicaltrials.gov/ct2/show/NCT04074460. [Last accessed February, 2025]
31. Hooijmans CR, Geessink FJ, Ritskes-Hoitinga M, Scheffer GJ. A Systematic Review of the Modifying Effect of Anaesthetic Drugs on Metastasis in Animal Models for Cancer. Plos One. 2016;11(5):e0156152.
32. Beilin B, Martin FC, Shavit Y, Gale RP, Liebeskind JC. Suppression of natural killer cell activity by high-dose narcotic anesthesia in rats. Brain Behav Immun. 1989; 3(2):129-37.
33. Singleton PA, Mirzapoiazova T, Hasina R, Salgia R, Moss J. Increased μ-opioid receptor expression in metastatic lung cancer. Br J Anaesth. 2014;113(Suppl 1):i103-8.

34. Koodie L, Yuan H, Pumper JA, Yu H, Charboneau R, Ramkrishnan S, et al. Morphine inhibits migration of tumor-infiltrating leukocytes and suppresses angiogenesis associated with tumor growth in mice. Am J Pathol. 2014; 184(4):1073-84.
35. Diaz-Cambronero O, Mazzinari G, Cata JP. Perioperative opioids and colorectal cancer recurrence: a systematic review of the literature. Pain Manag. 2018;8(5):353-61.
36. Page GG, Blakely WP, Ben-Eliyahu S. Evidence that postoperative pain is a mediator of the tumor-promoting effects of surgery in rats. Pain. 2001;90(1-2):191-9.
37. Soto G, Naranjo González M, Calero F. Intravenous lidocaine infusion. Rev Esp Anestesiol Reanim (Engl Ed). 2018;65:26974.
38. Chamaraux-Tran TN, Piegeler T. The amide local anesthetic lidocaine in cancer surgery-potential antimetastatic effects and preservation of immune cell function? A narrative review. Front Med (Lausanne). 2017;4:235.
39. Cata JP, Guerra C, Soto G, Ramirez MF. Anesthesia options and the recurrence of cancer: what we know so far? Local Reg Anesth. 2020;13:57-72.
40. Pandit JJ, McGuire N. Unlicensed intravenous lidocaine for postoperative pain: always a safer 'licence to stop' than to start. Anaesthesia. 2021;76:156-60.
41. O'Connor ME, Kirwan CJ, Pearse RM, Prowle JR. Incidence and associations of acute kidney injury after major abdominal surgery. Intensive Care Med. 2016;42:521-30.
42. Kotagal M, Symons RG, Hirsch IB, Umpierrez GE, Dellinger EP, Farrokhi ET, et al. Perioperative hyperglycemia and risk of adverse events among patients with and without diabetes. Ann Surg. 2015;261:97-103.
43. Vogt AP, Bally L. Perioperative glucose management: Current status and future directions. Best Pract Res Clin Anaesthesiol. 2020;34:213-24.
44. Yu J, Che L, Zhu A, Xu L, Huang Y. Goal-Directed Intraoperative Fluid Therapy Benefits Patients Undergoing Major Gynecologic Oncology Surgery: A Controlled Before-and-After Study. Front Oncol. 2022;12:833273.
45. Gómez-Izquierdo JC, Feldman LS, Carli F, Baldini G. Meta-analysis of the effect of goal-directed therapy on bowel function after abdominal surgery. Br J Surg. 2015;102(6):577-89.
46. Hacker NF, Rao A. Surgery for advanced epithelial ovarian cancer. Best Pract Res Clin Obstet Gynaecol. 2017;41:71-87.
47. Souki FG, Rodriguez-Blanco YF, Polu SR, Eber S, Candiotti KA. Survey of anesthesiologists' practices related to steep Trendelenburg positioning in the USA. BMC Anesthesiol. 2018;18:117.
48. Bujedo BM. Spinal opioid bioavailability in postoperative pain. Pain Pract. 2014;14(4):350-64.
49. Gehling M, Tryba M. Risks and side-effects of intrathecal morphine combined with spinal anaesthesia: a meta-analysis. Anaesthesia. 2009;64(6):643-51.
50. Pöpping DM, Elia N, Van Aken HK, Marret E, Schug SA, Kranke P, et al. Impact of epidural analgesia on mortality and morbidity after surgery: systematic review and meta-analysis of randomized controlled trials. Ann Surg. 2014; 259(6):105667.
51. Yousef NK. Quadratus Lumborum Block versus Transversus Abdominis Plane Block in Patients Undergoing Total Abdominal Hysterectomy: A Randomized Prospective Controlled Trial. Anesth Essays Res. 2018;12(3):742-7.
52. Khawaja ZH, Gendia A, Adnan N, Ahmed J. Prevention and Management of Postoperative Ileus: A Review of Current Practice. Cureus. 2022 Feb 27;14(2):e22652. doi: 10.7759/cureus.22652. PMID: 35371753; PMCID: PMC8963477.
53. Melnyk M, Casey RG, Black P, Koupparis AJ. Enhanced recovery after surgery (ERAS) protocols: Time to change practice? Can Urol Assoc J. 2011;5(5):342-8.
54. Meyer LA, Lasala J, Iniesta MD, Nick AM, Munsell MF, Shi Q, et al. Effect of an enhanced recovery after surgery program on opioid use and patient-reported outcomes. Obstet Gynecol. 2018;132:281-90.
55. Bisch SP, Wells T, Gramlich L, Faris P, Wang X, Tran DT, et al. Enhanced Recovery After Surgery (ERAS) in gynecologic oncology: System-wide implementation and audit leads to improved value and patient outcomes. Gynecol Oncol. 2018;151:117-23.
56. American Society of Anesthesiologists Task Force on Prevention of Perioperative Peripheral Neuropathies. Practice Advisory for the Prevention of Perioperative Peripheral Neuropathies 2018: An Updated Report by the American Society of Anesthesiologists Task Force on Prevention of Perioperative Peripheral Neuropathies. Anesthesiology. 2018;128(1):1126.
57. Ulm MA, Fleming ND, Rallapali V, Munsell MF, Ramirez PT, Westin SN, et al. Position-related injury is uncommon in robotic gynecologic surgery. Gynecol Oncol. 2014; 135(3):534-8.
58. Klauschie J, Wechter ME, Jacob K, Zanagnolo V, Montero R, Magrina J, et al. Use of anti-skid material and patient-positioning to prevent patient shifting during robotic-assisted gynecologic procedures. J Minim Invasive Gynecol. 2010;17(4):504-7.
59. Young CC, Harris EM, Vacchiano C, Bodnar S, Bukowy B, Elliott RRD, et al. Lung-protective ventilation for the surgical patient: international expert panel-based consensus recommendations. Br J Anaesth. 2019;123(6):898-913.
60. Nasioudis D, Albright BB, Haggerty AF, Ko EM, Kim SH, Morgan MA, et al. Survival following minimally invasive radical hysterectomy for patients with cervical carcinoma and tumor size ≤2 cm. Am J Obstet Gynecol. 2021;224: 317-8.e2.
61. Facer B, Wang F, Grijalva CG, Alvarez RD, Shu XO. Survival outcomes for robotic-assisted laparoscopy versus traditional laparoscopy in clinical stage I epithelial ovarian cancer. Am J Obstet Gynecol. 2020;222(5):474.e1-e12.

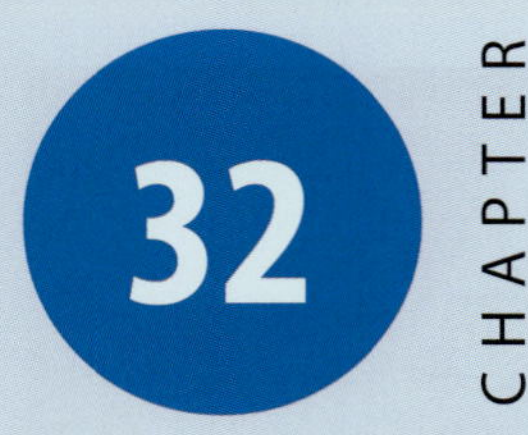

Anesthesia for Intracavitary and Interstitial Brachytherapy for Gynecological Cancers

Mithilesh Kumar Mishra, Sudeep Goyal, Anil Kumar Jain

INTRODUCTION

Most patients diagnosed with uterine malignancy after abnormal vaginal bleeding usually receive a surgical treatment by radical hysterectomy. Certain individuals, however, have high risk markers identified by surgical pathology that indicate an elevated chance of recurrence, necessitating additional adjuvant treatment with chemotherapy with or without radiation. In addition, a definitive strategy involving chemotherapy and radiation therapy is advised, especially in cases with locally advanced cancers. Brachytherapy may produce a fast dose fall-off to protect the surrounding organs at risk and the source can be placed close to the treatment target; it is an especially appealing method for treating gynecologic cancers with radiation.

It is important to note that brachytherapy (intraluminal, intracavitary, and multicatheter interstitial) is a part of standard of care for treating cervical malignancies that have progressed locally. If the sources are implanted within the tumor (permanently or temporarily), they are called interstitial brachytherapy and if the sources are placed close to the tumor, they are labeled as plesiotherapy. Novel developments in imaging modalities, three-dimensional adaptive treatment planning, and dose–volume reporting augment the accuracy and adaptability of this potent therapeutic instrument in the curative management of endometrial and cervical malignancies. Anesthesiologists comprise an integral part of this treatment module involving radiation oncologist, medical oncologist, and oncosurgeon. Anesthesia is required at all steps like examination under anesthesia, device placement, CT scan room, MRI suite, postprocedural pain relief, and immobilization.

BACKGROUND

The Greek word brakhus, which means "short", is where the word "brachytherapy" originates from. Target tissues are positioned close to or in direct contact with sealed radioactive sources in this radiation therapy technique. Source of brachytherapy is usually unstable gamma-emitting radioisotopes, such as isotopes of cesium or iridium, or traditionally radium (which is no longer used in medicine). The physics of the brachytherapy source provides a high dosage concentration right around the radioactive source, with a quick dose fall-off in the surrounding tissues. Brachytherapy can be delivered by using a number of techniques, such as interstitial delivery, which inserts the source directly into the tissue, and intracavitary delivery, which inserts the applicator inside an already-existing body cavity. The most treatable gynecologic malignancy with intracavitary brachytherapy are cervical and endometrial malignancies.[1]

In an attempt to treat a patient who had a locally advanced cervical squamous cell carcinoma with invasion of the bladder, rectal cavity and extension to the introitus, Margaret Cleaves, MD, reported the use of gynecologic intracavitary brachytherapy in 1903. Dr Cleaves decided to try applying radium bromide, which he had obtained from a nearby chemistry laboratory, in an effort to penetrate the tissues more deeply, following the conventional course of treatment with UV light and intravitreal X-rays. A strong reactivity of the mucosal membranes was observed after treatment for few days.[2] However, the tissues healed several days later and had a grossly normal look, free of bleeding, odor, and discharge.[2]

Role of anesthesoiologist an adequate anesthesia is if prime importance. Without adequate anesthesia, placement of applicator and needle insertion during cervix brachytherapy can cause pain, distress and hemodynamic instability (Tachycardia, HTN and ECG changes) in patient. The condition can become more worse during needle insertion in interstitial brachytherapy into the parametrium due to more severe pain as compared to intracavitary brachytherapy.

PROCEDURE

Knowing about the procedure not only helps the anesthesiologist understand the whole treatment plan but also improves support to oncologist colleague and patient care. Brachytherapy involves some equipment and applicators. In interstitial gynecologic brachytherapy, a plastic or metal applicator is placed within the target tissue, and loaded (computer controlled), automatic afterloading of a radioactive source for high-dose radiation to a tumor. Among the most recent equipment, for high-dose-rate (HDR) brachytherapy using high-energy radioisotopes, remote afterloading is frequently utilized. The high-activity radioactive source in a shielded safe is the component of a remote afterloader. It requires a specific protected space under video and audio supervision. Because of its extremely elastic nickel–titanium wire, the source can navigate curved paths without being trapped. The source can be moved by a fixed distance and at predetermined dwell durations with an accuracy of 1 mm thickness to the wire's attachment to a stepper motor. The source has a maximum velocity of 50 cm/s and a minimum dwell time of 0.1 second. Multiple indexed channels in the afterloader allow for the accommodation of multiple transfer tubes to the applicator.[3]

Patients with stage IB3-IVA disease would benefit from it, as it augments in conjunction with external beam radiation. In early-stage illness, brachytherapy alone might be considered if surgery is not approved. Depending on the clinical setting, multiple applicators can be employed for its delivery, which usually involves HDR. These consist of the Syed–Neblett template, the tandem and ring, the tandem and ovoid, and the cylinder with tandem. When given as a boost, standard dosage is based on the assumption that the patient has already received 45 Gy in the pelvis or will soon receive. 5.5 Gy × 5, 6 Gy × 5, 7 Gy × 4, and 5 Gy × 6 are some examples of fractionation systems. An EQD2 of 80–90 Gy should be the target for total radiation.[4]

MRI planning can also be done since it provides better soft-tissue delineation; however, CT planning is usually the basis for treatment planning. Although the results vary depending on the therapy's response and the initial stage, the majority of recent studies report 5-year local control rates of 98% for stage IB-IIA, 91% for IIB, 75% for III, and 76% for IVA. 82% of patients in stages I–II and 49% in stages III–IV survived for a full 5 years. Urinary tract infections, infertility, proctitis, vaginal stenosis, urethritis, rectal hemorrhage, urinary incontinence, fistula formation, uterine perforation, urgency in the bladder, and subsequent malignancy are among the complications.[5]

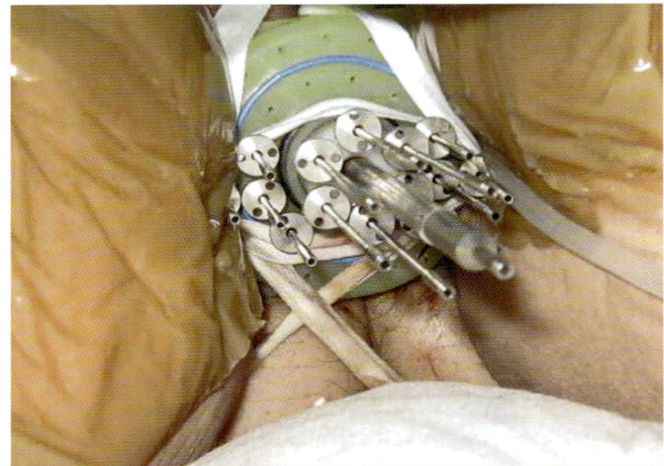

Fig. 1: Implant in situ (vaginal cylinder brachytherapy).

For patients with endometrial cancer, vaginal cylinder brachytherapy has become a standard adjuvant treatment **(Fig. 1)**. For many years, researchers have examined the use of radiation as an adjuvant treatment for endometrial cancer at high and intermediate risk. Whole pelvic radiation lowers the incidence of local recurrence in the pelvis by about 10% in early trials. 73% of these patients' recurrences were found to happen in the vaginal cuff. When vaginal cuff brachytherapy and total pelvic radiation were evaluated, PORTEC-2 found that the recurrence rates were similar. The parameters used to select adjuvant treatment are derived from the concept of a high-intermediate risk illness. This cohort is defined differently by the GOG-99 and PORTEC studies, although it is typically based on the patient's age, histologic grade, deep muscle invasion (>50%), and lymphovascular involvement.[6]

A single channel with different preset lengths and diameters (between 2.0 and 4.0 cm) usually serves as the vaginal cylinder applicator. One can also get segmented cylinders, which can be put together to the necessary length **(Fig. 2)**. Furthermore, the use of multichannel cylinders is made possible by their increased dosimetric control over rectal and bladder doses. To reduce the amount of vaginal wall dosage and minimize air gaps, it is advised to utilize the greatest diameter cylinder for the patient. One can use multiple dose fractionation strategies. Typically, in an adjuvant situation, 7 Gy × 3 administered to 5-mm depth or 6 Gy × 5 to the vaginal surface is used. It can be utilized with 6 Gy × 3 or 6 Gy × 2 surface prescriptions

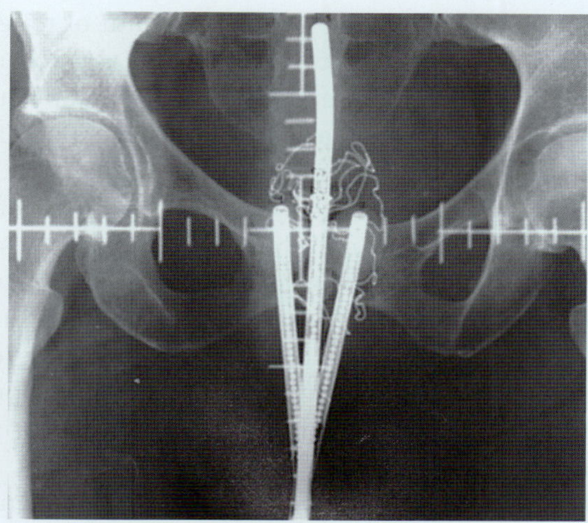

Fig. 2: X-ray of intrauterine applicator insertion.

when combined with external beam treatments. Low dose rate (LDR) can also be used, although HDR is the most popular. It is usually administered to the vaginal surface at a rate of 100 cGy/hr.[7]

Because CT-based planning makes it possible to visualize the cylinder in relation to the surrounding at-risk organs as well as bony pelvic architecture. Unless there is obvious lower vaginal involvement, American Brachytherapy Society (ABS) guidelines advise treating the upper vagina of 3–5 cm. Treatment-related side effects include dryness, vaginal shortening, stenosis, and cuff dehiscence. Brachytherapy may also be beneficial in the difficult case of endometrial cancer that is currently incurable. External beam radiation therapy can be utilized in conjunction with the Rotte "Y" applicator, a two-channel device that is positioned along the uterine wall. When combined with external beam radiation, HDR is often used to provide radiation at a dose of 20 Gy in 5 fractions and 35 Gy in 5 fractions when used alone. On the other hand, alternative fractionation schemes have been applied. Reference overall and cause-specific 5-year survival rates were 42% and 87%, respectively.[8]

ANESTHESIA CONCERNS AND MANAGEMENT

Brachytherapy for day-care cervical and endometrial cancer is mostly a short-duration procedure of 30–45 minutes but may involve multiple small sessions under anesthesia. Early ambulation and recovery post-procedural pain relief, and same day discharge are the plan of treatment.

Preoperative Evaluation

Most of these patients fall under ASA 2 and 3 with an average age group being 50 ± 10 years. Most frequent comorbidities are hypertension, diabetes, hypothyroid, anemia, pulmonary tuberculosis, coronary artery disease, chronic obstructive pulmonary disease (COPD), and epilepsy. Common electrolyte abnormalities are hypokalemia, hypomagnesemia because of gastrointestinal disturbances, volume depletion, chemotherapy and external beam radiation treatments. The nature of disease does not allow adequate time for optimization of comorbidities, although it is essential. Investigations based on the patient's profile and institutional protocol are applied. The effect of radiotherapy and chemotherapy on a patient's physiology and organs should be evaluated well.

Intraoperative

Many anesthesia options are available depending on the patient's profile and oncologist's requirement such as subarachnoid block (SAB), combination spinal and epidural (CSE), caudal block, general anesthesia (GA), IV sedation, GA with erector spinae plane block, and monitored anesthesia care (MAC). Remote location, restricted access to airway, scarcity of trained staff, darkness in USG, radiation in CT suite, and difficult monitoring in MRI are some concerns for the anesthesiologist.

Previously, neuraxial anesthesia was preferred due to longer surgical time, but now-a-days total intravenous anesthesia (TIVA) is preferred as surgical time is reduced drastically. Neuraxial anaestheisa also minimises the effects of systemic opioids and other anesthetic drugs and provides better pain relief. 95% of patients are managed with regional anesthesia for cancer of the cervix, and rest of the patients required GA/MAC with sedation. Reduced dosages of hyperbaric bupivacaine 0.5% (1–1.5 mL) produced enough immobility and painless conditions for the procedure, as well as ensured an early and safe discharge.[9] In a review of 1,622 anesthetics used for brachytherapy by Benrath et al.,[10] spinal anesthesia (single shot) was used in 30% of patients, spinal catheters in 53%, CSE in 7%, and epidural catheters in only 10%.

Since the patient is kept in lithotomy position for several hours, even when analgesia is obtained with an epidural or CSE, they still require sufficient comfort and sedation to undergo the surgery in the absence of a general anesthetic. Arranging the arms and legs correctly is crucial to prevent harm to the nerves. If sedation is required, midazolam can be given sporadically or continuously, along with propofol. An effective T10–L1 blockage is frequently necessary for applicators that are placed into the uterus and vagina. Supplied by sympathetic autonomic afferent causes central and lower abdominal cramping pain associated with nausea and vomiting. Due to the fact that the bladder is frequently dilated for imaging, abdominal cramping may occur even with neuraxial anesthesia, and a minimum of a T10 block is needed. Sacral blockage is typically necessary before inserting a rectal ultrasonography probe or applicator. S2–S4 blockade is required for cervix distension, upper vaginal packing, and labial sutures. Continuous epidural analgesia helps intraoperatively and postoperatively for subsequent radiation session as well.[11]

Nielsen AA provided data of their institute which showed that the anesthetic most often used was an epidural (53%), which was followed by a mixed spinal epidural (34%) and MAC with paracervical block (13%). The dosage most often employed for 0.75% bupivacaine was 1–1.5 mL with a spinal epidural. 0.25% bupivacaine divided into a total volume of 10–15 mL was the dose most often utilized for epidural anesthesia during implant procedures. 14% of the neuraxial anesthetics administered were intrathecal (also known as spinal) or epidural anesthetics. Fentanyl was added as a single dosage in 50% of these patients, and the remaining 50% had an epidural with hydromorphone or fentanyl continuously infused locally during and/or after the treatment. Epidural infusions were initiated at the time of implant placement and continued until the device was removed.[12]

In order to reduce the dose of opioids used, regional blocks were added whenever possible when administering general anesthesia. Propofol maintains immunological function and has a lower chance of inducing cancer recurrence, which makes TIVA a better option than inhalational anesthesia. A retrospective study done at AIIMS, Delhi, also concluded in favor of neuraxial anesthesia and if GA needed TIVA is preferred.[13]

In a retrospective study by Leong, intravenous midazolam, propofol, fentanyl, and oxycodone were used to induce moderate-to-deep drowsiness. A paracervical block with a combination of 1% ropivacaine, 2% lignocaine, and 1:1,000 adrenaline was used to induce local anesthesia. Nine patients underwent 35 brachytherapy insertions in total. The patients' ages ranged from 40 to 65 years, with a median age of 56 years. The American Society of Anesthesiologists classified eight of the patients' physical statuses as I or II, and one as III. 39 minutes was the average amount of time that the insertion took. For cervical cancer, combination of intracavitary and interstitial brachytherapy under sedation and local anesthesia is safe and practical. There may be large cost reductions as a result of this.[14]

During HDR intracavitary brachytherapy for cervical cancer, caudal epidural anesthesia is one of the safest and most effective options for regional anesthesia. In a study by Isoyama-Shirakawa et al. comprising 34 patients, it was found that using conscious sedation in addition to regional anesthesia decreased patient pain and discomfort during the treatment without increasing the risk of complications.[15]

After completion of the needle insertions, patient was returned to the supine position and shifted to computed tomography (CT) suite which is situated adjacent to the brachytherapy suite for confirmation of correct placement of needle and applicator.

Look for any hemodynamic instability and severe abdominal pain due to uterine perforation and bleeding from vessel injury, which can be detected in CT also.

Subsequently, patient were kept in post anesthesia recovery area for monitoring.

Postoperative

Following surgery, patients need admission for ongoing care with the applicators in situ for radiation after loading the following day. They are maintained in a strict bedrest state and require continuous analgesics.

Through its corresponding dorsal nerve branches, the pudendal nerve (S2–4) serves the penis or clitoris, as well as the inferior hemorrhoid and perineal branches, which supply the pelvic floor and perineum. However, there are other sensory nerves in the perineum besides the pudendal nerve. The terminal branches of the ilioinguinal (L1) and genitofemoral (L1–2) nerves innervate the labia majora, the base of the penis, and the scrotum with mixed sensory information. A sensory block up to a maximum height of L1.25 should be predicted following a 20 mL injection of 0.375% bupivacaine through the sacral hiatus. A smaller percentage of individuals whose tumor extends beyond the pudendal nerve's distribution experience insufficient analgesia since the block most frequently only reaches the lower lumbar roots. Continuous epidural infusion (with or without opioids), ultrasound-guided sacral analgesia, intravenous opioids, and/or supplementary painkillers are required in all cases.[16-19]

Postoperative nausea and vomiting (PONV) is common. Female sex, use of opioids, and gynecological procedure/manipulation make these patients a moderately high-risk group for PONV. Continuous epidural local anesthesia reduces total opioid consumption and risk of PONV. Adequate fasting, oral clear liquid till 2 hours preoperative, early oral feed postoperative, ondansetron prophylaxis, and addition of promethazine are known to reduce PONV.[20-22] In some institutions, they are able to perform the procedure with minimal sedation though larger studies are required to authenticate this.[23] At our centre we do almost all cases under TIVA.

Since there is no fixed anesthesia protocol for brachytherapy, we propose an anesthesia plan based on our review of literature **(Box 1)**.

BOX 1: Anesthesia algorithm.

Preoperative:
- Detailed history
- Airway assessment
- Clinical assessment of organ
- Comorbidities and optimization
- *Laboratory:* CBC, RFT, LFT, urine—routine and microscopy, S. electrolytes, coagulation studies, ECG, CXR, X-ray of spine
- Fasting—allow clear liquid till 2 hours preoperatively
- Premedication—anxiolytics

Intraoperative:
- Monitoring—ECG/NIBP/pulse oximetry
- Positioning and care of pressure points
- Anxiolytics
- CSE (first choice)/Epidural/SAB/GA/block
- Fluid management—balanced solution
- Pain relief—paracetamol/opioids/patient-controlled analgesia
- PONV prophylaxis

Postoperative:
- Pain relief—multimodal and procedure specific
- PONV—metoclopramide/ondansetron/dexamethasone
- Avoid opioids
- Delerium prophylaxis
- Early clear fluid postoperatively
- Anxiolytics
- Stop epidural after the last session
- Remove Foley's catheter 6 hours after epidural catheter removal

(CBC: complete blood count; KFT: kidney function test; LFT: liver function test; CXR: chest X-ray; GA: general anesthesia; NIBP: non-invasive blood pressure; CSE: combination spinal and epidural; PONV: postoperative nausea and vomiting; SAB: subarachnoid block)

CONCLUSION

The three main anesthetic methods for pelvic and gynecologic brachytherapy—general anesthesia, neuraxial anesthesia, and sedation—are discussed in earlier research and compiled in this chapter. Currently TIVA is the preferred choice of anesthesia. Adjuncts to the other elements of anesthesia therapy that were studied were nerve blocks, topical local anesthetics, premedications, and intravenous and oral analgesics. Multidisciplinary approach and team work are the cornerstone in managing these patients.

REFERENCES

1. Weiner AA, Schwarz JK. Intracavitary Brachytherapy for Gynecologic Malignancies: Applications and Innovations. Mo Med. 2015;112(5):366-72.
2. Aronowitz JN, Aronowitz SV, Robison RF. Classics in brachytherapy: Margaret Cleaves introduces gynecologic brachytherapy. Brachytherapy. 2007;6:293–7.
3. Whelan TJ, Aldrich JE, Voruganti SM, Wong OS, Filbee JF, Joseph PJ, et al. A comparison of manual and remote afterloading in the treatment of carcinoma of the cervix: increasing dose rate with a flexible applicator. Clin Oncol (R Coll Radiol). 1992;4(5):294-8.
4. Viswanathan AN, Beriwal S, De Los Santos JF, Demanes DJ, Gaffney D, Hansen J, et al., American Brachytherapy Society. American Brachytherapy Society consensus guidelines for locally advanced carcinoma of the cervix. Part II: high-dose-rate brachytherapy. Brachytherapy. 2012;11(1):47-52.
5. Pötter R, Tanderup K, Schmid MP, Jürgenliemk-Schulz I, Haie-Meder C, Fokdal LU, et al., EMBRACE Collaborative Group. MRI-guided adaptive brachytherapy in locally advanced cervical cancer (EMBRACE-I): a multicentre prospective cohort study. Lancet Oncol. 2021;22(4):538-47.
6. Abu-Rustum NR, Yashar CM, Bradley K, Campos SM, Chino J, Chon HS, et al. NCCN Guidelines® Insights: Uterine Neoplasms, Version 3.2021. J Natl Compr Canc Netw. 2021;19(8):888-95.
7. Coon D, Beriwal S, Heron DE, Kelley JL, Edwards RP, Sukumvanich P, et al. High-dose-rate Rotte "Y" applicator brachytherapy for definitive treatment of medically inoperable endometrial cancer: 10-year results. Int J Radiat Oncol Biol Phys. 2008;71(3):779-83.
8. Nag S, Erickson B, Parikh S, Gupta N, Varia M, Glasgow G. The American Brachytherapy Society recommendations for high-dose-rate brachytherapy for carcinoma of the endometrium. Int J Radiat Oncol Biol Phys. 2000;48(3): 779-90.
9. Petitt MS, Ackerman RS, Hanna MM, Chen L, Mhaskar RS, Fernandez DC, et al. Anesthetic and analgesic methods for gynecologic brachytherapy: A meta-analysis and systematic review. Brachytherapy. 2020;19:328-36.

10. Benrath J, Kozek-Langenecker S, Hüpfl M, Lierz P, Gustorff B. Anaesthesia for brachytherapy-5½ years of experience in 1622 procedures. Br J Anaesth. 2006;96:195-200.
11. Janaki MG, Nirmala S, Kadam AR, Ramesh BS, Sunitha KS. Epidural analgesia during brachytherapy for cervical cancer patients. J Can Res Ther. 2008;4:60-3.
12. Nielsen AA, Liyanage TA, Leiserowitz GS, Mayadev J. Optimal perioperative anesthesia management for gynecologic interstitial brachytherapy. J Contemp Brachytherapy. 2017;9(3):216-23.
13. Kumar V, Gulia A, Garg R, Gupta N, Bharati SJ, Mishra S, et al. Perioperative anesthesia management for brachytherapy in cancer patients: A retrospective observational study. J Anaesthesiol Clin Pharmacol. 2021;37(4):598-603.
14. Leong YH, Tan KHS, Choo BA, Koh VY, Tang JI. Novel anesthetic technique for combined intracavitary and interstitial brachytherapy for cervix cancer in an outpatient setting. J Contemp Brachytherapy. 2017;9(3):236-41.
15. Isoyama-Shirakawa Y, Nakamura K, Abe M, Kunitake N, Matsumoto K, Ohga S, et al. Caudal epidural anesthesia during intracavitary brachytherapy for cervical cancer. J Radiat Res. 2015;56:583-7.
16. Smith MD, Todd JG, Symonds RP. Analgesia for pelvic brachytherapy. Br J Anaesth. 2002;88:270-6.
17. Chen H, Leung SW, Wang C, Sun LM, Fang FM, Huang EY, et al. Local vaginal anaesthesia during high-dose-rate intracavitary brachytherapy for cervical cancer. Int J Radiat Oncol Biol Phys. 1998;42:541-4.
18. So W, Chui Y. Women's experience of internal radiation treatment for uterine cervical cancer. J Adv Nurs. 2007; 60:154-61.
19. Yang X, Li C, Li Z, Du D, Fu J. The clinical value of ultrasound-guided sacral anesthesia in Intracavitary and/or interstitial brachytherapy for cervical Cancer. Gynecol Oncol. 2024;191:31-6.
20. Lim KH, Lu JJ, Wynne CJ, Back MF, Mukherjee R, Razvi K, et al. A study of complications arising from different methods of anesthesia used in high-dose-rate brachytherapy for cervical cancer. Am J Clin Oncol. 2004;5:449-51.
21. Chanrachakul B, Likittanasombut L, O-Prasersawat P, Herabutya Y. Lidocaine versus plain saline for pain relief in fractional curettage: a randomized controlled trial. Obstet Gynecol. 2001;98:592-5.
22. Lim H, Doo AR, Son J, Kim JW, Lee KJ, Kim DC, et al. Effects of intraoperative single bolus fentanyl administration and remifentanil infusion on postoperative nausea and vomiting. Korean J Anesthesiol. 2016;69:51-6.
23. Mutyala S, Smith G, Ansinelli H, Thawani N. Feasibility of outpatient hybrid brachytherapy for cervical cancer with minimal sedation: Results from a single-institutional protocol. J Contemp Brachytherapy. 2023;15(1):43-7.

SECTION 8

Urological Onco-Anesthesia

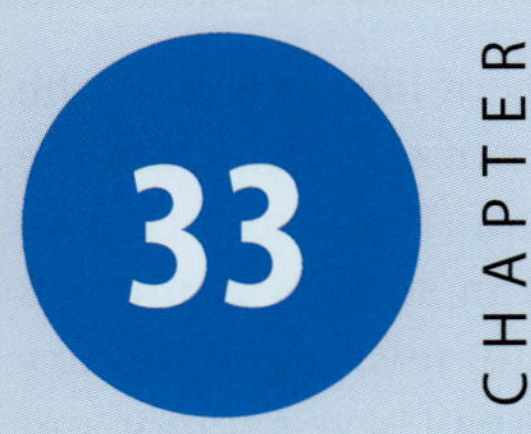

CHAPTER

Anesthesia for Renal Cancers (Radical and Nephron-sparing Nephrectomies)

Ajit Kumar, Ruma Thakuria

INTRODUCTION

The kidney represents a fundamental organ of the human body, fulfilling a multitude of critical physiological roles. Its primary function is to filter plasma and eliminate waste products while simultaneously maintaining water, osmolality, electrolyte, and acid–base homeostasis. This intricate system of processes is essential for the proper functioning of the body, and any disruption or dysfunction can lead to a host of adverse health outcomes. Therefore, a thorough understanding of the kidney's physiology and pathophysiology is crucial for medical professionals and researchers alike. In addition to secreting erythropoietin (EPO), they also secrete renin and play a part in blood pressure and fluid balance regulation. The kidneys are situated on the posterior abdominal wall, adjacent to the diaphragm and the 11th and 12th ribs. These vital organs are roughly 10 cm long, 5 cm wide, and 3 cm thick. The celiac and aortic renal ganglia provide sympathetic innervation to the kidneys from T8 to L1, and the vagus nerve provides parasympathetic input. Similarly, the aorticorenal, superior, and inferior hypogastric plexuses supply the ureters with sympathetic innervation from T10 to L2, while S2 to S4 supplies them with parasympathetic input. Pain is usually referred to the lower back, flank, ilioinguinal region, scrotum, or labia. Nociceptive fibers travel with the sympathetic to T10 to L1 (kidneys) and T10 to L2 (ureters) **(Fig. 1)**.

The renal blood flow (RBF) amounts to 20–25% of cardiac output (CO), with 80% flowing to the cortical nephrons and 20% to the medullary nephrons. Autoregulation of RBF occurs at a mean arterial pressure (MAP) of 80–180 mm Hg. It is crucial to maintain normal renal function during the perioperative period, as it is responsible for excreting anesthetics and medications, regulating fluid and acid–base balance, and controlling hemoglobin levels. The incidence of renal disease among patients seeking surgery is quite high and is known to be associated with a greater likelihood of poor postoperative outcomes. Even mild forms of renal dysfunction have been shown to increase the risk of postoperative complications. Therefore, it is important to carefully evaluate and manage renal function in these patients to minimize the risk of adverse events and promote optimal surgical outcomes.

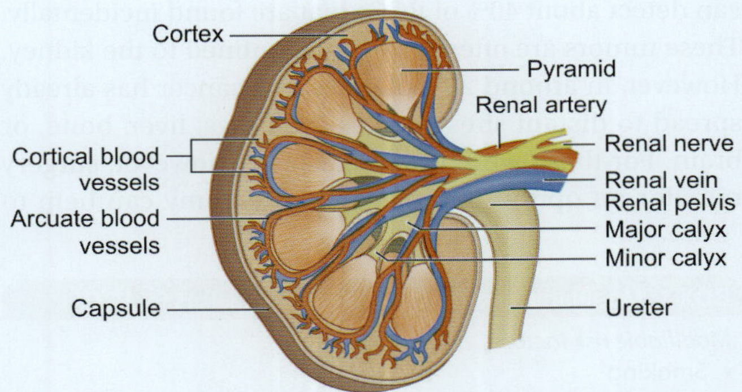

Fig. 1: Schematic diagram of kidney.

EPIDEMIOLOGY

Renal cell carcinoma (RCC) accounts for 2.2% of all new cancer cases worldwide, ranking ninth in men and fourteenth in women.[1] The International Agency for Research on Cancer (IARC) was created in 1965 by the World Health Assembly. It provides comprehensive information on global cancer epidemiology, using data from 343 population-based cancer registries in 65 countries.[2] RCC incidence has usually increased over time in both sexes and is expected to continue to rise over the next 15 years, with some variation across nations.[3] The regional distribution and increased prevalence of RCC have been largely linked to diversity in risk factors for the disease, as well as differences in healthcare delivery systems. Several modifiable and nonmodifiable risk factors for RCC have been identified **(Box 1)**. The prevalence of the disease is increasing due to the aging population and higher rates of risk factors like cigarette smoking (contributing to one-third of all cases), obesity, hypertension, asbestos exposure, and acquired polycystic kidney disease. Patients exhibiting symptoms typically have a palpable mass, loin pain, and hematuria. Nonspecific symptoms are fairly common and include fever, night sweats, weight loss, and malaise. Microscopic hematuria is often the first sign of small localized tumors, frequently detected by routine urinalysis and often asymptomatic. Abdominal imaging can detect about 40% of RCCs that are found incidentally. These tumors are often small and confined to the kidney. However, in around 25% of cases, the cancer has already spread to distant sites such as the lungs, liver, bone, or brain. For those who have metastases, however, surgery remains an option because a nephrectomy can help to reduce symptoms, enhance quality of life, and raise the likelihood of a better prognosis. Tumor extension into the renal vein and/or inferior vena cava (IVC) can occur in up to 25% of cases. This can result in serious symptoms such as pulmonary embolism and severe pulmonary congestion. Less than 2% of patients will have a tumor and thrombus at the right atrial border, and <10% will show up with a thrombus inside the IVC. Survival outcomes of RCC depend largely on the stage at diagnosis and are poor in late-stage disease.[4,5]

BOX 1: Modifiable and nonmodifiable risk factors for RCC.

Modifiable risk factors:
- Smoking
- Obesity
- Hypertension
- Diabetes
- Diet
- Occupation
- Drug exposure

Nonmodifiable risk factors:
- Age
- Sex
- Race
- Family history

(RCC: renal cell carcinoma)

Source: Rossi SH, Tanaka H, Usher-Smith JA, Bernhard JC, Fujii Y, Stewart GD. 2022 WUOF/SIU International Consultation on Urological Diseases: Kidney Cancer Screening and Epidemiology. Soc Int Urol J. 2022;3(6):371-85.

Nephrectomy was first described in 1969 for patients with RCC.[6] Surgical therapy differs according to the pathology. Simple nephrectomy is favored for people with non-neoplastic disease (e.g., trauma, nonfunctioning kidney with persistent infection), whereas radical nephrectomy is chosen for those with neoplastic disease. Radical nephrectomy entails the removal of Gerota's fascia, which includes the perinephric fat, lymphatics, and ipsilateral adrenal gland.

SURGICAL APPROACH

Various factors such as the location of the pathology, whether it is bilateral or multiple, history of a hereditary kidney cancer syndrome, baseline and differential renal function, baseline renal function, and the disease stage, all influence the surgical approach. The surgical approach is customized and mostly determined by the surgeon's preference.

Partial nephrectomy involves the removal of diseased part of the kidney with a margin of normal tissues. It is a nephron-sparing surgery where a large number of nephrons are spared **(Figs. 2A to C)**.[7] Partial nephrectomy is recommended for patients with kidney tumors that are smaller than 7 cm in diameter, those who are at risk of future renal impairment, tumors located in a peripheral

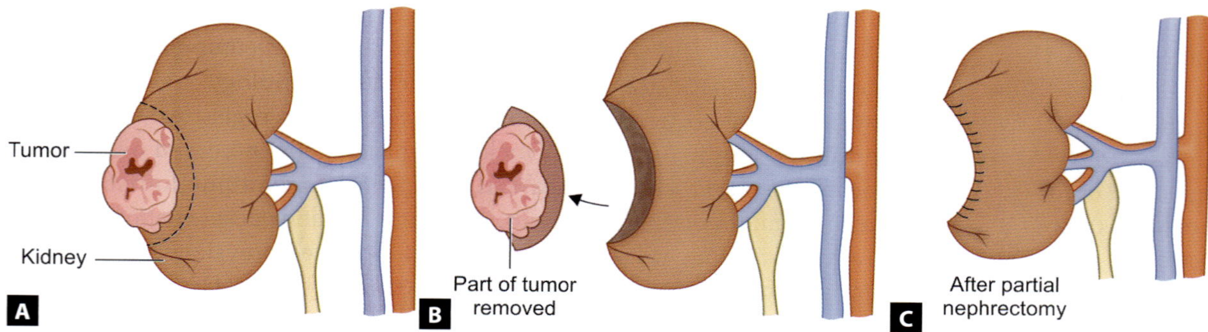

Figs. 2A to C: Partial nephrectomy.

position (such as at one pole), bilateral tumors, and those with a single kidney.

In selected cases, partial nephrectomy can be used for large or locally advanced RCC. In an ideal patient, a partial nephrectomy preserves kidney function without increasing the risk of recurrence.[8] Advanced laparoscopic techniques are often used for partial nephrectomy, which requires a high level of technical expertise. However, this technique can result in longer warm ischemic times, making open partial nephrectomy a better option in certain circumstances, such as when a patient has only one kidney. During surgery, if a synchronous tumor or extension into the renal vein is discovered, conversion from partial to radical nephrectomy is likely.

Radical nephrectomy is indicated for stages I, II, and III of RCC. Nephron-sparing surgery is a possibility for RCC patients with distant metastatic disease, bilateral tumors, and a high risk of developing severe renal impairment. Radical nephrectomy involves the removal of a significant number of nephrons **(Fig. 3)**.

The surgical incision in nephrectomy depends on the location of the tumor, the side of the kidney involved, body habitus, and the surgeon's preference. Commonly used incisions are flank, thoracoabdominal, and transabdominal (Chevron or anterior subcostal). In most cases, the kidney can be safely removed via the transperitoneal subcostal approach. The advantages of laparoscopic nephrectomy include reduced analgesic requirements, reduced hospital stay, and early discharge. Laparoscopic nephrectomy can be performed via either a transperitoneal

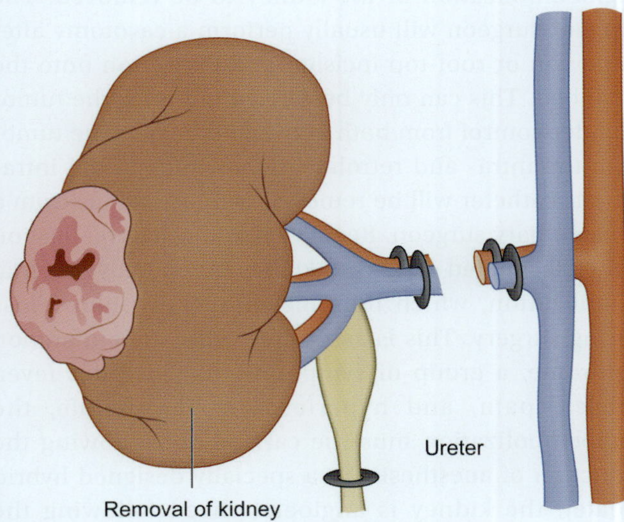

Fig. 3: Radical nephrectomy.

or retroperitoneal approach. Using the transperitoneal approach, three or four small abdominal incisions are made after the abdomen is insufflated with carbon dioxide using a trocar. Using the retroperitoneal approach, a retroperitoneal space is created by making a small incision in the back and inserting a dissecting balloon. Following the balloon's removal, the area is carbon dioxide-infused and two or three more tiny back incisions are made in preparation for the laparoscopic instruments. The kidney is released by laparoscopic dissection, after which it is either encased in a bag and removed through the suitable incision or placed in an impermeable sac, morcellated, and removed through one of the port sites. Sometimes, the kidney and ureter are removed together (laparoscopic radical nephroureterectomy).[9] For malignancies with a diameter of little >10 cm, a laparoscopic radical nephrectomy may be performed. Findings seem to show that mortality, recurrence, and rates of renal impairment are comparable, independent of surgical technique or strategy.

Given the hemodynamic instability or in patients with elevated intracranial pressure, a laparoscopic procedure might not be suitable for patients with severe ischemic or valvular heart disease. On the other hand, a low barrier for switching to open surgery after a laparoscopic try could be a reasonable strategy.[10]

PREOPERATIVE ASSESSMENT

In addition to a routine anesthetic assessment, a preoperative assessment should attempt to assess renal function and functional capacity and assess for cardiorespiratory disease severity and degree of urgency for intervention. Patients in their seventh decade of life should have significant occult cardiorespiratory disease excluded by the anesthetist, particularly those without a prior history. Hypertension is frequently associated with chronic renal failure and is believed to result from elevated renin/angiotensin system activity. Peripheral vascular disease and accelerated ischemic heart disease could follow. Edema may arise from heart failure, proteinuria, and hypoalbuminemia. Uremic patients may develop pericarditis. There could be autonomic and peripheral neuropathies. Patients with renal cell cancer may be anemic due to various reasons such as anemia of chronic disease, recurrent hematuria, and renal impairment, leading to reduced EPO production. It may be necessary to optimize hemoglobin levels preoperatively using oral or intravenous iron, EPO, and blood products. Anemia (normocytic, normochromic) may be detected by a complete blood cell count (CBC). The levels of urea and creatinine in plasma are useful indicators of overall renal health. Additionally, the glomerular filtration rate (GFR) can be precisely measured using creatinine clearance.

$$Creatinine\ clearance = u \times v / p$$

Where,
u = Urinary concentration of creatinine (mg/100 mL)
p = Plasma concentration of creatinine (mg/100 mL)
v = Urine volume (mL/min)

A 2-hour test is usually used for convenience; however, a 24-hour test is more accurate. Normal values are 85–125 mL/min in women and 95–140 mL/min in men. Creatinine clearance decreases with age.

Serum electrolyte concentrations should be measured in suspected cases of renal failure; however, these usually remain normal until severe renal disease is present. Arterial blood gas parameters can reveal metabolic acidosis in severe renal failure cases due to impaired acid excretion by the kidney.

Proper medication should be used to control hypertension. Appropriate antibiotics should be used to treat any urinary tract infection. Routine preoperative transfusion of anemic patients is usually unnecessary because these patients have chronic compensated anemia, and transfusion can exacerbate heart failure. Patients undergoing elective surgery may benefit from preoperative iron or EPO therapy to increase their hemoglobin levels. Due to the potential for intraoperative hemorrhage, prior blood grouping and cross-matching should be completed. It is crucial for management to monitor coagulation parameters using modalities such as activated clotting time, blood gas analysis, and thromboelastography.

Severe renal failure may result in fluid and electrolyte-related patient complications. These should be fixed to the greatest extent possible, as dialysis may be used.

Diabetes mellitus is a frequent cause of kidney issues, and it is essential to have a suitable plan in place for managing such patients during the perioperative period. Premedication may be used as necessary, and antacid prophylaxis should be considered for individuals with chronic kidney disease. Cardiac complications are particularly relevant, and at least electrocardiography and echocardiography should be performed. Apart from a chest X-ray and an ECG, consideration should also be given to stress echocardiography, coronary angiography, and static pulmonary function tests, if indicated.[11]

Anorexia, weight loss, and weakened immune system performance are the hallmarks of cachexia, a condition that affects about 50% of cancer patients.[12,13] Patients are often malnourished, which raises the risk of pressure sores, nosocomial infections, and delayed wound healing. Infections can worsen symptoms for cancer patients, and they can also be more challenging to treat. Nutritional supplements or enteral or parenteral feeding should be used to optimize nutritional status.

CAVOATRIAL DISEASE

Of all RCCs, 4–10% of cases will have an extension into the IVC. The stages have been described by Novick which helps to determine the surgical conduct and approach for extensive cases.[14] Individuals with cavoatrial involvement may exhibit significant thrombus-related morbidity and will require heparin medication for anticoagulation before, during, and following surgery. To assess the extent and stage of IVC involvement in the thrombus, comprehensive imaging is required. Typically, CT or magnetic resonance imaging (MRI) are used for this purpose. It is crucial to have current imaging since any thrombus expansion toward the heart during the preoperative period can drastically alter the course of treatment. When imaging retrohepatic tumor thrombus, transesophageal echocardiography (TEE) is very helpful and can provide more detailed information than CT or MRI.

In most cases, a saline-filled balloon will be inserted into the IVC (close to the tumor) to prevent embolization of the tumor and thrombus into the heart, along with angioembolization of the kidney to be removed. The vascular surgeon will usually perform a cavotomy after a chevron or roof-top incision and dissection onto the renal bed. This can only be carried out once the tumor is under control from both above and below. The tumor from the intra- and retrohepatic portions of the intra-venous catheter will be removed with assistance from a hepatobiliary surgeon. Renal vein and collateral ligation can be facilitated early with kidney preoperative arterial embolization, which minimizes excessive blood loss during surgery. This is associated with angioinfarction syndrome, a group of symptoms that includes fever, nausea, pain, and hypertension. If possible, the angioembolization must be carried out following the induction of anesthesia. In a specially designed hybrid theater, the kidney is angioembolized following the administration of anesthesia for the patient's comfort.

Many patients had IVC filters implanted in the past. This is still done for palliative patients who are not scheduled for surgical tumor removal, even though it is no longer standard procedure. If deemed essential, they ought to be installed 48 hours following the procedure to prevent thrombi from infiltrating the filter.

It is imperative to use a multispecialty approach that includes experts in radiology, anesthesia, urology, vascular, and hepatobiliary diseases. If there is a tumor thrombus that reaches the diaphragm, cardiothoracic input will be necessary. To enable the safe removal of the cancer, the patient will usually require cardiopulmonary bypass for tumors with a level 4 or possibly a level 3 extent. The risks of the procedure (namely, air emboli, stroke, and renal impairment) are balanced against the advantages of better surgical access, less bleeding, and decreased venous return when considering CPBP for level 3 disease. If the cancer adheres to the cava wall, deep hypothermic circulatory arrest may be used in patients with level 4 disease and those who require more technically complex surgery. Occasionally, a tiny sternotomy can be used to access a suprahepatic tumor if it has not progressed to the right atrial mouth. A small pericardial incision is used to control the IVC.[15]

EFFECTS OF DRUGS IN PATIENTS WITH REDUCED RENAL FUNCTION

Most anesthetic drugs are terminated through redistribution and metabolism, and they do not rely on renal excretion. When these drugs undergo biotransformation, they usually become inactive and are excreted in the urine as water-soluble forms of the parent compound. Even if renal excretion is impaired, the accumulation of these products is not harmful. Certain medications pass through the urine unchanged. The kidneys remove most medications, especially the nondepolarizing muscle relaxants. Such agents function by redistribution rather than elimination to cease their activity after a single small dose. Nonetheless, maintenance dosages should be administered with a greater gap between doses and be smaller than for patients with normal renal function. If one is available, a train-of-four nerve stimulator—a clinical monitor of neuromuscular function—should be employed. In contrast, atracurium and cisatracurium are broken down without the need for renal excretion through enzymatic ester hydrolysis and nonenzymatic alkaline degradation (Hofmann elimination), resulting in inactive compounds.[16]

Pseudocholinesterase is the enzyme that breaks down succinylcholine (suxamethonium). While uremia lowers the levels of this enzyme, they are rarely low enough to cause long-term blockage. Administering succinylcholine does raise serum potassium levels, which can be hazardous for patients who already have high potassium levels due to severe renal impairment. Neostigmine and other cholinesterase inhibitors must also be excreted from the body by the kidneys; in people with impaired kidney function, this excretion is postponed to the same extent as that of nondepolarizing muscle relaxants. Thus, "recurarization" should not happen unless there are special circumstances.

Certain drugs like atropine and glycopyrrolate are mostly eliminated from the body through urine without undergoing any changes. However, a one-time dose of these drugs will not cause any significant medical issues.[16] On the other hand, the maintenance dose of digoxin needs to be reduced based on the extent of kidney damage, and regular monitoring of blood levels is the best way to determine the effectiveness of the treatment. The decrease in albumin levels in uremic patients will have an impact on medications that are heavily bound to albumin, such as many induction agents. As a result, the amount of drug that is free in the body increases and the amount needed to cause anesthesia decreases.

Because inhaled anesthetic medicines are eliminated through the respiratory system, decreased kidney function will not affect the way these agents act on the body. This makes them the ideal choice for maintaining anesthesia. Both sevoflurane and enflurane biotransform to inorganic fluoride, although the amounts of fluoride that are created in the plasma are not nephrotoxic. Isoflurane, halothane, and, in particular, desflurane are metabolized by the liver to a much lesser extent and so have no nephrotoxic potential.

Since the liver is the primary site of opioid metabolism, renal disease should not significantly affect the pharmacokinetics or pharmacodynamics of opioids. But meperidine, also known as pethidine, and morphine both contain active metabolites that the kidney excretes and can build up in renal failure. Doses of these two drugs should, therefore, be reduced or limited.

ANESTHESIA

Intraoperative Management

Open or laparoscopic renal surgery typically requires general anesthesia combined with intermittent positive pressure ventilation (IPPV) and muscle relaxation. Because of the patient's posture and the increased intra-abdominal pressure resulting from laparoscopic surgery, endotracheal intubation is recommended. Intravenous or inhalational agents can be used to induce anesthesia; individuals with autonomic neuropathy should undergo a rapid sequence induction. For maintenance, inhalation agents such as halothane, isoflurane, or desflurane are advised. Atracurium and cisatracurium are the preferred long-acting nondepolarizing muscle relaxants of choice, especially for patients with impaired renal function.[17]

The surgical technique plays a role in determining the proper vascular access. A minimum of one wide gauge peripheral intravenous cannula is required for a standard radical nephrectomy (open, laparoscopic, partial, or full) in a patient without significant comorbidities. It is best to place an IV access in the ipsilateral limb to the kidney that is being removed if the patient is to be placed in the lateral position. Intravenous infusions must not be administered through any limb that has a functional arteriovenous fistula. Forearm veins should not be used for venous access in individuals who may eventually require dialysis because they are meant to be preserved for the formation of future fistulae. Invasive arterial cannula insertion enables early identification and management of variations in the patient's hemodynamic condition. A nephrectomy is one of the major surgeries for which many clinicians recommend additional noninvasive CO monitoring. It is becoming increasingly frequent practice to assist in optimizing intravascular fluid treatment through optimization of stroke volume. Real-time information about the existence and degree of IVC involvement is provided by intraoperative TEE in patients having radical nephrectomy for RCC.[18] If a patient undergoing surgery for RCC resection does not have a contraindication to TEE, and there is appropriate equipment and expertise, an intraoperative TEE should be considered in all patients with level II–IV tumor thrombus. The use of TEE can be more effective in patients with greater IVC tumor thrombus extension. Information from TEE frequently impacted surgical decision-making, especially in cases of intracardiac tumor extension.

Positioning

The surgical position for nephrectomy (radical and partial) is the "kidney position." After the administration of general anesthesia, a urinary catheter and orogastric tube are inserted, and the patient is positioned in a lateral, modified flank position at a 45° angle **(Fig. 4)**. The top of the iliac crest should rest at the top of the kidney, and the table should be flexed.[19] Positioning must be considered for open and laparoscopic nephrectomy, with varying degrees of tilt and flexion at the waist in the lateral position. Stretching or compression of the cervical plexus, brachial plexus, and common peroneal nerves can result in neuropathies when the nerves are positioned laterally. Axilla, knees, elbows, and ankles are suitable places with padding. Both shoulders should be in a neutral position, and caution should be used to prevent overly lateral neck stretching. Typically, the upper arm is supported by an armrest. Good padding is required in all pressure areas. To avoid unintentional harm, every functional arteriovenous fistula should be wrapped. The lower leg is often flexed and a pillow is positioned between the legs. To prevent rolling or shifting positions during surgery, the patient should be properly fastened to the table using strapping and back supports.

Position affects the respiratory system profoundly. There is a significant ventilation-perfusion mismatch because the lower lung's ventilation is reduced and its perfusion is raised. Additionally, there are reductions in

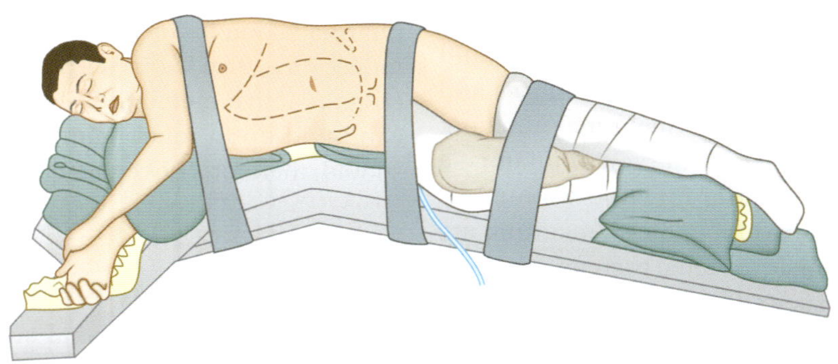

Fig. 4: Modified kidney position.

vital capacity, functional residual capacity, tidal volume, and thoracic compliance. Preexisting respiratory diseases may make these issues worse. Increasing the proportion of inspired oxygen or using a small amount of positive end-expiratory pressure (PEEP) can help patients who are having trouble maintaining low arterial oxygen saturation during the procedure. Lower lung postoperative atelectasis is not unusual. During a laparoscopic procedure, a pneumoperitoneum can worsen breathing and negatively impact the heart's output and venous return, especially if intra-abdominal pressure rises above 20 mm Hg.[10] Consequently, individuals with substantial systolic dysfunction or those with concomitant coronary artery disease and ventricular hypertrophies may not tolerate laparoscopic surgery successfully.

When utilizing a kidney bridge or "breaking" the table, the IVC can get kinked or compressed, especially when it is positioned right lateral, which can lower CO and venous return. Another factor that could reduce venous return is hepatic encroachment on the vena cava and mediastinal displacement. Cardiovascular indicators need to be closely monitored when placing patients.[20]

The basic principles of laparoscopic and robotic radical nephrectomy are similar. A retroperitoneal or intraperitoneal approach can be used for performing robotic-assisted laparoscopic nephrectomy. If a transperitoneal technique is to be used, the patient is positioned in a modified 45° flank position. For patients undergoing a retroperitoneal approach, a full flank position is used.[21]

Monitoring

It is crucial to regularly monitor cardiovascular and respiratory functions during medical procedures, especially due to the potential risks associated with patient positioning. In some cases, invasive monitoring of blood pressure and central venous pressure may be necessary, which depends on the patient's preoperative condition and the surgical risks involved. For tumors involving the IVC, the vessel may need to be cross-clamped to allow for resection.[22] Radical nephrectomy is the standard treatment for locally advanced tumors; however, it may also need venous thrombectomy, temporary blockage of the regional vasculature, and en bloc excision of surrounding organs.[23] Since these circumstances may lead to severe cardiovascular instability and extensive bleeding, it makes sense to establish large-bore peripheral venous access and central venous access. In cases where there is infiltration of the IVC, it may be necessary to use venovenous bypass. Therefore, it is important to involve a perfusionist in the planning of such cases. In addition, it is important to ensure that appropriate blood products are available, and that level 1 infusion equipment and vasopressor medications are prepared. Appropriate thromboprophylaxis should be undertaken.

Regular monitoring of patient temperature and warming is necessary since unintentional perioperative hypothermia (temperature ≤36°C) can lead to wound-healing complications, prolonged hospital stays, and intraoperative hemorrhage.[24] Active warming techniques such as using a forced-air warmer, heated mattress, and warmed IV fluids can be employed early on to help prevent hypothermia. It is essential to manage venous thromboprophylaxis thoroughly, which can be achieved using pneumatic calf compression devices, low molecular weight heparin treatment, and graded stockings.

Pain Management

A combination of general and regional methods is often effective in pain management. Various methods such as wound catheters, local infiltration, paravertebral block, low thoracic epidural analgesia (TEA), transversus abdominis plane block, rectus sheath blocks, quadratus lumborum blocks, and erector spinae blocks are commonly used for pain relief.

Thoracic epidural analgesia is considered the gold standard in upper abdominal surgery.[25-27] However, TEA may be a relative contraindication in open radical nephrectomy and IVC exploration for renal cancer with cavoatrial IVC tumor extension as these subsets of patients often require perioperative anticoagulation and risk developing coagulopathy secondary to massive intraoperative hemorrhage. Various alternative analgesic techniques have emerged recently, including continuous wound catheter analgesia, transversus abdominis plane analgesia, and erector spinae plane analgesia.[28-30] These methods often require the use of patient-controlled analgesia (PCA) with morphine because they are insufficient in providing enough visceral pain relief.[31]

While the efficacy of transversus abdominis plane block and paravertebral blocks in nephrectomy is not clear, they are known to reduce opioid doses without causing the hypotension that is often associated with epidurals.[32] Since the contralateral sympathetic nerve is unaffected by the thoracic paravertebral block, it produces more stable hemodynamics and has a unilateral epidural effect.[33,34]

POSTOPERATIVE CONSIDERATIONS

Critical Care Admission

Due to the complexity of these patients, it is recommended to schedule elective admission to the critical care unit. This will allow for close monitoring of cardiovascular and renal physiology after surgery.

Postoperative Renal Impairment

Chronic kidney disease is more common after radical nephrectomy than partial nephrectomy, even if the contralateral kidney and preoperative serum creatinine levels are normal.[35] Radical surgery increases the risk for chronic kidney disease compared to partial nephrectomy. It is recommended to use drugs that do not undergo renal excretion or metabolism in the perioperative period, regardless of preoperative serum creatinine concentration.

The management of patients before, during, and after a nephrectomy can vary significantly depending on the specific disease and patient group. As such, the anesthetist must be aware of the various surgical approaches available and ready to assist surgical colleagues and patients in deciding on the best approach based on the findings from preoperative assessment and staging of malignant disease. These findings help to guide preoperative optimization, referral to other specialized departments, determine the optimal timing of surgery, and allow the team to provide an individualized approach for each patient. Nephrectomy is still a potentially difficult case for the anesthesiologist since comprehensive imaging, MDT discussion, and preoperative preparation are typically required between various specialties.

CONCLUSION

In summary, a comprehensive understanding of the kidney's physiology and pathophysiology, the potential effects of the disease and surgical interventions on these functions, and the systemic effects of renal dysfunction are necessary for the difficult anesthetic management of patients undergoing renal cancer surgery, including radical and nephron-sparing nephrectomies. The necessity to take into account the effects of any medications that patients may be taking for RCC, the changed pharmacokinetics and pharmacodynamics of anesthetic agents in patients with RCC, and the effect of surgical stress on kidney function all add to this complexity. A thorough preoperative evaluation, accurate intraoperative treatment with careful monitoring and timely intervention for hemodynamic abnormalities, and attentive postoperative care—often in a critical care setting—are all necessary to provide the best possible patient outcomes. The anesthetist is central to ensuring familiarity with various surgical approaches and collaborating effectively with the surgical team to provide individualized care plans tailored to the individual patient, their RCC treatment regimen, and the surgical context.

REFERENCES

1. Ferlay J, Colombet M, Soerjomataram I, Parkin DM, Piñeros M, Znaor A, et al. Cancer statistics for the year 2020: An overview. Int J Cancer. 2021. Online ahead of print.
2. Bray F, Colombet M, Mery L, Piñeros M, Znaor A, Zanetti R, et al. Cancer Incidence in Five Continents, Vol. XI. IARC Scientific Publication No. 166. Lyon: International Agency for Research on Cancer; 2021.
3. Ervik M, Lam F, Laversanne M, Ferlay J, Bray F. Global Cancer Observatory: Cancer Over Time. Lyon, France: International Agency for Research on Cancer; 2020.
4. Nguyen MM, Gill IS, Ellison LM. The evolving presentation of renal carcinoma in the United States: trends from the Surveillance, Epidemiology, and End Results program. J Urol. 2006;176:2397-400.
5. Chow WH, Dong LM, Devesa SS. Epidemiology and risk factors for kidney cancer. Nat Rev Urol. 2010;7(5):245-57.
6. Robson CJ, Churchill BM, Anderson W. The results of radical nephrectomy for renal cell carcinoma. J Urol. 1969;101:297-301.
7. Haga N, Onagi A, Koguchi T, Hoshi S, Ogawa S, Akaihata H, et al. Perioperative Detection of Circulating Tumor Cells in Radical or Partial Nephrectomy for Renal Cell Carcinoma. Ann Surg Oncol. 2020;27(4):1272-81.
8. Mühlbauer J, Kowalewski KF, Walach MT, Porubsky S, Wessels F, Nuhn P, et al. Partial nephrectomy preserves renal function without increasing the risk of complications compared with radical nephrectomy for renal cell carcinomas of stages pT2-3a. Int J Urol. 2020;27(10):906-13.
9. NICE. (2005). Laparoscopic nephrectomy (including nephroureterectomy). [online] Available from https://www.nice.org.uk/guidance/ipg136. [Last accessed February, 2025]
10. Conacher ID, Soomro NA, Rix D. Anaesthesia for laparoscopic urological surgery. Br J Anaesth. 2004;93:859-64.
11. Cormier JN, Pollock RE. Principles of surgical cancer care. In: Shaw A, Riedel B, Burton A, Fields A, Feeley T (Eds). Acute Care of the Cancer Patient. London, UK: Taylor and Francis Group; 2005. pp. 17-30.
12. Nixon DW, Heymsfield SB, Cohen AE, Kutner MH, Ansley J, Lawson DH, et al. Protein-calorie undernutrition in hospitalized cancer patients. Am J Med. 1980;68:683-90.
13. Tisdale MJ. Biology of cachexia. J Natl Cancer Inst. 1997; 89:1763.
14. Novick AC, Kaye MC, Cosgrove DM, Angermeier K, Pontes JE, Montie JE, et al. Experience with cardiopulmonary

bypass and deep hypothermic circulatory arrest in the management of retroperitoneal tumors with large vena cava thrombi. Ann Surg. 1990;212(4):472-6.

15. Chapman E, Pichel AC. Anaesthesia for nephrectomy. BJA Educ. 2016;16:98-101.
16. Ofuru V, Abhulimen V. Surgical Haematuria: An Analysis of Causes in a Southern Nigerian State. Open J Urol. 2022; 12:401-9.
17. Rossi SH, Tanaka H, Usher-Smith JA, Bernhard JC, Fujii Y, Stewart GD. Kidney Cancer Screening and Epidemiology. Soc Int Urol J. 2022;3(6):371-85.
18. Kostibas MP, Arora V, Gorin MA, Ball MW, Pierorazio PM, Allaf ME, et al. Defining the Role of Intraoperative Transesophageal Echocardiography During Radical Nephrectomy with Inferior Vena Cava Tumor Thrombectomy for Renal Cell Carcinoma. Urology. 2017; 107:161-5.
19. Arain MR, Buggy DJ. Anaesthesia for cancer patients. Curr Opin Anaesthesiol. 2007;20:247-53.
20. Hart EM. (2006). Anaesthesia for Renal Surgery. [online] Available from https://resources.wfsahq.org/atotw/anaesthesia-for-renal-surgery/. [Last accessed February, 2025]
21. Krambeck AE, Gettman MT. Robotic renal surgery: radical and partial nephrectomy. Urol Robot Surg. 2007;60:462-70.
22. Munn J. Urological surgery. In: Allman KG, Wilson IH (Eds). Oxford Handbook of Anaesthesia, 2nd edition. Oxford, UK: Oxford University Press; 2007. pp. 566-86.
23. Rini BI, Campbell SC, Escudier B. Renal cell carcinoma. Lancet. 2009;373:1119-32.
24. Rajagopalan S, Mascha E, Na J, Sessler DI. The effects of mild perioperative hypothermia on blood loss and transfusion requirement. Anesthesiology. 2008;108:71-7.
25. Rawal N. Epidural technique for postoperative pain: gold standard no more? Reg Anesth Pain Med. 2012;37:310-7.
26. Weiss R, Pöpping DM. Is epidural analgesia still a viable option for enhanced recovery after abdominal surgery. Curr Opin Anesthesiol. 2018;31:622-9.
27. Ahn JH, Ahn HJ. Effect of thoracic epidural analgesia on recovery of bowel function after major upper abdominal surgery. J Clin Anesth. 2016;34:247-52.
28. Niraj G, Kelkar A, Jeyapalan I, Graff-Baker P, Williams O, Darbar A, et al. Comparison of analgesic efficacy of subcostal transversus abdominis plane blocks with epidural analgesia following upper abdominal surgery. Anaesthesia. 2011;66:465-71.
29. Liu SS, Richman JM, Thirlby RC, Wu CL. Efficacy of continuous wound catheters delivering local anesthetic for postoperative analgesia: a quantitative and qualitative systematic review of randomized controlled trials. J Am Coll Surg. 2006;203:914-32.
30. Tariq Z, Niraj G. Continuous erector spinae plane (ESP) analgesia in different open abdominal surgeries: a case series. J Anesth Surg. 2018;5:57-60.
31. Warusawitharana C, Tariq Z, Jackson B, Niraj G. Continuous erector spinae plane and intrathecal opioid analgesia: novel regimen avoiding thoracic epidural analgesia and systemic morphine in open radical cystectomy: a case series. A Pract. 2019;12:212-4.
32. Yin G, Li Y, Wei P, Ma X, Li B, Gan G, et al. Analgesic effect of the ultrasound-guided thoracolumbar paravertebral block in patients undergoing robot-assisted laparoscopic nephrectomy: a randomized controlled trial. BMC Anesthesiol. 2024;24:69.
33. Ardon AE, Lee J, Franco CD, Riutort KT, Greengrass RA. Paravertebral block: anatomy and relevant safety issues. Korean J Anesthesiol. 2020;73(5):394-400.
34. Zhen SQ, Jin M, Chen YX, Li JH, Wang H, Chen HX. Ultrasound-guided paravertebral nerve block anesthesia on the stress response and hemodynamics among lung cancer patients. World J Clin Cases. 2022;10(7):2174-83.
35. Huang WC, Levey AS, Serio AM, Snyder M, Vickers AJ, Raj GV, et al. Chronic kidney disease after nephrectomy in patients with renal cortical tumours: a retrospective cohort study. Lancet Oncol. 2006;7:735-40.

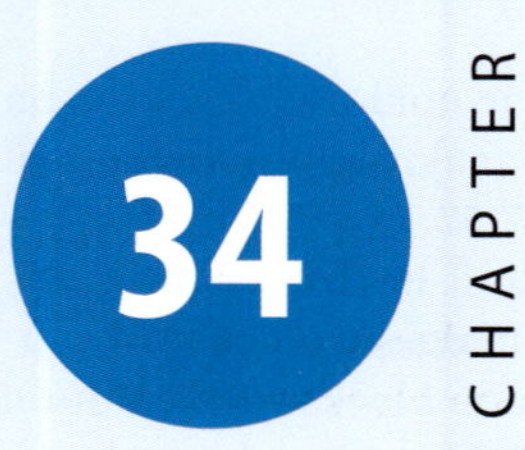

Anesthesia for Prostate Cancers (Robotic Prostatectomy)

Priyanka Sethi, Shayak Roy, Pradeep Kumar Bhatia

INTRODUCTION

Prostate cancer ranks as the primary solid organ malignancy among American men and stands as the second leading cause of cancer-related mortality. Globally, it ranks as the second most prevalent cancer, with an age-standardized rate of 28 per 100,000 males. Radical prostatectomy emerges as a standard treatment for localized prostate carcinoma, displaying a survival advantage over watchful waiting, as evidenced in the SPCG-4 (Scandinavian Prostate Cancer Group Study No. 4) trial. This surgical intervention exhibits a substantial reduction in cancer-specific mortality rates compared to passive monitoring, with decreases of 44% at 10 years, 35% at 12 years, and 38% at 15 years.

Nonetheless, open radical prostatectomy is associated with elevated rates of postoperative complications. Laparoscopic radical prostatectomy was introduced in 1997 with the intention of mitigating morbidity. Initial reports highlighted benefits such as decreased blood loss, shorter hospital stays, and earlier catheter removal compared to open surgery. However, its technical complexity limited widespread adoption among urologists. The advent of the da Vinci Surgical System revolutionized minimally invasive prostatectomy, offering improved ergonomics and a shorter learning curve. Robot-assisted radical prostatectomy (RARP) swiftly gained popularity due to its advantages over laparoscopic techniques. Studies suggest that the robotic system may significantly expedite the learning curve for experienced surgeons transitioning from open to minimally invasive procedures.

Since the Food and Drug Administration (FDA) approval in 2001, RARP has surpassed open prostatectomy as the preferred surgical approach, constituting approximately 80% of all prostatectomies in the US. Despite initial scepticism regarding clinical benefits, nationwide studies have demonstrated superior perioperative outcomes following RARP, including reduced transfusion rates, fewer complications, and shorter hospital stays.

However, robotic-assisted radical prostatectomy (RALP) poses several challenges for the anesthesiologists due to potential complications arising from the Trendelenburg position, pneumoperitoneum, and limited access to the patient during surgery.

PREOPERATIVE OPTIMIZATION OF THE PATIENTS

Preoperative optimization of patients with prostate cancer for robotic prostatectomy involves several steps aimed at maximizing the patient's overall health and reducing the risk of complications during and after surgery.

- *Medical evaluation and patient education:*
  - Conduct a thorough medical history review and physical examination.
  - Educate the patient about the procedure, potential risks, benefits, and postoperative expectations.
- *Diagnostic Workup:*
  - Confirm the diagnosis of prostate cancer through biopsy and staging with imaging studies (MRI, CT scan, and bone scan).
  - Assess the patient's baseline prostate-specific antigen (PSA) levels.
- *Cardiovascular assessment:*
  - Evaluate cardiovascular risk factors and optimize management (hypertension, diabetes, dyslipidemia).
  - Ensure adequate control of cardiac conditions such as coronary artery disease or arrhythmias.
- *Pulmonary evaluation:*
  - Assess respiratory function (PFT), especially in patients with a history of smoking or lung disease.
  - Optimize pulmonary function through smoking cessation, pulmonary rehabilitation, or bronchodilator therapy as necessary.

- *Nutritional assessment:*
  - Evaluate nutritional status and address deficiencies. In one study, it was found that patients who exhibited circulating 25(OH)D levels below 20 ng/mL, were associated with a heightened risk of both prostate-specific mortality and all-cause mortality, particularly within a population primarily of African descent. Interestingly, serum calcium levels did not seem to influence the impact of 25(OH)D on survival outcomes.[1]
  - Consider consultation with a nutritionist or dietitian for dietary optimization, especially in patients with malnutrition or obesity.
  - Prior research indicates a significant association between nutritional factors and the occurrence and progression of prostate cancer. The Geriatric Nutritional Risk Index (GNRI) stands as an objective measure for assessing the nutritional status of individuals aged 65 years and above. Studies have found out that GNRI is an effective and reliable tool for evaluating preoperative nutritional status of prostate cancer patients and it is correlated with postoperative recovery and complications.[2]
- *Medication review:*
  - Review current medications and adjust as necessary, especially anticoagulants and antiplatelet agents.
  - Discontinue medications that may increase bleeding risk, such as nonsteroidal anti-inflammatory drugs (NSAIDs) and herbal supplements.
- *Anemia management:*
  - Correct anemia preoperatively through iron supplementation, erythropoietin therapy, or blood transfusions, if indicated.
  - Optimize hemoglobin levels to reduce the risk of perioperative complications.
- *Infection control:*
  - Screen for and treat any active infections prior to surgery.
  - Consider perioperative antibiotic prophylaxis to reduce the risk of surgical site infections.
- *Urinary function assessment:*
  - Evaluate baseline urinary function and address any underlying issues such as benign prostatic hyperplasia (BPH) or urinary retention.
  - Consider urodynamic testing in patients with lower urinary tract symptoms (LUTS).
- *Psychosocial support:*
  - Assess the patient's psychosocial well-being and provide appropriate support and counseling.
  - Consider referral to a psychologist or support group for coping strategies and emotional support.
- *Prehabilitation:*
  - Implement preoperative exercise programs to improve physical fitness and enhance recovery.
  - Encourage smoking cessation, alcohol moderation, and stress-reduction techniques.
  - Initial evidence suggests that multimodal prehabilitation shows promise in preserving functional capacity following radical prostatectomy. However, the current literature indicates that outcomes such as complications and length of stay do not appear to be significantly impacted by prehabilitation interventions.[3]
- *Optimize diabetes control:* Ensure optimal glycemic control in diabetic patients through medication adjustments, dietary modifications, and close monitoring of blood glucose levels.
- *Thromboprophylaxis:* Assess the patient's risk of venous thromboembolism (VTE) and implement appropriate thromboprophylaxis measures, such as mechanical compression devices or pharmacological prophylaxis.
- *Multidisciplinary approach:* Collaborate with an interdisciplinary team including urologists, anesthesiologists, internists, and other specialists to optimize patient care.
- *Preoperative counseling:* Provide detailed preoperative counseling regarding the robotic prostatectomy procedure, including potential risks, benefits, and postoperative expectations.

By systematically addressing these aspects, the preoperative optimization process aims to improve patient outcomes, minimize complications, and enhance the overall success of robotic prostatectomy for prostate cancer.

INTRAOPERATIVE CONTINUATION OF OPTIMIZATION PROTOCOL

Enhanced recovery after surgery (ERAS) protocols aim to optimize perioperative care to facilitate faster recovery (shorter length of stay in hospitals) and reduce complications.[4] Here's an outline of intraoperative anesthesia management for robotic prostatectomy following ERAS criteria:

- *Preoperative optimization:*
  - Ensure preoperative assessment and optimization of comorbidities such as cardiovascular and pulmonary conditions as mentioned previously.
  - Preemptive management of pain and anxiety through patient education, multimodal analgesia, and anxiolytics is considered, if necessary.
- *Preoperative fasting:* Follow ERAS guidelines for preoperative fasting, allowing clear fluids up to 2 hours before induction of anesthesia to prevent dehydration and improve patient comfort.
- *Anesthetic technique:*
  - Utilize balanced anesthesia techniques combining inhalational agents (e.g., sevoflurane) or total intravenous anesthesia (TIVA) with short-acting opioids and adjunctive agents. However, recent literature fails to demonstrate which anesthetic technique is superior—TIVA or inhalational—with respect to perioperative outcomes in robotic prostate surgery.[5]
  - Consider regional anesthesia techniques such as epidural or spinal anesthesia for intraoperative and postoperative pain management. One meta-analysis found no association between the type of anesthesia/analgesia and oncologic outcomes, including biochemical recurrence-free survival. However, an interesting observation was made regarding the reduced risk of mortality associated with the use of regional anesthesia.[6]
  - During and after surgery, numerous factors contribute to whether tumor cells released during primary tumor resection will lead to cancer metastasis and progression. While regional anesthesia, analgesia, or both are unlikely to be the primary determinants of perioperative cancer progression, they can play a role as a small part of the overall equation, particularly for certain cancers. However, their use may help mitigate exposure to other factors that could contribute to cancer progression, such as stress hormone release, uncontrolled or poorly controlled pain, and exposure to volatile anesthetics and opioids. Implementing multimodal perioperative pain regimens that include regional anesthesia alongside other protective measures, such as nonsteroidal anti-inflammatory drugs (NSAIDs), may offer additional benefits. By combining regional anesthesia with other interventions known to reduce perioperative stress and inflammation, healthcare providers can potentially create a more conducive perioperative environment that minimizes the risk of cancer progression and optimizes patient outcomes.[7]
- *Positioning concerns:*
  - The Trendelenburg position during Robot-assisted laparoscopic prostatectomy (RALP) is associated with elevated intraocular pressure (IOP). There is a notable increase in IOP shortly after assuming the Trendelenburg position, with the magnitude of this increase decreasing to a moderate level 90 minutes afterward. Upon returning to the supine position, the IOP at 30 minutes post repositioning returns to levels observed before anesthesia induction.[8]
  - Low-quality evidence was found suggesting that an increase in intraocular pressure (IOP) after pneumoperitoneum and steep Trendelenburg positioning may be prevented by propofol compared with sevoflurane with increased IOP from baseline to 30 minutes in steep Trendelenburg. However, it is unclear whether this surrogate outcome translates directly to clinical avoidance of ocular complications during surgery. No studies addressed the secondary outcomes of adverse effects, all-cause mortality, respiratory or circulatory complications, cognitive dysfunction, length of stay, or cost.[5]
  - Intracranial pressure increases by impairing venous blood outflow due to robotic surgery and head-down tilt. Postoperative cognitive disorders are more likely to develop in elderly patients, who commonly undergo prostatectomy. Therefore, cognitive decline after surgery could be influenced significantly by increased intracranial pressure. After head-down tilt, intracranial compliance rapidly decreases despite normal vital signs, low lung pressure, and adequate anesthesia depth. The conclusion drawn is that intraoperative intracranial compliance monitoring is warranted since major changes in cerebral compliance occur during surgery, potentially enabling early identification and treatment of impaired cerebral compliance.[9]
- *Hemodynamic management:*
  - Maintain hemodynamic stability with careful titration of intravenous fluids and vasopressors

as needed to prevent hypotension and ensure adequate tissue perfusion.

- Utilize goal-directed fluid therapy to optimize intravascular volume status and minimize fluid overload.
- In a recent study, which compared outcomes between RARP and standard laparoscopic radical prostatectomy (LRP), RARP showed longer anesthesia, operation, and gas insufflation times, along with higher PCA bolus counts and analgesic volumes postoperatively compared to LRP. However, there were no significant differences in estimated blood loss. The findings suggest that while RARP may require more anesthesia and analgesia initially, LRP performs similarly in terms of anesthesia once operation time and port numbers are optimized.[10]
- In one study, it was observed that significant alterations in the hemodynamic parameters of 51 men undergoing robot-assisted laparoscopic prostatectomy (RALP), both intraoperatively and in the postoperative recovery room. The key findings include: (1) Notable changes in all hemodynamic parameters such as global end-diastolic volume index (GEDI), central venous pressure (CVP), systemic vascular resistance (SVR), Cardiac Index (CI), global ejection fraction (GEF), stroke volume variation (SVV), except extravascular lung water index (ELWI) during RALP compared to baseline; (2) increased cardiac contractility during RALP, peaking in the recovery room; (3) significant elevation in cardiac preload during RALP; and (4) 5.9% of patients experienced adverse cardiac events characterized by elevated troponin levels.[11]

- *Temperature management:* Employ active intraoperative temperature management strategies such as forced-air warming blankets or intravenous fluid warming to maintain normothermia and prevent perioperative hypothermia.
- *Pain management:* Implement multimodal analgesia techniques combining opioids with regional anesthesia (if applicable), nonsteroidal anti-inflammatory drugs (NSAIDs), acetaminophen, and/or local anesthetics to minimize opioid consumption and reduce postoperative pain.
    - Utilize epidural or regional nerve blocks for targeted pain relief and enhanced recovery.
- *Nausea and vomiting prophylaxis:*
    - Administer prophylactic antiemetic medications (e.g., ondansetron, dexamethasone) to reduce the incidence of postoperative nausea and vomiting.
    - Low-quality evidence suggests that postoperative nausea and vomiting (PONV) may be reduced over the short term (1–6 hours after surgery) after RARP by TIVA when compared with inhalational anesthesia (sevoflurane and desflurane).[5]
- *Neuromuscular blockade management:* Monitor neuromuscular blockade depth using train-of-four (TOF) monitoring and titrate neuromuscular blocking agents to achieve optimal muscle relaxation while minimizing residual blockade.
- *Optimization of fluid balance:* Employ restrictive fluid management strategies to minimize intraoperative fluid overload and reduce the risk of complications such as pulmonary edema and delayed recovery.
- *Minimizing opioid use:*
    - Emphasize opioid-sparing analgesic techniques to minimize opioid-related side effects such as respiratory depression, nausea, and ileus.
    - In a quality-improvement project to assess the feasibility of reducing or eliminating opioid use following RALP, it was noted that following the implementation of opioid-free pathway, the mean patient-reported pain score on each postoperative day was lower, indicating effective pain management without the need for opioids. Additionally, fewer postoperative complications were observed in the opioid-free pathway. Importantly, there was no statistically significant difference in the number of emergency room visits or readmissions within 3 weeks of surgery between the two pathways. These findings suggest that local anesthetic infiltration and non-narcotic pain medications can safely reduce or eliminate opioid use following RALP while maintaining adequate pain control. This approach not only benefits patients by minimizing opioid-related side effects but also potentially reduces the risk of opioid dependence and improves overall postoperative recovery.[12]
- *Perioperative normoglycemia:* Maintain perioperative euglycemia through careful glucose monitoring and insulin administration in diabetic patients to reduce the risk of surgical site infections and improve wound healing.

- *Postoperative extubation:* Aim for early extubation in the postanesthesia care unit (PACU) to facilitate early ambulation and expedite recovery.

By adhering to these intraoperative anesthesia management principles aligned with ERAS criteria, healthcare providers can contribute to optimized perioperative care and improved outcomes following robotic prostatectomy.

POSTOPERATIVE CRITICAL CARE MANAGEMENT IN ICU OR RECOVERY ROOM

Immediate Complications Monitoring

- Vigilant observation for postsurgical complications such as bleeding, infection, and adverse reactions to anesthesia.
- In 0.7% of patients undergoing longer procedures in the Trendelenburg position, there is a risk of developing airway edema and subsequent respiratory distress.
- Pressure support ventilation during emergence from general anesthesia demonstrated a reduced occurrence of postoperative atelectasis in comparison to spontaneous respiration with intermittent manual assistance in RALP.[13]
- The incidence of corneal abrasions (CA) has risen from 2000 to 2011 in radical prostatectomy procedures. Both laparoscopy and robotic assistance seem to independently contribute to this increased risk. Factors such as age, the presence of chronic conditions, and race influence the risk of CA. With the expanding utilization of robotic assistance, clinicians need to remain vigilant and implement strategies to reduce the occurrence of these eye injuries during the perioperative period. Additionally, efforts should be made to identify the underlying factors contributing to CA.[14]

Continuous Vital Signs Monitoring

Close monitoring is done for vital signs such as blood pressure, heart rate, and oxygen saturation to detect any signs of distress promptly.

Assessment for Surgical Complications

- Evaluation for potential complications specific to robotic prostatectomy, including nerve damage, urinary retention, and bowel dysfunction.
- Nerve-sparing technique is a viable option during RALP surgeries, particularly beneficial for long-term outcomes such as urinary continence and erectile function recovery, even in patients with high-risk prostate cancer. This approach is associated with improved oncological outcomes and enhances the quality of life for these patients up to 12 months postsurgery. The findings underscore the significance of nerve sparing in actively supporting the comprehensive treatment of high-risk prostate cancer.[15]

Effective Pain Management

Tailored pain management strategies are required to ensure patient comfort while minimizing the risk of complications such as respiratory depression. Postoperative pain following RALP can manifest as incisional discomfort, shoulder pain, and visceral pain. Despite its prevalence, the precise mechanism behind postoperative shoulder pain following laparoscopic surgery remains elusive. It is hypothesized that this pain may be linked to residual CO_2 remaining after pneumoperitoneum, although research indicates that warming the insufflation gas or utilizing lower insufflation pressures might help mitigate the incidence of shoulder pain. These interventions likely alleviate peritoneal irritation, consequently reducing shoulder discomfort.

PROcedure SPECific Postoperative Pain ManagemenT *(PROSPECT) guideline* for prostate surgery recommends as follows:

- Systemic analgesia should include paracetamol and either selective or nonselective nonsteroidal anti-inflammatory drugs. These should be administered preoperatively, intraoperatively, and postoperatively.
- Local wound infiltration should routinely be used for open surgery, provided intravenous lidocaine is not utilized, before other regional analgesia blocks.
- Continuous intravenous lidocaine is recommended during open surgery. Its use contraindicates concurrent infiltration with local anesthetics.
- Transversus abdominis plane (TAP) block is recommended as the primary choice for laparoscopic or robotic radical prostatectomy.
- Opioids should serve as rescue analgesics during the postoperative period.[16]

Early Mobilization

- Encourage early mobilization to prevent complications such as deep vein thrombosis and promote faster recovery.

- Laparoscopic prostatectomy has the potential to activate the clotting system, thereby influencing the risk of perioperative thrombosis in patients with prostate cancer. Additionally, Both total intravenous anesthesia with target-controlled infusion (TIVA-TCI) and balanced inhalational anesthesia patients exhibited a significant increase in procoagulant factors and a subsequent reduction in hemostatic system inhibitors during the early postoperative period. Furthermore, the use of robotics during surgery was associated with a notable increase in prothrombotic markers compared to laparoscopy alone. These findings support the adoption of perioperative thromboembolic prophylaxis in these patients.[17]

Hydration and nutrition support provide adequate hydration and nutrition support to facilitate healing and minimize postoperative complications.

Collaborative care: Regularly communicate and collaborate among surgical teams, anesthesia providers, and nursing staff to address concerns promptly and optimize patient outcomes.

RECENT EVIDENCES AND CONCERNS

- Mounting evidence indicates that ion channels and pumps are pivotal in regulating prostate cancer cell proliferation, evasion of apoptosis, invasion, and migration. These components emerge as potential targets for diagnosing, staging, and treating prostate cancer. Nevertheless, further research is required before these insights can be applied practically.[18]
- The integration of robotic technologies in urology presents both promise and ethical concerns. While accessibility, safety, and learning curve advancements make it feasible and economically viable, cost discrepancies and safety issues persist. Gender disparities in access require further investigation. Critical evaluation of evidence is essential to ensure ethical implementation and optimize outcomes in robotic urological surgery.[19]
- The viability of epidural anesthesia in patients undergoing transvesical single-port (SP) robotic radical and simple prostatectomy has also been assessed.[20] All procedures were completed successfully without additional ports, open conversion, or conversion to general anesthesia. There were no significant surgical interruptions, and movement-related interruptions were brief. No anesthesia-related complications were observed, and postoperative outcomes were favorable, with minimal opioid use and same-day discharges for most patients. The study suggests that epidural anesthesia without mechanical ventilation is safe and feasible for selected patients undergoing transvesical SP robotic prostatectomy, with no compromise in perioperative outcomes.[20]
- Tranexamic acid (TXA) effectively decreases intraoperative blood loss and transfusion requirements in prostate surgeries without raising the risk of deep vein thrombosis (DVT) and pulmonary embolism (PE).[21]
- Isoflurane enhances hypoxia-inducible factor-1a (HIF1a) expression in prostate cancer cells through the PI3K/AKT/mTOR pathway, resulting in heightened angiogenesis, proliferation, and chemoresistance markers. Conversely, the addition of propofol to isoflurane treatment counteracts these effects by inhibiting AKT phosphorylation. These findings contribute to the growing body of preclinical evidence suggesting that anesthetics directly impact cancer cell biology. Importantly, this research highlights the divergent effects of commonly used agents on HIF-1a and its associated actions, influencing malignant progression.[22]
- Biochemical recurrence rates and biochemical recurrence-free survival in patients with intermediate and high D'Amico risk after prostatectomy are not modified by opioids.[23]
- The association of perioperative allogeneic blood transfusion in patients with prostate cancer who underwent prostatectomy demonstrated that the use of allogeneic blood was not associated with systemic tumor progression, prostate cancer-specific death, or all-cause death.[24]
- Robotic-assisted perineal prostatectomy (RAPP) presents a novel surgical approach, particularly beneficial for prostate cancer patients with a history of intraabdominal surgery. A comparison between RAPP and RALP revealed shorter anesthesia, surgery, and insufflation times in RAPP patients. However, RAPP patients exhibited higher blood pCO_2 levels and a more pronounced decrease in pH 30 and 60 minutes after perineal CO_2 insufflation. Mean arterial pressures, driving pressure, and Ppeak and plateau values were significantly higher in RALP patients, particularly 60 minutes after insufflation, while static and dynamic lung compliance values were lower. These findings suggest that perineal CO_2 insufflation plays a pivotal

role in elevating CO_2 levels, despite the less pronounced impact on respiratory mechanics in RAPP patients due to their challenging lung position. Considering these alterations, especially the sudden rise in CO_2 levels, close monitoring and prompt intervention by anesthesiologists are crucial to maintain clinically safe conditions throughout the procedure.[25]

PRACTICE PRESCRIPTION (BASED ON EVIDENCE FROM PROTOCOLS/ GUIDELINE REFERENCES)

Prostate cancer surgery, particularly robotic prostatectomy, presents unique challenges and considerations in anesthesia management. Understanding the physiological mechanisms and scientific rationale behind anesthesia strategies is crucial for optimizing patient outcomes in this context.

Surgical Stress Response

Prostate cancer surgery triggers a significant stress response characterized by neuroendocrine, metabolic, and immune system activation. Anesthesia plays a pivotal role in modulating this response to minimize perioperative complications and improve patient recovery. Techniques such as balanced anesthesia, incorporating multimodal analgesia, and regional anesthesia help attenuate the stress response by reducing intraoperative opioid requirements and promoting early recovery.

Hemodynamic Stability

Maintaining hemodynamic stability during robotic prostatectomy is essential to ensure adequate tissue perfusion and oxygenation. Anesthesia techniques should aim to achieve smooth induction and maintenance of anesthesia while minimizing fluctuations in blood pressure and heart rate. Utilizing agents with rapid onset and offset, such as short-acting intravenous anesthetics and neuromuscular blockers, facilitates precise control of anesthesia depth and muscle relaxation, contributing to hemodynamic stability.

Pain Management

Effective pain management is paramount for optimizing patient comfort and facilitating early mobilization and recovery. A multimodal approach to analgesia, combining systemic opioids with local/regional techniques such as epidural analgesia or peripheral nerve blocks, offers superior pain control while minimizing opioid-related side effects. Regional anesthesia techniques, such as thoracic epidural analgesia or TAP blocks, provide targeted pain relief and may reduce the need for systemic opioids postoperatively.

Minimizing Complications

Anesthesia strategies should aim to minimize perioperative complications associated with robotic prostatectomy, including respiratory depression, postoperative nausea and vomiting (PONV), and urinary retention. Selecting appropriate anesthetic agents and techniques, optimizing fluid management, and implementing preventive measures such as antiemetic prophylaxis contribute to reducing the incidence of complications. Close collaboration between the anesthesia team, surgeons, and perioperative care providers is essential for comprehensive management and early detection of potential complications.

Neuroendocrine and Immunomodulatory Effects

Anesthesia has profound effects on the neuroendocrine and immune systems, which play key roles in the body's response to surgical stress and recovery. Strategies such as TIVA or volatile anesthetic agents may differentially influence neuroendocrine and immunomodulatory pathways, potentially impacting patient outcomes. Understanding the complex interplay between anesthesia, surgical stress and immune function is critical for optimizing perioperative care and long-term oncological outcomes in patients undergoing prostate cancer surgery.

CONCLUSION

The physiological responses to anesthesia during robotic prostatectomy are multifaceted, encompassing modulation of the stress response, maintenance of hemodynamic stability, effective pain management, complication prevention, and modulation of neuroendocrine and immunomodulatory pathways. Anesthesia strategies tailored to address these physiological considerations are essential for optimizing patient outcomes and facilitating successful perioperative management in this patient population.

REFERENCES

1. McGrowder D, Tulloch-Reid MK, Coard KCM, McCaw-Binns AM, Ferguson TS, Aiken W, et al. Vitamin D deficiency at diagnosis increases all-cause and prostate

cancer-specific mortality in jamaican Men. Cancer Control J Moffitt Cancer Cent. 2022;29:10732748221131225.

2. Shu W, Tao W, Chunyan H, Jie F, Yuan L, Yan X, et al. Preoperative nutritional evaluation of prostate cancer patients undergoing laparoscopic radical prostatectomy. PloS One. 2022;17(2):e0262630.
3. Minnella EM, Carli F, Kassouf W. Role of prehabilitation following major uro-oncologic surgery: a narrative review. World J Urol. 2022;40(6):1289-98.
4. Xu Y, Liu A, Chen L, Huang H, Gao Y, Zhang C, et al. Enhanced recovery after surgery (ERAS) pathway optimizes outcomes and costs for minimally invasive radical prostatectomy. J Int Med Res. 2020;48(6):300060520920072.
5. Herling SF, Dreijer B, Wrist Lam G, Thomsen T, Møller AM. Total intravenous anaesthesia versus inhalational anaesthesia for adults undergoing transabdominal robotic assisted laparoscopic surgery. Cochrane Database Syst Rev. 2017;4(4):CD011387.
6. Lee BM, Singh Ghotra V, Karam JA, Hernandez M, Pratt G, Cata JP. Regional anesthesia/analgesia and the risk of cancer recurrence and mortality after prostatectomy: a meta-analysis. Pain Manag. 2015;5(5):387-95.
7. Tedore T. Regional anaesthesia and analgesia: relationship to cancer recurrence and survival. Br J Anaesth. 2015;115 Suppl 2:ii34-45.
8. Kondo Y, Echigo N, Mihara T, Koyama Y, Takahashi K, Okamura K, et al. Intraocular pressure during robotic-assisted laparoscopic prostatectomy: a prospective observational study. Braz J Anesthesiol Elsevier. 2021; 71(6):618-22.
9. Saba GT, Quintão VC, Zeferino SP, Simões CM, Coelho RF, Fazoli A, et al. Noninvasive intracranial pressure real-time waveform analysis monitor during prostatectomy robotic surgery and Trendelenburg position: case report. Braz J Anesthesiol. 2021;71(6):656-9.
10. Lee D, Hwang BY, Kwon JY, Kim O, Hong JM, Kim HJ. A study of 57 patients with prostate cancer to compare outcomes of estimated blood loss and postoperative pain between robot-assisted laparoscopic radical prostatectomy and standard laparoscopic radical prostatectomy. Med Sci Monit Int Med J Exp Clin Res. 2023;29:e939584.
11. Pawlik MT, Prasser C, Zeman F, Harth M, Burger M, Denzinger S, et al. Pronounced haemodynamic changes during and after robotic-assisted laparoscopic prostatectomy: a prospective observational study. BMJ Open. 2020;10(10):e038045.
12. Horodyski L, Ball B, Emile C, Rhodes A, Miao F, Reis IM, et al. Safe transition to opioid-free pathway after robotic-assisted laparoscopic prostatectomy. J Robot Surg. 2022; 16(2):307-14.
13. Jeong H, Tanatporn P, Ahn HJ, Yang M, Kim JA, Yeo H, et al. Pressure support versus spontaneous ventilation during anesthetic emergence-effect on postoperative atelectasis: A randomized controlled trial. Anesthesiology. 2021;135(6):1004-14.
14. Sampat A, Parakati I, Kunnavakkam R, Glick DB, Lee NK, Tenney M, et al. Corneal abrasion in hysterectomy and prostatectomy: role of laparoscopic and robotic assistance. Anesthesiology. 2015;122(5):994-1001.
15. Liu Y, Deng XZ, Qin J, Wen Z, Jiang Y, Huang J, et al. Erectile function, urinary continence and oncologic outcomes of neurovascular bundle sparing robot-assisted radical prostatectomy for high-risk prostate cancer: A systematic review and meta-analysis. Front Oncol. 2023;13:1161544.
16. Lemoine A, Witdouck A, Beloeil H, Bonnet F; PROSPECT Working Group Of The European Society Of Regional Anaesthesia And Pain Therapy (ESRA). PROSPECT guidelines update for evidence-based pain management after prostatectomy for cancer. Anaesth Crit Care Pain Med. 2021;40(4):100922.
17. Sofra M, Antenucci A, Gallucci M, Mandoj C, Papalia R, Claroni C, et al. Perioperative changes in pro and anti-coagulant factors in prostate cancer patients undergoing laparoscopic and robotic radical prostatectomy with different anaesthetic techniques. J Exp Clin Cancer Res CR. 2014;33(1):63.
18. Sakellakis M, Chalkias A. The role of ion channels in the development and progression of prostate cancer. Mol Diagn Ther. 2023;27(2):227-42.
19. Esperto F, Prata F, Antonelli A, Alloni R, Campanozzi L, Cataldo R, et al. Bioethical implications of robotic surgery in urology: A systematic review. Minerva Urol Nephrol. 2021;73(6):700-10.
20. Kaouk J, Ferguson E, Ramos-Carpinteyro R, Chavali J, Geskin A, Cummings KC, et al. Transvesical percutaneous access allows for epidural anesthesia without mechanical ventilation in single-port robotic radical and simple prostatectomy. Urology. 2023;175:209-15.
21. Longo MA, Cavalheiro BT, de Oliveira Filho GR. Systematic review and meta-analyses of tranexamic acid use for bleeding reduction in prostate surgery. J Clin Anesth. 2018;48:32-8.
22. Huang H, Benzonana LL, Zhao H, Watts HR, Perry NJS, Bevan C, et al. Prostate cancer cell malignancy via modulation of HIF-1α pathway with isoflurane and propofol alone and in combination. Br J Cancer. 2014;111(7): 1338–49.
23. Rangel FP, Auler JOC, Carmona MJC, Cordeiro MD, Nahas WC, Coelho RF, et al. Opioids and premature biochemical recurrence of prostate cancer: a randomised prospective clinical trial. Br J Anaesth. 2021;126(5):931-9.
24. Yeoh TY, Scavonetto F, Weingarten TN, Karnes RJ, van Buskirk CM, Hanson AC, et al. Perioperative allogeneic nonleukoreduced blood transfusion and prostate cancer outcomes after radical prostatectomy. Transfusion (Paris). 2014;54(9):2175-81.
25. Emir NS, Akyol D, Sabaz MS, Karadağ S. Robotic assited perineal prostatectomy (RAPP) as a new era for anesthesiology: It's effects on hemodynamic parameters and respiratory mechanics. J Robot Surg. 2023;17(3):933-40.

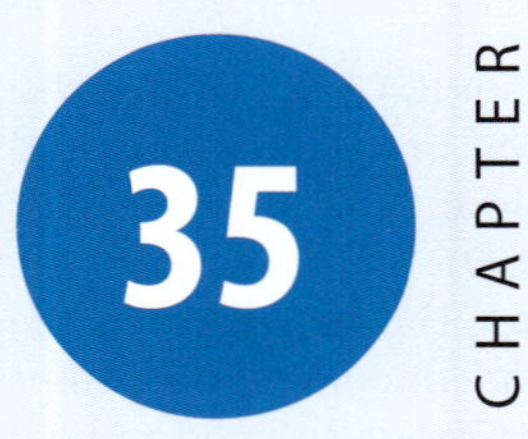

Anesthesia for Bladder Tumor Surgeries

Lalit Gupta, Lovenish Bains

INTRODUCTION

India faces a major health challenge in the form of cancer. In 2022, it was estimated that around 1.46 million new cases of cancer were reported in the country. Bladder cancer ranks as the 9th most prevalent type of cancer, as per the GLOBOCAN 2022 database.[1] Although bladder cancer is an uncommon malignancy among the Indian population, the burden and rates are considerably higher in men than in women, in whom the disease ranks as the 17th most common cancer and the 19th leading cause of cancer death. The 5-year prevalence rate of bladder cancer is approximately 1.8 per 100,000 people, leading to around 12,353 deaths every year due to this disease.[2] Management of bladder tumors often requires complex surgeries such as transurethral resection of bladder tumor (TURBT) or radical cystectomy (RC). During these operations, anesthesia is crucial for patient safety, comfort, and pain management. Anesthesiologists play a vital role by carefully planning the anesthesia based on the patient's overall health, tumor size, and potential risks. They must consider the type of anesthesia (general, spinal, or epidural), monitor fluids and vital signs, and ensure proper postoperative pain relief after surgery. This chapter will explore the critical role of anesthesia in bladder tumor surgeries and the various considerations anesthesiologists must take into account to ensure optimal patient care.

BLADDER ANATOMY AND PHYSIOLOGY

The urinary bladder is a hollow, muscular organ situated in the pelvic cavity. Its structure can be divided into several distinct layers, each contributing to its overall function. The innermost layer is the urothelium, a specialized epithelial lining that provides a barrier to urine. Beneath the urothelium lies the lamina propria, a submucosal layer composed of connective tissue, blood vessels, and nerves. The outermost layer is the detrusor muscle, a thick smooth muscle layer that contracts to expel urine during micturition.[3]

The bladder is innervated by parasympathetic, sympathetic, and somatic nerve fibers. These fibers help in regulating the bladder's function, including filling and emptying. Parasympathetic nerves originate from the sacral spinal cord levels S2-S4. These nerves come together to form the pelvic splanchnic nerves. The parasympathetic nerves stimulate the detrusor muscle to contract and the internal urethral sphincter to relax, while the sympathetic nerves promote bladder filling and constriction of the internal sphincter. Sympathetic nerves arise from the lower thoracic (T10–T12) and upper lumbar (L1–L2) levels of the spinal cord. They form the superior and inferior hypogastric plexuses and nerves. Sympathetic nerves promote relaxation of the detrusor muscle and contraction of the internal urethral sphincter, facilitating urine storage in the bladder. The pudendal nerve arises from the S2–;S4 levels of the sacral spinal cord as a branch of the sacral plexus. It provides somatic motor innervation to the striated muscle fibers of the external urethral sphincter, allowing voluntary control over this sphincter during urination. As the bladder fills, mechanoreceptors detect the stretch in the detrusor muscle and send signals to the spinal cord, stimulating the sympathetic response and inhibiting the parasympathetic response. When the bladder becomes fully distended, the parasympathetic response is stimulated, allowing for contraction of the detrusor muscle and relaxation of the internal sphincter.[4,5]

The nerve supply to the bladder can be impacted by bladder tumors, leading to various effects on bladder function. Some potential effects[4,6] are given in **Table 1**.

PATHOPHYSIOLOGY OF BLADDER TUMORS

Bladder tumors can be classified into several types, the most common being urothelial carcinoma. This type originates

TABLE 1: Impact of bladder tumors on nerve supply.

Effect	*Impact of bladder tumors*
Impaired bladder sensation	Damage or compression of sensory nerves can lead to decreased sensation of bladder fullness, making it difficult to recognize the need to urinate
Overactive bladder	Interference with nerves controlling bladder contraction and relaxation can cause sudden, involuntary bladder muscle contractions, leading to urgent and frequent urination
Urinary retention	Impaired nerve signals for bladder contraction and urethral sphincter relaxation can result in incomplete bladder emptying or urinary retention, increasing the risk of urinary tract infections
Neurogenic bladder dysfunction	Impingement on nerves supplying the bladder can cause either overactive or underactive bladder, depending on the specific nerves affected
Urinary incontinence	Damage to nerves controlling the external urethral sphincter can lead to involuntary leakage of urine
Pain or discomfort	Nerve compression or irritation can cause pain or discomfort in the pelvic region

from the urothelium, the bladder's innermost lining. Less common variants include squamous cell carcinoma and adenocarcinoma. Squamous cell carcinoma, frequently associated with chronic irritation and infections, and adenocarcinoma, arising from glandular tissues, both account for a smaller percentage of cases.[7]

Numerous risk factors contribute to the development of bladder tumors. Smokers face a three to four times higher risk of bladder cancer compared to nonsmokers, contributing to approximately 31% of bladder cancer deaths in men and 16% in women.[8] Occupational exposures to chemicals used in industries such as dye, rubber, leather, and paint have also been linked to increased tumor risk.[9] Additionally, chronic bladder infections, such as those caused by the *Schistosoma haematobium* parasite, can predispose individuals to squamous cell carcinoma.

The cellular and molecular mechanisms underlying bladder cancer involve a series of genetic mutations and alterations. These genetic changes ultimately lead to uncontrolled cell growth and the potential for metastasis.[10,11]

TABLE 2: Classification of bladder tumors.

Stage	*Description*
Ta	Noninvasive papillary tumor
T1	Tumor invades subepithelial connective tissue
Tis	Carcinoma in situ (flat tumor)
T2	Tumor invades muscle layer
T2a	Tumor invades superficial muscle (inner half)
T2b	Tumor invades deep muscle (outer half)
T3	Tumor invades perivesical tissue
T3a	Microscopically
T3b	Macroscopically (extravesical mass)
T4	Tumor invades any of the following: Prostate stroma, seminal vesicles, uterus, vagina, pelvic wall, abdominal wall
T4a	Tumor invades prostate stroma, seminal vesicles, uterus or vagina
T4b	Tumor invades pelvic wall or abdominal wall
N0	No regional lymph node metastasis
N1	Metastasis in a single lymph node in the true pelvis
N2	Metastasis in multiple regional lymph nodes in the true pelvis
N3	Metastasis in common iliac lymph node(s)
M0	No distant metastasis
M1a	Non-regional lymph nodes
M1b	Other distant metastases

Bladder tumors can be classified as nonmuscle invasive (NMIBC) or muscle-invasive (MIBC) based on their depth of invasion into the bladder wall. NMIBC includes Ta, T1, and carcinoma in situ (CIS), while MIBC includes T2, T3, and T4 tumors. Bladder tumors can also be classified based on their grade, with low-grade and high-grade tumors having different prognoses and treatment approaches.[12,13]

The primary types include urothelial carcinoma, squamous cell carcinoma, adenocarcinoma, and small cell carcinoma. Urothelial carcinoma, the most common type, can further be categorized into low-grade and high-grade tumors, each dictating different surgical approaches and prognoses. Lower-grade tumors are usually superficial and less aggressive, often managed with less extensive surgical procedures. High-grade tumors, on the other hand, are more invasive and may necessitate RC and lymph node dissection. Accurately classifying the tumor type is essential for planning the appropriate surgical strategy and anticipating possible complications **(Table 2)**.[14,15]

Bladder tumors can cause various symptoms, such as hematuria, dysuria, frequency, urgency, and incontinence, depending on their size, location, and stage. Advanced tumors may cause hydronephrosis, renal failure, and systemic symptoms such as weight loss, fatigue, and anorexia.[8] Understanding the pathophysiology of bladder tumors is essential for anesthesia management, as it helps in anticipating and managing potential complications related to the tumor itself, such as bleeding, obstruction, and metastatic disease.

PREOPERATIVE CONSIDERATIONS FOR BLADDER TUMOR SURGERIES

Patient Evaluation

Preoperative evaluation of patients scheduled for bladder tumor surgeries is very important to optimize outcomes and minimize risks. This comprehensive assessment includes a thorough patient history, physical examination, and a series of diagnostic tests to inform treatment planning and staging **(Table 3)**.[16,17] The staging system indicates the extent of tumor penetration and spread **(Table 2)**.

Comorbidities and Risk Factors

Assessment of comorbidities is crucial as these conditions may impact surgical outcomes and recovery for complex bladder surgery. Common comorbidities include cardiovascular diseases, diabetes, and pulmonary disorders. Each of these conditions requires careful preoperative optimization. Recognizing and addressing risk factors is also essential. Advanced age, obesity, and smoking are known to influence surgical outcomes adversely **(Table 4)**. These comorbidities, which are common due to the advanced age and coexisting diseases in many patients, can significantly influence survival rates, regardless of cancer stage. RC, a common surgical treatment, carries substantial risks, with 5-year overall and cancer-specific survival rates hovering around 50–70%.[18]

Various comorbidity indices are used to predict survival in bladder cancer patients undergoing RC. These indices, including the American Society of Anesthesiology (ASA) score, Adult Comorbidity Evaluation 27 (ACE-27), Charlson Comorbidity Index (CCI), Eastern Cooperative Oncology Group performance score (ECOG PS), Karnofsky Performance Status (KPS) scale, and the Elixhauser Index (EI), are not exclusive to bladder cancer but offer valuable insights into patient health. For instance, the ASA score, which ranges from 1 (healthy) to 6 (brain dead), assesses perioperative risk and has been widely applied in cancer surgery **(Table 5)**.[18-24]

The ASA score and CCI, in particular, have been linked to higher risks of major complications and mortality. The ACE-27, which classifies 27 conditions by severity, has demonstrated strong associations with early postoperative complications and overall survival in bladder cancer patients.

In addition to traditional comorbidity indices, factors such as sarcopenia (severe muscle wasting) and frailty have

TABLE 3: Preoperative evaluation of patients scheduled for bladder tumor surgeries.

Assessment	*Goal*
Patient history and physical examination	
Symptoms	Identify urinary symptoms, hematuria, pain, and other related issues
Medical history	Review previous illnesses, surgeries, and any history of bladder issues
Family history	Check for a family history of cancer, particularly bladder cancer
Diagnostic tests	
Urine cytology	Detects cancerous cells shed into the urine
Cystoscopy	Direct visualization of the bladder interior and any visible tumors
Imaging studies	Includes CT scans and MRIs to provide detailed information on tumor size, location, and spread

TABLE 4: Comorbidities and their impact on bladder tumors.

Comorbidities and risk factors	*Consideration*
Cardiovascular diseases	Requires medication adjustment and cardiologist evaluation before surgery
Diabetes	Needs careful preoperative optimization
Pulmonary disorders	Requires careful preoperative optimization
Advanced age	Known to influence surgical outcomes adversely
Obesity	Weight loss interventions should be considered preoperatively
Smoking	Smoking cessation programs should be considered preoperatively

TABLE 5: Comorbidity indices for bladder cancer survival.

Comorbidity index	*Description*	*Key features*	*Predictive value for bladder cancer survival*
American Society of Anesthesiology (ASA) Score	Assesses perioperative risk; ranges from 1 (healthy) to 6 (brain dead).	Oldest evaluation score, predicts mortality after general anesthesia	Strong predictor of major complications and perioperative mortality
Adult Comorbidity Evaluation 27 (ACE-27)	27-item instrument validated for adult oncology patients; conditions classified into three grades based on severity	Extensive use in cancer studies, detailed grading system	Associated with early postoperative complications and overall survival
Charlson Comorbidity Index (CCI)	Originally developed for general medical patients; includes an age-adjusted version	Most cited comorbidity index, includes multiple conditions	Associated with overall and high-grade complications, as well as survival outcomes
Eastern Cooperative Oncology Group Performance Status (ECOG PS)	Classifies performance status of cancer patients from 0 (full activity) to 5 (death)	Measures physical activity, not comorbidities	Significant predictor of perioperative mortality
Karnofsky Performance Status (KPS) Scale	Measures patient activity and medical care requirements; ranges from 0 (dead) to 100 (normal, no complaints)	Focuses on patient independence and performance activity	Does not measure comorbidity directly; related to overall survival
Elixhauser Index (EI)	Comprehensive set of 30 comorbidity measures for use with administrative data	Includes mental disorders, substance abuse, obesity, and other conditions	Predicts overall complications and perioperative mortality

emerged as significant predictors of adverse postoperative outcomes.[25,26] Nutritional status, including preoperative serum albumin levels, can enhance the predictive accuracy of comorbidity indices. Immunonutrition, involving arginine-enriched supplements, has shown promise in reducing postoperative complications and improving immune response.[27]

Preoperative Optimization before Bladder Tumor Surgery

Bladder tumor surgery is a complex and critical procedure that requires meticulous preoperative planning and optimization to enhance surgical outcomes and minimize complications of anesthesia. The process of preoperative optimization involves a comprehensive evaluation of the patient's overall health status and the implementation of interventions to address modifiable risk factors.[28,29]

Smoking Cessation

Encouraging smoking cessation before surgery is paramount in reducing perioperative and postoperative complications. Smoking adversely impacts respiratory function, impairs wound healing, and increases the risk of infections. Studies have shown that smokers are at a higher risk of complications such as pneumonia, myocardial infarction, and delayed wound healing post-surgery.[30,31] Without intervention, patients who smoke can experience significantly longer recovery times and poorer surgical outcomes.

Supporting patients in quitting smoking involves a multidisciplinary approach. Preoperative assessments can identify smokers and provide an opportunity to introduce smoking cessation programs. Strategies such as counseling, nicotine replacement therapy, and pharmacological aids—such as varenicline and bupropion—have proven effective in helping patients quit smoking. Preoperative preparations should begin well before the surgery date, ideally several weeks or months in advance, allowing sufficient time for the benefits of smoking cessation to manifest.

Glycemic Control

Optimizing blood glucose levels is crucial for diabetic patients undergoing bladder tumor surgery. Poor glycemic control is associated with an increased risk of

TABLE 6: Preoperative glycemic targets.

Glycemic control parameter	*Target range*
Preoperative glycemic control	
HbA1c level	<7% (up to 8% for certain patients)
Fasting blood glucose	80–130 mg/dL (4.4–7.2 mmol/L)
Postprandial blood	<180 mg/dL (10.0 mmol/L)
Intraoperative glycemic management	
Blood glucose	140–180 mg/dL (7.8–10.0 mmol/L)
Postoperative glycemic management	
Blood glucose	140–180 mg/dL (7.8-10.0 mmol/L)

postoperative complications, including infection rates, impaired wound healing, and longer hospital stays.[32] For instance, diabetic patients with elevated HbA1c levels face a higher risk of surgical site infections and other adverse outcomes. Managing blood glucose levels preoperatively involves close monitoring and adjustments to the patient's medical regimens **(Table 6)**. Strategies include tailoring insulin therapy, adjusting oral hypoglycemic agents, and ensuring dietary compliance.

Optimization of Chronic Medical Conditions

Management of chronic medical conditions such as hypertension, chronic obstructive pulmonary disease (COPD), and cardiovascular diseases is critical before bladder tumor surgery. Chronic illnesses can exacerbate perioperative risk and delays recovery if not well controlled.[33] For example, patients with poorly managed hypertension may face an elevated risk of intraoperative and postoperative cardiovascular events.

Interventions may involve medication adjustments, lifestyle changes, and targeted therapies. For hypertensive patients, ensuring blood pressure is within normal ranges through optimized antihypertensive therapy is essential. COPD patients may require preoperative pulmonary rehabilitation and optimization of their respiratory medications. The preoperative phase should include thorough evaluations to identify and manage these conditions, ensuring that patients are in the best possible condition for surgery.

Nutritional Assessment and Management

Malnutrition, prevalent in 21–55% of patients with muscle-invasive bladder cancer, is associated with increased morbidity and mortality.[34] Identifying and addressing malnutrition involves various tools and measures such as the Malnutrition Universal Screening Tool (MUST), Nutritional Risk Screening (NRS-2002), and evaluating preoperative laboratory values such as albumin and body mass index (BMI).[35] Effective nutritional interventions can enhance recovery and reduce complications.

Patients on Anticoagulation

For patients on anticoagulants undergoing bladder surgery, the following anesthesia considerations are important:[36]

- *Timing of anticoagulant administration:* Delay heparinization for at least 1 hour after nontraumatic needle placement to minimize bleeding risk.
- *Monitoring:* Monitor patients postoperatively for evidence of neurodeficits and assess coagulation status before resuming anticoagulation.
- *Catheter removal:* Remove neuraxial catheters 2–4 hours after the last heparin dose to minimize bleeding risk.
- *Local anesthetic concentration:* Use dilute concentrations of local anesthetics to minimize motor block and facilitate neurological evaluation.
- *Risk-benefit decision:* Conduct a risk-benefit decision with the surgeon and patient regarding the use of neuraxial techniques in patients on anticoagulants, considering the potential risks of bleeding and hematoma formation.
- *Oral coagulants:* For patients on oral coagulants such as aspirin or clopidogrel, consider the following:
    - *Timing of discontinuation*: Discontinue clopidogrel 7–10 days before surgery to minimize bleeding risk.
    - *Monitoring*: Monitor patients postoperatively for evidence of neural deficits and assess coagulation status before resuming anticoagulation.

Additionally, specific guidelines for managing aspirin and clopidogrel in different cardiac risk scenarios are as follows:

- *Not at a high risk for cardiac event (e.g., primary prevention setting):* Stop aspirin.
- *At a high risk of cardiac event (e.g., within 3 months post-myocardial infarction):* Continue aspirin.
- *Aspirin and clopidogrel:* Continue aspirin, stop clopidogrel.
- *Special high-risk situation (within 6 weeks of bare metal coronary stent insertion/12 months of drug eluting*

coronary stent insertion): Continue aspirin, continue clopidogrel.

Anesthesia Management

- Preoperative anesthesia considerations are based on the type and extent of bladder tumors. Patients with high-grade or muscle-invasive bladder tumors require more extensive surgical procedures, thus demanding comprehensive preoperative anesthesia planning.
- Preoperatively, evaluating the patient for potential anesthesia risks is crucial. This includes reviewing the patient's medical history, current medication, and any specific conditions that may affect anesthesia decisions. Intraoperative strategies must ensure hemodynamic stability, manage blood loss, and provide adequate pain control. Postoperative care includes monitoring for anesthesia-related complications and managing acute pain to facilitate recovery.
- Both general and regional anesthesia can be given to bladder tumors depending on type and nature of surgery **(Table 7)**.[37-42] For patients undergoing surgery for bladder cancer, using regional anesthesia, either alone or in combination with general anesthesia, is linked to a significant reduction in cancer recurrence. This is particularly evident in patients having TURBT for nonmuscle invasive bladder cancer.[40,41]
- The main limitation of a subarachnoid block is its incomplete blockade of the obturator nerve. This can lead to complications such as bladder rupture or injury due to adductor muscle contraction triggered by obturator nerve stimulation (known as the obturator reflex) during TURBT.[43]

TABLE 7: Anesthesia management for bladder tumor surgeries.

Bladder cancer type	***Management***	***Anesthesia***	***Intraoperative complications***	***Postoperative complications***
Superficial bladder cancer	Transurethral resection of bladder tumor (TURBT)	General or regional anesthesia	Bladder perforation, bleeding, incomplete resection	Urinary tract infection (UTI), recurrence of tumor
Muscle-invasive bladder cancer	Radical cystectomy	General anesthesia with or without epidural	Significant blood loss, long operative time, injury to adjacent organs	Prolonged intensive care unit (ICU) stay, thromboembolism, infection, urinary sepsis, electrolyte imbalances
Nonmuscle invasive bladder cancer	Intravesical therapy [e.g., Bacillus Calmette-Guérin (BCG) therapy, MITOMYCIN C]	Local anesthesia or sedation	Minimal intraoperative complications	Local irritation, allergic reactions, systemic absorption leading to toxicity
High-grade bladder cancer	Partial cystectomy	General anesthesia, often combined with epidural	Blood loss, injury to bladder and surrounding organs	Bladder leakage, infection, prolonged recovery, urinary sepsis
Invasive bladder cancer	Neobladder reconstruction (after radical cystectomy)	General anesthesia, often combined with epidural	Prolonged operative time, significant blood loss, anastomotic issues	Anastomotic leakage, infection, urinary incontinence, electrolyte imbalances, prolonged ICU stay
Urinary diversion post-cystectomy	Ileal conduit	General anesthesia, often combined with epidural	Bowel complications, blood loss, injury to surrounding structures	Stoma-related issues, bowel obstruction, infection, electrolyte imbalances
Localized bladder cancer	Bladder Preservation strategies [e.g., combined modality therapy (CMT)]	General anesthesia for surgery, sedation for chemoradiation sessions	Coordination of multiple treatments, potential for increased intraoperative bleeding	Increased risk of postoperative complications, close monitoring required
Low-grade bladder cancer	Laser ablation	General or local anesthesia	Bladder perforation, incomplete tumor ablation	Recurrence of tumor, UTI

Anesthesia Considerations for Common Urological Procedures for Bladder Carcinoma

- *Cystoscopy and biopsy procedures:* Local anesthesia is a common choice for cystoscopy and biopsy procedures due to its effectiveness in minimizing discomfort and pain. A local anesthetic gel is applied around the urethral opening to numb the area. The patient is positioned in a lithotomy position. A cystoscope is gently inserted into the urethra and moved through it into the bladder. A sterile saline solution is pumped into the bladder to inflate it, making it easier to see inside and perform any necessary procedures. While mild sedation may be used in combination, local anesthesia is generally preferred for outpatient procedures. It is essential for patients to follow proper postprocedure care and seek medical attention if they experience any complications or discomfort.
- For *TURBT*, the preferred anesthesia includes regional (spinal/epidural) or general anesthesia. The patient is positioned in the dorsal lithotomy position. If general anesthesia is required, a secure airway is necessary. The surgery is typically short, and fluid management involves monitoring for transurethral resection (TUR) syndrome and fluid absorption. Blood loss is minimal to moderate, and hemostasis is essential due to the risk of bleeding. Pain management involves mild-to-moderate pain, typically managed with oral analgesics or nonsteroidal anti-inflammatory drugs (NSAIDs). Postoperative considerations include mild pain and monitoring for bladder spasms. Antibiotic prophylaxis is administered for infection prevention.
- *Obturator nerve* (ON) stimulation during transurethral resection of lateral and posterolateral bladder wall tumor under spinal anesthesia can lead to complications. To prevent these complications, selective obturator nerve block (ONB) is used, which involves blocking the ON using ultrasound (US)-guided technique with or without nerve stimulation. The technique involves advancing an 80-mm stimulating insulated needle under US guidance to reach the anterior and posterior divisions of the ON, injecting 5 mL of bupivacaine 0.5% at each location, and monitoring the spread of the local anesthetic solution under real-time visualization.[44] This technique is used to provide pain relief and prevent obturator reflex during TURBT under spinal anesthesia, thereby reducing the risk of complications such as bleeding, bladder perforation, or incomplete tumor resection.
- For a *RC and ileal conduit or neobladder:* General anesthesia is preferred, with epidural anesthesia often used for pain control. The patient is positioned in a prolonged dorsal lithotomy or supine position, requiring endotracheal intubation for a controlled environment. The surgery is extended in duration, requiring careful fluid balance and anticipation of significant blood loss, with meticulous fluid and electrolyte monitoring. Hemostasis is critical due to the large surgical field. Pain management involves the use of epidural or patient-controlled analgesia (PCA) for postoperative pain. Postoperative considerations include monitoring for complications from the extensive surgery. Antibiotic prophylaxis is necessary due to the high infection risk.
- *Considerations for open surgery, laparoscopic surgery, and robotic surgery for cystectomy:* The anesthesia for open surgery, laparoscopic surgery, and robotic surgery for cystectomy differ in several key aspects **(Table 8)**:[37]

The key differences are:

- Open surgery has the longest duration and highest blood loss, requiring more invasive monitoring and fluid management.
- Laparoscopic and robotic surgeries require adjustments for pneumoperitoneum and steep Trendelenburg positioning.
- Robotic surgery has the longest duration and highest risk of hypothermia.
- Postoperative recovery is fastest for robotic surgery, with less pain and fewer complications.

Transurethral Resection Syndrome

- *Bladder perforation:*
  - Bladder perforation is a significant complication of TURBT, second only to bleeding.
  - Occurrence rates are relatively low, between 1.3% and 5%. However, systematic evaluation using cystograms before and after TURBT shows higher rates, potentially up to 58%.[45]
  - *Irrigation fluid:* Nonconducting, osmotically active solutions are required for TURBT when using a monopolar electric resectoscope.
  - *Causes:* Accumulation of hypotonic fluid in the peritoneal cavity and its excessive absorption can lead to TUR syndrome.
  - *Symptoms:*[46,47]
    - *Central nervous system:* Headache, nausea, vomiting, blurred vision, and confusion

TABLE 8: Considerations for open surgery, laparoscopic surgery, and robotic surgery for cystectomy.

Anesthesia considerations	*Open surgery*	*Laparoscopic surgery*	*Robotic surgery*
Preoperative evaluation	Comprehensive assessment for comorbidities	Similar to open surgery, focus on cardiopulmonary status	Similar to laparoscopic surgery, with additional emphasis on positioning
Duration of surgery	Longer	Moderate to long	Generally, longer than open or laparoscopic
Patient positioning	Supine, lithotomy	Supine, lithotomy	Steep Trendelenburg, lithotomy
Anesthetic technique	General anesthesia	General anesthesia, with potential regional anesthesia adjunct	General anesthesia, with potential regional anesthesia adjunct
Airway management	Standard intubation	Standard intubation	• Standard intubation, possible complications from steep • Trendelenburg position
Intraoperative monitoring	Standard monitoring, invasive lines often required	Standard monitoring, invasive lines often required	Enhanced hemodynamic monitoring, possible need for invasive lines
Ventilation considerations	Standard ventilation strategies	Adjustments for pneumoperitoneum	Increased inspiratory pressures due to pneumoperitoneum and steep Trendelenburg position
Hemodynamic management	Blood loss can be significant, requiring vigilance	Less blood loss than open surgery	Minimal blood loss, but risk of CO_2 embolism
Pain management	Epidural or Spinal anesthesia post operative, intravenous (IV) patient-controlled analgesia (PCA), multimodal analgesia	IV PCA, multimodal analgesia	IV PCA, multimodal analgesia, less pain postoperative compared to open surgery
Fluid management	Significant fluid shifts, requires careful management	Moderate fluid shifts	Minimal fluid shifts, but requires careful management in steep Trendelenburg
Temperature management	Risk of hypothermia, requires active warming	Risk of hypothermia, requires active warming	Higher risk of hypothermia due to longer duration and exposed body surface area, requires active warming
Postoperative considerations	Longer recovery, higher risk of complications such as ileus and infection	Faster recovery, fewer complications	Fastest recovery, minimal complications, enhanced recovery protocols
Postoperative pain	Higher, requires significant pain management	Moderate, easier to manage	Lower, less invasive nature of surgery

- *Circulatory system:* Hypotension, hypertension, bradycardia, arrhythmia, dyspnea, and pulmonary or cerebral edema
- *Hydroelectrolyte imbalance:* Hyponatremia, leading to hypovolemia, hypotension, oliguria, acute renal failure, metabolic acidosis, and potentially death.

- *Detection:* Acute changes in mental state, the common initial symptom, are more easily detected in conscious patients. The imbalance usually develops slower via extravascular absorption, with hyponatremia peaking 1–6 hours postprocedure.
- *Management of TUR syndrome:*[46,47]
  - *Initial medical management:* Plasma volume expansion, hypertonic saline solutions (3% or 5%), positive inotropic drugs, and respiratory support in severe cases
  - *Diuretic therapy:* Not routinely recommended; used for milder cases after normovolemia and hemodynamic stability are restored

- *Management of bladder perforation:*[48]
  - *Surgical intervention:* Immediate laparotomy or laparoscopic repair with peritoneal drainage is the gold standard.
  - *Conservative management:* Increasingly used for selected patients with favorable characteristics. This approach includes simple bladder drainage, systemic antibiotics, and percutaneous drainage, if necessary.

Postoperative Care and Pain Management for Complex Bladder Tumor Surgeries

- *Postoperative care:*[48]
  - *Monitoring:*
    - Continuous monitoring of vital signs (heart rate, blood pressure, oxygen saturation)
    - Regular assessments for signs of complications such as bleeding, infection, and urinary retention
    - Monitoring of fluid balance and electrolyte levels, especially in patients who underwent extensive surgery or experienced TUR syndrome
  - *Catheter care:*
    - Ensure proper function and maintenance of the urinary catheter.
    - Monitor urine output and appearance for signs of hematuria or obstruction.
  - *Mobilization:*
    - Encourage early ambulation to prevent thromboembolism.
    - Implement leg exercises and use compression stockings as needed.
- *Maintenance of normothermia*:
  - Use warming blankets or forced-air warming devices intraoperatively and postoperatively to maintain body temperature.
  - Monitor patient temperature regularly to prevent hypothermia, which can increase the risk of complications.
- *Nausea and vomiting prophylaxis*:
  - *Medications:*
    - *Ondansetron:* 4 mg IV every 6–8 hours as needed
    - *Metoclopramide:* 10 mg IV every 6 hours as needed
    - *Dexamethasone:* 4–8 mg IV as a single dose during surgery
    - *Scopolamine patch:* 1.5 mg transdermal patch applied preoperatively and worn for 72 hours
- *Prevention of thromboembolism after RC:*
  - Patients undergoing RC have a high risk of venous thromboembolism (VTE), with 3–12% developing VTE, over 50% of which occurs after hospital discharge.[49]
  - All patients undergoing RC should receive at least 4 weeks of pharmacologic VTE prophylaxis, with LMWH or oral anticoagulants, combined with early ambulation, to significantly reduce the high risk of postoperative thromboembolism.
- *Postoperative pain management:*[50,51]
  - *PCA:*
    - *Common medications:* Morphine, hydromorphone, and fentanyl
    - *Typical doses **(Table 9)***
  - *Epidural analgesia:*
    - *Medications:* A combination of a local anesthetic (e.g., bupivacaine, ropivacaine) and an opioid (e.g., fentanyl, morphine)
    - *Typical doses:*
      - *Bupivacaine:* 0.1–0.125% continuous infusion at 6–10 mL/hour
      - *Fentanyl:* 2–5 μg/mL added to the local anesthetic
  - *Oral and intravenous analgesics:*
    - *Nonopioid analgesics:* Acetaminophen, NSAIDs (e.g., ibuprofen, ketorolac)
      - *Acetaminophen:* 650–1,000 mg every 6 hours (maximum 4 g/day)
      - *Ibuprofen:* 400–600 mg every 6-8 hours (maximum 2400 mg/day)
      - *Ketorolac:* 15–30 mg IV every 6 hours (maximum 120 mg/day, typically limited to 5 days)
    - *Opioids for breakthrough pain:* Oral or IV opioids such as oxycodone, morphine
      - *Oxycodone:* 5–10 mg every 4–6 hours as needed
      - *Morphine:* 2–4 mg IV every 2–4 hours as needed

TABLE 9: Doses for patient-controlled analgesia (PCA) pump.

Medication	Bolus dose	Lockout interval	Continuous infusion
Morphine PCA	1–2 mg	6–10 minutes	0.5–1 mg/h
Hydromorphone PCA	0.2–0.4 mg	6–10 minutes	0.1–0.2 mg/h
Fentanyl PCA	10–20 μg	4–10 minutes	10–20 μg/h

- *Specific considerations for bladder surgeries:*
  - *TURBT:*
    - Pain is usually mild to moderate, managed with oral analgesics or NSAIDs.
    - Monitor for bladder spasms and manage with anticholinergics, if necessary.
  - *RC with ileal conduit or neobladder:*
    - Expect more intense and prolonged pain; use epidural analgesia or PCA for effective pain control.
    - Ensure close monitoring of the surgical site and any urinary diversions (e.g., ileal conduit) for complications.
    - Provide patient education on stoma care if an ileal conduit or other urinary diversion is performed.
    - Regular monitoring of electrolyte balance due to potential bowel manipulation during surgery.

ERAS in RC

Enhanced recovery after surgery (ERAS) protocols have been increasingly integrated into the treatment of patients undergoing RC for bladder cancer. RC, the standard treatment for muscle-invasive bladder cancer, involves significant morbidity and prolonged hospital stays. ERAS protocols aim to improve patient outcomes by incorporating multiple perioperative interventions. Studies indicate that ERAS protocols significantly enhance recovery, reduce complication rates, and shorten hospital stays post cystectomy of bladder.[52,53]

These interventions include preoperative patient counseling and education, nutritional optimization, avoiding mechanical bowel preparation, and carbohydrate loading before surgery. Intraoperative measures such as thromboembolic prophylaxis, goal-directed fluid therapy, and maintaining normothermia are also emphasized.[54] Postoperative strategies focus on early mobilization, early removal of urinary drains, prevention of ileus, and early oral feeding. Discharge planning includes detailed patient education on wound and stoma care, follow-up appointments, and psychosocial support to enhance recovery and reduce complications.[55]

Future research should aim to explore new strategies and interventions to enhance adherence to the ERAS protocol. This may involve patient education, promoting multidisciplinary teamwork, and implementing continuous quality improvement initiatives.

CONCLUSION

Anesthesiologists play a crucial role in the perioperative management of patients undergoing bladder cancer surgery. A thorough understanding of bladder anatomy and physiology, tumor classification, and the various surgical approaches is essential for providing safe and effective anesthetic care. By optimizing preoperative preparation, case-based intraoperative management, and ensuring appropriate postoperative care, anesthesiologists can contribute to improved patient outcomes and enhanced recovery after bladder cancer surgery. This comprehensive approach not only enhances the surgical experience but also promotes better recovery and long-term health for patients undergoing bladder tumor surgery.

REFERENCES

1. Bray F, Laversanne M, Sung H, Ferlay J, Siegel RL, Soerjomataram I, et al. Global cancer statistics 2022: GLOBOCAN estimates of incidence and mortality worldwide for 36 cancers in 185 countries. CA Cancer J Clin. 2024;74(3):229-63.
2. [online] Available from https://gco.iarc.who.int/media/globocan/factsheets/populations/356-india-fact-sheet.pdf. [Last accessed February, 2025].
3. Bolla SR, Odeluga N, Amraei R, Jetti R. Histology, Bladder. In: StatPearls [Internet]. Treasure Island (FL): StatPearls Publishing; 2025.
4. Yoshimura N, Chancellor MB. Neurophysiology of lower urinary tract function and dysfunction. Rev Urol. 2003;5 Suppl 8(Suppl 8):S3-S10.
5. Fowler CJ, Griffiths D, de Groat WC. The neural control of micturition. Nat Rev Neurosci. 2008 Jun;9(6):453-66.
6. Shermadou ES, Rahman S, Leslie SW. Anatomy, Abdomen and Pelvis: Bladder. In: StatPearls [Internet]. Treasure Island (FL): StatPearls Publishing; 2023..
7. Kaseb H, Aeddula NR. Bladder Cancer. In: StatPearls [Internet]. Treasure Island (FL): StatPearls Publishing; 2022.
8. Bourke L, Bauld L, Bullen C, et al. E-cigarettes and urologic health: A collaborative review of toxicology,epidemiology, and potential risks. Eur Urol. 2017; 71:915-23.
9. Reulen RC, Kellen E, Buntinx F, Brinkman M, Zeegers MP. A meta-analysis on the association between bladder cancer and occupation. Scand J Urol Nephrol Suppl. 2008;(218):64-78.
10. Martin C, Leiser CL, O'Neil B, Gupta S, Lowrance WT, Kohlmann W, et al. Familial cancer clustering in urothelial cancer: A population-based case-control study. J Natl Cancer Inst. 2018;110(5):527-33.
11. Noon AP, Martinsen JI, Catto JW, Pukkala E. Occupation and bladder cancer phenotype: Identification of workplace

patterns that increase the risk of advanced disease beyond overall incidence. Eur Urol Focus. 2018;4:725-30.
12. Iemura Y, Miyake M, Fukui S, Fujii T, Ohnishi S, Hori S, et al. Depth of invasion to the bladder wall as a prognostic factor and its association with circulating cell-free DNA levels in patients with muscle-invasive bladder cancer. Curr Urol. 2023;17(4):229-35.
13. EAU Guidelines. Edn. presented at the EAU Annual Congress Paris 2024. ISBN 978-94-92671-23-3.
14. Babjuk M, Burger M, Compérat EM, Gontero P, Mostafid AH, Palou J, et al. European association of urology guidelines on non-muscle-invasive bladder cancer (TaT1 and carcinoma in situ) - 2019 update. Eur Urol. 2019;76(5):639-57.
15. Kittler R, Shiang C, Hutchinson R, Kollipara RK, Kapur P, Franto F, Lotan Y. Grade progression in urothelial carcinoma can occur with high or low mutational homology: a first-step toward tumor-specific care in initial low-grade bladder cancer. Oncotarget. 2018;9(10):9415-24.
16. Guerra-Londono CE, Cata JP, Nowak K, Gottumukkala V. Prehabilitation in adults undergoing cancer surgery: A comprehensive review on rationale, methodology, and measures of effectiveness. Curr Oncol. 2024;31(4): 2185-200.
17. Hugen CM, Duddalwar V, Daneshmand S. Preoperative imaging for clinical staging prior to radical cystectomy. Curr Urol Rep. 2016;17(9):62.
18. Eisenberg MS, Boorjian SA, Cheville JC, Thompson RH, Thapa P, Kaushik D, et al. The SPARC score: A multifactorial outcome prediction model for patients undergoing radical cystectomy for bladder cancer. J Urol. 2013;190:2005-10.
19. Fairey AS, Jacobsen NE, Chetner MP, Mador DR, Metcalfe JB, Moore RB, et al. Associations between comorbidity, and overall survival and bladder cancer specific survival after radical cystectomy: results from the Alberta Urology Institute Radical Cystectomy database. J Urol. 2009;182:85-92.
20. Piccirillo JF, Tierney RM, Costas I, Grove L, Spitznagel EL Jr. Prognostic importance of comorbidity in a hospital-based cancer registry. JAMA. 2004;291:2441-7.
21. Oken MM, Creech RH, Tormey DC, Horton J, Davis TE, McFadden ET, et al. Toxicity and response criteria of the Eastern Cooperative Oncology Group. Am J Clin Oncol. 1982;5:649-55.
22. Mayr R, May M, Martini T, Lodde M, Comploj E, Pycha A, et al. Comorbidity and performance indices as predictors of cancer-independent mortality but not of cancer-specific mortality after radical cystectomy for urothelial carcinoma of the bladder. Eur Urol. 2012;62:662-70.
23. Elixhauser A, Steiner C, Harris DR, Coffey RM. Comorbidity measures for use with administrative data. Med Care. 1998;36:8-27.
24. Miller DC, Taub DA, Dunn RL, Montie JE, Wei JT. The impact of comorbid disease on cancer control and survival following radical cystectomy. J Urol. 2003;169:105-9.
25. Megwalu II, Vlahiotis A, Radwan M, Piccirillo JF, Kibel AS. Prognostic impact of comorbidity in patients with bladder cancer. Eur Urol. 2008;53:581-9.
26. Erdik A, Cimen HI, Atik YT, Gul D, Kose O, Halis F, et al. Sarcopenia is an independent predictor of survival in patients undergoing radical cystectomy for bladder cancer: a single-centre, retrospective study. Cent European J Urol. 2023;76(2):81-9.
27. Chappidi MR, Kates M, Patel HD, Tosoian JJ, Kaye DR, Sopko NK, et al. Frailty as a marker of adverse outcomes in patients with bladder cancer undergoing radical cystectomy. Urol Oncol. 2016;34:256, e1-6.
28. Maffezzini M, Gerbi G, Campodonico F, Parodi D, Capponi G, Spina A, et al. Peri-operative management of ablative and reconstructive surgery for invasive bladder cancer in the elderly. Surg Oncol. 2004;13(4):197-200.
29. Smelser WW, Tallman JE, Gupta VK, Al Hussein Al Awamlh B, Johnsen NV, et al. Implementation of a comprehensive prehabilitation program for patients undergoing radical cystectomy. Urol Oncol. 2023;41(2):108.e19-108.e27.
30. Bassett JC, Matulewicz RS, Kwan L, McCarthy WJ, Gore JL, Saigal CS. Prevalence and correlates of successful smoking cessation in bladder cancer survivors. Urology. 2021; 153:236-43.
31. Rink M, Crivelli JJ, Shariat SF, Chun FK, Messing EM, Soloway MS. Smoking and bladder cancer: A systematic review of risk and outcomes. Eur Urol Focus. 2015;1(1): 17-27.
32. Lee EK, Pirani K, Holzbeierlein JM, Martin P, Rangarajan P, Hamilton-Reeves J, et al. Glucose metabolism and bladder cancer. J Clin Oncol. 2017;35(6_suppl):359.
33. Mohammed T, Singh M, Tiu JG, Kim AS. Etiology and management of hypertension in patients with cancer. Cardiooncology. 2021;7(1):14.
34. Michel C, Robertson HL, Camargo J, Hamilton-Reeves JM. Nutrition risk and assessment process in patients with bladder cancer undergoing radical cystectomy. Urol Oncol Semi Orig Investig. 2020; 38: 719-24.
35. Ellis JL, Dalimov Z, Chew L, Quek ML. Preoperative optimization of the radical cystectomy patient: Current state and future directions. J Surg Oncol [Internet]. 2024;129(1):138-44.
36. Vasudeva P, Goel A, Sengottayan VK, Sankhwar S, Dalela D. Antiplatelet drugs and the perioperative period: What every urologist needs to know. Indian J Urol [Internet]. 2009;25(3):296-301.
37. Koo C-H, Ryu J-H. Anesthetic considerations for urologic surgeries. Korean J Anesthesiol. 2020;73(2):92-102.
38. Illias AM, Yu KJ, Wu SC, Cata JP, Tsai YF, Hung KC. Association of regional anesthesia with oncological outcomes in patients receiving surgery for bladder cancer: A meta-analysis of observational studies. Front Oncol. 2023;13:1097637.

39. Lenis AT, Lec PM, Chamie K, Mshs MD. Bladder cancer: A review. JAMA (2020) 324:1980-91.
40. Karadeniz MS, Mammadov O, Çiftci H, Usta SA, Pembeci K. Comparing the effects of combined General/Epidural anaesthesia and general anaesthesia on serum cytokine levels in radical cystectomy. Turkish J Anaesthesiol. (2017) 45:203-9.
41. Pei L, Tan G, Wang L, Guo W, Xiao B, Gao X, et al. Comparison of combined general-epidural anesthesia with general anesthesia effects on survival and cancer recurrence: a meta-analysis of retrospective and prospective studies. PloS One. 2014;9:e114667.
42. Dick A, Barnes R, Hadley H, Bergman RT, Ninan CA. Complications of transurethral resection of bladder tumors: Prevention, recognition and treatment. J Urol. 1980;124:810-1.
43. Kuo JY. Prevention of obturator jerk during transurethral resection of bladder tumor. JTUA. 2008;19:27-31.
44. Shah NF, Sofi KP, Nengroo SH. Obturator nerve block in transurethral resection of bladder tumor: A comparison of ultrasound-guided technique versus ultrasound with nerve stimulation technique. Anesth Essays Res. 2017;11(2):411-5.
45. Balbay MD, Cimentepe E, Unsal A, Bayrak O, Koç A, Akbulut Z. The actual incidence of bladder perforation following transurethral bladder surgery. J Urol. 2005; 174:2260-2.
46. Dorotta I, Basali A, Ritchey M, O'Hara JFJ, Sprung J. Transurethral resection syndrome after bladder perforation. Anesth Analg. 2003;97(5):1536-8.
47. Hahn RG. Transurethral resection syndrome from extravascular absorption of irrigating fluid. Scand J Urol Nephrol. 1993;27:387-94.
48. Oh SB, Ahn JH. Successful conservative management of a spontaneous intraperitoneal rupture of bladder diverticulum in a critical patient. Medicine (Baltim). 2020;99(7).
49. Klaassen Z, Arora K, Goldberg H, Chandrasekar T, Wallis CJD, Sayyid RK, et al. Extended venous thromboembolism prophylaxis after radical cystectomy: A call for adherence to current guidelines. J Urol. 2018;199(4):906-14.
50. The Urology Group of Virginia. Postoperative instructions for cystoscopy and transurethral bladder tumor resection (TURBT). [online] Available from: https://www.urologygroupvirginia.com/patient-resources/patient-instructions/postoperative-instructions/postoperative-instructions-for-cystoscopy-and-transurethral-bladder-tumor-resection-turbt. [Last accessed February, 2025].
51. Xu W, Daneshmand S, Bazargani ST, Cai J, Miranda G, Schuckman AK, et al. Postoperative pain management after radical cystectomy: Comparing traditional versus enhanced recovery protocol pathway. J Urol. 2015;194(5):1209-13.
52. Chen X, Yao J, Xin Y, Ma G, Yu Y, Yang Y, et al. Postoperative pain in patients undergoing cancer surgery and intravenous patient-controlled analgesia use: The first and second 24 h experiences. Pain Ther. 2023;12(1):275-92.
53. Mir MC, Zargar H, Bolton DM, Murphy DG, Lawrentschuk N. Enhanced recovery after surgery protocols for radical cystectomy surgery: review of current evidence and local protocols. ANZ J Surg. 2015;85(7-8):514-20.
54. Grilo N, Crettenand F, Bohner P, Rodrigues Dias SC, Cerantola Y, Lucca I. Impact of Enhanced Recovery after Surgery® Protocol Compliance on Length of Stay, Bowel Recovery and Complications after Radical Cystectomy. Diagnostics (Basel). 2024;14(3):264.
55. Sung LH, Yuk HD. Enhanced recovery after surgery of patients undergoing radical cystectomy for bladder cancer. Transl Androl Urol. 2020;9(6):2986-96.

36 CHAPTER

Anesthesia for Pheochromocytoma and Other Adrenal Tumor Excision

Pradeep Kumar Bhatia, Priyanka Sethi, Manoj Kamal

INTRODUCTION

The anesthesiologist's management of pheochromocytoma and other adrenal tumors poses a special challenge based on the complex physiological consequences of hypersecretion of catecholamines. These tumors, which are mainly derived from chromaffin cells, can result in profound hemodynamic instability and thus perioperative management is particularly challenging. Pheochromocytomas, although uncommon, have great impact on the outcome of surgery and thus careful preoperative planning, intraoperative caution, and postoperative monitoring are necessary.

Surgical resection is the definitive treatment of pheochromocytoma, though curative in the majority of cases, and risks catastrophic hypertensive emergencies, arrhythmias, and hemodynamic instability. Optimal anesthesia care can mitigate complications and make the operation safer. Careful knowledge of catecholamine kinetics, the pharmacologic mechanisms of adrenergic blockade, and judicious deployment of anesthetic drugs are the prerequisites for maximal perioperative benefit.

This chapter discusses the pathophysiology, diagnosis, and anesthetic considerations for pheochromocytoma and other adrenal tumors with a focus on the necessity of a multidisciplinary approach towards obtaining successful surgical results. Through attention to perioperative management, pharmacologic strategies, and intraoperative techniques, anesthesiologists can play an important role in enhancing patient safety and decreasing morbidity related to adrenal tumor removal.

DEFINITION AND EPIDEMIOLOGY OF PHEOCHROMOCYTOMA AND ADRENAL TUMORS

Pheochromocytoma is a functional catecholamine-secreting tumor of paraganglionic chromaffin cells. It is commonly found in the adrenal medulla and in approximately 10% in extra-adrenal sites. Pheochromocytomas are relatively uncommon tumors, with a prevalence of 0.3–0.95%.[1] In 4%, pheochromocytoma is diagnosed incidentally and is the cause of hypertension in 0.1% of hypertensive patients.[1] Pheochromocytomas occur equally in men and women, with approximately equal frequency in both adrenal glands. Around 10% of pheochromocytomas are either bilateral, multifocal, or malignant; occur in children; or are linked to a hereditary or familial syndrome. Pediatric pheochromocytomas are characterized by a slight male predominance and are less likely malignant than adult tumors. Approximately 30% of pediatric pheochromocytomas are bilateral, extra-adrenal, multiple, or familial.

IMPORTANCE OF ANESTHESIA MANAGEMENT IN SURGICAL OUTCOMES

The preferred treatment for pheochromocytomas is surgical removal of the tumor, which has a success rate exceeding 90%. However, due to end-organ damage resulting from excessive catecholamine secretion and labile hemodynamics from fluctuating catecholamine levels, it is one of the most complex and challenging tasks for the anesthesiologists. Proper preoperative optimization is essential to reduce perioperative morbidity and mortality.

OVERVIEW OF CATECHOLAMINE SECRETION AND EFFECTS

Catecholamines are produced in the chromaffin cells. The conversion of tyrosine to dihydroxyphenylalanine (DOPA) with the help of tyrosine hydroxylase (TH) is the rate-limiting step in the formation of DOPA.[2] Di-hydroxyphenylalanine is then converted into dopamine by the enzyme dopa decarboxylase, which is further transformed into norepinephrine (NE) by the enzyme dopamine β-hydroxylase. Phenylethanolamine-N-methyltransferase (PNMT) enzyme methylates the NE to epinephrine (E). These catecholamines are stored in vesicles and released into the bloodstream, with cardiac effects mediated through adrenoreceptors.

ANESTHESIA CONSIDERATIONS OF PHEOCHROMOCYTOMAS

Preoperative Assessment

Clinical Presentation and Diagnostic Workup

The clinical features of pheochromocytoma are dependent on the type and amount of catecholamine secreted by the tumor. The tumors may secrete E, NE, or dopamine in either a continuous manner (leading to sustained hypertension) or an episodic pattern (leading to paroxysms of symptoms). The classic symptoms, including paroxysmal hypertension, palpitations, and diaphoresis, are observed in only 40% of patients. Effects of long-standing and severe hypertension can be seen as damage to the end organs, especially heart, kidney, eyes, and central nervous system. Diabetes or deranged glucose metabolism may be present in up to 30–50% of the patients.[3] Within the chromaffin cells, NE and E are metabolized to normetanephrine and metanephrine. An increase in plasma metanephrines indicates heightened tumoral production of catecholamines, underpinning the high sensitivity and specificity of this diagnostic test. This is more reliable compared to measuring parent catecholamines in the plasma, which depends on their secretion from the tumor.

The imaging modalities for pheochromocytomas can be either morphological, that is, ultrasound (US), computed tomography (CT), and magnetic resonance imaging (MRI), or molecular, such as scintigraphy and positron emission tomography (PET), or a combination of both. In cases of clinically manifested pheochromocytomas, imaging is conducted after clinical and biochemical examinations to locate the tumor. CT is the most common imaging method used in the diagnosis of pheochromocytomas. The role of US is limited in the diagnosis of pheochromocytoma. The US of abdomen may incidentally detect an adrenal mass, especially on the right side because of the acoustic window of the liver.

Molecular imaging is a functional imaging modality which could be utilized to confirm the source of increased production of catecholamines. For most of the cases, one of the following methods is employed: 123I-MIBG scintigraphy, 18F-FDG, or 18F-DOPA PET/CT and somatostatin receptor imaging.[4]

The surgical approach to pheochromocytomas is based on imaging, identifying germline genetic mutations. The imaging enables assessment of malignancy and extent of disease. The laparoscopic approach or minimally invasive technique is preferred over open surgical technique for surgical excision of adrenal tumor. Minimally invasive techniques, approached either transabdominally or retroperitoneally, are the standard of care. Open surgical approaches are reserved for large tumors at risk for rupture and potentially malignant tumors.

Preoperative Optimization for Surgery

Preoperative evaluation should focus on assessing end-organ damage due to elevated catecholamine levels. These patients are at risk for catecholamine-induced cardiomyopathy and may present with arrhythmias, myocardial ischemia, and reduced ventricular ejection fraction. Preoperative preparation or optimization encompasses negation of the alpha-1-mediated vasoconstriction and beta-1-mediated tachycardia and inotropy.[5] The primary focus of "preparation" or "optimization" involves controlling hypertension and expanding blood volume. Hypertension in these patients can be paroxysmal with a normal baseline blood pressure, have an elevated baseline blood pressure with intermittent paroxysms, or be persistently high. The main cause of hypertension is the activation of alpha-receptors by catecholamines. Therefore, alpha-receptor antagonists are the initial choice of drugs for managing hypertension. The initiation of alpha-blockade can lead to severe orthostatic hypotension. To counteract this, hypotensive patients are advised to increase fluid and salt intake, or crystalloids and colloids may be given intravenously. A patient may require 5–15 days of preoperative preparation with optimal alpha-blocking drugs to optimize blood pressure, increased oral fluids and salt intake, and/or intravenous fluids before being "accepted" for surgery. Successful alpha blockade is indicated by normalized blood pressure with mild orthostasis. Other medications, such as beta-receptor antagonists and calcium channel blockers, also play a role in preoperative symptom control. Their use is warranted in the presence of arrhythmias, signs of myocardial ischemia, and cardiomyopathy due to excessive catecholamine secretion.

Pharmacological Considerations: Alpha and Beta-Adrenergic Blockade

Phenoxybenzamine is an irreversible, nonspecific alpha-adrenergic blocker used earlier for preoperative optimization of hypertension. It is long-acting and has a half-life of approximately 24 hours. It leads to smooth muscle relaxation in arterioles and venous capacitance vessels.

Orthostatic hypotension and reflex tachycardia, particularly in the context of hypovolemia, are potential side effects of alpha blockade, especially with long-acting phenoxybenzamine. Selective alpha-1-adrenergic blocking agents such as prazosin, terazosin, and doxazosin can be used to facilitate preoperative alpha blockade. These selective agents cause less reflex tachycardia than nonselective alpha-blockers because they leave alpha-2 inhibitory activity intact.[5]

Beta-receptor antagonists are effective in counteracting the tachycardia induced by alpha-blocking agents, a desired side effect indicating successful alpha blockade. Beta-blockers should be added to control tachycardia no earlier than 2–3 days after it appears. Cardioselective beta-antagonists such as metoprolol and atenolol are preferred due to fewer side effects compared to nonselective beta-antagonists.

Beta-blockers should never be used before initiating alpha blockade in patients with functioning tumors, as this could lead to unopposed alpha-adrenergic effects, causing severe vasoconstriction and potentially acute cardiac failure, hypertensive crisis, and pulmonary edema.

Timing and Titration of Preoperative Medication

Alpha-adrenergic blockade is administrated 10–14 days prior to the intervention to normalize the blood pressure and heart rate and to expand the blood volume. The period of alpha blockade should be extended in patients with organ damage from prolonged catecholamine excess. The initial dose of phenoxybenzamine is 10 mg taken orally once or twice daily, with an increase of 10–20 mg every 2–3 days as needed to control blood pressure. It takes about approximately 10–14 days for optimization. As the correct dose is reached, paroxysmal hypertensive episodes are controlled, and the patient becomes normotensive or even mildly hypotensive. If the initial dosage is too high, side effects occur more frequently. Patients should be warned about side effects, such as nasal stuffiness, tachycardia, dizziness, fatigue, orthostasis, and, in the case of males, retrograde ejaculation. The final dose is typically around 1 mg/kg/day, but it can vary widely, ranging from 20–100 mg/day up to a maximum of 240 mg/day.

The available selective alpha-1 adrenergic drugs preferentially act on the alpha-1 receptors and cause vasodilatation with less tachycardia. However, due to their short half-life, selective alpha-1 blocking agents may not sufficiently control the extra catecholamine release during surgery, potentially causing an intraoperative hypertensive crisis. Therefore, these drugs should be administered even on the day of surgery. The shorter half-life also makes these inhibitors less likely to cause hypotension after tumor removal. In some institutions, phenoxybenzamine is initially used and then replaced with selective alpha-1 adrenergic drugs 24–48 hours before surgery to minimize postoperative hypotension. Prazosin is usually initiated at 0.5–1 mg per dose every 4–6 hours and titrated to an average dose of 2–5 mg two or three times a day, up to a maximum total dose of 20–24 mg/day. Doxazosin, a longer-acting drug (12 hours), is typically administered once or twice daily. It starts at a dose of 1–2 mg/day and is titrated to control blood pressure, up to a maximum dose of 16 mg/day. Terazosin is also initiated at 1 mg/day, with an average dose of 2–5 mg/day, and can be increased to a maximum dose of 20 mg/day, depending on the treatment goals. It has a shorter life than doxazosin.

Metoprolol is administered in doses of 25–50 mg three to four times a day, while atenolol is given in doses of 12.5–25 mg two to three times a day. Propranolol, a nonselective beta-blocker, is prescribed in doses of 20–80 mg one to three times a day. Labetalol, which blocks both alpha and beta receptors, has been used preoperatively in some cases, but it should not be the first choice for blockade.

Calcium channel blockers, such as nicardipine, amlodipine, nifedipine, and verapamil, provide another option for preparing paraganglioma patients preoperatively. They inhibit NE-mediated transmembrane calcium influx into smooth muscle cells, thereby controlling hypertension and tachyarrhythmias without causing hypotension in normotensive individuals.

Calcium channel blockers have three main roles in the preparation of paraganglioma: (1) To supplement alpha blockade in patients with inadequate blood pressure control in order to limit the need of increasing the dosage of alpha blockers, (2) to provide an alternative option for patients with severe side effects due to alpha blockers, and (3) to treat patients with only intermittent hypertension.

Amlodipine is given at 10–20 mg/day, nicardipine at 60–90 mg/day, nifedipine at 30–90 mg/day, and verapamil at 180–540 mg/day.

Metyrosine is a TH inhibitor used in some centers to control excessive catecholamine production. TH plays a key role in the first step of catecholamine synthesis, and inhibiting this enzyme reduces the production of all catecholamine precursors and metabolites. Patients taking >2 g/day are advised to maintain high fluid intake to prevent crystalluria.

Intraoperative Management

General anesthesia is almost always preferred for pheochromocytoma resection. General anesthesia with epidural can prove to be an approach with better hemodynamics and postoperative pain control.[6]

Adequate anxiolysis should be done for pheochromocytoma patients to minimize stress and prevent catecholamine surges that could exacerbate their condition. An arterial line and a good IV access with two peripheral lines are necessary. Intraoperative transesophageal echocardiogram (TEE)/pulmonary artery catheter may be considered in patients with severe cardiomyopathy to guide fluid management/inotrope administration or to assess ventricular function. Central venous access for vasopressor/inotrope administration may be placed in patients with poor left ventricular (LV) function. Propofol is the agent of choice for the induction if the patient has good LV function. Patients with cardiomyopathy require a cardio-stable slow induction. The primary goal is a smooth induction of anesthesia with optimal depth to avoid a hypertensive response during laryngoscopy and endotracheal intubation.

Sevoflurane/isoflurane is a commonly used inhalational agent for the maintenance of anesthesia for pheochromocytomas resection as they have at least the arrhythmogenic potential with a favorable hemodynamic profile compared with other inhalational agents. Sympathomimetic drugs (such as ketamine and ephedrine) and drugs that cause histamine release (such as atracurium and morphine) should be avoided. Peritoneal insufflation during laparoscopic resection and tumor manipulation during surgery can cause an abrupt release of catecholamines, leading to severe hypertension and tachycardia.

This hypertensive crisis may result in myocardial ischemia or stroke. Short-acting and rapidly acting vasodilators, such as nitroprusside, nitroglycerine, or calcium channel blockers like nifedipine and clevidipine, are commonly used to control hypertension.

Ligation of the blood vessel of the tumor may follow a precipitous drop in blood pressure. This is usually due to the sudden drop in endogenous catecholamine levels in the setting of chronic downregulation of alpha-adrenergic receptors in patients with pheochromocytoma.

Fluid Management Strategies

Fluid therapy is a vital but complex component of the perioperative management of adrenal tumor patients.

While underhydration can cause severe hypotension after tumor resection, overhydration can result in pulmonary edema and congestive heart failure in an already compromised heart. Intraoperative attention to volume status and expertise in hemodynamic management are likely more crucial than specific preoperative rehydration. With the advent of various hemodynamic monitors, moving away from the empirical strategy of liberal fluid administration to prevent hypotension and adopting goal-directed fluid therapy can effectively reduce volume overload. If bilateral adrenalectomy is planned preoperatively, the patient should receive glucocorticoid stress coverage in the operating room.

Positioning and Surgical Access

Minimally invasive adrenalectomy, whether via the retroperitoneal or transperitoneal approach, is the gold standard for pheochromocytoma resection. This method is preferred because it results in lower postoperative pain, earlier ambulation, and faster recovery. Additionally, it has been associated with a reduced incidence of postoperative thromboembolic complications, shorter hospital stays, and greater cost-effectiveness. However, open procedures may be needed for larger masses and extra-adrenal tumors. Robot-assisted removal is also safe and feasible, but it does not seem to offer significant advantages over laparoscopic resection.

Collaboration with Surgical Team

Resecting a catecholamine-secreting tumor is a high-risk surgical procedure; even with optimal preoperative preparation, patients may still experience significant blood pressure fluctuations, irregular heart rhythms, and bleeding. Continuous communication between the surgical and anesthesia teams is crucial, particularly during the incision, venous supply division, and tumor manipulation.

Postoperative Care

Postoperative management typically necessitates admission to the intensive care unit. The most common complication is hypotension following tumor removal, with a prevalence between 20 and 70%. Fluid loading and vasopressor infusion are required to counteract this hypotension. In the event of hypotension, hemorrhagic complications should be ruled out first; however, the most likely cause is the prolonged effect of alpha-adrenoceptor blockers in the presence of reduced plasma catecholamine levels.[7]

Postoperative hypertension during the first 24 hours after surgery is most likely due to pain, volume overload, or autonomic instability, all of which should be treated symptomatically. If hypertension persists, it may be due to incomplete tumor resection, and the tumor should be analyzed for catecholamines and metanephrines in plasma and 24-hour urine samples.

Sudden catecholamine withdrawal after tumor removal can also lead to rebound hyperinsulinemia, which in turn can cause rebound hypoglycemia. Hourly blood sugar monitoring is mandatory for at least the first 12–24 hours of the postoperative period. Catecholamine secretion should return to normal levels within 1 week after tumor removal.

Long-term Follow-up and Surveillance

Patients with pheochromocytoma or paraganglioma are at risk of developing tumor recurrences or new tumors after successful resection of the primary tumor. The overall incidence exceeds 15%. Patients with inherited tumors have a higher probability of recurrence or new tumors. Most recurrences are metastatic, particularly in patients with *SDHB* mutations or nonhereditary tumors. The determination of plasma or urinary metanephrines (normetanephrine and metanephrine) 1 month after surgery is recommended to detect residual tumor. For patients with sporadic, single tumors ≤5 cm in diameter, clinical and biochemical follow-up should be conducted every 2 years. However, this follow-up period can be reduced to yearly if it is more convenient for patients and physicians. Patients with larger or multiple, but apparently benign tumors and/or those with inherited disease should be tested 6 months after surgery and then annually for the rest of their lives.

ANESTHESIA CONCERNS FOR OTHER ADRENAL TUMORS

Introduction

Besides pheochromocytoma, other surgical indications for adrenal gland are Conn syndrome and Cushing syndrome. Although they are rare, they pose challenges to the anesthesiologists. The adrenal cortex produces three types of hormones: (1) Glucocorticoids (cortisol), (2) mineralocorticoids (aldosterone and 11-deoxycorticosterone), and (3) androgens. The adrenal medulla secretes E and NE.

Cushing Syndrome

Excess circulating level of glucocorticoids, either due to overproduction or due to external supplementation at higher doses, may lead to characteristic features of weight gain and typical trio of "moon facies", "buffalo hump", and central obesity. In approximately 70% patients, the etiology of disease is pituitary in origin; in 15% cases, adrenocorticotropic hormone (ACTH) is produced from ectopic sites; and in the remaining 15%, the source is adrenal gland.[8,9] Cushing syndrome can be associated with other tumors or clinical situations such as pheochromocytoma, sarcoidosis, pancreatic acinar cell carcinoma, pre-eclamptic findings, malignant gastrinoma, bronchial carcinoid lung tumor, pancreatic neuroendocrine tumor, Hippel–Lindau disease, and mesenteric neuroendocrine carcinoma.[10]

The patients are diagnosed with an elevated level of blood and urinary cortisol. The differentiation of Cushing disease and Cushing syndrome is done by the dexamethasone suppression test. This test is helpful to know the source of glucocorticoid hypersecretion (pituitary or adrenal origin). On administration of high-dose dexamethasone, the cortisol and 17-hydroxycorticosteroid levels are depressed in the pituitary origin of glucocorticoid hypersecretion due to negative feedback control mechanism, while those in adrenal origin hypersecretion do not respond.

Ultrasonography, angio-CT, and MRI can also be helpful in confirming the diagnosis. Ectopic glucocorticoid-secreting tissues can also be detected using technetium-99m labeled octreotide scintigraphy examinations having receptors for somatostatin.[11]

Skin thinning and bruising associated with purple striae, proximal muscle weakness or fatigue, and spontaneous bone fractures due to osteopenia, sexual disorders (amenorrhea, infertility, menstrual irregularities, and decreased libido), hyperglycemia, metabolic alkalosis, and hypokalemia are common signs and symptoms. Cushing disease resulting from pituitary adenoma can manifest with visual disturbances, headache, and elevated intracranial pressure. Rarely, these patients present with psychiatric features and suicidal tendency.

Anesthetic Considerations

Extreme symptoms may require either open or laparoscopic adrenalectomy. The laparoscopic approach of adrenalectomy has minimum hemodynamic fluctuations and faster recovery, so this gold standard technique.

Preoperative optimization of hypercortisolism, hypertension, hyperglycemia, and hypokalemia and prevention of perioperative hypercoagulative state are necessary for safe surgical outcome. Preoperatively, these patients are on adrenal enzyme inhibitors, such as ketoconazole, metyrapone, mitotane, or aminoglutethimide, given alone or in combination.[12] These drugs should be continued in the preoperative period. All antihypertensive drugs, except the angiotensin-converting enzyme inhibitors (ACEIs) and angiotensin II receptor blockers (ARBs), must be continued till the morning of surgery, because of their exaggerated hypotensive effects after the anesthesia induction. Overexcretion of potassium can be minimized by potassium-sparing diuretics for control of water retention. Overproduction of cortisol is responsible for hyperglycemia. Just like other major surgeries, all patients should be shifted to insulin for better glycemic control in the perioperative period.[13] The goal is to maintain blood glucose levels within 120–180 mg/dL during the perioperative period. The perioperative venous thromboembolism and pulmonary thromboembolism can be reduced by using low-molecular-weight heparin (LMWH), lower-extremity compression devices, and early postoperative mobilization.

Fragile skin and osteopenia are taken care of during patient positioning and taping to avoid skin damages and bone fractures. Antiaspiration prophylaxis in the form of metoclopramide, ranitidine, and sodium citrate is necessary. The detailed anesthetic plan includes possible difficult airway management, rapid induction of anesthesia, standard and/or invasive monitoring, large-bore veins, central lines, and/or epidural catheter placement.

Mask ventilation and endotracheal intubation may be challenging. The ramp position, nasopharyngeal or oropharyngeal airway is helpful in preoxygenation and intubation. Central obesity is associated with reduced functional residual capacity (FRC) which in turn leads to atelectasis and hypoxia. The placement of an epidural catheter in the preoperative period will reduce postoperative respiratory complications. A large-bore intravenous canula is recommended similar to all major surgeries, to tackle sudden unexpected bleeding or fluid shift. Pulse oximetry, electrocardiography invasive blood pressure, temperature, end-tidal carbon dioxide, and central vein accesses are mandatory. Some cases with advanced cardiac diseases required Swan–Ganz pulmonary artery catheterization. Hydrocortisone succinate must be injected to prevent a possible glucocorticoid deficiency, especially in bilateral adrenalectomy.[14] In the postoperative period, the main concerns for anesthesiologists are pain management, control of hypertension, hyperglycemia, hypokalemia, and cortisol monitoring which are hallmarks of the anesthesiologist's role in treating a patient with Cushing disease.

HYPERALDOSTERONISM

Primary hyperaldosteronism is a rare disease of adrenal gland characterized with excessive secretion of aldosterone which causes retention of sodium and accumulation of water in the extracellular compartment which in turns lead to hypertension and hypokalemic alkalosis. The skeletal muscle weakness and fatigue are the other symptoms. The causes of hyperaldosteronism are primary and secondary. When the cause of excess production is adrenal itself, then it is labeled as primary form (Conn syndrome), while excess secretion of renin and activation of the renin–aldosterone axis are responsible for secondary hyperaldosteronism. It is also associated with severe liver diseases, nephritic syndrome, and cardiac failure.

Conn syndrome is diagnosed by hypokalemia, decreased renin level, high aldosterone blood level, high aldosterone to renin activity, CT scan, and potassium and sodium plasma concentration. The renin level is raised in secondary hyperaldosteronism. The aldosterone blocks the reuptake of noradrenaline, which might lead to myocardial fibrosis resulting in arrhythmias and myocardial ischemia.[15] Correction of hypokalemia and hypertension is the mainstay of medical optimization. The definitive treatment is the surgical removal of adenoma.

Anesthetic Considerations

The advantages associated with a laparoscopic approach made it the gold standard technique for surgical resection of tumor. The main concerns for anesthesia are intraoperative hemodynamic instability, hypokalemia, and metabolic alkalosis. Hypokalemia and metabolic alkalosis may prolong the action of neuromuscular-blocking agents, inducing bradycardia. Avoid intraoperative hyperventilation because it further worsens the hypokalemia. Conn syndrome can produce brisk and untreatable intraoperative hypertension, but it is less severe than pheochromocytoma.[16]

The control of cortisol level in the preoperative period is mandatory. Inhibition of cortisol synthetic property of etomidate mandates one to avoid etomidate for anesthesia induction.[17] Some cases may require hydrocortisone supplementation. Cortisol administration is helpful in perioperative hypoadrenocorticism or in chronic steroid administration.[18] Adrenal suppression induces hypotension, decreased cardiac output, hyponatremia, and hypoglycemia. A good cooperation between the anesthesiologist, endocrinologist, and surgeon is strongly recommended.

CONCLUSION

The anesthetic management of pheochromocytoma and other adrenal tumors is a special challenge because of the severe cardiovascular impact of excessive catecholamine release. Perioperative success depends on careful preoperative optimization, such as proper adrenergic blockade and fluid resuscitation, to reduce intraoperative hemodynamic instability. Intraoperative factors as blood pressure regulation, optimal choice of anesthetic agent, and close coordination with the surgical team, are mandatory to avoid complications like hypertensive crisis or abrupt hypotension after tumor resection. Besides pheochromocytoma, other adrenal pathologies such as Cushing syndrome and hyperaldosteronism also needs individualized anesthetic management. Postoperative management involves hemodynamic stabilization, vigilance for complications like hypoglycemia and adrenal insufficiency, and long-term monitoring for possible tumor recurrence. Multidisciplinary care, involving endocrinologists, anesthesiologists, and surgeons, is the key to best perioperative management. Through knowledge of the pathophysiology and anesthetic considerations of adrenal tumors, clinicians can improve perioperative patient safety and success of surgery.

REFERENCES

1. Hanna NN, Kenady DE. Pheochromocytoma. In: Holzheimer RG, Mannick JA (Eds). Surgical Treatment: Evidence-Based and Problem-Oriented. Munich: Zuckschwerdt; 2001. Available from: https://www.ncbi.nlm.nih.gov/books/NBK7002/
2. Bolander FF. Classical endocrinology. In: Bolander FF (Ed). Molecular Endocrinology, 3rd edition. San Diego: Academic Press; 2004. pp. 25-60.
3. Falhammar H, Kjellman M, Calissendorff J. Initial clinical presentation and spectrum of pheochromocytoma: a study of 94 cases from a single center. Endocr Connect. 2018;7(1):186-92.
4. Čtvrtlík F, Koranda P, Schovánek J, Škarda J, Hartmann I, Tüdös Z. Current diagnostic imaging of pheochromocytomas and implications for therapeutic strategy. Exp Ther Med. 2018;15(4):3151-60.
5. Kamath AS, Singh K. Perioperative Management of Pheochromocytoma. [Updated 2023 Jul 6]. In: StatPearls [Internet]. Treasure Island (FL): StatPearls Publishing; 2024 Jan-. Available from https://www.ncbi.nlm.nih.gov/books/NBK589634/ [Last accessed February, 2025].
6. Ramachandran R, Rewari V. Current perioperative management of pheochromocytomas. Indian J Urol. 2017;33(1):19-25.
7. Mamilla D, Araque KA, Brofferio A, Gonzales MK, Sullivan JN, Nilubol N, Pacak K. Postoperative Management in Patients with Pheochromocytoma and Paraganglioma. Cancers (Basel). 2019;11(7):936.
8. Williams GH, Dluhy RG. Disorders of the Adrenal Cortex. In: Fauci A, Braunwald E, Kasper D, Hauser S, Longo D, Jameson J, et al. Harrison's Principles of Internal Medicine, 17th edition. New York: McGraw Hill Professional Publishing; 2008. pp. 2259-60.
9. Michael FR, Fleisher LA. Anesthetic implications of concurrent diseases. In: Miller RD (Ed). Miller's Anesthesia, 7th edition. Philadelphia: Churchill Livingstone; 2009. pp. 1067-1150.
10. Domi R, Sula H, Kaci M, Paparisto S, Bodeci A, Xhemali A. Anesthetic considerations on adrenal gland surgery. J Clin Med Res. 2015;7(1):1-7.
11. Esfahani AF, Chavoshi M, Noorani MH, Saghari M, Eftekhari M, Beiki D, et al. Successful application of technetium-99m-labeled octreotide acetate scintigraphy in the detection of ectopic adrenocorticotropin-producing bronchial carcinoid lung tumor: a case report. J Med Case Rep. 2010;4:323.

12. Diez JJ, Iglesias P. Pharmacological therapy of Cushing's syndrome: drugs and indications. Mini Rev Med Chem. 2007;7(5):467-80.
13. Fasshauer M, Lincke T, Witzigmann H, Kluge R, Tannapfel A, Moche M, et al. Ectopic Cushing' syndrome caused by a neuroendocrine carcinoma of the mesentery. BMC Cancer. 2006;6:108.
14. Kissane NA, Cendan JC. Patients with Cushing's syndrome are care-intensive even in the era of laparoscopic adrenalectomy. Am Surg. 2009;75(4):279-283.
15. Winship SM, Winstanley JH, Hunter JM. Anaesthesia for Conn's syndrome. Anaesthesia. 1999;54(6):569-74.
16. Alseddeeqi E, Altinoz A, Ghashir NB. Seizure and coma secondary to Conn's syndrome: a case report. J Med Case Rep. 2020;14(1):100.
17. Absalom A, Pledger D, Kong A. Adrenocortical function in critically ill patients 24 h after a single dose of etomidate. Anaesthesia. 1999;54(9):861-7.
18. Shaikh S, Verna H, Yadav N, Jauhari M, Bullangowda J. Application of steroid in clinical practice: a review. ISRN Anesthesiol. 2012;985495.

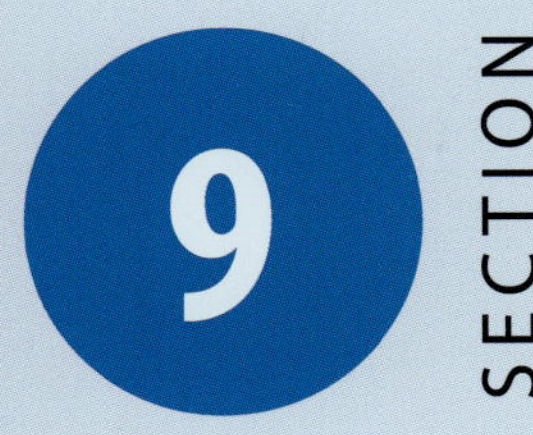

SECTION 9 Neurological Onco-Anesthesia

37 CHAPTER

Anesthesia for Supratentorial and Infratentorial Tumors

Devendra Gupta, Pragya Gupta

INTRODUCTION

Brain tumors represent a significant public health challenge, particularly in low- and middle-income countries, where their incidence is on the rise. Effective management necessitates a multifaceted interdisciplinary approach and the availability of adequate resources. The anesthetic management of patients undergoing craniotomy for intracranial tumor resection necessitates a comprehensive understanding of the impact of the brain tumor on cerebral physiology, as well as the effect of pharmacological agents on neurological function and oncological outcomes.

ANATOMY

Brain tumors are neoplasms that originate from diverse cell types within the central nervous system (CNS). These tumors are categorized as either primary, arising from the meninges, neuroepithelial tissues, pituitary gland, cranial nerves, and germ cells, or secondary, representing metastases from systemic cancers to the CNS. The supratentorial region, positioned above the tentorium cerebelli, is bordered superiorly and laterally by the skull and dura mater and is divided into two hemispheres by the falx cerebri. Each hemisphere comprises four lobes: frontal, temporal, parietal, and occipital. The insular cortex is considered as 5th distinct lobe of the cerebral cortex and forms the floor of the lateral sulcus (i.e., Sylvian fissure). In fact, the portions of parietal, frontal, and temporal lobes (called as the opercula) cover the insula. The posterior cranial fossa is the largest and deepest of the cranial fossae, accommodating critical structures including the brainstem (comprising the midbrain, pons, and upper medulla), cerebellum, cranial nerve nuclei III through XII, as well as ascending and descending neural tracts and the vertebrobasilar vascular system. Its floor is formed by the sphenoid, occipital, and temporal bones, with boundaries separating it from the middle cranial fossa, defined by the dorsum sellae of the sphenoid and the petrous portion of the temporal bone, and posteriorly by the foramen magnum. The tentorium cerebelli separates the posterior fossa from the supratentorial compartment, while the falx cerebelli divides the cerebellar hemispheres. Major venous sinuses within this region include the transverse and sigmoid sinuses. Most tumors of the posterior fossa are primary brain cancers and prevalent in pediatric age group.

EPIDEMIOLOGY

The 5th edition of the World Health Organization (WHO) classification of brain tumors (2021) builds upon the previous edition by emphasizing molecular markers in both the classification and grading of tumors, integrating many of the recommendations from the cIMPACT-NOW publications.[1] This molecular approach results in a somewhat heterogeneous classification depending on the tumor entity, as summarized in **Table 1**, which organizes brain tumors into distinct categories to ensure clarity and precision while preserving key information **(Table 1)**.

Supratentorial tumors account for approximately 80% of brain tumors in adults and 40% in children. In contrast, infratentorial tumors constitute 15–20% of brain tumors in adults and 54–70% in pediatric populations. Among malignant brain tumors, glioblastomas are the most common (47.7%), while meningiomas represent the most frequently occurring nonmalignant tumors (53.1%).[2]

In the posterior cranial fossa, tumors may be classified as intra-axial, originating within the brain parenchyma, or extra-axial, arising from surrounding structures. In the anterior compartment, intra-axial tumors predominantly include gliomas, while extra-axial tumors typically occur at the cerebellopontine angle, such as acoustic schwannomas, meningiomas, and epidermoid tumors.

TABLE 1: Classification of the brain tumor.

S. No.	Types of the brain tumor
A.	Gliomas, glioneuronal tumors, and neuronal tumors • Adult-type diffuse gliomas (astrocytoma, oligodendroglioma, and glioblastoma) • Pediatric-type diffuse low-grade gliomas • Pediatric-type diffuse high-grade gliomas • Circumscribed astrocytic gliomas (pilocytic astrocytoma, high-grade astrocytoma with piloid features, pleomorphic xanthoastrocytoma, subependymal giant cell astrocytoma, chordoid glioma, and astroblastoma) • Glioneuronal and neuronal tumors • Ependymal tumors • Choroid plexus tumors • Embryonal tumors (Medulloblastoma)
B.	Choroid plexus tumors example papilloma and carcinoma
C.	Embryonal tumors example medulloblastomas
D.	Pineal tumors
E.	Cranial and paraspinal nerve tumors (Schwannoma, neurofibroma, perineurioma, paraganglioma, etc.)
F.	Meningiomas
G.	Mesenchymal, nonmeningothelial tumors • Soft tissue tumors such as fibroblastic and myofibroblastic tumors • Vascular tumors such as hemangiomas and hemangioblastoma • Skeletal muscle tumors like rhabdomyosarcoma
H.	Chondro-osseous tumors like chondroma
I.	Melanocytic tumors
J.	Hematolymphoid tumors like lymphomas
K.	Germ cell tumors such as teratoma and germinoma
L.	Tumors of the sellar region such as pituitary adenoma and craniopharyngioma
M.	Metastases to the central nervous system (CNS) of brain, spinal cord, or meninges (mainly lungs, breast, or gastrointestinal tract)

In the posterior compartment, common intra-axial tumors include cerebellar astrocytomas, medulloblastomas, and ependymomas.[3]

PATHOPHYSIOLOGY

The supratentorial region is encased by the dura mater and skull, with balanced pressures between the left and right sides, as well as between the supratentorial and infratentorial compartments. According to the Monro–Kellie doctrine, the total intracranial volume within these compartments must remain constant **(Fig. 1)**.[4] This constraint limits the brain's capacity to compensate for an expanding mass, which can lead to increased intracranial pressure (ICP).[4] Supratentorial tumors disrupt intracranial homeostasis through multiple mechanisms:

- *Elevated ICP:* ICP typically ranges from 7 to 15 mm Hg in a supine adult. Within the rigid confines of the skull, key intracranial components include brain tissue, intravascular blood, and cerebrospinal fluid (CSF). In cases of intracranial tumors, the initial increase in volume is managed by redirecting CSF and venous blood. This translocation occurs to the spinal CSF space and extracranial veins, which helps maintain ICP during the early stages. However, when these compensatory mechanisms are exhausted (phase 2), even a minor volume increase can significantly elevate ICP **(Fig. 2)**. This can lead to ischemic injury due to impaired cerebral circulation and ultimately result in brain herniation (phases 3 and 4). Supratentorial tumors also increase ICP through peritumor edema.
- *Impaired autoregulation:* The presence of an intracranial tumor can adversely affect regional blood flow, disrupt autoregulation, and alter carbon dioxide (CO_2) reactivity in both ipsilateral and contralateral brain regions relative to the lesion **(Fig. 3)**.
- *Blood-brain barrier (BBB) disruption:* The BBB is often compromised in brain tumors, with alterations in permeability that vary depending on tumor type and stage. Significant increases in permeability typically occur in the later stages, as tumor mass expands. Additionally, functional changes in non-neoplastic brain cells are observed.[5]
- *Functional changes in adjacent brain cells:* Infiltrating tumor cells induce substantial alterations in non-neoplastic brain cells, especially neurons, contributing to clinical manifestations such as epilepsy. These changes are associated with modifications in the peritumoral microenvironment, including alterations in synaptic neurotransmitter release, reuptake, and the excitotoxic effects of glutamate.

The brain has a high metabolic demand and receives a disproportionate share of cardiac output, approximately 50 mL per 100 g of brain tissue per minute. Cerebral blood flow (CBF) is determined by the pressure gradient across the vessel wall, known as cerebral perfusion pressure (CPP), which is the difference between mean arterial pressure (MAP) and either ICP or central venous

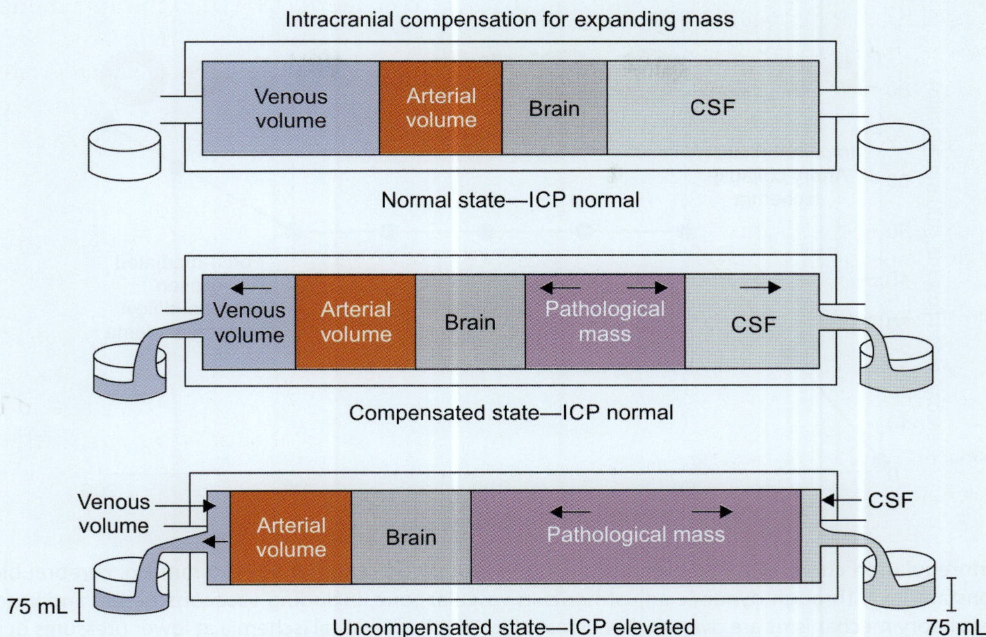

Fig. 1: The Monro-Kellie doctrine. Diagram illustrates the principle of volume constancy within the cranial cavity, emphasizing the compensatory relationship among brain tissue, intracranial blood, and cerebrospinal fluid (CSF). If the introduction of a mass, such as an intracranial tumor, displaces an equivalent volume of CSF and venous blood, intracranial pressure (ICP) remains within the normal range. However, once the compensatory mechanisms are exhausted, even minimal increase in pathological volume result in a rapid, exponential rise in ICP.

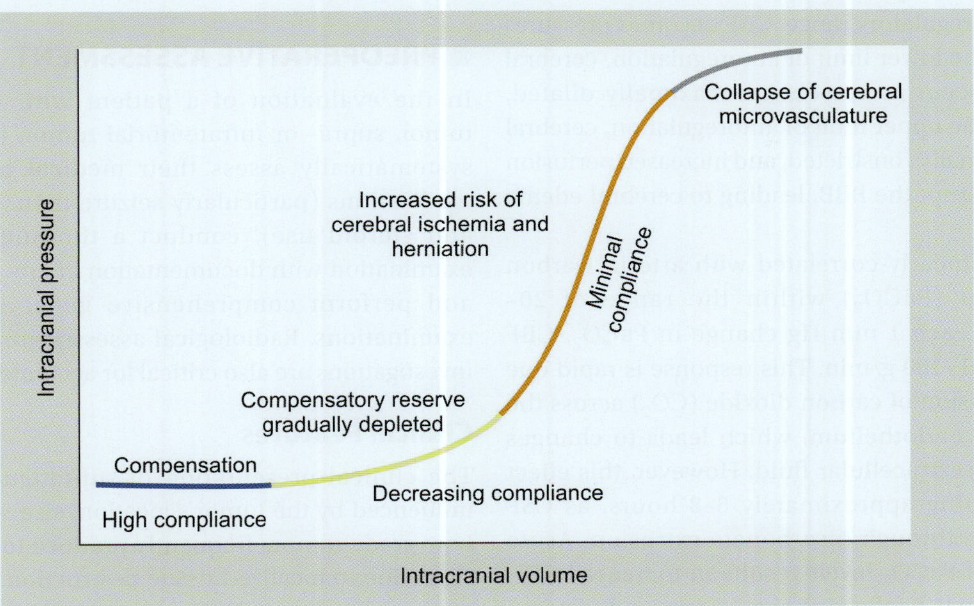

Fig. 2: Pressure-volume curve of intracranial pressure (ICP). The pressure-volume relationship of ICP is divided into four distinct phases: Phase 1 (Blue): Represents baseline intracranial volume with robust compensatory capacity and high compliance; Phase 2 (Yellow): Characterized by progressive depletion of compensatory reserves as intracranial volume increases; Phase 3 (Red): Indicates diminished compensatory reserve, with a heightened risk of cerebral ischemia and herniation; Phase 4 (Gray): Corresponds to critically elevated ICP, leading to collapse of cerebral microvasculature and impaired cerebrovascular reactivity.

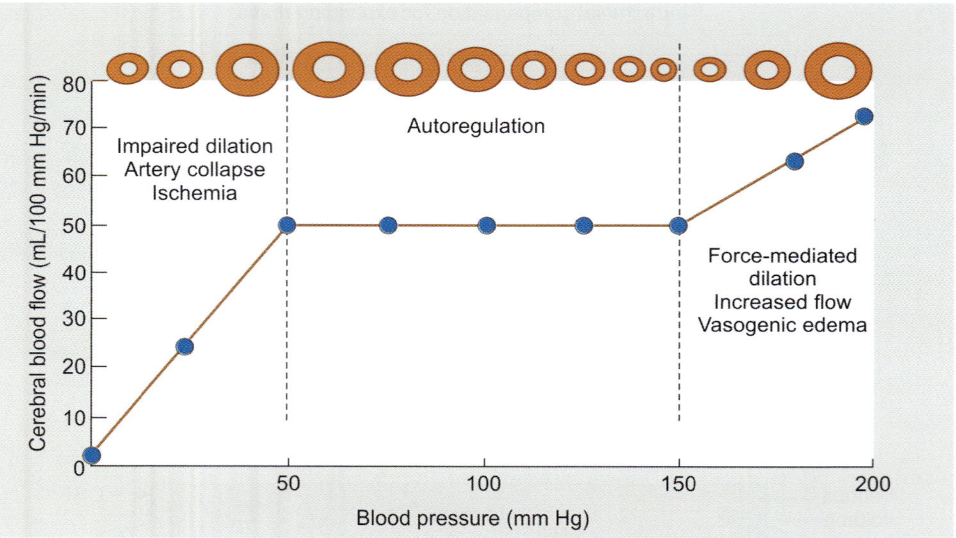

Fig. 3: Cerebral autoregulation curve. Within a mean arterial pressure (MAP) range of 50–150 mm Hg, cerebral blood flow (CBF) is maintained at a constant level through dynamic adjustments in vascular tone, including vasoconstriction and vasodilation. Beyond these limits, autoregulatory mechanisms are overwhelmed, resulting in either cerebral ischemia at lower pressures or vasogenic edema at higher pressures.

pressure (CVP), depending on which is higher. Cerebral autoregulation maintains CBF within a relatively constant range across MAP values between 65 and 150 mm Hg, assuming normal venous pressure. When MAP falls outside this autoregulatory range, CBF becomes pressure-passive. Below the lower limit of autoregulation, cerebral ischemia may occur as vessels are maximally dilated, whereas above the upper limit of autoregulation, cerebral vessels are maximally constricted, and increased perfusion pressure may disrupt the BBB, leading to cerebral edema or hemorrhage.

The CBF is linearly correlated with arterial carbon dioxide tension ($PaCO_2$) within the range of 20–80 mm Hg. For each 1 mm Hg change in $PaCO_2$, CBF adjusts by 1–2 mL/100 g/min. This response is rapid due to the swift diffusion of carbon dioxide (CO_2) across the cerebrovascular endothelium, which leads to changes in the pH of the extracellular fluid. However, this effect is transient, lasting approximately 6–8 hours, as CSF pH renormalizes through bicarbonate extrusion. Acute normalization of $PaCO_2$ levels results in increased CBF, which can elevate ICP following hypocapnia and increase the risk of cerebral ischemia after hypercapnia. Thus, both hyperventilation and hypoventilation significantly influence CBF. In contrast, changes in arterial oxygen tension (PaO_2) within the range of 60–300 mm Hg have minimal impact on CBF. However, when PaO_2 falls below 60 mm Hg, CBF increases markedly, whereas PaO_2 levels exceeding 350 mm Hg may induce mild cerebral vasoconstriction.

PREOPERATIVE ASSESSMENT

In the evaluation of a patient with an intracranial tumor, supra- or infratentorial tumor, it is essential to systematically assess their medical history, current medications (particularly seizure management efficacy and steroid use), conduct a thorough neurological examination with documentation of any existing deficits, and perform comprehensive general and systemic examinations. Radiological assessments and laboratory investigations are also critical for accurate diagnosis.

Clinical Features

The clinical presentation of supratentorial tumors is influenced by the tumor's location, size, and growth rate. Low-grade tumors frequently produce focal neurological signs due to localized tissue destruction or compression of specialized regions. For example, lesions in the motor cortex may result in contralateral hemiparesis, those near the language centers can lead to aphasia, and tumors affecting the optic apparatus may cause visual disturbances. Involvement of the hypothalamic-pituitary axis can lead to endocrinopathies. These site-specific manifestations provide critical insights into the tumor's characteristics and prompt us about diagnosis and therapeutic strategies. As the tumor enlarges, patients may develop generalized symptoms such as headache, nausea, projectile vomiting, cognitive decline, and altered consciousness attributed to increased ICP. Elevated ICP can reduce CPP consequently causing cerebral ischemia. Tumors that grow slowly often present with a gradual, progressive symptom onset, while hemorrhage within the tumor may precipitate an acute clinical presentation.[6]

Symptoms of posterior cranial fossa lesions differ from those of supratentorial tumors, frequently presenting with signs of increased ICP, such as headache, nausea, vomiting, and papilledema. These symptoms can escalate rapidly, particularly in cases of acute hydrocephalus. Localized manifestations at the lesion site may include movement disorders, alterations in muscle tone, and ocular signs such as nystagmus, strabismus, diplopia, and abnormal pupillary reactions. Additional symptoms may include cranial nerve deficits, bulbar palsy, bradycardia, respiratory distress, and in severe cases, sudden brainstem herniation, which can be fatal. The classic triad associated with a posterior fossa mass comprises headache, vomiting, and ataxia, whereas seizures are uncommon compared to supratentorial tumors. Certain genetic diseases are characterized by the development of multiple intracranial tumors **(Table 2)**. A detailed patient history is essential to identify these conditions, as they often present with a range of symptoms and may lead to early detection of associated tumors, guiding appropriate management.

TABLE 2: Genetic syndromes and associated brain tumors.

Syndromes	*Associated brain tumors*
Neurofibromatosis type 1	Astrocytoma, optic glioma, neurofibroma
Neurofibromatosis type 2	Vestibular schwannoma, meningioma, astrocytoma
Von Hippel–Lindau syndrome	Hemangioblastoma
Turcot syndrome	Glioblastoma multiforme, medulloblastoma
Tuberous sclerosis	Astrocytoma
Li-Fraumeni syndrome	Choroid plexus carcinoma, medulloblastoma, astrocytoma
Cowden syndrome	Meningioma, gangliocytomas

Neurologic Evaluation

Neurologic evaluation in brain tumor cases is essential for identifying the location and extent of the disease, documenting nervous system dysfunction, and assessing the patient's physical status, and neurological reserve **(Table 3)**. This evaluation helps in formulating a comprehensive anesthetic plan tailored to the patient. It is critical to establish a baseline of the patient's neurological function and note any deficits. Additionally, signs and symptoms of increased ICP, such as headache or altered mental status, should be monitored. Tumor size and location are crucial for anesthesia planning as well such as positioning, postoperative ventilation, and predicting potential complication and prognosis.

Cardiovascular Evaluation

Preoperative evaluation of cardiac status is crucial in patients with intracranial tumors, particularly through cardiac studies such as electrocardiograms (ECGs) and echocardiograms (ECHO), especially in those with underlying heart disease. These assessments should be tailored to the patient's specific condition and potential intraoperative risks. Cardiac abnormalities, such as dysrhythmias, tachycardia, bradycardia, and hypertension, can significantly impact anesthesia management. It is essential to assess for a patent foramen ovale (PFO) in patients undergoing craniotomy in a sitting position, as its presence may represent a relative contraindication.

Respiratory System Evaluation

Respiratory complications are a significant concern in patients undergoing elective craniotomy for brain tumor surgery, particularly in posterior fossa tumor surgeries involving lesions near the brainstem. Prolonged surgical duration and challenging positioning can place substantial stress on the cardiorespiratory system. The incidence of postoperative pulmonary complications is notably higher in patients with a history of smoking, previous pulmonary disease, or the American Society of Anesthesiologists (ASA) classification greater than II. Additionally, approximately 40% of brain metastases originate from the lungs, which may exacerbate preexisting respiratory compromise due to the primary pathology itself.[7] A history of obstructive sleep apnea (OSA) can significantly impact both intraoperative and postoperative care in neurosurgical patients. Certain populations, such as those with acromegaly and Cushing's disease, have a high prevalence of OSA due to anatomical

TABLE 3: Preoperative clinical examination.

Systems	*Performing a quick neurological examination*
Higher mental functions	During patient assessment, key factors such as appearance, mood, thought processes, and speech should be evaluated. Altered mental status can be assessed using the "AVPU" scale (A: Alert, V: responds to verbal stimuli, P: responds to painful stimuli, U: Unresponsive) and the Glasgow Coma Scale (GCS) to quantify the level of consciousness
Motor system	Patient's gait and assessment of their ability to perform toe and heel walks should be observed carefully. Upper limb weakness using the pronator drift test and hand grasp test on the ulnar side should be evaluated. For lower limb weakness, assessment of drift and test dorsiflexion and plantar flexion should be done. If any motor tests yield abnormal results, proceed with formal extremity testing. Motor strength should be graded on a 0–5 scale, with 0 indicating no movement and 5 indicating full movement against gravity and resistance. Reflexes should be tested for the biceps (C5, C6), triceps (C7, C8), patellar (L2, L3, and L4), tendo-achilles (S1, S2), and plantar reflex (Babinski sign for upper motor neuron lesions), with responses graded from 0 (no response) to 4+ (hyperreflexia)
Sensory system	The sensory examination evaluates pain and light touch sensation bilaterally on the hands, feet, and limbs. Simultaneous sensory extinction testing is employed to detect subtle central nervous system deficits. Posterior column testing is specifically reserved for patients with suspected neuropathies or those presenting with sensory abnormalities
Cranial nerve examination	Cranial nerve examination is conducted through patient history and observation, with particular attention to nerves II, III, IV, and VI in individuals presenting with neurological complaints: • *Cranial nerve II:* Assess visual acuity, visual fields, and perform an ophthalmoscopic examination • *Cranial nerve III:* Evaluate pupil size and symmetry, as well as adduction and vertical gaze • *Cranial nerve IV:* Test internal depression of the eye via the superior oblique muscle • *Cranial nerve VI:* Assess abduction of the eye using the lateral rectus muscle
Cerebellar function (coordination and balance)	Balance involves integrating inputs from the cerebellum, visual system, vestibular system, and proprioception. The Romberg test evaluates balance. Swaying with eyes open or closed indicates a cerebellar lesion that other sensory systems cannot compensate for

and physiological changes associated with these conditions. Recognizing and managing OSA is essential, as it may necessitate adjustments in anesthesia techniques and postoperative monitoring to prevent complications related to airway obstruction, hypoventilation, and respiratory depression.

Airway Examination

Airway management in neurosurgical patients requires specialized considerations due to conditions that can complicate intubation and risk neurological compromise. Certain patient populations, such as those with pituitary tumors presenting with Cushing's disease or acromegaly, are particularly vulnerable to challenges in ventilation, tracheal obstruction, and intubation difficulty. In addition to difficult mask ventilation and intubation, challenging extubation is also a critical factor. Following pituitary surgery, nasal packing is often applied, which can cause significant discomfort and distress during emergence from anesthesia. A comprehensive preoperative airway assessment is therefore vital, encompassing evaluation for difficult mask ventilation, difficult laryngoscopy and/or intubation, and accessibility of the front of neck for emergency airway access if required.

Laboratory Investigations

Baseline hemoglobin (Hb) levels have been shown to predict the likelihood of transfusion in patients undergoing cranial surgery with significant blood loss, thus aiding in the planning of perioperative transfusion requirements. The patients with glioblastoma multiforme, which carries risks of both iatrogenic bleeding and thrombosis due to the release of procoagulants, coagulation profiling is essential to evaluate and manage these risks effectively. Hyperglycemia is commonly observed in neurosurgical patients, primarily due to steroid administration. Pituitary adenomas are often associated with diverse endocrine abnormalities, including Cushing's syndrome, acromegaly, and hypothyroidism, each of which may impact perioperative management. While primary brain tumors generally exert minimal direct effects on the gastrointestinal system, patients may experience nausea, vomiting, and stress-related gastric ulcers as a result of elevated ICP or steroid use.

Renal function may be adversely affected due to reduced oral intake and the frequent administration of diuretics, such as mannitol or furosemide, as well as the use of contrast agents. These factors can contribute to dehydration and increased renal workload, heightening the risk of acute kidney injury and necessitating careful monitoring of fluid balance and renal function.

The ECG and chest X-ray (CXR) are recommended for most brain surgeries, to assess baseline cardiac and pulmonary status. Additionally, in cases of compromised cardiac function or anticipated significant blood loss, a 2-D ECHO and stress ECHO should be performed to evaluate cardiac reserve and optimize perioperative management.

Diagnostic Evaluation/Imaging Techniques

Neuroimaging is a standard diagnostic tool in patients with suspected intracranial lesions, aiding in accurate localization and differentiation of lesion types. Magnetic resonance imaging (MRI) is particularly favored for patients with slowly progressing neurological symptoms, given its superior sensitivity over computed tomography (CT) in detecting and characterizing intracranial lesions. Imaging is used to assess the tumor's size and location, its proximity to eloquent brain regions or major vessels, vascularity, presence of peritumoral edema, and signs of elevated ICP, such as midline shift, ventricular compression, and temporal lobe herniation **(Figs. 4A and B)**.

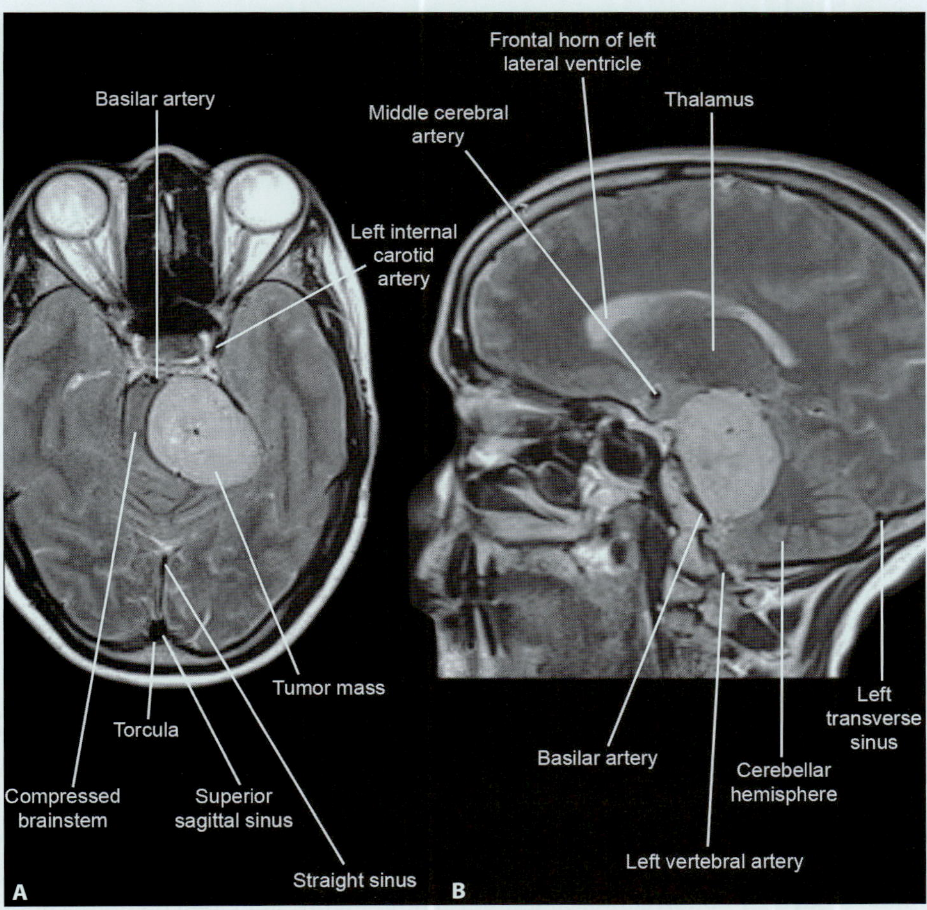

Figs. 4A and B: (A) The axial cut of the T2WI of the magnetic resonance imaging (MRI) brain suggests a globular mass lesion which is hyperintense located in left crural cistern. The major portion of the lesion is infratentorial and causing significant compression and distortion of the brainstem. The basilar artery is pushed toward the right side; (B) The T2WI sagittal cut of the MRI brain suggests the lesion in left crural cistern causing compression over the midbrain laterally, vermis with buckling of the left cerebellar folia in the posterior aspect. The lesion has pushed the left posterior cerebral artery superiorly and compression of the basilar artery. The 4th ventricle is not visualized clearly.

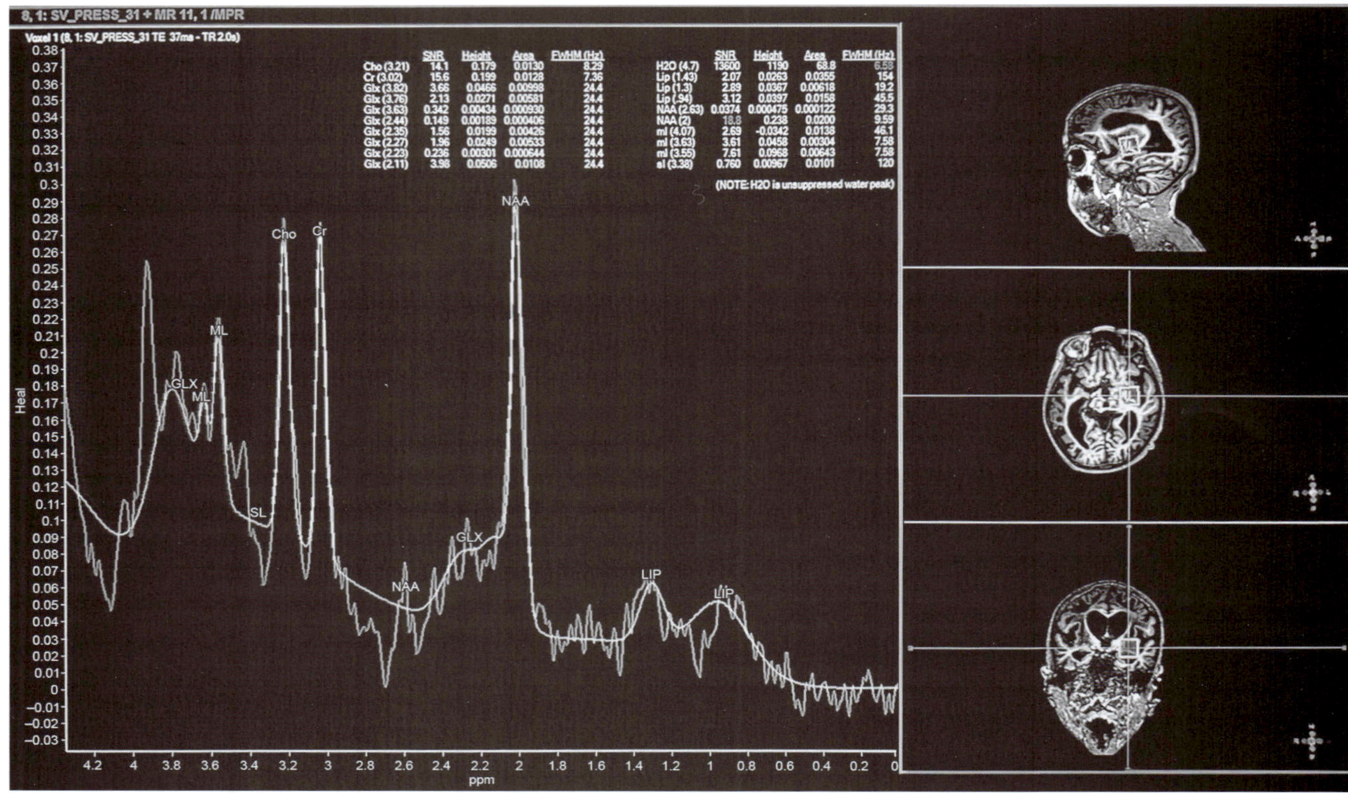

Fig. 5: Magnetic resonance (MR) spectroscopy. MR spectroscopy of brain showing various metabolites in graphical representation, most noticeable are N-acetyl Aspartate (NAA), Choline (Cho), and Creatinine (Cr).

Magnetic resonance spectroscopy (MRS) integrates the molecular differentiation capabilities of nuclear magnetic resonance (NMR) with the spatial localization features of MRI **(Fig. 5)**. Key metabolites analyzed in brain tumor spectroscopy include choline, N-acetyl aspartate, creatine, lipids, myo-inositol, and lactate. Evaluating the relative changes in these metabolites, alongside other imaging features, can aid in distinguishing primary brain tumors from metastases, grading gliomas, and differentiating recurrence from radiation necrosis. Metabolite ratios, such as choline-to-creatine (Cho/Cr) or choline-to-N-acetyl aspartate (Cho/NAA), are often used to enhance diagnostic sensitivity and are widely applied in clinical practice. CT angiography is now routinely performed for large or complex tumors to identify abnormal vasculature or arteriovenous malformations within or surrounding the lesion. Detailed assessment of the tumor's location and size aids in planning surgical approach, estimating potential blood loss, and evaluating the risk of air embolism, particularly in cases like convexity meningiomas near the dural sinus. Although MRI is generally more sensitive than CT in tumor evaluation, patients presenting with acute neurological deterioration may initially undergo CT imagining for quick diagnosis of hemorrhage or herniation. Positron emission tomography (PET) provides quantitative data on metabolic activity within the brain, enabling differentiation of tumors from inflammatory lesions.

PREOPERATIVE OPTIMIZATION

Effective preoperative planning requires a thorough discussion with the surgical team to address critical details such as tumor size and location, diagnosis, surgical approach, the need for ICP management, neuromonitoring requirements, anticipated complications, expected blood loss and the surgical objectives—whether for radical excision or decompression.

Premedication should generally include all regular medications, particularly steroids like dexamethasone, as patients with significant tumor-related mass effect and edema often benefit from preoperative steroid therapy. While a 48-hour regimen is optimal, clinical improvements are commonly seen within 24 hours. For patients with elevated ICP, preoperative sedatives or anxiolytics should be minimized or avoided to prevent CO_2 retention, as even low doses of benzodiazepines or opioids can exacerbate neurological deficits. In patients with posterior fossa lesions, sedative premedication is especially limited due to the risks of hypoventilation and increased ICP. Antiepileptic medications should be continued unless seizure focus mapping is planned.[8] Blood thinners must be discontinued, and all home medications should be reviewed to determine safe continuation.

SURGICAL APPROACHES AND POSITIONING

The traditional and most common surgical approach for brain tumor removal is craniotomy, which involves opening the skull to access and resect the tumor. Various approaches are (1) Frontal craniotomy, (2) Pterional craniotomy (frontotemporal), (3) Temporal and subtemporal craniotomy, (4) Anterior parasagittal and subfrontal approach, (5) Posterior parasagittal craniotomy, (6) Midline suboccipital craniotomy, (7) Lateral suboccipital approach, (8) Trans-sphenoidal approach, (9) Endoscopic approach, and (10) Keyhole surgery.

In neurosurgical procedures, the extended duration and requirement for precise localization of brain tumor areas necessitate positioning the patient in a manner that is physiologically optimal, safe, and comfortable. Optimal positioning in brain tumor surgery is essential and is determined by factors such as the tumor's anatomical location, type, and the selected surgical approach. Common positions include supine (for frontal, temporal, or parietal tumors), prone (for occipital lobe and posterior fossa tumors), sitting, semisitting, lateral, semilateral (Jannetta), and park bench (for posterior parietal, occipital, or cerebellopontine angle tumors). Each positioning technique is tailored to provide optimal access to the target area while minimizing the risk of injury to surrounding brain tissue. Effective positioning allows the neurosurgeon precise access to the area of interest, facilitating tumor resection with minimal disruption to adjacent structures.

Positioning begins promptly following the induction of anesthesia and the establishment of sufficient venous access and necessary monitoring devices. The placement of skull pins during positioning can cause significant nociceptive stimulation, potentially leading to hemodynamic fluctuations. To mitigate these effects, it is recommended to increase the depth of anesthesia and augment analgesia with a prepinning bolus of remifentanil (0.25–1 μg/kg), fentanyl (1–2 μg/kg), esmolol (0.25–0.5 mg/kg), or propofol (0.5–1 mg/kg).[9] Local anesthetic infiltration at the pin sites can further attenuate adverse CNS and hemodynamic responses. Additionally, performing a scalp nerve blockade prior to pin application can help maintain intraoperative hemodynamic stability and provide effective postoperative analgesia. Proper patient positioning is essential to ensure comfort, minimize injury risk, and facilitate optimal surgical conditions. Adequate padding should be applied at all pressure points to prevent tissue injury. A slight head-up tilt is often beneficial across positions to promote venous drainage. Avoid excessive neck flexion, extension, or rotation to preserve cerebral venous outflow, maintaining a two-finger distance between the chin and sternum to prevent airway compromise. Slight knee flexion helps reduce the risk of lumbosacral strain. For lateral positioning, an axillary roll is recommended to prevent brachial plexus stretch injury.[10] Finally, all tubes and monitoring devices should be securely fastened to maintain a clear and unobstructed surgical field.

ANESTHETIC MANAGEMENT

The primary goals of anesthetic care during brain tumor surgery include:

- *Optimization of cerebral physiology:* Ensuring optimal cerebral perfusion and oxygenation while preventing secondary systemic insults.
- *Brain relaxation and neuroprotection:* Providing a relaxed brain to facilitate surgical access, along with implementing strategies for neuroprotection.
- *Patient positioning for surgical access and safety:* Achieving ideal patient positioning to enhance surgical accessibility while minimizing positioning-related risks.
- *Adequate anesthetic depth:* Maintaining an adequate depth of anesthesia to prevent hemodynamic instability.
- *Conditions for intraoperative neurophysiological monitoring (IONM):* Optimizing intraoperative conditions to support reliable neurophysiological monitoring.
- *Prevention and management of complications:* Vigilantly preventing, promptly identifying, and

effectively managing potential complications, such as venous air embolism (VAE).

- *Facilitated postoperative recovery:* Finally, enabling a smooth recovery with early awakening to allow for timely neurological assessment, minimize postoperative pain, and enhance neurological outcomes.[11]

Induction

Induction of anesthesia in neurosurgical patients typically involves intravenous anesthetics combined with opioids to maintain hemodynamic and cerebral stability. Propofol (1.25–2.5 mg/kg) and thiopental (3–6 mg/kg) are the preferred agents for induction for their effects on cerebral vasculature and cerebral metabolic rate of oxygen ($CMRO_2$), while etomidate (0.3 mg/kg) may be chosen in patients with frailty, advanced age, or poor cardiac reserve due to its hemodynamic stability.[12] Ketamine is generally avoided due to its potential to elevate ICP and induce postoperative hallucinations. For muscle relaxation and intubation, rocuronium, vecuronium, atracurium, and cisatracurium are commonly used, with rocuronium preferred for its rapid onset of intubating conditions. Succinylcholine is typically avoided, as it may increase ICP. Opioids such as fentanyl and morphine are frequently administered due to their minimal impact on CBF, metabolism, and ICP, provided normocapnia and normotension are maintained. Most intravenous anesthetics—excluding ketamine—reduce CBF, $CMRO_2$, and ICP, thus supporting optimal conditions for neurosurgery.

Monitoring

Comprehensive monitoring is essential during brain tumor surgery to ensure patient safety and stability. Standard monitoring includes ECG, pulse oximetry (SpO_2), noninvasive blood pressure (NIBP), temperature, end-tidal carbon dioxide ($EtCO_2$), and urine output. Arterial line insertion is often preferred to enable continuous beat-to-beat blood pressure recording and facilitate arterial blood gas analysis, as well as electrolyte and osmolality assessment. For patients at risk of significant intraoperative fluid shifts, VAE, or requiring prolonged mechanical ventilation, CVP catheter placement is advisable. In cases where CVP is used for air aspiration during VAE events, its position at the superior vena cava–right atrium junction should be confirmed via P-wave monitoring on ECG or through transesophageal echocardiography (TEE).

Depth of anesthesia monitoring using processed electroencephalogram (EEG)-based monitors, such as bispectral index (BIS) or entropy, is now routine to enhance anesthetic control. Additionally, neuromuscular monitoring is advised when muscle relaxants are not used, particularly when intraoperative neurophysiological monitoring is conducted to preserve neurological function integrity during surgery.

Tumor resections near eloquent brain regions often require brain mapping and evoked potential monitoring to enable precise localization and safe dissection. For procedures with a risk of cerebral hypoperfusion, EEG and evoked potential monitoring are crucial. Intraoperative neuromonitoring (IONM) techniques, such as somatosensory evoked potentials (SSEPs), transcranial electrical motor evoked potentials (MEPs), brainstem auditory evoked responses (BAERs), direct electrical stimulation, and free-running electromyography (EMG), play a vital role in safeguarding critical neural structures during neurosurgery.[13]

The facial nerve (CN VII) and vestibulocochlear nerve (CN VIII) are highly susceptible to injury during cerebellopontine angle and brainstem surgeries, making continuous facial nerve monitoring essential. Standard techniques for facial nerve monitoring include direct electrical stimulation to elicit compound muscle action potentials (CMAP) and the use of transcranial facial nerve motor evoked potentials (FNMEP) to assess nerve integrity throughout the procedure.[14]

Maintenance

An ideal anesthetic agent for maintenance of anesthesia should stabilize systemic hemodynamics, preserve CBF, and reduce $CMRO_2$ and ICP. In patients with large tumors or intracranial hypertension (ICH), reducing brain volume enhances surgical exposure and minimizes ischemia. Short-acting, titratable agents are preferred for their precise control and rapid onset. Intravenous anesthetics are often chosen for their ability to reduce brain swelling and limit increases in CBF and ICP.[12] Caution is needed with volatile anesthetics, as they may worsen elevated ICP. Short-acting opioids, such as fentanyl and remifentanil are commonly used in neurosurgical procedures. These opioids have minimal impact on CBF, $CMRO_2$, and ICP, as long as normocapnia and normotension are maintained. The choice of agent for the maintenance of anesthesia is either propofol or an inhalational agent. A 2015 study comparing propofol, sevoflurane, and desflurane along with nitrous oxide found all the three agents similar and acceptable for the conduct of anesthesia in patients undergoing craniotomy for supratentorial tumors.[15] Remifentanil is often administered with propofol and has the advantage of being easily titratable.

Hemodynamics

Maintaining stable hemodynamics is crucial in neurosurgery to ensure adequate CPP, which is the difference between MAP and ICP. Cerebral perfusion is essential for sustaining brain tissue metabolism, and any reduction in CPP can lead to ischemia. Avoiding intraoperative hypotension is therefore critical, as it can significantly compromise perfusion. The perilesional area suffers from compromised perfusion due to mass effect and elevated ICP. This can lead to impairing neuronal oxygenation and resulting in neuronal injury. A modest increase in MAP may enhance cerebral perfusion, trigger, decrease cerebral blood volume, decrease ICP, and help minimize cerebral ischemia. Furthermore, intraoperative undue hypertension poses additional risks, as it can elevate cerebral blood volume and potentially exceed the brain's autoregulatory capacity, thereby increasing ICP. Common triggers for hypertensive responses include skull pin insertion and periosteum elevation. Through proactive hemodynamic control, perioperative cerebral stability can be maintained, reducing the risk of adverse neurological outcomes.

Anesthetic management aims to create a relaxed brain environment that facilitates optimal surgical access while minimizing brain retraction and perilesional neuronal injury. A practical checklist is suggested to help with the differential diagnosis of unsatisfactory brain relaxation **(Table 4)**. The literature demonstrates that hyperosmolar solutes enhance brain elastance and reduce brain volume during craniotomies by creating an osmotic gradient across the blood-brain barrier, which promotes water movement from brain tissue to the intravascular space. A good, relaxed brain improves surgical access and widens the surgical view for the surgeon. It minimizes retraction, reduces local hypoperfusion and cerebral ischemia, and, therefore, minimizes the risk of complication and postoperative neurological deficit. Hypertonic saline and mannitol, the primary osmotic agents, have been widely utilized for decades in both elective and emergency craniotomies. Higher doses of mannitol improve brain

TABLE 4: A practical checklist of the factors related with poor brain relaxation or tense brain.

Factor	Description
Oxygenation	Hypoxia induces an increase in CBF and CBV
Hemoglobin	Low arterial blood oxygen content results in an increase in CBF and CBV
Body position	Head-down position impedes cerebral venous drainage, with resultant increase of CBV. The head-down position also impedes the movement of CSF from the intracranial space to the extracranial intrathecal compartment
Anesthesia depth, analgesia, and muscle relaxation	Light plane of anesthesia (BIS >60), decreased analgesia, and less muscles relaxation many a times cause brain bulge
Carbon dioxide	Raised $PaCO_2$ increases CBF and CBV
Airway pressure	Elevated airway pressure raises intrathoracic pressure, which in turn impedes cerebral venous return, leading to increased ICP and contribute to brain bulging
Blood pressure	In brain regions with impaired autoregulation, such as tumor-affected areas, hypertension leads to increase in CBF and CBV, whereas hypotension can result in ischemia
Neck position	Lateral flexion or torsion may obstruct venous drainage, with resultant increase of CBV hence poor brain relaxation
Masses	Many a times additional masses (e.g., contralateral subdural hematoma due to headframe pin trauma, enlarging pneumocephalus)
Volatile anesthetics	High-MAC volatile anesthetics cause cerebral vasodilatation, with resultant increase in CBF and CBV
Other factors	Fever/hyperthermia, hyperglycemia, subclinical seizures, urinary retention
Imaging study	Careful evaluation of CT and MRI studies may predict possibility of poor brain relaxation on craniotomy

(BIS: bispectral index; CT: computed tomography; CBF: cerebral blood flow; CBV: cerebral blood volume; CSF: cerebrospinal fluid; ICP: intracranial pressure; MAC: minimum alveolar concentration; $PaCO_2$: arterial carbon dioxide tension)

relaxation but are associated with an increased likelihood of adverse effects; thus, a dose of 1.0 g/kg is recommended intraoperatively to achieve optimal brain relaxation with minimal side effects. Similarly, the administration of a 3 mL/kg infusion of 3% NaCl (1.027 mOsm/mL) over 30 minutes is recommended, as it achieves satisfactory brain relaxation while preserving stable hemodynamic status.[16] Loop diuretics like furosemide as an additional measure for lowering ICP may be implied in refractory cases. Steroids reduce perilesional interstitial edema by minimizing fluid leakage from surrounding neocapillaries and are typically started upon tumor diagnosis and should be continued perioperatively.

Ventilation should be adjusted to maintain normocapnia targeting a $PaCO_2$ of 30–35 mm Hg, while keeping intrathoracic pressures low. While hyperventilation can decrease brain tension but poses a risk of cerebral hypoperfusion resulting in cerebral ischemia.[17] Careful management of positive end-expiratory pressure (PEEP) is critical, with levels below 10 cmH_2O typically having minimal impact on CBF or ICP in neurosurgical patients. Low PEEP helps prevent increase in intrathoracic and ICP, thereby minimizing the risk of compromised cerebral perfusion. However, individualized adjustments based on patient-specific factors, such as lung compliance and ICP, may be necessary to optimize respiratory support while maintaining optimum CBF.

Despite the careful following of the checklists, if the brain appears tense prior to dural opening, it is advisable to switch to intravenous anesthetic agents, such as propofol, and increase the depth of anesthesia. Additional management may include the substantial use of osmotic diuretics, controlled hyperventilation to maintain $PaCO_2$ between 28 and 32 mm Hg, and maintaining slightly elevated blood pressure (MAP 90–100 mm Hg). CSF drainage via a ventricular catheter, if placed preoperatively, can also help relieve ICP.

Maintaining glycemic control between 110 and 160 mg/dL is essential, as hyperglycemia and hypoglycemia can trigger anaerobic metabolism, leading to acidosis and impaired cerebral function, which negatively impacts neurological recovery and outcomes.[18] Maintaining optimal hematocrit levels is critical, since anemia impairs oxygen delivery and neuronal preservation in the penumbral zone. Intraoperative blood transfusions should be guided by expected blood loss, physiological markers (e.g., base deficit, bicarbonate, and pH), and hemodynamic status. Hematocrit readings may be unreliable due to dehydration or excessive fluid administration. Normothermia must be maintained, with correction of hyperthermia to prevent increased $CMRO_2$, which can worsen outcomes in elevated ICP conditions.[19] Seizures are common in patients with supratentorial lesions, particularly near the cortex. Typically, these patients are on anticonvulsants, phenytoin sodium is the standard perioperative anticonvulsant, with alternatives including phenobarbital or sodium valproate. However, newer second-generation antiepileptics, such as levetiracetam, may be preferred due to their lower side effect profile.

Emergence

The planning of recovery and extubation will be guided by multiple factors, including the patient's preoperative status (particularly their neurological and physiological condition), the ease of airway management, the intraoperative course (metabolic and hemodynamic changes) and events, and the postoperative clinical status. Additionally, careful consideration of hemodynamic stability, ventilatory requirements, and the risk of postoperative complications is essential to ensure a smooth transition to spontaneous breathing and optimize overall patient outcomes.

Early extubation in neurosurgical patients offers several advantages, including enabling timely postoperative neurological evaluation for early detection of complications such as cerebral edema, hemorrhage, or new deficits; reducing the risk of ventilator-associated complications, minimizing hemodynamic fluctuations and stress responses associated with prolonged intubation; decreasing the likelihood of ICU delirium; and shortening the duration of ICU stay. Thus, patients who are preoperatively conscious, cooperative, and neurologically intact, with uncomplicated airway management and an uneventful intraoperative course, are expected to have a favorable recovery. In such cases, tracheal extubation is performed once the established criteria for extubation are met. In such cases, efforts should focus on maintaining normothermia, normotension, normoglycemia, normocarbia, and adequate Hb levels from the time the patient is transferred to the operating room (OR), as these factors are critical for smooth recovery and successful extubation. Extubation should be performed when the patient is fully awake and demonstrates adequate spontaneous breathing efforts. In most patients, extubation is uneventful, however a wide array of issues can be encountered ranging from minor to life-threatening. While coughing and bucking may not have direct long-term consequences, they are associated with a range of secondary issues including cardiovascular complications (myocardial ischemia and arrhythmias), disruption of the surgical site and bleeding, and an increased intracranial and intraocular pressure. In order to facilitate a smooth extubation, the principal aims are to suppress severe cough, hypertension, tachycardia, breath-holding, and laryngospasm. Dexmedetomidine appeared to be the most effective medication for decreasing the frequency of moderate-to-severe emergence cough followed by remifentanil and fentanyl, however, β-blockers, labetalol, and lidocaine, have been utilized in different doses and administration techniques to attenuate the hemodynamic responses associated with extubation.[20]

Delayed emergence and extubation in neurosurgical patients is planned for those with preoperative unconsciousness or reduced Glasgow Coma Scale (GCS) scores due to raised ICP or neurological deficits, significant intraoperative events such as complex surgeries, brain swelling, major blood loss, or hemodynamic instability, difficult airway cases, persistent airway edema, poor postoperative respiratory effort, or severe systemic illnesses such as cardiac, pulmonary, or metabolic disorders.

Complications

Post-tumor resection craniotomy patients should be managed in a specialized neuro-ICU for continuous neurological and physiological monitoring. Postoperative complications following intracranial surgery depend on the tumor's site and type. Major complications occur in 13–27% of patients,[21] including neurologic (hematomas, cerebral edema, and seizures), hemodynamic, metabolic, and respiratory issues. Minor complications such as postoperative nausea and vomiting (PONV), postcraniotomy pain, and hyperglycemia may also signal underlying major complications.

Constant vigilance and prompt detection of postoperative complications are essential for favorable outcomes. Postoperative hypertension can cause intracranial bleeding or hematoma.[22] Postoperative care includes managing fluid and electrolyte balance, ensuring adequate nutrition, and continuing seizure prophylaxis, corticosteroids, and antiedema measures. Adequate sedation with fast-acting, titratable agents is crucial for patients on elective mechanical ventilation to ensure tolerance and allow timely neurological assessment.

SPECIAL CONSIDERATION

Posterior Fossa Surgery

The posterior fossa, the deepest of the cranial fossae, is anatomically bordered by the dorsum sellae and the basilar portion of the occipital bone (clivus) anteriorly. Laterally, it is enclosed by the petrosal and mastoid segments of the temporal bone, while superiorly, it is delineated by the dural tentorium cerebelli. Posteriorly and inferiorly, it is bounded by the occipital bone. The posterior fossa contains critical neurological structures, including the cerebellum, midbrain, pons, medulla, and several cranial nerves, within a compact and rigid bony compartment. Tumors represent the most prevalent pathology affecting the posterior fossa, constituting over 60% of all brain tumors in children. In adults, though less common than in children, these typically include primary tumors such as vestibular schwannomas, meningiomas, hemangioblastomas, and ependymomas, as well as metastatic lesions.[3] These tumors often present with symptoms related to increased ICP, cranial nerve dysfunction, or cerebellar ataxia due to the confined nature of the posterior fossa and its vital structures. The involvement of lower cranial nerve palsy suggests invasion or compression of the brainstem and helps to plan tracheal extubation at end of surgery **(Fig. 4)**.

Two primary techniques are commonly employed to access posterior fossa pathologies: the midline suboccipital approach and the retromastoid approach. The midline suboccipital approach targets conditions involving the cerebellum, fourth ventricle, brainstem, and foramen magnum, focusing on adequate exposure and avoiding venous sinus or neural damage. The retromastoid approach is suited for cerebellopontine angle tumors, vascular lesions, and cranial nerve V–XII pathologies, aiming to ensure sufficient access while avoid injury to the dura or venous sinuses, and minimizing complications. The prone and sitting positions provide midline access but require care to avoid abdominal compression and reduce bleeding. The lateral and modified lateral positions (park-bench position) enhance unilateral access and gravity-assisted drainage, with careful attention to securing lines, the tracheal tube, and pressure areas. Muscle relaxants should be avoided if MEP or facial nerve monitoring is planned. Intraoperative neurophysiologic monitoring necessitates a total intravenous anesthesia plan, with depth of anesthesia monitoring offering additional benefits. The detection of VAE during surgery is critical, particularly in posterior fossa tumor resection in sitting. The recommended monitoring techniques, ranked by sensitivity, include TEE as the most sensitive method, followed by precordial Doppler ultrasound, which provides real-time detection of air bubbles within the venous system.[23] $EtCO_2$ monitoring serves as an additional measure, as sudden and sustain decrease in $EtCO_2$ by 2–4 mm Hg may indicate compromised pulmonary circulation due to VAE. Combining these techniques can enhance the likelihood of early VAE detection, enabling prompt intervention and minimizing the risk of adverse outcomes.[23] Promptly notifying the surgeon of VAE facilitates immediate interventions such as saline irrigation of the surgical field, bone wax application, and bilateral jugular compression to prevent further air entry. Discontinuation of N_2O and aspiration of air or blood via a central venous catheter help reduce the VAE burden. Administering 100% oxygen provides hemodynamic support. In severe cases, repositioning the patient to lower the surgical site relative to the heart or adopting the left lateral decubitus position, also known as the Durant maneuver may be necessary.

Intraoperative Magnetic Resonance Imaging

The distinction between tumor and normal brain tissue is one of the main challenges in achieving the maximum extent of resection without compromising functional areas. This challenge is particularly pronounced in primary brain tumors which exhibit a diffuse growth pattern resulting in a transitional zone at the tumor margins where malignant and normal cells intermingle. Intraoperative MRI (iMRI) offers near-real-time imaging, providing precise guidance to enhance the accuracy of brain tumor resection. While anesthetic management for iMRI is largely similar to that of other neurosurgical procedures, strict adherence to MRI safety protocols and regular staff training are essential to prevent accidents and life-threatening emergencies. All ferromagnetic objects must be removed and kept outside the OR, and only MRI-compatible equipment, including anesthesia machines, carts, intubation tools, monitors, stethoscopes, intravenous (IV) poles, and body warmers, are permitted. Similarly, all surgical instruments must be MRI-compatible. Absolute contraindications to entering the MRI suite include the presence of pacemakers, cochlear implants, certain cranial aneurysm clips, and metallic joints or implants.

Minimally Invasive Endoscopic Surgery

Minimally invasive brain tumor surgery, or keyhole surgery, utilizes advanced neuroendoscopic techniques to remove tumors with minimal disruption to surrounding healthy brain tissue. This approach involves accessing the tumors through small incisions (Keyhole craniotomy) or natural openings like the nostrils or mouth, using flexible, lighted endoscopes to navigate and operate within the brain, ventricles, skull base, or orbits. Anesthesia for pituitary surgery through transsphenoidal approach has been dealt in separate chapter.

For a neoplasm as diverse in location and invasiveness as meningioma, the surgical team must be adept at utilizing multiple surgical approaches with both microscopic and endoscopic techniques. The use of total intravenous anesthesia (TIVA), smaller scalp and muscle incisions, limited monopolar cautery, and targeted craniotomies to reduce brain exposure, are associated with accelerated healing, reduced postoperative pain, and enhanced patient mobility, facilitating earlier hospital discharge.[24] Comparative studies of standard versus minimally invasive skull base approaches have demonstrated that reducing the average craniotomy size by 3–5 times does not compromise the risk of postoperative complications or the likelihood of complete tumor resection. These findings support the efficacy and safety of minimally invasive techniques for patients.[25]

Awake Craniotomy

Awake craniotomy is the gold standard for resecting brain tumors located in or near eloquent areas. Both the asleep-awake-asleep technique and monitored anesthesia care are effective approaches, with the choice of anesthetic strategy largely determined by the preferences and expertise of the anesthesiologist and surgical team. Preoperative administration of antiepileptics and benzodiazepines may be omitted if intraoperative electrocorticography (ECoG) is planned. In the OR, patient comfort should be prioritized by maintaining an ambient temperature of 22–24°C and minimizing noise levels. Propofol, remifentanil, dexmedetomidine, and scalp nerve block provide reliable conditions for intraoperative brain mapping. There were no statistically significant differences between propofol and dexmedetomidine in terms of intraoperative adverse events, patient satisfaction, or procedure duration. However, surgeon satisfaction was significantly higher in the dexmedetomidine group.[26] Optimal patient selection, comprehensive perioperative psychological support, and individualized anesthetic management at each stage of surgery are essential to ensure procedural safety, efficacy, and patient satisfaction. Seizures, hypertension, respiratory depression, nausea, vomiting, and mild brain swelling are potential complications during awake craniotomy. The primary risk factors for intraoperative seizures include a history of preoperative seizures and the presence of frontal lobe tumors.[27] Airway obstruction is another serious complication but can often be managed with simple interventions such as a jaw thrust, insertion of a nasopharyngeal airway, and administration of supplemental oxygen. To address potential airway emergencies, a full range of airway equipment, including a laryngeal mask airway, video laryngoscope, and endotracheal tube, should be readily available.[28]

CONCLUSION

Brain tumors represent a small incidence of global cancers, yet they carry a significant risk of long-term morbidity and mortality. Anesthetic considerations for brain tumor surgery are highly dependent on the tumor's location within the cranial cavity and the associated clinical presentation. Key anesthetic objectives include maintaining cerebral homeostasis by ensuring normovolemia, normoglycemia, normotension, and preserving CPP. Precise regulation of systemic blood pressure within the cerebral autoregulatory range is crucial to prevent ischemic injury or hemorrhage and a thorough understanding of cerebrovascular physiology is essential for anesthesiologists to deliver optimal perioperative care in brain tumor patients.

REFERENCES

1. Louis DN, Perry A, Wesseling P, Brat DJ, Cree IA, Figarella-Branger D, et al. The 2021 WHO Classification of Tumors of the Central Nervous System: a summary. Neuro Oncol. 2021;23(8):1231-51.
2. Kohler BA, Ward E, McCarthy BJ, Schymura MJ, Ries LA, Eheman C, et al. Annual report to the nation on the status of cancer, 1975-2007, featuring tumors of the brain and other nervous system. J Natl Cancer Inst. 2011;103(9):714-36.
3. Ostrom QT, Gittleman H, Fulop J, Liu M, Blanda R, Kromer C, et al. CBTRUS statistical report: primary brain and central nervous system tumors diagnosed in the United States in 2008-2012. Neuro Oncol. 2015;17 Suppl 4(Suppl 4):iv1-iv62.
4. Wilson MH. Monro-Kellie 2.0: The dynamic vascular and venous pathophysiological components of intracranial pressure. J Cereb Blood Flow Metab. 2016;36(8):1338-50.
5. Liubinas SV, O'Brien TJ, Moffat BM, Drummond KJ, Morokoff AP, Kaye AH. Tumour associated epilepsy and glutamate excitotoxicity in patients with gliomas. J Clin Neurosci. 2014;21(6):899-908.
6. Zwetnow NN, Schrader H, Löfgren J. Effects of continuously expanding intracranial lesions on vital physiological parameters. An experimental animal study. Acta Neurochir (Wien). 1986;80(1-2):47-56.
7. Chu H, Dang BW. Risk factors of postoperative pulmonary complications following elective craniotomy for patients with tumors of the brainstem or adjacent to the brainstem. Oncol Lett. 2014;8(4):1477-81.
8. Paquin-Lanthier G, Subramaniam S, Leong KW, Daniels A, Singh K, Takami H, et al. Risk factors and characteristics of intraoperative seizures during awake craniotomy: A retrospective cohort study of 562 consecutive patients with a space-occupying brain lesion. J Neurosurg Anesthesiol. 2023;35(2):194-200.
9. Kuo YW, Chen YT, Lieu AS, Lee MS, Su YF, Lai HC, et al. Predicting the optimal concentration of remifentanil for skull pin fixation with hemodynamic and analgesia nociception index monitoring. Sci Rep. 2024;14(1):6441.
10. Rath GP, Bithal PK, Chaturvedi A, Dash HH. Complications related to positioning in posterior fossa craniectomy. J Clin Neurosci. 2007;14(6):520-5.
11. Kumaresan A, Kasper E, Bose R. Anesthetic management of supratentorial tumors. Int Anesthesiol Clin. 2015;53(1): 74-86.
12. Chui J, Mariappan R, Mehta J, Manninen P, Venkatraghavan L. Comparison of propofol and volatile agents for maintenance of anesthesia during elective craniotomy procedures: systematic review and meta-analysis. Can J Anaesth. 2014;61(4):347-56.
13. Deinsberger W, Christophis P, Jödicke A, Heesen M, Böker DK. Somatosensory evoked potential monitoring during positioning of the patient for posterior fossa surgery in the semisitting position. Neurosurgery. 1998;43(1):36-40; discussion 40-2.
14. Topsakal C, Al-Mefty O, Bulsara KR, Williford VS. Intraoperative monitoring of lower cranial nerves in skull base surgery: technical report and review of 123 monitored cases. Neurosurg Rev. 2008;31(1):45-53.
15. Bastola P, Bhagat H, Wig J. Comparative evaluation of propofol, sevoflurane and desflurane for neuroanaesthesia: A prospective randomised study in patients undergoing elective supratentorial craniotomy. Indian J Anaesth. 2015;59(5):287-94.
16. Wu CT, Chen LC, Kuo CP, Ju DT, Borel CO, Cherng CH, et al. A comparison of 3% hypertonic saline and mannitol for brain relaxation during elective supratentorial brain tumor surgery. Anesth Analg. 2010;110(3):903-7.
17. Gelb AW, Craen RA, Rao GS, Reddy KR, Megyesi J, Mohanty B, et al. Does hyperventilation improve operating condition during supratentorial craniotomy?

A multicenter randomized crossover trial. Anesth Analg. 2008;106(2):585-94.
18. Sieber F, Smith DS, Kupferberg J, Crosby L, Uzzell B, Buzby G, et al. Effects of intraoperative glucose on protein catabolism and plasma glucose levels in patients with supratentorial tumors. Anesthesiology. 1986;64(4):453-9.
19. Dietrich WD. The importance of brain temperature in cerebral injury. J Neurotrauma. 1992;9 Suppl 2:S475-85.
20. Fan Q, Hu C, Ye M, Shen X. Dexmedetomidine for tracheal extubation in deeply anesthetized adult patients after otologic surgery: a comparison with remifentanil. BMC Anesthesiol. 2015;15:106.
21. Bruder NJ. Awakening management after neurosurgery for intracranial tumours. Curr Opin Anaesthesiol. 2002;15(5):477-82.
22. Basali A, Mascha EJ, Kalfas I, Schubert A. Relation between perioperative hypertension and intracranial hemorrhage after craniotomy. Anesthesiology. 2000;93(1):48-54.
23. Ganslandt O, Merkel A, Schmitt H, Tzabazis A, Buchfelder M, Eyupoglu I, et al. The sitting position in neurosurgery: indications, complications and results. a single institution experience of 600 cases. Acta Neurochir (Wien). 2013;155(10):1887-93.
24. Mallari RJ, Avery MB, Corlin A, Eisenberg A, Hammond TC, Martin NA, et al. Streamlining brain tumor surgery care during the COVID-19 pandemic: A case-control study. PLoS One. 2021;16(7):e0254958.
25. Feigl GC, Staribacher D, Britz G, Kuzmin D. minimally invasive approaches in the surgical treatment of intracranial meningiomas: An analysis of 54 Cases. Brain Tumor Res Treat. 2024;12(2):93-9.
26. Viderman D, Nabidollayeva F, Bilotta F, Abdildin YG. Comparison of dexmedetomidine and propofol for sedation in awake craniotomy: A meta-analysis. Clin Neurol Neurosurg. 2023;226:107623.
27. Spena G, Roca E, Guerrini F, Panciani PP, Stanzani L, Salmaggi A, et al. Risk factors for intraoperative stimulation-related seizures during awake surgery: an analysis of 109 consecutive patients. J Neurooncol. 2019;145(2):295-300.
28. Gruenbaum SE, Bilotta F, Bertasi TGO, Bertasi RAO, Clifton WE, Gruenbaum BF, et al. Emergency airway management during awake craniotomy: Comparison of 5 techniques in a Cadaveric Model. J Neurosurg Anesthesiol. 2022;34(1):74-8.

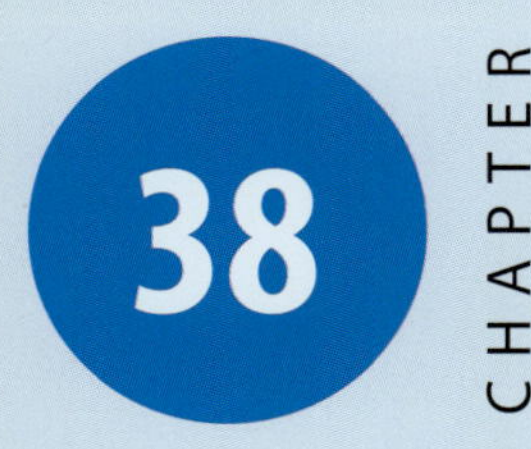

Anesthesia for Transsphenoidal Pituitary Tumor Surgeries

Swati Chhabra, Ruchi Pathak, Manbir Kaur

INTRODUCTION

The pituitary gland, physiologically known as the master gland, is responsible for secretion of hormones that regulate other glands in the body **(Table 1)**. Anatomically, it is referred to as "hypophysis" cerebri (from the Greek for "lying under") due to the gland's position on the underside or base of the brain within the sella turcica. Previously thought to be accessible only through open surgery requiring craniotomy, pituitary surgeries have evolved to be fully endoscopic procedures through the sphenoid

TABLE 1: Hormones secreted by the pituitary gland.

Hormones	***Produced by***	***Functions***
Hormones from anterior pituitary (adenohypophysis)		
Growth hormone (GH)/ somatotropin	Somatotroph cells	• Stimulates liver, muscle, cartilage, bone, and other tissues to synthesize and secrete insulin-like growth factors (IGFs) that promote growth of body cells • Promotes protein synthesis, tissue repair, and lipolysis
Thyroid-stimulating hormone (TSH)	Thyrotroph cells	Stimulates synthesis and secretion of thyroid hormones by thyroid gland
Follicle-stimulating hormone (FSH)	Gonadotroph cells	• In males, stimulates testes to produce sperm • In females, initiates development of oocytes and induces ovarian secretion of estrogens
Luteinizing hormone (LH)	Gonadotroph cells	• In males, stimulates testes to produce testosterone • In females, stimulates secretion of estrogens and progesterone: – Ovulation – Formation of corpus luteum
Prolactin (lactotrophs)	Lactotroph cells	Together with other hormones, promotes milk production by mammary glands
Adrenocorticotropic hormone (ACTH)	Corticotroph cells	Stimulates secretion of glucocorticoids (mainly cortisol) by adrenal cortex, mineralocorticosteroids such as aldosterone, and adrenal androgens such as testosterone
Melanocyte stimulating hormone (MSH)	Corticotroph cells (secreted by intermediate zone of pituitary)	Regulates the production of the skin pigment melanin
Hormones from posterior pituitary (neurohypophysis)		
Antidiuretic hormone (ADH)	Supraoptic and paraventricular nuclei	• Decreases urine production and causes the kidneys to return more water to the blood, thus decreasing urine volume • Decreases the water lost through sweating and causes constriction of arterioles, which increases blood pressure
Oxytocin	Supraoptic and paraventricular nuclei	• Contraction of smooth muscle cells in the wall of the uterus during labor • Promotes expulsion of the placenta and stimulates milk ejection ("letdown") from the mammary glands

sinus. The transsphenoidal approach was first described in 1907 and subsequently modified and popularized by Harvey Cushing, thereby revolutionizing approach to skull-base surgery.[1,2]

Transsphenoidal approaches consist of microscopic approach via transnasal or sublabial route and endoscopic transnasal transsphenoidal approach. Modifications such as expanded endoscopic endonasal approach (EEEA) and combined transsphenoidal transmaxillary approaches are also described.[3-6] Computer-assisted navigation and guidance have further improved this technique. Magnetic resonance imaging (MRI) with facial makers used to identify key anatomic features are obtained prior to surgery. Intraoperative coregistration of the facial markers with the MRI aids in directing the angle of approach and ensuring thorough resection of the tumor during surgery.[7] Transsphenoidal surgeries have peculiar anesthetic considerations related to the hormonal imbalance and related comorbidities, access to the surgical site, visualization of field of surgery, and concerns of shared airway, which will be discussed in the subsequent sections of this chapter.

Indications of transsphenoidal approach to surgery include pituitary tumors and other sellar lesions such as Rathke's cyst, craniopharyngiomas, meningiomas, chordomas, or metastatic lesions. The transsphenoidal approach is contraindicated in sphenoid sinusitis, intrasellar vascular anomalies like ectatic midline carotid arteries, or significant lateral suprasellar extension of tumor.[8]

Pituitary surgeries are usually elective cases unless patient is diagnosed with acute hemorrhagic infarction of the pituitary also known as pituitary apoplexy in which the patient presents with sudden onset hormonal shutdown and visual loss requiring urgent decompression of hematoma to relieve the symptoms and prevent permanent damage.

RELEVANT ANATOMY AND PHYSIOLOGY

The pituitary gland lies within the sella turcica, a saddle-shaped depression in the sphenoid bone. The gland is fully surrounded by sphenoid bone except for the opening of the thin diaphragma sellae overlying it through which the pituitary stalk passes that connects the gland to hypothalamus. The pituitary gland is divided into two main lobes: (1) The anterior pituitary (adenohypophysis) and (2) the posterior pituitary (neurohypophysis). Both the lobes have distinct origin, structure, and function. The anterior pituitary develops from the Rathke's pouch (an invagination of the oral ectoderm) and is mainly composed of glandular epithelial tissue that secretes hormones. The posterior pituitary originates from the neuroectoderm, as a downward extension of the hypothalamus and consists of neural tissue. The hormones of posterior pituitary are synthesized in the hypothalamus and transported to the axon terminals to be stored and released from posterior pituitary. Arterial supply is derived from the superior and inferior hypophyseal artery and hypophyseal plexus and veins drain into the cavernous sinus that lies on either side of the gland.[9,10] The cavernous sinus houses important structures like the cavernous part of internal carotid artery (ICA) and cranial nerves III, IV, VI, and V (some divisions) that can be damaged during the surgery **(Figs. 1 and 2)**.

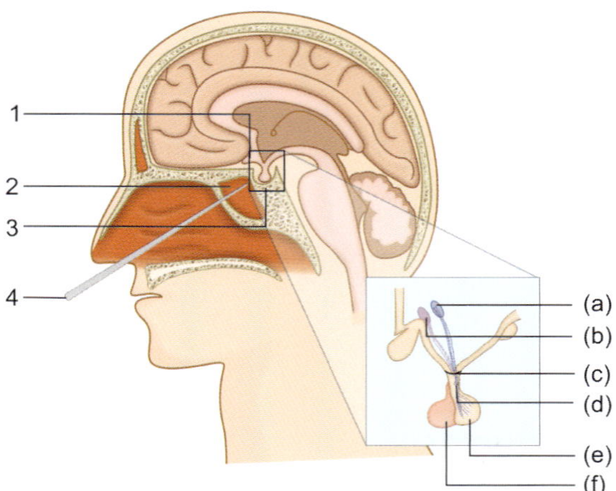

Fig. 1: Midsagittal section of brain showing location of pituitary gland (1) and its relations to sella turcica (2) and sphenoid sinus (3). Trajectory of the instruments (4) in transnasal transsphenoidal surgeries. Inset shows hypothalamus and pituitary gland with neurons from paraventricular hypothalamic nucleus (a) and the supraoptic hypothalamic nucleus (b) forming hypothalamophyseal tract (d) along the infundibulum (c). Two lobes of pituitary namely, anterior lobe (e) and posterior lobe (f).
Source: Image drawn by Dr Kshama Jain, Associate Consultant, Neurosurgery, Asian Institute of Medical Sciences, Faridabad.

CLASSIFICATION OF PITUITARY TUMORS

Based on the tumor size, pituitary tumors are classified into microadenomas (<10 mm), macroadenomas (≥10 mm), and giant macroadenomas (≥40 mm). Pituitary tumors may locally invade one or both cavernous sinuses and/or the bone by breaching into the sphenoid sinus. Pituitary carcinomas with metastasis, however, are rare and account for about 0.1% of pituitary tumors.[11]

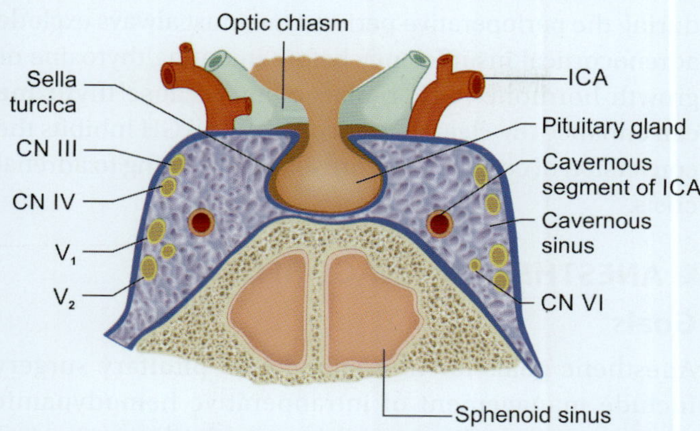

Fig. 2: Coronal section of brain showing relations of pituitary gland with optic chiasm, internal carotid artery (ICA), and cavernous sinus with its contents namely cavernous segment of ICA, cranial nerves (CN) III, IV, VI, and V (1st and 2nd divisions).
Source: Dr Kshama Jain, Department of Neurosurgery, AIIMS Jodhpur.

Clinically, the tumors are divided into functional and nonfunctional tumors based on the endocrinological profile. Patients with functional tumors present early with symptoms of hormonal hypersecretion, whereas those with nonfunctional tumors often present later and have symptoms resulting from mass effects of the tumor, such as headache, visual loss due to compression of the optic chiasm or hydrocephalus, hypopituitarism from compression of the anterior pituitary, or hyperprolactinemia because of hypothalamic dysfunction. Many patients are asymptomatic and report for surgery if tumor is found incidentally during intracranial imaging.[12]

Pituitary tumors can be grouped into the following categories based on the hormones secreted.

Prolactinomas

Prolactinomas are the most common secretory tumors of the pituitary gland accounting for 30–40% of total pituitary adenomas, with a peak prevalence in women aged 25–34 years. They are mostly benign. Symptoms are either due to mass effect or hypersecretion of prolactin. Hyperprolactinemia causes growth arrest and pubertal delay in adolescents. In males, hyperprolactinemia may present with decreased libido, impotence, erectile dysfunction, and oligozoospermia (due to secondary hypogonadism). In females, it causes oligomenorrhea, amenorrhea, infertility, loss of libido, and galactorrhea. Medical therapy for prolactinomas includes dopamine agonists namely, bromocriptine and cabergoline. These drugs suppress the synthesis and release of prolactin and lactotroph cellular proliferation, causing shrinkage of the tumor by fibrosis. Patients presenting for surgery after medical therapy may have increased risk of intraoperative blood loss from the fibrotic tumor. Bromocriptine has more side effects than cabergoline like nausea, vomiting, nasal stuffiness, and postural hypotension. Of note, studies indicate increased prevalence of subclinical cardiac valve fibrosis in patients with prolactinomas on long-term bromocriptine and cabergoline treatment.[13-15]

Acromegaly

Oversecretion of growth hormone before puberty causes chronic progressive increase in height as well as soft-tissue overgrowth, a condition known as gigantism. The increase in growth hormone secretion after the fusion of epiphyseal growth plates is known as acromegaly. Soft-tissue growth manifests as increased size of hands, feet, and lower jaw with coarsening of facial features. There is a higher incidence of difficult mask ventilation and intubation due to presence of macroglossia, enlarged epiglottis, narrow glottic opening, and subglottic narrowing. The clinical features including neuropathies (recurrent laryngeal nerve palsy, carpal tunnel syndrome, etc.) and cardiovascular changes (hypertension, ventricular hypertrophy, diastolic dysfunction, cardiomyopathy, coronary artery disease, preexisting arrhythmias, congestive heart failure, and right ventricular dysfunction) are common. These patients are also prone to obstructive sleep apnea (OSA) and pulmonary hypertension. Diabetes mellitus/hyperglycemia may coexist requiring control and close monitoring of blood glucose levels.[16-18]

Cushing's Disease

Cushing's disease is a condition developing from long-term exposure to excess endogenous glucocorticoid leading to multiple systemic effects including higher incidence of cardiovascular comorbidities like hypertension, dyslipidemia, premature atherosclerosis, coronary artery disease, and increased risk of stroke. Immunosuppression, diabetes mellitus, and paper-thin skin with easy bruising contribute to poor wound healing. Difficult peripheral intravenous cannulation is expected due to fragile skin. Difficult mask ventilation and intubation can be attributed to increased fat deposition in neck, buffalo hump, truncal obesity, decreased compliance of chest wall, and increased occurrence of gastroesophageal reflux.

Myopathy of proximal muscle groups may contribute to delayed recovery from anesthesia.[19] Hypercortisolism also fosters a prothrombotic state by altering regulators of fibrinolysis, platelet function, and chronic endothelial damage. This leads to increased risk of venous thromboembolism.[20] Symptomatic treatment includes preoperative administration of adrenal steroidogenesis inhibitors (ketoconazole, metyrapone, and osilodrostat) but their major drawback is worsening of hypokalemia, hypertension, and peripheral edema in some patients. Uncontrolled hypertension and an abnormal glucose metabolism are the major predictors of morbidity and mortality in these patients. Correcting dyselectrolytemia is of prime importance.

Thyrotropin-secreting Tumors

Thyrotropin-secreting tumors are relatively rare. These tumors present with features of hyperthyroidism (palpitations, tremor, weight loss, insomnia, tachycardia, and cardiac arrhythmias). Thyroid enlargement is a common finding, which may be large enough to compress the trachea.[21] Medical management of hyperthyroidism includes antithyroid drugs like propylthiouracil and symptomatic treatment with propranolol, which should be continued before surgery.

Pituitary Hyposecretion

Hormone hyposecretion occurs due to pressure effect of tumor on other secretory cells, pituitary apoplexy, or rarely Sheehan syndrome. Patients can present with adrenocortical insufficiency, hypothyroidism, or diabetes insipidus (DI).

Secondary or central hypothyroidism occurs because of reduced secretion of thyroid-stimulating hormone (TSH) due to hypothalamus or pituitary dysfunction leading to reduced secretion of thyroid hormones. Clinical features include bradycardia, weight gain, fatigue, constipation, dry skin, and cold intolerance. Thyroxine is initiated preoperatively and is continued on the morning of surgery.

Adrenocortical insufficiency can present as a life-threatening condition with fatigue, muscle weakness, low blood sugar, and low blood pressure. In acute presentation, patients require intravenous hydrocortisone replacement together with fluid resuscitation. Measurement of baseline serum cortisol levels enables to find out the approximate supplementation dose of corticosteroids during the perioperative period. One must always exclude adrenocortical insufficiency before initiating thyroxine or growth hormone (GH) replacement because thyroxine can enhance the clearance of cortisol, and GH inhibits the conversion of cortisone to cortisol, both leading to adrenal crisis.[22]

ANESTHETIC MANAGEMENT

Goals

Anesthetic goals for transsphenoidal pituitary surgery include management of intraoperative hemodynamic responses, providing conditions to facilitate surgical exposure like induced hypotension along with maintenance of cerebral perfusion and oxygenation, and allowing for rapid smooth emergence for immediate postoperative assessment with intact upper airway reflexes to prevent silent aspiration, if at all postnasal drip is present in the postoperative period.

Preoperative Assessment and Optimization

History with detailed evaluation of presenting symptoms and their progression, followed by elaborate examination of all systems are required due to the multisystem involvement.

Visual-field blurring is a common presenting complaint yet sometimes, a reduction in temporal field vision may not be noticed by the patient and is revealed only on examination; therefore, ophthalmic evaluation with a baseline perimetry is mandatory for documentation and to see any recovery or deterioration in the postoperative period. Also, pituitary tumors may present with signs of elevated intracranial pressure (ICP), such as papilledema, either because of their size or obstruction of the third ventricle, which can be ruled out by an ophthalmological examination.

A meticulous airway examination is mandatory, especially in patients presenting with acromegaly or Cushing's disease. Airway ultrasound may be helpful in screening for narrowing of supraglottic and subglottic regions and predicting difficult airway.[23] Hoarseness of voice may indicate a recurrent laryngeal nerve palsy, which can be confirmed on indirect laryngoscopic examination. Preoperative overnight polysomnography can be helpful to assess the severity of OSA and plan for awake intubation. All equipment including oropharyngeal and nasopharyngeal airway, laryngeal mask airway (LMA), video laryngoscope, and fiberoptic intubation aids should be kept handy. Elective awake fiberoptic intubation can be opted in predicted difficult mask ventilation with increased risk of pharyngeal collapse. A history of nasal surgery, deviated nasal septum, or nasal turbinate enlargement (in acromegaly) should be taken into account.

Laboratory workup includes complete blood count, coagulation profile, electrolytes including Na^+, K^+, and renal function tests. Pituitary tumors can be a part of multiple endocrine neoplasia-1 (MEN1) syndrome and baseline serum Ca^{2+} should also be evaluated to rule out any parathyroid involvement.[24] Thorough endocrine evaluation is done to ascertain the secretory or nonsecretory nature of the tumor and to demarcate preoperative baseline functioning of pituitary gland. Routinely, serum levels of prolactin, thyroid function test, luteinizing hormone, follicle-stimulating hormone, testosterone (in men), adrenocorticotropic hormone, cortisol, and insulin-like growth factor-1 (IGF-1), a surrogate marker for growth hormone, are measured. An endocrinologist's opinion is crucial to gain insight into the requirement of replacement therapy perioperatively. Usually, thyroid hormone and glucocorticoids are replaced preoperatively only if they are found to be below the normal range. Some institutes practice prophylactic administration of glucocorticoids in the perioperative period followed by testing for hypothalamo–pituitary–adrenal axis several weeks after the surgery. In general, with preoperatively intact adrenal function, there is less risk of development of adrenal insufficiency in the postoperative period. However, few patients might experience early transient adrenal insufficiency and regain function in the subsequent weeks. Some patients show late recovery up to months, and therefore, require proper long-term follow-up with an endocrinologist to prevent unnecessary preoperative and postoperative supplementation of glucocorticoid in order to reduce morbidity due to adverse effects of steroid therapy.[25-29]

Fasting blood sugar and postprandial blood sugar for screening of diabetes and regular charting to be maintained if patient is a known case of diabetes. Glycemic control may require insulin supplementation.

Echocardiogram and 2D echocardiography should be obtained as risk of arrhythmias and cardiac abnormalities are common in patients with acromegaly, hyperthyroidism, and Cushing's syndrome.

Arterial blood gas analysis can be used to rule out hypokalemic metabolic alkalosis in Cushing's disease and for evaluation of baseline CO_2 in patients with OSA. Spirometry is initiated in the preoperative phase for obese patients who are at a higher risk of basal atelectasis and other postoperative pulmonary complications, especially in patients requiring continuous positive airway pressure (CPAP) support.

Prolactinomas commonly increase in size during pregnancy to cause symptoms in a previously asymptomatic patient. Amenorrhea may be due to the pregnancy or hyperprolactinemia, hence pregnancy test for women of childbearing age presenting with amenorrhea should be obtained.

Optimization of rhinitis, if present, is necessary to prevent respiratory tract hyperactivity or ascent of infection toward dura. A nasal swab is taken for documentation of commensals or ruling out any pathogens and antibiotic nasal drops are initiated according to the antibiotic sensitivity.

Radiological evaluation to look for the size, extent, vascularity, and spatial relation to the nearby vital structures like ICA, anterior cerebral artery (ACA), and cavernous sinus helps the anesthesiologist in predicting the duration of surgery, planning venous access for intraoperative fluid resuscitation, ionotropic supplementation, or blood transfusion if necessary.

Positioning and Venous Access

The patient is laid supine with 20–30° head-up position with mild flexion at neck. Head is secured in a Mayfield head holder or rested upon a horseshoe depending on the convenience of the surgeon. The abdomen or thigh is prepared for harvesting fat or tensor fascia lata for sellar defect reconstruction after surgery. Peripheral neuropathies are common in acromegaly and extra care must be taken in such patients to pad pressure points adequately. Patients with Cushing's disease may have osteoporosis and fragile skin thus, positioning should be done very carefully to prevent fractures and bruising. In patients with exophthalmos (hyperthyroidism or Cushing's disease), the eyes should be taped and padded properly.

Good intravenous access is ensured for cases with large tumors with extension into cavernous sinus. Venous access may be difficult for patients with Cushing's and acromegaly (coarse thickened skin), sometimes necessitating central venous access.

Premedication

Antacid prophylaxis (H_2 blockers or proton pump inhibitors) is given especially in patients with Cushing's disease (higher incidence of peptic ulcer and gastroesophageal reflux disease). Sedative premedication like benzodiazepines or opioids are avoided in patients with OSA.

Induction and Maintenance

For induction of anesthesia, propofol is commonly used. Titrated doses of induction agents are used in hypothyroidism. Etomidate can be used in cases with cardiac comorbidities, but caution should be exercised while inducing patients with preexisting adrenocortical insufficiency. Depolarizing or nondepolarizing muscle relaxants are administered to facilitate intubation. In situations with anticipated difficult airway, faster onset and short-acting muscle relaxants are preferred like succinylcholine or rocuronium with sugammadex reversal, if required. Titrated doses of anesthetic agents are used for induction and maintenance in patients with clinical hypothyroidism. Sympathetic response to intubation can be blunted by short-acting agents like lignocaine, esmolol, or fentanyl. Endotracheal tube (ETT) is secured with tapes fixed away from nasal area to reduce chances of dislodgement/malpositioning due to soiling by fluids used for irrigation. The ETT is preferably fixed on the left side to allow access of endoscope from right side. Consider smaller ETT to avoid injury in patients with expected glottic or subglottic narrowing. To prevent silent aspiration of irrigation fluid, blood, or cerebrospinal fluid (CSF) into the trachea, a throat pack is usually placed in the oropharynx.

For maintenance of anesthesia, inhalational agents like sevoflurane are preferred; similarly, short-acting opioids like fentanyl and remifentanil are favored to minimize postoperative sedation and permit neurologic examination immediately after surgery. Some studies aimed to assess the time to recovery from anesthesia have compared total intravenous anesthesia (TIVA) with propofol to inhalational agents like sevoflurane and found them to be comparable.[30-32]

Intraoperative neuromonitoring may be required in selected cases if the tumor is invading the cavernous sinus to involve the cranial nerves. Such cases are conducted in TIVA because inhalational agents interfere with nerve monitoring modalities. Depth of anesthesia is maintained with propofol infusion along with fentanyl or dexmedetomidine infusions to ensure hypnosis, analgesia, and immobility during the surgery. Bispectral index (BIS) is used for monitoring the depth of anesthesia. Motor evoked potential (MEP) or somatosensory evoked potentials (SSEP) are assessed for cranial nerves III, IV, VI, V1, and V2. In MEP analysis, neuromuscular blocking agents (NMBA) are avoided, and monitoring is performed to detect the density of neuromuscular blockade and evaluate the need for reversal of residual effects of NMBA. Visual evoked potential (VEP) monitoring is also performed for optic nerve function, but it is very sensitive to the anesthetic agents and results may not be reliable.

Monitoring

Standard American Society of Anesthesiologists (ASA) monitoring includes pulse oximetry, electrocardiography, noninvasive blood pressure, end-tidal carbon dioxide, and temperature. Additionally, invasive blood pressure (IBP) monitoring is advisable for better control of blood pressure more so in patients with coexisting cardiovascular comorbidities. Radial artery is commonly used for arterial catheterization. Of note, acromegalic patients may suffer from ulnar artery compression due to carpal tunnel syndrome; therefore, modified Allen's test should be performed preoperatively and perfusion of hand should be checked at regular intervals intraoperatively. Arterial catheter also aids in intraoperative sampling for blood gas analysis, measuring blood glucose for assessing glycemic control, serum electrolytes, and serum osmolarity for diagnosing intraoperative diabetes insipidus (DI) or syndrome of inappropriate antidiuretic hormone secretion (SIADH).

Temperature monitoring is of importance as patients are susceptible to both hypothermia from the irrigation fluid and hyperthermia due to manipulation of hypothalamus.[33] A pharyngeal or esophageal temperature probe may not be ideal for this surgery because of the risk of dislodgement and inaccurate readings on exposure to warm irrigation fluid. Alternative sites of temperature monitoring like skin probe placed in axilla (peripheral body temperature) or tympanic membrane temperature monitoring (core temperature) can be used.

Patient is catheterized for accurate fluid management, especially with the risk of DI during stalk manipulation. Insensible loss is less in such endoscopic/microscopic surgeries. The use of type and quantity of irrigation fluid should be noted. Blood loss is usually predictable unless vascular complications occur such as injury to the sphenopalatine artery and its branches and injury to the carotid artery. Detailed study of preoperative imaging is essential to avoid this complication. In situations where intraoperative hemostasis cannot be achieved by direct vascular repair or endovascular clamps/clips, interventions such as stenting, balloon occlusion, or coiling may be required urgently.

Hemodynamic Responses and Field of Surgery

Intraoperatively, sympathetic hemodynamic response is seen when adrenaline (1:10,000) is injected into the nasal mucosa to prepare the nares for endoscopic surgery, during the nasal dissection phase, and while incising the dura. Ensuring adequate depth of anesthesia and analgesia with short-acting opioids or dexmedetomidine can help overcome the hemodynamic changes, improve endoscopic vision, and hence, shorten the duration of surgery. The sympathetic stimulation is intense at times and may require rescue with short-acting beta blockers like esmolol or vasodilators like nitroglycerine. Dexmedetomidine has recently gained popularity due to its property of providing good hemodynamic stability and short contact sensitivity half-life. It has been used as nebulization and infusions with or without lignocaine to reduce the sympathetic response in nasal phase of transsphenoidal surgery as well as overall.[34-37]

Visualization and access to tumor can also be enhanced by controlled hypercapnia ($PaCO_2$ of 40–45 mm Hg) or injection of isotonic saline/air into a lumbar intrathecal catheter placed usually at L4–L5 space, which can temporarily increase intracranial pressure and enhance exposure of the tumor by pushing it inferiorly into the sella. For large tumors, CSF can be drained from the lumbar catheter to prevent intraoperative arachnoid breach. The lumbar drain may be left in place following surgery if a CSF leak is present. Post-tumor resection hemostasis is achieved at baseline blood pressure and CSF leak is ruled out by performing Valsalva maneuver.

Extubation

Smooth extubation to prevent rise in blood pressure is essential for reducing risk of CSF leak or hematoma formation at surgical site. Any inadvertent movement like bucking in lighter plane of anesthesia risks dislodgement of graft, and hence should be completely avoided. Bailey's maneuver can be employed for this after thorough suctioning and removal of throat pack as LMA is better tolerated in lighter planes of anesthesia than ETT. The LMA is removed when the patient is awake. Patients with clinical hypothyroidism may require postoperative respiratory support because of reduced metabolism of drugs, an obtunded ventilatory response to hypercapnia and hypoxia, and increased risk of hypothermia that contribute to delayed recovery from anesthesia.

Postoperative Care

Postoperatively, monitoring in an intensive care unit (ICU) is advised. Head-up position is maintained, and patient should be comforted and asked to breathe from mouth. Close observation for neurological deterioration, epistaxis, visual dysfunction, DI, and hypotension secondary to acute hypocortisolism, is required.

The incidence of postoperative nausea vomiting (PONV) is higher in presence of intraoperative CSF drainage/leak and subsequent fat grafting or presence of silently trickled blood in stomach. Antiemetic prophylaxis should be given to all patients before extubation and continued in the postoperative period. Ondansetron (5HT3 antagonist) is used on a regular basis. Some studies now suggest that dexamethasone does not interfere with the postoperative cortisol assays and can be used for PONV prophylaxis.[38]

Patients may have discomfort in breathing due to nasal packing, which is usually left in situ for 48–72 hours after surgery. This can be overcome, to an extent, by proper preoperative counseling. Mucosal damage during surgery can impair ciliary function and presence of packing impedes the drainage of mucous, both contributing to risk of sinusitis. Nasal congestion and mild nasal bleeding are also anticipated in 1–2 weeks after surgery. Postoperative analgesia is usually achieved by paracetamol and fentanyl. Opioids should be used with caution in obese and hypothyroid patients who are at increased risk of sedation. The use of bilateral infraorbital nerve blocks and sphenopalatine nerve blocks have been described for reducing both intraoperative and postoperative pain and may also help in tolerating the nasal pack better.[39,40] The CSF leak and subsequent meningitis are usually prevented by a multilayer closure at the end of surgery and smooth extubation. In the occurrence of a leak in the postoperative period, the patient is advised bed rest, and a lumbar drain is placed to reduce ICP and promote healing. If the leak does not improve, exploration and closure of the defect are to be done. In event of reexploration, the patient is induced with rapid sequence induction to prevent ascent of infection through the defect.

Injury to optic nerve may cause worsening of the visual field. Treatment includes observation, intravenous high-dose steroids, or optic nerve decompression. Intraoperative injury to olfactory nerve can cause postoperative hyposmia and anosmia and injury to cranial nerves III, IV, and VI can cause ophthalmoplegia.

Pneumocephalus can ensue due to air entrapment in cranial cavity during surgery. Also, early CPAP resumption is believed to increase size of pneumocephalus post-transsphenoidal surgery. Optimal timing for resumption of CPAP has not been defined and requires prior planning and discussion with the surgeon. Recent studies suggest that early resumption of CPAP may benefit the patient more than causing harm.[41-43] Diagnosis of pneumocephalus is aided by postoperative CT scan. It can present as nausea, vomiting, irritability, and sometimes seizures, all these can cause raised ICP and increased incidence of postoperative CSF leak. Mild pneumocephalus treated conservatively with oxygen supplementation in fowlers position is used to facilitate resorption. Whereas a large pneumocephalus or tension pneumocephalus may require burr hole and evacuation.

Endocrine complications following pituitary surgery are fairly common with incidence ranging from 5–25%. Certain complications, such as DI, SIADH, and adrenal insufficiency, can be life-threatening if not treated promptly. Postsurgical hypopituitarism may be partial, affecting either the anterior or posterior pituitary, or total, impacting both. This condition can be transient and self-limiting or may develop into permanent dysfunction, necessitating lifelong hormone replacement therapy **(Tables 2 and 3)**. Regular follow-up and hormonal evaluations by an endocrinologist can significantly enhance the quality of life.

TABLE 2: Postoperative endocrine complications arising from anterior pituitary.

Endocrine complications	***Diagnosis***	***Management***
Adrenal insufficiency	Low serum cortisol and plasma ACTH	Hydrocortisone supplementation
Hypothyroidism	Low serum TSH, T3, and T4	Thyroxine supplementation (titrated up to a maintenance dose)
Hypogonadism	• Exclude hyperprolactinemia • Normal menses in a premenopausal woman, rule out hypogonadism • Low serum LH, FSH, testosterone (in men), and estradiol (in premenopausal women)	• *Males:* Testosterone supplementation when fertility is not desired • *Females:* Estrogen supplementation when fertility is not desired • *Gonadotropins:* To be used when the patient desires to be fertile
Decreased GH secretion	Low serum IGF-1	Recombinant human growth hormone (rhGH) (started with low doses and titrated up to a maintenance dose)

(ACTH: adrenocorticotropic hormone; FSH: follicle-stimulating hormone; GH: growth hormone; IGF: insulin-like growth factors; LH: luteinizing hormone; T3: triiodothyronine; T4: thyroxine; TSH: thyroid-stimulating hormone)

TABLE 3: Postoperative endocrine complications arising from posterior pituitary.

Endocrine complications	***Incidence***	***Cause***	***Onset***	***Diagnosis***	***Management***	***Prognosis***
Diabetes insipidus (DI)[22,44-46]	8–24%	Inadequate secretion of ADH resulting from manipulation/ compression of pituitary stalk/ hypothalamus	Preoperative, intraoperative, or post-operative	• Hypotonic polyuria >4 mL/kg/h for 3 consecutive hours or >50 mL/kg/24 h • Urine osmolality <280 mOsm/Kg • Urine specific gravity <1.005 • Hypernatremia >140–145 mmol/L • Serum osmolarity >300	• Mild DI with intact thirst mechanism is managed conservatively with oral fluid replacement • *Unresolved/impaired thirst:* 0.45% NS or 5% dextrose with or without administration of synthetic ADH analog (desmopressin)	Transient (resolves in 24 hours in most cases), permanent, or remits and then recurs postoperatively (triphasic response)

Contd...

Contd...

Endocrine complica-tions	*Incidence*	*Cause*	*Onset*	*Diagnosis*	*Management*	*Prognosis*
Syndrome of inappro-priate ADH secretion (SIADH)[22,44-46]	4–5%	Impairment in regulatory mechanisms secreting ADH leads to increased secretion of ADH	Postoperative day 5–7	• High urinary sodium > 40 mmol/L • Urine osmolality >100 mOsm/kg • Hyponatremia <135 mEq/L • Serum Osmolarity <280 mOsm/L	• Treatment depends on the degree of hyponatremia • Fluid restriction and occasionally salt administration are the mainstay of therapy • Symptomatic patients are hospitalized and managed with intravenous 3% saline	• May be transient or permanent • It may present as a part of triphasic response and progresses to permanent DI

(ADH: antidiuretic hormone; DI: diabetes insipidus; SIADH: syndrome of inappropriate antidiuretic hormone secretion)

CONCLUSION

Anesthetic management of pituitary tumor patients involves addressing hormonal imbalances, multiorgan involvement, and being cognizant of the specific concerns in different surgical approaches. Transsphenoidal pituitary surgery presents numerous advantages over transcranial resection, such as the absence of an external incision, the elimination of frontal lobe retraction, a comprehensive panoramic view through angled scopes, significantly reduced postoperative pain, and a notably shorter hospital stay. Recent advances like neuronavigation and intraoperative MRI aid the surgeon in guiding complete resection with minimal damage to surrounding structures. However, in some cases, transcranial surgery may be necessary if the tumor extends beyond the reach of the transsphenoidal approach. Patients presenting with pituitary tumors require a holistic approach with a team of doctors comprising of neurosurgeon, endocrinologist, anesthesiologist, pathologist, and radiation oncologist for diagnosis, perioperative care, and regular follow-up.

REFERENCES

1. Liu JK, Das K, Weiss MH, Laws ER Jr, Couldwell WT. The history and evolution of transsphenoidal surgery. J Neurosurg. 2001;95(6):1083-96.
2. Schmidt RF, Choudhry OJ, Takkellapati R, Eloy JA, Couldwell WT, Liu JK. Hermann Schloffer and the origin of transsphenoidal pituitary surgery. Neurosurg Focus. 2012;33(2):E5.
3. Dai W, Zhuang Z, Ling H, Yang Y, Hang C. Systematic review and network meta-analysis assess the comparative efficacy and safety of transsphenoidal surgery for pituitary tumor. Neurosurg Rev. 2021;44(1):515-27.
4. Jankowski R, Auque J, Simon C, Marchal JC, Hepner H, Wayoff M. Endoscopic pituitary tumor surgery. Laryngoscope. 1992;102(2):198-202.
5. Li K, Zhang J, Wang XS, Ye X, Zhao YL. A systematic review of effects and complications after transsphenoidal pituitary surgery: Endoscopic versus microscopic approach. Minim Invasive Ther Allied Technol. 2020;29(6):317-25.
6. Castaño-Leon AM, Paredes I, Munarriz PM, Jiménez-Roldán L, Hilario A, Calatayud M, et al. Endoscopic transnasal trans-sphenoidal approach for pituitary adenomas: A comparison to the microscopic approach cohort by propensity score analysis. Neurosurgery. 2020;86(3):348-56.
7. Campisi BM, Costanzo R, Gulino V, Avallone C, Noto M, Bonosi L, et al. The role of augmented reality neuronavigation in transsphenoidal surgery: A systematic review. Brain Sci. 2023;13(12):1695.
8. Miller BA, Ioachimescu AG, Oyesiku NM. Contemporary indications for transsphenoidal pituitary surgery. World Neurosurg. 2014;82(6 Suppl):S147-51.
9. Renn WH, Rhoton AL Jr. Microsurgical anatomy of the sellar region. J Neurosurg. 1975;43(3):288-98.
10. Barkhoudarian G, Kelly DF. The pituitary gland: Anatomy, physiology, and its function as the master gland. Cushing's Disease. Netherlands: Elsevier; 2017. pp. 1-41.
11. Dekkers OM, Karavitaki N, Pereira AM. The epidemiology of aggressive pituitary tumors (and its challenges). Rev Endocr Metab Disord. 2020;21(2):209-12.
12. Tahara S, Hattori Y, Suzuki K, Ishisaka E, Teramoto S, Morita A. An overview of pituitary incidentalomas: diagnosis, clinical features, and management. Cancers (Basel). 2022;14(17):4324.
13. dos Santos Nunes V, El Dib R, Boguszewski CL, Nogueira CR. Cabergoline versus bromocriptine in the

treatment of hyperprolactinemia: A systematic review of randomized controlled trials and meta-analysis. Pituitary. 2011;14(3):259-65.
14. Castinetti F, Albarel F, Amodru V, Cuny T, Dufour H, Graillon T, Morange I, et al. The risks of medical treatment of prolactinoma. Ann Endocrinol (Paris). 2021;82(1):15-9.
15. De Vecchis R, Esposito C, Ariano C. Cabergoline use and risk of fibrosis and insufficiency of cardiac valves. Meta-analysis of observational studies. Herz. 2013;38(8):868-80.
16. Lee HC, Kim MK, Kim YH, Park HP. Radiographic predictors of difficult laryngoscopy in acromegaly patients. J Neurosurg Anesthesiol. 2019;31(1):50-6.
17. Sharma D, Prabhakar H, Bithal PK, Ali Z, Singh GP, Rath GP, et al. Predicting difficult laryngoscopy in acromegaly: A comparison of upper lip bite test with modified Mallampati classification. J Neurosurg Anesthesiol. 2010;22(2):138-43.
18. Ali Z, Bithal PK, Prabhakar H, Rath GP, Dash HH. An assessment of the predictors of difficult intubation in patients with acromegaly. J Clin Neurosci. 2009;16(8):1043-5.
19. Domi R. Cushing's surgery: Role of the anesthesiologist. Indian J Endocrinol Metab. 2011;15(Suppl 4):S322-8.
20. Feelders RA, Nieman LK. Hypercoagulability in Cushing's syndrome: Incidence, pathogenesis and need for thromboprophylaxis protocols. Pituitary. 2022;25(5):746-9.
21. Dyer MW, Gnagey A, Jones BT, Pula RD, Lanier WL, Atkinson JLD, et al. Perianesthetic management of patients with thyroid-stimulating hormone-secreting pituitary adenomas. J Neurosurg Anesthesiol. 2017;29(3):341-6.
22. Prete A, Corsello SM, Salvatori R. Current best practice in the management of patients after pituitary surgery. Ther Adv Endocrinol Metab. 2017;8(3):33-48.
23. Carsetti A, Sorbello M, Adrario E, Donati A, Falcetta S. Airway ultrasound as predictor of difficult direct laryngoscopy: A systematic review and meta-analysis. Anesth Analg. 2022;134(4):740-50.
24. Syro LV, Scheithauer BW, Kovacs K, Toledo RA, Londoño FJ, Ortiz LD, et al. Pituitary tumors in patients with MEN1 syndrome. Clinics (Sao Paulo). 2012;67(Suppl 1):43-8.
25. Pofi R, Gunatilake S, Macgregor V, Shine B, Joseph R, Grossman AB, et al. Recovery of the hypothalamo-pituitary-adrenal axis after transsphenoidal adenomectomy for non-ACTH-secreting macroadenomas. J Clin Endocrinol Metab. 2019;104(11):5316-24.
26. Buttan A, Mamelak AN. Endocrine outcomes after pituitary surgery. Neurosurg Clin N Am. 2019;30(4):491-8.
27. Wentworth JM, Gao N, Sumithran KP, Maartens NF, Kaye AH, Colman PG, et al. Prospective evaluation of a protocol for reduced glucocorticoid replacement in transsphenoidal pituitary adenomectomy: Prophylactic glucocorticoid replacement is seldom necessary. Clin Endocrinol. 2007;68(1):29-35.
28. Rajaratnam S, Seshadri M, Chandy M, Rajshekhar V. Hydrocortisone dose and postoperative diabetes insipidus in patients undergoing transsphenoidal pituitary surgery: A prospective randomized controlled study. Br J Neurosurg 2003;17(5):437-42.
29. Regan J, Watson J. Selective use of peri-operative steroids in pituitary tumor surgery: Escape from dogma. Front Endocrinol (Lausanne). 2013;4:30.
30. Kim DH, Min KT, Kim EH, Choi YS, Choi SH. Comparison of the effects of inhalational and total intravenous anesthesia on quality of recovery in patients undergoing endoscopic transsphenoidal pituitary surgery: A randomized controlled trial. Int J Med Sci. 2022;19(6):1056-64.
31. Gollapudy S, Poetker DM, Sidhu J, Riess ML. Total intravenous versus inhaled anesthesia in transsphenoidal tumor surgery. Am J Otolaryngol. 2018;39(5):567-9.
32. Ali Z, Prabhakar H, Bithal PK, Dash HH. Bispectral index-guided administration of anesthesia for transsphenoidal resection of pituitary tumors: a comparison of 3 anesthetic techniques. J Neurosurg Anesthesiol. 2009;21(1):10-5.
33. Osilla EV, Marsidi JL, Shumway KR, Sharma S. Physiology, temperature regulation. In: StatPearls [Internet]. Treasure Island (FL): StatPearls Publishing; 2024. Available from https://www.ncbi.nlm.nih.gov/books/NBK507838/ [Last accessed February, 2025]
34. Liu Z, Gao C, Liu C, Liu W, Xu X, Ma T, et al. Supplementation with dexmedetomidine for transsphenoidal resection of pituitary adenoma: A meta-analysis of randomized controlled trials. Clin Neuropharmacol. 2021;44(1):17-20.
35. Aldosari N, Alrashid S, Alshareeda AH, Alenezi A, Alenezi MY, Almutairi A, et al. Dexmedetomidine in patients undergoing transsphenoidal resection of pituitary adenoma: An updated systematic review and meta-analysis of randomized placebo-controlled trials. Cureus. 2023;15(8):e44132.
36. Praveen R, Sethuraman M, Vimala S, Prathapadas U, Hrishi AP, Nair P, et al. A prospective-randomized placebo-controlled trial comparing the effects of nebulized dexmedetomidine v/s dexmedetomidine-lignocaine mixture on intraoperative hemodynamics and surgical field quality in patients undergoing endoscopic transnasal transsphenoidal pituitary tumor surgery. Surg Neurol Int. 2023;14:431.
37. Kang R, Jeong JS, Ko JS, Lee SY, Lee JH, Choi SJ, et al. Intraoperative dexmedetomidine attenuates norepinephrine levels in patients undergoing transsphenoidal surgery: A randomized, placebo-controlled trial. BMC Anesthesiol. 2020;20(1):100.
38. Burkhardt T, Rotermund R, Schmidt NO, Kiefmann R, Flitsch J. Dexamethasone PONV prophylaxis alters the hypothalamic-pituitary-adrenal axis after transsphenoidal pituitary surgery. J Neurosurg Anesthesiol. 2014;26(3):216-9.
39. Jonnavithula N, Padmaja D, Abhishek K, Dilipkumar K, Gopinath R, Manas P. Bilateral infraorbital nerve block for post operative analgesia following transsphenoidal pituitary surgery. Br J Anaesth. 2011;107.

40. Ali AR, Sakr SA, Rahman ASM. Bilateral sphenopalatine ganglion block as adjuvant to general anaesthesia during endoscopic trans-nasal resection of pituitary adenoma. Egypt J Anaesth. 2010;26(4):273-80.
41. Chaskes MB, Rabinowitz MR. Safety of restarting continuous positive airway pressure (CPAP) therapy following endoscopic endonasal skull base surgery. World J Otorhinolaryngol Head Neck Surg. 2022;8(1):61-5.
42. Risbud A, Kuan EC, Wu AW, Mamelak AN, Tang DM. Postoperative obstructive sleep apnea management following endoscopic pituitary surgery: A systematic review. World Neurosurg. 2023;176:143-8.
43. White-Dzuro GA, Maynard K, Zuckerman SL, Weaver KD, Russell PT, Clavenna MJ, et al. Risk of post-operative pneumocephalus in patients with obstructive sleep apnea undergoing transsphenoidal surgery. J Clin Neurosci. 2016;29:25-8.
44. de Vries F, Lobatto DJ, Verstegen MJT, van Furth WR, Pereira AM, Biermasz NR. Postoperative diabetes insipidus: How to define and grade this complication? Pituitary. 2021;24(2):284-91.
45. Brooks EK, Inder WJ. Disorders of salt and water balance after pituitary surgery. J Clin Endocrinol Metab. 2022; 108(1):198-208.
46. Woodmansee WW, Carmichael J, Kelly D, Katznelson L; AACE Neuroendocrine and Pituitary Scientific Committee. American Association of Clinical Endocrinologists and American College of Endocrinology Disease state clinical review: Postoperative management following pituitary surgery. Endocr Pract. 2015 ;21(7):832-8.

CHAPTER 39

Anesthesia for Awake Craniotomy in Brain Tumor Resections

Siddharth Chavali, Jayanth Ranganathan Seshan, Girija Prasad Rath

INTRODUCTION

Awake craniotomy (AC) is an anesthetic technique primarily used to facilitate the safe resection of brain tumors located in eloquent regions, responsible for critical functions such as motor control, language, and sensory perception.[1,2] By allowing the patient to remain awake during specific phases of surgery, AC enables intraoperative functional mapping, aiding the surgeon in distinguishing tumor tissue from the healthy brain. This real-time feedback is critical in ensuring that the maximal extent of the tumor is removed without impairing neurological function.[3]

Awake craniotomy was initially developed for epilepsy surgery but has since gained widespread use in the resection of brain tumors in eloquent cortex areas.[4] While advancements in neuroimaging have enhanced preoperative planning, functional mapping during surgery remains the gold standard in avoiding permanent neurological deficits. The anesthetic management of AC presents unique challenges, demanding a precise interplay among sedation, analgesia, and patient monitoring, with an emphasis on maintaining the patient's ability to participate in intraoperative neurological assessments.

HISTORICAL CONTEXT AND EVOLUTION OF AWAKE CRANIOTOMY

The concept of AC dates back to the late 19th century when Sir Victor Horsley performed brain surgeries on patients with epilepsy, mapping seizure foci with primitive cortical stimulation techniques.[5] This method was refined by Wilder Penfield, who developed the "Montreal procedure" in the 1930s.[6] Penfield's technique involved stimulating specific regions of the brain in awake patients to map cortical functions, which helped guide the resection of epileptogenic tissue. The development of functional brain mapping revolutionized epilepsy surgery and paved the way for its application in brain tumor resections.

In the modern era, AC has become the standard approach for resecting tumors in eloquent areas, such as those controlling language or motor functions. Advances in neuroimaging techniques, such as functional magnetic resonance imaging (fMRI) and diffusion tensor imaging (DTI), have facilitated more precise preoperative planning.[7] However, intraoperative functional mapping remains indispensable for maximizing tumor resection while minimizing postoperative deficits.

INDICATIONS FOR AWAKE CRANIOTOMY IN BRAIN TUMOR RESECTIONS

Awake craniotomy is primarily indicated for the resection of tumors located in or near eloquent brain regions where damage to functional areas could lead to permanent neurological deficits. Common indications include:

- *Low-grade gliomas:* Low-grade gliomas often invade critical brain regions, particularly those associated with motor or language function. Since these tumors tend to have diffuse borders and slow growth patterns, the ability to map functional areas during surgery is crucial in determining the extent of safe resection.[8]
- *High-grade gliomas*: Although high-grade gliomas (e.g., glioblastomas) are more aggressive and typically require extensive resection, AC is still valuable for preserving neurological function when these tumors are located near eloquent cortex.[9] Even in the setting of malignant gliomas, functional preservation is key to maintaining the patient's quality of life postoperatively.
- Metastatic tumors
- *Epilepsy surgery:* Although not tumor-related, AC remains the gold standard for mapping for epileptogenic foci involving the eloquent cortex. In this setting, intraoperative mapping helps localize seizure foci while preserving critical brain function, particularly in cortical areas responsible for speech or motor control.[10]

SURGICAL STEPS UNIQUE TO AWAKE CRANIOTOMY

Cortical Mapping

During AC, cortical mapping is a critical technique used to identify functional areas of the brain before resection. The surgeon employs a bipolar or monopolar stimulator probe to stimulate specific cortical regions while the patient is awake, allowing for real-time assessment of brain function.[11]

- *Motor mapping:* The patient is monitored for involuntary movements or disturbances in the contralateral side of the body, including the face, arm, and leg. This process helps to delineate areas responsible for motor function, ensuring that essential pathways are preserved during surgery.
- *Sensory mapping:* Patients are asked to report any abnormal sensations, such as tingling or numbness, elicited by stimulation. This feedback aids in identifying sensory pathways and minimizes the risk of postoperative sensory deficits.
- *Language mapping:* Language-related areas are assessed by engaging the patient in tasks such as picture naming, counting, reading words, or repeating complex sentences. While picture naming is the most common intraoperative language mapping task, the monitoring includes the identification of deficits like paraphasia (semantic or phonological), circumlocutions, neologisms, slurred or stuttered responses, or speech arrest.[12]
- *Visual mapping:* This aspect involves monitoring for any abnormal visual experiences, such as hallucinations or visual field cuts, during cortical stimulation. By identifying and preserving visual pathways, the risk of postoperative visual impairment can be significantly reduced.

The involvement of the anesthesiologist in these mapping procedures varies by institutional practice. For complex mapping, especially of language and visual areas, collaboration with neuropsychologists or speech-language therapists is often essential to ensure comprehensive evaluation and patient safety.

Electrocorticographic Recordings

In patients undergoing surgery for epilepsy, electrocorticographic (ECoG) recordings are performed to localize epileptogenic foci accurately.[13,14]

- *Electrode placement:* Electrodes are placed on the surface of the brain over suspected epileptogenic areas. This placement is crucial for capturing electrical activity directly from the cortical surface.
- *Recording conditions:* For optimal ECoG recording, it is vital to discontinue any anesthetic infusions at least 20 minutes before starting the procedure, as medication can interfere with the quality of the recordings.
- *Stimulation for localization:* In cases where precise localization is necessary, small doses of anesthetic agents, such as methohexital (10–50 mg), thiopental (25–50 mg), or etomidate (2–4 mg), may be administered to stimulate the epileptogenic focus.

Preoperative Preparation and Patient Selection

The selection of appropriate candidates for awake craniotomy is crucial for the success of the procedure. Preoperative preparation includes a comprehensive assessment of the patient's neurological, psychological, and physical fitness to tolerate the surgery.

Patient Selection

Ideal candidates for AC must be cooperative and able to follow instructions during the awake portions of surgery.[15] Critical factors to consider include:

- *Psychological readiness:* Patients should be mentally prepared for the procedure and must be able to tolerate the awake phases without excessive anxiety or distress. Those with significant psychiatric disorders, high levels of anxiety, or claustrophobia may not be suitable candidates for AC.
- *Cognitive ability:* Patients must have the cognitive capacity to understand and comply with intraoperative instructions, such as performing motor tasks, naming objects, or following verbal commands during functional mapping.
- *Medical fitness:* Patients with respiratory comorbidities (e.g., obstructive sleep apnea) or significant obesity (BMI >40) may present additional challenges due to the increased risk of airway compromise during sedation.
- *Other considerations:* Though patient refusal should be the only absolute contraindication, due consideration must be given to other issues like patients' anticipated difficult airways, expected difficulty in resection of deep-seated tumors, severe cardiac conditions,

or uncontrolled seizures. It is feasible to initiate anticonvulsants and achieve high-normal target plasma concentrations (20 mg/dL for phenytoin) prior to surgery. From a surgical point of view, deep-seated lesions or imaging features suggestive of impending herniation are likely to pose intraoperative mass effects and may be avoided.[16]

Preoperative Counseling

Preoperative counseling plays a vital role in preparing patients for awake craniotomy.[17] Patients must understand the surgery sequence, including when they will be awake and what tasks they must perform. The neurosurgeon, the neuroanesthesiologist, and the neuropsychologist should be involved together in evaluating and counseling the patient preoperatively. The patient's cognition and psychological status should be evaluated first and then the patient is prepared for awake neurosurgery. This includes exposure of the patient to the operating room (OR) environment, explanation of the patient's position and the relative position of the anesthesiologist and the neurosurgeon, possible painful stimuli, and how the patient can communicate any discomfort to the OR team. Alternatively, leaflets or videos containing such information can be distributed. This counseling helps alleviate anxiety and ensures the patient's cooperation during critical phases of the operation.

The anesthesia and surgical teams must develop a clear communication strategy with the patient to ensure they respond appropriately to brain mapping instructions.

Preoperative Medication Management

Most patients undergoing AC continue their usual medications, particularly antiepileptic drugs, to minimize the risk of intraoperative seizures. Sedative premedication, such as benzodiazepines, should generally be avoided as they may interfere with the patient's ability to remain responsive during the awake phases. However, agents like dexmedetomidine may be used judiciously to manage anxiety without overly sedating the patient.

Anesthetic Techniques for Awake Craniotomy

The anesthetic plan for AC must strike a balance between adequate analgesia, sedation, and patient cooperation during critical phases of the surgery. Two main approaches are used for AC are: *Conscious sedation* and the *asleep-awake-asleep (AAA)* technique.[18]

Conscious Sedation

Conscious sedation involves keeping the patient in a lightly sedated state while allowing them to remain awake and responsive during functional mapping. This technique is suitable for shorter surgeries or when functional testing is required for most of the procedure.[19] The main agents used include:

- *Propofol:* Propofol is administered as an infusion (50–150 μg/kg/min) to maintain light sedation.[20] Its rapid onset and short duration of action make it ideal for maintaining a controlled, easily adjusted level of sedation.
- *Remifentanil:* This ultra-short-acting opioid provides excellent analgesia with minimal residual effects, making it particularly useful during painful parts of the surgery (e.g., skull pinning or craniotomy).[21] Typical infusion rates range from 0.01 to 0.05 cg/kg/min.
- *Dexmedetomidine*: Increasingly used in ACs, dexmedetomidine offers sedative and analgesic properties without significant respiratory depression, which allows for spontaneous ventilation.[22] Infusions typically range from 0.2 to 1 μg/kg/h. Its ability to provide rousable sedation makes it especially useful in maintaining patient cooperation during functional mapping.

Role of target-controlled infusion (TCI) pumps and monitoring of sedation: Propofol and remifentanil sedation can be administered through TCI pumps with target plasma/effect site concentrations based on different pharmacokinetic models. The dose can be titrated based on depth of anesthesia (DoA) monitoring using bispectral index (BIS) or entropy. Ideally, sedative agents should be withheld during the period of monitoring. Remifentanil can be used in low doses during the planned awake phase to manage nociception. **Table 1** enlists the common anesthetic drugs used in AC.

Asleep–Awake–Asleep Technique

The AAA technique is commonly used for more complex or lengthy surgeries, where the patient needs to be fully anesthetized for parts of the procedure.[25] In this approach, the patient is put under general anesthesia for the craniotomy and then awakened for functional mapping. After mapping, general anesthesia is reinduced for the resection and closure.

- *Initial asleep phase:* General anesthesia is induced using agents such as propofol and remifentanil.

TABLE 1: Common anesthetic drugs and dosage for awake craniotomy.[23,24]

Drug	*Dose*	*Complications*
Propofol	• 50–150 µg/kg/min • *TCI:* 2–4 µg/mL	Oversedation, airway obstruction, and hypoxia
Remifentanil	• 0.01–0.05 µg/kg/min • *TCI:* 2–3 ng/mL (sedation) • *TCI:* 1.5–2 ng/mL (mapping)	Bradycardia, hypotension, and postoperative shivering
Dexmedetomidine	• *Loading dose:* 1 µg/kg/min over 10 minutes • *Maintenance:* 0.2–0.7 µg/kg/min	Bradycardia and hypotension and hypertension (with loading doses)

(TCI: target-controlled infusion)

A laryngeal mask airway (LMA) is often used to secure the airway while avoiding the need for tracheal intubation. Muscle relaxants are typically avoided to facilitate spontaneous ventilation once the patient is awakened.

- *Awake phase:* Once the brain is exposed and functional mapping is ready to begin, the patient is awakened by discontinuing the sedative infusions. Sedation is lightened to the point where the patient can respond to commands and perform tasks such as speaking or moving their limbs.
- *Final asleep phase:* After functional mapping, anesthesia is reinduced using propofol and remifentanil, allowing the surgeon to complete tumor resection and wound closure.

The AAA technique provides the advantage of maximizing patient comfort during the more invasive parts of the surgery while still allowing for critical functional testing during the awake phases. However, it requires precise management of transitions between sedation and wakefulness to avoid airway or hemodynamic instability.

Scalp Blocks and Local Anesthesia

Effective local anesthesia is essential for various aspects of AC, including skull pinning, incision management during procedures performed under conscious sedation, and minimizing discomfort during emergence in cases utilizing an asleep-awake anesthetic technique.[26]

Local infiltration with 1–2% lidocaine is commonly employed for pinning sites. The scalp can be anesthetized using a regional field block technique, which involves infiltrating local anesthetic around the incision and at the pin sites or by performing a scalp block. The specific nerve blocks utilized in a scalp block depend on the incision and craniotomy location. A comprehensive scalp block typically necessitates bilateral injections targeting six major nerves and a large volume of local anesthetic solution **(Fig. 1)**. **Table 2** enlists the various nerves and the landmarks for injection. General principles for scalp block are that vascular injection needs to be prevented by negative aspiration before drug delivery and limiting the volume of drug deposited to 1–2 mL at each site. The use of ultrasound at the landmarks mentioned and the identification of nerves can also help avoid complications.[27]

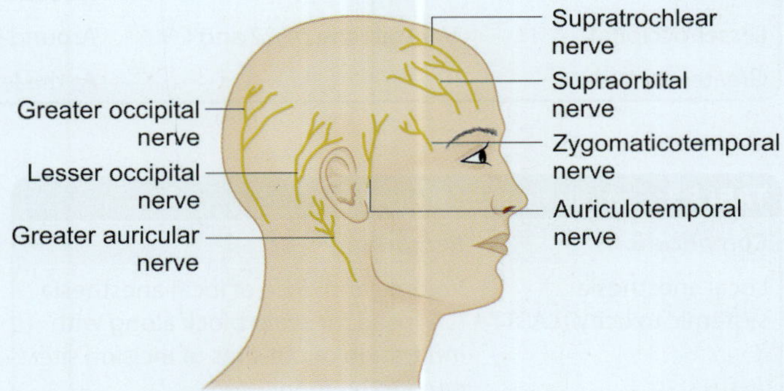

Fig. 1: Describes the anatomy of scalp nerves for blockade. The greater auricular nerve provides sensory innervation behind the ear and the mastoid process; blockade of this nerve contributes to a comprehensive scalp block.

It is recommended to use a long-acting local anesthetic, such as 0.25% bupivacaine, 0.2% ropivacaine, or 0.25% levobupivacaine, often combined with epinephrine at a concentration of 1:200,000. This combination helps to prolong the duration of the block and reduces systemic absorption. Though considered safe, complications have been reported and precautions must be taken **(Table 3)**.

Despite adequate scalp anesthesia, patients may still experience discomfort during the procedure unless supplemental opioids are provided. Studies indicate that up to 30% of patients report significant pain during

TABLE 2: Various nerves to be blocked for regional scalp block and relevant landmarks.

Nerve	Origin	Landmarks/Technique
Supraorbital	Ophthalmic division (V1) of trigeminal nerve	Injection 0.5–1 mm below the supraorbital rim at the level of the supraorbital ridge
Supratrochlear		1 cm medial to the injection of the supraorbital nerve
Zygomaticotemporal	Maxillary division (V2) of trigeminal nerve	Injection over the groove on the zygomatic arch, 1–2 cm lateral to the lateral canthus
Auriculotemporal	Mandibular division (V3) of trigeminal nerve	Palpate the superficial temporal artery 1 cm anterior to the tragus; insert needle posterior to the artery and anticipate loss of resistance from the temporalis fascia at a depth of 1–2 cm and inject drug at this point
Greater occipital	Dorsal ramus of C2	Palpate occipital artery midway between occipital protuberance and the mastoid process. Insert needle medially and inject.
Lesser occipital	Ventral rami of C2 and C3	Around 2–3 cm lateral to the injection point for the greater occipital nerve
Greater auricular		At the level of the tragus, 2 cm posterior to the auricle

TABLE 3: Complications of scalp block.

Complications	Remarks
Local anesthesia systemic toxicity (LAST)	Volume and dose of local anesthesia (LA) used for scalp block along with infiltration of pin sites of incision site need to be monitored
Hematoma/ intravascular absorption	Injury to superficial temporal, supraorbital, or occipital artery must be prevented by careful injection. The high vascularity of scalp can also lead to intravascular absorption
Transient facial nerve palsy	
Transient ptosis	
Trigeminocardiac reflex	

the procedure.[28] Potential causes include inadequate coverage of the incision site, pain originating from adjacent structures, or the wearing off of the block during extended surgical procedures. Manipulating the dura mater can elicit severe pain, particularly during dissection near meningeal vessels.[29] Additionally, local anesthetic infiltration of the temporalis muscle might be necessary to manage pain during dissection for pterional craniotomy. Finally, local anesthetic may also be required for scalp closure at the end of the surgical procedure.

Intraoperative Monitoring and Management

During AC, the anesthesia team is responsible for continuously monitoring the patient's physiological and neurological status. This involves managing sedation and analgesia while maintaining the patient's ability to cooperate during functional testing.

Hemodynamic Monitoring

Hemodynamic stability is crucial during AC to avoid brain swelling, maintain cerebral perfusion, and ensure optimal surgical conditions. Monitoring tools are standard, including electrocardiography (ECG), pulse oximetry, and noninvasive blood pressure (NIBP). In patients with significant cardiovascular risk or anticipated hemodynamic instability, invasive arterial pressure monitoring may be necessary to provide continuous readings and allow frequent blood sampling.

Dexmedetomidine is particularly valuable in maintaining hemodynamic stability.[30] However, it may cause bradycardia, which can be managed with atropine or glycopyrrolate if needed. Blood pressure fluctuations are often managed with vasoactive agents, such as phenylephrine or ephedrine, for hypotension and beta-blockers or esmolol for hypertension.

Respiratory Monitoring

Maintaining spontaneous ventilation is essential in conscious sedation techniques. The patient's respiratory status is monitored using end-tidal CO_2 ($EtCO_2$), preferably attached to nasal prongs to ensure adequate ventilation. Nasopharyngeal airways, or LMAs, may be used to address airway obstruction during sedation. During the asleep phases of the AAA technique, mechanical ventilation is provided typically using an LMA to avoid the complications associated with tracheal intubation.

Neurological Monitoring

Functional mapping is the cornerstone of awake craniotomy and the anesthesia team must ensure that the patient is awake and responsive during this phase. Neurological monitoring includes:

- *Cortical mapping:* The neurosurgeon uses direct electrical stimulation to map eloquent brain areas. The patient is asked to perform tasks such as naming objects, counting, or moving their limbs to identify and avoid critical regions.[31]
- *Evoked potentials:* In some cases, motor-evoked potentials (MEPs) and somatosensory-evoked potentials (SSEPs) are used to monitor the integrity of motor and sensory pathways during surgery.[32]

Processed electroencephalogram (EEG) monitoring (e.g., BIS or entropy) can also guide sedation depth, ensuring that the patient remains appropriately awake during functional testing while minimizing discomfort.[33] The level of sedation can be monitored clinically with the use of the modified observer's assessment of alertness/sedation scale (MOASS) score or the Ramsay sedation scale (RSS) score. The modified RSS is currently used in intraoperative clinical practice with a target score of 2–4.[34] **Table 4** provides a comprehensive description of the modified RSS and compares it to the American Society of Anesthesiologists (ASA) definitions of general anesthesia (GA) and levels of sedation/analgesia.[35]

TABLE 4: Sedation scores: ASA and modified Ramsay sedation score.

ASA continuum of sedation	***Modified Ramsay sedation score***
Minimal sedation/ anxiolysis	*1:* Awake and alert, no cognitive impairment
Moderate sedation/ analgesia *(conscious sedation)*	*2:* Awake but tranquil, conversational response to verbal commands
	3: Asleep but purposeful, conversational response to verbal commands
	4: Asleep, purposeful responses to commands *louder* than conversational level or glabellar tap, or both
Deep sedation/ analgesia	*5:* Asleep, sluggish purposeful response to commands *louder* than conversational level or *strong* glabellar tap, or both
	6: Asleep, sluggish purposeful response to painful stimulus
General anesthesia	*7:* Asleep, only reflex withdrawal to painful stimulus
	8: Unresponsiveness to external stimulus

(ASA: American Society of Anesthesiologists)

Intraoperative Complications

Awake craniotomy carries specific intraoperative risks that must be anticipated and managed by the anesthesia team:

Airway Compromise

Airway obstruction is a common challenge during the awake phases, particularly in patients with preexisting airway issues or obesity.[36] Nasopharyngeal airways may be used to manage mild airway obstructions, while more severe cases may require the insertion of an LMA. If airway compromise cannot be adequately managed, conversion to GA may be necessary.

Seizures

Seizures can occur during cortical stimulation, particularly in patients with a history of epilepsy.[37-39] Focal seizures are typically managed by irrigating the brain with cold saline, while generalized seizures may require intravenous antiepileptic drugs. Seizure management is critical to prevent movement that could lead to surgical complications or brain injury.

Brain Swelling (Cerebral Edema)

Intraoperative brain swelling, or cerebral edema, can occur due to surgical manipulation or changes in cerebral perfusion. Brain swelling can obstruct the surgeon's view and increase the risk of neurological injury.[40] Management strategies include:

- *Mannitol or hypertonic saline:* These osmotic agents reduce intracranial pressure (ICP) by drawing fluid out of brain tissue.
- *Corticosteroids:* Dexamethasone is commonly used to reduce inflammation and cerebral edema in the perioperative period.
- *Hyperventilation:* Short periods of hyperventilation can reduce ICP by inducing vasoconstriction and decreasing cerebral blood volume.

Hemodynamic Instability

Blood pressure fluctuations are common during AC due to surgical manipulation or anesthesia-related effects.[41] Dexmedetomidine can help maintain hemodynamic stability, but vasoactive agents may be required to manage hypotension or hypertension. Excessive hemodynamic fluctuations should be avoided to reduce the risk of increased ICP or hemorrhage.

Patient Agitation or Anxiety

Patient agitation or anxiety can complicate the awake phases of surgery.[17] Mild sedation can reduce anxiety without oversedating the patient. Clear communication and reassurance from the anesthesia and surgical teams are also essential for maintaining patient cooperation. Xerostomia is also a cause of patient anxiety and loss of cooperation, which can be addressed by intermittently applying moist cotton or gauze to the patients' lips.

Nausea/Vomiting

Nausea and vomiting are expectedly more common with the AAA technique after the awakening of the patient for monitoring. Opioid administration may predispose patients to increased risk. Use of propofol as the anesthetic agent and of LMA to secure the airway can reduce the risk partially. Dexamethasone use is associated with a lesser incidence of nausea/vomiting over 5-HT3 receptor antagonists as antiemetic prophylaxis.[42]

Conversion to General Anesthesia

Any of the complications discussed earlier may necessitate conversion to GA, although uncontrolled seizures and airway obstruction may need a lower threshold for conversion to GA.

Operating Room Considerations

Preparation of the OR includes positioning the anesthesia workstation and the neurophysiology monitoring equipment by the side of the patient table and ensuring that the patient's face and airway remain accessible at all times. It is essential to restrict the movement of personnel and noise inside the OR to ensure a calm environment for the patient. Information about *AC in progress* must be displayed to avoid unnecessary personnel/equipment movement. Regulation of OR temperature needs to be done even before the patient entry. The use of forced-air warming blankets and fluid warmers can help prevent hypothermia.

Intraoperative Positioning

Proper patient positioning during AC is crucial for both surgical access and patient comfort. The patient will be required to remain in the same position for several hours, making optimal positioning essential to avoid discomfort, pressure injuries, or airway compromise.[43,44]

- *Head position:* The head is typically secured in a Mayfield head holder to prevent movement during the procedure. Careful attention should be paid to avoid excessive neck flexion, extension, or rotation, which could impede venous return or cause airway obstruction. The position should allow the surgical team access to the tumor while maintaining a comfortable position for the patient.
- *Body positioning:* Depending on the tumor location, patients are usually positioned in a supine, lateral, or semisitting position. Adequate padding must be placed under pressure points, such as the heels, elbows, and sacrum, to prevent pressure sores. Arm boards should be used to support the arms and avoid brachial plexus injury.
- *Padding and support:* Padding should also be placed under the knees to prevent hyperextension of the legs. In lengthy procedures, leg position should be adjusted to maintain circulation and avoid compartment syndrome.

Patients should be positioned as comfortably as possible since they will remain in the same position for an extended period, and discomfort may lead to increased anxiety or movement during the awake phases.

POSTOPERATIVE CARE

The principles of postoperative care are similar to those of managing patients after GA. Positioning, hemodynamic, respiratory, and neurological monitoring follow similar guidelines to any neurosurgical procedure. Focus should be on early enteral nutrition, ambulation, and removal of invasive catheters. Admission to intensive care units or discharge after a postanesthesia care unit (PACU) stay depend on institutional guidelines.

CURRENT RESEARCH AND FUTURE DIRECTIONS

Recent research in AC has focused on optimizing anesthetic techniques to improve patient outcomes. The integration of *neuroimaging techniques*, such as fMRI and DTI, with AC has improved preoperative planning, allowing surgeons to identify and map functional areas with greater precision. However, intraoperative mapping remains the most reliable method for ensuring the safe resection of tumors in eloquent brain regions.[45]

The availability of advanced neuronavigation techniques has resulted in possible avoidance of skull pin insertion that can contribute to significantly lesser requirement of anesthetic agents and scalp blocks.[46] Low- and low-to-middle-income countries (LIC and LMICs) provide significant opportunities for learning and research in AC for brain tumor surgeries, but the challenges include standardization and validation of techniques for preoperative evaluation, surgical techniques, and neuromonitoring methods.[47] Recent evidence points toward reduced incidence of intraoperative complications with safer anesthetic drugs available currently. The fast-changing landscape of neurosurgery and neuroanesthesia has resulted in a recent focus on the applicability of these techniques in the pediatric population. Future research will likely explore the role of advanced imaging in combination with real-time cortical mapping to enhance surgical precision.

CONCLUSION

Awake craniotomy is a highly specialized procedure that requires meticulous anesthetic management to balance patient comfort, safety, and cooperation during functional mapping. The anesthesiologist's role is critical in ensuring that the patient remains sedated enough to tolerate the procedure while being awake and cooperative for brain mapping. As neuroanesthetic techniques continue to evolve, AC will remain an essential tool for maximizing tumor resection while preserving critical neurological functions.

REFERENCES

1. Paldor I, Drummond KJ, Awad M, Sufaro YZ, Kaye AH. Is a wake-up call in order? Review of the evidence for awake craniotomy. J Clin Neurosci. 2016;23:1-7.
2. Dziedzic T, Bernstein M. Awake craniotomy for brain tumor: indications, technique and benefits. Expert Rev Neurother. 2014;14(12):1405-15.
3. Chowdhury T, Gray K, Sharma M, Mau C, McNutt S, Ryan C, et al. Brain cancer progression: a retrospective multicenter comparison of awake craniotomy versus general anesthesia in high-grade glioma resection. J Neurosurg Anesthesiol. 2022;34(4):392-400.
4. Moniz-Garcia D, Bojaxhi E, Borah BJ, Dholakia R, Kim H, Sousa-Pinto B, et al. Awake craniotomy program implementation. JAMA Network Open. 2024;7(1):e2352917.
5. Sahjpaul RL. Awake craniotomy: controversies, indications, and techniques in the surgical treatment of temporal lobe epilepsy. Can J Neurol Sci. 2000;27(Suppl 1):S55-63; discussion S92-6.
6. Ladino LD, Rizvi S, Téllez-Zenteno JF. The montreal procedure: the legacy of the great Wilder Penfield. Epilepsy Behav. 2018;83:151-61.
7. Shalan ME, Soliman AY, Nassar IA, Alarabawy RA. Surgical planning in patients with brain glioma using diffusion tensor MR imaging and tractography. Egypt J Radiol Nucl Med. 2021;52(1):110.
8. Albuquerque LAF, Macêdo Filho LJM, Borges FS, Pessoa FC, Diógenes GS, Rocha CJV, et al. Awake craniotomy for diffuse low grade gliomas in a resource limited setting: lessons learned with a consecutive series of 51 surgeries. World Neurosurg. 2023;177:e563-79.
9. Ramakrishnan PK, Saeed F, Thomson S, Corns R, Mathew RK, Sivakumar G. Awake craniotomy for high-grade gliomas: a prospective cohort study in a UK tertiary-centre. Surgeon. 2024;22(1):e3-12.
10. Sitnikov AR, Grigoryan YA, Mishnyakova LP. Awake craniotomy without sedation in treatment of patients with lesional epilepsy. Surg Neurol Int. 2018;9:177.
11. Fernández Coello A, Moritz-Gasser S, Martino J, Martinoni M, Matsuda R, Duffau H. Selection of intra-operative tasks for awake mapping based on relationships between tumor location and functional networks. J Neurosurg. 2013;119(6):1380-94.
12. Morshed RA, Young JS, Lee AT, Berger MS, Hervey-Jumper SL. Clinical pearls and methods for intraoperative awake language mapping. Neurosurgery. 2020;89(2):143-53.
13. Chui J, Manninen P, Valiante T, Venkatraghavan L. The anesthetic considerations of intraoperative electrocorticography during epilepsy surgery. Anesth Analg. 2013; 117(2):479-86.
14. Erickson KM, Cole DJ. Anesthetic considerations for awake craniotomy for epilepsy and functional neurosurgery. Anesthesiol Clin. 2012;30(2):241-68.
15. Santini B, Talacchi A, Casagrande F, Casartelli M, Savazzi S, Procaccio F, et al. Eligibility criteria and psychological profiles in patient candidates for awake craniotomy: a pilot study. J Neurosurg Anesthesiol. 2012;24(3):209-16.
16. Kayama T; Guidelines committee of the Japan awake surgery conference. The guidelines for awake craniotomy guidelines committee of The Japan Awake Surgery Conference. Neurol Med Chir (Tokyo). 2012;52(3):119-41.
17. Nossek E, Matot I, Shahar T, Barzilai O, Rapoport Y, Gonen T, et al. Failed awake craniotomy: a retrospective analysis in 424 patients undergoing craniotomy for brain tumor. J Neurosurg. 2013;118(2):243-9.
18. Stevanovic A, Rossaint R, Veldeman M, Bilotta F, Coburn M. Anaesthesia management for awake craniotomy: systematic review and meta-analysis. PLoS One. 2016;11(5):e0156448.
19. Danks RA, Aglio LS, Gugino LD, Black PM. Craniotomy under local anesthesia and monitored conscious sedation for the resection of tumors involving eloquent cortex. J Neurooncol. 2000;49(2):131-9.
20. Hans P, Bonhomme V, Born JD, Maertens de Noordhoudt A, Brichant JF, Dewandre PY. Target-controlled infusion of

propofol and remifentanil combined with bispectral index monitoring for awake craniotomy. Anaesthesia. 2000; 55(3):255-9.
21. Goettel N, Bharadwaj S, Venkatraghavan L, Mehta J, Bernstein M, Manninen PH. Dexmedetomidine vs propofol-remifentanil conscious sedation for awake craniotomy: a prospective randomized controlled trial. Br J Anaesth. 2016;116(6):811-21.
22. Bekker AY, Kaufman B, Samir H, Doyle W. The use of dexmedetomidine infusion for awake craniotomy. Anesth Analg. 2001;92(5):1251-3.
23. Chui J. Anesthesia for awake craniotomy: an update. Rev Colomb Anestesiol. 2015;43:22–8.
24. Komatsu R, Turan AM, Orhan-Sungur M, McGuire J, Radke OC, Apfel CC. Remifentanil for general anaesthesia: a systematic review. Anaesthesia. 2007;62(12):1266-80.
25. Rajan S, Cata JP, Nada E, Weil R, Pal R, Avitsian R. Asleep-awake-asleep craniotomy: a comparison with general anesthesia for resection of supratentorial tumors. J Clin Neurosci. 2013;20(8):1068-73.
26. Osborn I, Sebeo J. “Scalp Block” during craniotomy: a classic technique revisited. J Neurosurg Anesthesiol. 2010;22(3):187-94.
27. Zetlaoui PJ, Gauthier E, Benhamou D. Ultrasound-guided scalp nerve blocks for neurosurgery: a narrative review. Anaesth Crit Care Pain Med. 2020;39(6):876-82.
28. Milian M, Tatagiba M, Feigl GC. Patient response to awake craniotomy - a summary overview. Acta Neurochir (Wien). 2014;156(6):1063-70.
29. Fontaine D, Almairac F, Santucci S, Fernandez C, Dallel R, Pallud J, et al. Dural and pial pain-sensitive structures in humans: new inputs from awake craniotomies. Brain. 2018;141(4):1040-8.
30. Garavaglia MM, Das S, Cusimano MD, Crescini C, Mazer CD, Hare GMT, et al. Anesthetic approach to high-risk patients and prolonged awake craniotomy using dexmedetomidine and scalp block. J Neurosurg Anesthesiol. 2014;26(3): 226-33.
31. Kim SS, McCutcheon IE, Suki D, Weinberg JS, Sawaya R, Lang FF, et al. Awake craniotomy for brain tumors near eloquent cortex: correlation of intraoperative cortical mapping with neurological outcomes in 309 consecutive patients. Neurosurgery. 2009;64(5):836-45.
32. Saito T, Muragaki Y, Tamura M, Maruyama T, Nitta M, Tsuzuki S, et al. Awake craniotomy with transcortical motor evoked potential monitoring for resection of gliomas in the precentral gyrus: utility for predicting motor function. J Neurosurg. 2019;132(4):987-97.
33. Soehle M, Wolf CF, Priston MJ, Neuloh G, Bien CG, Hoeft A, et al. Propofol pharmacodynamics and bispectral index during key moments of awake craniotomy. J Neurosurg Anesthesiol. 2018;30(1):32-8.
34. Sheahan CG, Mathews DM. Monitoring and delivery of sedation. Br J Anaesth. 2014;113(suppl_2):ii37-47.
35. American Society of Anesthesiologists. (2024). Statement on continuum of depth of sedation: Definition of general anesthesia and levels of sedation/analgesia. [online]. Available from https://www.asahq.org/standards-and-practice-parameters/statement-on-continuum-of-depth-of-sedation-definition-of-general-anesthesia-and-levels-of-sedation-analgesia [Last accessed March, 2025].
36. Sivasankar C, Schlichter RA, Baranov D, Kofke WA. Awake craniotomy: a new airway approach. Anesth Analg. 2016; 122(2):509-11.
37. Paquin-Lanthier G, Subramaniam S, Leong KW, Daniels A, Singh K, Takami H, et al. Risk factors and characteristics of intraoperative seizures during awake craniotomy: a retrospective cohort study of 562 consecutive patients with a space-occupying brain lesion. J Neurosurg Anesthesiol. 2023;35(2):194-200.
38. Roca E, Pallud J, Guerrini F, Panciani PP, Fontanella M, Spena G. Stimulation-related intraoperative seizures during awake surgery: A review of available evidences. Neurosurg Rev. 2020;43(1):87-93.
39. Yuan Y, Peizhi Z, Xiang W, Yanhui L, Ruofei L, Shu J, et al. Intraoperative seizures and seizures outcome in patients undergoing awake craniotomy. J Neurosurg Sci. 2019;63(3):301-7.
40. Khu KJ, Ng WH. Intraoperative swelling leading to neurological deterioration: an argument for large craniotomy in awake surgery for glioma resection. J Clin Neurosci. 2009;16(7):886-8.
41. Sinha PK, Koshy T, Gayatri P, Smitha V, Abraham M, Rathod RC. Anesthesia for awake craniotomy: a retrospective study. Neurol India. 2007;55(4):376-81.
42. Sato T. Dexamethasone versus 5-HT3 receptor antagonists in preventing nausea during awake craniotomy: a propensity score matching study. JA Clin Rep. 2024;10(1):63.
43. Wahab SS, Grundy PL, Weidmann C. Patient experience and satisfaction with awake craniotomy for brain tumours. Br J Neurosurg. 2011;25(5):606-13.
44. Potters JW, Klimek M. Awake Craniotomy: improving the patient's experience. Curr Opin Anaesthesiol. 2015; 28(5):511-6.
45. Picht T, Kombos T, Gramm HJ, Brock M, Suess O. Multimodal protocol for awake craniotomy in language cortex tumour surgery. Acta Neurochir (Wien). 2006;148(2):127-37; discussion 137-8.
46. Hall S, Kabwama S, Sadek AR, Dando A, Roach J, Weidmann C, et al. Awake craniotomy for tumour resection: The safety and feasibility of a simple technique. Interdiscip Neurosurg. 2021;24:101070.
47. Pascual JSG, de Lotbiniere-Bassett M, Khu KJO, Starreveld YP, Lama S, Legaspi GD, et al. Challenges and opportunities in awake craniotomy for brain tumor surgery in low- and lower-middle-income countries: a narrative review and perspective. World Neurosurg. 2024;189:118-26.

40 CHAPTER

Anesthesia for Spinal Tumors

Sanjay Agrawal, Sharmishtha Pathak, Veena Asthana

INTRODUCTION

The type of surgery performed on the spine encompasses operations for trauma, deformity, and myelopathy. The majority of these surgeries are performed on trauma patients and spinal tumors form a very small part of surgeries undertaken on the spine. Spinal tumors constitute 15–20% of all central nervous system tumors.[1] These tumors can be incapacitating, leading to significant morbidity and mortality. Primary spine tumor accounts for 5% of all cases and the commonest tumor is secondary metastasis.[2,3]

Patients present with pain, typically long-standing, localised, dull in nature and potentially aggravated by supine positioning. Nerve root or spinal cord compression by tumor mass may lead to motor symptoms (weakness or paralysis, loss of sphincter function) and sensory symptoms (paresthesia). In malignant lesions, systemic symptoms, including weight loss or fatigue, may be present.[4,5]

The patients with spinal tumors are being considered for surgery, primarily to relieve pain and prevent the occurrence or further neurological deterioration, and stabilize the vertebral column.

With the advancement in imaging technologies, and anesthesia and surgical practices increasing older patients with significant comorbidities are being offered ever more major procedures for which they would have previously not been considered. Increasing numbers of decompressive procedures for metastatic spinal cord compression are being performed as a result of improved oncological therapies. With this the number of patients with comorbidities, coming for spinal surgeries is also increasing and the challenges faced by the anesthesiologist like prone positioning, prolonged duration of surgery, and blood loss also increase. Understanding the anatomy of the spine and the origin of spinal tumors helps in understanding the risks and perioperative complications, thus reducing postoperative morbidity and mortality.

ANATOMY OF SPINE AND SPINAL CORD

The spine is constituted of 33 individual bones and 31 pairs of spinal nerves. It provides the main support for the body, allowing us to stand upright, bend, and twist while protecting the spinal cord from injury. The vertebrae are numbered and divided into regions: Cervical, thoracic, lumbar, sacrum, and coccyx.[6,7]

The spinal cord begins at the medulla oblongata, runs in the spinal canal, and ends in the lower back, as it tapers to form conus medullaris. In relation to the spine, the spinal cord runs from the top of the C1 vertebra to approximately the level of the L1 vertebra in adults and the L3 vertebra in children. It is about 45 cm in length and is cylindrical in shape. A fibrous band called the *filum terminale* begins at the tip of the conus medullaris and extends to the pelvis. At the end of the spinal cord, the cord fibers separate into the cauda equina, which is a collection of nerves and derives its name from the Latin translation of "horse's tail."[8]

Any interruption of spinal cord function by disease or injury at a particular level may result in a loss of sensation and motor function below that level. Depending on the severity of the disease or injury, the loss of function may be permanent.

EPIDEMIOLOGY AND CLINICAL PRESENTATION OF SPINAL TUMORS

Primary spinal cord tumors comprise 5% of all primary central nervous system (CNS) tumors in adults. Age-adjusted incidence is slightly higher in males (0.67 compared with 0.59 per 100,000 population). The incidence is higher in non-Hispanic whites compared to Hispanics or non-Hispanic blacks.[2] Most of these tumors present as extramedullary masses (70%); 15–25% of spinal tumors involve the cervical spine, 50–55% thoracic spinal canal, and 25–30% lumbosacral spine.[9] Most common histologic subtypes in adults include meningeal tumors, nerve sheath tumors, and ependymal tumors. Common primary intramedullary spinal cord tumors are astrocytomas or ependymomas. Intradural extramedullary tumors —including schwannomas, neurofibromas, and meningiomas—that affect the paravertebral area may spread and compress the cord through expansion.[10-12] Hemangiomas (benign tumors of the blood vessels) are usually discovered incidentally and usually do not produce symptoms. However, symptoms can emerge if pathologic vertebral fractures or epidural extension occurs.

In the pediatric population, spinal cord tumors are slightly more common, representing 4–5% of all primary CNS tumors. Ependymal tumors, gliomas, and nerve sheath tumors are the most common histologic subtypes in children. Pilocytic astrocytomas comprise the majority of gliomas.[13,14]

The etiology of spinal cord tumors is largely unknown. Prior exposure to radiation therapy may increase the risk of developing secondary malignancies such as sarcomas and gliomas as well as benign tumors, such as meningiomas. Depending on the histologic type, tumors may be associated with genetic syndromes such as neurofibromatosis (NF) 1 and 2 as well as von Hippel-Lindau disease.[15]

Metastatic lesions are responsible for 85% of neoplastic spinal cord compression cases. Systemic cancers with the likelihood of spinal metastasis include breast cancer, prostate, renal, lung, lymphoma, sarcoma, and multiple myeloma.

Metastatic spinal cord compression usually follows arterial hematogenous dissemination of malignant cells to the vertebral bodies, with subsequent expansion into the epidural space. Spread into the epidural space may also occur by means of tumor extension through the intervertebral foramina or hematogenous spread to the vertebral bodies by way of the Batson venous plexus (particularly with prostate cancer).

Most frequently, metastatic seeding involves the thoracic spine (accounting for about 70% of cases), with the lumbar spine being the second most involved site (20% of cases). The cervical spine is affected in approximately 10% of cases. Multiple spinal levels are affected in 30% of patients. Gastrointestinal and pelvic malignancies tend to affect the lumbosacral spine. Lung and breast cancers are more likely to affect the thoracic spine.[4,16]

Intramedullary metastases are rare. Signs and symptoms resemble epidural compression; however, if motor weakness is present, it is more likely to be unilateral. Leptomeningeal metastases spread by means of diffuse or multifocal seeding of the meninges from advanced systemic cancer (e.g., lung or breast cancer, melanoma, and lymphoma). Leptomeningeal metastasis presents as *multifocal neurological* deficits referable to the spinal cord. The clinical presentation in compression caused by metastatic lesions is indistinguishable from that caused by primary disease.[16]

PREOPERATIVE ANESTHETIC CONSIDERATIONS AND CHALLENGES

Special considerations include:
- Cervical spine range of motion.
- Assessment of restrictive lung disease due to spinal malformation.
- Assessment of preoperative neurological deficit and its documentation.
- Autonomic hyperreflexia.
- Frailty assessment and prehabilitation.

When assessing patients before spinal surgery, particular care should be given to the respiratory, cardiovascular, and neurological systems; all may be affected by the pathology for which the spinal surgery is proposed.

The details of the assessment required and investigations to assess each system are detailed in **Table 1**. Besides the systemic assessment, it is also important for the anesthesiologist to understand that a maximum number of these patients have pain as their presenting complaint with some degree of neurological deficit. The pain associated with spinal cord tumors may be acute, chronic, or acute-on-chronic. When eliciting a history, the anesthesiologist should inquire regarding duration, location, and quality. Use of pain medications should be noted, including current medications and medications used previously. This will influence the intraoperative approach, particularly for narcotic usage, and will assist in managing acute postoperative pain. All the pain medications should be continued preoperatively as per the usual schedule. Continuation of adjunctive medications like gabapentin is recommended; however, the use of nonsteroidal anti-inflammatory drugs (NSAIDs) is controversial, because of the potential for postoperative bleeding.[5,17]

Patients undergoing spinal surgery may be at increased risk of thromboembolic disease as a result of

TABLE 1: Preoperative assessment of a patient with spinal tumor—systemwise approach.

System	*Assessment required*	*Minimum investigation*	*Optional investigation*
Airway	Previous difficulty in intubation, restriction of neck movement, and the stability of the cervical spine	Cervical spine lateral X-rays with flexion/ extension views (for patients with rheumatoid arthritis)	CT scan and MRI
Cervical spine	Presence of pain, neurological deficit	X-ray and CT scans	MRI
Respiratory system	History, physical examination, bedside pulmonary function tests, use of continuous positive airway pressure (CPAP) at night	Plain chest radiograph	Pulmonary function test (if one-lung ventilation is required), pulmonary diffusion capacity
Cardiovascular system	History of breathlessness on exertion, assessment of functional capacity, coronary artery disease, and use of antiplatelet therapy and new-onset breathlessness, especially in patients receiving cardiotoxic chemotherapeutic agents	Arterial blood gas analysis, ECG, and echocardiography	Dobutamine stress test
Neurological system	History of onset of symptoms, sensory or motor neurological deficit	CT scan and MRI	Nerve function tests and electromyography
Hematological system	History of nutritional deficiency	Complete blood count, coagulation profile, blood grouping and cross-matching, urea, electrolytes, albumin, and calcium	LFT

(CT: computed tomography; ECG: electrocardiogram; MRI: magnetic resonance imaging; LFT: liver function test)

prolonged surgery, prone positioning, malignancy, and extended periods of postoperative recumbency. The use of compression stockings and pneumatic boots is recommended.[18] Many surgeons prefer not to administer anticoagulants because their use may be associated with hemorrhagic complications, including increased blood loss and epidural hematoma.[19-21]

CHOICE OF ANESTHESIA TECHNIQUE

Premedication

The use of bronchodilating agents may be of value in optimizing respiratory function preoperatively. In patients with a high spinal cord lesion, or those in whom fiberoptic intubation is to be undertaken, administration of anticholinergic agent glycopyrrolate (200 ± 400 μg by IV or IM injection) should be considered.[22] Many patients will have factors that increase the risk of regurgitation and aspiration of gastric contents, such as recent opioid administration, high spinal cord injury, and incompetence of the upper esophageal sphincter, such patients should receive aspiration prophylaxis prior to induction.[23,24]

Induction

The choice of induction technique, intravenous (IV) or inhalation, is guided primarily by the patient's condition, age, and consideration of the ease of tracheal intubation Preoxygenation is advisable in all patients. Unless there are concerns over the stability of the cervical spine or airway maintenance, IV induction is suitable. IV induction agent usage reduces the amplitude of evoked potential responses, and in particular, cortical responses, but these effects do not prevent useful intraoperative recording of cortical somatosensory evoked potential (SSEP) and transcranial electrical motor evoked potentials (MEP).[25] Inhalational agents reduce the amplitude of potential responses to a greater degree compared to IV induction agents, but no studies have compared an inhalation induction technique with an IV technique in this respect.

Intubation

The decision to intubate the patient awake or asleep depends on pathology and clinical manifestation The patient must be counseled if awake fiberoptic intubation is planned.

Flowchart 1: Algorithm for intubation of patients with cervical spine pathology.

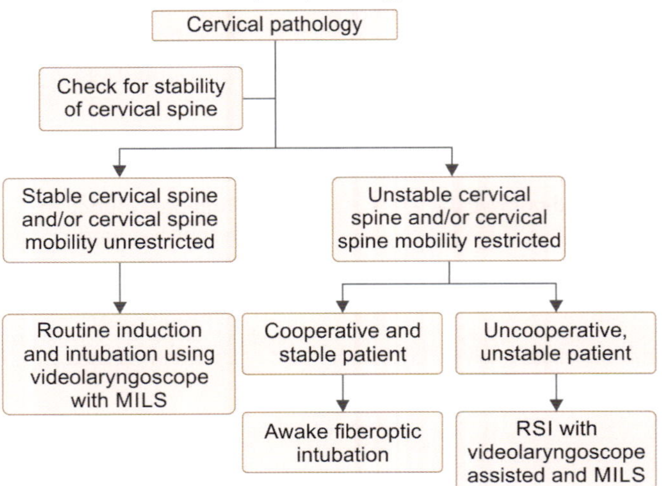

(MILS: manual in-line stabilization; RSI: rapid sequence intubation)

Flowchart 1 illustrates the intubation of patients with cervical spine pathology

Maintenance of Anesthesia

The type of monitoring chosen to assess spinal cord integrity has a bearing on the anesthetic technique used for maintenance. A stable anesthetic depth is required for reliably assessing the changes in SSEPs or MEPs. A technique involving nitrous oxide 60% and isoflurane/sevoflurane <0.5 MAC is compatible with neuromonitoring, but MAC >0.5 may impair the potential recording and thus propofol may be preferred.[26]

Neurophysiologists monitoring evoked potentials should be made aware of any sudden decrease in arterial pressure, or the need to administer a bolus of opioids or change the anesthetic depth. Sudden cardiovascular instability during anesthesia may result from the spinal cord and brainstem reflexes, from mediastinal distortion as a result of surgical manipulation, or more commonly from blood loss.

Induced Hypotension

Hypotensive anesthesia may be used to improve the surgical field and to reduce blood loss during major spinal surgery. Mean arterial pressure (MAP) is typically maintained at 60 mm Hg. There is little evidence that any particular agent is superior, but the avoidance of tachycardia is an essential part of a good anesthetic technique.

Muscle Relaxation

When myogenic motor evoked responses are to be recorded, the neuromuscular block must be carefully monitored and a constant depth of block maintained. It is advisable to administer a nondepolarizing neuromuscular blocking agent such as atracurium using a continuous IV infusion device during major spinal surgery.

Intraoperative Monitoring and Positioning of the Patient

Cardiovascular Monitoring

Prolonged anesthesia in unusual positions, combined with significant blood loss, the hemodynamic effects of thoracic surgery, and the use of controlled hypotension, necessitates continuous and comprehensive monitoring of the cardiovascular system. Invasive arterial pressure monitoring comes to the rescue of the anesthesiologist in such scenarios.[27,28] In the prone position, central venous pressure (CVP) may be a misleading indicator of right and left ventricular end-diastolic volume. High CVP values may be misleading indicators of adequate cardiac filling in the prone position.[5,22] The changes are probably a result of raised intrathoracic pressure causing reduced ventricular compliance and compression of the inferior vena cava. Dependent lower limbs cause a reduced venous return to the heart.

Respiratory Monitoring

Respiratory system monitoring should always include end-tidal carbon dioxide concentration and peak airway pressure. In major surgery, serial measurements of arterial oxygen tension are recommended.

Temperature Monitoring

Thermoregulation may already be impaired in patients who have spinal cord lesions before surgery. Prolonged anesthesia causes significant heat loss. The use of temperature monitoring, warming of all IV fluids, and a warm air mattress device is recommended.

Positioning

The patient's position for spinal surgery varies depending on the level of the spine to be operated upon and the nature of the proposed surgery. Patients may be repositioned intraoperatively. It is important that venous pressures at the surgical site are kept low to reduce bleeding (reverse

Trendelenburg tilt and a free abdomen), and peripheral nerves, bony prominences, and the eyes are protected.[29]

Lumbar Surgery

Anterior approaches require a laparotomy, and general surgical input may be required in difficult cases. Posterior surgery requires a prone patient with a free abdomen to keep epidural venous pressure low (the patient supported on a Wilson frame, for example, or a raised mattress with a hole for the abdomen).

Thoracic Surgery

Anterior approaches to the thoracic spine are via a thoracotomy with the patient supported in a lateral position. If a double-lumen endobronchial tube is used to allow deflation of one lung for surgical access, a fiberoptic bronchoscope should always be used to check tube placement after the patient is finally positioned. Posterior approaches to the thoracic spine require a prone patient with an uncompressed abdomen.

Cervical Surgery

Patients are usually positioned with their feet close to the anesthetic machine. This allows surgical access to the head and neck. Extensions are needed for breathing circuits and IV lines, and it may be useful to place an IV cannula in the patient's foot. Tracheal tubes must be carefully secured without impinging on the surgical field so as to prevent accidental extubations. For anterior surgery, a reinforced tracheal tube will reduce the risk of airway obstruction as tracheal retraction occurs during surgery. The head is supported on a padded head ring or the "horseshoe" of a Mayfield neurosurgical operating table attachment. Reverse Trendelenburg positioning minimizes venous bleeding. Venous pooling in the lower limbs and intraoperative retraction of the carotid artery make an arterial line advisable for most patients. For posterior approaches to the cervical spine, the head of the prone patient can be supported on the gel-padded horseshoe of the Mayfield table attachment or placed in a skull clamp.[30] The orbits, the superior orbital nerve, and the skin over the maxilla are at particular risk of ischemic injury if positioning is incorrect. These problems are avoided by using a skull clamp. The head height and degree of neck flexion may be adjusted intraoperatively, and pressure areas must be rechecked after such maneuvers. Support for the tracheal tube and breathing circuitry is difficult; care must be taken if equipment has been taped to the operating table, and that tubes are not dislodged as the head position is altered. Venous air embolism is a risk for these patients because veins at the operative site are above the level of the heart. Unfortunately, methods to reduce blood loss such as reduced venous pressure increase the risk of this complication.[31]

Prone Position

The key to safe prone positioning is the appropriate selection of the many types and sizes of support that are available **(Table 2) (Figs. 1A and B)**. Foam bolsters are commonly used, at the level of the chest below the axillae and at the anterior superior iliac spines. The arms should not be abducted > 90°s, in order to reduce the risk of brachial plexus injury. The ulnar nerve at the elbow is at risk of pressure-related injury when the arms are flexed in the prone position, thus special care should be taken for padding at the elbow joint. If the arms remain by the patient's side, then the thumbs should be positioned pointing downward, maintaining the normal anatomy.

Special care should be taken to prevent pressure on the abdomen as this will be transmitted to the venous system and cause increased bleeding from the valveless epidural veins. The eyes are kept closed to protect the tear film and padding should be avoided.[29,32] A number of headrests **(Fig. 1A)** are available that are designed to avoid pressure on the eyes while maintaining the neck in a neutral position. Some include a mirror to facilitate easier intraoperative checking. External pressure on the eyes may also be completely avoided by the use of devices such as the Mayfield head fixator **(Fig. 1B)**. The head is held in a clamp by pins which are inserted into the outer table of the skull. It affords excellent control of the head and neck and is commonly used during operations on the posterior cervical spine. **Table 2** lists the commonly used body, and head supports for prone positioning.

Blood Conservation

Blood loss during single-level procedures is not excessive, but during more extensive spinal surgery, it can be considerable; typically, losses are 10–30 mL/kg, a result of loss from decorticated bone and disruption of rich vascular networks.[33] The degree of blood loss is associated with: Body weight, type and extent of tumors, raised intra-abdominal pressure in a prone position, and associated comorbidities.

TABLE 2: Various types of frames/tables and head support used for prone positioning during spinal surgery.

Body support	***Use***	***Advantages***	***Disadvantages***
Pillows	Small cases	Quick to set-up	• Limited chest support • Difficult to ensure a free abdomen • Not fixed, amenable to movement during positioning
Chest roll		Ensures free abdomen	Direct and indirect pressure injury, associated with hepatic failure when poorly positioned
Pelvic roll	Elevates the lower spine		Direct and indirect pressure injury, bladder compression when improperly positioned
Thoracic support/ Montreal mattress	Cervical and thoracic spinal surgery	Easy to place on a table, allows free abdominal movement, arms can be positioned by the side or flexed and abducted	Direct pressure injury to the groin if incorrectly positioned
Wilson frame	Lumbar spine surgery	Loss of lumbar lordosis, pressure distributed to patient's sides, pelvis and chest are supported while abdomen hangs free	• Only the width of support can be increased, may be too long for short-statured patients. • Difficult to place arms by the side
Allen table/ Jackson table	Spine surgery, good radiological access	• Abdomen and chest free • Arm supports and mirrors to permit an easy view of the face and endotracheal tube. • Permit wide range of rotation of the patient, movable supports help in positioning for all body structure types in patients, permits 360° rotation without change of table	Large piece of equipment, airway access is difficult, difficult to control the height of table
Cambridge frame/ Relton–Hall frame	Scoliosis surgery	Can be adjusted for each patient	Patient rests on pressure points only, skin necrosis common in prolonged surgery
Andrew's frame (knee-chest position)	Occipital, cervical, lumbar surgery	Loss of lumbar lordosis	Increased venous pooling in legs, decreased stroke volume, pressure injury on knees common, increased chances of lower limb nerve injury
		Head support	
Head support	***Use***	***Advantages***	***Disadvantages***
Mayfield Clamp and pins	Cervical spine surgery	No direct pressure on eyes, easy access to ETT	Risk of scalp laceration, pin site bleeding, EDH, no support for ETT
Preformed foam	All spine cases	Easy view of the eyes	One size does not fit all, difficult to access ETT, not reusable
Gel Support	All spine cases	Different sizes, with different profiles, reusable	Shape is easily distortable, high chances of pressure injuries
Horseshoe	Quick procedures	Easily available	Can change position when the patient is moved due to spinal instrumentation
Gel ring	Short cases	Easily available	Head is turned, risk of vessel, nerve, or bony injury

(EDH: extradural hematoma; ETT: endotracheal tube)

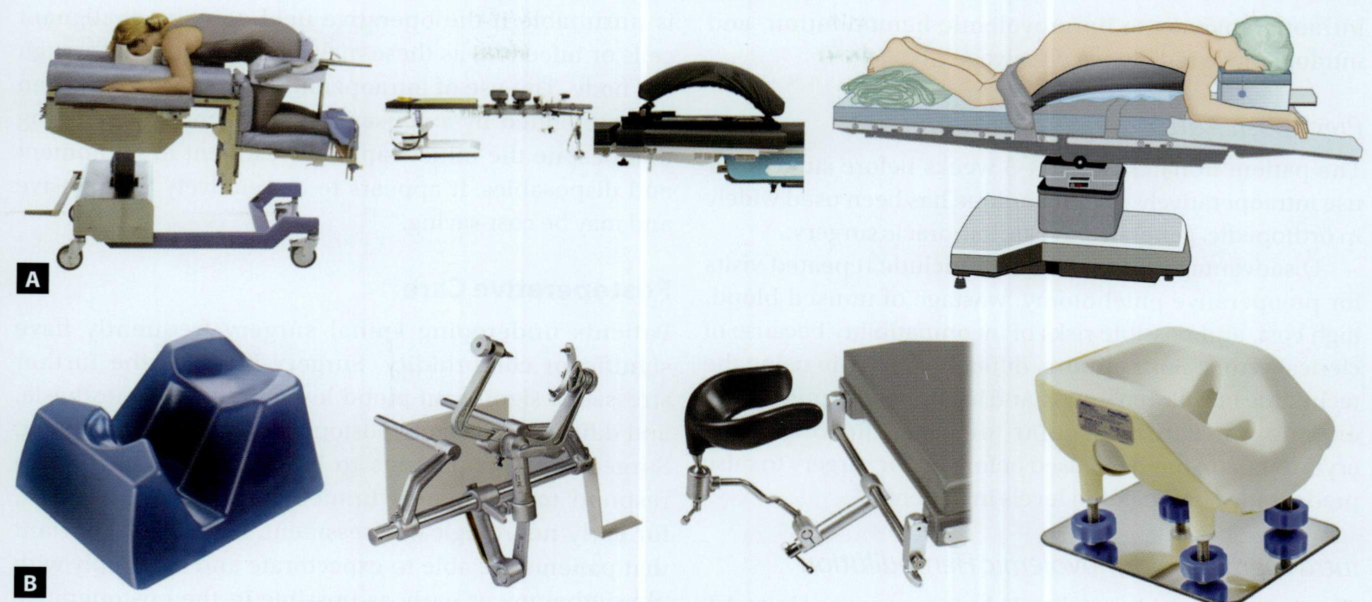

Figs. 1A and B: (A) Various types of tables and supports for prone positioning (From left to right—Andrew's frame, Jackson table, Wilson frame, and Wilson frame in use with patient positioned); (B) Various types of head support for prone positioning (From left to right—gel foam, Mayfield skull clamp, Horseshoe, Foam headrest with mirror).

Blood loss is associated with increased operative time, delayed wound healing, wound infections, and increased requirement for blood transfusion. The risks of allogeneic blood transfusion include hypothermia, impairment of coagulation, hyperkalemia, hypocalcemia, transfusion reactions, acute lung injury, immunomodulation, and viral and bacterial infection. Allogeneic blood transfusion should therefore be reduced to a minimum. This can be accomplished by techniques to reduce blood loss and by autologous blood transfusion.[34]

Reducing Blood Loss

Blood loss can be minimized by careful patient positioning, good surgical technique, controlled hypotensive anesthesia, and by the use of agents such as antifibrinolytics. When patients are placed in the prone or knee-chest positions, care must be taken to minimize intra-abdominal pressure. It has been shown that positioning devices, such as the Relton–Hall frame, which allows the abdominal viscera to hang freely, reduce inferior vena cava (IVC) pressure by one-third. Raised IVC pressure is associated with lumbar venous engorgement and increased blood loss. One study has shown minor changes to patient positioning on the Wilson frame can reduce blood loss per vertebral level by approximately 50%.[35,36]

Hypotensive Anesthesia

Hypotensive anesthesia has long been established as a safe and effective method for reducing blood loss by up to 58% during spinal surgery.

Antifibrinolytic Agents

Drugs such as synthetic lysine analogs, tranexamic acid, and aminocaproic acid, and the protease inhibitor, aprotinin have been used to reduce blood loss during spinal surgery. Only aprotinin, however, has been shown to cause a statistically significant reduction in intraoperative blood loss. Aprotinin is a polypeptide derived from bovine lung, which is an inhibitor of plasmin and kallikrein, forming a reversible complex with the serine binding site on the enzyme. It also preserves platelet function.

Desmopressin has been shown to reduce bleeding times in patients with platelet disorders. In spinal surgery, it may have a tendency to reduce blood loss.[37]

In major spinal surgery, it is good practice to ensure adequate patient positioning, use a controlled hypotensive anesthesia technique, and to use an infusion of aprotinin.

Provision of Autologous Blood

Autologous blood can be made available to the patient by three methods; predeposit autologous transfusion, intraoperative acute normovolemic hemodilution, and intraoperative red blood cell salvage.

Predeposit Autologous Transfusion

The patient donates blood 3–5 weeks before surgery for use intraoperatively. This technique has been used widely in orthopedic, general, and cardiothoracic surgery.

Disadvantages of this method include repeated visits for preoperative phlebotomy, wastage of unused blood, high cost, and possible risks of incompatibility because of clerical errors. Furthermore, difficulties arise in using the technique in children < 30 kg and in adults with preexisting anemia or cardiovascular disease. Recombinant erythropoietin has been used before major surgery to raise preoperative hemoglobin levels in patients.[38]

Intraoperative Normovolemic Hemodilution

This is performed immediately before surgery. Up to 1 L of whole blood is removed, and stored in bags with anticoagulant according to the formula:

$$\text{Volume to be removed} = \text{EBV3 (initial Hct} \pm \text{target Hct)/ mean Hct}$$

where EBV = estimated blood volume, Hct = hematocrit, mean Hct = arithmetic mean of initial Hct and the target Hct.

The removed blood is replaced by an IV infusion of colloid or crystalloid to achieve normovolemia with a reduced hematocrit. During surgery, less red cell mass is lost for a given volume of blood. The donated whole blood may be retransfused once hemostasis is achieved, or a critical value of hemoglobin is reached. The technique has been shown to reduce blood requirements in spinal surgery.[39]

Intraoperative Cell Salvage

Blood lost during surgery is collected using commercially available equipment and is then anticoagulated, filtered for clots and debris, centrifuged, and resuspended in saline before re-infusion to the patient. Many liters of blood can be salvaged. It is a good practice to use cell-salvaged blood where blood loss is anticipated to be >15 mL/kg. Disadvantages are that reinfused red cells may contain residual anticoagulant, and also that coagulation factors and platelets are consumed at the wound site. Clotting factors may therefore need to be replaced using donor-fresh frozen plasma. Only approximately half of the blood lost during surgery can be salvaged, and the technique is unsuitable if the operative field contains malignant cells or infection, as these may be disseminated through the body. The use of intraoperative cell salvage has been recommended by a consensus conference, concluding that despite the initial capital investment in equipment and disposables, it appears to be relatively inexpensive and may be cost-saving.[40-42]

Postoperative Care

Patients undergoing spinal surgery frequently have significant comorbidity. Surgery imposes the further stresses of significant blood loss, prolonged anesthesia, and difficulties in acute postoperative pain management. Surgeons prefer patients to be conscious and able to respond to commands immediately after anesthesia, for early neurological assessment. It is also important that patients are able to expectorate and to comply with physiotherapy as early as possible in the postoperative period.

Indications for Postoperative Ventilation

The decision to provide a period of postoperative artificial ventilation should have been made before surgery commences and explained to the patient. The need for postoperative ventilation is suggested by patient and surgical factors. Patient factors include the presence of a pre-existing neuromuscular disorder, severe restrictive pulmonary dysfunction with a preoperative vital capacity of <35% of predicted, a congenital cardiac abnormality, right ventricular failure, and obesity. Surgical factors include a prolonged procedure, surgical invasion of the thoracic cavity, and blood loss >30 mL/kg.[43] Frequently, it is necessary only to provide artificial ventilation for a few hours in postoperative care.

Postoperative Analgesia

Pain management can be a considerable challenge. Patients undergoing spinal surgery, particularly through a thoracic approach, may have a large incision extending over several dermatomes. Many patients have preexisting chronic pain conditions, may be cognitively impaired (some neuromuscular disorders), or be very young (children). A multimodal approach to analgesia is recommended, using a combination of simple primary analgesics, opioids, and regional anesthesia techniques where appropriate.[44] For initial postoperative analgesia, it is useful to restart, if possible, all the analgesics the patient was receiving preoperatively. Undoubtedly, the patient's requirements will be increased postoperatively and additional therapy will be required.

Parenteral Opioids

The use of parenteral opioids has been the mainstay of analgesia for all patients undergoing spinal surgery. Opioids can be administered via intramuscular (IM), IV (continuous infusion and patient-controlled analgesia devices with or without background infusions), intrapleural, epidural, and intrathecal routes. Their use, via the IV route in particular, is associated with side effects such as respiratory depression, nausea and vomiting, sedation, and gastrointestinal ileus. The latter may be, especially disadvantageous after major spinal surgery when some degree of paralytic ileus is common.

Patients with cancer may not be naive to opioid drugs and such individuals must be assumed to have acquired a degree of opioid tolerance. For patients who have received long-term opioids preoperatively by other routes (e.g., enteral and transdermal), these should also be restarted as early as possible postoperatively and gradually reduced over subsequent days or weeks.

Nonsteroidal Anti-inflammatory Drugs

Simple analgesics alone afford inadequate analgesia even for relatively minor spinal surgery. NSAIDs, both non-selective cyclo-oxygenase inhibitors, and selective cyclo-oxygenase 2 (COX-2) inhibitors, have however been used successfully after spinal surgery.

The use of NSAIDs may increase bleeding time by 30–35%, cause gastritis, and be associated with acute renal failure, particularly in the presence of hypovolemia and hypotension. The safety profile of selective COX-2 inhibitors in major spinal surgery is yet to be fully evaluated. If, however, patients have been taking NSAIDs to help relieve pain without complication preoperatively, it is useful to restart the medication in the immediate postoperative period for its opioid-sparing effects.[45]

Epidural Analgesia

The use of local anesthetic agents, alone or in combination with opioids by the epidural route after spinal surgery has been described, as the epidural catheter being placed intraoperatively by the surgeon.

Epidural anesthesia with local anesthetic agents can make neurological assessment difficult. Concerns over the rare but serious risks of epidural hematoma and infection associated with indwelling catheters have hindered its widespread use. The incidence of local superficial infection after routine epidural catheter placement has been quoted to be as high as 12%. However, the incidence of epidural abscess related to epidural catheter placement, although difficult to determine precisely, is rare.

Other Techniques

Intrapleural infusions of local anesthetic and/or opioids may be considered after a thoracotomy. Intrapleural infusions of local anesthetic agents have been reported to reduce systemic opioid requirements in such circumstances. A number of studies, however, have found intrapleural analgesia with local anesthetic agents to offer inferior analgesia to epidural opioids, and there remains concern over the blood levels of local anesthetic agents achieved, and the risk of local anesthetic toxicity.

Late Complications

A retrospective study of 1,223 anterior thoracic and lumbar spinal procedures found a respiratory complication rate of 7% (adult respiratory distress syndrome, pneumonitis, atelectasis, and infection), pulmonary embolism of 0.8%, cerebral vascular accident of 0.25%, and death of 0.33% [four patients: One died of acute respiratory distress syndrome (ARDS) on day 31, one myocardial infarction on day 1, and two died of fatal pulmonary emboli on days 3 and 8)].[46]

Screening studies for thromboembolic complications after spinal surgery have quoted varied incidences between 0.395 and 15.5%. One partially randomized study found an incidence of 0.3% when Doppler ultrasonography was used postoperatively to detect venous thrombosis in patients treated with either mechanical (compression stockings and pneumatic boots) or pharmacological (warfarin) methods of prophylaxis. If; however, no methods of thromboprophylaxis are used and venography is the screening method, incidences of venous thrombosis of 15.5% have been quoted. In one prospective study, symptomatic pulmonary emboli occurred in 2.2% of all spinal fusions, and these were more common after combined anterior/posterior approach procedures (6%) than posterior approach procedures alone (0.5%).[30]

There has been a paucity of well-conducted randomized controlled trials comparing methods of thromboprophylaxis. Few would argue against the use of compression stockings and pneumatic boots, the use of which is relatively free of complications. However, the use of pharmacological methods of thromboprophylaxis (using heparin, for example) is contentious. Their use may be associated with hemorrhagic complications such as increased intraoperative and postoperative blood loss, and epidural hematoma. Treatment of thromboembolism produces the risk of major heparin-related complications (44%) such as epidural hematoma, gastrointestinal bleeding, and wound infection. Insertion of an IVC filter may be appropriate in these circumstances.

CONCLUSION

Spinal surgery presents a number of challenges to the anesthetist. Patients are now undergoing major spinal surgery for conditions such as malignancy, scoliosis, and trauma, which would not have been contemplated 20 years ago. Despite this, postoperative neurological morbidity has been reduced by advances in spinal cord monitoring techniques. The anesthetist has an important role to play in facilitating the use of these new techniques. They must also manage the relief of postoperative pain in these patients, who have frequently been receiving several analgesics preoperatively.

REFERENCES

1. Stier GR, Vandse R, Cole DJ. Neurosurgical Diseases and Trauma of the Spine and Spinal Cord: Anesthetic Considerations. In: Cottrell JE, Patel PM, Soriano SGBT-C& PN (Eds). New Delhi: Elsevier; 2025. pp. 390-449.
2. Kumar N, Tan WLB, Wei W, Vellayappan BA. An overview of the tumors affecting the spine-inside to out. Neurooncol Pract. 2020;7(Suppl_1):i10-7.
3. Clarke MJ, Mendel E, Vrionis FD. Primary spine tumors: Diagnosis and treatment. Cancer Control. 2014;21(2):114-23.
4. Arshad MA, Russo A, Holmes K. [Online] Available from Metastatic spinal disease. https://resources.wfsahq.org/atotw/metastatic-spinal-disease/ [Last accessed March, 2025].
5. Walha S, Fairbanks SL. Spinal cord tumor surgery. Anesthesiol Clin. 2024;39(1):139-49.
6. Devereaux MW. Anatomy and examination of the spine. Neurol Clin. 2007;25(2):331-51.
7. Bogduk N. Functional anatomy of the spine. Handb Clin Neurol. 2016;136:675-88.
8. Williams A, Newell RLM, Collins P. Back and macroscopic anatomy of spinal cord. In: Standring S (Ed). Gray's Anatomy: The Anatomical Basis of Clinical Practice, 39th edition. London: Churchill Livingstone; 2005. pp. 769-70.
9. Koeller KK, Shih RY. Intradural extramedullary spinal neoplasms: radiologic-pathologic correlation. Radiographics. 2019;39(2):468-90.
10. Schellinger KA, Propp JM, Villano JL, McCarthy BJ. Descriptive epidemiology of primary spinal cord tumors. J Neurooncol. 2008;87(2):173-9.
11. Henson JW. Spinal cord gliomas. Curr Opin Neurol. 2001; 14(6):679-82.
12. Houten JK, Cooper PR. Spinal cord astrocytomas: presentation, management and outcome. J Neurooncol. 2000;47(3):219-24.
13. Benesch M, Frappaz D, Massimino M. Spinal cord ependymomas in children and adolescents. Child's Nerv Syst. 2012;28(12):2017-28.
14. Arora RS, Alston RD, Eden TOB, Estlin EJ, Moran A, Birch JM. Age–incidence patterns of primary CNS tumors in children, adolescents, and adults in England. Neuro Oncol. 2009;11(4):403-13.
15. Zadnik P, Gokaslan Z, Burger P, Bettegowda C. Spinal cord tumours: advances in genetics and their implications for treatment. Nat Rev Neurol. 2013;9(5):257-66.
16. Choi D, Crockard A, Bunger C, Harms J, Kawahara N, Mazel C, et al. Review of metastatic spine tumour classification and indications for surgery: the consensus statement of the Global Spine Tumour Study Group. Eur Spine J. 2010;19(2):215-22.
17. Shetty AP, Shetty AP, Subramanian B, Kanna RM, Rajasekaran S. A prospective randomized study to analyze the efficacy of balanced pre-emptive analgesia in spine surgery. Spine J. 2019;19(4):569-77.
18. Nazareth A, D'Oro A, Liu J, Schoell K, Heindel P, Jakoi A, et al. Risk Factors for Postoperative Venous Thromboembolic Events in Patients Undergoing Lumbar Spine Surgery. Glob Spine J. 2019;9(4):409-16.
19. Patel D, Best S, Ziino C. Venous thromboembolism prophylaxis following degenerative spine surgery: a narrative review. AME Med J. 2024;9:13.
20. Sansone JM, del Rio AM, Anderson PA. The Prevalence of and Specific Risk Factors for Venous Thromboembolic Disease Following Elective Spine Surgery. JBJS. 2010;92(2): 304-13.
21. Buchanan IA, Lin M, Donoho DA, Ding L, Giannotta SL, Attenello F, et al. Venous Thromboembolism After Degenerative Spine Surgery: A Nationwide Readmissions Database Analysis. World Neurosurg. 2019;125:e165-74.
22. Raw DA, Beattie JK, Hunter JM. Anaesthesia for spinal surgery in adults. BJA Br J Anaesth. 2003;91(6):886-904.
23. Hambly PR, Martin B. Anaesthesia for chronic spinal cord lesions. Anaesthesia. 1998;53(3):273-89.
24. Engelhardt T, Webster NR. Pulmonary aspiration of gastric contents in anaesthesia. Br J Anaesth. 1999;83(3):453-60.
25. Wang AC, Than KD, Etame AB, La Marca F, Park P. Impact of anesthesia on transcranial electric motor evoked potential

monitoring during spine surgery: a review of the literature. Neurosurg Focus. 2009;27(4):E7.
26. Sloan TB. Anesthesia effects and evoked potentials. In: Reisin RC, Nuwer MR, Hallett M, Medina CBT-S to CN (Eds). Advances in Clinical Neurophysiology. Amsterdam: Elsevier; 2002. pp. 325-8.
27. Dulfer S, Sahinovic M, Lange F, Wapstra F, Postmus D, Potgieser A, et al. The influence of depth of anesthesia and blood pressure on muscle recorded motor evoked potentials in spinal surgery. A prospective observational study protocol. J Clin Monit Comput. 2021;35(5):967-77.
28. Ma R, Qiao R, Xu M, Li R, Hu Y. Application of Controlled Hypotension During Surgery for Spinal Metastasis. Technol Cancer Res Treat. 2022;21:15330338221105718.
29. Cunha P, Barbosa T, Correia G, Silva R, Cruz Oliveira N, Varanda P, et al. The ideal patient positioning in spine surgery: a preventive strategy. EFORT Open Rev. 2023; 21(8):63-72.
30. Kwee M, Ho Y, Rozen W. The prone position during surgery and its complications: a systematic review and evidence-based guidelines. Int Surg. 2015;100(2):292-303.
31. Edgcombe H, Carter K, Yarrow S, Berkshire R, Foundation NHS, Road L, et al. Anaesthesia in the prone position. Br J Anaesth. 2008;100(2):165-83.
32. Garg B, Bansal T, Mehta N, Sharan A. Patient positioning in Spine Surgery: What Spine Surgeons should know? Asain Spine J. 2023;17(4):770-81.
33. Urban M, Beckman J, Gordon M, Urquhart B, Boachie-Adjei O. The efficacy of antifibrinolytics in the reduction of blood loss during complex adult reconstructive spine surgery. Spine (Phila Pa 1976). 2001;26(10):1152-6.
34. Zheng F, Cammisa FPJ, Sandhu HS, Girardi FP, Khan SN. Factors Predicting Hospital Stay, Operative Time, Blood Loss, and Transfusion in Patients Undergoing Revision Posterior Lumbar Spine Decompression, Fusion, and Segmental Instrumentation. Spine (Phila Pa 1976). 2002; 27(8):818-24.
35. Lee T-C, Yang L-C, Chen H-J. Effect of Patient Position and Hypotensive Anesthesia on Inferior Vena Caval Pressure. Spine (Phila Pa 1976). 1998;23(8):941-7;discussion 947-8.
36. Park CK. The Effect of Patient Positioning on Intraabdominal Pressure and Blood Loss in Spinal Surgery. Anesth Analg. 2000;91(3):552-7.
37. Yuan L, Zeng Y, Chen Z, Zhang X, Mai S, Song P, et al. Efficacy and safety of antifibrinolytic agents in spinal surgery: a network meta-analysis. Chin Med J (Engl). 2019;132(5):577-88.
38. Cha CW, Deible C, Muzzonigro T, Lopez-Plaza I, Vogt M, Kang JD. Allogeneic Transfusion Requirements After Autologous Donations in Posterior Lumbar Surgeries. Spine (Phila Pa 1976). 2002;27(1):99-104.
39. Epstein NE. Bloodless spinal surgery: a review of the normovolemic hemodilution technique. Surg Neurol. 2008;70(6):614-8.
40. Cheriyan J, Cheriyan T, Dua A, Goldstein JA, Errico TJ, Kumar V. Efficacy of intraoperative cell salvage in spine surgery: a meta-analysis. J Neurosurg Spine SPI. 2020; 33(2):261-9.
41. Kumar N, Chen Y, Zaw AS, Nayak D, Ahmed Q, Soong R, et al. Use of intraoperative cell-salvage for autologous blood transfusions in metastatic spine tumour surgery: a systematic review. Lancet Oncol. 2014;15(1):e33-41.
42. Kumar N, Tan JYH, Chen Z, Ravikumar N, Milavec H, Tan JH. Intraoperative cell-salvaged autologous blood transfusion is safe in metastatic spine tumour surgery: early outcomes of prospective clinical study. Eur Spine J. 2023;32(7):2493-502.
43. Jaipanya P, Lertudomphonwanit T, Chanplakorn P, Pichyangkul P, Kraiwattanapong C, Keorochana G, et al. Predictive factors for respiratory failure and in-hospital mortality after surgery for spinal metastasis. Eur Spine J. 2023;32(5):1729-40.
44. Berardino K, Carroll AH, Kaneb A, Civilette MD, Sherman WF, Kaye AD. An Update on Postoperative Opioid Use and Alternative Pain Control Following Spine Surgery. 2021;13(1):1-12.
45. Bongiovanni T, Lancaster E, Ledesma Y, Whitaker E, Steinman M, Allen I, et al. Systematic Review and Meta-Analysis of the Association Between Non-Steroidal Anti-Inflammatory Drugs and Operative Bleeding in the Perioperative Period. J Am Coll Surg. 2021;232(5):765-90.e1.
46. Faciszewski T, Winter R, Lonstein J, Denis F, Johnson L. The surgical and medical perioperative complications of anterior spinal fusion surgery in the thoracic and lumbar spine in adults. A review of 1223 procedures. Spine (Phila Pa 1976). 1995;20(14):1592-9.

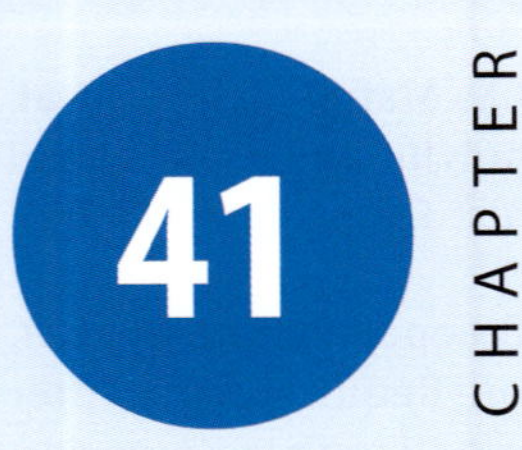

Neurophysiological Monitoring for Brain and Spine Tumor Surgeries

Anjana Sagar Wajekar

INTRODUCTION

Neurosurgical patients are always at risk for hypoxic, ischemic, or traumatic injury to neural tissues. The use of intraoperative neurophysiological monitors enables early detection of these insults and thereby helps improve patient outcomes by facilitating early correction before injury becomes permanent.[1-3] Monitoring involves near-continuous assessment of the functional integrity of neural pathways. Despite conflicting evidence in the improvement of neurological outcomes, the use of intraoperative neurophysiological monitoring (IONM) is recommended for neurosurgeries, especially in eloquent areas.[3]

NEUROPHYSIOLOGICAL MONITORS

There are numerous neurophysiological monitors targeting the function, perfusion, oxygenation, and metabolism of the brain **(Table 1)**. Not all of them can be utilized intraoperatively.

ROLE OF INTRAOPERATIVE NEUROPHYSIOLOGICAL MONITORING IN BRAIN AND SPINE TUMOR SURGERIES

Traditionally, intraoperative wake-up tests in spine surgeries or awake craniotomy have been routinely practiced in patients posted for neurosurgical procedures

TABLE 1: Neurophysiological monitors.

Function	Electroencephalogram (EEG)	• Raw EEG • Computerized processed • Compressed spectral assay • Density spectral assay • Aperiodic analysis • Bispectral analysis (BIS)	
	Evoked potentials (EPs)	*Sensory:* • Somatosensory EP • Brainstem auditory EP • Visual EP	*Motor:* • Transcranial magnetic MEP • Transcranial electric MEP • Direct spinal cord stimulation
	Electromyography (EMG)	Cranial nerves (V, VII, IX, X, XI, and XII)	
Cerebral perfusion and intracranial pressure		*Cerebral blood flow:* • Nitrous oxide wash-in • Radioactive xenon clearance • Laser Doppler blood flow • Transcranial Doppler USG • Microvascular Doppler USG • Indocyanine green video-angiography	*Intracranial pressure:* • Intraventricular catheter • Fiberoptic intraparenchymal catheter • Subarachnoid bolt • Epidural catheter
Metabolism		*Intracerebral:* Intracerebral PO_2 electrode	*Noninvasive:* • Transcranial cerebral oximetry (NIRS) • Jugular venous oximetry

(MEP: motor evoked potential; NIRS: near-infrared spectroscopy; USG: ultrasonography)

at risk of neurological injury. Over the past few years, this has largely been replaced by neurophysiological monitors.[3] The most commonly employed monitors are the monitors of functional integrity, which include the electroencephalogram (EEG), sensory and motor evoked potentials (MEPs), and electromyography.[1,2] Brain and spine tumor surgeries generally employ multimodal monitoring as they have been shown to give superior results.[4,5]

- *Electroencephalogram:* Raw EEG is the summation of the excitatory postsynaptic action potential generated by the pyramidal cells of the cerebral cortex. The EEG contains components of different frequencies and harmonics. These are volume conducted and can be recorded from the scalp and forehead utilizing surface or needle electrodes. The electrode arrangement uses bipolar active recording with arbitrary designation of the recording and the reference electrode.

Although the 16-channel EEG recording (8 channels in each hemisphere) is the gold standard, it is rarely performed intraoperatively due to the complexity and inaccessibility of recording sites during neurosurgeries. Most intraoperative EEG machines utilize a two- to four-channel recording with computer processing to simplify the output. These raw EEGs are displayed in various ways as enumerated in **Table 2**. Alternately, direct electrocorticography (ECoG) can also be obtained from the cerebral surface with the help of strip electrodes placed intraoperatively. This is utilized for monitoring seizure activity. Deep brain stimulators (DBSs) performed for movement disorders capture the electrical activity via microelectrodes placed in the thalamic and subthalamic nuclei.

Electroencephalogram reflects the state of arousal and metabolic activity of the brain. Cerebral electrical activity generation requires adequacy of perfusion combined with an adequate supply of substrates such as glucose and oxygen. Depression of EEG is caused by significant reductions in cerebral blood flow (CBF), glucose, and oxygen levels.

- *Bispectral analysis (BIS):* It is a derived EEG parameter that is used to monitor the depth of anesthesia and not a neurological insult. The placement of an external BIS electrode, although feasible for spine tumor surgeries, may be restricted by inaccessibility during neurosurgery. A processed BIS value can directly be obtained from the processing of raw EEG recorded as part of neurophysiological monitoring during brain surgeries. A value between 40 and 60 is considered adequate depth to prevent intraoperative awareness. A value of >80 indicates imminent emergence from anesthesia. Intraoperative use of evoked potential (EP) monitoring necessitates the use of total intravenous anesthesia (TIVA) with or without target-controlled infusion (TCI). Monitoring depth of anesthesia with BIS is strongly recommended during TIVA without muscle relaxant and mandatory when TIVA with muscle relaxants is administered.[6] Also, BIS monitoring facilitates depth monitoring during awake craniotomies, especially asleep—awake anesthesia.
- *Electromyography:* Irritation of peripheral nerves or spinal nerve roots can lead to spontaneous motor movement even under general anesthesia. This is sometimes used in cervical and lumbar spine surgery. It necessitates complete or partial withholding of the use of intraoperative muscle relaxants.

TABLE 2: Electroencephalogram (EEG) waveforms.

Waveforms	*Speed (Hz)*	*Mental state*	*EEG recording*
Beta	12–30	Focused	
Alpha	8–12	Relaxed	
Theta	4–8	Drowsy	
Delta	1–4	Deep sleep	

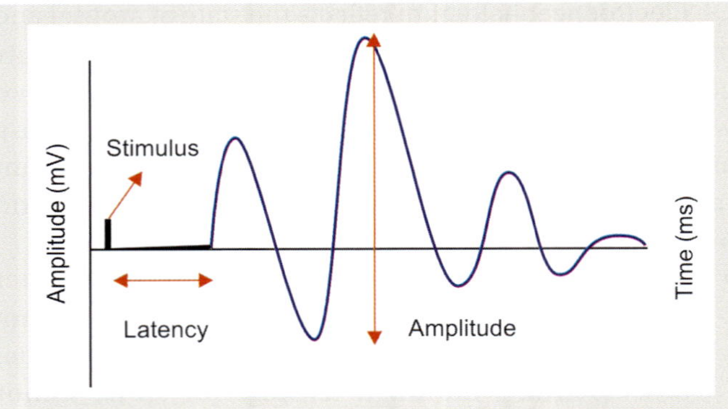

Fig. 1: Latency and amplitude of wave after evoked potential stimulus.

- *Evoked potential monitoring:* These include event-related, anatomical pathway-specific monitoring where the EEG or EMG waves are observed after an evoked stimulus (mostly electrical). Cortical EP are monitored for brain surgeries, whereas EP for spine surgeries can be recorded from both cortical and epidural/subdural space.[5] The EP recorded from epidural space are more robust than the cortical EPs **(Fig. 1)**.
- *Sensory EP:* These assess the functionality of any sensory nerve, either cranial or peripheral, and are hence utilized in both brain and spine surgeries. Any sensory nerve can be stimulated and the waves observed for typical peaks and troughs, as described by the polarity and latency. The amplitude of these EP is small as compared to raw EEG and needs computer averaging of repetitive stimuli for interpretation. The common modalities used in clinical practice include somatosensory EP (SSEP), brainstem auditory EP (BAEP), and visual EP (VEP).
  - *Somatosensory EP:* Most commonly used sensory EP. It records the response to stimulating the median nerve, ulnar nerve, or posterior tibial nerve. It monitors the integrity of the respective pathway from the peripheral receptors to the cerebral cortex. They are used for sensory function monitoring in both brain and spine tumor surgeries. A 50% decline in amplitude or a 10% increase in latency after a specific surgical step warrants a change in surgical strategy to prevent potential postoperative neurodeficit.[1]
  - *Brainstem Auditory EP:* Stimulation of the auditory (VIII) nerve typically with repetitive clicks administered to the ear via headphones or ear-induced transducers leads to a series of seven short latency period peaks (named with Roman numerals). BAEP is used in acoustic neuroma surgery. Rarely, it may be used for general assessment of the brain stem during posterior fossa surgery. An increase in latency of >1 ms, especially in wave V, is clinically significant. A 50% reduction in amplitude and loss of wave V is strongly predictive of postoperative hearing loss. BAEP, unlike cortical SSEP, can be recorded with high-dose inhalational anesthetics.
  - *Visual EP:* It measures the electrical activity in the visual cortex in response to the visual stimulus delivered through a specialized goggle. It tests the functionality of the visual pathway, from the eyes, optic nerves, optic chiasma, and optic tract up to the visual cortex. It is rarely used intraoperatively. It can only be performed under TIVA. VEPs are used in craniopharyngioma and pituitary adenoma surgeries.[15]
- *Motor EP:* Since SSEP can assess only the integrity of sensory pathways, MEP complements them by assessing the integrity of motor pathways. MEP is an electromyographic wave recorded over the muscles of the hand or leg in response to the motor cortical stimulus. The stimulus is delivered in the form of a depolarization using transcranial magnetic or electric stimulus. The large voltage of MEP negates the need of averaging. Only electric stimulus is recordable under anesthesia. D-wave monitoring is a highly reproducible and another accurate monitor but cannot be done below the 10th–11th thoracic level due to an insufficient number of corticospinal tracts below this level. A 50% decrease in amplitude up to a complete loss of signal indicates a high probability of severe neurodeficit, for example, paraplegia. It can be used in both brain and spine surgeries.
- *Monitoring of cranial nerve function:* Posterior fossa surgeries, especially around the lower brainstem, have the potential to injure cranial nerves V, VII, IX, X, XI, and XII **(Table 3)**. Both spontaneous and EP-based electromyographic monitoring can be done in posterior fossa surgeries.
- *Others:* The role of other neurophysiological monitors depends on the type and extent of tumor, major vascular invasion, etc. Intraoperative transcranial ultrasonography and Doppler (over the zygomatic arch) provide a noninvasive continuous measurement

TABLE 3: Cranial nerves for monitoring with their innervated muscles.

Cranial nerve	*Innervated muscle*
V	Masseter, temporalis
VII	Orbicularis oculi, orbicularis oris, mentalis, and frontalis
IX	Stylopharyngeus
X	Pharyngeal and laryngeal muscles
XI	Sternocleidomastoid, Trapezius
XII	Tongue

of middle cerebral artery (MCA) velocity. It can provide a qualitative assessment of cerebral perfusion pressure and detection of particulate emboli. Jugular bulb venous oximetry or noninvasive near-infrared spectroscopy (NIRS) may be used as monitors of global brain oxygenation in major surgeries. These monitors are not specific to spine and brain tumor surgeries.

The common contraindications to the use of monitors of functional integrity are the presence of cardiac arrhythmias, implantable cardiac devices or pacemakers, intracerebral aneurysm clips or other metal implants, epilepsy, and loose teeth.[3]

INTRAOPERATIVE MANAGEMENT

Special attention should be paid to the positioning of the patient during IONM, especially the prone position. Properly secured endotracheal intubation is paramount. Bite block should be placed between the molar teeth during MEP monitoring in any position, under anesthesia. The electrical stimulus used for MEP can cause forceful masseter contraction leading to endotracheal tube damage and intraoral injury.[1,2] Lower cranial nerve monitoring necessitates the placement of electrodes in the uvula and tongue after intubation. Care should be taken to prevent displacement in the event of any further intraoral procedures and these should be removed and checked prior to extubation.[1] Proper padding and measures to prevent pressure sores due to the electrode wires should be taken.

The anesthesia technique plays a crucial role during neurosurgeries under IONM.[1,2] The effect of the choice and dose of anesthesia agents on the different modalities of IONM, interference with their result interpretation needs to be thoroughly understood. Almost all anesthetics may cause a decrease in amplitude and an increase in latency. Inhalational anesthetic agents affect the different IONM modalities more than intravenous agents. It is reported that cortical SSEP can be recorded even during deep barbiturate coma when the EEG is isoelectric.[1] In contrast, inhalational anesthetics cause a significant dose-dependent reduction in amplitude and increase in latency. Both MEP and SSEP become unrecordable with high doses of inhalational anesthetics [minimum alveolar concentration (MAC) >0.5–1]. The use of inhalational agents (MAC <1) is safe only in cases of peripheral electromyographic monitoring such as those used for spine nerve root monitoring. Inhalational agents are inadvisable for use in brain tumor surgeries under IONM. Nitrous oxide is a profound depressant of the amplitude of SSEP, especially in combination with inhalational agents. The use of TIVA is preferred for intraoperative monitoring of SSEP. Propofol is the drug of choice for TIVA as it has a clinically insignificant effect on IONM signals. It is essential to titrate the dose and avoid sudden large bolus doses of propofol to minimize disruption in IONM signals. The steady plasma and effect site concentrations can easily be achieved with propofol infusions, especially with TCIs. Various pharmacokinetic–pharmacodynamic models are available, of which the Eleveld general-purpose model is the most recently developed model. The Eleveld model (effect site concentration 3–6 μg/mL) has been validated in a wide range of populations from adult to pediatric. Short-acting benzodiazepines such as midazolam do not impede EPs and can be used. Opioids have negligible effects on SSEP. Opioids by virtue of synergistic action with propofol, thereby reducing the dose of propofol and hemodynamic stability, are the cornerstone of TIVA management. Remifentanil infusion (Minto or Eleveld TCI model) or fentanyl (bolus or manual infusion) is frequently used. Ketamine and etomidate have an amplitude augmentation effect on SSEP. Dexmedetomidine can be added as required to the propofol–remifentanil/fentanyl regimen as interference with IONM signals is not significant. MEP also requires the use of TIVA with dose adjustment so as to prevent burst suppression activity. Although best MEPs are recorded only in the complete absence of muscle relaxation, some authors advocate the use of partial relaxation to minimize patient movement to stimulus. Neuromuscular blocking agents routinely only have a role for smooth endotracheal tube insertion and may be administered after completion of IONM. In some

TABLE 4: Effects of various anesthetic agents on SSEP and MEP.

Anesthetic agent	*SSEP*	*MEP*
Inhalational agents	Suppressed if MAC >1	Suppressed
Propofol	Unchanged	Unchanged
Barbiturates	Unchanged	Suppressed
Benzodiazepine (short acting and premedication dose)	Unchanged	Unchanged
Ketamine	Enhanced	Enhanced
Etomidate	Enhanced (only cortical)	Enhanced
Opioids	Unchanged	Unchanged
Dexmedetomidine	Unchanged	Unchanged
Muscle relaxants	Unchanged	Suppressed

(MAC: minimum alveolar concentration; MEP: motor evoked potential; SSEP: somatosensory evoked potential)

scenarios, partial neuromuscular relaxation can help SSEP and D-wave monitoring by eliminating spontaneous electromyographic activity **(Table 4)**.

Scalp block can help not only to reduce the pin insertion and incision response but also helps to reduce the overall dose of propofol. Addition of an additive such as clonidine or dexmedetomidine (1mcg/kg) to local anesthetic in scalp block will help prolong the duration of block.

Hypothermia (<35°C), severe hypocapnia (arterial CO_2 <20 mm Hg), anemia (hematocrit <25%), and fall in mean arterial pressure (below autoregulatory limits mean arterial pressure <60 mm Hg) can lead to false-positive IONM findings.[1,2] Every alert on the IONM finding should lead to confirmation of the maintenance of intraoperative physiological homeostasis in the form of euvolemia, normotension, normothermia, normocapnia, normoxia, anemia prevention, and depth of anesthesia to limit the effects of hypoxic or ischaemic insult on the quality of IONM signals. Postoperatively, rapid recovery and extubation facilitate immediate neurological evaluation and early detection of postoperative neurological sequelae.

The anesthesia technique remains the same for awake craniotomy with or without IONM since IONM is used only during the awake phase. In the event that the asleep-awake technique with a muscle relaxant is utilized, then adequate reversal of the neuromuscular blocking agent should be confirmed with a quantitative train of four monitors.

UTILITY OF INTRAOPERATIVE NEUROPHYSIOLOGICAL MONITORING IN SPINE AND BRAIN TUMOR SURGERIES

Recent advances in both anesthesia techniques and monitoring devices have greatly improved the accuracy and reliability of IONM. It has become the standard of care in several centers due to both potential favorable outcomes and as a safety net for clinical and medicolegal concerns. An understanding of the inherent limitations of IONM as well as the increased cost and duration of surgery also needs to be kept in mind. A gamut of studies have investigated the use of IONM during spine and brain tumor surgeries. Several studies and reviews have reported favorable outcomes and benefits to the use of IONM during spine cord tumor surgeries.[7-11] A study in the use of IONM in spinal cord hemangioblastomas has reported that pathological IONM changes are associated with poorer neurological outcomes both new onset and long term.[7] Another study has demonstrated the loss of IONM signals in cervical spine patients even during head positioning which were restored with changes made to the position of the head.[8] Some studies have reported cases where there has not been a demonstrable improvement in outcomes with the use of IONM, and the rate of complications and length of hospital stay are shown to be equivalent to surgery without IONM. In the absence of any adverse effects of the use of IONM, authors preferred the use of IONM for "peace of mind," medicolegal considerations, and easy data retrieval.[12,13] Unlike spine surgeries, IONM is considered a gold standard for intracranial surgery, especially in eloquent areas. IONM is used in both adult and pediatric brain tumor surgery.[14,15] The use in pediatric patients is challenging due to the impact of variability in patient age and size on the IONM signals.[14] Literature has shown that multimodal IONM is superior to unimodal IONM to maximize tumor resection in eloquent areas.[4,5,15]

CONCLUSION

The use of IONM necessitates a multidisciplinary team of neurosurgeons, anesthesiologists, and neurophysiologists. Communication is the foundation for optimal functioning regarding the need for any type of IONM, administration of suitable anesthesia techniques to minimize their effect on IONM, and prompt intervention in the event of changes in IONM signals. The use of proper protocols and checklists for intraoperative loss of IONM signals is paramount.

REFERENCES

1. Wing-hay HY, Chun-kwong EC. (2019). Introduction to intraoperative neurophysiological monitoring for anaesthetists. In: StatPearls. [online] Available from https://resources.wfsahq.org/atotw/introduction-to-intraoperative-neurophysiological-monitoring-for-anaesthetists/ [Last accessed March, 2025].
2. Ghatol D, Widrich J. (2024). Intraoperative neurophysiological monitoring. In: StatPearls. Treasure Island (FL): StatPearls Publishing. [online] Available from: https://www.ncbi.nlm.nih.gov/books/NBK563203/ [Last accessed March, 2025].
3. Gruenbaum BF, Gruenbaum SE. Neurophysiological monitoring during neurosurgery: anesthetic considerations based on outcome evidence. Curr Opin Anaesthesiol. 2019; 32(5):580-4.
4. Rabai F, Mohamed B, Seubert CN. Optimizing intraoperative neuromonitoring: anesthetic considerations. Current Anesthesio Rep. 2018;8:306-17.
5. Verla T, Fridley JS, Khan AB, Mayer RR, Omeis I. Neuromonitoring for intramedullary spinal cord tumor surgery. World Neurosurg. 2016;95:108-16.
6. Nimmo AF, Absalom AR, Bagshaw O, Biswas A, Cook TM, Costello A, et al. Guidelines for the safe practice of total intravenous anaesthesia (TIVA): joint guidelines from the Association of Anaesthetists and the Society for Intravenous Anaesthesia. Anaesthesia. 2019;74(2):211-24.
7. Siller S, Szelenyi A, Herlitz L, Tonn JC, Zausinger S. Spinal cord hemangioblastomas: significance of intraoperative neurophysiological monitoring for resection and long-term outcome. J Neurosurg Spine. 2017;26:483-93.
8. Appel S, Korn A, Biron T, Goldstein K, Rand N, Millgram M, et al. Efficacy of head repositioning in restoration of electrophysiological signals during cervical spine procedures. J Clin Neurophysiol. 2017;34:174-8.
9. Appel S, Biron T, Goldstein K, Ashkenazi E. Effect of intra- and extraoperative factors on the efficacy of intraoperative neuromonitoring during cervical spine surgery. World Neurosurg 2019;123:e646-51.
10. Park JH, Lee SH, Kim ES, Eoh W. Analysis of multimodal intraoperative monitoring during intramedullary spinal ependymoma surgery. World Neurosurg. 2018;120:e169-80.
11. Ghadirpour R, Nasi D, Iaccarino C, Romano A, Motti L, Sabadini R, et al. Intraoperative neurophysiological monitoring for intradural extramedullary spinal tumors: predictive value and relevance of D-wave amplitude on surgical outcome during a 10-year experience. J Neurosurg Spine. 2018;30:259-67.
12. Kahraman S, Gocmen S, Alpsan Gokmen MH, Acka G, Pusat S. Intraoperative neurophysiologic monitoring for lumbar intradural schwannomas: does it affect clinical outcome? World Neurosurg. 2019;124:e789-92.
13. Pusat S, Kural C, Solmaz I, Temiz C, Kacar Y, Tehli O, et al. Comparison of electrophysiological outcomes of tethered cord syndrome and spinal intradural tumors: a retrospective clinical study. Turk Neurosurg. 2017;27:797-803.
14. Kim K, Cho C, Bang MS, Shin HI, Phi JH, Kim SK. Intraoperative neurophysiological monitoring: a review of techniques used for brain tumor surgery in children. J Korean Neurosurg Soc. 2018;61:363-75.
15. Brandmeier S, Taskiran E, Bolukbasi FH, Sari R, Elmaci I. Multimodal intraoperative neurophysiological monitoring in neurosurgical oncology. Turk Neurosurg. 2018;28:204-10.

SECTION

Pediatric Onco-Anesthesia

42 CHAPTER

Anesthesia for Wilms Tumor

Sravya Adda, Vibhavari Naik

INTRODUCTION

Wilms tumor (WT), also referred to as nephroblastoma, is the second most prevalent intra-abdominal cancer and the fifth most common pediatric malignancy.[1,2] It affects approximately 1 in 10,000 children. With long-term survival rates exceeding 90% for localized disease and 75% for metastatic cases, WTs represent a significant success story in pediatric oncology. This has been attributed to early detection and optimal multidisciplinary care.[3] The tumor was first reported by German anatomist and surgeon Max Wilms in a series of 7 cases in 1899.[3] The "Rule of 10" as depicted in **Box 1** has traditionally been used to describe associations with WT, though variations in incidences have been observed in the literature.

The management of WT includes a multidisciplinary approach involving medical oncology, radiation oncology, pathologists, and surgeons. Anesthesiologists also play a crucial role in managing these cases, participating in diagnostic radiological procedures, the placement of long-term vascular access for chemotherapy, and providing anesthesia for surgery and sedation for radiotherapy if required. In this chapter, we aim to provide an overview of WT management and the associated anesthetic considerations.

EPIDEMIOLOGY

Wilms tumor is the most common renal tumor in children accounting for 90% of cases.[2] According to the World Health Organization, the age-standardized incidence rate of WT among children aged 0–14 years in India is 4.4 age-standardized rate per million.[4] The majority of children are diagnosed between the ages of 1 and 5 years, with the peak incidence at age 3.[5] Epidemiologically, WT is classified into sporadic, genetic, and familial with familial accounting for up to 1–2%.[6] Familial tumors are mainly due to mutation at one of two loci—FWT-1 on chromosome 17q and FWT-2 on 19. While the majority occur sporadically, 10–15% are associated with genetic malformation syndromes[7] and require active surveillance as these children belong to the high-risk group. The associated genetic syndromes are listed in **Table 1**.

BOX 1: Rule of 10 in Wilms tumor.

- 10% are bilateral
- 10% have vascular invasion
- 10% have calcifications on computed tomography
- 10% have unfavorable histology
- 10% have pulmonary metastases at presentation

TABLE 1: Genetic syndromes associated with Wilms tumor.

Syndrome	*Characteristic features of the syndrome*	*Incidence of Wilms tumor*
Overgrowth syndromes		
Beckwith–Wiedemann syndrome	Macroglossia, hemi hyperplasia, omphalocele, neonatal hypoglycemia, macrosomia, and embryonal tumors (e.g., Wilms tumor, hepatoblastoma, neuroblastoma, and rhabdomyosarcoma)	10–20%
Isolated hemihypertrophy	Unilateral bone and soft tissue hypertrophy without any syndromic association	3–5%
Frasier syndrome	Ambiguous genitalia, streak gonads, and focal segmental glomerulosclerosis	Low
Perlman syndrome	Macrocephaly, macrosomia, up-sweeping anterior scalp line, deep-set eyes, depressed nasal bridge, everted upper lip, and hypotonia	75%

Contd...

Contd...

Syndrome	**Characteristic features of the syndrome**	**Incidence of Wilms tumor**
Nonovergrowth syndromes		
Denys–Drash syndrome	Triad: Pseudo-hermaphroditism, glomerulopathy, and Gonadoblastoma	95%
WAGR syndrome	Wilms' tumor, aniridia, genitourinary malformations, and mental retardation	50%
Trisomy 18 (Edwards syndrome)	Congenital heart defect, underdeveloped lungs, joint and bone abnormalities, hearing loss, cleft lip, and eye defects	Low
Golabi–Behmel syndrome	Macrocephaly, macroglossia, widened nasal bridge, thick lips, hypoplastic or absent index fingernails, enlarged liver, spleen, kidneys, abdominal wall defects, diaphragmatic or inguinal hernia, extra nipples, and intellectual disability	5–10%

PATHOLOGY

Wilms tumor is a type of renal carcinoma that arises from embryonal cells, which resemble primitive epithelial cells. It is characterized by a triphasic pattern that includes blastemal, stromal, and epithelial cells. Kidney development in fetal age is contributed by two main components: The ureteric bud, which forms collecting ducts, and the metanephric mesenchyme or blastema, which aids in forming other kidney structures. Typically, the blastema disappears by 36 weeks of gestation, but, in approximately 1% of cases, remnants of metanephric blastema persist, known as nephrogenic rests. These rests are precursors of WT and are found in approximately 40% of cases[3,8] as described in **Figure 1**.

CLINICAL PRESENTATION

Children with WT often present with a painless abdominal lump. When present, abdominal pain is the most prevalent symptom, occurring in roughly 40% of cases, while 25–30% of patients present with hematuria.[6] Other symptoms include fever, anorexia, nausea, and vomiting. In children with a predisposing clinical syndrome, renal tumors may be detected during routine screening. There have been reports in the literature of acute pain accompanied

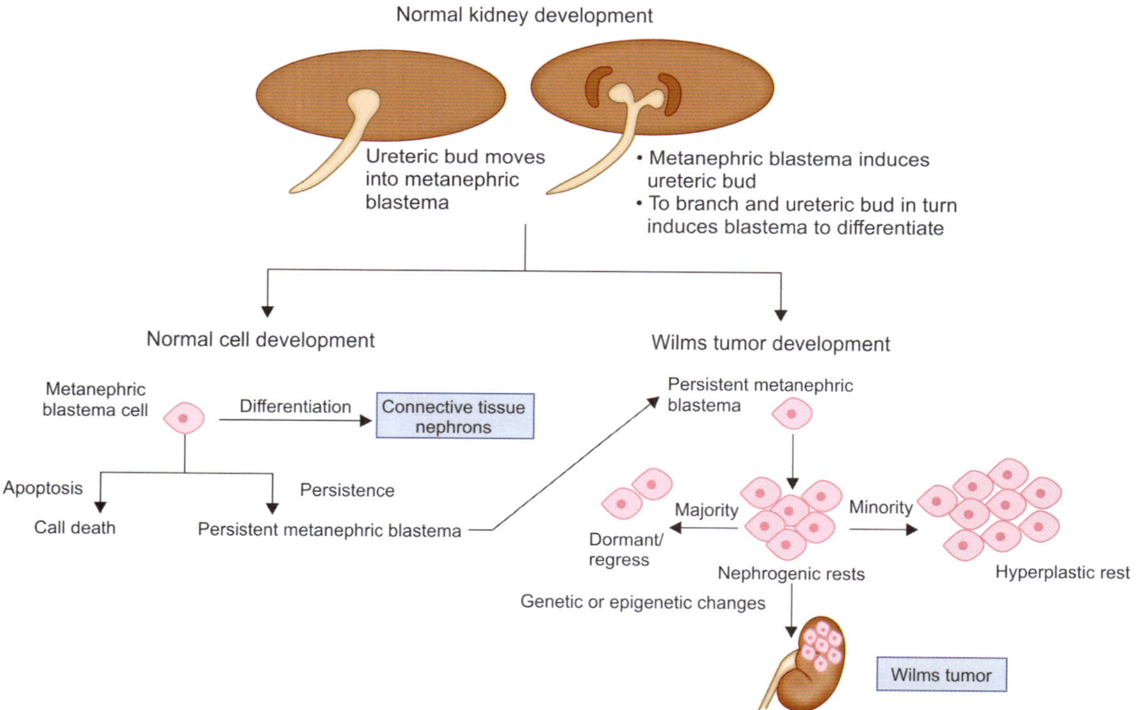

Fig. 1: Embryogenesis of Wilms tumor.

by fainting episodes due to tumor capsule rupture and intraabdominal bleeding.[3,9] This condition manifests as a rapidly enlarging mass, anemia, pain, and fever. Atypical manifestations seen in <10% of cases include ascites, congestive cardiac failure, and hepatomegaly in patients with inferior vena cava (IVC) thrombus extending beyond hepatic veins.[6,10] Additionally, the tumor can produce hormonal substances that lead to paraneoplastic syndromes[3] such as hypertension due to renin secretion, polycythemia, and acquired von Willebrand disease each of which has implications as discussed later. It is crucial to rule out association with congenital syndromes based on the clinical features mentioned in **Table 1**.

DIAGNOSIS

Advancements in radiological techniques have significantly improved the early detection of nonpalpable WTs and their metastasis, playing a crucial role in diagnosis and staging. Ultrasonography (USG) is the initial diagnostic tool typically revealing the tumor as an echogenic mass with distinct hypoechoic necrotic areas and calyceal distortion with renal displacement, classically known as the "claw sign".[5] This imaging method is advantageous for distinguishing between renal and extrarenal masses, assessing caval patency, and identifying tumor thrombus.[11] While USG is an effective starting point, all patients with renal masses should undergo cross-sectional imaging with computed tomography (CT) or magnetic resonance imaging (MRI) which often provide crucial additional information. Research indicates that contrast-enhanced computed tomography (CECT) and MRI are more sensitive than USG for diagnosing tumor thrombus.[5] CT scans are essential for tumor staging, assessing the presence of thrombus, lymph node status,[12] and evaluating lung metastasis, which occurs in 10% of cases. MRI is vital for illustrating the tumor's relationship to surrounding organs and is more sensitive than CT in detecting nephrogenic rests, which appear as homogeneous lesions after gadolinium enhancement.[12] **Figures 2A and B** depict CT scan images of large WT in both sagittal and transverse cross-sections. Echocardiography is recommended for patients who have received neoadjuvant chemotherapy (NACT) to assess cardiac function as well as in the presence of a tumor thrombus extending into the atrium. Additional investigations may be considered to screen for tumor-associated anemia, thrombocytopenia, kidney dysfunction, abnormal liver enzymes in cases with liver metastasis, and coagulation disorders like WT-acquired von Willebrand disease. Urine analysis for catecholamine is advised in situations where imaging is not able to differentiate neuroblastoma from WT or in cases presenting with hypertension.[7]

STAGING

Staging in WT is done prechemotherapy using the International Society of Paediatric Oncology (SIOP) and postchemotherapy using the Children's Oncology Group (COG) staging. **Table 2** presents a summary of the same.

TREATMENT PROTOCOL

Surgery is the mainstay of treatment for early-stage disease and can be combined with chemotherapy and

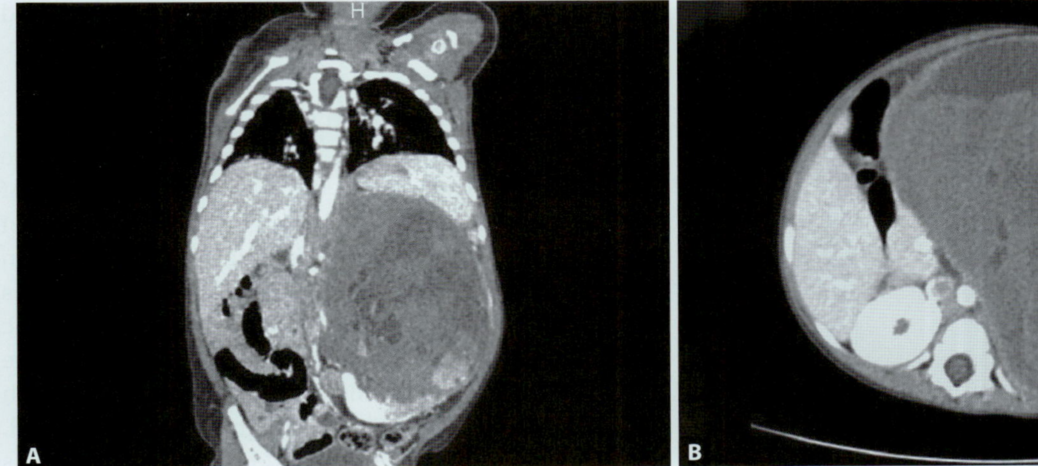

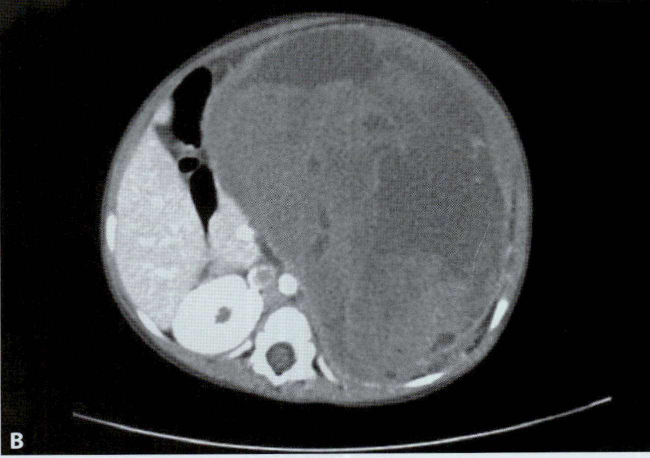

Figs. 2A and B: CT scan showing a large heterogenous hypodense solid mass in the left renal fossa.

TABLE 2: Wilms tumor staging.

Stage 1	Tumor limited to the kidney with capsule intact and resectable
Stage 2	The tumor extends beyond the kidney involving the renal capsule or renal vein but is resectable
Stage 3	Residual tumor, involvement of abdominal nodes, peritoneal spillage, tumor biopsy before preoperative chemotherapy, or surgery
Stage 4	Hematogenous metastasis
Stage 5	Bilateral renal tumors

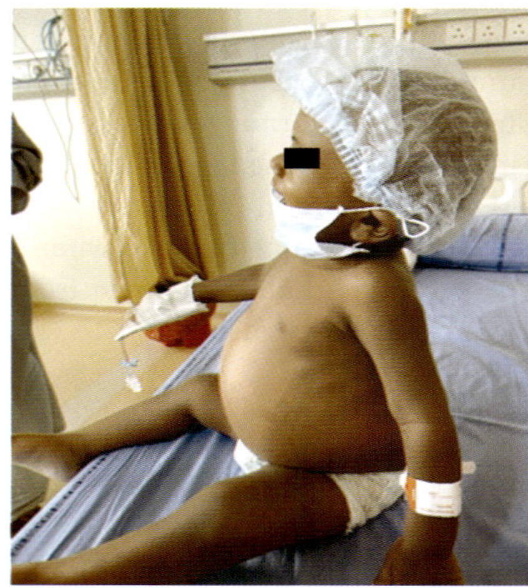

Fig. 3: Child presenting with a large abdominal mass.

radiotherapy in advanced disease. Though WTs respond well to both chemotherapy and radiotherapy, the optimal timing for chemotherapy is still under debate. The North American National WT Study/Children's Oncology Group protocol (NWTS/COG) recommends initial nephrectomy followed by chemoradiotherapy, whereas the European SIOP protocol advocates for NACT followed by surgery[12] and clinical outcomes are comparable between the two groups. In resource-limited settings like India, where patients present with larger tumors as depicted in **Figure 3**, NACT followed by surgery is a preferred choice to reduce the tumor burden for surgery.

Chemotherapy

Chemotherapy is often the first treatment modality. For unilateral WT, the duration of NACT typically ranges from 4 to 6 weeks, depending on the presence of metastasis. In cases of bilateral WT, NACT usually lasts about 6–12 weeks.[12] Certain scenarios[12,13] where NACT has shown to have better outcomes include:

- Extension of tumor thrombus above the level of the hepatic veins
- Direct tumor invasion requiring organ removal
- Excessive tumor burden resulting in patients being poor candidates for surgery
- Concern for surgical morbidity, intraoperative tumor spill, and/or residual disease following resection

The chemotherapeutic drugs commonly used in various protocols include vincristine, actinomycin D, and doxorubicin, while in some cases, cyclophosphamide, carboplatin, and etoposide are also being used. **Table 3** outlines the anesthetic-relevant side effects associated with each of these chemotherapeutic drugs.

TABLE 3: Side effects of chemotherapeutic drugs.

Chemotherapeutic drug	*Adverse effects of anesthetic relevance*
Vincristine	Peripheral neuropathy (reversible), myelosuppression, SIADH, convulsions, and toxicity enhanced by liver impairment
Actinomycin D	Myelosuppression, deranged LFTs, and veno-occlusive disease
Doxorubicin	Reduced cardiac contractility, may cause cardiac failure, and thrombocytopenia
Cyclophosphamide	Hemorrhagic cystitis, SIADH, pulmonary fibrosis, and cardiomyopathy
Etoposide	Myelosuppression
Carboplatin	Nephrotoxicity, peripheral neuropathy, and thrombocytopenia

(LFT: liver function test; SIADH: syndrome of inappropriate antidiuretic hormone secretion)

Surgery

Surgery is the cornerstone of WT treatment, with the primary objective being the complete removal of the tumor without rupture along with assessment of disease extent. The timing of surgery differs between nonmetastatic and metastatic WTs. Typically, surgery is performed post-NACT in the fifth week for nonmetastatic cases and in the seventh week for metastatic cases.[12] The preferred procedure is radical nephrectomy with lymph node sampling, performed through a transabdominal, or thoracoabdominal incision. En-bloc resection is preferred to prevent tumor spill, which is more likely in the right-sided and large tumors.[6] There is an emerging trend in performing nephron-sparing surgery (NSS) whenever feasible, to prevent renal dysfunction later in life. NSS is particularly indicated in patients with a solitary kidney, syndromic patients at higher risk of bilateral disease, those with bilateral disease, and those with tumors < 300 mL.[14,15] Intraoperative ultrasound may help in the identification of precise margins when NSS is done. NSS requires cross-clamping of renal vessels to reduce bleeding during renal parenchymal incision which is later sutured after tumor resection.[14] A warm ischemia time of around 20–30 minutes can be safely used.[14] If anticipating longer clamp time, local ice slush application may be considered. Lymph node sampling of seven areas is recommended, including the paracaval suprahilar node, paracaval infrahilar node, para-aortic suprahilar node, paraaortic infrahilar node, mesenteric lymph node, and both iliac nodes.[12]

Radiotherapy

Wilms tumor is highly radiosensitive, which makes radiotherapy highly effective to enhance local control and treat metastatic sites. Typically, radiation therapy begins 9–14 days after surgery if there are no medical contraindications.[12,13] Children with Stage III disease are offered flank or whole-body radiation based on the extent of resection, nodal involvement, presence of positive margins, and tumor histology.[12] Furthermore, in cases of tumor spillage, rupture, or lung metastases, whole-body irradiation is advised. Generally, a total dose of 10.8 Gy over 6 fractions at 1.8 Gy per fraction is offered to the patients.[12]

ROLE OF ANESTHESIOLOGIST

Children with WT might require anesthesia at various points throughout their long-duration treatment. It is crucial to personalize their evaluation to the specific procedure they are scheduled for and their current clinical condition. Procedures requiring anesthesia expertise include:

- Imaging studies (CT and MRI)
- Ultrasound-guided renal tumor biopsy
- Long-term venous access device placement
- Radiotherapy
- Surgical tumor resection

Anesthesia Considerations

Children with WT requiring short procedures such as imaging, biopsy, venous access device placement, and radiotherapy are typically managed with intravenous sedation. Since these procedures are often performed outside of operating rooms, it is important to consider the specific requirements and constraints of these locations. During MRI and radiotherapy, absolute immobility is essential to ensure good-quality images and optimal delivery of radiation to target tissues with minimal damage to surrounding healthy tissues, respectively. The need for anesthesia is highly age-dependent: All patients under 3 years of age require anesthesia, while it is rarely needed for patients over 7 years of age.[16] An anesthesiologist may use a single drug or a combination of drugs, including propofol, ketamine, dexmedetomidine, and fentanyl. Propofol infusion alone or with dexmedetomidine maintains spontaneous breathing and allows faster recovery.[17] Painful procedures like biopsy and venous device placement, along with local anesthetic infiltration may require the addition of fentanyl or ketamine to propofol or inhalational anesthesia. Children undergoing surgical tumor resection may present with several perioperative challenges. These include managing issues related to thermoregulation, fluid balance, ventilation due to increased intra-abdominal pressure (IAP), intermittent IVC compression, and the potential for major hemorrhage.[18] Furthermore, concerns related to NACT **(Table 3)**, paraneoplastic phenomena, large tumors, and intravascular extension of tumor thrombus when present add to the challenges. These are discussed below.

Preoperative Assessment and Optimization

The preoperative assessment should include a detailed history, physical examination, and treatment review. The anesthesiologist should be fully informed about the tumor's extent and any adherence to surrounding structures as it implicates higher blood loss. Along with the routine, history should include any family history of WT, prior diagnosis of syndromes, any symptoms related to paraneoplastic syndromes or advanced disease, details of NACT if received, and the complications if any.[18,19]

The patient's history should guide the physical examination. In cases of syndrome-associated WT, it is crucial to look for syndrome-associated features outlined in **Table 1**. These patients may present with macroglossia, hypotonia, micrognathia, congenital heart diseases, and other conditions that may necessitate the requirement of special care including a difficult airway cart. For patients with advanced disease, signs of respiratory involvement should be sought for. Blood pressure measurement should always be done in these children as increased renin secretion may be present in 25% of these patients, presenting as hypertension.[6] Selecting the appropriate cuff size is crucial for the accurate measurement of blood pressure in children. The cuff length should be 80–100% of the arm's circumference, and the width should be 40% of the arm's circumference. Hypertension in these patients results from increased renin secretion, making them responsive to angiotensin-converting enzyme (ACE) inhibitors, which can be initiated preoperatively. Usually, 2.5 mg of Enalapril is started once daily which can be adjusted as per response. Another important aspect to consider during the examination is nutritional assessment. Up to 30% of cancer children experience malnutrition due to reduced oral intake, the effects of cancer itself, the toxicity of therapies, and increased physiological requirements.[20] Nutritional assessment should include weight, height, body mass index (BMI), and midupper arm circumference (MUAC), all plotted on WHO growth charts.[21] A structured approach like the ABCD method—anthropometric, biochemical, clinical, and dietary assessment can be considered. As required, hematinics and protein diet should be started as a part of prehabilitation.

Preoperative investigations help to identify comorbidities, risk stratify, and guide perioperative management. Complete blood count may reveal anemia secondary to occult hematuria, neutropenia, and thrombocytopenia following NACT. Baseline renal function tests may be considered in large and bilateral tumors. Coagulation profile and viral screening can be ordered as per hospital policy. Chest X-ray (CXR) and CT chest help identify pulmonary metastasis in advanced disease. Patients who have received NACT may need to be further evaluated for adverse effects of chemotherapy drugs as depicted in **Table 3**. Serum electrolytes to rule out syndrome of inappropriate antidiuretic hormone (SIADH) secretion, liver function tests if suspecting liver toxicity, and two-dimensional (2D) echocardiography for chemo-induced cardiotoxicity.

Oncosurgical procedures are time-sensitive. Time to surgery (TTS) refers to the interval between the start of preoperative treatment, such as chemotherapy, to the surgical removal of WT. Literature indicates that in patients with unilateral WT, with or without metastasis, who require approximately 4–5 weeks of NACT, a TTS of up to 60 days does not affect outcomes. Similarly, in patients with bilateral tumors without metastasis, who require 6–12 weeks of NACT, TTS should not be delayed beyond 120 days as it can result in poorer outcomes.[12] Therefore, preoperative optimization should be completed within these time frames.[22]

Anesthetic Management

The preoperative evaluation and findings help guide the choice of anesthesia. For a child scheduled for surgical resection, it is essential to adhere to the basic principles of pediatric anesthesia.[19] General anesthesia with endotracheal intubation is preferred **(Fig. 4)**. The analgesic options are discussed separately. Premedication may be given according to institutional protocol. It should be avoided in children with large tumors with abdominal distension, which can lead to respiratory compromise, and in syndromic children with an anticipated difficult airway.

Induction can be intravenous or inhalational with sevoflurane, depending on the availability of vascular access. Rapid sequence induction may be necessary for patients with a large tumor and the presence of diaphragmatic splinting. Lateral position or IVC tilt using a folded sheet may be employed if a large mass compresses the IVC. For airway management, general anesthesia with cuffed endotracheal tube (ETT) is recommended. Pressure-controlled ventilation can be used to offset high IAPs due to large mass and then peak pressure can be lowered after the abdomen is opened.

For vascular access, it is recommended to have either one central venous access and one wide-bore peripheral

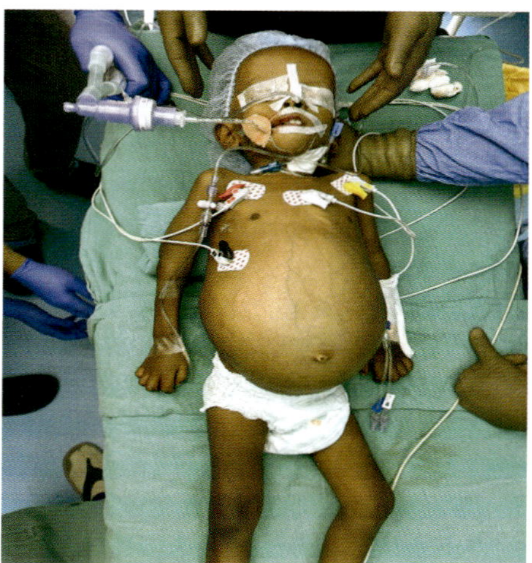

Fig. 4: Child with large Wilms tumor anesthetized with monitoring lines in situ.

line or two peripheral lines of which one is wide bore—one for administering maintenance fluids and the other for rapid infusion of blood and blood products if required. The central line or long-term venous access device is useful for repeated blood sampling postoperatively, as in large tumors and after massive fluid shifts. Intravenous access above the diaphragm should be considered in cases involving IVC incision. During surgery, careful excision of the tumor without spillage is crucial. However, this can lead to intraoperative IVC compression and reduced venous return during manipulation, which may impact hemodynamics during surgery, necessitating hemodynamic monitoring in large tumors.[18]

Thermoregulation is crucial to prevent hypothermia in pediatric patients due to large incisions and third-space fluid loss. Utilizing table warmers and warm fluids and covering the limbs and head with insulating material can be helpful. Standard practices also include careful positioning, padding of pressure areas, and eye protection. Smaller tumors are resected using minimally invasive techniques, which provide benefits such as faster recovery, reduced postoperative pain, early ambulation, and a lower incidence of postoperative ileus. It is commonly advised to utilize slower insufflation rates <1 L/min and to maintain IAP at 6–8 cm H_2O for infants and up to 12 cm H_2O for younger children having laparoscopic procedures. IAPs >12 cm H_2O should be avoided because they can compress the IVC, reducing preload and causing hemodynamic instability. Additionally, ventilatory settings should be adjusted to maintain end-tidal CO_2 ($ETCO_2$) levels between 30 and 35 mm Hg to avoid hypercarbia.[23]

The impact of anesthetic selection on tumor recurrence has been scarcely studied in WT. In a study by Muller et al., no significant association was observed between either regional anesthesia or the choice of anesthetic and tumor recurrence. However, the use of regional anesthesia was found to be beneficial as it reduced both hospital stay and the postoperative neutrophil–lymphocyte ratio.[24]

Perioperative Analgesic Considerations

Perioperative pain management is a critical aspect of surgical care, and multimodal analgesia including regional anesthesia is essential for reducing perioperative opioid use. Epidural analgesia is preferred for pain management during and after open nephrectomy, though its role in enhanced recovery after surgery (ERAS) protocols with minimally invasive techniques is debated. A well-placed epidural at the lower thoracic level between T9 and T12 provides optimal coverage for the surgical area.[18] In patients with large tumors and intravascular thrombus extension, we should be careful during epidural placement owing to the risk of encountering veins in expanded retroperitoneal venous collaterals, which communicate with the epidural venous plexus. **Figure 5** gives us an overview of dermatomes that need to be blocked for different surgical incisions. For the laparoscopic approach, port-site local infiltration can be considered. Other regional analgesic techniques include the use of paravertebral blocks with 0.5 mL/kg of 0.2% bupivacaine or ropivacaine, often combined with additives. When covering more than two to three dermatomes, it is necessary to administer the block at multiple levels. An infusion of 0.3 mL/kg/h (up to a maximum of 0.5 mg/kg/h) is recommended in children. Additionally, studies have explored the use of erector spinae blocks[25] and quadratus lumborum blocks[26] for pain management. **Figures 6A and B** show the probe position and sonoanatomy of the erector spinae plane block. These techniques have the added benefit of

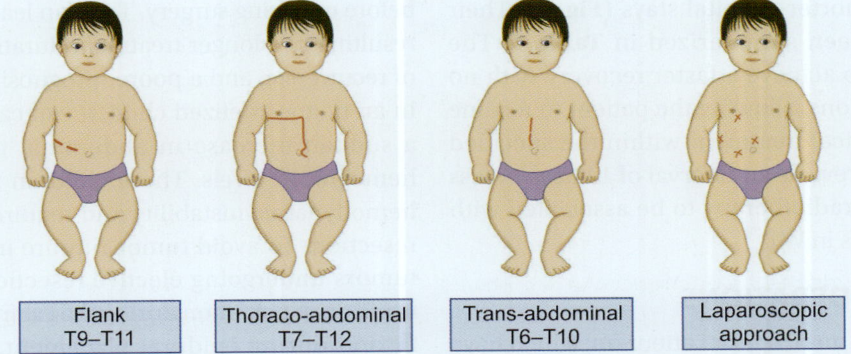

Fig. 5: Common surgical incisions for Wilms tumor resection depicting dermatomal levels.

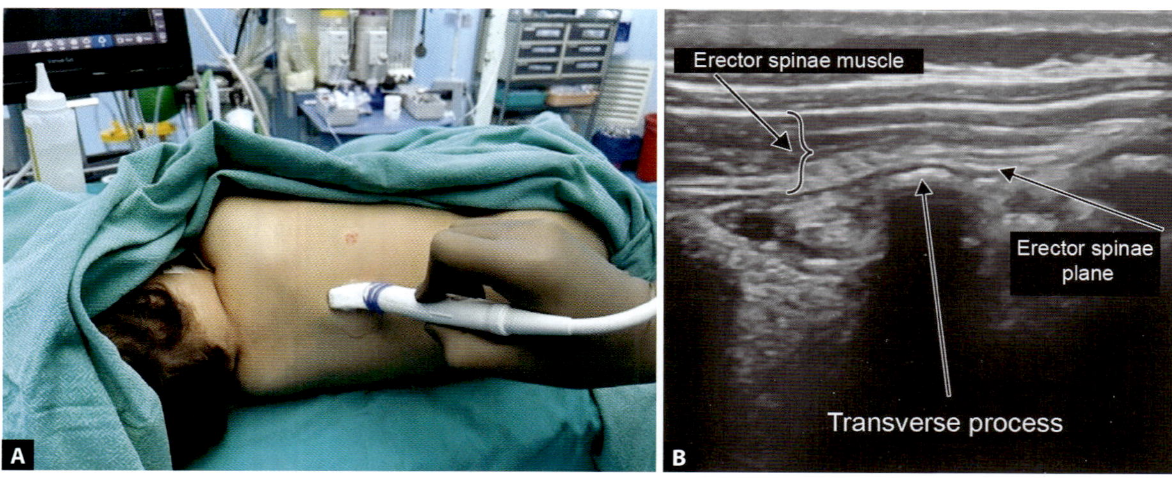

Figs. 6A and B: Erector spinae plane block for analgesia. (A) The ultrasound probe position; (B) Labeled sonoanatomy.

avoiding perioperative hypotension as compared to the epidural technique. Other intravenous analgesics include paracetamol at a dose of 15 mg/kg three times a day and opioids such as fentanyl or morphine administered as intermittent boluses. Although nonsteroidal anti-inflammatory drugs (NSAIDs) were traditionally avoided, ERAS literature now supports their use for analgesia after nephrectomies.[27]

Enhanced Recovery After Surgery Protocol

Enhanced recovery after surgery is a multidisciplinary approach aimed at improving patient care, expediting surgical recovery, and reducing postoperative complications. While the ERAS protocols for adults are well established and effective at reducing postoperative complications, the application of ERAS in pediatric patients is still evolving. Nevertheless, several studies have shown promising results in pediatric patients. In a study by Moon et al.,[27] implementing the ERAS protocol in 66 children with WT undergoing nephrectomy resulted in faster recovery and shorter hospital stays **(Fig. 7)**. Their ERAS protocol has been summarized in **Table 4**. The objective should be to achieve a faster recovery with no or minimal complications, allowing the patient to resume the intended oncological treatment within the specified time frame. Research reveals an interval of 14 days or less between surgery and radiotherapy to be associated with improved survival rates in WT.[28]

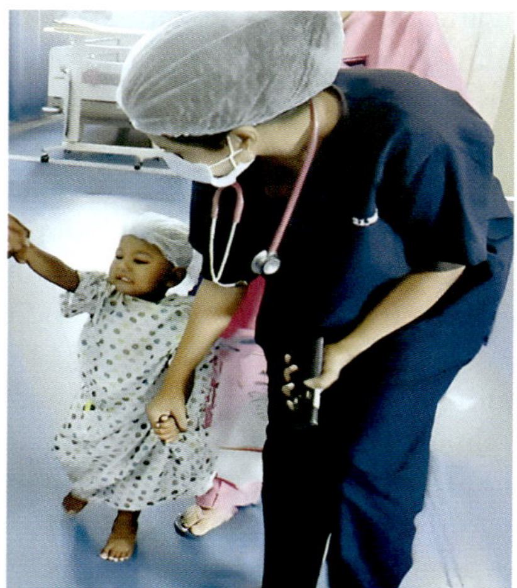

Fig. 7: Early mobilization according to ERAS protocol. (ERAS: enhanced recovery after surgery)

SPECIAL CONSIDERATIONS

Several circumstances merit special attention, which have been detailed in the subsequent subsections.

Tumor Rupture

Tumor rupture is a serious complication that can occur before or during surgery. This can lead to tumor upstaging, resulting in a longer treatment duration, an increased risk of recurrence, and a poorer prognosis. If a tumor ruptures in an unanesthetized child, it can cause abdominal pain, a sudden increase in abdominal girth, and a drop in hemoglobin levels. These children may also experience hemodynamic instability and require emergency surgical resection. To avoid tumor rupture in children with large tumors undergoing elective resection, it is important to avoid deep palpation during the examination, and extreme flexion during epidural placement, and to be cautious during positioning, as even minor trauma can lead

TABLE 4: CHOP (Children's Hospital of Philadelphia) ERAS protocol.[27]

Preoperative	*Intraoperative*	*Postoperative*
• Preadmission counseling • Family education regarding discharge criteria • Clear liquids for 2 hours preoperatively • Nutritional optimization	• Avoid thoracoabdominal incision • Avoid routine use of nasogastric tubes • Avoid epidurals • Minimize usage of arterial lines unless indicated	• No routine ICU stays • Clear liquids on POD 0 • Early starting of regular diet • Early mobilization • Avoid narcotic drug usage • Routine use of IV ketorolac • Early removal of Foley catheter

(ERAS: enhanced recovery after surgery; ICU: intensive care unit; IV: intravenous; POD: postoperative day)

to tumor rupture in large tumors. During surgical resection, the utmost care is taken to ensure en-bloc removal of the tumor and to prevent spillage. The ratio of tumor area to the abdominal area in preoperative CT scans of >0.5 has been observed to be associated with intraoperative tumor rupture.[29] Additionally, it was observed that right-sided tumors and those larger than 12 cm are at a higher risk of rupture.[29,30]

Preprocedural Embolization

Preprocedural embolization is not routinely performed in WT. In literature, it has been used as an adjunct to chemotherapy to reduce tumor size and vascularity before surgery in large tumors at risk of intraoperative spill or those not responsive to NACT.[31] It is also indicated in patients with gross hematuria and those with significant tumor bleed.[31] Anesthetic considerations for these patients are similar to nonoperating room anesthesia (NORA) procedures, where location-specific factors must be taken into account. The duration of these vascular procedures can vary widely, lasting up to 8 hours. Meticulous attention to positioning is crucial as access to the patient may be impossible during the procedure.[32] These patients are at an increased risk for radiation exposure, which can elevate the likelihood of future cancer. Efforts to minimize radiation exposure should be implemented, such as reducing the number of studies, opting for ultrasound and MRI scans when feasible, adhering to pediatric-specific dose-limiting protocols, and shielding patients with lead.

Bilateral Tumors

Bilateral WT, also known as synchronous bilateral nephroblastoma (stage V), occurs when tumors are present in both kidneys simultaneously and is observed in about 5–10% of cases.[33] It is commonly observed in syndromic children, such as those with Beckwith–Wiedemann, Denys–Drash, and WAGR. Research revealed that patients with bilateral WT have a significantly higher risk of developing end-stage renal disease (ESRD) within 20 years after treatment, with a cumulative incidence of 12% compared to <1% in patients with unilateral WT.[7] Surgical management often involves newer techniques like NSS after administering NACT 12 weeks' duration to shrink tumor size.

Intravascular Extension of Tumor

According to the National Wilms Tumor Study, intravascular extension is observed in 4.5–6% of patients,[34] with the majority of cases limited to the IVC; however, in 1% of cases, the extension can reach the atrium. This condition is more commonly seen on the right side due to the smaller renal vein compared to the left. Preoperative evaluation with echocardiography is crucial in assessing valvular function and chamber involvement as well as evaluating the cardiac function of the patient. Various classifications based on the extent of tumor thrombus have been proposed, with the first one introduced by Daum et al.[35] In 2013, Abdullah et al.[36] suggested a modification of Daum's classification, creating a more comprehensive tool that categorizes the upper extent of the tumor thrombus **(*see* Fig. 8)**.

Anesthetic considerations for patients with intravascular thrombus vary depending on the thrombus level. First, the free end of the thrombus is visualized using ultrasound **(Figs. 9A and B)**. For a level 1 thrombus, the IVC is mobilized and clamped both above and below the renal vein which can cause hemodynamic instability.[18] This instability is even more pronounced with a level 2 thrombus, where the IVC clamp is placed further away. After clamping cavotomy is performed and thrombus is retrieved **(Fig. 9C)**. Patients with a level 3 thrombus, where the thrombus extends to the hepatic veins, may exhibit additional symptoms such as hepatic vein congestion and ascites. It is crucial to evaluate their liver function tests preoperatively. During surgery, retraction of the liver is required for more proximal clamping of the IVC, which can lead to significant hypotension due to both the IVC

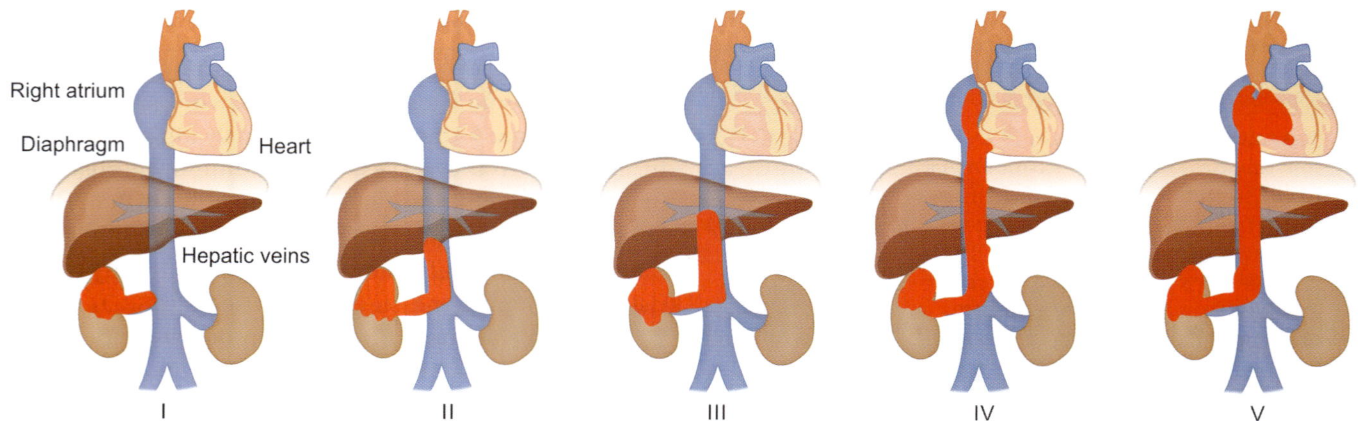

Fig. 8: Abdullah's classification of intracaval extension of Wilms tumor.[36] (I—thrombus <5 cm below hepatic veins; II—thrombus >5 cm below hepatic veins; III—thrombus extending to hepatic veins; IV—thrombus extending up to right atrium; V—thrombus extending up to right ventricle.)

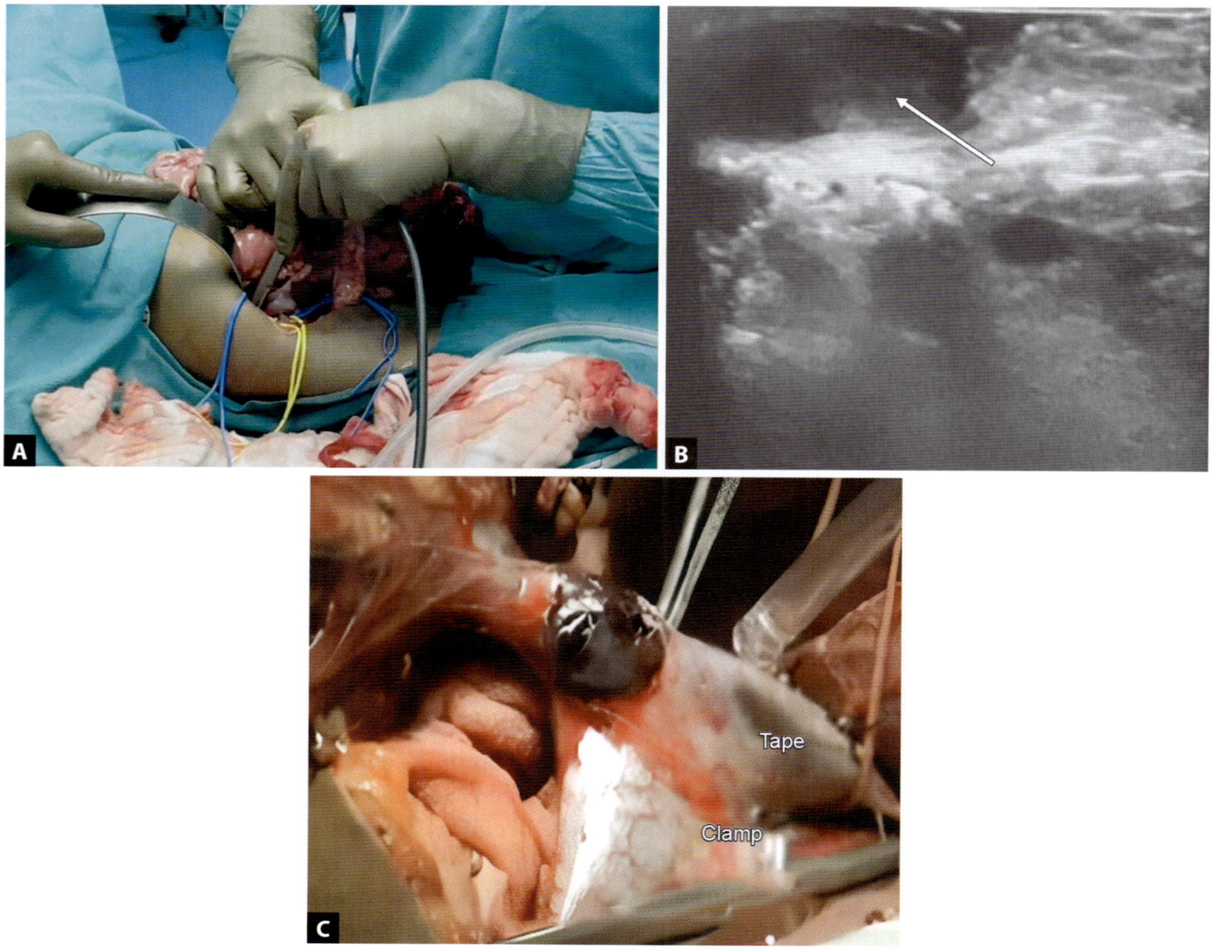

Figs. 9A to C: Intravascular extension of Wilms tumor. (A) The use of ultrasound probe for intravascular tumor localization; (B) The yellow arrow shows the ultrasound image of the tumor thrombus in the IVC; (C) Intraoperative tumor retrieval.

clamping and major blood loss. For patients with level 4 and 5 thrombus, tricuspid valve dysfunction and pleural effusion are common, reducing their respiratory reserves. Surgical management for these patients often necessitates cardiopulmonary bypass with deep hypothermic arrest to mobilize the tumor from the atrium and ventricles.[34]

Perioperative Tumor Lysis Syndrome

Tumor lysis syndrome is a life-threatening oncological emergency typically observed in rapidly proliferating tumor cells. Though tumor lysis may occur spontaneously, some of the described triggers are chemotherapy, radiation, large tumor, and tumor manipulation during surgery. Although it is more frequently associated with hematological malignancies, its occurrence in solid tumors has also been reported including during the excision of WT.[37] High index of suspicion and knowledge of the diagnosis and management of this syndrome can prevent life-threatening consequences.

Paraneoplastic Phenomena

Various paraneoplastic phenomena are observed secondary to WT which include hypertension, polycythemia, acquired von Willebrand disease, and Cushing syndrome.

- *Hypertension:* Hypertension is observed in 25% of cases due to increased plasma renin secretion produced by the renal cortex trapped within the tumor.[38] In some cases, the precursor prorenin is secreted, not resulting in hypertension. Hypertension associated with WT can be labile and severe. Due to the vasoconstrictor action of angiotensin II, these patients may experience intravascular volume contraction and left ventricular hypertrophy, along with potential electrolyte disturbances. Because of this mechanism, patients are often started on preoperative ACE inhibitors such as captopril and enalapril. Renin levels return to baseline after surgical resection, although blood pressure may take up to a month to normalize, reflecting the gradual resolution of arteriolar medial and left ventricular hypertrophy. Antihypertensive treatment can usually be discontinued within 1–3 weeks after resection.
- *Polycythemia:* Although reported in very few cases, it is primarily associated with male gender, favorable histology, and older age. It may or may not be linked to elevated erythropoietin levels.[39] Assessment of hematocrit is crucial, and when above 50, it increases blood viscosity and reduces oxygen delivery, potentially leading to tissue hypoxia. Anesthetic considerations for these patients also include the perioperative risk of thrombosis and bleeding diathesis.[40] Successful anesthetic management hinges on phlebotomy, adequate hydration, and the recognition and management of thrombotic and bleeding issues.
- *Acquired von Willebrand syndrome* (AvWS)*:* Observed in about 5–10% of cases,[38] Von Willebrand factor is a plasma protein essential for platelet adhesion and is a component of coagulation factor VIII. AvWS associated with Wilms tumor is characterized by bleeding due to platelet dysfunction and coagulation disturbances, including an elevated partial thromboplastin time (PTT). Initial therapy should include DDAVP; if this is not successful, cryoprecipitate (concentrated Von Willebrand factor) can be used.[38] Preoperatively, it is necessary to check platelet count and APTT. Neuraxial techniques and deep peripheral nerve blocks are contraindicated in patients with altered coagulation function due to the risk of epidural hematoma formation. Other analgesic options, such as wound infiltration with local anesthesia or a catheter for continuous wound infiltration, should be considered.[41]
- *Cushing's syndrome:* Ectopic ACTH-secreting tumors have been observed in children, with a few reported cases of Wilms' tumor associated with Cushing's syndrome showing elevated ACTH levels. These levels typically normalize after tumor resection. Patients with Cushing's syndrome, as part of a paraneoplastic syndrome, exhibit symptoms like those of Cushing's disease, such as moon facies and truncal obesity, and males may develop gynecomastia. Perioperatively, these patients may require glucocorticoid supplementation until the hypothalamic–pituitary–adrenal (HPA) axis recovers.[42]

Postoperative Considerations

Complications can be categorized into postsurgical and long-term complications. Postsurgical complications include bleeding, acute renal failure, bowel obstruction (4–5.1%), sepsis, and peritonitis.[43,44] Long-term complications, which are late iatrogenic sequelae of therapy, are observed in two thirds of patients who received treatment for Wilms tumor. These include the following[5]:

- *Renal dysfunction:* It is more commonly observed in syndromic patients, those with bilateral Wilms tumor, and those who underwent abdominal irradiation. The risk of renal failure in unilateral Wilms tumor is very low, at 0.25%.[5] These patients require long-term monitoring of renal function.

- *Lung damage:* It can occur due to chemotherapy or total lung irradiation for metastasis.
- *Congestive heart failure (CHF):* May be caused by anthracyclines. Dose-related cardiomyopathy from doxorubicin is reported in approximately 5% of patients receiving a cumulative dose of 400–500 mg/m^2. Frequent scans and timely cessation of the drug can help avoid this complication. Other complications: These include liver damage, an increased risk of secondary neoplasms (1.5–5.6%) in the irradiated field, and musculoskeletal defects secondary to inadvertent exposure to radiation.

Palliative Concerns in Wilms Tumor

Palliative care is a holistic approach aimed at improving the quality of life for both the child and the family, focusing on symptom management and emotional support. In patients with WT, key concerns include pain, fatigue, breathing difficulties, nausea, and vomiting. As palliative physicians, our goal should be to provide adequate pain relief using age-appropriate doses of opioid analgesics and to ensure adequate hydration and nutrition. It is also important to have sensitive conversations with parents about their goals and preferences for their child's care, including palliative and end-of-life care when necessary.

Anesthetic Implications in Wilms Tumor Survivors

With long-term survival rates exceeding 90% in patients with WT, these patients may undergo additional procedures in the future either in form of follow-up or may be posted for an entirely different surgical procedure. After completion of therapy, all patients are reviewed every 3 months during the first year, and then every 6 months for the following 2 years. Each follow-up in the first 3 years includes a radiological evaluation, such as an ultrasound or CECT scan, along with a CXR.[5] Anesthesia may be required for these patients for NORA procedures. During their assessment, we should take into account the long-term implications of treatment as mentioned above, that is, renal dysfunction, lung damage due to irradiation, and chemotherapy-induced cardiomyopathy.

CONCLUSION

Wilms tumor is a pediatric malignancy with a favorable prognosis due to advances in early detection, multidisciplinary treatment, and optimized anesthetic management. Anesthesiologists play a crucial role throughout the patient's journey—from diagnosis to surgery and postoperative recovery—ensuring safety and minimizing perioperative complications. Associated syndromes, large tumors, and IVC thrombus present unique challenges that require careful management. Surgical advancements, including laparoscopic procedures and the ERAS protocols, have facilitated faster recovery, permitting timely continuation of oncological treatments and improving overall outcomes.

REFERENCES

1. Davidoff AM. Wilms tumor. Adv Pediatr. 2012;59(1):247-67.
2. Nakata K, Colombet M, Stiller CA, Pritchard-Jones K, Steliarova-Foucher E; IICC-3 contributors. Incidence of childhood renal tumours: an international population-based study. Int J Cancer. 2020;147(12):3313-27.
3. Szychot E, Apps J, Pritchard-Jones K. Wilms' tumor: biology, diagnosis and treatment. Transl Pediatr. 2014;3(1):12.
4. Srinivasan S, Ramanathan S, Prasad M. Wilms tumor in India: a systematic review. South Asian J Cancer. 2023;12(02):206-12.
5. Bhutani N, Kajal P, Sharma U. Many faces of Wilms tumor: recent advances and future directions. Ann Med Sur. 2021;64:102202.
6. Board PP. Wilms tumor and other childhood kidney tumors treatment (PDQ®): health professional version. PDQ Cancer Information Summaries [Internet]. 2002.
7. Theilen TM, Braun Y, Bochennek K, Rolle U, Fiegel HC, Friedmacher F. Multidisciplinary treatment strategies for Wilms tumor: recent advances, technical innovations and future directions. Front Pediatr. 2022;10:852185.
8. Breslow NE, Beckwith JB, Perlman EJ, Reeve AE. Age distributions, birth weights, nephrogenic rests, and heterogeneity in the pathogenesis of Wilms tumor. Pediatr Blood Cancer. 2006;47(3):260-7.
9. Huang JL, Liao Y, An Y, Qiu MX. Spontaneous rupture of adult Wilms' tumor: a case report and review of the literature. Can Urol Assoc J. 2015;9(7-8):E531-4.
10. Nicodemus. Diagnosis and Management of Wilms Tumor. OAIJMR. 2022;2(2):172-8. Available from https://hmpublisher.com/index.php/OAIJMR/article/view/178 [Last accessed March, 2025].
11. Dumba M, Jawad N, McHugh K. Neuroblastoma and nephroblastoma: a radiological review. Cancer Imaging. 2015;15(1):5.
12. Prasad M, Vora T, Agarwala S, Laskar S, Arora B, Bansal D, et al. Management of Wilms tumor: ICMR consensus document. Indian J Pediatr. 2017;84(6):437-45.
13. Pater L, Melchior P, Rübe C, Cooper BT, McAleer MF, Kalapurakal JA, et al. Wilms tumor. Pediatr Blood Cancer. 2021;68 Suppl 2:e28257.

14. Milford K, DeCotiis K, Lorenzo A. Wilms tumor: a review of current surgical controversies. Transl Androl Urol. 2020;9(5):2382-92.
15. Murphy AJ, Davidoff AM. Nephron-sparing surgery for Wilms tumor. Front Pediatr. 2023;11:1122390.
16. Li LW, Chua GW, Wenjun K, Bong CL. Anaesthesia for radiotherapy in paediatric oncology-a retrospective observational study in an Asian population. Chin Clin Oncol. 2021;10(3):24.
17. Guimaraes Ferreira Fonseca L, Garbin M, Bertolizio G. Anesthesia for pediatric magnetic resonance imaging: a review of practices and current pathways. Curr Opin Anaesthesiol. 2023;36(4):428-34.
18. Whyte SD, Mark Ansermino J. Anesthetic considerations in the management of Wilms' tumor. Paediatr Anaesth. 2006;16(5):504-13.
19. Zeigler LN, Modes KB, Deshpande JK. Anesthesia for pediatric urological procedures. In: Andropoulos DB, Gregory GA (Eds). Gregory's Pediatric Anesthesia, 6th edition. New York: Wiley; 2020. pp. 813-33.
20. Pedretti L, Massa S, Leardini D, Muratore E, Rahman S, Pession A, et al. Role of nutrition in pediatric patients with cancer. Nutrients. 2023;15(3):710.
21. Viani K, Trehan A, Manzoli B, Schoeman J. Assessment of nutritional status in children with cancer: a narrative review. Pediatr Blood Cancer. 2020;67 Suppl 3:e28211.
22. Meier CM, Furtwängler R, Mergen M, Welter N, Melchior P, Schenk JP, et al. Impact of time to surgery on outcome in Wilms tumor treated with preoperative chemotherapy. Cancers. 2023;15(5):1494.
23. Goyal R, Powell WF. Anaesthesia for paediatric laparoscopic surgery. Paediatr Anaesth. 2020;417:1-6.
24. Müller SD, Both CP, Sponholz C, Voelker MT, Christiansen H, Niggli F, et al. Association between intraoperative blood transfusion, regional anesthesia and outcome after pediatric tumor surgery for nephroblastoma. Cancers. 2022;14(22):5585.
25. Aksu C, Gürkan Y. Ultrasound guided erector spinae block for postoperative analgesia in pediatric nephrectomy surgeries. J Clin Anesth. 2018;45:35-6.
26. Chakraborty A, Goswami J, Patro V. Ultrasound-guided continuous quadratus lumborum block for postoperative analgesia in a pediatric patient. A A Case Rep. 2015;4(3):34-6.
27. Moon JK, Hwang R, Balis FM, Mattei P. An enhanced recovery after surgery protocol in children who undergo nephrectomy for Wilms tumor safely shortens hospital stay. J Pediatr Surg. 2022;57(10):259-65.
28. Stokes CL, Stokes WA, Kalapurakal JA, Paulino AC, Cost NG, Cost CR, et al. Timing of radiation therapy in pediatric Wilms tumor: a report from the National Cancer Database. Int J Radiat Oncol Biol Phys. 2018;101(2):453-61.
29. Fukuzawa H, Shiima Y, Mishima Y, Sekine S, Miura S, Yabe K, et al. Predictive factor for intraoperative tumor rupture of Wilms tumor. Pediatr Surg Int. 2017;33(1):91-5.
30. Barber TD, Derinkuyu BE, Wickiser J, Joglar J, Koral K, Baker LA. Wilms tumor: preoperative risk factors identified for intraoperative tumor spill. J Urol. 2011;185(4):1414-8.
31. Marra P, Di Fazio B, Dulcetta L, Carbone FS, Muglia R, Bonaffini PA, et al. Embolization in pediatric patients: a comprehensive review of indications, procedures, and clinical outcomes. J Clin Med. 2022;11(22):6626.
32. Nelson O, Bailey PD. Pediatric anesthesia considerations for interventional radiology. Anesthesiol Clin. 2017;35(4):701-14.
33. Murphy AJ, Davidoff AM. Bilateral Wilms tumor: a surgical perspective. Children. 2018;5(10):134.
34. Kajal K, Munirathinam GK, Mandal B, Gandhi K, Singh H, Kanojia R. Wilm's tumor with intracardiac extension causing dynamic tricuspid valve obstruction: an anesthetic challenge. Saudi J Anaesth. 2018;12(2):321-3.
35. Daum R, Roth H, Zachariou Z. Tumor infiltration of the vena cava in nephroblastoma. Eur J Pediatr Surg. 1994;4(1):16-20.
36. Abdullah Y, Karpelowsky J, Davidson A, Thomas J, Brooks A, Hewitson J, et al. Millar AJ. Management of nine cases of Wilms' tumour with intracardiac extension—a single centre experience. Journal of pediatric surgery. 2013;48(2):394-9.
37. Dhar M, Prakash S, Pandey V, Pai VK. Intraoperative tumor lysis syndrome in a child with Wilms' tumor. Anesth Essays Res. 2016;10(1):145-7.
38. Leslie SW, Sajjad H, Murphy PB. Wilms tumor. In: StatPearls. Treasure Island (FL): StatPearls Publishing; 2023. PMID: 28723033.
39. Lal A, Rice A, al Mahr M, Kern IB, Marshall GM. Wilms tumor associated with polycythemia: case report and review of the literature. J Pediatr Hematol Oncol. 1997;19(3):263-5.
40. Kamat S, Deepa C, Priolkar S, Nazareth M. A case of polycythemia vera for orthopedic surgery: perianesthetic considerations. Saudi J Anaesth. 2012;6(1):87-8.
41. Kedir H, Tumin D, Veneziano G, Tobias JD. Acquired von Willebrand disease in a child with Wilms' tumor: implications for postoperative regional anesthesia. J Med Cases. 2018;9(10):345-7.
42. Faizan M, Manzoor J, Saleem M, Anwar S, Mehmood Q, Hameed A, et al. Paraneoplastic cushing syndrome due to Wilm's tumor. J Coll Physicians Surg Pak. 2017;27(5):313-5.
43. Chapman E, Pichel A. Anaesthesia for nephrectomy. BJA Educ. 2015;16(3):98-101.
44. Ritchey ML, Shamberger RC, Haase G, Horwitz J, Bergemann T, Breslow NE. Surgical complications after primary nephrectomy for Wilms' tumor: report from the National Wilms' Tumor Study Group. J Am Coll Surg. 2001;192(1):63-8.

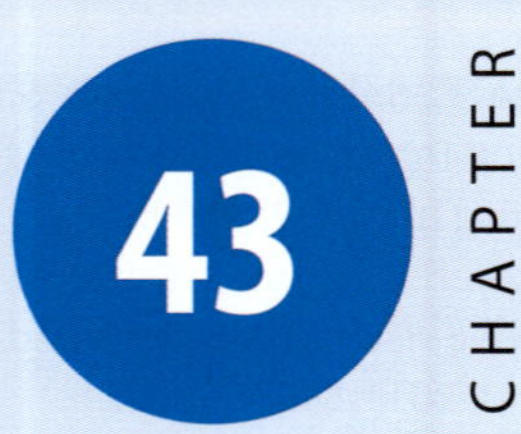

CHAPTER

Anesthesia for Pediatric Neuroblastoma Surgery

Pascal Owusu-Agyemang

BACKGROUND

Neuroblastomas are extracranial tumors which develop in the sympathetic nervous system.[1] Neuroblastomas can originate anywhere the neural crest cells migrate to. However, about 50% arise from the adrenal medulla.[2] Overall, neuroblastomas are the most common abdominal tumor in children and account for 5–8% of all pediatric malignancies.[3,4] Histologically, neuroblastomas are small, round, blue cell tumors, with distinguishing neuritic processes and Homer Wright rosettes.[3]

CLINICAL PRESENTATION

The clinical symptoms of neuroblastomas depends on the anatomic site.[3] Tumors located in the region of the cervical spine may present with Horner syndrome. Tumors arising in the thoracic cavity may initially be asymptomatic but may progress to dyspnea and difficulty feeding after increase in tumor size.[5,6] Abdominal and pelvic tumors may also be incidentally discovered by palpation. However, larger tumors may be associated with abdominal distention, obstructive symptoms including partial rectal obstruction, or neurogenic bladder.[7-9] In some instances, bony metastases could be the first clinical manifestation of neuroblastoma.[10,11] The most frequent sites of bony metastases are cortical bone and bone marrow, which may lead to bone pain. Spinal involvement may lead to compression fractures and paraparesis.[12]

Adequate planning for the anesthetic management of children undergoing neuroblastoma surgery requires a thorough understanding of the location and extent of the disease, as well as the potential surgical challenges.[2] The current staging system for neuroblastoma is the International Neuroblastoma Risk Group Staging System (INRGSS). The INRGSS quantifies the extent of disease by image defined risk factors (IDRFs) and the presence of metastatic disease.[13] IDRFs are identified with computed tomography and magnetic resonance imaging and help identify tumor involvement with vital structures. Thus, characterization of IDRFs is critical to surgical planning.

Although the amplification of biological factors is generally associated with advanced stages of disease, rapid tumor progression, and poor outcomes, age at diagnosis remains the primary patient-related risk factor, with studies showing that children diagnosed before 18 months of age to be at lower risk.[14]

In accordance with the INRGSS system, tumors are categorized as follows:[2]

- *L1:* Localized tumor not involving vital structures as defined by the list of image-defined risk factors and confined to one body compartment
- *L2:* Locoregional tumor with presence of one or more image-defined risk factors.
- *M:* Distant metastatic disease (except stage MS)
- *MS:* Metastatic disease in children younger than 18 months with metastases confined to skin, liver, and/or bone marrow

Based on staging, age, histology, and tumor biology, patients are grouped into:[2]

- *Very low risk:* Differentiated tumors, localized disease L1 or MS disease without MYN-amplifications or SCAs
- *Low risk:* L2 disease without concerning biologic factors and M disease <18 months, who do not meet criteria for MS disease, with no concerning biologic factors, and hyperdiploid tumors
- *Intermediate risk:* L2 patients of any age with SCA but without unfavorable histology or MYC-N amplification and metastatic patients less than 18 months without higher risk biologic factors
- *High risk:* MYC-N amplification or L2/M disease >12 months of age with unfavorable biology

PATIENT MANAGEMENT

Very low-risk disease is usually managed with surgical resection alone. Low-risk disease is managed with biopsy, neoadjuvant chemotherapy, and subsequent surgical resection. The majority of patients with intermediate-risk disease are treated with a combination of surgery and chemotherapy.

Treatment of children with high-risk disease is usually carried out in phases which include chemotherapy, surgery, radiotherapy, myeloablative therapy with stem cell transplant, isotretinoin, and immunotherapy.[2]

Most chemotherapy regimens for children with neuroblastoma may include doxorubicin, cyclophosphamide, carboplatin, etoposide, and cyclophosphamide. In addition, combinations of various chemotherapy regimens with immunotherapies have been described.[15] The side effects of these agents include doxorubicin-associated cardiac toxicity, and renal and hepatic toxicity from cyclophosphamide and carboplatin. Immunotherapies have also been associated with various side effects including but not limited to tachycardia, hypertension, chronic pain, capillary leak syndrome, and nausea.[15] In addition, myeloablative chemotherapy may lead to anemia or thrombocytopenia.

Preoperative Assessment

Multidisciplinary planning with the surgical and oncology teams is often encouraged. In addition to a general preoperative assessment which includes an evaluation of the complete blood count, electrolyte, coagulation, hepatic, and renal profiles, knowledge of the levels of the tumor markers—vanillylmandelic acid (VMA), and homovanillic acid (HMA)—are important to the anesthesiologist. The significance of these catecholamine metabolites (VMA and HMA) is their potential association with hypertension. Furthermore, an understanding of the IDRF and knowledge of chemotherapy regimens undergone will guide the anesthesiologist in anticipating potential risks associated with surgery and the side effects of chemotherapy.[15]

An assessment of chemotherapy-related side effects may warrant further evaluation. For example, an echocardiogram may be necessary to assess doxorubicin-associated cardiac toxicity.[16] In addition, high levels of circulating catecholamines (VMA and HMA) have been associated with structural myocardial changes.[17]

Anesthetic Concerns

To improve the chances of survival, surgical resection of neuroblastoma aims for >90% resection of gross disease.[2] However, neuroblastomas with IDRFs often involve major vessel encasement **(Table 1)**. Thus, major hemorrhage is a significant risk, especially in high-risk neuroblastoma, where encasement of major blood vessels are not uncommon. In addition, many tumors have their own arterial supply and venous drainage and present a significant challenge to surgeons in attaining hemostasis.

High-risk neuroblastoma often present in the abdomen or pelvis. It is not uncommon for these tumors to encase the aorta, inferior vena cava, portal vein, renal vessels, celiac artery, and superior mesenteric vessels.[2]

Anesthetic Management

To date, there is no standardized or recommended anesthetic management for children undergoing neuroblastoma surgery. After careful consideration of the risk factors involved, most commonly used anesthetics and analgesics may be safely used during neuroblastoma surgery.[4,18] The most critical aspect of anesthetic management is an awareness of the extent of the disease and the risks involved with the surgical procedure. Thus, for high-risk cases, invasive hemodynamic monitoring, and adequate intravenous access in the form of central venous lines may be necessary. A multimodal approach to pain management with the inclusion of opioid and non-opioid analgesics, epidural analgesia, or regional anesthetic blocks may be useful for large tumor resections.[19]

For the resection of thoracic neuroblastomas, thoracotomy is most used. Thus, lung isolation with bronchial blockers or double-lumen tubes may be required.[20] For smaller tumors, a thoracoscopic approach has been described.[21]

As a result of the upregulation of the renin–angiotensin–aldosterone system and excess catecholamine (epinephrine and dopamine) production from tumor, approximately ~19% of children with neuroblastoma are diagnosed with hypertension.[3,18] Chemotherapy-related side effects as well as the need for concurrent hyperhydration have also been shown to contribute to hypertension.[3]

There is a lack of data on the incidence of intraoperative hypertension during pediatric neuroblastoma surgery. The few available studies report an incidence to be rare <3.5%.[3,18] However, in a recent study by Liu and colleagues, the overall incidence of intraoperative hypertension in

TABLE 1: Definition of image defined risk factors (IDRF).

Anatomic region	*Description*
Multiple body compartments	Ipsilateral tumor extension within two body compartments (i.e., neck and chest, chest and abdomen, or abdomen and pelvis)
Neck	• Tumor encasing carotid artery, vertebral artery, and/or internal jugular vein • Tumor extending to skull base • Tumor compressing trachea
Cervicothoracic junction	• Tumor encasing brachial plexus roots • Tumor encasing subclavian vessels, vertebral artery, and/or carotid artery • Tumor compressing trachea
Thorax	• Tumor encasing aorta and/or major branches • Tumor compressing trachea and/or principal bronchi • Lower mediastinal tumor infiltrating costovertebral junction between T9 and T12 vertebral levels
Thoracoabdominal junction	Tumor encasing aorta and/or vena cava
Abdominal and pelvis	• Tumor infiltrating porta hepatis and/or hepatoduodenal ligament • Tumor encasing branches of superior mesenteric artery at mesenteric root • Tumor encasing origin of celiac axis and/or origin of superior mesenteric artery • Tumor invading one or both renal pedicles • Tumor encasing aorta and/or vena cava • Tumor encasing iliac vessels • Pelvic tumor crossing sciatic notch
Intraspinal tumor	Intraspinal tumor extension (whatever the location) provided that more than one-third of spinal canal in axial plane is invaded, the perimedullary leptomeningeal spaces are not visible, or the spinal cord signal intensity is abnormal
Infiltration of adjacent organs and structures	Pericardium, diaphragm, kidney, liver, duodenopancreatic block, and mesentery

Source: Adapted from Monclair T, Brodeur GM, Ambros PF, Brisse HJ, Cecchetto G, Holmes K, et al. The International Neuroblastoma Risk Group (INRG) staging system: An INRG Task Force report. J Clin Oncol. 2009;27:298-303.

a cohort of 102 children was 13%.[3,18] In this study, all patients who experienced intraoperative hypertension had elevated preoperative urine catecholamine levels. This suggests that the incidence of hypertension during neuroblastoma surgery may be higher than previously thought, and the contribution of increased levels of circulating catecholamines may be significant. However, the presence of intraoperative hypertension was not associated with the need for postoperative intensive care monitoring.

Hypertension may be exacerbated during induction of anesthesia and/or intraoperative tumor manipulation. Thus, it is imperative for the anesthesiologist to have an assessment of the risk for hypertension and to have rapidly acting antihypertensive drugs available. It may be reasonable to start with the administration of shorter-acting antihypertensives such as esmolol before administering longer-acting agents. This may allow the anesthesiologist to assess the response to antihypertensive agents and avoid prolonged hypotension in instances where hypertension is caused by brief tumor manipulation. Laryngotracheal analgesia with lidocaine spray may help reduce the stress response to intubation.

The disposition of patients after surgery depends on the extent of the surgical procedures and any complications or concerns over the intraoperative period.

CONCLUSION

Involvement in the multidisciplinary planning process could provide significant information about the severity of disease, comorbidities, and goals of surgical resection. The most critical aspect of anesthetic management is the awareness of the extent of the disease and constant communication with the surgical teams.

REFERENCES

1. Wienke J, Dierselhuis MP, Tytgat GAM, Künkele A, Nierkens S, Molenaar JJ. The immune landscape of neuroblastoma: Challenges and opportunities for novel therapeutic strategies in pediatric oncology. Eur J Cancer. 2021;144:123-50.
2. Shaffiey SA, Le HD, Christison-Lagay E, Fialkowski EA, Aldrink JH, Grant CN, et al. Critical elements of pediatric neuroblastoma surgery. Semin Pediatr Surg. 2023;32(5):151338.
3. Croteau N, Nuchtern J, LaQuaglia MP. Management of neuroblastoma in pediatric patients. Surg Oncol Clin N Am. 2021;30(2):291-304.

4. Tognon C, Pulvirenti R, Fati F, De Corti F, Viscardi E, Volpe A, et al. Anesthesia in children with neuroblastoma, perioperative and operative management. Children (Basel). 2021;8(5).
5. Rudolf JW, Thapa M. Thoracic neuroblastoma. Radiol Case Rep. 2011;6(2):440.
6. Feki J, Boudawara O, Makni S, Sellami-Boudawara T, Khanfir A. An uncommon breast metastasis of mediastinal neuroblastoma within a child: A case report. Breast J. 2021;27(4):377-9.
7. Cronin EM, Coffey JC, Herlihy D, Romics L, Aftab F, Keohane C, et al. Massive retroperitoneal ganglioneuroma presenting with small bowel obstruction 18 years following initial diagnosis. Ir J Med Sci. 2005;174(2):63-6.
8. Selvaratnam R, Karger AB. A newborn with distended abdomen. Clin Chem. 2016;62(8):1061-4.
9. Han LA, Khine W, Lin TM, Thu M. Neuroblastoma involving urinary bladder: A rare type of tumor with diagnostic ambiguity. IJU Case Rep. 2019;2(4):229-31.
10. Özger NH, Sağlam Y, Kebudi R, Dikici F. A neuroblastoma case presenting with pathologic femur fracture. Acta Orthop Traumatol Turc. 2013;47(1):60-4.
11. Soliman H, El-Noueam K, Ettaby A, Fadel S, Abougabal AM. Whole-body three-dimensional short tau inversion recovery and T1-weighted in/opposed phase MRI in the detection of neuroblastoma bone marrow metastasis: comparative study with PET/CT utilising bone marrow biopsy as the reference standard. Clin Radiol. 2023;78(7):e535-41.
12. Jasiewicz B, Helenius I. Tumors and infections of the growing spine. J Child Orthop. 2023;17(6):556-72.
13. Brisse HJ, McCarville MB, Granata C, Krug KB, Wootton-Gorges SL, Kanegawa K, et al. Guidelines for imaging and staging of neuroblastic tumors: Consensus report from the International Neuroblastoma Risk Group Project. Radiology. 2011;261(1):243-57.
14. London WB, Castleberry RP, Matthay KK, Look AT, Seeger RC, Shimada H, et al. Evidence for an age cutoff greater than 365 days for neuroblastoma risk group stratification in the Children's Oncology Group. J Clin Oncol. 2005;23(27):6459-65.
15. Pieniazek B, Cencelewicz K, Bzdziuch P, Mlynarczyk L, Lejman M, Zawitkowska J, et al. Neuroblastoma: A review of combination immunotherapy. Int J Mol Sci. 2024; 25(14).
16. Armenian S, Bhatia S. Predicting and preventing anthracycline-related cardiotoxicity. Am Soc Clin Oncol Educ Book. 2018;38:3-12.
17. Sethi P, Peiris CD. A review of catecholamine associated cardiomyopathies and channelopathies. Cureus. 2020; 12(2):e6957.
18. Liu J, Zurakowski D, Weldon C, Umaretiya P, Holzman R, Lin YC. Perioperative hypertension and anesthetic management in patients undergoing resection of neuroblastoma. Paediatr Anaesth. 2023;33(7):577-82.
19. Moon JK, Hwang R, Balis FM, Mattei P. An enhanced recovery after surgery protocol in children who undergo nephrectomy for Wilms tumor safely shortens hospital stay. J Pediatr Surg. 2022;57(10):259-65.
20. Mayer BFB, Schunn MC, Urla C, Schäfer JF, Fideler F, Neunhoeffer F, et al. Trap-door thoracotomy and clamshell thoracotomy as surgical approaches for neuroblastoma and other thoracic tumors in children. Cancers (Basel). 2024;16(2).
21. Lecompte JF, Sarnacki S, Irtan S, Piolat C, Scalabre A, Talon I, et al. Thoracoscopy for pediatric thoracic neurogenic tumors-a European multi-center study. Cancers (Basel). 2023;15(22).

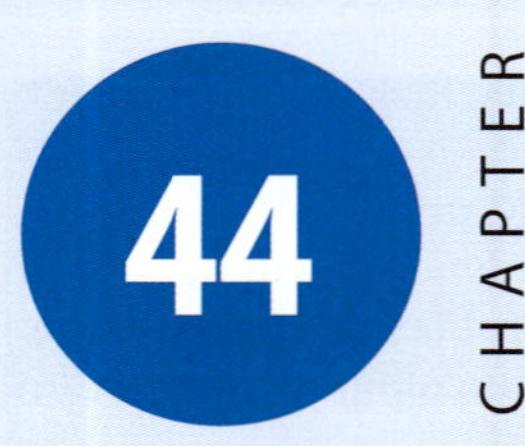

Anesthesia for Pediatric Hepato-Pancreato-Biliary Surgeries

Jeson R Doctor, Veer D Thakkar

INTRODUCTION

Children under the age of 18 years comprise an important subset of patients undergoing various procedures and major surgeries under anesthesia. Pediatric patients presenting with tumors of the liver, pancreas, and the biliary tree require anesthesia for various diagnostic and therapeutic procedures. These include anesthesia for procedures in nonoperating room locations such as upper gastrointestinal (GI) endoscopies and endoscopic retrograde cholangiopancreatography (ERCP) in the endoscopy suites; computed tomography (CT)—guided biopsies, radiofrequency ablation (RFA) procedures, peripherally inserted central catheter (PICC) line and chemoport insertions in the intervention radiology suite; MRIs, etc. Major surgeries such as hepatectomies, surgeries involving the hepatobiliary tree, splenectomy and Whipple's procedure are what we will be focusing on in this chapter.

Apart from the usual challenges and concerns in pediatric patients, children with malignancies have their own unique set of problems. Repeated diagnostic and therapeutic procedures, difficult intravenous access, anxiety, malnutrition states including cancer cachexia, systemic and immunosuppressive side effects of radio-therapy and chemotherapy, major blood loss are some of the challenges that a pediatric oncoanesthesiologist has to anticipate and manage.

TYPES OF PEDIATRIC HEPATO-PANCREATO-BILIARY TUMORS

Tumors Affecting the Liver

Two thirds of hepatic tumors in the pediatric age group are malignant. In 2014, the international consensus classification of pediatric liver tumors classified these lesions into epithelial tumors, mixed epithelial and mesenchymal tumors.[1] Hepatoblastoma is the most common tumor in the pediatric age group and is discussed here.

Hepatoblastoma

Hepatoblastoma and hepatocellular carcinoma are the two most common malignant primary hepatic tumors in children, with the former accounting for 90% malignant tumors in children younger than five years of age.[2] Overall, hepatoblastoma is the third most common intra-abdominal malignancy in children after neuroblastomas and Wilm's tumor. The survival rates for children with hepatoblastomas ranges from 60% to >75%, yet it is lower than the overall survival of pediatric malignancies which about 80%.[3-6] In recent years, there has been growing evidence to suggest a relationship between the incidence of hepatoblastomas and very low birth weight (VLBW). The increase in the numbers of hepatoblastoma may be related to increased survival rates of premature babies due to better medical care.[7] Other risk factors include infertility treatment, preeclampsia, high maternal pregnancy weight, oligo/polyhydramnios, parent's tobacco use or occupational exposure to petroleum, paint and pigment products, iron, lead, tin and copper.[7,8] Oxygen therapy and the use of furosemide in the perinatal period have been reported as risk factors for development of hepatoblastomas in VLBW infants.[9] A few syndromes are associated with a higher frequency of hepatoblastoma, viz., Beckwith-Wiedemann syndrome, hemihypertrophy, Trisomy 18 (Edward's syndrome), and familial adenomatous polyposis.[10]

Clinical presentation: A palpable abdominal mass and abdominal distension are the most common presenting features of a hepatoblastoma. Nonspecific symptoms such as loss of appetite, nausea, vomiting, and weight loss are also common. Jaundice is rarely a presenting feature. Ascites, gastrointestinal bleed, splenomegaly and pruritus may be seen in occasional cases. Precocious puberty may be seen due to high levels of beta-human chorionic gonadotropin.[11] About 20% of patients with hepatoblastomas present with distant metastasis at presentation with lung being the most common site for metastasis.[12,13]

Preoperative investigations:

- >90% of cases have high blood alpha-fetoprotein (AFP) levels. Several studies have confirmed that AFP is an important surveillance marker in children who have undergone hepatectomy for malignancies, those with unfavorable tumor histopathology, poor response to chemotherapy, and poor outcomes. Children with low AFP levels at diagnosis tend to have a more aggressive course, with widespread disease, chemoresistance and a 2-year survival rate of only 24%.[14]
- Abdominal ultrasound and CT of the thorax and abdomen are useful in staging the disease, assessing the resectability, assessing the response to systemic chemotherapy, calculation of future liver remnant (FLR) and CT volumetric assessment.
- Liver function test such as serum bilirubin and liver enzymes are usually normal unless the patient has been on hepatotoxic chemotherapy regimens.
- Complete blood count may show anemia, thrombocytopenia, and leukocytosis in case of bone marrow suppression due to recent chemotherapy.
- Baseline coagulation profile is used to assess the synthetic function of the liver and rule out underlying coagulopathy secondary to impaired absorption of vitamin K in obstructive jaundice. The vitamin-K dependent coagulation factors may not be synthesized as a result of this. It can be corrected by preoperative administration of vitamin K.
- Two-dimensional echocardiography is indicated in syndromic children, patients with poor nutritional status, huge abdominal masses, and in children who have received doxorubicin-based chemotherapy.

Treatment options: The survival rates of children with hepatoblastomas have improved dramatically over the last three decades largely due to improvements in treatment, including chemotherapy, surgical techniques, supportive care, and the introduction of orthotopic liver transplantation for locally advanced and unresectable disease. The overall 5-year event-free survival of patients treated with chemotherapy and surgery ranges from 75% to 90%.[15-19]

Standard-risk hepatoblastomas include tumors that are confined to the liver and involve not more than three hepatic sectors. High-risk hepatoblastomas are the ones that involve the entire liver; the portal vein, the right and left branches or all three hepatic veins, or the inferior vena cava.

- *Surgery:* Complete surgical resection of the tumor is essential to ensure long-term survival. Consensus is, however, lacking as to the actual timing for surgery. Some patients undergo upfront surgery followed by chemotherapy and some receive neoadjuvant chemotherapy (NACT) before liver resection. Irrespective of the timing of surgery, the liver of a pediatric patient has an excellent capacity to regenerate even after aggressive resections. The residual liver in a child is essentially normal (unlike in adults in whom the liver may be cirrhotic) decreasing the chances of post hepatectomy liver failure. Therefore, 70–80% of the liver can be safely resected.[20,21] The right lobe of the liver consists of segments 5, 6, 7, and 8 whereas the left lobe consists of segments 1, 2, 3, and 4.[22] Depending on the number of segments involved and the extent of resection, the surgical plan could vary with nonanatomical resection, sectionectomy, right, central or left hepatectomy, and right- or left-extended hepatectomy.
- *Chemotherapy:* Standard-risk hepatoblastomas may undergo upfront surgery or may receive two to four cycles of cisplatin-based chemotherapy followed by surgery. High-risk hepatoblastomas receive NACT before surgery. These may be PLADO – cisplatin and doxorubicin, or C5V – cisplatin, 5- FU and vincristine or SUPERPLADO – alternating cycles of carboplatin/doxorubicin and cisplatin. Preoperative chemotherapy is usually given with the aim of making unresectable and borderline tumors resectable.
- *Other modalities:* Transarterial chemoembolization (TACE) and transarterial radioembolization (TARE) have been used to decrease the size of the tumor by giving higher doses of chemotherapy or radioactive particles locally with lower systemic effects.[20] Portal vein embolization (PVE) is done by particle embolization of the portal vein supplying the diseased segments. It helps by diverting the portal blood flow to

the normal segments causing preferential hypertrophy of the normal liver, thereby increasing the future liver remnant (FLR). These strategies have been applied mainly in patients with a liver remnant that was predicted to be too small for resection.[23] The role of other modalities such as radiofrequency ablation and cryoablation (that are useful in adults) have not been documented in children.

Tumors Affecting the Biliary Tract and Pancreas

Pancreatic tumors are rare in children with an estimated age-adjusted incidence of 0.19 cases per million pediatric population in North America.[24] According to the 2019 World Health Organization (WHO) classification of tumors of the digestive tract, pancreatic tumors are divided into three categories including benign epithelial tumors, malignant epithelial tumors, and neuroendocrine tumors (NETs) with an additional group of rare non-epithelial tumors.[25] Various types of pediatric pancreatic tumors are enumerated in **Table 1**.

The differentiation of pancreatic tumors in children is often difficult due to nonspecific and overlapping clinical features and radiological characteristics. Unlike adults, these lesions tend to be well circumscribed and are noninvasive, making them amenable to surgical resection and longer expected survival. The most common ones—pancreatoblastoma, solid pseudopapillary neoplasm, and NET—are described in the following text.

TABLE 1: Pediatric pancreatic tumors.

Tumor	*Origin*	*Malignant potential*
Serous cystadenoma	Epithelial	Benign
Mucinous cystic neoplasm	Epithelial	Premalignant
Solid pseudo-papillary neoplasm	Epithelial	Usually benign
Neuroendocrine tumor	Epithelial, ectodermal	Usually benign
Pancreatoblastoma	Epithelial	Malignant
Ductal adenocarcinoma	Epithelial	Malignant
Acinar cell carcinoma	Epithelial	Malignant
Inflammatory myofibroblastic tumor	Mesenchymal	Usually benign
Ewing's sarcoma, primitive neuroectodermal tumor	Mesenchymal	Malignant
Kaposiform hemangioendothelioma	Mesenchymal	Locally invasive
Leukemia, lymphoma	Mesenchymal	Malignant
Secondary (metastasis)	Variable	Malignant

Pancreatoblastoma

Pancreatoblastoma is the most common pancreatic solid tumor in children. It accounts for about 25% of all pancreatic solid lesions in children <10 years of age. It has a strong association with Beckwith–Wiedemann syndrome, with a prevalence of up to 50%. These tumors are generally located in the head and body of the pancreas. They vary in size from 5 to 20 cm. They are soft and well circumcised.

Clinical presentation: Children with pancreatoblastoma are usually asymptomatic except for a large palpable abdominal mass. Presenting symptoms are usually nonspecific such as abdominal pain, anorexia, weight loss, vomiting, diarrhea, and fatigue. Jaundice is usually not a presenting symptom. AFP is a reliable tumor marker in 70–80% patients and its levels usually correlate well with the size of the tumor. An ultrasound of the abdomen demonstrates a solitary lesion with solid and cystic components. A CT or an MRI is required to assess the locoregional extent of the disease.

Treatment options: Complete surgical resection is the mainstay treatment of pancreatoblastoma, with 5-year survival rates of >70% in patients without metastases who underwent complete resections without any residual disease. Neoadjuvant chemotherapy is recommended for patients with locally invasive disease and in patients who have distant metastases to achieve complete surgical resection.

Solid Pseudopapillary Neoplasm

Solid pseudopapillary neoplasm (SPN) is an exocrine pancreatic tumor. The median age of presentation of this neoplasm is 13–15 years with girls being affected by it more than boys.[26,27] The origin of SPN remains unknown; however, they are postulated to arise from embryonal pancreatic pluripotent cells. These tumors are usually indolent low-grade, but sometimes focal high-grade malignancies are reported. They are large at the time of diagnosis, with median reported diameters varying from

5–6.8 cm and can go up to 20 cm. Most often, they are well circumscribed.[26-29] SPN can be present throughout the pancreas, but are most commonly found in the pancreatic tail.[27,30]

Clinical presentation: SPN may be detected incidentally on scans performed for other indications. Abdominal pain, a palpable abdominal mass, and vomiting are the most common presenting features. Jaundice may or may not be present, depending upon the location of the tumor. In case, the tumor is located at the head of the pancreas, jaundice is the presenting symptom due to biliary obstruction. Tumor markers such as AFP, carcinoembryonic antigen (CEA) and carbohydrate antigen (CA 19-9) are not raised.

Treatment options: Complete surgical resection is the treatment of choice for SPN, irrespective of the size of the tumor or presence of metastasis. Surgery entails a distal pancreatosplenectomy for tumors arising from the tail and body while a Whipple's procedure may be required in tumors originating from the head of the pancreas. Enucleation surgery should be avoided which may lead to incomplete resection and high chances of recurrence. The prognosis following a complete resection is excellent with overall survival rates ranging from 89 to 98%.[26-28] Adjuvant chemotherapy is not recommended in patients where complete surgical resection has been achieved.

Neuroendocrine Tumors

Pediatric NETs are benign tumors and mostly affect teenagers. They originate in the islet cells of the pancreas and classified as functional or non-functional depending on hormone secretion. Non-functioning NETs are asymptomatic and found incidentally. Functional NETs manifest symptoms based on the hormone secreted by them. Insulinoma and gastrinoma are the two most common type of functional pediatric NETs.

Insulinomas, due to uncontrolled secretion of insulin, present with symptoms of hypoglycemia, palpitations, tremors, perspiration, and sometimes seizures. In severe cases, insulinomas may present as persistent hyperinsulinemic hypoglycemia, which presents as behavioral changes, seizures and coma in children.

Gastrinomas, derived from gastrin-secreting G cells, cause hypersecretion of hydrochloric acid in the stomach. Clinical manifestations include peptic ulcer disease, gastroesophageal reflux disease (GERD), and most commonly, diarrhea. Unlike insulinomas, gastrinomas are larger in size and 60% are malignant.

Treatment options: Surgical resection is the curative treatment for pancreatic NETs. Lesions in the pancreatic head are treated with pancreaticoduodenectomy, while distal lesions undergo a distal pancreatectomy. Gland-preserving procedures such as duodenum-preserving pancreatic head resections, central pancreatectomy, and enucleation may be an option for functional NETs depending upon its size and whether it is malignant or not. Patients with pancreatic NETs may be on octreotide for symptom control prior to surgery.

ANESTHETIC MANAGEMENT OF PEDIATRIC HPB TUMORS

Children posted for excision of HPB tumors are often challenging with respect to challenges posed by major abdominal surgery superadded to the pediatric concerns. The Enhanced Recovery Pathway after Surgery (ERAS) is gaining widespread importance in children.[31] More adherence to the elements of this pathway needs some dedication and an extra effort on the part of the perioperative care team. Preoperative evaluation and investigations and treatment options have been discussed in the earlier section of this chapter above and are specific to the type of diseases.

Goals of Anesthesia and Surgery in Major Abdominal Surgeries in Children

- Maximize safe resection with minimal residual disease
- Minimize blood loss and coagulopathy and optimize blood therapy
- Avoid liver failure in the postoperative period by leaving enough healthy liver post resection
- Optimal fluid balance to prevent hypovolemia and hypervolemia. Hypovolemia can decrease tissue perfusion and cause acute kidney injury. Hypervolemia can lead to bowel edema compromising high risk bowel anastomoses such as pancreatojejunostomy and hepaticojejunostomy in a Whipple's procedure. Overzealous fluid administration can lead to decreased lung compliance, fluid overload, and paralytic ileus in an edematous bowel.
- Maintain normoglycemia especially in cases of Insulinomas.
- Maintain normothermia and optimal tissue perfusion.
- In case a splenectomy is planned, relevant vaccination for pneumococcus and meningococcus should be given

Anesthetic Management

General anesthesia with epidural anesthesia is the anesthetic of choice for patients undergoing hepato-pancreato-biliary tumor resection surgeries. Fasting guidelines of 8 hours for fatty meals, 6 hours for solids, 4 hours for breast milk, and 2 hours for clear liquids should be advocated.[32] Clear fluids till 2 hours prior to the procedure prevents dehydration, hypoglycemia, and makes the child less irritable.[32]

Separation anxiety can be dealt with by giving adequate premedication such as oral midazolam (0.5 mg/kg) or by parental presence during induction of anesthesia. Intravenous induction, in case a venous access, is in situ or inhalational induction with sevoflurane can be performed.

Intraoperative monitoring should be done with ECG, capnography, pulse oximetry, appropriately sized blood pressure cuff, and hourly urine output. Temperature and blood sugars should also be monitored.

Hepatobiliary surgeries can have torrential blood loss and fluid shifts so atleast two wide-bore intravenous accesses are recommended, preferably in the upper limbs. The venous return from the lower limbs may be reduced in cases of cross-clamping of the inferior vena cava (IVC).

Adequate preoxygenation in propped-up position will help in prolonging the apnea time during endotracheal intubation in children with large intra-abdominal tumors. Intubation with pediatric microcuffed endotracheal tubes with controlled ventilation is recommended. Care should be taken that the cuff of the endotracheal tube is just beyond the vocal cords so as to avoid inadvertent endobronchial migration of the tube during upper abdominal retraction and application of Thompson, Bookwalter, or similar retractors.

The position is usually supine for abdominal tumors with midline or transverse incisions depending on the location and extent of the mass. A nasogastric tube should be inserted to decompress the stomach and should be kept on continuous drainage to prevent regurgitation and collection of gastric secretions in the oral cavity during surgical retraction of the stomach.

Antibiotic surgical prophylaxis should be given well in advance due to a higher incidence of perioperative infections and sepsis in these children.

Analgesia: Thoracic epidural analgesia at the T6–T9 level is recommended after discussing the extent of surgical incision. The risk–benefit ratio of epidural is to be assessed with coagulopathy, hypotension, and bleeding. If the coagulation profile is normal, analgesia with an epidural catheter inserted congruent to the surgical incision is preferred. A 19G/18G-epidural catheter set is often used. Care should be taken that the epidural catheter is fixed well to avoid accidental dislodgements and migrations. The toxic dose of local anesthetics should be borne in mind while using epidural analgesia. The infusion dose for levobupivacaine is 0.3 mg/kg/h.[33] Shorter-acting opioids such as fentanyl and remifentanil can be used intravenously for multimodal analgesia. The risk–benefit ratio of paracetamol (PCM) and nonsteroidal anti-inflammatory drugs (NSAIDs) should be weighted.

Intraoperative invasive hemodynamic monitoring is desirable due to extensive resections which may lead to blood loss and hemodynamic instability. Invasive arterial blood pressure monitoring is mandatory in view of the hemodynamic changes that may occur due to extensive resections, blood loss and cross clamping of porta hepatis or IVC. It is also helpful for intraoperative monitoring of arterial blood gases and arterial lactate as a guide for adequate fluid resuscitation. Pulse pressure variation (PPV) is a helpful parameter that is derived from the arterial pressure waveform for adequacy of fluid therapy. The trend can be a useful guide to indicate whether the child will benefit with fluids or vasopressors. A central venous catheter may be reserved for large tumors, major resections, requirement of high doses of vasopressors, children with poor cardiac function, and in kids with difficult peripheral venous access. Using the central venous catheter for monitoring the CVP is very institute specific and is not mandatory.[21]

Anesthesia is maintained with oxygen and air (50:50) with low flows and an inhalational agent with closed circuit on controlled ventilation and a muscle relaxant. During liver resections, N_2O should be avoided keeping in mind a theoretical risk of venous air embolism and bowel distention.

Fluid therapy: A balanced crystalloid such as Ringer's lactate with or without dextrose (1–2% DRL) should be used as maintenance fluid depending on the blood sugars. Maintenance fluid can be given according to the Holliday Segar formula. Replacement of blood loss needs to be done as per the maximum allowable blood loss. Fluid therapy can be titrated with the use of mean arterial pressure, PPV, urine output, arterial pressure waveform, arterial lactate, etc. Overhydration with crystalloids should be avoided to prevent bowel edema as this can lead to compromise of bowel anastomosis such as pancreatojejunostomy, hepaticojejunostomy, gastrojejunostomy, or jejunostomy. In cases where there is hypotension with adequate fluid resuscitation a small dose of vasopressor such as noradrenaline may be used to maintain the mean arterial pressure (MAP) and ensure adequate end organ perfusion.

4 or 5% albumin may be tried in cases of extensive dissection and retroperitoneal handling for maintaining the intravascular volume and oncotic pressure and reduction of interstitial and bowel edema.

Blood loss should be assessed and replaced with packed cells, fresh frozen plasma (FFP), cryoprecipitate, and platelets due to a lower circulating blood volume and a lower maximum allowable blood loss in children.

Hourly urine output should be monitored and maintained at 0.5–1 mL/kg/h.

Blood glucose and electrolyte monitoring: Maintain normoglycemia, especially in cases of insulinomas and NET of pancreas.

Thermoregulation: Maintenance of normothermia is essential with the use of forced air warmers with blankets and fluid warmers. Hypothermia can have a number of deleterious effects such as coagulopathy, increased myocardial irritability, prolonged action of opioids, muscle relaxants, delayed recovery from anesthetics, and vasoconstriction with inadequate end-organ perfusion to name a few.[34]

Intraoperative Challenges

Hemodynamical instability is anticipated at the following time points during the intraoperative period:

- The hepatic pedicle (Pringle maneuver) is clamped to achieve complete or partial inflow control. This maneuver reduces the blood loss but significantly decreases the cardiac output due to decrease in the preload and increase in the afterload **(Figs. 1A to C)**.
- *Total vascular occlusion/total hepatic vascular exclusion (THVE):* Complete clamping of the portal vessels and the infra- and suprahepatic parts of the IVC is done **(Figs. 1A to C)**. The venous return decreases approximately by 40–60% and the systemic vascular resistance increases by as high as 80% leading to significant fall in the cardiac output. The heart rate increases by up to 50%.[35] The liver can tolerate up to 60 minutes of continuous clamping and up to 120 minutes of intermittent clamping.[21,36]

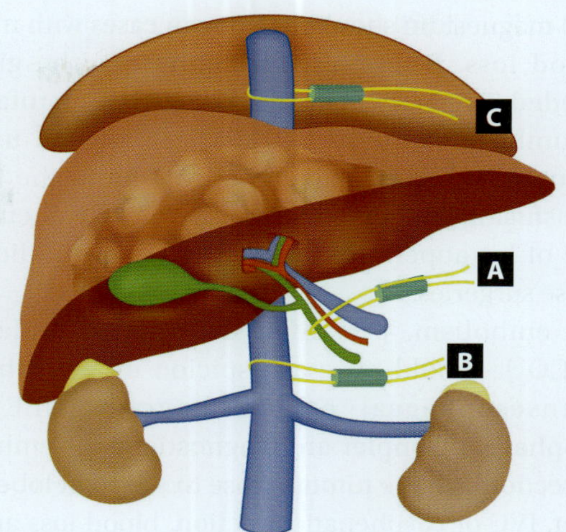

Figs. 1A to C: Partial and total hepatic occlusion. (A) Pringle's maneuver; (B and C) Infrahepatic and suprahepatic IVC cross-clamping; (A + B + C) Total hepatic vascular exclusion (THVE).

A test occlusion prior to formal clamping is generally done to check if the child tolerates the clamping.[21] If the child develops severe hemodynamic instability secondary to the test clamping, the child may require more preloading, high-dose vasopressors or a venovenous bypass in order to bypass the liver and maintain the preload to the heart. Aiming for a higher CVP (approximately 14 cm of water) by adequately correcting the volume deficit may mitigate the precipitous fall in preload but lead to a higher blood loss due to back-leak from the hepatic veins.

- Venous return and in turn cardiac output may also decrease if the IVC is kinked or tented while handling the liver or the periportal structures.

Intraoperative Complications

- *Massive blood loss and coagulopathy:* Optimal surgical techniques including adequate use of inflow and outflow control, using newer equipment such as ultrasonic cutting and coagulation [Cavitro Ultrasonic Surgical Aspirator (CUSA)], Liga Sure, harmonic scalpel, endoscopic staplers, and pressurized water jets should be employed to minimize blood loss. Intravenous tranexamic acid may help in reducing blood loss.

  Blood and blood products such as packed cells, FFP, cryoprecipitates, and platelets should be used to maintain circulating volume and prevent coagulopathy. Correction with intravenous calcium and magnesium should be done in cases with massive blood loss. Recombinant factors may be given if needed. Thromboelastography (TEG) or rotational thromboelastometry (ROTEM) should be used to identify and treat coagulopathy. Due to the fear of transfusing malignant cells back into the circulation, use of intraoperative cell salvage is contradicted in these surgeries.

- Air embolism, a sudden drop in end-tidal CO_2 ($EtCO_2$), should raise a suspicion of air embolism. Transesophageal echocardiogram (TEE) and esophageal Doppler are diagnostic of air embolism. Resection of large tumors close to the right lobe of the liver, IVC or cavohepatic junction, blood loss and low CVP technique puts the patients at risk of air embolism.
- Damage to the portal vein, branches of the celiac trunk, hepatic duct and the kidney.

Reversal and extubation: Postoperatively these children should be reversed and extubated in the operating room if they are alert, warm, comfortable with stable hemodynamics, and adequately resuscitated. One may decide to ventilate the child in case of major resections, fluid shifts, massive blood loss, and hemodynamic instability.

Postoperative Analgesia

- Postoperative pain management can be done using variable-rate elastomeric pumps through the epidural catheters using 0.1 or 0.05% solution of levobupivacaine. Care must be taken so that the toxic dose of local anesthetic is not exceeded. Epidural analgesia is routinely used for 4–5 days postoperatively. Postoperative coagulation profile must be checked prior to removal of epidural catheters. Pain relief can be assess using tools such as the FLACC (Face, Legs, Activity, Cry, Consolability) scale, Wong–Baker faces scales, or the visual analog score (VAS) depending on the child's age.[37]
- Regional truncal blocks such as subcostal transversus abdominis plane (TAP) block or rectus sheath catheters have been tried in children in whom epidural analgesia is contraindicated.[38]
- Parent- or nurse-controlled analgesia (PCA/NCA) with intravenous short-acting opioids are helpful but need a monitored environment. A longer lockout interval is usually recommended.
- Coanalgesics such as paracetamol, tramadol, and NSAIDs need to be titrated judiciously for their risk–benefit ratio.

Postoperative Recovery Care

- *Intravenous fluid therapy:* This needs to be titrated till the child is nil by mouth. Dextrose supplementation may be needed to avoid catabolism and hypoglycemia. A good guide to fluid therapy is 2 mL/kg for the first 10 kg, 1 mL/kg for the next 10 kg, and 0.5 mL/kg for each kg above 20 kg.[39]
- Start enteral feeding as soon as possible and feasible.
- Remove tubes such as nasogastric tubes and urinary catheters as soon as possible.
- Care of intravenous lines with splints should be taken.
- Keep the child warm.
- Parental presence with toys in the postoperative care area is helpful to keep the child calm and entertained.
- Monitor the child for postsurgical problems and treat them early.
- Physiotherapy and early mobilization are helpful.

Postoperative Complications

- *Postoperative liver failure and liver dysfunction*[35]*:* The predisposing factors are previously diseased liver, low volume liver remnant, liver ischemia, massive blood loss, and reperfusion injury due to free radicals.[40]

  The proposed methods to avoid this are ischemic preconditioning, infusion of NAC intraoperatively and postoperatively, avoiding hypotension, careful case selection, and minimizing blood loss.

  The patient may present with encephalopathy, deteriorating liver function, and persistent increase of liver enzymes. The goals of treatment are management of hypoglycemia, management of salt and water retention (due to secondary hyperaldosteronism) along with therapies such as proton-pump inhibitors, enteral feeding, lactulose, NAC infusion, and correction of dyselectrolytemia and coagulation abnormality.
- *Bleeding and coagulation abnormalities:* There may be a cause for concern while considering removal of the epidural catheter on postoperative days 4–5 if the international normalized ratio (INR) is >1.4.[21]
- Renal dysfunction and acute kidney injury (AKI)
- *Sepsis and infections* need prolonged antibiotic cover and prophylactic vaccinations post splenectomy.
- Respiratory failure and acute respiratory distress syndrome (ARDS)

- *Postoperative anastomotic leak, pancreatic or biliary leak* need draining/pig tailing and surgical re-exploration. Interventions such as percutaneous transhepatic biliary drainage (PTBD) may be needed to divert the bile from the anastomotic site and allow healing.
- Postoperative pancreatitis
- Hyperglycemia and dyselectrolytemia in NET resections.

CONCLUSION

Hepatobiliary and pancreatic surgeries in children are challenging with fluid shifts, extensive surgical resections and blood loss adding to the challenges of pediatric anesthesia.

It involves meticulous planning and careful precision based management to ensure successful and favorable outcomes.

REFERENCES

1. López-Terrada D, Alaggio R, de Dávila MT, Czauderna P, Hiyama E, Katzenstein H et al.; Children's Oncology Group Liver Tumor Committee. Towards an international pediatric liver tumor consensus classification: Proceedings of the Los Angeles COG liver tumors symposium. Mod Pathol. 2014;27:472-91.
2. Darbari A, Sabin KM, Shapiro CN. Epidemiology of primary hepatic malignancies in US children. Hepatology. 2003;38:560-6.
3. Agarwala S. Primary malignant liver tumors in children. Indian J Pediatr. 2012;79:793–800.
4. American Childhood Cancer Organization. (2013). Childhood Cancer Statistics. [online] Available from https://www.acco.org/us-childhood-cancer-statistics/. [Last accessed on February, 2025].
5. Ismail H, Broniszczak D, Kalicinski P, Dembowska-Baginska B, Perek D, Teisseyre J, et al. Changing treatment and outcome of children with hepatoblastoma: analysis of a single center experience over the last 20 years. J Pediatr Surg. 2012;47:1331-9.
6. Kim T, Kim DY, Cho MJ, Kim SC, Seo JJ, Kim IK. Surgery for hepatoblastoma: from laparoscopic resection to liver transplantation. Hepatogastroenterology 2011;58:896-9.
7. Janitz AE, Ramachandran G, Tomlinson GE, Krailo M, Richardson M, et al. Maternal and paternal occupational exposures and hepatoblastoma: Results from the HOPE study through the Children's Oncology Group. J Expo Sci Environ Epidemiol. 2017;27: 359-64.
8. Buckley JD, Sather H, Ruccione K, Rogers PC, Haas JE, Henderson BE et al. A case-control study of risk factors for hepatoblastoma. A report from the Childrens Cancer Study Group. Cancer. 1989;64:1169-76.
9. Tomasz C, Marcin H, Natalia F, Dominik G, Ewelina B, Karolina W, et al. Hepatoblastoma in a one month infant – a case report. J Educ Health Sport. 2018;8:90-5.
10. Thomas D, Pritchard J, Davidson R, McKiernan P, Grundy RG, de Ville de Goyet J. Familial hepatoblastoma and APC gene mutations: Renewed call for molecular research. Eur J Cancer. 2003;39:2200-4.
11. McArthur JW, Toll GD, Russfield AB, Reiss AM, Quinby WC, Baker WH. Sexual precocity attributable to ectopic gonadotropin secretion by hepatoblastoma. Am J Med. 1973;54:390-403.
12. Schnater JM, Köhler SE, Lamers WH, von Schweinitz D, Aronson DC. Where do we stand with hepatoblastoma? A review. Cancer. 2003;98:668-78.
13. Fabre M, Yilmaz F, Buendia MA. Les tumeurs hépatiques de l'enfant: expérience à propos de 245 tumeurs et revue de la littérature [Hepatic tumors in childhood: experience on 245 tumors and review of literature]. Ann Pathol. 2004;24:536-55. French.
14. De Ioris M, Brugieres L, Zimmermann A, Keeling J, Brock P, Maibach R, et al. Hepatoblastoma with a low serum alpha-fetoprotein level at diagnosis: The SIOPEL group experience. Eur J Cancer. 2008;44:545-50.
15. Katzenstein HM, Langham MR, Malogolowkin MH, Krailo MD, Towbin AJ, McCarville MB, et al. Minimal adjuvant chemotherapy for children with hepatoblastoma resected at diagnosis (AHEP0731): a Children's Oncology Group, multicentre, phase 3 trial. Lancet Oncol. 2019; 20:719-27. Erratum in: Lancet Oncol. 2019;20:e243.
16. Brown J, Perilongo G, Shafford E, Keeling J, Pritchard J, Brock P, et al. Pretreatment prognostic factors for children with hepatoblastoma-results from the International Society of Paediatric Oncology (SIOP) study SIOPEL 1. Eur J Cancer. 2000;36:1418-25.
17. Feng J, He Y, Wei L, Chen D, Yang H, Tan R, et al. Assessment of survival of pediatric patients with hepatoblastoma who received chemotherapy following liver transplant or liver resection. JAMA Netw Open. 2019;2:e1912676.
18. Hiyama E, Hishiki T, Watanabe K, Ida K, Ueda Y, Kurihara S, et al. Outcome and late complications of hepatoblastomas treated using the japanese study group for pediatric liver tumor 2 protocol. J Clin Oncol. 2020;38:2488-98.
19. Ehrlich BS, McNeil MJ, Pham LTD, Chen Y, Rivera J, Acuna C, et al. Treatment-related mortality in children with cancer in low-income and middle-income countries: a systematic review and meta-analysis. Lancet Oncol. 2023;24:967-77.
20. Herzog CE, Andrassy RJ, Eftekhari F. Childhood cancers: Hepatoblastoma. Oncologist. 2000;5:445-53.
21. Loveland JA, Krog F, Beale P. A review of pediatric liver resections in Johannesburg: experiences and preferred technique. S Afr Med J. 2012;102:881-3.

22. Shoup M, Gonen M, D'Angelica M, Jarnagin WR, DeMatteo RP, Schwartz LH, et al. Volumetric analysis predicts hepatic dysfunction in patients undergoing major liver resection. J Gastrointest Surg. 2003;7:325-30.
23. Clavien PA, Petrowsky H, DeOliveira ML, Graf R. Strategies for safer liver surgery and partial liver transplantation. N Engl J Med. 2007;356:1545-59.
24. Perez EA, Gutierrez JC, Koniaris LG, Neville HL, Thompson WR, Sola JE. Malignant pancreatic tumors: incidence and outcome in 58 pediatric patients. J Pediatr Surg. 2009;44:197-203.
25. Nagtegaal ID, Odze RD, Klimstra D, Paradis V, Rugge M, Schirmacher P, et al. WHO Classification of Tumours Editorial Board. The 2019 WHO classification of tumours of the digestive system. Histopathology. 2020;76:182-8.
26. Hwang J, Kim DY, Kim SC, Namgoong JM, Hong SM. Solid-pseudopapillary neoplasm of the pancreas in children: can we predict malignancy? J Pediatr Surg. 2014;49:1730-3.
27. van den Akker M, Angelini P, Taylor G, Chami R, Gerstle JT, Gupta A. Malignant pancreatic tumors in children: a single-institution series. J Pediatr Surg. 2012;47:681-7.
28. Laje P, Bhatti TR, Adzick NS. Solid pseudopapillary neoplasm of the pancreas in children: a 15-year experience and the identification of a unique immunohistochemical marker. J Pediatr Surg. 2013;48:2054-60.
29. Speer AL, Barthel ER, Patel MM, Grikscheit TC. Solid pseudopapillary tumor of the pancreas: a single-institution 20-year series of pediatric patients. J Pediatr Surg. 2012; 47:1217-22.
30. Mao C, Guvendi M, Domenico DR, Kim K, Thomford NR, Howard JM. Papillary cystic and solid tumors of the pancreas: a pancreatic embryonic tumor? Studies of three cases and cumulative review of the world's literature. Surgery. 1995;118:821-8.
31. Rafeeqi T, Pearson EG. Enhanced recovery after surgery in children. Transl Gastroenterol Hepatol. 2021;6:46.
32. Frykholm P, Disma N, Andersson H, Beck C, Bouvet L, Cercueil E, et al. Pre-operative fasting in children: a guideline from the European Society of Anaesthesiology and Intensive Care. Eur J Anaesthesiol. 2022;39:4-25.
33. https://www.nysora.com/topics/sub-specialties/pediatric-anesthesia/pediatric-epidural-spinal-anesthesia-analgesia/ (last accessed on 9-12-2024).
34. Reynolds L, Beckmann J, Kurz A. Perioperative complications of hypothermia. Best Pract Res Clin Anaesthesiol. 2008;22:645-57.
35. Hartog A, Mills G. Anaesthesia for hepatic resection surgery. Contin Educ Anaesth Crit Care Pain. 2009;9:1-5.
36. Mogane P, Motshabi-Chakane P. Anaesthetic considerations for liver resections in paediatric patients. South Afr J Anaesth Analg. 2013;19:290-4.
37. Sansone L, Gentile C, Grasso EA, Di Ludovico A, La Bella S, Chiarelli F, et al. Pain evaluation and treatment in children: a practical approach. Children (Basel). 2023;10:1212.
38. Bakshi SG, Doctor JR, Trivedi BD, Qureshi SS. Transversus abdominis plane catheters for postoperative pain relief in pediatric patients. J Anaesthesiol Clin Pharmacol. 2017;33:121-2.
39. Lee H, Kim JT. Pediatric perioperative fluid management. Korean J Anesthesiol. 2023;76:519-530.
40. Li K, Jiang F, Aizpuru M, Larson EL, Xie X, Zhou R, et al. Successful management and technical aspects of major liver resection in children: a retrospective cohort study. Medicine 2021;100:6 (e24420).

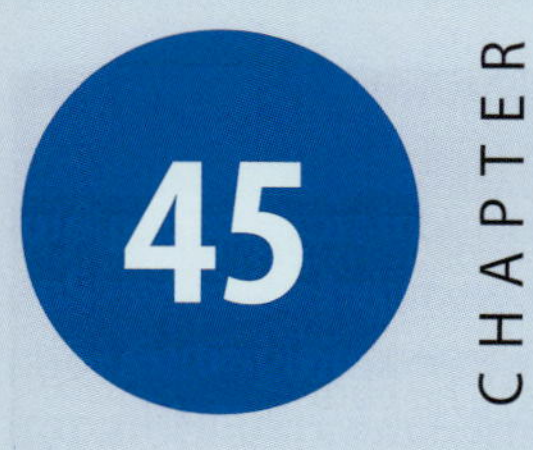

CHAPTER 45

Fluid Therapy and Hemodynamic Monitoring in Pediatric Major Abdominal Cancer Surgeries

Preethy J Mathew, Vighnesh Ashok

INTRODUCTION

Pediatric solid abdominal tumors encompass a heterogenous group of neoplasms arising from various tissues of the abdominal viscera. Most of the solid abdominal tumors in children arise from the kidneys (nephroblastoma), liver (hepatoblastoma), adrenal glands (neuroblastoma), or ovaries (germ cell tumors and teratomas).[1] While solid abdominal tumors are relatively rare compared to other childhood cancers, they still constitute a significant proportion of pediatric oncology cases. The exact incidence varies by tumor type, age, and gender. For instance, nephroblastoma typically occurs in children aged 2–5 years of age, while neuroblastomas occur much earlier in infancy and are more common in boys.[2] Surgery plays a crucial role in the management of these childhood cancers, with a primary aim to completely resect the tumor, while preserving organ function whenever possible. These surgeries are major involving considerable surgical time, large fluid shifts, significant blood loss, and the need for intraoperative fluid resuscitation. Thus, a clear understanding of fluid therapy and hemodynamic monitoring is essential for anesthesiologists providing for the perioperative care of these complex patients.

In this chapter, we aim to give a brief outline of pediatric fluid compartments and how children are different from adults in their perioperative fluid needs, before going into details about the principles and practices of intraoperative fluid therapy and hemodynamic monitoring in these children during surgery. We will also explain, briefly, the dynamic parameters available for intraoperative hemodynamic monitoring and guiding fluid therapy in children undergoing these complex surgeries.

PEDIATRIC FLUID COMPARTMENTS

The total body water (TBW) is predominantly distributed between the intracellular and extracellular compartments, with the transcellular fluid compartment (cerebrospinal fluid, peritoneal fluid, and synovial fluid) contributing a minor fraction.[3] Children have a higher percentage of TBW, comprising up to 90% of body weight in neonates, which decreases significantly during the first year of life and reaches adult levels of 60% after infancy.[4] TBW is primarily distributed in the extracellular compartment, and this proportion decreases from 40% in term neonates to adult levels of 20–25% during childhood.[5] As children grow, there is a gradual shift in fluid distribution, with a relative decrease in extracellular fluid and a concomitant increase in the intracellular fluid compartment reaching adult proportions in late childhood.

Besides the higher percentage of TBW, pediatric patients differ significantly from adults in their fluid requirements in the perioperative period for the following reasons:[6,7]

- Children have higher basal metabolic rates per unit of body weight compared to adults, thereby having greater fluid needs.
- The increased basal metabolism is also responsible for greater fluid losses through respiration, evaporation, and urine.
- Children possess a greater body surface area relative to their body weight compared to adults, increasing their insensible fluid losses during the perioperative period.
- Neonates and infants have immature kidneys with reduced ability to handle sodium loads and concentrate urine, leading to higher urine output per unit weight.

Understanding these crucial differences is essential for appropriate intraoperative fluid management in children with solid abdominal tumors undergoing surgery.

COMPONENTS OF PERIOPERATIVE FLUID THERAPY

The Association of Pediatric Anaesthetists guidelines describe pediatric perioperative fluid therapy as having three components.[8] The same principles would apply to children undergoing surgery for solid abdominal tumors resections, as well. The overall aim of perioperative fluid therapy is to maintain an optimal hydration status, ensure adequate intravascular volume to meet organ perfusion needs and tissue oxygenation, maintain normal electrolyte balance, and support ongoing metabolic requirements and calorie goals, through the administration of isotonic fluids.

The three components of perioperative fluid therapy are given in the following text:

1. *Correction of preexisting fluid deficits due to preoperative fasting (either due to the disease condition or due to mandated fasting before induction of general anesthesia), dehydration, and gastrointestinal fluid losses.*

   Current guidelines for preoperative fasting recommend ad-lib clear fluids until 2 hours before surgery to minimize preoperative deficits.[9] Nevertheless, children with abdominal tumors may have reduced oral intake due to loss of appetite or chemotherapy-induced nausea and vomiting. Hence, preoperative fasting duration should be estimated meticulously to replace this deficit by multiplying the number of hours of fasting with the maintenance fluid requirements per hour. It is recommended to administer half of this calculated volume in the first hour and the remaining half over the next 2 hours.[10] Considering that the abdominal tumors are usually resected as part of a planned treatment, it is imperative to (p)re-hydrate children with poor oral intake and dehydration before surgery. Such (p)re-hydration may require intravenous fluid therapy for 24–48 hours preceding the scheduled surgery. Dehydration, if present in the immediate preoperative period, would need an aggressive fluid replacement with 20–40 mL/kg of a balanced salt solution till the time the child appears well or is hemodynamically stable.[7]

2. *Administration of maintenance fluids to meet ongoing metabolic requirements for water, glucose, and electrolytes.*

   The volume of fluid administered is traditionally estimated using the Holliday and Segar 4-2-1 regimen **(Table 1)** to calculate the hourly fluid requirement, namely 4 mL/kg for children <10 kg, 40 mL + 2 mL/kg above 10 kg for children between 10–20 kgs, and 60 mL + 1 mL/kg above 20 kg for children weighing >20 kg.[11]

TABLE 1: Holliday–Segar 4:2:1 rule for calculation of the volume of intraoperative maintenance fluids.

Weight (kg)	*Fluid requirement per hour intraoperatively*
<10	4 mL/kg
10–20	40 mL + 2 mL/kg for each kg above 10 kg
>20	60 mL + 1 mL/kg for each kg above 20 kg

   The composition of maintenance fluid is discussed in the next section.

3. *Replacement of ongoing losses during surgery:* Ongoing losses include surgical bleeding, insensible water loss into the respiratory circuit and from exposed body surfaces, and evaporative losses from exposed visceral surfaces, as applicable.[4] The occurrence and significance of "third-space" losses described in earlier studies and literature are currently a matter of debate, particularly in the pediatric population. The evaporative losses from visceral surfaces can be significant during abdominal surgery and require replacement at varying rates depending on the extent of surgery. Most major abdominal surgeries in children would require around 5–10 mL/kg/hr of fluid replacement intraoperatively.[12]

CHOICE OF INTRAOPERATIVE FLUID THERAPY

Hypotonic Versus Isotonic Fluids

Historically, hypotonic solutions were suggested as maintenance fluids in the pediatric population due to concerns about renal immaturity in neonates and early infancy.[13] Over the years, clinical evidence has consistently demonstrated the significant risk of postoperative hyponatremia with perioperative administration of hypotonic solutions.[14,15] The mechanism for the development of hyponatremia is two-fold. While dilutional hyponatremia occurs initially due to the administration of hypotonic solutions, the subsequent osmotic and nonosmotic triggers during surgery result in the release of antidiuretic hormone that further leads to active water retention worsening hyponatremia.[14] Thus, most current guidelines from national and international organizations recommend the routine use of isotonic balanced salt solutions during pediatric surgery.[16]

While normal saline is the cheapest and the most widely used isotonic crystalloid solution, studies have shown that large-volume resuscitation with normal saline can lead to the development of hyperchloremic metabolic acidosis,

TABLE 2: Composition and osmolarity of commonly available intravenous fluids in pediatrics.

Electrolytes	*Normal saline*	*Ringer's lactate*	*Isolyte P*	*PlasmaLyte*	*D5*	*Albumin 5%*	*Hetastarch 6%*
Na^+	154	130	26	140	–	145 + 15	154
K^+	–	4	21	5	–	<2.5	–
Cl^-	154	109	21	98	–	100	154
Mg^{2+}	–	–	3	–	–	–	–
Acetate	–	–	24	27	–	–	–
Lactate	–	28	–	–	–	–	–
Glucose (g%)	–	–	5	–	5	–	–
Phosphate (mg%)	–	–	3	–	–	–	–
Osmolarity (mOsm/L)	308	274	340	295	252	330	310

which can have negative perioperative consequences.[17] On the other hand, balanced salt solutions closely mimic the electrolyte composition of human plasma, thereby minimizing disturbances in acid–base balance and electrolyte levels when administered to patients. Ringer's lactate, Hartmann's solution, Isolyte P, and PlasmaLyte are some of the commonly used balanced salt solutions used in pediatric patients and have been shown to maintain better acid–base status in children undergoing major abdominal surgery.[18,19] **Table 2** describes the composition and osmolarity of some of the commonly used fluids perioperatively. Currently, there is not enough evidence to recommend any one BSS over the other for major pediatric cancer surgeries, and the choice of BSS used would depend on the availability, anesthesiologist preference, and institute protocols.

Role of Dextrose-containing Fluids Intraoperatively

Supplementation of glucose is usually not necessary in otherwise healthy children undergoing a major cancer surgery. Unnecessary glucose supplementation can cause iatrogenic hyperglycemia, which can have negative patient consequences.[20] Beyond the neonatal timeframe, pediatric patients have sufficient reserves to meet their metabolic requirements during surgery. However, children with significant malnutrition, hypermetabolic states, critical illness, and mitochondrial disorders would require glucose supplementation intraoperatively. When indicated, the addition of 1–2.5% dextrose to the intraoperative maintenance fluid is sufficient to provide body glucose requirement and prevent hypoglycemia and ketoacidosis, without an added risk of hyperglycemia.[16] In prolonged cancer surgery, it could be reasonable to monitor blood glucose concentrations periodically and correct hypoglycemia if it occurs.

Role of Colloids

Colloids contain noncrystalline particles suspended in a balanced salt solution and remain within the intravascular compartment following infusion, resulting in better expansion of plasma volume.[21] Colloids either can be synthetic (hydroxyethyl starch, dextran, gelatin) or can be derived from blood (human albumin). While the use of dextran and gelatin in pediatric surgical patients is limited due to the risk of anaphylaxis, hydroxyethyl starch has been used in pediatric surgical patients with no serious adverse effects.[22] However, just as in adults, the use of hydroxyethyl starch is cautioned in children with preexisting renal impairment. Albumin remains the main colloid for rapid volume expansion in neonates and infants. While being less allergic than synthetic colloids, albumin is more expensive to produce and store. 5% albumin is isotonic to plasma and a good intraoperative plasma volume expander in hypotensive infants under general anesthesia and can be used intraoperatively in hemodynamically unstable infants during abdominal cancer surgery.[23]

Blood Component Therapy

The need for transfusion of blood products in the intraoperative period is a highly individualized decision depending on the child's age, baseline hemoglobin, severity and rapidity of blood loss, and the patient's hemodynamic status.[24] The maximum allowable blood loss is a useful parameter to calculate for every pediatric patient undergoing major cancer surgery, to guide anesthesiologists regarding the need for intraoperative transfusion of packed cells. The transfusion trigger for major abdominal surgeries is usually accepted around 7–8 g/dL.[25] Excessive administration of intravenous fluids can lead to dilution of platelets and coagulation factors, leading to thrombocytopenia and coagulopathy, respectively. In this context, the transfusion of other blood components such as fresh frozen plasma and platelets would be dictated by clinical factors and point-of-care testing.

Vasoactive Drugs

In case of acute hemodynamic instability or persistent hypotension unresponsive to intravenous fluid resuscitation, it would be prudent to start vasoactive medications to ensure adequate microcirculation and tissue perfusion to mitigate the development of metabolic acidosis. Vasoactive drugs could be either vasopressors (phenylephrine, norepinephrine) or inotropes (dopamine, dobutamine, epinephrine). While the evidence to guide the appropriate choice of vasoactive drug in pediatric hemorrhagic shock is limited, dopamine and, to a lesser extent, dobutamine are used in clinical practice to augment blood pressure and stabilize hemodynamics in the intraoperative period.

HEMODYNAMIC MONITORING TO GUIDE FLUID THERAPY

Liberal Versus Restrictive Fluid Therapy

Liberal and restrictive fluid therapies represent two contrasting approaches in intraoperative fluid administration.[26] The traditional approach has been a liberal fluid therapy based on concerns to prevent hypovolemia and aimed to administer intravenous fluids more freely to maintain hemodynamic stability while reducing the incidence of hypotension and improving tissue perfusion. This approach has been found to be associated with increased risks of fluid overload, pulmonary complications, bowel edema, and longer postoperative recovery times.[27] Thus, more restrictive strategies for intraoperative fluid administration were developed to minimize fluid overload and its antecedent risks while ensuring adequate tissue perfusion.[28] However, the clinical evidence base for either of the two strategies in pediatric surgery is still conflicting in terms of the real impact of these contrasting strategies on intraoperative fluid management.

Goal-directed Fluid Therapy

There is growing emphasis on goal-directed fluid therapy (GDFT) where fluid administration is guided by real-time monitoring of specific hemodynamic parameters to optimize tissue perfusion while at the same time minimizing the risk of under-resuscitation or fluid overload.[29,30] Indeed, individualized fluid management based on patient-specific factors, the surgical procedure being performed, and ongoing assessment of the patient's fluid status rather than strict adherence to either liberal or restrictive therapy protocols is recommended. A key feature of such individualized and goal-directed administration of intraoperative fluids is the careful assessment of the pediatric patient's "fluid responsiveness" to guide further resuscitative efforts.[31]

Fluid Responsiveness

Fluid responsiveness describes the ability of intravenous fluids to improve cardiovascular function, tissue perfusion, and cellular metabolic physiology and is defined as an increase in cardiac output (or stroke volume) by a certain predefined magnitude (usually 10–15%) in response to a fluid bolus (fluid challenge).[32] Several hemodynamic variables have been studied as potential predictors of fluid responsiveness, with varying clinical values and usefulness. The goal of intraoperative hemodynamic monitoring is to optimize tissue perfusion and oxygen delivery while avoiding both under- and overhydration.[33]

Fluid administration is conventionally monitored using parameters such as heart rate, systolic or mean arterial blood pressure, central venous pressure, and urine output. Since these parameters are not directly influenced by cardiopulmonary interactions and therefore do not reflect changes in cardiac output, these are technically classified as static parameters and have poor predictive values for determining fluid responsiveness in children.[34] In contrast, dynamic assessment of fluid responsiveness utilizes variables that reflect cardiopulmonary interactions and are derived from either the arterial waveform, plethysmographic tracing, or Doppler echocardiographic tracings and have shown to be more useful in gauging pediatric fluid responsiveness.[35] The following sections will describe briefly the physiological basis of these parameters and summarize the evidence base for their use in children undergoing surgery.

DYNAMIC PREDICTORS OF FLUID RESPONSIVENESS

Unlike static predictors which are hemodynamic parameters at a particular point in time, dynamic predictors quantify the effect of a specific preload-altering maneuver (for instance, mechanical breath) on a cardiovascular response (change in stroke volume or cardiac output).[36] The increase in intrathoracic pressure during a mechanical breath causes a transient decrease in venous return. Approximately three heartbeats later (reflecting the pulmonary transit time), the effect of this decreased venous return is seen as a decrease in the left ventricular end-diastolic volume and the stroke volume.[35] This change is further reflected downstream as variations in aortic blood flow, arterial blood pressure, and plethysmographic waveforms from which are derived most of the commonly used dynamic predictor variables.[37] The degree of variation observed is greater in hypovolemic patients functioning in the steep portion of Frank–Starling curve (fluid responders) **(Fig. 1)**.[38,39] Thus, dynamic predictors reflect the variation in preload (venous return) induced by mechanical ventilation to identify responders for fluid boluses.

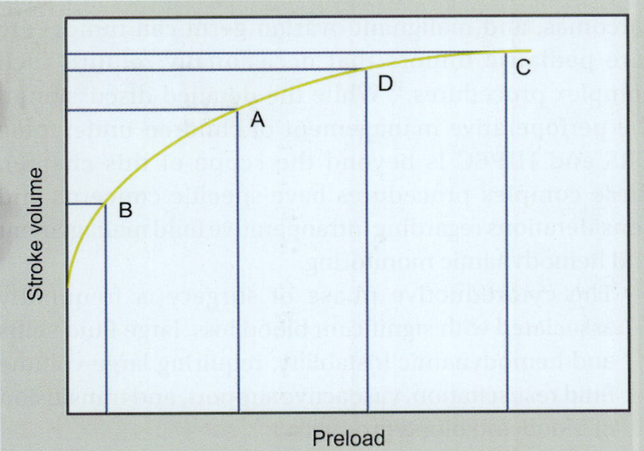

Fig. 1: Left ventricular function curve describing the effect of changes in preload on the stroke volume (Frank–Starling mechanism). The decrease in venous return during a positive pressure breath causes a significant decrease in stroke volume (A to B) when the patient is on the steep portion of the curve (fluid responder) compared to a small decrease in stroke volume (C to D) in a fluid nonresponder.

Variables Derived from the Arterial Pressure Waveform

Systolic pressure variation (SPV), pulse pressure variation (PPV), and stroke volume variation (SVV) are the three parameters derived from the arterial pressure waveform that have been studied as dynamic predictors of fluid responsiveness in pediatric patients.[40-42] While SPV and PPV can be measured using an indwelling arterial catheter, SVV has been measured using pulse contour analysis technology with the help of monitors such as PiCCO (Pulsion Medical Systems SE, Feldkirchen, Germany), Vygon (Vytech, Ecouen, France), and Flotrac (Edwards Lifesciences, California, United States). However, in contrast to the strong evidence in adult surgical patients, the reliability of these indices as dynamic predictors of fluid responsiveness in children has been poor, and the reasons are multiple.

The arterial pressure waveform tracing is dependent not just on the stroke volume, but also on the arterial elastance (or recoil property) which is a parameter that is different in the pediatric population, as compared to adults. Furthermore, the elastance properties of the vascular tree also change depending on the age of the pediatric population being studied. Moreover, the pulse-wave velocity of the limb arteries has been shown to increase nonlinearly with age.[43] Finally, the basis behind these dynamic predictors is the cardiopulmonary interaction which is subjective to lung compliance, chest wall elastance, and airway resistance, which are all significantly different in children compared to adults, limiting the perioperative use of SPV, PPV, and SVV in pediatric patients.[44]

Variables Derived from the Plethysmography Waveform

The plethysmographic variability index (PVI) is measured as the dynamic changes in the perfusion index (PI) during a single respiratory cycle and is derived from the plethysmographic waveform. The PVI is calculated as the difference between the maximum and minimum values of the PI (the ratio of pulsatile to nonpulsatile infrared absorption) during a single mechanical breath divided by the maximum PI.

$$PVI = \frac{PI_{max} - PI_{min}}{PI_{max}} \times 100$$

Several studies have evaluated the utility of PVI to determine fluid responsiveness in pediatric patients, with varying results. The cutoff of PVI in mechanically ventilated pediatric patients has been reported to be between 11 and 17%.[45]

Overall, as the plethysmographic waveform is derived from changes in vessel volume rather than pressure, PVI appears to be more independent of the effect of lung compliance, chest wall elastance, and vessel recoil, thereby having a better utility to predict fluid responsiveness in pediatric surgical patients, compared to SPV, PPV, and SVV. However, obtaining an accurate and stable pulse oximetry trace may be challenging in smaller children and could also be influenced by concomitant use of electrocautery and regional blood flow in the fingers (hypothermia, use of vasopressors, etc.).

Echocardiography-based Variables

Aortic blood flow peak velocity (ΔVPeak), aortic velocity and time integral (ΔVTI) are flow-based variables that can be measured either transthoracic or transesophageal at the left ventricular outflow tract or the ascending aorta by Doppler echocardiography.[42] Of these, the respiratory variation of peak velocity of aortic blood flow (ΔVPeak), measured as the difference between the maximum peak velocity and the minimum peak velocity divided by the mean peak velocity over a single respiratory cycle, is the most consistent predictor of fluid responsiveness in mechanically ventilated pediatric patients.[42]

Unlike the other dynamic predictors, ΔVPeak is not affected by changes in peripheral perfusion or arterial compliance. A wide range of cutoffs to distinguish between fluid responders and nonresponders has been described in children, ranging from 7 to 20%.[42] The use of these variables in clinical practice is, however, limited by the need for expensive equipment and skilled expertise to interpret the echocardiographic findings. Furthermore, unlike parameters derived from the arterial waveform and the plethysmographic trace which are continuous hemodynamic data, flow-based variables are measured intermittently. Intermittent dynamic predictors, understandably, identify hemodynamic changes later than continuous dynamic predictors impacting their clinical utility.

Other Dynamic Predictors

Other dynamic predictors of fluid responsiveness have very low to no utility in pediatric surgical patients.[41]

- The classical passive leg raise test has very limited applicability in the intraoperative period, due to interruption of surgery and potential disruption of the sterile surgical field.
- While respiratory variations in inferior vena cava diameter have been studied in adults to have good predictive value, the results in children have been far less encouraging. Furthermore, from a practical standpoint, measuring changes in the diameter of the inferior vena cava is unfeasible in abdominal surgeries for solid organ tumor resection.
- Noninvasive cardiac output monitors based on thoracic electrical bioimpedance (NICOM, Cheetah Medical Inc, Baxter, Deerfield, United States; Physioflow, Neumedx Inc, Manatec Biomedical, France) have been used to measure changes in thoracic blood velocity through the cardiorespiratory cycle. Studies in the pediatric population are, so far, limited with varying results. Furthermore, their use in the intraoperative period may be limited by motion artifacts and interference from electrocautery.

SPECIAL SITUATIONS

Cytoreductive Surgery and Hyperthermic Intraperitoneal Chemotherapy

Pediatric patients with peritoneal carcinomatosis require more complex cytoreductive surgery (CRS) with or without the intraoperative use of hyperthermic intraperitoneal chemotherapy (HIPEC) to reduce the disease burden. Desmoplastic small, round cell tumor, sarcomas, and malignant ovarian germ cell tumors are rare pediatric tumors that occasionally require such complex procedures.[46] While the detailed discussion of the perioperative management of children undergoing CRS and HIPEC is beyond the scope of this chapter, these complex procedures have specific concerns and considerations regarding intraoperative fluid management and hemodynamic monitoring.

- The cytoreductive phase of surgery is frequently associated with significant blood loss, large fluid shifts and hemodynamic instability, requiring large-volume fluid resuscitation, vasoactive support, and transfusion of blood and blood products.
- Hyperthermia during the heated chemotherapy phase leads to hyperdynamic circulation with vasodilatation, tachycardia, and an increased cardiac output. There is also greater insensible fluid loss in this phase due to hyperthermia.
- Transperitoneal absorption of carrier fluid (usually normal saline with/without dextrose) used during the

instillation of chemotherapy can result in intravascular volume overload, dilutional dyselectrolytemia, blood glucose fluctuations, and pulmonary edema.

- Hemodynamic fluctuations, use of cytotoxic drugs, and hyperthermia increase the risk of acute kidney injury, which can be worsened due to inadvertent fluid under-resuscitation.

While earlier recommendations favored liberal fluid therapy in adult patients undergoing HIPEC procedures as part of CRS, the recognition of subsequent complications of fluid overload on patient morbidity and mortality has led to a less liberal approach. On the other hand, the use of a very restrictive fluid approach could be associated with a higher risk of hemodynamic instability, acute kidney injury, and metabolic acidosis. While the optimal fluid therapy strategy for these procedures in children is still unclear, it is reasonable to use some form of GDFT using dynamic predictors of fluid responsiveness to individualize and optimize intraoperative fluid administration and patient outcomes.[47] Further work needs to be done and reported in this area before more concrete recommendations can be made.

CONCLUSION

Surgery for resection of abdominal tumors in children is a complex procedure with unique challenges. Due to the significant risk of blood loss and large fluid shifts, these children require careful management of their intraoperative fluid requirements. While liberal and restrictive fluid therapies have their advantages and disadvantages, using a more individualized and goal-directed hemodynamic strategy with the incorporation of dynamic predictors of fluid responsiveness could benefit patient outcomes postoperatively. A clear understanding of the various available parameters and the required technology is crucial for anesthesiologists to provide optimum perioperative care for these challenging patient populations. Currently, parameters derived from respiratory changes in the plethysmographic waveform and aortic blood flow peak velocity offer the best strategies to guide intraoperative fluid management in these patients. More work is needed to identify suitable cutoffs and validate patient outcomes.

REFERENCES

1. Allen-Rhoades W, Whittle SB, Rainusso N. Pediatric solid tumors in children and adolescents: an overview. Pediatr Rev. 2018;39:444-53.
2. Dumba M, Jawad N, McHugh K. Neuroblastoma and nephroblastoma: an overview and comparison. Cancer Imaging. 2014;14:O15.
3. Bhardwaj N. Perioperative fluid therapy and intraoperative blood loss in children. Indian J Anaesth. 2019;63:729-36.
4. Meyers RS. Pediatric fluid and electrolyte therapy. J Pediatr Pharmacol Ther. 2009;14:204-11.
5. Sümpelmann R, Vennari M, Agrò FE. Fluid management in pediatric patients. In: Agrò FE (Ed). Body Fluid Management. Milano: Springer; 2013. pp. 165-73.
6. Sümpelmann R, Becke K, Zander R, Witt L. Perioperative fluid management in children: Can we sum it all up now? Curr Opin Anesthesiol. 2019;32:384-91.
7. Jain A. Body fluid composition. Pediatr Rev. 2015;36:141-52.
8. Murat I, Dubois M-C. Perioperative fluid therapy in pediatrics. Pediatr Anesth. 2008;18:363-70.
9. Thomas M, Morrison C, Newton R, Schindler E. Consensus statement on clear fluids fasting for elective pediatric general anesthesia. Paediatr Anaesth. 2018;28:411-4.
10. Smith I, Kranke P, Murat I, Smith A, O'Sullivan G, Søreide E, et al. Perioperative fasting in adults and children: Guidelines from the European Society of Anaesthesiology. Eur J Anaesthesiol. 2011;28:556-69.
11. Holliday MA, Segar WE. The maintenance need for water in parenteral fluid therapy. Pediatrics. 1957;19:823-32.
12. Mathew A, Rai E. Pediatric perioperative fluid management. Saudi J Anaesth. 2021;15:435-40.
13. McNab S, Ware RS, Neville KA, Choong K, Coulthard MG, Duke T, et al. Isotonic versus hypotonic solutions for maintenance intravenous fluid administration in children (review). Cochrane Database Syst Rev. 2014;12:CD009457.
14. Halberthal M, Halperin ML, Bohn D. Lesson of the week: acute hyponatremia in children admitted to hospital: retrospective analysis of factors contributing to its development and resolution. BMJ. 2001;322:780-2.
15. Arieff A. Postoperative hyponatraemic encephalopathy following elective surgery in children. Pediatr Anesth. 1998;8:1-4.
16. Eaddy N, Watene C. Perioperative management of fluids and electrolytes in children. BJA Educ. 2023;23:273-8.
17. Eisenhut M. Adverse effects of rapid isotonic saline infusion. Arch Dis Child. 2006;91:797.
18. Semler MW, Kellum JA. Balanced crystalloid solutions. Am J Respir Crit Care Med. 2019;199(8):952-60.
19. Disma N, Mameli L, Pistorio A, Davidson A, Barabino P, Locatelli BG, et al. A novel balanced isotonic sodium solution vs normal saline during major surgery in children up to 36 months: a multicenter RCT. Paediatr Anaesth. 2014;24:980-6.
20. Nishina K, Mikawa K, Maekawa N, Asano M, Obara H. Effects of exogenous intravenous glucose on plasma glucose and lipid homeostasis in anaesthetized infants. Anesthesiology. 1995;83:258-63.

21. Saudan S. Is the use of colloids for fluid replacement harmless in children? Curr Opin Anaesthesiol. 2010;23:363-7.
22. Sümpelmann R, Kretz FR, Luntzer R, de Leeuw TG, Mixa V, Gäbler R, et al. Hydroxyethyl starch 130/0.42/6:1 for perioperative plasma volume replacement in 1130 children: results of a European Prospective Multicenter Observational Postauthorization Safety Study (PASS). Paediatr Anaesth. 2012;22:371-8.
23. Van der linden P, De Ville A, Hofer A, Heschl M, Gombotz H. Six percent hydroxyethyl starch 130/0.4 (Voluven®) versus 5% human serum albumin for volume replacement therapy during elective open-heart surgery in pediatric patients. Anesthesiology. 2013;119:1296-309.
24. Morley SL. Red blood cell transfusions in acute pediatrics. Arch Dis Child Educ Pract. 2009;94:65-73.
25. Dehmer JJ, Adamson WT. Massive transfusion and blood product use in the pediatric trauma patient. Semin Pediatr Surg. 2010;19:286-91.
26. Nisanevich V, Felsenstein I, Almogy G, Weissman C, Einav S, Matot I. Effect of intraoperative fluid management on outcome after intraabdominal surgery. Anesthesiology. 2005;103:25-32.
27. Holte K, Sharrock NE, Kehlet H. Pathophysiology and clinical implications of perioperative fluid excess. Br J Anaesth. 2002;89:622-32.
28. Brandstrup B, Tonnesen H, Beier-Holgersen R, Hjortso E, Ording H, Lindorff Larsen K, et al. Effects of intravenous fluid restriction on postoperative complications: comparison of two perioperative fluid regimens. Ann Surg. 2003;238:641-8.
29. Kendrick JB, Kaye AD, Tong Y, Belani K, Urman R, Hoffman C, et al. Goal-directed fluid therapy in the perioperative setting. J Anaesthesiol Clin Pharmacol. 2019;35:S29-S34.
30. Miller TE, Roche AM, Mythen M. Fluid management and goal-directed therapy as an adjunct to enhanced recovery after surgery (ERAS). Can J Anaesth. 2015;62:158-68.
31. Marik PE, Lemson J. Fluid responsiveness: an evolution of our understanding. Br J Anaesth. 2014;112:617-20.
32. Messina A, Pelaia C, Bruni A, Garofalo E, Bonicolini E, Longhini F, et al. Fluid challenge during anesthesia: a systematic review and meta-analysis. Anesth Analg. 2018;127:1353-64.
33. Vincent JL, Weil MH. Fluid challenge revisited. Crit Care Med. 2006;34:1333-7.
34. Marik PE, Monnet X, Teboul JL. Hemodynamic parameters to guide fluid therapy. Ann Intensive Care. 2011;1:1.
35. Cherpanath TGV, Geerts BF, Lagrand WK, Schultz MJ, Groeneveld ABJ. Basic concepts of fluid responsiveness. Neth Heart J. 2013;21:530-6.
36. Geurin L, Monnet X, Teboul JL. Monitoring volume and fluid responsiveness: from static to dynamic indicators. Best Pract Res Clin Anaesthesiol. 2013;27:177-85.
37. Cavallaro F, Sandroni C, Antonelli M. Functional hemodynamic monitoring and dynamic indices of fluid responsiveness. Minerva Anestesiol. 2008;74:123-35.
38. Frank O. On the dynamics of cardiac muscle. Am Heart J. 1959;58:282-317.
39. Starling EH. The Linacre Lecture on the Law of the Heart Given at Cambridge, 1915. Nature. 1918;101:43.
40. Gan H, Cannesson M, Chandler JR and Ansermino JM. Predicting fluid responsiveness in children: a systematic review. Anesth Analg. 2013;117(6):1380-92.
41. Lee JH, Kim EH, Jang YE, Kim HS, Kim JT. Fluid responsiveness in the pediatric population. Korean J Anesthesiol. 2019;72(5):429-40.
42. Pereira de Souza Neto E, Grousson S, Duflo F, Ducreux C, Joly H, Convert J, et al. Predicting fluid responsiveness in mechanically ventilated children under general anaesthesia using dynamic parameters and transthoracic echocardiography. Br J Anaesth. 2011;106(6):856-64.
43. Michard F, Boussat S, Chemla D, Anguel N, Mercat A, Lecarpentier Y, et al. Relation between respiratory changes in arterial pulse pressure and fluid responsiveness in septic patients with acute circulatory failure. Am J Respir Crit Care Med. 2000;162:134-8.
44. Chemla D, Hebert JL, Coirault C, Zamani K, Suard I, Colin P, et al. Total arterial compliance estimated by stroke volume-to-aortic pulse pressure ratio in humans. Am J Physiol. 1998;274:500-5.
45. Cannesson M, Attof Y, Rosamel P, Desebbe O, Joseph P, Metton O, et al. Respiratory variations in pulse oximetry plethysmographic waveform amplitude to predict fluid responsiveness in the operating room. Anesthesiology. 2007;106:1105-11.
46. Durnford S, Boss L, Bell J. Cytoreductive surgery and hyperthermic intraperitoneal chemotherapy. BJA Educ. 2021;21:187-93.
47. Gupta N, Kumar V, Garg R, Bharti SJ, Mishra S, Bhatnagar S. Anesthetic implications in hyperthermic intraperitoneal chemotherapy. J Anaesthesiol Clin Pharmacol. 2019; 35:3-11.

SECTION 11

Bone and Soft Tissue Onco-Anesthesia

46 CHAPTER

Anesthesia for Hemipelvectomy

Gauri Raman Gangakhedkar, Bhuvaneswari Balasubramanian, Unmesh Pramod Bedekar

INTRODUCTION

Hemipelvectomy, a complex major surgical procedure involving the removal of "part or all" of the pelvis, is relatively rare. It is typically performed in cases of malignancies such as sarcomas, metastatic cancers, or severe trauma. With regards to pelvic tumors, the prognosis is poorer than other tumors, since these tumors are larger at presentation than most tumors and their proximity to neurovascular structures, gastrointestinal tract, and urinary tract potentiates the possibility of their involvement.[1] Bone and soft tissue sarcomas of the musculoskeletal system are rare and account for 0.16% and 0.3% of all newly diagnosed tumors.[2]

The procedure is associated with high rates of complications, including infection, wound healing problems, and significant blood loss. Functional impairment is also a major concern, as the surgery often results in the loss of limb function and necessitates extensive rehabilitation. Given the complexity and risks associated with hemipelvectomy, a multidisciplinary approach is essential. Effective collaboration between oncologists, orthopedic surgeons, plastic surgeons, anesthesiologists, rehabilitation specialists, and nursing staff is essential for optimizing surgical outcomes, managing complications, and ensuring effective postoperative rehabilitation and support for the patient. Furthermore, the psychological impact of such a major surgery necessitates ongoing mental health support.

SURGICAL PERSPECTIVE

Hemipelvectomy-level amputations are generally carried out at major tertiary medical centers for the management of soft tissue and bone tumors. Chondrosarcoma is the most prevalent primary tumor of the pelvis, with Ewing's sarcoma and osteosarcoma ranking as the subsequent most common tumors.[3] However, additional indications for this procedure consist of infection, ischemia, prior myelopathy with persistent nonhealing wounds, and extensive trauma.[4]

TABLE 1: Types of hemipelvectomy with extent.[6]

Type of hemipelvectomy	*Zone of involvement*
Type 1	Ilium
Type 2	Acetabulum/periacetabular region
Type 3	Pubis
Type 4 (extended type 1)	Hemisacrum

Over the past two decades, the development and use of advanced diagnostic and adjuvant therapies have allowed orthopedicians to offer limb preserving (internal hemipelvectomy) surgeries, thus allowing a better return of functionality.[5] The indications of an external hemipelvectomy are now limited to tumors that cannot be removed using limb-sparing methods, with safe margins and to offer palliative care for patients experiencing pain or discomfort that cannot be alleviated by less invasive treatments.[6] Surgical classifications of hemipelvectomies, i.e., Enneking's classification, is based on the region of the pelvis involved and is given in **Table 1**. One or more of the pelvic zones are resected, size, and extent of lesion.[7]

PREOPERATIVE IMAGING

Before planning a patient for local surgery, assessment of distal metastasis using positron emission tomography-computed tomography (PET-CT), magnetic resonance imaging (MRI), or CT thorax-abdomen and three-phase skeletal scintigraphy should assessed to understand prognosis. The extent of surgery is decided after reviewing compartment MRI imaging with contrast medium, no older than 4 weeks. In addition to the MRI, a CT is helpful in bony tumors, such as osteosarcomas and chondrosarcomas.

ANESTHETIC CONCERNS

The anesthetic concerns that arise in patients undergoing hemipelvectomies are diverse and span from the preoperative to the postoperative period. A summary of these concerns is enlisted as **Box 1**.

PREOPERATIVE CONCERNS

Patient Factors

The mean age of patients presenting for surgery was found to be 49 years in a study by Guder et al.[2] Since, patients who have bone or soft tissue malignancies, undergo neoadjuvant chemotherapy and radiation, finding issues such as significant anemia and thrombocytopenia are not uncommon.[8] These patients might thus need preoperative exogenous erythropoietin administration and blood and blood product transfusion.[9]

Preoperative evaluation for these patients usually includes a basic hematological work-up, imaging of the lesion, cardiorespiratory fitness, assessment of comorbidities, and functional evaluation to assess for tolerance to sustain massive, anticipated blood loss. This would include blood tests including complete blood count, renal, and liver function tests, serum electrolytes, and coagulation profile. From the perspective of cardiorespiratory fitness, electrocardiogram, echocardiography, and pulmonary function tests may be required, depending on the nature of chemotherapy provided. The names, side effects, and anesthetic implications of the various chemotherapeutic agents are mentioned in **Table 2**.

Depending on the extent of the disease, a preoperative consultation with surgical oncologists, urologists, and plastic surgeons are recommended.[10] Preoperative imaging also helps in determining the vascularity of the tumor and enables possible radiological intervention in the form of angioembolization in highly vascular tumors. Preoperative bowel preparation using laxatives should be undertaken to improve intraoperative visibility and minimize the risk of bacterial contamination from potential bowel injuries. A large number of patients are poorly nourished and require nutrition consultations with parenteral nutrition to ensure better outcomes. Additionally, placing a diverted ureteral stent can be advantageous for large tumors on the pelvic side, as it helps prevent ureteral injury. The role of multidisciplinary involvement is highlighted in **Table 3**.

Additionally, the preoperative evaluation period is used to investigate and optimize other comorbidities that the patient may have. Once the risk stratification is complete, a written informed consent with documentation of possible risks is taken and adequate blood and blood products are reserved.

BOX 1: Summary of anesthetic concerns.

Preoperative concerns:
- Multidisciplinary evaluation for the extent of surgery
- Concerns regarding chemotherapy
- Prehabilitation
- Optimization of comorbidities
- Written informed consent with documentation of risks

Intraoperative concerns:
- SSI prophylaxis
- GA + epidural/MMA
- *Monitoring:* ASA + POC monitor+ IBP ± TEE + CO
- Positioning concerns
- Adequate fluid replacement
- Blood loss estimation
- MTP
- Blood loss and transfusion-reducing strategies

Postoperative concerns:
- ICU/HDU for close monitoring
- Continue blood loss correction
- Thromboprophylaxis
- PONV treatment
- Analgesia
- Physiotherapy and rehabilitation

(ASA: American Society of Anesthesiologists; CO: cardiac output; IBP: intraoperative blood pressure; GA: general anesthesia; HDU: high-dependency unit; ICU: intensive care unit; MMA: middle meningeal artery; MTP: massive transfusion protocol; PONV: postoperative nausea and vomiting; SSI: surgical site infection; TEE: transesophageal echocardiogram)

Prehabilitation

Prehabilitation forms a crucial aspect of ensuring better patient outcomes. It focuses on improving the patient's physical and psychological condition before surgery and using a three-pronged approach including, physical therapy to boost strength and endurance, nutritional support to optimize body weight and nutrient reserves, and psychological support to prepare the patient mentally for the procedure and recovery. Evidence indicates that prehabilitation effectively reduces postoperative complications and shortens hospital stays.[11]

Physical therapy aims at increasing strength and conditioning the muscles so rehabilitation and mobilization become easier. Preoperative counseling and psychotherapy are crucial due to the profound impact of

TABLE 2: Chemotherapeutic agents and their implications.[8]

Class of chemotherapeutic agent	*Name of specific chemotherapeutic agents*	*Anticipated side effects*	*Anesthetic implications*
Anthracyclines	• Doxorubicin • Daunorubicin	ECG changes such as ST-T changes, bundle branch blocks, QT-prolongation, and dysrhythmias. Pericarditis, myocardial dysfunction, pericardial effusion	Anticipate exaggerated myocardial depression with anesthesia, and preoperative echocardiography to evaluate cardiac function, serum electrolytes
Platinum analogs	• Cisplatin • Carboplatin	Peripheral neuropathy, nephrotoxicity, neurotoxicity, ototoxicity, hepatotoxicity	• Liver function and renal function test, electrolyte monitoring, pre-operative neurological assessment • Possibility of neuropathy with regional anesthesia
Taxanes	• Paclitaxel • Docetaxel	Cardiac toxicity-bradyarrhythmia/tachyarrhythmia, autonomic and peripheral neuropathy	• Electrolyte monitoring, preoperative neurological assessment • Possibility of neuropathy with regional anesthesia
Antimetabolites	• Methotrexate	Mucositis, reversible encephalopathy, lung toxicity-interstitial pneumonitis, lung fibrosis, hepatic fibrosis, and acute renal failure	Avoid NSAIDs, monitor lung and liver functions
Alkylating agents	• Cyclophosphamide • Ifosfamide	Encephalopathy, hepatotoxicity, renal impairment, hemorrhagic cystitis, pseudocholinesterase inhibition with cyclophosphamide	Monitor serum electrolytes, liver, renal functions, ensure hydration and diuresis, duration of action of succinylcholine can be prolonged

(ECG: electrocardiogram; NSAIDs: nonsteroidal anti-inflammatory drugs)

TABLE 3: Role of multidisciplinary team management from the preoperative period.

Faculty	*Role*	*Possible preoperative intervention*
Pain Medicine	Addressing and optimizing preoperative pain	–
Surgical oncology	Mobilizations of bowel, bowel resection, and stoma formation	Proper bowel preparation to aid visualization and prevent injury
Urology	Cystography, partial cystectomy, and ileal conduit	Cystoscopy—assessment of postvoid urine volume, ureteric stent, or percutaneous nephrostomy
Plastic surgery	Assessment of defect and reconstruction of bony and soft tissue defects	–
Interventional radiology	Evaluation of vascularity of large pelvic tumors	Preoperative angioembolization to prevent intraoperative bleeding
Nutrition	Evaluation of nutritional deficits	Initiation of enteric or parenteral nutrition to enhance outcomes
Physiotherapy	Assessment of baseline functions, provision of education on the role of occupational therapy and physiotherapy	Strength and conditioning exercises to aid rehabilitation after surgery
Psychology	Aiding self-image issues and addressing mental health issues	Understand mindset, expectations and setting realistic of what to expect from the perioperative course and long-term recovery

Source: Guder WK, Hardes J, Nottrott M, Streitbürger A. Hemipelvectomy for pelvic sarcomas. Orthopade. 2019;48(9):760-7.

hemipelvectomy. These interventions aid patients and their families in understanding the procedure, managing expectations, and addressing the psychological effects. By tackling concerns related to body image, functionality, and quality of life, these measures can significantly enhance the patient's mental readiness for surgery.[12]

Pain management is also a critical component, as around one-third of patients with pelvic tumors, typically experience substantial pain preoperatively.[13] An integrated pain service team is necessary for effective management, employing strategies such as preemptive analgesia to mitigate postoperative pain and multimodal analgesia to improve pain control and minimize opioid use. Effective pain management also helps ensure that patients are in better shape to participate in strengthening exercises.

Nutritional optimization consists of aggressive anemia correction, starting high protein diets, and the use of parenteral nutrition if the bowel is involved.[2,11]

INTRAOPERATIVE CONCERNS

The major intraoperative concerns associated with patients undergoing hemipelvectomies, stem from prolonged surgery in the lateral position, major blood loss, risk of hypothermia, and need for institution of appropriate analgesia strategies in the intraoperative period. Before making the anesthetic plan, a discussion with the surgeons is essential to understand the extent of the surgical plan, estimate the anticipated blood loss, stratify patient-specific risks, and evaluate the need for postoperative monitoring in the high-dependency unit versus the intensive care unit (ICU).[10]

Positioning

This prolonged, complex surgery is carried out in a lateral decubitus position. As with all positions, anatomical positioning is preferred, i.e., no joint must be positioned in a manner that would be unnatural. Eyes, ears all pressure points are to be padded, and head and neck should be cushioned to keep it in neutral position. A soft roll must be placed on the dependent side, to prevent compression of the axillary neurovascular bundle. The dependent upper arm should be monitored for the adequacy of perfusion.[8]

To prevent intraoperative mishaps, a circuit must be examined for stretching, kinks, and the possibility of disconnection. Auscultation after repositioning and evaluation of airway pressures, will also reveal any migration of the endotracheal tube. The possibility of laryngeal and pharyngeal edema due to prolonged lateral position, leading to difficulty in extubation of the patient must be kept in mind.[14]

Monitoring

In addition to the standard American Society of Anesthesiologists (ASA) monitoring, which consists of electrocardiography, pulse oximetry, temperature, noninvasive blood pressure, and end-tidal carbon dioxide; having invasive blood pressure measurement with an arterial line, is considered standard for patients undergoing hemipelvectomy. Cardiac output monitors and transesophageal echocardiography should be used when the comorbidities of the patient demand the same.

Adequate intravenous peripheral access, consisting of multiple wide-bore peripheral cannula, for transfusion and central venous access for inotropic support must be instituted. It must be borne in mind that obtaining adequate intravenous (IV) access and invasive monitors may prove challenging secondary to ongoing oncologic treatments.

Monitoring in hemipelvectomies also consists of point-of-care systems such as blood gas analysis to detect acid-base changes and hemoglobin, and thromboelastography (TEG) to guide blood product transfusions when needed.

Anesthesia Management

General anesthesia with endotracheal intubation and skeletal muscle relaxants is anesthetic of choice. Maintenance of anesthesia is usually done using inhalational agents. In the past few years, there has been emerging evidence to suggest that total intravenous anesthesia, and propofol in particular, with its anti-inflammatory and antioxidant properties and maintenance of natural killer cell function, shows antiproliferative properties.[15] These properties seem particularly lucrative in patients who undergo neoadjuvant chemotherapy and radiotherapy which already suppresses the bone marrow. However, given the frequent need for massive blood transfusion, and requirement of inotropic supports, and the penchant that propofol has, to cause hypotension, its utility in such surgeries remains underexplored.

Patients undergoing hemipelvectomies are already at a high risk of developing infections, prevention of surgical site infection, by using antibiotic prophylaxis and continuing the same in the postoperative period, is essential.[1]

Fluid Management

A large volume of blood loss is anticipated through pelvic surgeries and needs replacement. Fluid replacement is usually done with balanced salt solutions with a replacement rate of 3–4 mL/kg/h. Additional fluid boluses can be administered, using dynamic fluid status using parameters, such as pulse pressure variation and systolic pressure variation, which are obtained from invasive blood pressure monitoring.

Management of Blood Loss

A 2017 study pegged the mean blood loss at 3,000 mL (range: 2,500–4,200 mL), where the mean duration of surgery was 6.5 hours (range: 5–8 hours).[16] The current definition of *major blood loss* is "50% blood loss within 3 hours or a rate >150 mL/min." As can be seen by the data from the abovementioned study, patients undergoing hemipelvectomy fit the description of major blood loss. As a result, addressing this large volume of blood loss during the intraoperative period forms the most crucial area of concern for anesthetists. External hemipelvectomies, involvement of sacrum or acetabulum, tumor volume >400 cm,[2] and tumors located close to internal iliac vessels, are factors that predispose higher blood losses, which can be predicted by good imaging strategies and discussion with the surgeons.[17,18] In addition to these factors, surgical factors, such as dissection along the bone margins, method of reconstruction and total operative time also influence intraoperative blood loss.

Real-time assessment of the said blood loss forms another area of concern since the blood loss remains concealed in the drapes and potential for hidden hematomas leading to frequent underestimation of losses. Keeping a hawk-eyed watch over the suction, and measuring the drains and drapes, when possible, helps in accurate estimation of losses. Since the estimation of the loss done in this manner may delay resuscitative efforts, it may be advisable to increase the reliance on point-of-care techniques to aid replacements, such as TEG and rotational thromboelastometry (ROTEM).[18,19] These techniques offer valuable insight into what blood components require replacement and potentially allow early recognition, and hence treatment, of consumptive coagulopathy.

Blood loss estimation and volume status can also be surmised using point-of-care hemoglobin testing and regular arterial blood gas analysis, which are both rapid and fairly accurate. However, they would limit the anesthetists' understanding of coagulopathy.[20,21]

Massive Transfusion Protocol

Given the predilection for bleeding, keeping adequate blood products, blood warming devices, and rapid infusors available is advisable. Additionally, having and knowing the institutional MTPs is crucial. Components of the MTP are summarized in **Table 4**, which must be instituted rapidly once massive is identified. Complications of rapid blood transfusion such as hypothermia, dilutional coagulopathy, dilutional thrombocytopenia, metabolic acidosis, electrolyte abnormalities, citrate toxicity, transfusion-related acute lung injury (TRALI), transfusion-associated circulatory overload and allergic reactions, must be borne in mind. Massive blood transfusion in hemipelvectomies can also trigger complications including anemia, coagulopathy, and hyperbilirubinemia.

Minimizing Surgical Blood Loss

Surgical cross-clamping has been advocated in bleed of >3 L. One novel modality of blood loss mitigation strategy described in traumatic hemipelvectomies is the endovascular balloon occlusion of the aorta (REBOA) which helps as a "non-invasive clamp" of the infrarenal aorta to help reduce blood loss. Its utility in oncologic hemipelvectomies, even as a last resort, needs to be utilized further.[10,22]

Blood Transfusion Mitigation Strategies

The use of antifibrinolytics such as tranexamic acid, epsilon aminocaproic acid (EACA), and aprotinin can prolong the integrity of the clot, by inhibiting fibrinolysis of the thrombus by plasmin.[14,23] A few RCTs have explored the safety of these agents in oncosurgery and found that they have not found any added risks.[23]

Among the various nonpharmacological strategies for reducing blood transfusion, autologous blood donation in well-optimized patients forms a good alternative. Normovolemic hemodilution can also help in reducing blood loss substantially.

The use of intra-operative cell salvage has recently been gaining some traction in literature. However, in spite of the purported benefit of leukocyte depletion filters in reducing the risk of metastasis, the theoretical risk that the salvaged blood will contain malignant cells from the operative field and allow metastasis still weighs heavily.[24]

TABLE 4: Massive transfusion protocol.

Step	*Action*	*Details*
1	Activate the massive transfusion protocol (*Trigger:* ongoing massive blood loss identified, 4–10 units of PRBC transfused)	• Insert extra wide-bore lines • Intimate the blood bank regarding the need for MTP • Intimate the ICU regarding the evolving situation • Arrange for extra manpower in OT to help through the situation • Ensure the presence of adequate amounts of colloids, crystalloids, infusion sets, and IV calcium in OT • Connect the rapid infusion pumps or pressure bags to speed the fluid infusion rate
2	Stop bleeding	Use packs, clamps, or REBOA in rare instances
3	Restore circulating volume	Rapidly perfuse with crystalloids or colloids, until blood/blood products that would increase oxygen-carrying capacity arrive
4	Mobilize and transfuse MTP packs	Kits or packs with the redefined ratio of packed red blood cells, FFP/ cryoprecipitate, and platelets units (random donor platelets) in each pack (e.g., 1:1:1 or 2:1:1 ratio) for transfusion
5	Continue resuscitation till targets are met	• MAP around 60 mm Hg, systolic arterial pressure 80–100 mm Hg (in hypertensive patients one may need to target higher MAP) • Hb 7–9 g/dL • INR <1.5; activated PTT <42 s • Fibrinogen >1.5–2 g/L • Platelets >50 × 10^9/L • pH 7.35–7.45 • Core temperature >35.0°C • Base deficit <3.0/lactates <2 mEq/L
6	Liaise with the hematology laboratory to ensure rapid reporting	Send baseline investigations of hematologic parameters, coagulation profile, serum fibrinogen, and biochemistry
7	Watch for and manage complications	• Citrate toxicity—calcium supplementation • Hyperkalemia • Hypothermia—ensure active warming • Hypomagnesemia—supplement magnesium • Acidosis • TRALI • SIRS • Sepsis • Thrombotic complications

(FFP: fresh frozen plasma; Hb: hemoglobin; MAP: mean arterial pressure; ICU: intensive care unit; INR: international normalized ratio; PRBC: packed red blood cells; SIRS: systemic inflammatory response syndrome; REBOA: Resuscitative Endovascular Balloon Occlusion of the Aorta; OT: operation theater; TRALI: transfusion-associated lung injury)

Sources:

1. Patil V, Shetmahajan M. Massive transfusion and massive transfusion protocol. Indian J Anaesth. 2014;58(5):590-5.
2. Rao S, Martin F. Guideline for management of massive blood loss in trauma. Anaesthesia. 2012;28(1):125-9.

Analgesia[10]

Since a large number of patients are already suffering from chronic pain, a proper plan for analgesia has to be made. Central neuraxial blockade, with an epidural catheter, is the intraoperative analgesic technique of choice, particularly, if there are no contraindications on account of extensive resection or neurovascular dissection. Effective epidurals work brilliantly, particularly since they can continue to be used in the postoperative period.

If epidurals cannot be used for some reason, multimodal analgesia must be instituted. The conduct of anesthesia can include opioids and analgesic adjuncts, such as ketamine, dexmedetomidine, and lidocaine infusions. Perineural catheters can also be considered to reduce the postoperative opioid requirements.

Pulmonary Embolism and Other Complications

Long-bone surgeries are inherently high-risk procedures, where there is an increased likelihood of pulmonary embolism. During surgical manipulation, the release of thrombogenic, inflammatory, and vasoactive substances into open circulation, can lead to a sudden cardiovascular collapse, decline in end-tidal carbon dioxide ($EtCO_2$), desaturation, and even drive a need for vasopressor support. Perioperative blood transfusion and antineoplastic agents also lead to thromboembolism and hence predispose to embolism.[25]

Early detection by a vigilant anesthetist, symptomatic management, and an adequately filled right heart will help overcome this situation. Sensitive monitoring devices such as transesophageal echocardiography will help quantify and correlate the embolus shower with clinical symptoms. Routine use in hemipelvectomy; however, is not yet recommended.

With the increasing use of allografts another potential problem that arises, is that of bone cement implantation syndrome (BCIS).[26,27] BCIS is a known complication with joint arthroplasties (incidence 16–37%) but is poorly understood. The symptoms include hypotension, hypoxia, cardiac arrhythmias, and even cardiac arrest.[28] BCIS is a diagnosis of exclusion, and as the symptoms overlap grossly with those of a pulmonary embolism, the diagnostic and management modalities remain the same. Where it differs is its complete reversibility, which can occur in minutes to hours.

POSTOPERATIVE CONCERNS

The postoperative period for patients who have undergone hemipelvectomies, either internal or external, is quite stormy and requires vigilant monitoring. Hence, shifting these patients to the high-dependency unit or ICU is advisable.

Monitoring

Early postoperative care constitutes continuing to monitor electrocardiography, pulse oximetry, invasive blood pressure measurement, temperature, and urine output measure measurement, which have been instituted in the intraoperative period, to ensure well-being and accurate ongoing fluid and electrolyte correction. Given the potential for hemodynamic instability secondary to ongoing blood loss, continuing ventilatory support during the postoperative period is not uncommon.[14] One of the most important aspects of postoperative care is to continue hawk-eyed vigilance over ongoing blood loss by monitoring the drain outputs. Drain output can be high-colored and the use of packs to achieve hemostasis and subsequent surgical procedures for pack removal are also known to be performed.[14]

Fluid Therapy

Patients being shifted to the postanesthesia care unit usually still require fluid resuscitation without inotropic supports to compensate for the drain output and correct surgical losses. Continuing the invasive blood pressure monitoring allows early pick up and prompt address of IV fluid requirements. Balanced salt solutions are the ideal choice for both maintenance and resuscitation. Since the patients are usually young, transfusion triggers can be safely set up between 7 and 9 g/dL.[29] Frequent estimation of hematological and biochemical parameters, and use of point-of-care coagulation testing, go a long way in accurately predicting the need for postoperative transfusion.

Thromboprophylaxis

Venous thromboembolism is a significant postoperative complication associated with major orthopedic surgery, particularly when associated with prosthetic reconstructions, and malignancies. In hip surgeries, the incidence of deep vein thrombosis has been found to be as high as 45–69%.[9] In addition to these risk factors, patients recuperating from internal hemipelvectomies are required to use a hip abduction brace which prevents hip flexion >75°, and maintains the hip at 20° abduction, while limiting hip rotation.[10] Nonweight bearing gait training usually only begins by postoperative day 3–5. As a result, it is crucial to start thromboprophylaxis as soon as surgical hemostasis is achieved, using prophylactic doses of low molecular weight heparin (LMWH).[8]

Postoperative Nausea Vomiting

Postoperative nausea vomiting (PONV) is an unfortunately common outcome after hemipelvectomy on account of multiple factors including, but not limited to, long duration of surgery, use of inhalational agents, extensive bone manipulation, and need for use of high doses of opioids during the perioperative period.[30] Preoperative use of opioids increases the need for post-operative opioids and thus, the incidence of PONV increases even further.[9] 5-hydroxytryptamine type 3 receptors (5HT-3) or serotonin antagonists form the mainstay of PONV prophylaxis. Other agents that work on dopaminergic pathways such as metoclopramide and dexamethasone can be used as adjuvants.

Postoperative Analgesia

Effective management of acute postoperative pain following hemipelvectomy is crucial to ensure optimal recovery. The ideal solution is to make a preoperative plan, keeping in mind the patients' pre-operative pain scores. The use of regional anesthetic techniques such as central neuraxial blockade, and perineural catheters help in early mobilization and increase analgesic efficacy. Intravenous patient-controlled analgesia (IV PCA) pumps are used to cover the immediate postoperative period in patients where regional anesthesia has not been used. Multimodal analgesia using the World Health Organization (WHO) step ladder approach, forms the cornerstone of pain management, combining opioids with nonopioid medications such as nonsteroidal anti-inflammatory drugs (NSAIDs) and acetaminophen to enhance pain control and reduce opioid requirements.[31] The doses of nonopioid analgesics are elucidated in **Table 5**.

REHABILITATION AFTER HEMIPELVECTOMY

The recovery in terms of both healing and functionality can be a challenge for the treating team. Various studies have documented the average length of stay as ranging between 6 and 20 days, with significantly longer hospital stays being documented for external hemipelvectomies.[32,33] The course of physical rehabilitation is described in the table given below. The patients also have to be retrained to sit, using a posture that takes the weight off the surgical site. Physiotherapy is also necessary to prevent gait deviations secondary to limb-length discrepancy, that can occur after an internal hemipelvectomy without reconstruction. The gait training includes the use of a shoe insert, and eventually an external shoe lift, to help reduce the risk of acquired scoliosis and back pain.

Patients in whom prostheses are implanted receive rehabilitation that focuses on function, comfort, and cosmesis. The process for "prosthesis training" includes not only gait training, but also donning and doffing, functional training, and fall recovery strategies.[4] Goals of physiotherapy in the postoperative period are given in **Table 6**.

TABLE 5: Postoperative use of analgesics.[8]

Class	*Drug*	*Doses*
Acetaminophen		• PO 4 hourly/QID 325–650 mg • IV TDS/QID 10–15 mg/kg
Nonsteroidal anti-inflammatory drugs (NSAIDs) and cyclo-oxygenase-2 (COX-2) inhibitors	Diclofenac	• *PO:* 100–200 mg/day in two to three divided doses • IV BD/TDS 1–1.5 mg/kg
	Ibuprofen	• *IV:* 400 mg first dose, followed by 100–200 mg q4–6 hours • *PO:* TDS/QID 1,200–3,200 mg per day
	Ketorolac	*PO:* 7.5–15 mg daily
	Meloxicam	*PO:* 50–200 mg daily in a single dose or two divided doses
	Celecoxib	IV BD 200 mg (adults)
Alpha-2-agonists	Clonidine	• PO 0.2 mg BD • *Epidural:* 30–40 μg/h
	Dexmedeto-midine	• IV loading 0.5–1.0 μg/kg over 10 minutes • Infusion 0.2–1.0 μg/kg/h
N-methyl-D-aspartate (NMDA antagonists)	Ketamine	• IV bolus 0.3–0.5 mg/kg • Infusion 0.1–0.2 mg/kg/h
	Magnesium sulfate	• Loading dose 30–50 mg/kg • Maintenance 8–15 mg/kg/h
Local anesthetics	Lignocaine	• IV bolus 1.5 mg/kg • Infusion 1–2 mg/kg/h
Anticonvulsants	Pregabalin	PO 150–600 mg/day in two to three divided doses
	Gabapentin	PO 300–1,200 mg TDS

TABLE 6: Goals of physiotherapy in the postoperative period.

Time frame	*Rehabilitation goals*
Up to 6 weeks	Neutral hip position using cast
POD 0–1	In bed mobility
POD 2–3	Transfers without weight-bearing
POD 3–5	Gait training without weight-bearing
6 weeks	Gradual weight bearing with weaning from assistive device
6–9 months	Successful weaning with no device

Occupational therapy is also instituted to re-train the patients to independently perform activities of daily living such as dressing, bathing, and bowel and bladder management. Additionally, occupational therapists and psychologists form valuable members of the perioperative team and help address body image issues, facilitate psychosocial adaptation, and encourage the patients to indulge in meaningful leisure interests, thus helping promote an overall sense of well-being and inclusion in society.

COMPLICATIONS AFTER HEMIPELVECTOMY

These patients appear to be at a high risk of various types of complications, with the incidence rate as high as 50–61%, being indicative of the need for specialized and vigilant monitoring and care of these patients extending further on into the postoperative period.[33] The complications include deep vein thrombosis, vascular spasm, seroma, neurologic deficit, bowel, bladder, and sexual dysfunction, and complications associated with the prosthesis such as loosening, displacement, breakage or autograft fracture, and leg-length discrepancy.[10]

One of the most frequent complications after hemipelvectomy is wound complications with an incidence ranging from 20 to 80%.[4] Extensive tumors with extraosseous extension, extensive resection, reconstruction with metallic prosthesis, prolonged surgical time, massive blood transfusion, and use of a structural allograft have been associated with an increased risk of such wound complications.[10]

IMPLEMENTATION OF ENHANCED RECOVERY PATHWAYS IN PATIENTS UNDERGOING HEMIPELVECTOMY

Since the introduction of enhanced recovery after surgery (ERAS) protocols for colorectal surgeries, the protocols have been modified and adapted to accommodate a vast number of surgeries. Given that implementation of ERAS protocols has shown improved patient outcomes by shortening the length of hospital stay, reducing postoperative complications, and improving patient outcomes and satisfaction, implementation of these protocols in patients undergoing hemipelvectomies seems to be the way forward.[34] However, while established protocols are available for enhanced recovery after total joint arthroplasties and spinal fusion surgeries, none are presently available for patients undergoing hemipelvectomies.[35] Though this may be attributable in part, to how infrequently these surgical procedures are carried out, most components of the established ERAS programs can be duplicated to hemipelvectomy surgeries in an effort to emulate the success of other ERAS programs.

Each element of the pathway is not only interlinked but also has a synergistic effect with the other elements; for example, to ensure early mobilization, pain optimization, prevention of PONV, early removal of urinary catheters, and appropriate fluid and blood management, are essential.[36] As a result, the successful implementation of enhanced recovery pathways requires a multidisciplinary effort from surgery, anesthesia, nursing, and physical therapy teams.

CHRONIC PAIN AFTER HEMIPELVECTOMY

Chronic pain after hemipelvectomy affects 30–90% of the patients. It manifests as residual limb pain, phantom limb pain, and neuromas.[37] Effective management is essential and involves both preventive and therapeutic strategies. The role of anesthetists is crucial to ensure appropriate use of multimodal analgesia, and regional nerve blocks and thus prevent the transition of acute to chronic pain. In a study that assessed chronic pain in posthemipelvectomy, 30% of the patients suffered from moderate pain, and 50% had numbness around the surgical site. They found no correlation between the type of surgery and the neuropathic pain scores recorded ($p = 1.0$).[37]

LONG-TERM FOLLOW-UP OF PATIENTS UNDERGOING HEMIPELVECTOMY

Though survival after hemipelvectomies has increased in recent years due to an improvement in surgical, and anesthetic techniques and rehabilitation strategies, the ability of these individuals to get assimilated into their societal roles is still debatable. Wido et al. assessed the need for such patients to access healthcare.[38] When patients who had undergone hemipelvectomies were followed up for a period of two years, though their need for healthcare support appeared to have gradually spent lesser amounts of time seeking healthcare, the number still remained very high. (0–12 months: mean 105.9 (SD: 98.8), 13–24 months: mean 48.9 (SD: 68.5).[38] When evaluated at a median interval of 27 months after the primary surgery, patients undergoing hemipelvectomies were found to still have a significant level of dependence with regard to bladder function. (17.4% of the patients with internal hemipelvectomy and 47.4% with external hemipelvectomy).[39] Another study assessed the quality of life using the Musculoskeletal Tumor Society (MSTS) score, where the MSTS score was 24 (±5) (on a scale of 0–30, higher scores indicating better function, indicating moderate to good scores in the whole cohort.[37] While the patients appeared to be generally satisfied with their quality of life, the patients who underwent internal hemipelvectomies had significantly higher scores for pain ($p = 0.0028$).[39]

NEWER HORIZONS IN HEMIPELVECTOMY

The morbidity after a hemipelvectomy and the return of functionality has been an area of concern. One of the pioneer steps in improving functional capacity has been the advent of prostheses after hemipelvectomy, particularly for tumors arising from the acetabulum.[40] With the advent of three-dimensional (3D) printing, it is now possible to create modular prostheses that allow better biological stability and early resumption of function with better long-term functional capacity.[41] The new polycentric hip joints reduce gait abnormalities even further, by 3D movement of the hip joint during walking. They are used with motion sensor knees and carry out automatic adjustments that allow for real-time adaptation during walking.[4] Studies have demonstrated reduced visual analog scale (VAS) scores and functionality good enough to allow patients to have a squatting function too.[42]

CONCLUSION

In summary, hemipelvectomies are rare and intricate procedures marked by massive blood loss, requiring challenging rehabilitation, exceptional expertise, and precision. The complexity of this surgery necessitates a meticulous approach to anesthesia, with special emphasis on effective blood loss management, maintaining hemodynamic stability, and providing optimal pain control. The perioperative course for these patients is often fraught with complications and the path to recovery involves not only addressing immediate surgical demands but also supporting long-term rehabilitation. Successful outcomes hinge on seamless coordination among the surgical, anesthesia, and rehabilitation teams, each of which plays a vital role in managing the intricate balance of care. Continued research and refinement in anesthetic techniques and perioperative strategies are essential to improve patient safety and recovery in this high-risk surgical context.

REFERENCES

1. Benatto MT, Hussein AM, Gava NF, Maranho DA, Engel EE. Complications and cost analysis of hemipelvectomy for the treatment of pelvic tumors. Acta Ortop Bras. 2019;27(2):104-7.
2. Guder WK, Hardes J, Nottrott M, Streitbürger A. Hemipelvectomy for pelvic sarcomas. Orthopade. 2019;48(9):760-7.
3. Banskota N, Yang H, Fang X, Yuan D, Zhang W, Duan H. Comparative study of pelvic sarcoma patients undergoing internal and external hemipelvectomy: a meta-analysis study. Front Surg. 2022;9:988331.
4. Houdek MT, Kralovec ME, Andrews KL. Hemipelvectomy: high-level amputation surgery and prosthetic rehabilitation. Am J Phys Med Rehabil. 2014;93(7):600-8.
5. Arnal-Burró J, Calvo-Haro JA, Igualada-Blazquez C, Gil-Martínez P, Cuervo-Dehesa M, Vaquero-Martín J. Hemipelvectomy for the treatment of high-grade sarcomas: pronostic of chondrosarcomas compared to other histological types. Rev Esp Cir Ortop Traumatol. 2016; 60(1):67-74.
6. Griesser MJ, Gillette B, Crist M, Pan X, Muscarella P, Scharschmidt T, et al. Internal and external hemipelvectomy or flail hip in patients with sarcomas: quality-of-life and functional outcomes. Am J Phys Med Rehabil. 2012; 91(1):24-32.
7. Revuri VR, Moody K, Lewis V, Mejia R, Harrison DJ, Ahmad AH. Pain and analgesia in children with cancer after hemipelvectomy: a retrospective analysis. Children (Basel). 2022;9(2):237.
8. Kumar A, Bhargava T. Perioperative Management of Patients Undergoing Orthopaedic Oncological Surgeries. [Online] Available from https://resources.wfsahq.org/atotw/perioperative-management-of-patients-undergoing-orthopaedic-oncological-surgeries/ [Last accessed March, 2025].
9. Anderson MR, Jeng CL, Wittig JC, Rosenblatt MA. Anesthesia for patients undergoing orthopedic oncologic surgeries. J Clin Anesth. 2010;22(7):565-72.
10. Lewis VO, Kemp A, Roubaud MJ, Ajay D, Westney OL, Ajay D, Westney OL, Smith T 3rd, et al. Multidisciplinary Approach to Hemipelvectomy for Pelvic Sarcomas. JBJS Rev. 2022;10(5).
11. Waterland JL, McCourt O, Edbrooke L, Granger CL, Ismail H, Riedel B, et al. Efficacy of prehabilitation including exercise on postoperative outcomes following abdominal cancer surgery: a systematic review and meta-analysis. Front Surg. 2021;8:628848.
12. Roşca AC, Baciu CC, Burtăverde V, Mateizer A. Psychological Consequences in Patients With Amputation of a Limb. An interpretative-phenomenological analysis. Front Psychol. 2021;12:537493.
13. Zhang Q, Wu Y, Hong S, Feng Y. Trajectory of worst pain within the first two weeks following pelvic and sacral tumor surgery and long-term outcome: a pilot observational prospective cohort study. BMC Anesthesiol. 2023;23(1):73.

14. Molnar R, Emery G, Choong PF. Anaesthesia for hemipelvectomy—a series of 49 cases. Anaesth Intensive Care. 2007;35(4):536-43.
15. Ng VY, Hollander KN, Carr SR, Tanaka K. Total Intravenous Anesthesia and Acute Normovolemic Hemodilution for Sarcoma Surgery. Cureus. 2020;12(11):e11319.
16. Salunke AA, Shah J, Warikoo V, Chakraborty A, Sahijwani H, Sharma M, et al. Surgical management of pelvic bone sarcoma with internal hemipelvectomy: oncologic and functional outcomes. J Clin Orthop Trauma. 2017; 8(3):249-53.
17. Tang X, Guo W, Yang R, Tang S, Ji T. Evaluation of blood loss during limb salvage surgery for pelvic tumours. Int Orthop. 2009;33(3):751-6.
18. Nates JL, Price KJ. Oncologic Critical Care: Orthopedic surgery and femoral/humeral fracture repairs. Germany: Springer; 2019.
19. Whiting D, DiNardo JA. TEG and ROTEM: technology and clinical applications. Am J Hematol. 2014;89(2):228-32.
20. Patil V, Shetmahajan M. Massive transfusion and massive transfusion protocol. Indian J Anaesth. 2014;58(5):590-5.
21. Rao S, Martin F. Guideline for management of massive blood loss in trauma. Anaesthesia. 2012;28(1):125-9.
22. Herold J, Notov D, Reeps C, Schaser KD, Kamin K, Mäder M, et al. Limb salvage in traumatic hemipelvectomy: case series with surgical management and review of the literature. Arch Orthop Trauma Surg. 2023;143(10):6177-92.
23. Sampaio AM, Guimarães GMN, Medeiros GP, Damasceno GMM, Silva RMA, Nunes RR, et al. Efficacy and safety of antifibrinolytics in oncological surgery: a systematic review and meta-analysis. Braz J Anesthesiol. 2019;69(5):484-92.
24. Klein AA, Bailey CR, Charlton AJ, Evans E, Guckian-Fisher M, McCrossan R, et al. Association of anaesthetists guidelines: cell salvage for peri-operative blood conservation 2018. Anaesthesia. 2018;73(9):1141-50.
25. Zec T, Di Napoli R, Fievez L, Ben Aziz M, Ottaiano A, Vittori A, et al. Efficacy and Safety of Tranexamic Acid in Cancer Surgery. An Update of Clinical Findings and Ongoing Research. J Multidiscip Healthc. 2022;15:1427-44.
26. Campanacci D, Chacon S, Mondanelli N, Beltrami G, Scoccianti G, Caff G, et al. Pelvic massive allograft reconstruction after bone tumour resection. Int Orthop. 2012; 36(12):2529-36.
27. Lowe M, Jeys L, Grimer R, Parry M. Pelvic reconstruction using pedestal endoprosthesis—experience from Europe. Annals of Joint. 2019;4:34.
28. Al-Husinat L, Jouryyeh B, Al Sharie S, Al Modanat Z, Jurieh A, Al Hseinat L, et al. Bone cement and its anesthetic complications: a narrative review. J Clin Med. 2023; 12(6):2105.
29. Carson JL, Stanworth SJ, Dennis JA, Trivella M, Roubinian N, Fergusson DA, et al. Transfusion thresholds for guiding red blood cell transfusion. Cochrane Database Syst Rev. 2021;12(12):CD002042.
30. Tran VN, Fitzpatrick BJ, Das S. Antiemetics and Apfel Scores in Orthopedic Surgery. Hosp Pharm. 2022;4(5):01-8.
31. Anekar AA, Hendrix JM, Cascella M. WHO Analgesic Ladder. In: StatPearls: Treasure Island (FL): StatPearls Publishing; 2024.
32. Couto AG, Araújo B, Torres de Vasconcelos RA, Renni MJ, Da Fonseca CO, Cavalcanti IL. Survival rate and perioperative data of patients who have undergone hemipelvectomy: a retrospective case series. World J Surg Oncol. 2016;14(1):255.
33. Ogura K, Boland PJ, Fabbri N, Healey JH. Rate and risk factors for wound complications after internal hemipelvectomy. Bone Joint J. 2020;102-B(3):280-4.
34. Choi YS, Kim TW, Chang MJ, Kang SB, Chang CB. Enhanced recovery after surgery for major orthopedic surgery: a narrative review. Knee Surg Relat Res. 2022;34(1):8.
35. ERAS® Society. Orthopaedics. [Online] Available from https://erassociety.org/specialty/orthopaedics [Last accessed March, 2025].
36. Ljungqvist O, Scott M, Fearon KC. Enhanced recovery after surgery: a review. JAMA Surg. 2017;152(3):292-8.
37. Bakshi S, Rana M, Gulia A, Puri A, Harsha TS, Tiwari S, Gotur A. Prevalence of chronic pain following resection of pelvic bone tumours: a single centre prospective observational survey. Br J Pain. 2022;16(3):263-9.
38. Wido D, Harrington CJ, Schulz RN, Jannace KC, Smith DG, Pasquina PF. Healthcare utilization following hemipelvectomy or hip disarticulation in the military health system. Mil Med. 2024;189(1-2):e235-41.
39. Beck LA, Einertson MJ, Winemiller MH, DePompolo RW, Hoppe KM, Sim FF. Functional outcomes and quality of life after tumor-related hemipelvectomy. Phys Ther. 2008; 88(8):916-27.
40. Holzapfel BM, Pilge H, Prodinger PM, Toepfer A, Mayer-Wagner S, Hutmacher DW, et al. Customised osteotomy guides and endoprosthetic reconstruction for periacetabular tumours. Int Orthop. 2014;38(7):1435-42.
41. Li J, Liu Z, Peng D, Chen X, Yu C, Shen Y. New adjustable modular hemipelvic prosthesis replacement with 3D-print osteotomy guide plate used in periacetabular malignant tumors: a retrospective case series. J Orthop Surg Res. 2022;17(1):259.
42. Wang J, Min L, Lu M, Zhang Y, Wang Y, Luo Y, et al. What are the complications of three-dimensionally printed, custom-made, integrative hemipelvic endoprostheses in patients with primary malignancies involving the acetabulum, and what is the function of these patients? Clin Orthop Relat Res. 2020;478(11):2487-501.

47

CHAPTER

Anesthesia for Bone and Soft Tissue Tumors

Mamta Dubey, Soumi Pathak, Amit Kumar Mittal

INTRODUCTION

Musculoskeletal tumors are benign or malignant growths which develop within the bone or soft tissue. Bone sarcomas account for 0.2% of all malignancies with an incidence of 0.9 per 100,000 persons per year.[1] The peak age of incidence of primary bone tumors is the second decade and metastatic bone tumors is the sixth decade of life.[2] Most commonly occurring bone tumors are osteosarcoma, osteoblastoma, Ewing's sarcoma, and chondrosarcoma. With advances in diagnosis and treatment modalities, the 5-year survival rates have increased significantly: 54% for osteosarcoma, 75% for chondrosarcoma, and 50% for Ewing's sarcoma.[3] Secondary causes of lesions in bone are metastasis from cancers of the breast, lung, prostate, etc. Multiple myeloma is a tumor arising in bone marrow that causes lytic lesions in the bones leading to pathological fractures.

PREOPERATIVE ASSESSMENT

The presenting complaints in osteosarcoma are usually pain, swelling, or pathological fractures. Sometimes evidence of metastasis to the lungs, soft tissue, and lymph nodes is present at the time of diagnosis.[4] In Ewing's sarcoma, back pain indicates the pelvic location of the tumor. Systemic symptoms such as fever and weight loss indicate metastatic disease. About 20% of patients presenting with metastatic disease have lung and pleura involvement. Chondrosarcomas are the third group of primary bone tumors and may present as bony or joint pain that is worse at night, palpable mass, or pathological fractures.

Preanesthetic Evaluation

The goals of preanesthetic evaluation are as follows:

- To educate the patient and organize resources for perioperative care
- To formulate plans for intraoperative care, postoperative recovery, and perioperative pain management
- To take informed consent

During the preanesthesia evaluation, the patient's performance status to withstand the surgery should be evaluated in terms of nutritional status, preexisting comorbidities, the effect of metastasis, and the impact of therapies such as neoadjuvant chemotherapy or radiotherapy.[5] Clinical characteristics to consider include smoking, recent upper respiratory infection, and cardiac disease. Enquire for previous exposure to anesthesia. Physical examination should include airway assessment, intravenous access (expected difficult cannulation) or in-situ peripherally inserted central venous catheters, spine examination, lungs, heart, and any other system involved due to the distant metastasis, with documentation of vital signs. Patients should also be assessed for the presence of deep vein thrombosis (DVT), if, there is a history of prolonged immobilization. Patients with metastatic bone lesions may have significant pain, requiring multiple analgesics. Details of these medications should be elicited carefully. Preoperative investigations and consultations should be ordered based on clinical findings and preexisting medical comorbidities, received adjuvant therapies, and the invasiveness of the planned procedure. At a minimum, hemoglobin, coagulation studies, serum biochemistries, electrocardiogram (ECG), and chest X-ray should be ordered in every patient. Neoadjuvant chemotherapy regimens can cause nephrotoxicity, hepatotoxicity, or cardiotoxicity; hence, mandating serum glucose, sodium, potassium, calcium, renal and liver function studies, and transthoracic echocardiography. Chemotherapy-induced myelosuppression should be optimized preoperatively and adequate blood and its products arranged. Preoperative embolization may be required in tumors with increased vascularity. Communication with the surgeon regarding the extent of resection, expected duration, and patient positioning allows the anesthesiologist to plan for appropriate monitoring and access. Psychoemotional issues due to diagnosis of malignancy or functional disability are quite common and preanesthesia visit is the heightened time to address all these issues, referral for psychosocial counseling, and prescribing anxiolytic medications. Anesthesiologists should establish a rapport with the patient and explain the planned anesthesia technique, means of perioperative pain management, and postoperative care.

Commonly performed surgical procedures for orthopedic malignancies:

- *Minor procedures*: Bone biopsy, curettage and bone cementing and radiofrequency ablations, and preoperative embolization of highly vascular bone tumors
- *Amputation (depending on the site involved)*: Below knee/above knee/above elbow/forequarter, hip disarticulation, etc.
- Wide local excision of soft tissue mass and/or reconstruction with myocutaneous free flap or neurovascular reconstruction and placement of brachytherapy catheters
- Limb salvage surgery (LSS) for sarcomas of bone and soft tissue
- Nailing and internal fixation in impending fractures
- Hemipelvectomy and sacrectomy

Many of these surgeries require multidisciplinary team involvement; hence, a good communication with all concerned teams helps in the seamless conduct of anesthesia.

POSITIONING

Orthopedic surgeries require varied patient positions such as supine, lateral, prone, or beach chair depending on the location of the tumor.[6] There are specific concerns regarding airway, ventilation, and nerve injuries with each of these positions. Precautions should be taken to prevent airway edema, nerve injuries, or pressure sores. These concerns have been discussed in the subsequent section.

Lateral Position

The concerns in the lateral position include suboptimal airway access, ventilation-perfusion mismatch, and tube malpositioning; hence, tube position should be confirmed after positioning. When the blood pressure cuff is placed on the dependent arm, inaccuracies in measurement are possible due to compression, hence, if possible place the BP cuff on nondependent arm. Adequate padding should be done to prevent radial nerve or common peroneal nerve injury and limit abduction at the shoulder to <90°. Head should be kept in a neutral position and folding of ears avoided. Patients should be strapped adequately to prevent sliding down of patient while tilting the table.

Prone Position

Airway access is difficult in the prone position, so utmost care should be taken to secure the endotracheal tube and recheck the tube position, once the patient is positioned prone. Respiratory mechanics improve in the prone position due to an increase in functional residual capacity. However, hemodynamic parameters deteriorate due to a decrease in cardiac output (12–24%) related to a reduction in venous return, decreased left ventricular (LV) compliance, and compression on inferior vena cava (IVC) from inappropriately placed bolsters. If the possibility of hemodynamic instability or any cardiac event is high, preparedness to make the patient supine and resuscitation measures (such as placing defibrillator paddles) should be ready beforehand, as resuscitation is difficult in this position.

Cannulation sites should be carefully selected, avoiding antecubital fossa to prevent kinking. During the change of position from supine to prone or vice versa, disconnect lines and monitoring cables to prevent inadvertent disconnection or dislodgement of lines. Maintain head and neck in a neutral position and avoid pressure on eyes, nose, breast, genitalia, or bony prominences. To avoid the possibility of postoperative visual loss, retinal ischemia and ischemic optic neuropathy arterial pressure should be maintained.

Beach Chair Position

Ensure the endotracheal tube is properly secured as access to the airway is limited due to surgical drapes. For correct BP measurement, avoid cuff placement on legs, place cuff on the nonoperative arm, and in case of invasive BP measurement, place transducer at the level of the tragus. Maintain the mean arterial pressure within normal limits, to preserve renal and cerebral perfusion. If hypotension ensues during beach-chair position, it should be treated with vasopressors and fluids.

ORTHOPEDIC ONCOLOGY AND ENHANCED RECOVERY AFTER SURGERY

The aim of implementing enhanced recovery after surgery (ERAS) protocols in patients undergoing major orthopedic oncosurgery is to promote early recovery, reduce perioperative stress, and pain management with multimodal analgesia, and reduce postoperative stay, complications, hospital costs and return to intended oncology therapy (RIOT).[7] The following interventions are proposed to achieve the above-mentioned goals **(Table 1)**.

Adequate pain management, reduced swelling, and normal mobilization with walking aids are the criteria for discharge from the hospital. Following knee surgery, the patient should be able to lift their limb with a stretched knee and achieve pain-free flexion to 90° and after hip surgery controlled walking to and from bed should be possible.

ANESTHESIA AND SURGICAL OUTCOME

Outcome after orthopedic oncosurgery depends on various factors, such as patient factors, the extent of surgery, and anesthesia-related techniques. Studies suggest that anesthetic techniques, such as regional anesthesia (RA), total intravenous anesthesia, and minimizing the use of volatile anesthetics,[8] opioids and allogenic blood transfusion may prevent cancer recurrence.[8] The proposed mechanism of action is suppression of cellular immunity, directly promoting apoptosis and reducing both proliferation and invasion of cancer cells. Regional/neuraxial anesthesia suppresses surgical stress response, decreases blood loss and need for transfusion, and reduces the incidence of deep venous thrombosis. Simultaneously, it provides superior analgesia and better patient satisfaction and decreases the incidence of chronic postsurgical pain (CPSP) or phantom limb sensations.[9] However, spinal anesthesia because of hypotension, intrathecal opioid additives, or sympathetic blockade can result in a vagally mediated overactivity of the gastrointestinal system and may cause PONV.

Regional anesthesia has a manifold influence on the surgical outcome.[10] Firstly, it facilitates earlier physiotherapy and joint mobilization by reducing acute pain. Secondly, it reduces the frequency of regrafting or thrombectomy after lower-limb arterial reconstruction surgery. Thirdly, in free flap reconstruction surgeries, it increases fistula blood flow and reduces vasospasm. It also reduces the chances of surgical site infections. Hypothermia and optimal patient positioning are other factors influencing the outcome of surgery.

LIMB SALVAGE SURGERY

The limb salvage surgical technique involves the wide resection of malignant bone tumors along with adjoining soft tissue and biopsy tract, and placement of prostheses with either primary closure of the wound or free flap reconstruction. Sometimes, the resected bone receives intraoperative radiation, the irradiated bone is reinserted and secured with plating and is further strengthened by a vascularized bone graft. Rotational arthroplasty is another major limb salvage surgical procedure opted in selected patients depending on the site of tumors.

TABLE 1: Perioperative interventions to be implemented for achieving the desired enhanced recovery after orthopedic oncological surgical procedures.

Preoperative measures	*Intraoperative measures*	*Postoperative measures*
Counseling and prehabilitation	Supplement neuraxial/regional anesthesia	Early ambulation
Correction of anemia (iron replacement, erythropoietin, and blood transfusion)	Individualized fluid therapy, preferably goal directed	Thromboprophylaxis
Informed consent	• Prevent hypothermia • Warm fluids, and patient warmer	Muscle strengthening exercise and physiotherapy
Cessation of smoking for 4 weeks	Early removal of Ryles tube, catheter, and drains	Assisted ambulation to prevent falls
Preoperative muscle strengthening by Limb physiotherapy, if not contraindicated	• Prevention of postoperative nausea and vomiting • Avoidance of tourniquets or drains if possible	Multimodal analgesia with regional blocks, paracetamol, NSAIDs, low-dose or short-acting opioids
Carboload and restrict preoperative fasting to 2 hours for clear fluids and 6 hours for solid food	Prophylactic antimicrobials (first- or second-generation cephalosporin 30–60 minutes prior to surgery	Psychological support from an interdisciplinary team

The recommended safe margin of bone resection is 3 cm with a sleeve of normal muscle and soft tissue. The resected area is reconstructed by any of the described methods, such as, tumor endoprosthesis, autograft bone or large segment allograft bone reconstruction, or a fibula transplantation.

Anesthetic Consideration for Limb Salvage Surgery

Preoperative Visit and Optimization

The main aim of a preoperative visit is to counsel the patient, ease out patient's anxiety and apprehension, to inform about various anesthesia options such as general anesthesia alone or supplemental regional anesthesia. It is the time to prescribe appropriate premedication, antibiotics or antiemetic or other relevant medication and arrangement of adequate amount of blood components.

Intraoperative Anesthesia Management

Strict aseptic precaution and antibiotic prophylaxis should be practiced, as most of the patients are immune-compromised. A large-bore intravenous cannula should be inserted and standard monitoring should be applied in all patients and insertion of a central venous catheter and arterial line should be decided depending upon patient factors and the extent of surgery. If not contraindicated, general anesthesia (GA) should be supplemented with regional blocks or epidural. For induction and maintenance of anesthesia, any combination of anesthetic drugs can be used. Propofol is the drug of choice, as it has a rapid onset of hypnosis, smooth and complete amnesia, and rapid recovery. Additionally, it has antiemetic and antineoplastic effects. During maintenance, a balanced anesthesia technique is preferable, which includes a combination of intravenous propofol, an inhalation agent [with or without nitrous oxide (N_2O)], along with a muscle relaxant and analgesic agent and/or regional anesthesia.[11] Though various drawbacks of N_2O such as diffusion hypoxia, increased PONV, and bowel distension have been defined, it can be used as part of balanced anesthesia in the absence of contraindications.[12] Despite numerous side effects, opioids remain an integral component of a total intravenous anesthesia (TIVA) technique and perioperative pain relief; however, in the era of ERAS, the lowest possible dose of opioids should be used. Concomitant administration of nonopioid analgesics such as acetaminophen, nonsteroidal anti-inflammatory drugs (NSAIDs), or cyclooxygenase (COX)-2 specific inhibitors, and adjuvant agents (dexamethasone, dexmedetomidine, ketamine, or lignocaine) and regional anesthesia has been found to have opioid sparing-effect.[13] Some nonpharmacologic analgesic techniques such as cold packs, acupuncture, meditation, and distraction are also proposed.[14]

Anesthesia Adjuncts

Various drugs that have opioid-sparing effects can be used as adjuncts in balanced anesthesia technique.

- Dexmedetomidine due to its analgesic, sedative, anxiolytic, antiemetic, and sympatholytic properties reduces the requirement of sedative-hypnotic and opioid. It also reduces the incidence of postoperative nausea and vomiting (PONV) and the emergence of delirium.[15]
- Ketamine has excellent analgesic effects, preserves airway reflexes and respiratory drive, and has broncho-dilator properties. As it causes an increase in blood pressure, heart rate, cardiac output, pulmonary artery pressure, and intracranial pressure, it is preferable to avoid in cardiac patients. Psychotomimetic effects such as hallucinations, nightmares, and vivid dreams are another potential drawbacks. Thus, ketamine should be typically reserved for use in opioid-tolerant patients.[16]
- Lidocaine infusion has been found effective in reducing the requirement of opioid and sedative-hypnotic agents, and it improves postoperative pain, particularly if regional anesthetic techniques cannot be employed.[17]

Regional anesthesia for LSS: Details of regional and blocks have been discussed in post-operative pain section.

Intraoperative fluid management aims to maintain euvolemia in major orthopedic surgeries, a zero-balance or restrictive fluid therapy (fluid transfusion at 3 mL/kg/h) for minimally or moderately invasive surgery and goal-directed fluid therapy in patients undergoing major surgical procedures (e.g., >500 mL blood losses and/or fluid shifts are expected) using one or more invasive dynamic hemodynamic parameters to achieve a prespecified goal.[18,19]

Intraoperatively, a restrictive transfusion threshold should be followed with the transfusion threshold being 7–8 g/dL in otherwise healthy adults. For intraoperative blood conservation, if not contraindicated, deliberate hypotension, autologous blood donation, and or acute normovolemic hemodilution can be practiced along with some surgical blood conservation techniques; such as the application of tourniquets, use of small incisions, use of electrosurgery devices, or the use of topical hemostatic agents, tissue adhesives, fibrin sealants, and autologous platelet gels. Tranexamic acid and Epsilon-aminocaproic acid are antifibrinolytic agents which can be used as systemic hemostatic agents.

Postoperative Course and Follow-up

The main pearls in postoperative management include pain management, prophylaxis against venous thromboembolism (VTE), minimization of postoperative morbidity, and appropriate physical therapy (PT) to achieve the best possible joint movement and return to full function as safely as possible. After an uneventful immediate postoperative course, RIOT is the next goal to be achieved.

Tourniquets

Tourniquets are aids that help in providing a bloodless field in surgeries of limbs (orthopedic and plastic surgery).[20] The limb is exsanguinated and adequately padded before inflating the tourniquet. Usually, the tourniquet is inflated 100 mm Hg above systolic pressure for the upper arm and 100–150 mm Hg above systolic pressure for the thigh. The safe duration of tourniquet inflation is described as 1–3 hours depending on the limb selected, but if the duration of inflation is likely to exceed 2 hours, then it should be deflated every 30 minutes for 5 minutes. Contraindications to the use of tourniquets are DVT, peripheral neuropathy, peripheral vascular disease, and patients with poor cardiac reserve. Reperfusion following deflation of the tourniquet leads to the release of metabolites from the ischemic limb resulting in a fall in mean arterial pressure, a decrease in peripheral vascular resistance, and a transient increase in end-tidal carbon dioxide ($EtCO_2$).

Bone Cement Implantation Syndrome

Bone cement implantation syndrome (BCIS) is a potentially fatal complication of LSS, observed in <5% of patients due to the use of polymethylmethacrylate cement.[21] Embolization of fat and marrow debris is supposed to be the main cause of BCIS, other contributing factors may be cement monomer toxicity, anaphylatoxin release, prostaglandin release, or the use of a long-stem femoral component. Clinical signs and symptoms of BCIS comprise a variety of clinical features including hypoxia, hypotension, neurologic symptoms, cardiac arrhythmia, and possibly cardiac arrest. A significant drop in systolic blood pressure (20 mm Hg or more) during the insertion of a cemented femoral component is an alarming sign of BCIS. Aggressive volume resuscitation, supplemental oxygen, and supportive care are the main pillars of management. Preventive measures for BCIS include pulse lavage of the femoral canal, slow introduction of the stem, providing a vent hole in the bone for long-stem component insertion, and minimal pressurization of cement.

AMPUTATION

In oncological malignancies of extremities, amputation surgeries are mainly offered to those patients, when it is not possible to achieve tumor-free margins, local recurrence after LSS, and failure of adjuvant chemotherapy. Although preservation of limb length is desirable even during amputations, achieving a free margin after tumor resection, the healing potential of the stump, and the rehabilitation potential of the patient are the main factors for deciding the level of the amputation. The target is 3–4 inches of normal bone margin to provide better functional outcomes. Like LSS, amputation surgeries should be headed by preoperative evaluation and preparation of the patient, which includes evaluation of medical risk, nutrition assessment, preoperative antibiotics, and thromboembolism prophylaxis. However, detailed counseling regarding prosthetics, rehabilitation, and psychological consultation is required in amputation patients compared to LSS patients. Posttraumatic stress disorder due to the disability, young age at the time of the amputation, and pain necessitate psychological counseling. To speed up postoperative ambulation and self-care activities, training exercises for isometric strengthening of the muscles of the uninvolved extremities, trunk, and the muscles spared in the affected limb to be started preoperatively. Major amputations are almost always performed under general anesthesia. Epidural/neural sheath catheters/regional blocks should be a part of the anesthesia regimen to reduce the incidence of postoperative pain.[22] However, minor amputations (toe/finger) are occasionally performed using local anesthesia or blocks. A multidisciplinary approach is advocated in the postoperative care of amputation patients, including acute or chronic pain services, rehabilitation medicine, physical therapy, and psychiatry services. The postoperative care should ensure optimal wound healing, minimize limb swelling, prevent joint contractures, and improve muscle strength and function.

Phantom Limb Pain

Perception of pain in a detached body part (limb) is referred to as phantom limb pain and should be distinguished from other causes of stump pain. The phantom limb pain is commonly seen in both upper and lower extremity amputations. The exact mechanism of phantom limb pain is not defined, and it is related to the reorganization of the primary somatosensory and motor cortices of the brain.[23] Risk factors which influence the development of chronic phantom limb pain include extremity pain before the amputation, male sex, site and level of amputation, and psychological factors such as stress and depression. Various pain management strategies and treatments have been used such as pharmacologic agents (e.g., opioids and ketamine), regional anesthesia (e.g., epidural for acute phantom pain), and nonpharmacological means (mirror therapy or brain-computer interface training to create visual-proprioceptive dissociation in the brain). These modalities can be used solely or in combination, without any consensus on the best treatment strategy.

SOFT TISSUE TUMORS

Soft tissue sarcoma (STS) could be benign or malignant tumors that arise from muscle, tendons, fat, lymph, blood vessels, or nerves. Several types of STS have been identified including, angiosarcoma, dermatofibrosarcoma protuberant, gastrointestinal stromal tumor (GIST), Kaposi's sarcoma, leiomyosarcoma, liposarcoma, rhabdomyosarcoma, peripheral nerve sheath tumor, synovial sarcoma, and undifferentiated pleomorphic sarcoma. The ratio for an STS to be benign or malignant is 150:1. Though the exact etiology is not known, possible reasons for an STS include a genetic predisposition or a previous history of radiotherapy. STS is commonly seen in adults (40 years or more); however, synovial sarcoma and epithelioid sarcomas are more frequently seen in young adults, but, rhabdomyosarcoma commonly affects children. Lower extremity STS is twice more common than the upper extremity.[24] Radiotherapy and/or chemotherapy are given preoperatively to reduce tumor size, but surgery remains the mainstay of treatment. Mostly these tumors present as painless lumps. Superficial lumps can be diagnosed early; however, deep-seated tumors can only be identified when they grow to 10 cm or more in size. Pressure symptoms and difficulty in mobility are the usual presentation of patients when an STS is in proximity to a joint. Referred pain, paresthesia, and focal neurological deficit are the other presenting symptoms. Very large tumors may result in DVT, and a Doppler scanning is advised to rule out DVT.

Magnetic resonance imaging (MRI) is the imaging modality of choice to detect, localize, and study the relation of STS with neurovascular structures and for staging of tumors. For patients in whom MRI is contraindicated, a computed tomography (CT) scan can be used. Positron emission tomography (PET) CT scan can be used to assess treatment response after surgical and systemic therapy or to detect distant metastasis or bony involvement. Fine needle or core needle/incision biopsy/excision biopsy can be used to establish the histological diagnosis.

Surgical resection of STS remains the mainstay of treatment.[25] Four commonly performed approaches for resection are intralesional, marginal, wide local, and radical. Reconstruction of defects can be completed either by primary closure (90–95% of patients),[26] or a rotation or a free flap. Neurovascular bundle embedded in tumor may require neurovascular reconstruction. In patients who require a free flap reconstruction, plastic surgeons should be consulted before surgery and intravenous access and invasive lines planned accordingly.

A surgical plan could influence anesthesia planning; so, a communication between the surgical and anesthesia team facilitates anesthesia planning, regarding the choice of anesthesia, patient positioning, airway management, and regional anesthesia. Adjuvant therapies for STS include cryotherapy, radiofrequency ablation, chemotherapy, and radiotherapy (external beam or brachytherapy).

FREE FLAP RECONSTRUCTION

The primary indication of free flaps in STS are wide defects created after the resection of large parts of bone and soft tissue in which primary closure of soft tissue defects may not be possible. Additionally, free flaps are the first choice for soft tissue coverage in distal leg defects. Free tissue transfer includes preparation of the recipient site, harvesting of the flap, and revascularization of the flap. To ensure tissue perfusion pressure and thus the viability of free flap, hemodynamic parameters, $ETCO_2$, pH, blood glucose, temperature, arterial blood gas should be maintained in the physiological range. The goal of fluid transfusion is to maintain hemodynamic stability while avoiding flap edema. Overzealous blood transfusion should be discouraged, unless hematocrit falls below 30, as this value is often considered to optimally balance blood viscosity and oxygen transfer to the flap. Regional anesthesia is beneficial because of the sympathetic blockade and subsequent vasodilation.

SPINE SURGERY

In a paradigm-shifting of technological advancements, such as stereotaxis, navigation, endoscopy, and percutaneous instrumentation, robot-assisted surgery has emerged as the future of spine surgery. The use of CT-guided 3D navigation systems reduces radiation exposure.[27] Depending upon the vertebral levels involved, extent of surgery, and expected blood loss spinal surgical procedures are categorized into three groups:-Minor, major, and complex.

1-2 level anterior cervical discectomy (ACDF) and decompression or microdiscectomy without instrumentation are minor surgeries and do not require placement of invasive lines and can be managed with one large bore IV cannula. Major surgeries such as 3–4 level ACDF, 1–2 level anterior lumbar body fusion, 1–2 level transforaminal lumber body fusion, 1–2 level anterior/posterior fusion will require arterial BP monitoring in addition. Complex surgeries involving 6–8 level of instrumentation, ≥3 level anterior/posterior fusion, pedicle subtraction osteotomy, tumor corpectomy or debulking will need placement of at least 2 large bore IV cannulae, arterial line, and a central line.[28]

General anesthesia is preferred for all spine surgeries as it provides a secure airway, better surgical exposure under muscle relaxants, and better control of intraoperative hemodynamic changes. The essential components for minimally invasive surgeries include conscious sedation and long-acting local analgesia; and the advantages are less blood loss, early ambulation, lesser pain, and shorter hospital stays. Fluoroscopy-guided epidural along with conscious sedation for lumbar surgery may be a feasible approach while treating patients undergoing lumbar spinal surgery in <4 hours.[29] Awake endoscopic transforaminal spine surgeries are a newer innovation.

The advantages and disadvantages of the different modes of anesthesia for various spine surgeries are mentioned in **Table 2**.

Perioperative Anesthesia Concerns in Spine Surgery[31]

The preoperative assessment of the airway, respiratory system, cardiovascular system, laboratory investigations, and preoperative fasting as per ERAS protocols have already been covered in previous sections (preanesthetic evaluation and ERAS) **(Table 3)**.

Intraoperative Concerns

The details of intraoperative concerns for spine surgeries including preemptive analgesia , minimally invasive techniques , blood loss reduction , monitoring and positioning have been discussed in **Table 3**. Post operative management including pain is also described in **Table 3**.

TABLE 2: Advantages and disadvantages of mode of anesthesia for various spine surgeries.

Spine surgery	*Mode of anesthesia*	*Advantage*	*Disadvantage*
Endoscopic transforaminal lumbar interbody fusion (TLIF)	Conscious sedation	↓ Surgical duration ↓ Blood loss ↓ Duration of hospital stay	• Maintenance of Patent airway may be challenging • Nausea • Vomiting
Lumbar discectomy and laminectomy	Regional anesthesia (spinal or epidural anesthesia)	↑ Analgesia ↓ Blood Loss ↓ Rise in intraocular pressure in the prone position	• Not suitable in the anticipated difficult airway, severe spinal stenosis, history of intracranial hypertension, coagulopathy, systemic infection, and skin infection • Poor control of intraoperative hemodynamic changes • May hamper the postoperative neurological examination

Source: Khanna P, Sarkar S, Garg B.[30]

TABLE 3: Perioperative anesthesia concerns during spine surgery and strategies to resolve them.

Preemptive analgesia	Paracetamol, gabapentin 20 mg, ketorolac, and pregabalin 75 mg
Minimally invasive techniques with small incision	• Total intravenous anesthesia (i.e., intravenous ketamine or Propofol) • Regional anesthesia • Normovolemia and normothermia • Spinal cord perfusion pressure must be maintained to prevent ischemia, and MAP of 80 – 90 mm Hg should be maintained • Opioid-limited or opioid-free analgesia • OLV may be required in thoracic spine surgeries, which can be achieved with the use of double-lumen endotracheal tubes and bronchial blockers
Blood loss reduction techniques	• Erythropoietin 100–300 IU/kg/day, subcutaneus • Autologous blood donation • Preoperative embolization • Tranexamic acid, aprotonin • Controlled hypotension • Cell saver • TEG-guided transfusion
Position-related concerns[32,33]	• Visual loss, peripheral nerve injury • Careful selection of equipment, utilization of checklists for careful positioning, padding, and periodic assessment • Suboptimal prone positioning may increase the intra-abdominal and intrathoracic pressure, leading to a rise in transmitted venous pressure to the inferior vena cava and epidural veins, thereby causing unexpected surgical bleeding
Pain management	• Epidural steroid 5–10 mg dexamethasone per level, intrathecal morphine 75–150 μg • Ketamine bolus of 0.15–10 mg/kg ± a continuous infusion of 0.1–0.5 mg/kg/h • Dexmedetomidine bolus of 0.3–1 mg/kg over 10–15 minutes, followed by a continuous infusion of 0.2–0.6 mg/kg/h • Erector spinae block
Monitoring	Somatosensory evoked potentials (SSEPS) and motor evoked potentials (MEPS)
Postoperative management	• Early mobilization • Prompt nutrition • Cessation of intravenous fluids • Postoperative monitoring and follow-up with enhanced recovery after surgery team • Nonopioid pain management

(MAP: mean arterial pressure; OLV: one-lung ventilation; TEG: thromboelastography)
Source: Brown JM.[31]

PAIN MANAGEMENT IN BONE AND SOFT TISSUE SARCOMA

Orthopedic surgery results in moderate to severe pain, and various treatment modalities have been described to manage it.

Mechanism and Transmission of Pain Pathway

Apart from the soft tissue, pain fibers have been found in the periosteum, cambium, bone matrix, Haversian canals, and bone marrow in the medullary cavity of the bone. The Aδ-fibers transmit acute pain, whereas C-fibers transmit slower, dull pain **(Fig. 1)**.

Analgesic Techniques for Perioperative Pain Management

Both pharmacological and nonpharmacological analgesic techniques have been described for perioperative pain management.

Pharmacological techniques include central neuraxial techniques, regional anesthesia, and systemically administered medications.[34] While, nonpharmacological techniques include acupuncture, aromatherapy, music therapy, hot and cold compresses, the elevation of surgical extremities, transcutaneous nerve stimulation, peripheral nerve stimulation, and hypnosis.

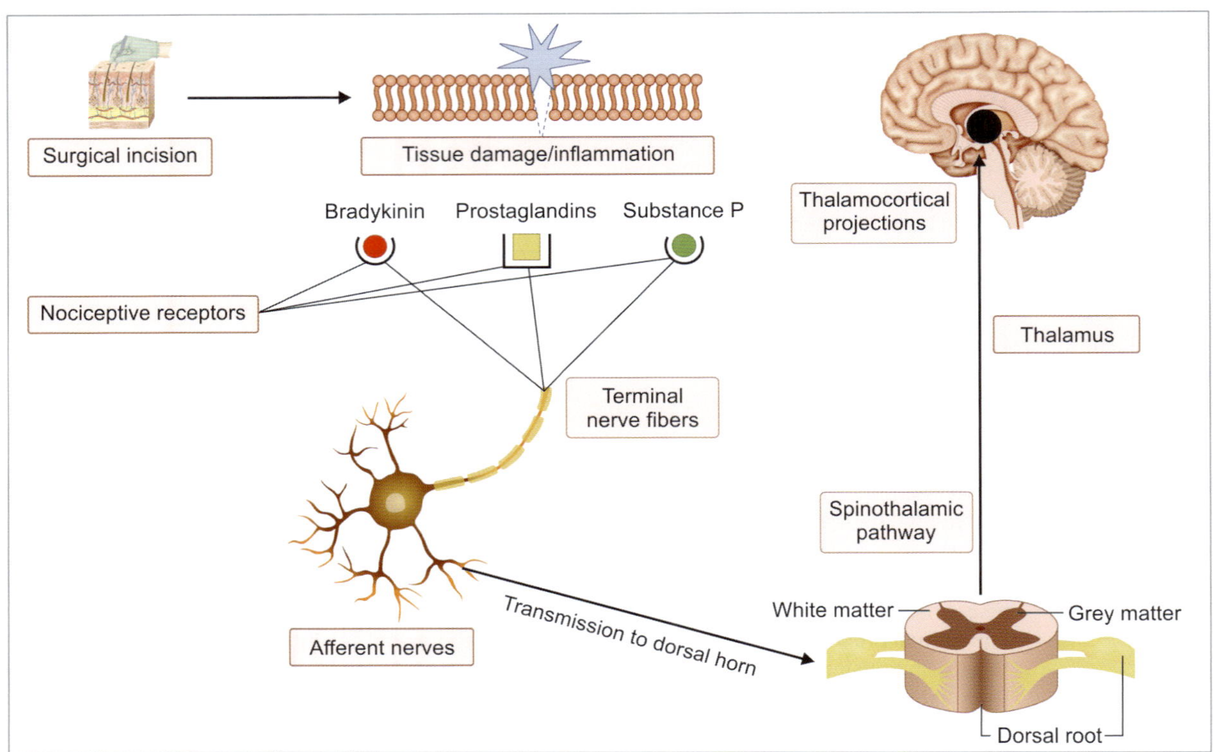

Fig. 1: Mechanism and transmission of pain at surgical site.[9]
Source: Hebl JR, Dilger JA, Byer DE, Kopp SL, Stevens SR, Pagnano MW, et al.[9]

Central Neuraxial Techniques[35]

Epidural analgesia: The advantages of epidural analgesia are decreased surgical stress response and the requirement for opioids. It also reduces the incidence of cancer recurrence, thromboembolic phenomenon, cardiac arrhythmias, and pulmonary complications and facilitates the earlier return of bowel function.

Spinal analgesia: Low doses of intrathecal administration of local anesthetics and various adjuvants are effective in providing precise and controlled pain relief by directly blocking the pain pathway in the spinal cord. However, neuraxial analgesia is not ideal for early ambulation and outpatient procedures. Precaution should be exercised, whenever the patient is receiving anticoagulants.

Somatic nerve blocks: Somatic nerve blocks can be a valuable alternative or adjuvant to general or neuraxial anesthesia. The advantages of these blocks include excellent analgesia and minimize systemic opioid requirements with minimal change in hemodynamic and respiratory parameters, phantom limb pain management, and reduction of cancer recurrence. Contraindications includes preexisting peripheral nerve lesions, mechanical compression or infiltration by tumors, and damage caused by chemotherapy/radiotherapy. Sometimes, disturbances in axonal flow kinetics and neurofilament architecture associated with peripheral nerve blockade may aggravate nerve function, a complication known as "*Double crush phenomenon*".

Regional Blocks

Peripheral nerve blocks are used to supplement analgesia for procedures on upper or lower limbs. These may be given as per anatomical landmarks or ultrasound and peripheral nerve stimulator guided.

Upper Limb Blocks (Table 4)[36]

The details of various regional blocks for upper limb surgery are discussed in **Table 4**. **Figure 2** shows the anatomical landmarks for scalene nerve block and **Figures 3A and B** show the sonoanatomy. 3B also shows the separation of planes on injecting the local anesthetic. **Figure 4A and B**

TABLE 4: Anatomical details, indications, and complications associated with various upper limb nerve blocks.

Block	*Indications*	*Nerve root blocked*	*Landmark*	*Complications*
Interscalene nerve block	Surgeries over the shoulder, proximal aspect of the humerus, and distal aspect of the clavicle	• Supraclavicular nerve (C3-C4) • Brachial plexus (C5- C7)	LA injected between anterior and middle scalene muscles lateral to the carotid artery and internal jugular vein	• Phrenic nerve palsy • Horner syndrome, and hoarseness
Supraclavicular nerve block	Surgeries over arm, elbow, forearm, and hand	C5-T1	LA injected above the clavicle between the anterior and middle scalene muscles at the level of the first rib, where the subclavian artery crosses over it	Pneumothorax, phrenic nerve palsy, and hoarseness
Infraclavicular nerve block	Surgeries over the elbow, forearm, and hand	C5-T1	LA injected around the axillary artery below the clavicle, medial to coracoid process	Pneumothorax
Axillary nerve block	Surgeries over the elbow, forearm, and hand	Median nerve, ulnar nerve, radial nerve, and musculocutaneous nerve	LA injected around the axillary artery at the medial aspect of proximal arm	Hematoma formation and intravascular injection

Source: Mehrkens H, Geiger PM.[36]

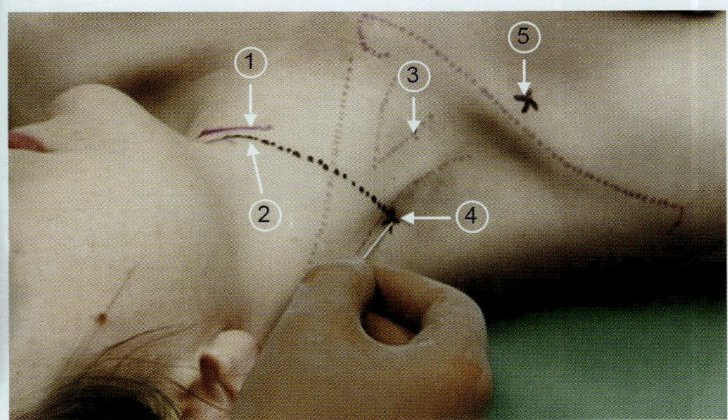

Fig. 2: Anatomical landmarks for interscalene nerve block.[36] (1) Cricoid, (2) Superior thyroid notch, (3) Sternocleidomastoid muscle, (4) Puncture site for anterior access, (5) Vertical, infraclavicular puncture site.
Source: Mehrkens H, Geiger PM.[36]

shows the sonoanatomy of axillary nerve block and **Figure 5** shows the anatomical landmarks for infrclavicular nerve block.

Lower Limb Blocks (Table 5)

The details of commonly used lower limb blocks are mentioned in **Table 5** while **Figures 6A and B** show the anatomical landmarks and sonoanatomy for femoral nerve block respectively. **Figure 7** shows the anatomical landmarks for sciatic nerve block .

Opioids and other adjuvants are used as analgesics to supplement regional blocks or as sole analgesics when regional analgesia is contraindicated. **Table 6** lists the various opioids and their dosing intervals while **Table 7** lists the adjuvants which can be used.

RADIATION SAFETY

Continuous radiation exposure related to intraoperative imaging in minimally invasive orthopedic procedures is a significant concern for patients, surgeons, and operative room personnel. The staff and patients are exposed to both direct and scatter radiation.

Direct radiation (predominant source of radiation exposure) is the radiation directly absorbed from the beam projected from the source. However, scatter radiation (deflected off a surface) affects the personnel who stand further away from the surgical table. This ionizing radiation causes cellular damage by the production of reactive oxygen species.[39] The pathologic effects of ionizing radiation exposure are further classified as stochastic or deterministic where the risk of developing cancer is independent of the radiation dose received or increases beyond a threshold dose, respectively.

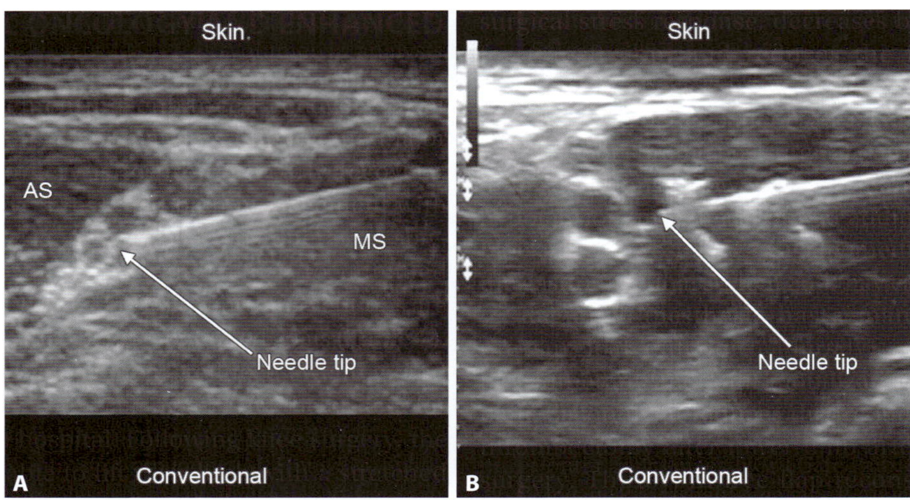

Figs. 3A and B: Sonoanatomy—interscalene block.
Source: Nysora.[37]

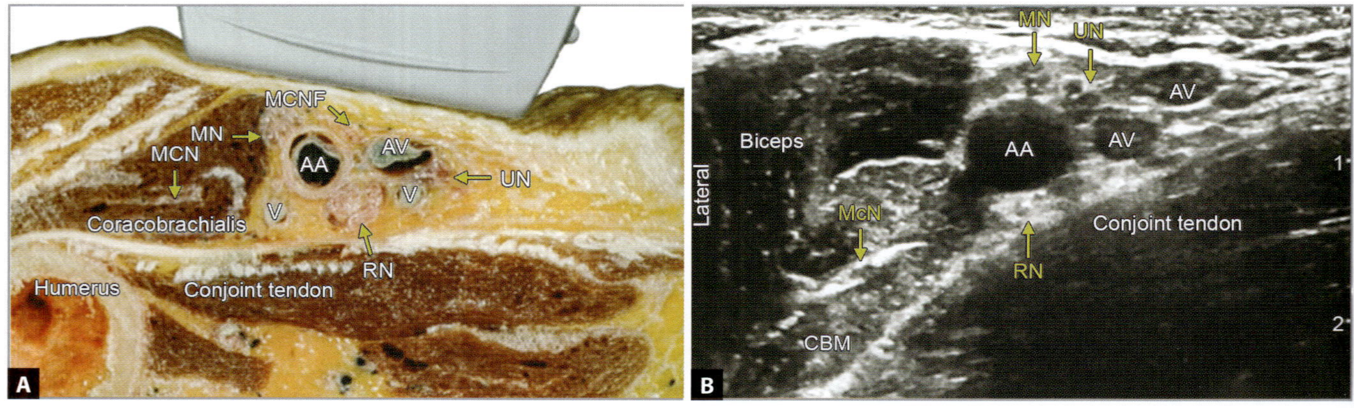

Figs. 4A and B: Sonoanatomy of axillary nerve block. (AA: axillary artery; AV: axillary vein; CBM: coracobrachialis muscle; MN: median nerve; MCN: musculocutaneous nerve; MCNF: medial cutaneous nerve of forearm; RN: radial nerve; UN: ulnar nerve)
Source: Nysora.[37]

General Strategies for Reducing Radiation Exposure

As the exposure rate from a radiation source drops off by the inverse of the distance squared, hence, a safe distance between 46–200 cm from radiation sources is recommended. Also, maximizing the distance between the source and the patient's skin and minimizing the distance between the image intensifier and the patient's skin lessen scatter radiation. Appropriate personal shielding such as lead aprons with the lead-equivalent minimum, front and back, of 0.25 mm (the standard is 0.5 mm) and thyroid collar, lead glasses/goggles, radiation shielding pads/hats, and personal dosimetry monitors should be worn by all operators and staff.[40] Reducing frame rates to 7.5 frames per second for fluoro and 15 for cine, and limiting the annual dose between 50 and 20 mSv for radiation officers and 5 mSv for patient relatives are other safety measures. Inspection of lead aprons for damage should be done at least annually. Lastly, newer imaging technologies such as neuronavigation and O-Arm can be used to limit radiation exposure.

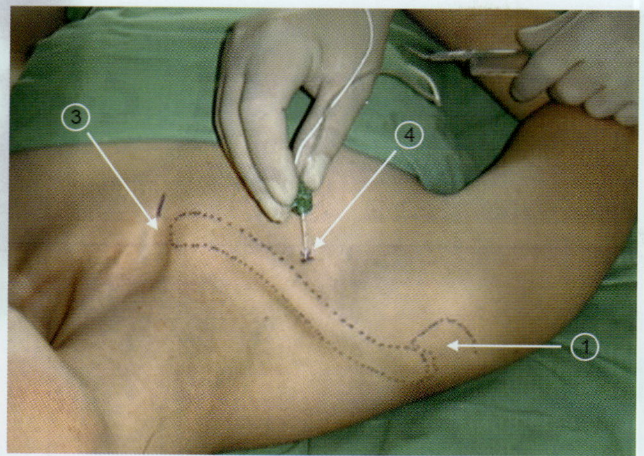

Fig. 5: Anatomical landmarks for vertical infraclavicular nerve block.[36] (1) Acromion process, (3) Medial head of clavicle, (4) Vertical, infraclavicular puncture site.
Source: Mehrkens H, Geiger PM.[36]

RECENT ADVANCES IN ORTHOPEDICS

Research and advancement is the necessity for the improvement of an existing technique, and orthopedic oncology is not an exception. The newer advances are as follows:

- 3-D printing or CAD-CAM (computer-aided design, computer-aided manufacturing) used for the production of customized implants and patient-specific prostheses, especially in challenging positions such as sacrum and pelvis[41]
- *Cobots:* Surgical robots collaborate with humans. Implant position and orientation can be adjusted via the interface, while the surgeon maintains control of the surgery.
- Computer-assisted navigation systems facilitate resection for bone tumors, but they cannot ensure negative soft tissue margins.

TABLE 5: Anatomical details, indications, and complications associated with various lower limb nerve blocks.

Block	*Indication surgeries*	*Nerves blocked*	*Landmark*	*Complication*
Femoral nerve block	Anterior aspect of the thigh and medial aspect of the leg below the knee	Femoral nerve	Inguinal crease; located lateral to femoral artery	Lower limb weakness and falls, bleeding, infection, and nerve damage
Fascia iliaca block	Anterior aspect of the thigh and medial aspect of the leg below the knee	Femoral nerve and lateral femoral cutaneous nerve of the thigh	Inguinal crease, LA injected under fascia iliaca	Lower limb weakness and falls, bleeding, infection, and nerve damage
Popliteal block	Foot, ankle, and posterior knee	Sciatic nerve	Popliteal fossa, located cephalad to the knee near popliteal artery	Motor blockade
Adductor canal block	Medial aspect of the knee, foot, and ankle	Saphenous nerve and nerve to vastus medialis (branch of femoral nerve)	The medial thigh, located deep to the sartorius muscle, adjacent to the femoral artery and vein	Bleeding, infection, nerve damage, and potential lower extremity weakness at high dose

Source: Mehrkens H, Geiger PM.[36]

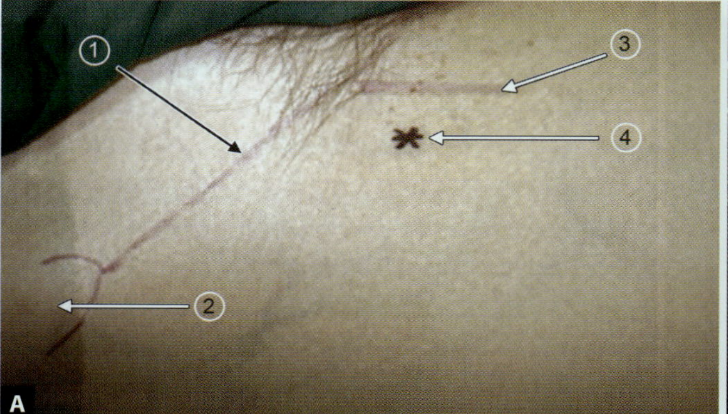

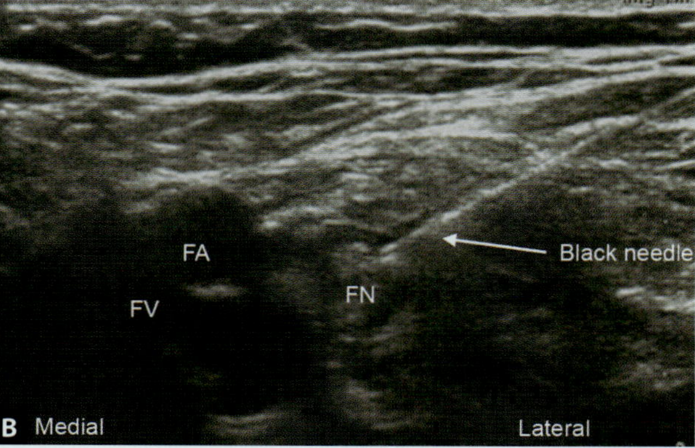

Figs. 6A and B: (A) Anatomical landmarks for femoral nerve block. (1) Inguinal ligament, (2) Femoral artery, (3) Anterior superior iliac spine (4) Puncture site for femoral nerve block; (B) Sonoanatomy of femoral nerve. (FA: femoral artery; FV: femoral vein; FN: femoral nerve).
Source: Nysora.[37]

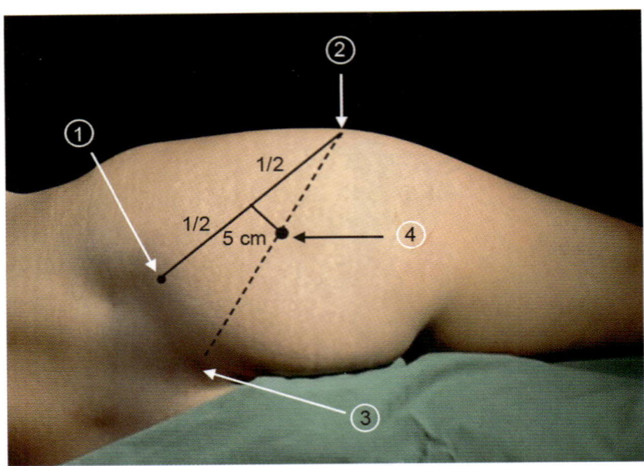

Fig. 7: Anatomical landmarks for sciatic nerve block.[36] (1) Posterior superior iliac spine, (2) Greater trochanter, (3) Sacral notch, (4) Puncture site for sciatic nerve block.
Source: Mehrkens H, Geiger PM.[36]

TABLE 6: Onset, duration and route of administration of commonly used opioids analgesics.

Drug	Route	Dose	Onset	Duration
Morphine	PO IV	15–60 mg 5–15	45 minutes 10 minutes	4–5 hours 3.5–4 hours
Fentanyl	IV Sublingual TTS	5–150 µg 100–400 µg 25–100 µg	3–5 minutes 5–10 minutes 17–24 hours	30 minutes 60 minutes 72 hours
Oxycodone	PO	5–10 mg	5–10 minutes	3–4 hours
Methadone	PO IV	5–15 mg 5–10 mg	15–45 minutes 3–6 minutes	6–8 hours 4–6 hours
Buprenorphine	TD patch	5, 10, 20 µg	26–36 hours	1 week
Tramadol	IV PO	50–100 mg 50–200 mg	10–15 minutes 40 minutes	3–4 hours 4–6 hours

(IV: intravenous; PO: per oral; TD: transdermal; TTS: transdermal therapeutic system)
Source: El-Tallawy SN, Nalamasu R, Salem GI, LeQuang JAK, Pergolizzi JV, Christo PJ.[38]

TABLE 7: Onset, duration, and route of administration of commonly used adjuvants.

Drug	*Route*	*Dose*	*Duration*
Antidepressants: • Amitriptyline • Nortriptyline	 PO PO	 10–150 mg 25–100 mg	 24 hours 24 hours
Duloxetine	PO	60 mg	24 hours
Gabapentin Pregabalin Carbamazepine	PO PO PO	200–400 mg 75–300 mg 400–1,200 mg	
Dexamethasone	IV/PO	4–8 mg	4–8 hours
Prednisolone	PO		12 hours
lidocaine	TD	5% patch	12 hours
Capsaicin		8% patch	Days–weeks

(IV: intravenous; PO: per oral; TD: transdermal)
Source: El-Tallawy SN, Nalamasu R, Salem GI, LeQuang JAK, Pergolizzi JV, Christo PJ.[38]

- Percutaneous cryoablation is a new treatment option for extra-abdominal desmoid tumors. The procedure requires mild sedation and is performed as a care procedure in a radiology suite.[42]
- Pazopanib and sorafenib are orally administered chemotherapeutic agents used in the treatment of soft tissue sarcomas. Though they have very few side effects during treatment, long-term treatment can cause hypertension and hypothyroidism.

CONCLUSION

Musculoskeletal tumors are benign or malignant. Malignant tumors can be primary or metastatic and involve varying age group of patients , from adolescents to elderly. These surgeries range from minor procedures to extensive surgeries requiring vascular reconstruction , free tissue transfer and massive blood transfusion. Patients often have multiple comorbidities and after effects of chemotherapy and radiotherapy . Preoperative risk assessment and medical optimization influence perioperative outcomes.

These surgeries may require different positions and careful padding of pressure points should be done to avoid nerve injuries. Careful attention should be paid to blood loss and fluid management. Awareness of potential for bone cement implantation syndrome and fat embolism helps in mitigating the complications.

Regional nerve block techniques are useful to provide perioperative analgesia and use of ultrasound for this purpose improves the success and safety. Thromboprophylaxis and effective multimodal pain management ensures, rehabilitation and optimal patient outcomes.

REFERENCES

1. Franchi A. Epidemiology and classification of bone tumors. Clin Cases Miner Bone Metab. 2012;9(2):92-5.
2. Jain K, Sunila, Ravishankar R, Mruthyunjaya, Rupakumar CS, Gadiyar HB, et al. Bone tumors in a tertiary care hospital of south India: A review 117 cases. Indian J Med Paediatr Oncol. 2011;32(2):82-5.
3. Karmaniolou, Iosifina, Makris, Alexandros, Lamprou, et al. Perioperative management of patients with bone and soft tissue tumors: A narrative review. Acta Anaesth Belg. 2017;68:1-12.
4. Odri GA, Tchicaya-Bouanga J, Yoon DJY, Modrowski D. Metastatic Progression of Osteosarcomas: A Review of Current Knowledge of Environmental versus Oncogenic Drivers. Cancers (Basel). 2022;14(2):360.
5. West H, Jin JO. Performance Status in Patients with Cancer. JAMA Oncol. 2015;1(7):998.
6. Hartley J. (2020). Patient Positioning During Anaesthesia. WFSA Resource Library. [online] Available from https://resources.wfsahq.org/atotw/patient-positioning-during-anaesthesia/ [Last accessed March, 2025].
7. Bourazani M, Asimakopoulou E, Magklari C, Fyrfiris N, Tsirikas I, Diakoumis G, et al. Developing an enhanced recovery after surgery program for oncology patients who undergo hip or knee reconstruction surgery. World J Orthop. 2021;12(6):346-59.
8. Sekandarzad MW, van Zundert AAJ, Lirk PB, Doornebal CW, Hollmann MW. Perioperative anesthesia care and tumor progression. Anesth Analg. 2017;124:1697-708.
9. Hebl JR, Dilger JA, Byer DE, Kopp SL, Stevens SR, Pagnano MW, et al. A pre-emptive multimodal pathway featuring peripheral nerve block improves perioperative outcomes after major orthopedic surgery. Reg Anesth Pain Med. 2008;33:510-7.
10. Kamel I, Ahmed MF, Sethi A. Regional anesthesia for orthopedic procedures: What orthopedic surgeons need to know. World J Orthop. 2022;13(1):11-35.
11. Irwin MG, Chung CKE, Ip KY, Wiles MD. Influence of propofol-based total intravenous anaesthesia on peri-operative outcome measures: a narrative review. Anaesthesia. 2020;75(Suppl 1):e90-100.
12. Buhre W, Disma N, Hendrickx J, DeHert S, Hollmann MW, Huhn R, et al. European Society of Anaesthesiology Task Force on Nitrous Oxide: a narrative review of its role in clinical practice. Br J Anaesth. 2019;122(5):587-604.
13. Veyckemans F. Opioid-free anaesthesia: Still a debate? Eur J Anaesthesiol. 2019;36:245.
14. Komann M, Weinmann C, Schwenkglenks M, Meissner W. Non-Pharmacological methods and post-operative pain relief an observational study. Anesth Pain Med. 2019;9(2):e84674.
15. Duan X, Coburn M, Rossaint R, Sanders RD, Waesberghe JV, Kowark A. Efficacy of perioperative dexmedetomidine on postoperative delirium: systematic review and meta-analysis with trial sequential analysis of randomised controlled trials. Br J Anaesth. 2018;121:384-97.
16. Schwenk ES, Viscusi ER, Buvanendran A, Hurley RW, Wasan AD, Narouze S, et al. Consensus Guidelines on the Use of Intravenous Ketamine Infusions for Acute Pain Management From the American Society of Regional Anesthesia and Pain Medicine, the American Academy of Pain Medicine, and the American Society of Anesthesiologists. Reg Anesth Pain Med. 2018;43:456-66.
17. Weibel S, Jelting Y, Pace NL, Helf A, Eberhart LH, Hahnenkamp K, et al. Continuous intravenous perioperative lidocaine infusion for postoperative pain and recovery in adults. Cochrane Database Syst Rev. 2018;6:CD009642.
18. Joshi GP, Kehlet H. CON: Perioperative Goal-Directed Fluid Therapy Is an Essential Element of an Enhanced Recovery Protocol? Anesth Analg. 2016;122:1261-3.

19. Miller TE, Roche AM, Mythen M. Fluid management and goal-directed therapy as an adjunct to Enhanced Recovery After Surgery (ERAS). Can J Anaesth. 2015;62:158.
20. Sharma JP, Salhotra R. Tourniquets in orthopedic surgery. Indian J Orthop. 2012;46(4):377-83.
21. Saleh KJ, Kassim R, Yoon P, Vorlicky LN. Complications of total hip arthroplasty. Am J Orthop (Belle Mead NJ). 2002;31(8):485-8.
22. Lans J, Hoftiezer Y, Lozano-Calderón SA, Heng M, Valerio IL, Eberlin KR. Risk Factors for Neuropathic Pain Following Major Upper Extremity Amputation. J Reconstr Microsurg. 2021;37:413-20.
23. MacIver K, Lloyd DM, Kelly S, Roberts N, Nurmikko T. Phantom limb pain, cortical reorganization and the therapeutic effect of mental imagery. Brain. 2008; 131:2181-91.
24. Church DJ, Krumme J, Kotwal S. Evaluating Soft-Tissue Lumps and Bumps. Mo Med. 2017;114(4):289-94.
25. Blazer DG, III, Chang AE. Operative Management of Soft Tissue Sarcoma. In: Minter RM, Doherty GM (eds). CURRENT Procedures: Surgery. The McGraw-Hill Companies; 2010.
26. Malawer MM, Price WM. Gastrocnemius transposition flap in conjunction with limb-sparing surgery for primary bone sarcomas around the knee. Plast Reconstr Surg. 1984; 73:741-50.
27. Cui GY, Tian W, He D, Xing YG, Liu B, Yuan Q, et al. [Effects of robot-assisted minimally invasive transforaminal lumbar interbody fusion and traditional open surgery in the treatment of lumbar spondylolisthesis]. Zhonghua Wai Ke Za Zhi. 2017;55(7):543-8.
28. Zheng K, Angst M. (2020). Guidelines for the intraoperative management of patients undergoing spine surgery - ether - resources for anesthesia research and education - Stanford University. [online] Available from Ether.stanford.edu [Last accessed March, 2025].
29. Kang SY, Kashlan ON, Singh R, Rane R, Adsul NM, Jung SC, et al. Advantages of the Combination of Conscious Sedation Epidural Anesthesia Under Fluoroscopy Guidance in Lumbar Spine Surgery. J Pain Res. 2020;13:211-9.
30. Khanna P, Sarkar S, Garg B. Anesthetic considerations in spine surgery: What orthopaedic surgeon should know! J Clin Orthop Trauma. 2020;11(5):742-8.
31. Brown JM. (2020). UpToDate. [online] Available from https://www.uptodate.com/contents/anesthesia-for-elective-spine-surgery-in-adults?source=history_widget [Last accessed March, 2025].
32. Lee LA, Roth S, Posner KL, Cheney FW, Caplan RA, Newman NJ, et al. The American Society of Anesthesiologists Postoperative Visual Loss Registry: analysis of 93 spine surgery cases with postoperative visual loss. Anesthesiology. 2006;105(4):652-9; quiz 867-8.
33. Chui J, Murkin JM, Posner KL, Domino KB. Perioperative peripheral nerve injury after general anesthesia: a qualitative systematic review. Anesth Analg. 2018;127:134-43.
34. Chunduri A, Aggarwal AK. Multimodal Pain Management in Orthopedic Surgery. J Clin Med. 2022;11(21):6386.
35. Moraca RJ, Sheldon DG. The role of Epidural anaesthesia and analgesia in surgical practice. Ann Surg. 2003;238: 663-73.
36. Mehrkens H, Geiger PM. Peripheral Regional Anaesthesia Tutorial. Ulm Rehabilitation Hospital. Braun Tutorial, 3rd edition.
37. Nysora. https://www.nysora.com/pain-management/ultrasound-guided-upper-extremity-blocks/ [Last accessed March, 2025].
38. El-Tallawy SN, Nalamasu R, Salem GI, LeQuang JAK, Pergolizzi JV, Christo PJ. Management of Musculoskeletal Pain: An Update with Emphasis on Chronic Musculoskeletal Pain. Pain Ther. 2021;10(1):181-209.
39. Vozenin-Brotons MC. Tissue toxicity induced by ionizing radiation to the normal intestine: understanding the pathophysiological mechanisms to improve the medical management. World J Gastroenterol. 2007;13:3031-2.
40. Kern M. (2018). Novel Radiation Protection Devices: An Update on Radiation Safety in the Cath Lab. Cath Lab Digest. [online] Available from https://www.hmpgloballearningnetwork.com/site/cathlab/article/novel-radiation-protection-devices-update-radiation-safety-cath-lab [Last accessed March, 2025].
41. Jeyaraman M, Nallakumarasamy A, Jeyaraman N. Industry 5.0 in Orthopaedics. Indian J Orthop. 2022;56(10):1694-702.
42. Errani C, Mavrogenis AF, Tsukamoto S. What's new in musculoskeletal oncology. BMC Musculoskelet Disord. 2021;22:704.

Section 12 Oncocritical Care

48

CHAPTER

Tumor Lysis Syndrome and its Management

Shikha Sachan, Deepti Gupta, Ashish Mani Tripathi

INTRODUCTION

Tumor lysis syndrome (TLS) is a common and life-threatening oncological emergency. It is a metabolic disorder due to the rapid breakdown of highly divisible cancerous cells in response to chemotherapeutic agents. With the surge of new and highly effective novel cytotoxic therapies, the condition is now seemingly more prevalent. The most commonly associated malignancies are hematological cancers and solid tumors.[1,2] Lysis of proliferating tumor cells leads to the release of nucleic acids and subsequent increase in urates as well as potassium and phosphate. The classic tetrad present in TLS is hyperuricemia caused by a breakdown of nucleic acids, hyperkalemia, hyperphosphatemia, and hypocalcemia.

The most worrisome feature of TLS is acute kidney injury (AKI) mainly due to the deposition of urate crystals in renal tubules. The electrolyte derangements (hyperkalemia, hyperphosphatemia, and hypocalcemia) can cause life-threatening derangements of the cardiovascular as well as central nervous system.

EPIDEMIOLOGY

Hematological malignancies such as acute lymphoblastic leukemia, acute myeloid leukemias, and poorly differentiated lymphomas (e.g., Burkitt's lymphoma) and high-grade non-Hodgkin's lymphoma are more sensitive to cytotoxic chemotherapy and have the highest association with TLS. It may also be present with solid tumors (hepatocellular carcinoma, hepatoblastoma, testicular tumors, breast malignancies) as well as chronic leukemia. TLS has a rapid development course which can occur during or 1 week after initiation of chemotherapy.[1,2]

PATHOPHYSIOLOGY

Tumor lysis syndrome occurs when there is a rapid breakdown of tumor cells and leakage of intracellular metabolites after initiation of cytotoxic chemotherapy in a chemosensitive malignancy. The intracellular metabolites are nucleic acids, potassium, and phosphorous. The metabolism of nucleic acids released from the tumor deoxyribonucleic acid (DNA) into the systemic circulation occurs in the liver and is catalyzed through the enzyme xanthine oxidase.

Flowchart 1 shows the metabolism of nucleic acids.

The final product in the metabolism pathway is the relatively poorly soluble uric acid which is excreted through the kidneys. An excess production of uric acid exhausts this excretion capacity and leads to the precipitation of urate crystals in the renal tubules and renal failure. The nonprimate mammals have a unique enzyme called *urate oxidase* which can convert excess uric acid to allantoin which is much more soluble. Humans, however, lack this enzyme.

The exorbitant release of intracellular phosphorous from the lysis of tumor cells has its own consequences. Once the renal excretion capacity of this ion is exhausted, there is a rise in serum phosphorous levels. Hyperphosphatemia in turn leads to secondary hypocalcemia due to precipitation of calcium phosphate which can get deposited in renal tubules leading to nephrocalcinosis.[3]

Flowchart 1: Metabolism of nucleic acid.

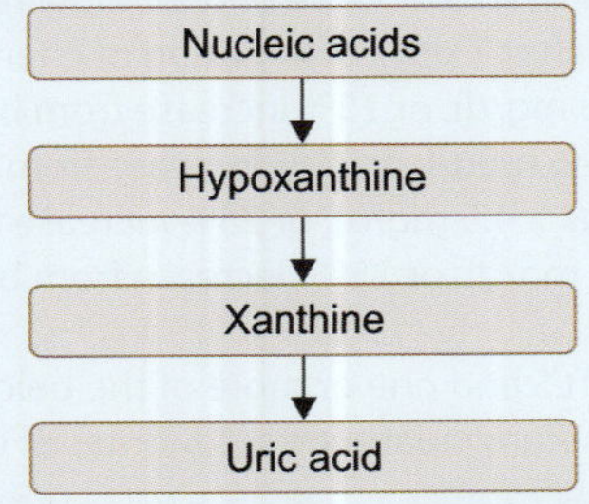

Source: Murray RK, Granner DK, Mayes PA, Rodwell VW. In: Harper's Illustrated Biochemistry, 26th edition. New York: Tata McGraw-Hill Education; 2003.

The breakdown of tumor cells leads to the rapid expulsion of intracellular potassium into the circulation and can cause significant hyperkalemia and can cause further complications, such as arrhythmia, and cardiac arrest because of the AKI.

It is to be noted that cell lysis also leads to a release of metabolic byproducts, such as pyruvate, lactate, and glucose thus causing metabolic acidosis and hyperglycemia.

CLINICAL FEATURES

Tumor lysis syndrome can be a life-threatening condition. Patients usually present with features of metabolic derangements, i.e., hyperuricemia, hyperphosphatemia, hypocalcemia, and hyperkalemia. Common features are nausea, vomiting, diarrhea, abdomen pain, anorexia, lethargy, muscle cramps, tetany, heart failure, arrythmias, confusion, seizures, syncope, and possible sudden death.

The most notorious complication is renal failure which is a result of hyperuricemia and nephrocalcinosis. Hyperkalemia can cause ventricular arrythmias, paresthesia, muscle weakness, and gastrointestinal disturbances. Hyperphosphatemia can present as altered consciousness, hypotension, and atrial arrythmias. Hypocalcemia can lead to cardiac disturbances, hypotension, and coagulopathy.

DIAGNOSIS

Cairo–Bishop classification is often used for the purpose of classification and attempts to classify TLS on the basis of laboratory values and clinical presentation **(Box 1)**.

BOX 1: Cairo and Bishop criteria for tumor lysis syndrome (TLS).

- *Laboratory TLS*
  - Abnormality in two or more of the following before 72 hours or after 7 days of initiation of chemotherapy
  - Uric acid > 8 mg/dL or 25% increase from baseline
  - Potassium > 6 mEq/L or 25% increase from baseline
  - Phosphorous > 4.5 mg/dL or 25% increase from baseline
  - Calcium < 7 mg/dL or 25% decrease from baseline
- *Clinical TLS*
  - Laboratory TLS and one or more of the below criteria.
  - Increase in serum creatinine > 1.5 times of upper limit of normal
  - Seizure
  - Cardiac arrhythmia or sudden death

RISK FACTORS

- High-risk cancers **(Table 1)**
- High cell proliferative state.
- High chemosensitive tumors
- Large tumor burden or bulky disease
- Highly effective chemotherapy
- Organ infiltration by tumor
- Preexisting oliguria due to dehydration
- Acidic urine
- Nephropathy

Elevated serum lactate dehydrogenase (LDH) >1,500 IU is an important biomarker of rapid cell turnover and is important for risk assessment of TLS.

PREVENTION

Patients who are at greatest risk of developing TLS can be prevented by continuous monitoring, hydration, and to a much lesser extent the use of certain hypouricemic agents.[4]

Adequate hydration with crystalloids is the key to the prevention of TLS as it maintains glomerular filtration and renal perfusion. The choice of intravenous fluids should be based on the serum levels of potassium, calcium, and phosphate levels of in patients with hypovolemia and Hyponatremia choice of fluid is isotonic saline. One should be careful to avoid volume overload in patients

TABLE 1: Risk of tumor lysis syndrome (TLS) as per tumor type.

Degree of risk	*Tumor type*
High	• Burkitt's lymphoma • High-grade non-Hodgkin's lymphoma • T-cell acute leukemia • Lymphoblastic lymphoma
Moderate	• Low-grade lymphoma treated with chemotherapies • Multiple myeloma • Breast carcinoma treated with hormonal therapy • Small cell lung carcinoma • Germ cell tumors, such as seminoma and ovarian tube
Low	• Low-grade lymphoma treated with interferons • Merkel's cell carcinoma • Medulloblastoma • Adenocarcinoma of the gastrointestinal tract

Source: Jeha S. Tumour lysis syndrome. Semin Hematol. 2001;38(Suppl 10):4-8.

with preexisting renal and cardiac dysfunction. Fluid therapy should be continued till tumor load decreases or LDH normalizes.

The use of diuretics can be considered in patients who are not hypovolemic and do not have obstructive uropathy.

Uric acid excretion may be promoted by using acetazolamide or sodium bicarbonate for alkalizing urine, but it can lead to precipitation of calcium phosphate leading and worsening kidney function.[5,6]

HYPOURICEMIC THERAPY FOR THE PREVENTION OF TUMOR LYSIS SYNDROME

Allopurinol blocks the enzyme xanthine oxidase which catalyzes the conversion from hypoxanthine to xanthine and xanthine to uric acid. The net result is overall reduced production of uric acid. This however may lead to accumulation of hypoxanthine and xanthine resulting in xanthine nephropathy. The recommended dose is 300–600 mg/day. It should be started 24–48 hours before chemotherapy and can be continued for a week to 10 days. Rare but possible side effects are hypersensitivity reactions, bone marrow depression, and liver derangement.

Rasburicase is a recombinant urate oxidase enzyme that converts uric acid to allantoin which is highly soluble.[7,8] It is usually administered intravenously every 24 hours for 5–7 days. The dose of rasburicase is 0.2 mg/kg once daily for 5–7 days.[9,10] Dose adjustment is required in patients with AKI. Rasburicase is contraindicated in patients with glucose-6-phosphate dehydrogenase (G6PD) deficiency, pregnancy, and breastfeeding.[11] Side effects include infusion reactions (fever, chills, and hypertension), nausea, vomiting, fatigue, dizziness, and rarely anaphylaxis and hypersensitivity reactions.

Febuxostat

It is a new orally used hypouricemic agent that inhibits xanthine oxidase and may be used in patients who are allergic to allopurinol or who cannot tolerate allopurinol.[3]

Typically administered dose is 40–80 mg oral daily.

TREATMENT

Emergency Dialysis

- *Indications:* Initiate when there is severe hyperkalemia (>6 mmol/L), persistent hyperphosphatemia, symptomatic hypocalcemia, or AKI with oliguria or anuria despite adequate hydration and medical management.
- *Options:*
  - *Intermittent hemodialysis (IHD):* Preferred for rapid correction of metabolic disturbances.
  - *Continuous renal replacement therapy (CRRT):* Beneficial for hemodynamically unstable patients as it allows gradual correction and fluid management.
- *Goals:* Rapidly lower uric acid, potassium, and phosphorus levels to mitigate organ damage.

Rasburicase

- *Mechanism:* Rasburicase converts uric acid to allantoin, which is more soluble and easily excreted via the kidneys.
- *Indications:* Administer to patients with hyperuricemia or those at high risk for TLS.
- *Administration:*
  - *Dose:* Typically, 0.2 mg/kg IV once daily for 1–3 days, based on uric acid levels and renal function.
- *Advantages:* More effective and faster acting than allopurinol for reducing uric acid levels.
- *Caution:* Avoid deficiency in patients with glucose-6-phosphate dehydrogenase (G6PD) deficiency due to the risk of hemolysis.

Fluid Management

- *Goals:* Maintain urine output of 2–3 mL/kg/hour to enhance the excretion of uric acid and electrolytes.
- *Fluids:* Use isotonic saline for hydration; avoid potassium-containing fluids.
- *Caution:*
  - Monitor for fluid overload, especially in patients with cardiac or renal dysfunction.
  - Adjust fluid rates based on urine output and hemodynamic status.

Electrolyte Management

- *Hyperkalemia:*
  - Use calcium gluconate for cardiac membrane stabilization if electrocardiogram (ECG) changes occur.
  - Administer insulin with dextrose, sodium bicarbonate, or beta-agonists to shift potassium intracellularly.
  - Use potassium-binding agents (e.g., sodium polystyrene sulfonate) or dialysis for removal.

- *Hyperphosphatemia:*
  - Restrict dietary phosphate.
  - Administer phosphate binders (e.g., calcium acetate or sevelamer).
- *Hypocalcemia:* Treat symptomatic hypocalcemia cautiously, as calcium administration can exacerbate metastatic calcification.
- *Metabolic acidosis:* Use sodium bicarbonate in severe cases but avoid overcorrection.

Cardiac Monitoring

- *Rationale:* Electrolyte imbalances, particularly hyperkalemia, can precipitate arrhythmias or cardiac arrest.
- *Methods:*
  - Continuous ECG monitoring for arrhythmias.
  - Promptly address life-threatening rhythms with appropriate interventions (e.g., antiarrhythmics and defibrillation).

Supportive Care

- *Hyperkalemia and hyperphosphatemia:* Manage aggressively as described above.
- *AKI:* Support with fluids, dialysis, and avoidance of nephrotoxic agents.
- *Pain and symptom control:* Address associated symptoms, such as muscle cramps, nausea, and fatigue.

Chemotherapy

- *Modification:* In patients with established TLS or high risk of progression:
  - Delay initiation until metabolic imbalances are corrected.
  - Reduce doses temporarily to minimize tumor burden and subsequent lysis.
- *Rationale:* Reducing tumor lysis prevents exacerbation of electrolyte disturbances.

Bisphosphonates

- *Use:* Administer in cases of hypercalcemia associated with malignancy.
- *Agents:* Zoledronic acid or pamidronate can be used to reduce calcium levels and prevent calcification.
- *Caution:* Monitor for potential nephrotoxicity, especially in patients with compromised renal function.

Plasma Exchange

- *Indications:* Considered in refractory cases of hyperuricemia or when dialysis is not feasible.
- *Benefits:* Removes circulating tumor cells, uric acid, and other metabolic waste products.
- *Challenges:* Limited availability and resource intensive.

Monitoring

- *Parameters to track:*
  - Uric acid, potassium, calcium, phosphorus, and creatinine levels.
  - Acid–base status and hydration status.
  - Cardiac function and urine output.
- *Frequency*: Initially every 4–6 hours; adjust based on clinical stability.
- *Long-term follow-up:* Monitor for complications, such as chronic kidney disease and recurrent TLS.

Effective management of TLS requires a multidisciplinary approach focused on prompt recognition, aggressive correction of metabolic disturbances, and continuous monitoring to prevent complications. Early initiation of prophylactic measures and treatment can significantly improve outcomes. It is essential to note that treatment should be individualized based on the patient's specific needs and medical history. In some cases, additional treatments may be necessary. Consultation with a nephrologist, oncologist, and other specialists is crucial to ensure comprehensive management.

CONCLUSION

Tumor lysis syndrome is a life-threatening oncological emergency. As more and more highly effective cancer drugs are introduced, the incidence of TLS is anticipated to increase even more. Patients who are at higher risk of developing TLS should have a multidisciplinary approach with the involvement of an oncologist, a nephrologist, and an intensivist. Prompt identification and aggressive management are essential to avoid the life-threatening consequences of TLS.

REFERENCES

1. Cairo MS, Bishop M. Tumour lysis syndrome: new therapeutic strategies and classification. J Haematol. 2004; 127(1):3-11.
2. Howard SC, Jones DP, Pui CH. The tumor lysis syndrome. N Engl J Med. 2011;364 (19):1844-54. [Erratum: N Engl J Med. 2018;379(11):1094.]

3. Mayer MD, Khosravan R, Vernillet L, Wu JT, Joseph-Ridge N, Mulford DJ, et al. Pharmacokinetics and pharmacodynamics of febuxostat, a new non-purine selective inhibitor of xanthine oxidase in subjects with renal impairment. Am J Ther. 2005;12(1):22-34.
4. Jeha S. Tumor lysis syndrome. Semin Hematol. 2001; 38(Suppl 10):4-8.
5. Abu-Alfa AK, Younes A. Tumor lysis syndrome and acute kidney injury: evaluation, prevention, and management. Am J Kidney Dis. 2010;55(5 Suppl 3):S1-19.
6. Van den Berg H, Reintsema AM. Renal tubular damage in rasburicase: risks of alkalinisation. Ann Oncol. 2004;15(1):175-6.
7. Lopez-Olivo MA, Pratt G, Palla SL, Salahudeen A. Rasburicase in tumor lysis syndrome of the adult: a systematic review and meta-analysis. Am J Kidney Dis. 2013;62(3):481-92.
8. Bose P, Qubaiah O. A review of tumour lysis syndrome with targeted therapies and the role of rasburicase. J Clin Pharm Ther. 2011;36(3):299-326.
9. Coiffier B, Altman A, Pui CH, Younes A, Cairo MS. Guidelines for the management of pediatric and adult tumor lysis syndrome: an evidence-based review. J Clin Oncol. 2008;26(16):2767-78. [Erratum: J Clin Oncol. 2010; 28(4):708].
10. Jones GL, Will A, Jackson GH, Webb NJ, Rule S; British Committee for Standards in Haematology. British committee for standards in haematology. Guidelines for the management of tumour lysis syndrome in adults and children with haematological malignancies on behalf of the British committee for standards in haematology. Br J Haematol. 2015;169(5):661-71.
11. Sonbol MB, Yadav H, Vaidya R, Rana V, Witzig TE. Methemoglobinemia and hemolysis in a patient with G6PD deficiency treated with rasburicase. Am J Hematol. 2013;88(2):152-4.

CHAPTER 49

Febrile Neutropenic Patient in the Intensive Care Unit

Sukhada Savarkar, Atul Prabhakar Kulkarni

INTRODUCTION

Febrile neutropenia (FN) is a common and life-threatening complication encountered in cancer patients undergoing cytoreductive chemotherapy. Since these neutropenic patients may not mount the normal neutrophil-mediated inflammatory response, a fever may be the earliest and only sign of infection. Therefore, recognizing neutropenic fever early and initiating empirical therapy promptly is critical to prevent progression to sepsis and potential fatality. Since these patients can deteriorate very rapidly, and go into multiorgan failure due to septic shock it should be treated as an emergency.

The association between neutropenia and increased mortality was first described by Bodey and colleagues in 1966 in patients with acute myeloid leukemia (AML).[1] Although substantial progress has been made in understanding the pathophysiology and management of FN, it continues to be a clinical challenge, associated with high morbidity, mortality, and significant financial burden.

Patients with FN are frequently admitted to intensive care due to organ dysfunction, sepsis, or septic shock. Due to availability of better treatments for cancer, improved survival of cancer patients, and increased number of hematopoietic stem cell transplant (HSCT); more and more patients with FN are getting admitted to critical care unit. Despite prompt treatment, mortality due to FN in critically ill patient can be as high as 50%.[2] Increasing incidence of resistant gram-negative pathogens make the treatment of FN even more challenging. Therefore, FN in critical care unit should be treated as a medical emergency and a thorough understanding of the FN process and its management is the need of the hour for an intensivist.

In this chapter, we summarize the etiology, pathophysiology, diagnosis, and management of FN in critically ill patients.

DEFINITION

According to Infectious Diseases Society of America (IDSA) guidelines;[3] FN is defined as "a one-time oral temperature of >38.3°C or a sustained temperature of >38°C for ≥1 hour in a patient who has an absolute neutrophil count (ANC) of <500 cells/μL or an ANC that is expected to decrease to <500 cells/mm^3 during the next 48 hours.

Profound neutropenia refers to neutropenia in which the ANC is <100 cells/mm^3, while "functional neutropenia" describes cases where hematologic malignancies cause qualitative defects in circulating neutrophils, such as impaired phagocytosis and pathogen killing. These patients are at increased infection risk even with a "normal" neutrophil count.

Critically ill FN patients get admitted to intensive care unit (ICU) primarily due to neutropenic sepsis or septic shock with organ dysfunction. There is no universal definition for neutropenic sepsis. Sepsis in a patient having neutropenia can be considered as neutropenic sepsis. Sepsis itself is defined as "life-threatening organ dysfunction caused by a dysregulated host response to infection". Therefore, any sign of organ dysfunction with neutropenia should be treated as sepsis.

Several guidelines are commonly used to manage FN patients which are National Comprehensive Cancer Network (NCCN) guidelines, European Society for Medical Oncology (ESMO) practical guidelines, IDSA guidelines, joint American Society of Clinical Oncology (ASCO)/IDSA guidelines for outpatient management guidelines and, Fourth European Conference on Infections in Leukaemia (ECIL-4) guidelines.[3-7] While these guidelines differ slightly from each other in terms of management, definition, treatment duration, and de-escalation policy; their rationale behind the management remains similar.

EPIDEMIOLOGY

Fever occurs frequently during cytotoxic chemotherapy. 10–50% of patients with solid tumors and >80% of those with hematologic malignancies or undergoing HSCT will develop FN during the course of chemotherapy.[3] Standard chemotherapy regimens are associated with 6–8 days of neutropenia, and FN is observed in around 8 cases per 1,000 patients receiving chemotherapy.[8]

The FN is associated with significant morbidity with 20–30% of patients requiring hospital admission for management of complications. The overall in-hospital mortality of FN is around 10% which can increase up to 15% for patients with leukemia.[9]

Data on the incidence of neutropenic sepsis or neutropenic septic shock is limited. Studies suggest that nearly 50% of patients with neutropenic fever develop sepsis, and up to 10% of patients with neutropenic fever progress to septic shock.[10] Mortality in excess of 50% despite prompt antibiotic treatment has been reported in neutropenic patients presenting with septic shock or pneumonia.

ETIOLOGY

Most patients will have no infectious etiology documented. Bacteremia is seen in 10–25% of all patients, whereas clinically documented infections occur in 20–30% of febrile episodes with intestinal tract, lung, and skin being the common sites of infection.[3]

Most of the infections are bacterial in origin. During the 1960s and 1970s, infections were mainly caused by gram-negative organisms. Later, gram-positive organisms became more common in 1980s and 1990s. Increased prophylaxis against gram-negative organisms and increased use of indwelling central venous catheter were probably responsible for this shift.

In the recent decades, this shift from gram-negative bacteria to gram-positive bacteria is again changing toward an increase in incidence of gram-negative infections globally. In particular, there is increased incidence of drug-resistant gram-negative infections such as extended-spectrum beta-lactamase producing (ESBL) Enterobacterales, carbapenemase-producing pathogens in FN patients which are associated with higher risk of mortality.[8,11,12]

In contrast to the western data, gram-negative bacteremia is much more common than gram-positive bacteremia in febrile neutropenic patients in Indian population. Pathogens isolated from studies done in India suggest Enterobacteriaceae (*E. coli* and *Klebsiella* species) and *Pseudomonas aeruginosa* be the most common among gram-negative organisms. Among gram-positive isolates, *Staphylococcus aureus* and coagulase-negative *Staphylococcus* (CoNS) are most common isolates.[13]

Fungal infections can be seen commonly in high-risk patients but are uncommon in low-risk patients. Fungal infections are rarely identified as a cause of fever in the early period of neutropenia. They are usually seen in patients with prolonged or profound neutropenia. *Candida* and *Aspergillus* are the most frequent pathogens responsible for most invasive fungal infections during neutropenia.

Viral infections, especially human herpesviruses, are common in high-risk patients. Commonly seen viral pathogens include reactivated or de novo herpes viruses (e.g., herpes simplex, cytomegalovirus, and Epstein-Barr virus) and respiratory viruses (influenza virus, respiratory syncytial virus, parainfluenza virus types I to IV, human adenovirus, human rhinoviruses, human coronaviruses, and human metapneumovirus).

Despite best efforts, in majority of FN patients; no causative organism or identifiable site of infection can be identified.

PATHOPHYSIOLOGY

Neutropenia can occur either due to direct effect of malignancy as seen in leukemia or more commonly as an effect of cytotoxic chemotherapy. For majority of chemotherapy regimens, the nadir of neutropenia occurs 5–10 days after the last dose.

Cytotoxic chemotherapy or cytotoxic radiation induces neutropenia by injuring or destroying hematopoietic precursor cells within the bone marrow and by injuring the bone marrow structure itself.[14] Neutropenia develops when the circulating neutrophils reach the end of their life span and are not replaced. Some regimens destroy the circulating neutrophils and other white blood cells as well in addition to the precursor cells causing a more rapid leukopenia than regimens which only affect the marrow.

Normally, when there is a localized infection, neutrophils are rapidly recruited at the site, and they have a key role in controlling localized infections. Neutrophils also contribute to tissue repair and regulation of the adaptive immune response. Hence, neutropenic patients are not only deficient in the immediate response to infection but also have an altered physiology in the regulation of the immune response to injury and tissue repair. As the cytotoxic chemotherapy is not selective, neutropenic patients also have lymphopenia, thrombocytopenia, and anemia further impairing the normal immune response.

Another detrimental effect of cytotoxic chemotherapy is that damages the mucosal linings of the gastrointestinal, sinopulmonary, and genitourinary tracts which can lead to increased mucosal permeability and translocation of bacteria and fungi colonizing the mucosal surfaces. This is an important source of gram-positive, gram-negative, and fungal infections in neutropenic patients.

RISK FACTORS

Any oncologic patient receiving myelosuppressive chemotherapy is at risk of developing neutropenia, opportunistic infections, and associated complications. But certain factors which place the patients at higher risk of developing complications from FN. Several clinical studies have identified and tried to classify patients into high versus low risk for developing severe infection and complications. Factors that can place these patients at high risk of developing severe infections typically include sustained severe neutropenia anticipated to last >1 week, clinical instability (e.g., altered mental status or hypotension), presence of significant medical comorbidities, uncontrolled progressive cancer, poor functional status, grade 3 or 4 mucositis, or advanced age. Patients with acute leukemia or patients undergoing induction phase of acute leukemia or HSCT are also at high risk for complications.

In addition to the clinical factors and criteria, there are many scoring systems available for categorizing FN patients. MASCC scoring system **(Table 1)**, Clinical Index of Stable Febrile Neutropenia (CISNE) scoring **(Table 2)**, and Talcott's rule are some risk stratifying tools that can be used to stratify patients and identify patients at high risk. MASCC risk index score is used widely to assess the risk of complications in FN. It divides patients into high-risk patients (MASCC >21) and low risk patients (MASCC <21). The CISNE is an upcoming prognostic score for predicting serious complications in outpatients with solid tumors and stable FN episodes.[7]

These scoring systems help the clinician to decide the type of antibiotic regimen, appropriate location for delivery of empirical antibiotics, as well as the timing of hospital discharge in FN patients. In general, low-risk patients can be managed on outpatient basis with oral antibiotics and high-risk patients should receive empiric IV antibiotics and hospitalization.

TABLE 1: MASCC risk index score.

Patient characteristics	***Points***
Burden of FN with no or mild symptoms	5
No hypotension (SBP >90 mm Hg)	5
Absence of COPD	4
Solid organ or hematological malignancies with no previous fungal infection	4
No dehydration requiring volume expansion	3
Outpatient status	3
Burden of febrile neutropenia with moderate symptoms	3
Age <60 years	2

(COPD: chronic obstructive pulmonary disease; FN: febrile neutropenia; MASCC: Multinational Association for Supportive Care in Cancer; SBP: systolic blood pressure)

TABLE 2: CISNE score.

Characteristic	***Points***
Performance status ≥2 (ECOG)	2
Stress-induced hyperglycemia	2
Chronic obstructive pulmonary disease	1
Chronic cardiovascular disease	1
Grade ≥2 mucositis (National Cancer Institute)	1
Monocytes <200 per mcL	1

Note:
- *Low risk:* 0 points
- *Intermediate risk:* 1–2 points
- *High risk:* >3 points

(CISNE: Clinical Index of Stable Febrile Neutropenia; ECOG: Eastern Cooperative Oncology Group)

These high-risk patients are more likely to require ICU admission due to complications. Respiratory complications requiring ventilator support and hemodynamic compromise requiring fluid and vasopressors for sepsis and septic shock are common reasons for ICU admission in these patients.[15]

Febrile neutropenic patients generally present to the ICU with following clinical or laboratory parameters of organ failure (but not limited to):[13]

- Tachypnea requiring oxygen therapy >4 L/min to maintain saturation >90%

- Hypotension
- Altered mental status (without focal neurological deficit)
- Oliguria or rising creatinine

In the past, there has been some degree of hesitation for admitting FN patients who have cancer to ICU due to very high mortality in these patients. These patients have been considered "too ill" to benefit from critical care and severe neutropenia at the time of ICU admission has often been identified as an adverse prognostic factor for survival in cancer patients. However, neutropenia might not be impacting survival in these patients in the setting of septic shock. Almost similar ICU mortality rates have been observed among neutropenic and non-neutropenic patients with cancer and septic shock. In fact, literature suggests that the presence of comorbidities may have a greater influence on hospital mortality in febrile neutropenic patients with cancer and severe sepsis or septic shock.[15,16] Therefore, presence and degree of neutropenia should not be considered as triage factor for ICU admission. In addition, delayed ICU admission ranging from hours to days has been independently associated with increased mortality. Hence early ICU admission should be considered in this subgroup of patients.

INITIAL ASSESSMENT AND WORK-UP

Once the patient gets admitted to ICU, the initial assessment should include a detailed history and physical examination to identify the potential sources of infection (e.g., mouth sores, skin lesions, pulmonary findings, abdominal tenderness or pain, and infected indwelling catheters), systematic analysis of severity and duration of neutropenia, underlying immunosuppression, and ongoing antibiotic treatment. Laboratory studies at presentation should include complete blood count with differential, electrolytes, and markers of renal and hepatic function (creatinine, blood urea nitrogen, and transaminases), C-reactive protein or procalcitonin, an arterial blood gas, coagulation studies, and lactate levels.

Blood cultures are crucial for evaluation of neutropenic patients with fever. A minimum of two sets of blood cultures should be collected preferable before starting empirical therapy. Blood cultures should be collected from peripheral sites and from lumen of indwelling catheters if present.

Othe investigations can be targeted toward specific signs and symptoms of patients. For example, urine cultures should be obtained if patient presents with urinary symptoms. Diarrhea, especially in a patient treated with antibiotics, should prompt evaluation for *Clostridium difficile* colitis. Respiratory symptoms or abnormalities on chest imaging should be evaluated with testing for respiratory viruses and sputum culture.

In patients with persistent or prolonged FN or worsening clinical symptoms, following studies can be considered:

- HRCT if fever despite 72 hours of antibiotics (for invasive pulmonary aspergillosis)
- CT sinuses for fungal infections, e.g., mucormycosis
- CT abdomen for hepatosplenic candidiasis
- *Bronchoalveolar lavage (BAL):* Stains, cultures, and biomarkers
- To Look for noninfectious causes of fever, e.g., venous thromboembolism

TREATMENT

Neutropenic fever is a medical emergency, and appropriate empiric antibiotics must be started without delay, preferably within 60 minutes of presentation. As mentioned earlier, it is desirable to obtain blood cultures if possible before antibiotic initiation or change in antibiotic regimen, as long as this does not delay antibiotic administration.

There are many treatment guidelines available for prevention and treatment of FN. However, there is limited literature and guidelines for management of FN in ICU setting. An expert panel from the French Intensive Care Society has formulated recommendations for FN management in critically ill patients;[17] however, many of the recommendations are based on low-grade evidence suggesting the need for further studies. Recently, "Indian Antimicrobial Prescription Guidelines in Critically Ill Immunocompromised Patients" have been formulated which includes recommendations for treatment of critically ill FN patients in ICU.[13]

General principles for management of FN patients who are critically ill and require ICU admission are as follows:

- In majority of FN patient who present to ICU, an antibiotic regimen will already be in place started from the ward. This regimen may need escalation depending on the clinical status of the patient.
- Local antimicrobial susceptibility, prevalence of multidrug-resistant strains and the severity of disease are important factors to consider before staring or escalating the empirical treatment in ICU. The aim of

empiric therapy is to cover the most likely and most virulent pathogens that may cause rapid deterioration in patients' clinical condition.

- Even with appropriate antibiotics, fever in neutropenic patients typically persists for a period of 5 days. Therefore, ongoing fever without clinical instability, should not always be viewed as failure of antibiotic therapy.
- Although gram-positive bacteria are frequently identified during neutropenic fever episodes, it is important to cover for gram-negative pathogens because of their increasing prevalence, virulence, and association with sepsis.
- The use of combination antibiotic regimens [dual gram-negative coverage with an antipseudomonal beta-lactam (BL) and an aminoglycoside] in neutropenic fever is controversial. The literature shows conflicting results regarding the benefit of combination therapy. Therefore, current available guidelines for the management of neutropenic fever and sepsis recommend monotherapy unless the clinical situation demands combination therapy.
- Appropriate empiric antibiotics choices include a fourth-generation antipseudomonal cephalosporin (cefepime), β-lactam/β-lactamase combination (e.g., piperacillin/tazobactam), or a carbapenem (imipenem and meropenem). However, recent studies from the Indian subcontinent indicate that many gram-negative pathogens isolated from initial blood cultures in patients are resistant to noncarbapenem antibiotics.
- Due to this increased prevalence of multidrug-resistant organisms, it is reasonable to start or escalate to a broad-spectrum carbapenem such as imipenem or meropenem in critically ill FN patients as initial therapy.
- Empiric combination of meropenem and colistin/polymyxin B can be considered in the following patients having high risk of infection with resistant gram-negative organisms.
  - Critically ill patients with underlying acute leukemia presenting to the ICU
  - Patients of leukemia/lymphoma on BL/beta-lactamase inhibitor (BLI) ± aminoglycosides, shifted to ICU from ward
  - Previous exposure to broad-spectrum antibiotics such as carbapenems or BL/BLI combination in last 1 month
  - Hypotensive patients requiring vasopressor infusions (refractory septic shock)
  - Patient shifted to the ICU on carbapenem therapy
- For carbapenem-resistant gram-negative organisms, treatment options include ceftazidime-avibactam plus aztreonam or polymyxins as a single agent or in combination with another agent demonstrating in vitro susceptibility.[18]
- Antibiotics such as fosfomycin, tigecycline, and minocycline may be considered in infection with multidrug-resistant bacteria after confirming in vitro susceptibility and after considering the in vivo penetration at the source of sepsis.
- Vancomycin is not a standard part of empirical antibiotic therapy for the febrile neutropenic patient. Vancomycin/teicoplanin should be added as empiric therapy in following patients with:
  - Suspected indwelling vascular catheter infection
  - Skin and soft-tissue infection
  - Previous colonization/infection with MRSA
  - *Blood culture:* Gram positive cocci awaiting identification
  - Severe mucositis
  - Hemodynamic instability in patients admitted from home/OPD
- Daptomycin/linezolid should be used for vancomycin resistant strains.
- Antifungal therapy is recommended when patients get admitted to ICU with shock or respiratory failure and their fever persists or recurs or they have clinical deterioration after >3 days of broad-spectrum antibiotics. Risk factors for predisposing these patients to fungal infections are allogenic HSCT, presence of severe mucositis with diarrhea, prolonged neutropenia >10 days, worsening on broad spectrum antibiotics, prior history of steroids, history of invasive fungal infection, and new-onset lung infiltrate.
- For patients who have no obvious source of infection, *Candida* infection should be suspected. Echinocandins (caspofungin) are favored over azoles for empiric therapy as some *Candida* species are resistant to azoles.
- For persistently febrile patients with pulmonary nodules or nodular pulmonary infiltrates, invasive mold infections (aspergillus) should be strongly suspected and treated. Voriconazole is the drug of choice for proven, probable or possible aspergillosis.

Liposomal amphotericin B is the drug of choice for suspected or confirmed mucor mycosis.

- Empirical use of antiviral drugs is indicated only in patients with clinical or laboratory evidence of viral infection.
- Sulfamethoxazole/trimethoprim should be started in patients who are at high risk for developing Pneumocystis carinii pneumonia and present to ICU with hypoxemic respiratory failure (high-risk patients are patients undergoing allogeneic HSCT, autologous HSCT, patients on high-dose corticosteroid therapy, and patients receiving T-cell-depleting agents such as fludarabine, purine analogs, and rituximab).
- There is no role for routine empirical antimicrobial therapy against tropical infections such as malaria and leptospirosis.
- Antimicrobial de-escalation should be implemented in the following situations:
  - Once the organism is identified, de-escalation should be done to an antibiotic that the organism is sensitive to.
  - In patients without microbiologically documented infection, empirical antibiotics should be continued till the patient is afebrile for at least 48 hours and there is evidence of marrow recovery (neutrophil count ≥500 cells/mm^3) after which de-escalation can be considered.

CONCLUSION

Febrile neutropenia in the ICU is a medical emergency that demands prompt identification, risk stratification, and targeted treatment. Improved survival rates in cancer patients, advancements in treatments, and the introduction of new regimens have led to an increase in ICU admissions for patients with FN. Effective management relies on a multidisciplinary approach involving oncologists and intensivists to ensure optimal patient outcomes. Although outcomes for critically ill FN patients have improved, the increasing prevalence of antimicrobial resistance highlights the need for novel therapies, timely de-escalation, and early recognition of causative organisms. Further research into the pathophysiology of neutropenic sepsis is essential for earlier diagnosis and management of febrile neutropenic patients.

REFERENCES

1. Bodey GP, Buckley M, Sathe YS, Freireich EJ. Quantitative relationships between circulating leukocytes and infection in patients with acute leukemia. Ann Intern Med. 1966;64(2):328-40.
2. Legrand M, Max A, Peigne V, Mariotte E, Canet E, Debrumetz A, et al. Survival in neutropenic patients with severe sepsis or septic shock. Crit Care Med. 2012;40(1):43-9.
3. Freifeld AG, Bow EJ, Sepkowitz KA, Boeckh MJ, Ito JI, Mullen CA, et al. Clinical practice guideline for the use of antimicrobial agents in neutropenic patients with cancer: 2010 Update by the Infectious Diseases Society of America. Clin Infect Dis. 2011;52(4):427-31.
4. Averbuch D, Orasch C, Cordonnier C, Livermore DM, Mikulska M, Viscoli C, et al. European guidelines for empirical antibacterial therapy for febrile neutropenic patients in the era of growing resistance: Summary of the 2011 4th European Conference on Infections in Leukemia. Haematologica. 2013;98(12):1826-35.
5. Baden LR, Swaminathan S, Angarone M. Prevention and treatment of cancer-related infections, version 2.2022, NCCN clinical practice guidelines in oncology. J Natl Compr Canc Netw. 2016;14:882-913.
6. Klastersky J, de Naurois J, Rolston K, Rapoport B, Maschmeyer G, Aapro M, et al. Management of febrile neutropaenia: ESMO Clinical Practice Guidelines. Ann Oncol. 2016;27(suppl 5):v111-8.
7. Taplitz RA, Kennedy EB, Flowers CR. Outpatient management of fever and neutropenia in adults treated for malignancy: American society of clinical oncology and infectious diseases society of America clinical practice guideline update summary. J Oncol Pract. 2018;14(4):250-5.
8. Boccia R, Glaspy J, Crawford J, Aapro M. Chemotherapy-induced neutropenia and febrile neutropenia in the US: A beast of burden that needs to be tamed? Oncologist. 2022;27(8):625-36.
9. Kuderer NM, Dale DC, Crawford J, Cosler LE, Lyman GH. Mortality, morbidity, and cost associated with febrile neutropenia in adult cancer patients. Cancer. 2006;106(10):2258-66.
10. Heinz WJ, Buchheidt D, Christopeit M, Von Lilienfeld-Toal M, Cornely OA, Einsele H, et al. Diagnosis and empirical treatment of fever of unknown origin (FUO) in adult neutropenic patients: guidelines of the Infectious Diseases Working Party (AGIHO) of the German Society of Hematology and Medical Oncology (DGHO) Ann Hematol. 2017;96:1775-92.
11. Gudiol C, Bodro M, Simonetti A, Tubau F, González-Barca E, Cisnal M, et al. Changing aetiology, clinical features, antimicrobial resistance, and outcomes of bloodstream infection in neutropenic cancer patients. Clin Microbiol Infect. 2013;19(5):474-9.
12. Trecarichi EM, Pagano L, Candoni A, Pastore D, Cattaneo C, Fanci R, et al. Hemabis Registry-Seifem Group, I Current epidemiology and antimicrobial resistance data for bacterial bloodstream infections in patients with hematologic

malignancies: an Italian multicentre prospective survey. Clin Microbiol Infect. 2015;21:337-43.
13. Kulkarni AP, Sengar M, Chinnaswamy G, Hegde A, Rodrigues C, Soman R, et al. Indian antimicrobial prescription guidelines in critically ill immunocompromised patients. Indian J Crit Care Med. 2019;23(Suppl 1):S64-96.
14. Stephens RS. Neutropenic Fever in the Intensive Care Unit. Oncologic Critical Care. Oncologic Critical Care. 2009; 1297-311.
15. Bow EJ. Infection in neutropenic patients with cancer. Crit Care Clin. 2013;29(3):411-41.
16. Taccone FS, Artigas AA, Sprung CL, Moreno R, Sakr Y, Vincent JL. Characteristics and outcomes of cancer patients in European ICUs. Crit Care. 2009;13(1):R15.
17. Schnell D, Azoulay E, Benoit D, Clouzeau B, Demaret P, Ducassou S, et al. Management of neutropenic patients in the intensive care unit (NEWBORNS EXCLUDED) recommendations from an expert panel from the French Intensive Care Society (SRLF) with the French Group for Pediatric Intensive Care Emergencies (GFRUP), the French Society of Anesthesia and Intensive Care (SFAR), the French Society of Hematology (SFH), the French Society for Hospital Hygiene (SF2H), and the French Infectious Diseases Society (SPILF). Ann Intensive Care. 2016;6(1):90.
18. Indian Council of Medical Research. (2025). *Guidance on Diagnosis & Management of Carbapenem Resistant Gram-negative Infections*. [online] Available from https://www.icmr.gov.in/guidelines [Last accessed March, 2025].

CHAPTER

Postoperative Critical Care after Major Cancer Surgeries

Deepa Chandramohan, Dileep Damodaran

INTRODUCTION

Postoperative management, following major oncological surgeries, is challenging. The radical and ultraradical cancer surgeries of varying organ sites are associated with profound hemodynamic and biochemical derangements leading to increased incidences of Clavien–Dindo grade III–V postoperative complications. These major surgeries involve prolonged operative time with extensive dissection, multiviscera resections and major blood loss leading to hypothermia acid–base disturbances, severe dyselectrolytemia, increased requirement of blood product transfusions, and need of postoperative mechanical ventilation. The acute phase response due to the surgical stress results in colossal cytokine release with widespread capillary leak leading to systemic inflammatory response syndrome (SIRS), loss of gut integrity, and thereby, higher propensity for sepsis and multiorgan dysfunction.[1] The systemic inflammatory and endocrine disturbances associated with this stress response lead to a multitude of manifestations such as coagulopathy, respiratory failure, major adverse cardiac events (MACEs), renal, adrenal or hepatic insufficiency or failure, to name a few, during the postoperative period. The magnitude of this response is proportional to the surgery-related tissue trauma and the complexity of the procedure, which is further modified by factors such as pain, stress, or a secondary insult. The inflammatory mediators peak at around day 1–2 and then return to baseline levels by days 6–7.[1] A delicate balance between the systemic proinflammatory and anti-inflammatory mediators is important for the return of homeostasis postsurgery. This initial critical period, hence, is the tempestuous phase that requires stringent monitoring and intensive care for a good postoperative outcome.

In this chapter, we will discuss the postoperative critical care management following major and supramajor thoracic, abdominopelvic, and retroperitoneal cancer surgeries. The components of postoperative critical care are listed in **Box 1**.

POSTOPERATIVE ANALGESIA

Adequate postoperative analgesia is an integral component of the critical care pathway that leads to a good postoperative outcome. The ideal analgesic used in the postoperative period must provide excellent pain relief, facilitate early mobilization and physiotherapy, and must have the minimal adverse effects on gut motility.[2] Higher pain scores have been noted to be associated with a multitude of postoperative complications such as major pulmonary and cardiac events, delirium, anastomotic failures, metabolic disturbances, delayed recovery, prolonged hospital stay, and development of chronic pain syndromes.[3] Adequate analgesia during the immediate postoperative period leads to lesser incidence of postoperative pulmonary complications (PPCs), MACEs and postoperative delirium, prevents worsening of metabolic acidosis, mitigates the colossal flare-up of proinflammatory mediators, and facilitates early ambulation.[2] This allows a smooth transition of physiological functions back to near normal, which translates to shorter length of intensive care unit (ICU) and hospital length of stay (LOS), reduced costs,

BOX 1: Components of postoperative critical care.

- Postoperative mechanical ventilation and oxygen therapy
- Intravenous fluid therapy
- Correction of dyselectrolytemia and acid-base imbalance
- Transfusion of blood products
- Prophylaxis against venous thromboembolism
- Nutrition and glycemic control
- Physiotherapy
- Postoperative antibiotic therapy
- Monitoring and prevention of vital organ dysfunction

emotional well-being of patients and better patient and family satisfaction. Multimodal analgesia (MMA) strategy provides good quality pain relief during the postoperative period by deftly intertwining various techniques and medications such as epidural analgesia, nerve blocks, local anesthetics (LAs), opioids and non-opioids [i.e., nonsteroidal anti-inflammatory drugs (NSAIDs) and acetaminophen].[4,5] This strategy provides superior analgesia through the additive or synergistic effects of drugs (with varied mechanisms of action) while minimizing the adverse effects of individual drugs and reducing the use of opioids.[5,6] Chronic opioid use develops in about 6% of patients following surgery and these figures are presumed to be higher in patients undergoing cancer surgery.[7] The opioid-sparing strategies used in MMA can help in reducing the need for opioid prescription upon discharge.

Epidural analgesia, using a mixture of LAs and short-acting opiates or other adjuvants, is one of the optimal techniques for providing excellent pain relief during the first 72 hours following major cancer surgeries. In addition to providing comprehensive pain control, it aids in facilitating gut recovery and resultant anastomotic stability, reducing pulmonary complications and shortening the LOS, with acceptable complication rates.[8,9] Management of hypotension and breakthrough pain and meticulous neurologic monitoring for the timely detection of epidural hematoma and epidural abscess are of paramount importance during this period. Patient-controlled epidural analgesia is gaining more popularity lately, compared to conventional epidural infusion. Following removal of the epidural catheter, opioids, NSAIDs, and acetaminophen are recommended.[2,5,6]

Ultrasound-guided nerve blocks (NBs), both single-shot and continuous, are gaining popularity as a vital component of MMA for postoperative somatic pain management. Transversus abdominis plane (TAP), rectus sheath, erector spinae plane, quadratus lumborum, and paravertebral blocks are being increasingly used for providing both intraoperative and postoperative analgesia in patients undergoing major cancer surgeries. NBs, involving LAs with or without adjuvants, aid to reduce systemic opioid consumption, reduce postoperative nausea and vomiting (PONV), improve pain control, decrease postoperative complications, shorten the LOHS, and improve patient outcomes. The potential adverse effects of NBA include nerve damage, infection, hematoma, LA toxicity and inadequate analgesia.[10-12]

Wound infiltration analgesia (WIA), either as a single-shot injection at the end of surgery or as continuous infusion via a catheter is an approach that administers LAs (with or without adjuvants) directly to the site of incision. WIA in association with TAP block has been observed to achieve good postoperative pain relief while diminishing the need for opioids, reducing PONV, and promoting faster recovery of bowel function.[12,13] Although WIA is less effective than epidural analgesia in terms of analgesic efficacy and functional recovery and poses a higher risk of wound infection, it is associated with a lower risk of other adverse events such as hypotension.

Opioids and NSAIDs provide excellent postoperative analgesia, but they are associated with a vast array of undesirable adverse effects, especially in elderly patients and those with preexisting organ dysfunction. Dipyrone (metamizole) is an alternative with no risk of renal dysfunction unlike NSAIDs, but at the cost of agranulocytosis. The Enhanced Recovery After Surgery (ERAS) guidelines do not recommend the use of systemic ketamine, lidocaine, or gabapentin for postoperative analgesia following major cancer surgeries.[2,5,6]

Electroacupuncture and transcutaneous electrical acupoint stimulation (TEAS) are intriguing adjunctive tools for acute postoperative pain management, especially following colorectal cancer surgery in the elderly. These techniques has been demonstrated to reduce the incidence and duration of postoperative ileus, improve ambulation, decrease the incidence of PONV, reduce postoperative pain scores, and reduce the LOHS in patients undergoing colorectal surgery for cancer.[14,15] Novel controlled-drug delivery systems such as hydrogels and nanoparticles are engineered to precisely regulate the distribution of drugs. These innovative agents which are expected to optimize the therapeutic efficacy and mitigate the incidence of side effects, will be the future of MMA.[16,17]

POSTOPERATIVE MECHANICAL VENTILATION AND OXYGEN THERAPY

Major and prolonged surgeries are associated with major fluid shifts and altered vascular permeability.[1] The perioperative infusion of intravenous (IV) fluids and blood products, the altered body fluid constitution and fluid dynamics, and the resultant uneven Starling forces result in third-space fluid loss and interstitial edema, despite the hypovolemia that may persist during the postoperative period.[18] Increased extravascular lung water (EVLW) culminates in "wet lungs," low pulmonary compliance, and increased work of breathing. Additionally, the residual effects of general anesthetics, impaired mucociliary clearance, weak cough reflex, and postoperative respiratory muscle weakness result in inefficient sputum clearance, reduced lung compliance, inadequate ventilation, and impaired oxygenation. These perturbations predispose these patients to postoperative pulmonary complications (PPCs) that include basal pulmonary atelectasis, pneumonia, pulmonary edema, postextubation respiratory failure, transfusion-related acute lung injury and acute respiratory distress syndrome (ARDS). This, in turn, leads to poor outcomes in terms of increased duration of mechanical ventilation, increased lengths of ICU and hospital LOS, and increased hospital costs.[19]

Postoperative pulomnary complications constitute 10–40% of the postoperative complications following major surgeries. The most severe form of PPC is postoperative respiratory failure (PRF), which is defined as mechanical ventilation longer than 48 hours with or without unplanned postoperative reintubation.[19,20] The various risk factors for PRF are enumerated in **Box 2**.[21,22]

BOX 2: Risk factors for postoperative respiratory failure.

- *Patient factors:*
  - Advanced age (above 65 years)
  - Higher frailty index
  - Poor nutritional status
  - History of smoking or reactive/obstructive airway disease
  - Obesity with or without obstructive sleep apnea
  - Poor cardiopulmonary reserve
- *Surgical factors:*
  - High surgical complexity scores
  - Emergency surgery
  - Thoracic surgeries and upper abdominal surgeries
  - Major surgical procedures involving the airway or the diaphragm
- *Intraoperative and postoperative factors:*
  - Surgical procedures lasting >3 hours
  - Major intraoperative blood loss
  - Massive transfusion of blood products
  - Intraoperative hemodynamic instability
  - Intraoperative major adverse cardiac events
  - Poorly controlled pain
  - Severe dyselectrolytemia
  - Severe metabolic acidosis
  - End-of-surgery serum lactate >3.5 mmol/L
  - Inadequate ventilatory drive after reversal of neuromuscular blockade with or without hypercapnia
  - Fluid overload with or without oxygenation failure

These subset of patients will benefit from prophylactically continuing mechanical ventilation postoperatively in the ICU, giving adequate time for gradual weaning and extubation. This strategy will also buy time for redistribution of the accumulated interstitial fluid, return of capillary integrity, IV fluid stewardship, fluid deresuscitation and reduce the chance of postextubation respiratory failure.

The patients at risk of developing PRF are appropriate candidates for prophylactic use of high-flow nasal oxygen (HFNO) therapy or noninvasive ventilation (NIV) following extubation in the operating room (OR) or later in the ICU.[22,23] HFNO can also be initiated preemptively in those showing early signs of postoperative respiratory distress. Monitoring the postoperative patients following extubation as well as on HFNO/NIV with the help of scores such as ROX index [the ratio of peripheral oxygen saturation (SpO_2) divided by fraction of inspired oxygen (FiO_2) to the respiratory rate] can help in escalating oxygen therapy as needed. Use of HFNO has been found to reduce the incidence of PPCs, atelectasis, reintubation rates, and NIV requirement, along with the added advantages of better patient compliance and reduced work of breathing.[22,24] NIV is associated with poor patient tolerance as well as skin breakdown. However, there has been no significant mortality benefit in postoperative patients when the use of HFNO was compared with NIV or conventional oxygen therapy.[24,25]

INTRAVENOUS FLUID THERAPY

Postoperative IV fluid therapy following major cancer surgery is an integral component of postoperative critical care protocols in an oncocritical care unit. In the perioperative setting, fluid management should be appropriate to maintain adequate organ perfusion and peripheral oxygen delivery, while avoiding the consequences of fluid overload. The art and science of deciding the drug (which IV fluid), its dose, its duration, and its de-escalation must be carefully carried out during the postoperative period for each patient on an "individual" basis, abiding by the institutional fluid stewardship protocols. Fluid stewardship should focus on the 4 questions (when to start IV fluids, when to stop IV fluids, when to start fluid removal, and when to stop fluid removal), and on the conceptual ROSE model that describes the four phases during fluid therapy (resuscitation, optimization, stabilization, and evacuation).[26]

In the surgical ICUs, the major fraction of IV fluids administered is not for resuscitation (6%), but for maintenance (25%), nutrition (33%), and fluid creep (33%), with the rest being blood product transfusions.[27] The fluid management during the postoperative period depends on multiple factors such as the technique of surgery (laparoscopic or open), complexity of the surgical procedure, intraoperative blood and fluid losses, volume of blood products transfused, acid-base disturbances, serum albumin levels, hemodynamic indices, cardiopulmonary reserve, organ dysfunctions, and comorbidities. Postoperative hypervolemia as well as hypovolemia are associated with high postoperative morbidity and mortality.[18,27,28] A "liberal" fluid approach leads to tissue edema, anastomotic failure, organ dysfunction, and increased lengths of ICU stay and hospital stay, whereas an excessively "restrictive" fluid approach causes tissue hypoperfusion and tissue hypoxia leading to increased postoperative organ dysfunction, particularly acute kidney insufficiency (AKI). A higher cumulative fluid balance (CFB) during the immediate postoperative period has been found to be associated with poorer outcomes such as increased incidence of postoperative surgical complications, increased duration of mechanical ventilation, increased LOHS, increased risk of PPCs, delayed return of bowel motility, and increased mortality.[28] In patients undergoing surgery for esophageal cancer, fluid overload was positively associated with poor outcome and higher incidence of anastomotic leakage.[29,30] A balanced perioperative fluid therapy on the day of surgery is noted to be associated with a faster recovery, lower morbidity, shorter LOHS, and lesser 30-day re-admission rate.[31]

Choice of Fluids

Balanced salt solutions, such as RL (lactated Ringer's solution) and Plasmalyte P that cause minimal alteration of the physiological milieu are the fluids of choice during the postoperative period.[27] The newer balanced salt solutions or RL is preferred to normal saline (NS) as prolonged infusion of the NS can result in hyperchloremic metabolic acidosis and renal dysfunction. Colloids, such as IV 20% human albumin, are being increasingly used in surgical ICUs to reduce the postoperative requirement of crystalloids and also to reduce the chances of bowel wall edema and consequent anastomotic dehiscence, especially in those with hypoalbuminemia.[18,26-28] Although other colloids such as starches and dextrans have the advantages of higher plasma-expansion capacity, and reduction of vasopressor requirement, they are not commonly advocated during postoperative period due to documented higher incidence of renal dysfunction and coagulopathy. However, there are opposing views about the use of starches in the postoperative period, and pending the results of various ongoing trials, a consensus about its use in surgical ICU is not yet ready. Supplementing IV 20% albumin can aid in maintaining intravascular volume and vital organ perfusion pressures and reduce IV crystalloid requirement.[18,22,27] Nevertheless, the role of albumin as a resuscitation fluid remains controversial. The ERAS Society recommendations for postoperative management of patients undergoing gynecological or abdominal oncology surgery include a discontinuation of IV fluids within 24 hours after surgery. Early initiation of oral/enteral feeds helps in tapering off IV fluid administration.[2,6]

Resuscitation Strategy—Dynamic and Personalized

All phases of IV fluid therapy, i.e., resuscitation phase, optimization phase, stabilization phase, and evacuation phase will have to be "personalized" as per the hemodynamic parameters (both static and dynamic), fluid responsiveness (FR), and fluid tolerance (FT) of the patient.[32] Additionally, serial values of serum lactate and cardiac output monitoring can guide the alterations in the fluid administration rate, rather than relying on parameters such as heart rate, blood pressure, CVP, and urine output that will relay only inconclusive and delayed information. Inotropes and vasopressors may be required depending on the clinical condition and cardiac indices. Stroke volume-guided fluid therapy that takes into account the FR and FT status of the patient along with other cardiac indices can reduce the risk of fluid overload, vasopressor use and renal dysfunction during the postoperative stay.[32-34]

In patients who have undergone major cancer surgeries that involve extensive peritonectomy, multivisceral resections and hyperthermic intraperitoneal chemotherapy (HIPEC), the increased capillary permeability consequent to the massive cytokine release and endothelial glycocalyx dysfunction necessitates close monitoring of EVLW while administering IV crystalloids during the postoperative period. A "restrictive" continuous fluid administration with intermittent fluid boluses as per the static and dynamic hemodynamic indices is preferable in such patients.[18,27] A study by Chandramohan et al. describes the strategy of dynamic multiparameter-based IVF therapy, especially in ultraradical surgeries such as cytoreductive surgery (CRS) with HIPEC.[22] It took into consideration multiple factors including intraoperative PCI, extent of peritonectomy, blood loss, volume of blood products transfused, serial serum lactate values, static and dynamic hemodynamic indices, fluid responsiveness, and thoracic fluid content monitoring using noninvasive cardiac output monitor in addition to standard parameters assessed in goal-directed fluid therapy. FR- and FT-guided fluid therapy helps the ICU team to understand if the fluid requirement of the surgical patient has plateaued over time and also about the need of initiation of fluid deresuscitation with diuretics during the postoperative period. Optimal fluid therapy improves postoperative outcome and hence, IV fluids, like other medications, must be administered as per well-defined protocols and on a "personalized" basis.

Correction of Dyselectrolytemia and Acid-base Imbalance

Dyselectrolytemia is common in postoperative patients due to multiple factors such as fluid shifts, third-space and insensible fluid losses, inadequate intake, hemodilution, and drug interactions. Maintaining normal levels of serum electrolytes is important in postoperative critical care. Serum sodium levels need to be maintained within normal limits to avoid postoperative neurological disturbances. Serum potassium levels are to be monitored at least twice daily during the first 24 hours, and thereafter daily during the next 72 hours. Cardiac arrhythmias are frequent following extensive mediastinal dissection in complicated esophageal surgeries and maintaining serum potassium levels above 4 mEq/L have been found to reduce the incidence and severity of arrhythmias by maintaining cardiac membrane potential stability. Ionized calcium levels also need to be normalized to maintain stable cardiac rhythms and to improve myocardial contractility. Calcium is an inopressor that improves the ventricular stroke volume index without causing tachycardia. It reverses the myocardial depression caused by volatile anesthetics, hyperlactatemia, and hypocalcemia.[22,35] Magnesium levels need to be monitored daily during postoperative stay as majority of patients have hypomagnesemia right from the preoperative period. Uncorrected hypomagnesemia is one of the common causes for refractory hypokalemia. Serum phosphate levels tend to drop with the initiation of parenteral nutrition during the postoperative period in about 50% of patients. Magnesium and phosphate, being integral components of ATP, require to be maintained within normal limits as hypomagnesemia and hypophosphatemia are two common, but avoidable reasons for ICU readmission.

Metabolic acidosis is common during postoperative period, the usual reasons being hyperlactatemia, diabetic ketoacidosis, AKI, and hyperchloremia. Certain major surgeries such as liver resections, parenchyma-sparing liver metastatectomy, and CRS with HIPEC are associated with significant hyperlactatemia and metabolic acidosis during the immediate postoperative period.[22,36] Persistent hyperlactatemia of >4 mmol/L and lactate clearance of <40% at 24 hours during the postoperative course have been associated with worse patient outcomes.[36-38] Early postoperative lactate values following hepatectomy are markers for clinically relevant posthepatectomy liver failure.[39] Persistent hyperlactatemia and metabolic acidosis can lead to irreversible myocardial depression and propensity for cardiac arrhythmias. Also, hyperlactatemia can result in significant drop in ionized calcium levels that can adversely affect the cardiovascular dynamics.[22]

Serial serum lactate levels and lactate kinetics can help in guiding postoperative IV fluid therapy.[22] Persistent hyperlactatemia beyond 12 hours of postoperative period, despite correcting hypovolemia should prompt looking into other contributory factors such as: (1) Early sepsis, (2) postoperative pulmonary complications as evidenced by drop in PaO_2/FiO_2 ratios, (3) low hemoglobin causing decreased tissue oxygen delivery, (4) acute postoperative cardiac dysfunction, e.g., stress cardiomyopathy, (5) ongoing use of vasopressors, (6) hypothermia causing increased peripheral vascular resistance, and (7) mesenteric ischemia.[22] Diabetic ketoacidosis and AKI are common causes of high anion gap (AG) metabolic acidosis during postoperative stay. Hyperchloremia secondary to infusion of IV normal saline is also a major cause of normal AG metabolic acidosis in postoperative patients.

Transfusion of Blood Products

Patients undergoing major cancer surgery at a higher risk of severe bleeding and coagulopathy due to the tumor biology, preoperative chemoradiation, immunotherapy, surgical complexity, and perioperative factors such as hemodilution, hypothermia, and metabolic disturbances.[40] Postoperatively, blood products are usually administered to improve oxygen delivery and/or to correct clinically significant coagulopathy. However, transfusion-related immune modulation which is a complication of blood product transfusion can result in cancer recurrence, progression and shorter recurrence-free survival.[40]

A "restrictive" transfusion trigger of 7–8 g/dL of hemoglobin (Hb) for postoperative packed red blood cell (PRBC) transfusion is being widely practiced. However, factors such as patient's age, frailty, comorbidity burden, cardiopulmonary dysfunction, acute myocardial ischemia, severe hypoxemia, ongoing blood loss, and overall clinical scenario should be considered and transfusion triggers may be amended upto Hb of 10 g/dL. However, unlike the previous landmark trials, the TRICOP trial noted a significantly lower mortality rate in the "liberal" (Hb of 9 g/dL) transfusion-strategy group, in oncology patients with septic shock.[41] A few authors have opined that the "timely" correction of blood losses might prevent hyperlactatemia, by reversing the impaired oxygen delivery. On the contrary, multiple authors have observed the association between perioperative blood transfusion and postoperative SIRS with poor outcome following pelvic exenteration for colorectal cancer. Further studies are required to pinpoint the specific PRBC transfusion trigger in postoperative period following cancer surgery. Intraoperative autologous blood cell salvage had been previously associated with the concern of tumor cell dissemination. However, the recently published papers support its safety and efficacy and find it to be a suitable option with advantages such as no cancer recurrence risk and reduced requirement for postoperative allogenic transfusion.[42]

Dilutional thrombocytopenia and disseminated intravascular coagulation (DIC) are the most common causes of thrombocytopenia during and after cancer surgery. Most guidelines recommend a threshold platelet count of 40,000–50,000/μL for performing major invasive procedures. In the absence of associated coagulation abnormalities, platelet transfusion triggers of 40,000–50,000/μL can be used to control or prevent bleeding after major cancer surgeries. Maintaining platelet counts between 50,000/μL and 100,000/μL would be preferred following most major surgeries, except neurosurgical ones that demand higher thresholds of 100,000/μL. Dilutional coagulopathy and DIC are the most common reasons that necessitate transfusion of FFP or cryoprecipitate during the postoperative period. Use of viscoelastic tests such as thromboelastography (TEG) and rotational thromboelastometry (ROTEM), rather than the conventional coagulation tests (INR, PTT, PT, platelet count) can provide better insights to choose "the right" blood product for the "right reasons" during the postoperative period.[43]

Till date, no clear indications or consensus guidelines exist on the postoperative blood product transfusions following major oncological surgeries. Oncology centers should institute blood product transfusion protocols with the help of a multidisciplinary team of perioperative physicians. Strategies to minimize perioperative blood loss, and the use of modern technology to guide personalized IV fluid administration and to single out the exact site of abnormality in the coagulation pathway will help to individualize blood product transfusions and minimize the ill-effects of transfusion in oncology patients.

PROPHYLAXIS AGAINST VENOUS THROMBOEMBOLISM

Venous thromboembolism (VTE) has been reported as the most common cause of 30-day mortality following surgery in cancer patients. The presence of malignancy itself predisposes these patients to high risk of VTE due to various poorly understood multifaceted direct as well as indirect molecular mechanisms.[44] The different risk factors for VTE in cancer patients have been enlisted in **Box 3.**[44,45]

Whenever feasible, out-of-bed ambulation as early as POD-1 is advised. The ERAS and European Society for Medical Oncology (ESMO) guidelines recommend the use of mechanical thromboprophylaxis (MTP) until complete mobilization, in association with pharmacological prophylaxis (PTP), instead of PTP alone following major cancer surgeries.[2,6,45] Intermittent pneumatic compression or graduated compression stockings provide reasonable MTP in the postoperative periods. MTP is advised until the patient is completely mobilized. MTP can also be used as monotherapy or as an alternative, if PTP is contraindicated.[2,45]

Unless contraindicated, PTP with low molecular weight heparin (LMWH) or unfractionated heparin (UFH) is recommended in all patients undergoing major cancer surgery. LMWH once daily and UFH three times daily administered subcutaneously have comparable efficacies.[2,44,45] LMWH is associated with a lower incidence of wound hematoma, lower risk of heparin-induced thrombocytopenia and a more convenient administration schedule compared to UFH even though both show no difference with respect to mortality, pulmonary embolism and bleeding.[45] No specific LMWH has been proven to be

BOX 3: Risk factors for venous thromboembolism in cancer patients.

- *Patient factors:*
  - Advanced age (above 65 years)
  - *Comorbidities:* Renal failure, respiratory disease, heart disease, and acute infection
  - Higher body mass index
  - Immobility for more than 3 days
  - Previous history of venous thromboembolism (VTE)
- *Disease factors:*
  - Site of cancer, e.g., higher incidence of VTE in cancers of pancreas, lung, gastrointestinal, kidney ovary, breast and prostate
  - Advanced stage of cancer—with regional or distant metastases
  - Histology of cancer—adenocarcinomas and high-grade solid tumors
  - First year following cancer diagnosis—highest risk period due to multiple therapeutic interventions
  - Hypercoagulable states, e.g., multiple myeloma
- *Treatment-related factors:*
  - *Prior chemotherapy:* Cisplatin, L-asparginase, thalidomide, lenalidomide, and tamoxifen
  - *Surgery:* Gynecological, major abdominopelvic and retroperitoneal
  - High surgical complexity scores
  - High peritoneal carcinomatosis index
  - Major blood loss and massive blood transfusion
  - Longer operating hours
  - Prolonged mechanical ventilation
  - Prolonged ICU stay and hospital stay
  - Lack of administration of anticoagulation at discharge

superior to the other yet. PTP with LMWH or UFH should be commenced within 2–12 hours preoperatively. The highest recommended prophylactic dose is LMWH once daily or UFH 5,000 IU thrice daily.

The ESMO guidelines recommend PTP for all patients undergoing major cancer surgery, for at least 7–10 days postoperatively.[2,45] In those undergoing major open or laparoscopic abdominal or pelvic cancer surgery or laparoscopic colorectal cancer surgery, who have high-risk factors such as restricted mobility, obesity, or history of VTE, or any additional risk factor, extended postoperative PTP for upto 4 weeks with LMWH is recommended.[2,6,45] In low-risk cancer surgeries, the appropriate duration of thromboprophylaxis should be decided on a case-to-case basis. There are only limited data on the efficacy and safety of fondaparinux or direct oral anticoagulants (DOACs) during the postoperative period in cancer patients.

Prevention of Postoperative Ileus

Major cancer surgeries that involving exploratory laparotomy, extensive bowel manipulation, multiple visceral resections, bowel resection and anastomoses, and postoperative opioid use are associated with a higher incidence of prolonged postoperative ileus (POI). Peritoneal carcinomatosis, colonic surgery, HIPEC, and higher perioperative CFB are additional predictive elements for POI. Epidural analgesia, electroacupuncture, and TEAS in addition to improving pain scores, have been associated with decreased incidence of POI following major surgeries.[14,15,46] Postoperative ERAS interventions such as immediate postoperative removal of the nasogastric tube, MMA, removal of the bladder catheter on POD-1, early initiation of oral feeds and early ambulation help to reduce POI.[2,6,46] Coffee consumption and chewing gum, though controversial, have been noted to reduce the time to bowel movement and flatus.[46] Drugs such as alvimopan and IV magnesium sulfate have demonstrated a decrease in the interval to resumption of transit (ROT). A recent animal study demonstrated mosapride and levosulpiride to be associated with improvement of gastric motility and intestinal transit rate and good glycemic control.[47] Other prokinetic agents such as diatrizoate meglumine, ulimorelin, erythromycin, neostigmine, metoclopramide, and cisapride have failed to show benefit for ileus.

Nutrition and Glycemic Control

Preoperative malnourishment is associated with an increased risk of postoperative complications, mortality, and worse long-term oncology outcomes. Routine preoperative nutritional screening and assessment, and nutritional support in the malnourished patient is recommended by the ERAS society.

The ERAS guidelines recommend an early initiation of enteral nutrition (EN) in patients who have undergone major cancer surgeries as early postoperative nutritional support is associated with shorter LOHS, reduced anastomotic dehiscence, earlier resumption of bowel function as well as reduced morbidity and mortality.[48,49] Early oral feeding (a low-residue diet preferred to clear liquids) along with measures to reduce POI, is associated with earlier return of bowel function, shorter LOHS and does not pose a higher risk of anastomotic leaks and other complications.[48-50]

Parenteral nutrition (PN) using all-in-one three-chamber bag needs to be considered in patients where gastrointestinal complications or POI prevents oral intake. Early supplemental PN needs to be considered for patients with postoperative complications impairing gastrointestinal function in whom the energy and nutrient requirements cannot be met by oral and enteral intake alone (<50% of caloric requirement) for >7 days.[49] In critically ill patients after abdominal or esophageal surgery and unable to eat orally, the ESPEN recommends early EN via feeding tubes (rather than PN) unless discontinuity or obstruction of gastrointestinal tract, or abdominal compartment syndrome is present. In the case of an unrepaired anastomotic leak, internal or external fistula, or if distal feeding access is not achieved, EN should be withheld and PN may be commenced.[50] The guidelines have recommended up to 2 g of protein/kg/day and 25–30 kcal/kg/day.[49,50] Daily recording of nutritional intake during postoperative stay in order to identify patients with insufficient intake is recommended routinely.

Uncontrolled hyperglycemia as well as severe hypoglycemia during postoperative period have been associated with poor outcomes and high mortality. There is no universally accepted insulin regimen for glycemic control in patients undergoing major cancer surgery. Intravenous insulin infusions and intermittent short-acting insulin, in order to maintain postoperative blood glucose levels at 140–180 mg/dL (7.8–10 mmol/L), are recommended to reduce postoperative mortality.[2,6]

Physiotherapy

Prolonged bed rest and immobilization following major surgeries are associated with increased risk of PPCs, decreased skeletal muscle strength, POI and delayed ROT, VTE, insulin resistance and prolonged hospital stay. Factors that lead to delayed mobilization following major cancer surgery include prolonged ICU stay, ongoing IV fluid therapy, presence of abdominal or intercostal drains, indwelling urinary catheter, obesity, and high frailty index. All major thoracic and upper abdominal surgeries, especially done through the open technique, are associated with some degree of postoperative respiratory muscle weakness. This, along with poorly tackled postoperative pain, immobilization and residual effects of general anesthesia can adversely affect ventilatory efforts, diaphragmatic function and chest wall compliance. Pneumonectomy can result in diaphragmatic dysfunction due to costophrenic obliteration, intercostal space reduction, and paradoxical diaphragmatic movement resulting from phrenic nerve injury.

Physiotherapy during the postoperative period following major cancer surgeries involve early mobilization and ambulation, limb physiotherapy and chest physiotherapy. Mobilization and physiotherapy, as early as the day of surgery, are recommended in the ERAS protocols to improve the capacity to perform out-of-bed activities, facilitate resumption of gastrointestinal function, and reduce the incidence of postoperative complications. Limb mobilization exercises under supervision during the postoperative period will prevent general muscle weakness and shorten the otherwise prolonged postoperative hospital stay. Post-thoracotomies and upper abdominal surgeries, breathing exercises for pulmonary expansion and bronchial hygiene, inspiratory muscle training, postural correction, and shoulder range of motion activities can improve inspiratory muscle strength and endurance, functional exercise capacity, dyspnea, and quality of life. MMA is also very important in that, it not only renders patient comfort, but also assures better cooperation with physiotherapy, and thereby helps in preventing atelectasis and other PPCs. Physiotherapy programs must be "individualized" according to the type of surgery, and according to each patient's needs.

Postoperative Antibiotic Therapy

Postoperative surgical site infections (SSI) and sepsis are troublesome complications after major cancer surgery leading to prolonged hospital stay and higher mortality rates. Antibiotic prophylaxis is usually institution-based taking into account the institutional antibiogram, extent of oncologic disease, the surgical complexity, and the risk of postoperative neutropenia. Risk factors for postoperative abdominal sepsis include the extensive cytoreduction, colorectal resections, splenectomy, intraoperative peritoneal cavity contamination, major blood loss, prolonged surgery, advanced age and poor preoperative nutritional status. Penicillins and cephalosporins with or without metronidazole are the common choice for perioperative antibiotic prophylaxis following major cancer surgeries. 1-day administration of first-generation cephalosporins has been found to be adequate for preventing postoperative wound infections, UTIs, and vaginal cuff cellulitis following gynecologic cancer surgery.[51] The incidence of SSIs after CRS and HIPEC ranges between 11 and 46%. Bacterial translocation during HIPEC has been hypothesized in these patients who are at high risk of postoperative abdominal infections and septic complications.[52] Use of biomarkers such as serum procalcitonin, cultures from suspected sites, use of rapid diagnostic tests such as nucleic acid amplification tests (NAATs), rapid escalation of antibiotic therapy, and a watchful postoperative eye have all been proposed for early detection and tackling of possible infectious complications following CRS and HIPEC.[22,52] Preoperative administration of oral antibiotics in addition to perioperative IV antibiotics in patients undergoing elective colorectal surgery has been shown to significantly reduce the incidence of postoperative SSIs.[53]

There are very few studies or guidelines specifically for cancer patients regarding the optimal duration of postoperative antibiotic prophylaxis. Short-term prophylactic antibiotics has been found to be effective in reducing the incidence of SSIs in stomach cancer surgery, especially in cases without serious comorbidities or significant combined resection.[54] A systematic review in head and neck cancer surgery patients observed that long-course does not provide any advantage over short-course antibiotic prophylaxis.[55] The Centers for Disease Control and Prevention (CDC) guideline recommends antibiotic therapy for 24 hours or less in clean/uncontaminated surgery.

Monitoring and Prevention of Vital Organ Dysfunction

Postoperative multiorgan dysfunction is a serious and fatal complication, classified as Clavien–Dindo Grade IV following major cancer surgery. Acute coronary syndrome, acute pulmonary thromboembolism, acute respiratory failure, acute kidney insufficiency, acute liver failure, sepsis, multiple organ dysfunction syndrome (MODS), and coagulopathies including DIC are among the major causes of mortality following major cancer surgeries. Hence, stringent monitoring of these patients is important during the postoperative period especially during the first 48–72 hours. A high index of suspicion for early sepsis is required in postoperative cancer patients due to their already disheveled immune status. Morbidity risk factors such as advanced age, severe comorbidities, poor nutritional status, prolonged surgery, high surgical complexity score, major intraoperative blood loss, massive transfusion of blood products, intraoperative hemodynamic instability and cardiac arrhythmias, severe dyselectrolytemia, major acid–base disturbances and continued requirement of mechanical ventilation are a few among the list of indications for postoperative surgical ICU admission. Vitals parameters, dynamic cardiac indices, blood gases, biochemical values, biomarkers, microbiological clues, and hematological parameters need to be regularly and meticulously monitored in these patients for prevention as well as early recognition of postoperative complications and vital organ dysfunction.

CONCLUSION

"Closure is not the end of everything...it is always the beginning of something new". This holds true after any major surgery due to the physiological and biochemical derangements that ensue. Postoperative critical care management is a dynamic process. A judicious combination of tending to ever-changing individual needs and adherence to guidelines is the key. Development of standardized institutional protocols for the postoperative management of patients undergoing major cancer surgeries is vital to ensure consistency and reproducibility, as well as to improve the failure-to-rescue index. These critical care protocols are not meant to be rigid dictums, rather they serve as signposts to guide the team during the immediate postoperative care of patients. A multidisciplinary team that includes critical care physicians, surgical oncologists, infectious disease physicians, critical care nurses, laboratory personnel, physiotherapists, and nutritionists need to work in harmony to ensure a good postoperative outcome.

KEY POINTS

- This immediate postoperative tempestuous period following major cancer surgeries, associated with profound hemodynamic and biochemical derangements, requires stringent monitoring and intensive care for a good postoperative outcome.
- Multi-modal analgesia using various analgesic techniques and medications provides excellent analgesia through the additive or synergistic effects of drugs, while minimizing the adverse effects of individual drugs and reducing the use of opioids.
- Patients at high risk of PRF benefit from continuing postoperative overnight mechanical ventilation and gradual weaning. HFNO or NIV can be used prophylactically in such patients following extubation.
- Dynamic multi-parameter-based administration of IV fluids combining well-defined protocols and taking into account static and dynamic hemodynamic

parameters, fluid responsiveness and fluid tolerance of the patient on a personalised basis is always advisable.

- Supplementing IV 20% H. albumin can aid in maintaining intravascular volume and vital organ perfusion pressures, and reduce IV crystalloid requirement during the postoperative period.
- Correction of dyselectrolytemia and acid-base disturbances is recommended to prevent organ dysfunction. Persistent hyperlactatemia of >4 mmol/L and lactate clearance of <40% at 24 hours during the immediate postoperative period have been associated with worse patient outcomes.
- A PRBC transfusion trigger of 7–9 g/dL of hemoglobin is being practiced in multiple centers, with triggers rising to 10 g/dL in scenarios such as cardiopulmonary dysfunction, acute myocardial ischemia, severe hypoxemia, and ongoing blood loss.
- Use of viscoelastic tests rather than the conventional coagulation tests can provide better insights in choosing 'the right blood product for the "right reasons" during the postoperative period.
- PTP with LMWH or UFH is recommended in all patients undergoing major cancer surgery for at least 7–10 days postoperatively. In those patients at high-risk of VTE, extended postoperative PTP for upto 4 weeks with LMWH is recommended.
- Interventions such as immediate postoperative removal of the nasogastric tube, multimodal analgesia, removal of the bladder catheter on POD-1, early initiation of oral feeds and early ambulation help to reduce POI. Coffee consumption and chewing gum, and drugs such as alvimopan and IV magnesium sulfate have been noted to reduce the time to ROT.
- Whenever feasible, EN should be preferred over PN due to its beneficial effects on maintaining bowel integrity.
- Physiotherapy during the postoperative period following major cancer surgeries should be initiated, as early as the day of surgery and must be "individualized" according to the type of surgery, and patient's needs.
- Perioperative antibiotic prophylaxis is usually based on institutional antibiogram, extent of oncologic disease, the surgical complexity, and the risk of postoperative neutropenia.
- Striving to attain reasonable compliance to the ERAS protocol is known to reduce morbidity and mortality. Developing standardized institutional protocols leads to consistent and reproducible delivery of care.

REFERENCES

1. Albaugh VL, Breitman I, and Abumrad NN. Metabolic and inflammatory responses to trauma and infection. In: Fischer JE. Fischer's Mastery of Surgery, 7th edition. Philadelphia: Wolters Kluver; 2019. pp. 104-61.
2. Hübner M, Kusamura S, Villeneuve L, Al-Niaimi A, Alyami M, Balonov K, et al. Guidelines for Perioperative Care in Cytoreductive Surgery (CRS) with or without hyperthermic IntraPEritoneal chemotherapy (HIPEC): Enhanced Recovery After Surgery (ERAS®) Society Recommendations — Part II: Postoperative management and special considerations. Eur J Oncol Surg. 2020; 46(12):2311-23.
3. Ireland KC, Lalkhen AG. Postoperative analgesia. Anaesth Intensive Care Med. 2022;23(1):29-36.
4. Huang L, Zhang T, Wang K, Chang B, Fu D, Chen X. Postoperative multimodal analgesia strategy for enhanced recovery after surgery in elderly colorectal cancer patients. Pain Ther. 2024;13(4):745-66.
5. Batchelor TJP, Rasburn NJ, Abdelnour-Berchtold E, Brunelli A, Cerfolio RJ, Gonzalez M, et al. Guidelines for enhanced recovery after lung surgery: recommendations of the Enhanced Recovery After Surgery (ERAS®) Society and the European Society of Thoracic Surgeons (ESTS). Eur J Cardiothorac Surg. 2018;55(1):91-115.
6. Nelson G, Bakkum-Gamez J, Kalogera E, Glaser G, Altman A, Meyer LA, et al. Guidelines for perioperative care in gynecologic/oncology: Enhanced Recovery After Surgery (ERAS) Society recommendations—2019 update. Int J Gynecol Cancer. 2019;29(4):651-68.
7. Lawal OD, Gold J, Murthy A, Ruchi R, Bavry E, Hume AL, et al. Rate and risk factors associated with prolonged opioid use after surgery. JAMA Netw Open. 2020;3(6):e207367.
8. Popping DM, Elia N, Marret E, Remy C. Tramer MR. Protective effects of epidural analgesia on pulmonary complications after abdominal and thoracic surgery: a meta-analysis. Arch Surg. 2008;143:990-9.
9. Owusu-Agyemang P, Soliz J, Hayes-Jordan A, Harun N, Gottumukkala V. Safety of epidural analgesia in the perioperative care of patients undergoing cytoreductive surgery with hyperthermic intraperitoneal chemotherapy. Ann Surg Oncol. 2014;21:1487- 93.
10. Black KA, Nelson G, Goucher N, Foley J, Pin S, Chong M, et al. Effect of transversus abdominis plane block on postoperative outcomes in gynecologic oncology patients managed on an enhanced recovery after surgery pathway. Gynecol Oncol. 2023;178:1-7.
11. Korgvee A, Junttila E, Koskinen H, Huhtala H, Kalliomaki ML. Ultrasound-guided quadratus lumborum block for postoperative analgesia. Eur J Anaesthesiol. 2020;38(2):115-29.
12. Hamel J-F, Joris J, Slim K, Régimbeau JM, Cotte E, Léger M, et al. Transversus abdominis block or wound infiltration should be performed in colorectal surgery patients in an

enhanced recovery setting: a propensity score analysis of a national database. J Gastrointest Surg. 2023;27(4):798-802.
13. Ventham NT, O'Neill S, Johns N, Brady RR, Fearon KCH. Evaluation of novel local anesthetic wound infiltration techniques for postoperative pain following colorectal resection surgery: a meta-analysis. Dis Colon Rectum. 2014;57(2):237-50.
14. Wang Y, Yang J-W, Yan S-Y, Lu Y, Han J-G, Pei W, et al. Electroacupuncture vs sham electroacupuncture in the treatment of postoperative ileus after laparoscopic surgery for colorectal cancer: a multicenter randomized clinical trial. JAMA Surg. 2023;158(1):20-7.
15. Chen HT, Hung KC, Huang YT, Wu JY, Hsing CH, Lin CM. Efficacy of electroacupuncture in improving postoperative ileus in patients receiving colorectal surgery: a systematic review and meta-analysis. Int J Surg. 2024;110(2):1113-25.
16. Li J, Mooney DJ. Designing hydrogels for controlled drug delivery. Nat Rev Mater. 2016;1(12):16071.
17. Liu L, Yao W, Xie X, Lu X. pH-sensitive dual drug loaded janus nanoparticles by oral delivery for multimodal analgesia. J Nanobiotechnol. 2021;19(1):235.
18. Dull RO, Hahn RG. Hypovolemia with peripheral edema: What is wrong? Crit Care. 2023;27(1):206.
19. Karamchandani K, Khorsand S, Ebeling C, Yan L, Nakonezny PA, Carr ZJ. Predictors of failure to rescue after postoperative respiratory failure: a retrospective cohort analysis of 13,047 patients using the ACS-NSQIP dataset. J Surg Res. 2024;293:482-9.
20. Gupta H, Gupta PK, Fang X, Miller WJ, Cemaj S, Forse RA, et al. Development and validation of a risk calculator predicting postoperative respiratory failure. Chest. 20;140(5):1207-15.
21. Kulkarni AP, Agarwal V. Extubation failure in intensive care unit: predictors and management. Indian J Crit Care Med. 2008;12(1):1-9.
22. Chandramohan D, Mohamed F, Vikram S, Damodaran D, Shamsudeen S, Rahman F, et al. Standardised critical care strategies improve outcomes following cytoreductive surgery with hyperthermic intraperitoneal chemotherapy in an Indian peritoneal malignancy centre. Indian J Surg Oncol. 2023;14(4):920-27.
23. Oczkowski S, Ergan B, Bos L, Chatwin M, Ferrer M, Gregoretti C, et al. ERS clinical practice guidelines: high-flow nasal cannula in acute respiratory failure. Eur Respir J. 2022;59(4):2101574.
24. Papachatzakis Y, Nikolaidis PT, Kontogiannis S, Trakada G. High-flow oxygen through nasal cannula vs. non-invasive ventilation in hypercapnic respiratory failure: a randomized clinical trial. Int J Environ Res Public Health. 2020;17(16):5994.
25. Ovtcharenko N, Ho E, Alhazzani W, Cortegiani A, Ergan B, Scala R, et al. High-flow nasal cannula versus non-invasive ventilation for acute hypercapnic respiratory failure in adults: a systematic review and meta-analysis of randomized trials. Crit Care. 2022;26(1):348.
26. Malbrain MLNG, Martin G, Ostermann M. Everything you need to know about deresuscitation. Intensive Care Med. 2022;48(12):1781-86.
27. Malbrain MLNG, Langer T, Annane D, Gattinoni L, Elbers P, Hahn RG, et al. Intravenous fluid therapy in the perioperative and critical care setting: Executive summary of the International Fluid Academy (IFA). Ann Intensive Care. 2020;10(1):64.
28. Malbrain MLNG, Wilkinson J, Malbrain L, Nasa P, Wong A. Fluid accumulation and deresuscitation. In: Malbrain ML, Wong A, Nasa P, Ghosh S, (Eds). Rational Use of Intravenous Fluids in Critically Ill Patients, 1st edition. pp. 495-526.
29. Kubo Y, Tanaka K, Yamasaki M, Yamashita K, et al. The impact of perioperative fluid balance on postoperative complications after esophagectomy for esophageal cancer. J Clin Med. 2022;11(11):3219.
30. Takahashi M, Toyama H, Takahashi K, Kaiho Y, Ejima Y, Yamauchi M. Impact of intraoperative fluid management on postoperative complications in patients undergoing minimally invasive esophagectomy for esophageal cancer: a retrospective single-center study. BMC Anesthesiol. 2024;24(1):29.
31. Pisarska-Adamczyk M, Torbicz G, Gajewska N, Małczak P, Major P, Pędziwiatr M, et al. The impact of perioperative fluid therapy on the short-term outcomes after laparoscopic colorectal cancer surgery with ERAS protocol: a prospective observational study. Sci Rep. 2023;13(1):22282.
32. Melo RH, Santos MHCD, Ramos FJDS. Beyond fluid responsiveness: The concept of fluid tolerance and its potential implication in hemodynamic management. Crit Care Sci. 2;35(2):226-9.
33. Douglas IS, Alapat PM, Corl KA, Exline MC, Forni LG, Holder AL, et al. Fluid response evaluation in sepsis hypotension and shock: a randomized clinical trial. Chest. 2020;158(4):1431-45.
34. Latham HE, Bengtson CD, Satterwhite L, Stites M, Subramaniam DP, Chen GJ, Simpson SQ. Stroke volume guided resuscitation in severe sepsis and septic shock improves outcomes. J Crit Care. 2017;42:42-6.
35. Aguilera IM, Vaughan RS. Calcium and the anaesthetist. Anaesthesia. 2000;55(8):779-90.
36. Veličković J, Palibrk I, Miličić B, Veličković D, Jovanović B, Rakić G, et al. The association of early postoperative lactate levels with morbidity after elective major abdominal surgery. Bosn J Basic Med Sci. 2019;19(1):72-80.
37. Vincent JL, Quintairos E Silva A, Couto L Jr, Taccone FS. The value of blood lactate kinetics in critically ill patients: a systematic review. Crit Care. 2016;20(1):257.
38. Chaudhari M, Agarwal N. Study of significance of serum lactate kinetics in sepsis as mortality predictor. Indian J Crit Care Med. 2022;26(5):591-5.

39. Niederwieser T, Braunwarth E, Dasari BVM, Pufal K, Szatmary P, Hackl H, et al. Early postoperative arterial lactate concentrations to stratify risk of post-hepatectomy liver failure. Br J Surg. 2021;108(11):1360-70.
40. Cata JP, Gottumukkala V. Blood transfusion practices in cancer surgery. Indian J Anaesth. 2014;58(5):637-42.
41. Bergamin FS, Almeida JP, Landoni G, Galas FRBG, Fukushima JT, Fominskiy E, et al. Liberal versus restrictive transfusion strategy in critically ill oncologic patients: The transfusion requirements in critically ill oncologic patients randomized controlled trial. Crit Care Med. 2017;45(5):766-73.
42. Abou Daher L, Heppell O, Lopez-Plaza I, Guerra-Londono CE. Perioperative blood transfusions and cancer progression: a narrative review. Curr Oncol Rep. 2024;26(8):880-9.
43. Ramanujam V, DiMaria S, Varma V. Thromboelastography in the perioperative period: a literature review. Cureus. 2023;15(5):e39407.
44. Abdol Razak NB, Jones G, Bhandari M, Berndt MC, Metharom P. Cancer-associated thrombosis: an overview of mechanisms, risk factors, and treatment. Cancers (Basel). 2018;10(10):380.
45. Falanga A, Ay C, Di Nisio M, Gerotziafas G, et al. ESMO Guidelines Committee. Venous thromboembolism in cancer patients: ESMO Clinical Practice Guideline. Ann Oncol. 2023;34(5):452-67.
46. Venara A, Neunlist M, Slim K, Barbieux J, Colas PA, Hamy A, Meurette G. Postoperative ileus: Pathophysiology, incidence, and prevention. J Visc Surg. 2016;153(6):439-46.
47. Akrab SNA, Al Gawhary NE, Shafik AN, Morcos GNB, Wissa MY. The role of mosapride and levosulpiride in gut function and glycemic control in diabetic rats. Arab J Gastroenterol. 2023;24(2):109-16.
48. Herbert G, Perry R, Andersen HK, Penfold C, Lewis SJ. Early enteral nutrition within 24h of lower gastrointestinal surgery versus later commencement for length of hospital stay and postoperative complications. Cochrane Database Syst Rev. 2019;7:CD006506.
49. Weimann A, Braga M, Carli F, Higashiguchi T, Hübner M, Klek S, et al. ESPEN practical guideline: clinical nutrition in surgery. Clin Nutr. 2021;40(7):4745-61.
50. Singer P, Blaser AR, Berger MM, Calder PC, Casaer M, Hiesmayr M, et al. ESPEN practical and partially revised guideline: Clinical nutrition in the intensive care unit. Clin Nutr. 2023;42(9):1671-89.
51. Byun JM, Jeong DH. Antibiotic prophylaxis for gynecologic cancer surgery. Taiwan J Obstet Gynecol. 2020;59(4): 514-519.
52. Vallicelli C, Coccolini F, Sartelli M, Ansaloni L, Bui S, Catena F. Antibiotic prophylaxis for surgical site infection in general surgery: oncological treatments and HIPEC. Antibiotics (Basel). 2021;11(1):43.
53. Woodfield JC, Clifford K, Schmidt B, Turner GA, Amer MA, McCall JL. Strategies for antibiotic administration for bowel preparation among patients undergoing elective colorectal surgery: a network meta-analysis. JAMA Surg. 2022;157(1):34-41.
54. Lee JS, Lee HH, Song KY, Park CH, Jeon HM. The feasibility of short term prophylactic antibiotics in gastric cancer surgery. J Gastric Cancer. 2010;10(4):206-11.
55. Iocca O, Copelli C, Ramieri G, Zocchi J, Savo M, Di Maio P. Antibiotic prophylaxis in head and neck cancer surgery: systematic review and Bayesian network meta-analysis. Head Neck. 2022;44(1):254-61.

CHAPTER

Airway Management for Oncological Patients in the Intensive Care Unit

Malini P Joshi, Shilpushp J Bhosale, Atul Prabhakar Kulkarni

INTRODUCTION

Cancer patients require intensive care unit (ICU) admission due to effects of cancer, complications arising from the cancer treatment, or underlying malignancy.[1]

Airway management for critically ill cancer patients is complex and it is associated with unique challenges due to compromised physiological reserve, aspiration risk, hemodynamic instability, and increased morbidity and mortality.

The goals of management should be to establish a secure airway, ensure adequate oxygenation, and ventilation with hemodynamic stability, at all times throughout the procedure.

CHALLENGES IN AIRWAY MANAGEMENT IN ONCOLOGICAL CRITICAL CARE

The National Audit Projects (NAP4) findings indicated that approximately one-fourth major airway hospital mishaps take place in the ICU leading to adverse outcomes.[2] This report showed that 40% cases were related to the head, neck, or tracheal cancers. Approximately, 70% adverse outcomes were associated with obstructed airway, with poor management being implicated in one-third of cases.

The most common causes for these events were poor identification and incomplete planning of at-risk patients with difficult airway, inadequate provision of skilled staff and equipment to manage these events, delayed recognition of events, and failure to rescue the airway.

The NAP4 recommendations are described in **Box 1**.

BOX 1: NAP4 recommendations

- Have an "airway management strategy" with timely implementation of these plans
- Assess for possible difficult airway early and plan for securing the airway
- Keep difficult airway trolley in the ICU
- Use capnography for all airway interventions and in ventilated patients
- Train all staff for difficult airway management and encourage simulation exercises for improved outcomes

(ICU: intensive care unit; NAP4: 4th National Audit Project)

AIRWAY EMERGENCIES IN AN ONCOLOGICAL INTENSIVE CARE UNIT

Airway cancers such as head, neck, and mediastinal cancers and those with previous surgery can develop obstruction, have compression of airway, and may have distorted airway anatomy. This is worsened by edema and inflammation due to the disease and therapy. All these factors result in challenges in airway assessment and difficulty in ventilation, laryngoscopy, and intubation.

Successful management involves anticipation and management of difficult airway scenarios with individually tailored primary and backup plans. A multidisciplinary team involving the intensivists, radiologists, ear-nose-throat (ENT) surgeons, anesthesiologists, oncologists, and interventional pulmonologists and thoracic surgeons are necessary for management of patients with high-risk airway.

AIRWAY ASSESSMENT IN A DIFFICULT AIRWAY PATIENT IN CANCER INTENSIVE CARE UNIT

Each ICU patient must be assessed and evaluated for difficulty in securing or salvaging airway.

Questions to be asked include:

- Is there an actual or potential airway obstruction?
    - What is the likelihood of development of airway obstruction?
- Will there be difficulty in mask ventilation, laryngoscopy, or intubation?

TABLE 1: Effects of radiation on the airway.

Face and buccal mucosa	Mucositis, dry mouth
TM joint	Fibrosis, trismus, and ankylosis due to pterygoid and masseter muscle fibrosis
Dentition	Loss of teeth
Tongue	Glossitis, tongue enlargement
Floor of mouth	Fibrosis
Mandible	Radio-osteonecrosis
Suprahyoid region	Fibrosis and edema
Larynx	Necrosis, fibrosis, and vocal cord oedema
Lower airway	Glottic/epiglottis edema—difficult laryngeal exposure

Look for the predictors of potential difficult airway such as reduced mouth opening, Mallampati score, reduced thyromental distance, inadequacy of mandibular space for intubation, neck mobility, history of previous airway surgeries, and radiation therapy.

Previously irradiated airway is a risk factor for difficult airway **(Table 1)**. Advanced imaging, such as computed tomography (CT) scans and magnetic resonance imaging (MRI), provides valuable information about neck anatomy and airway patency and predicts intubation challenges.

Management strategy in high-risk airway patients includes:
- Awake and asleep intubation
- Invasive or noninvasive technique
- In critical airway stenosis, consider awake tracheal intubation and awake tracheostomy.

MACOCHA Score is a validated airway assessment scoring system for ICU patients **(Table 2)**.

It has a sensitivity of 73%, although it has not been validated for video laryngoscopy.[3]

IMAGING FOR DIAGNOSIS OF DIFFICULT AIRWAY

These modalities are attractive options for the diagnosis of difficult airway and allow precise diagnose, we are unlikely to be able to obtain these in an emergency. However, imaging may have been performed prior to ICU admission while being assessed for extent of cancer to decide therapeutic modalities by the primary surgeon or physicians.

TABLE 2: MACOCHA score components.

Score components	***Points assigned***
Factors related to patient:	
Mallampati score III and IV	5
Obstructive sleep apnea syndrome	2
Reduced mobility of cervical spine	1
Mouth opening <3 cm	1
Factors related to pathology:	
Coma	1
Severe hypoxemia	1
Factors related to operator:	
Nonanesthesiologists	1

Score—0 (easy) to 12 (very difficult)
Score ≥3—predictor of difficult intubation in ICU patients

Radiographs of the Neck[4]

Advantages of radiographs of the neck are given here.
- Quick, inexpensive, and easily accessible in resource-limited settings[5]
- X-ray anteroposterior (AP) and lateral view to see presence of soft tissue swelling, tracheal compression/deviation distal obstruction, and airway collapse.
- Reduced space (<5 mm) between C1 spinous process and occiput on lateral neck radiograph in neutral position for predicting inability to position patient for intubation.

Computed Tomography and Magnetic Resonance Imaging

These allow better assessment than radiography to pick up complex airway pathologies such as tracheal deviation, compression, intratracheal extension, retrosternal extension, and intrathoracic lesions. MRI is more effective in diagnosing soft tissue pathology.

Ultrasound plays an important role in difficult airway management in ICU. It helps in identifying intubation landmarks, such as cricothyroid membrane or tracheal rings, helps in confirming correct endotracheal tube placement, and can help in predicting postextubation laryngeal edema, etc.[6]

AIRWAY OBSTRUCTION AT PRESENTATION TO THE ICU

Patients can present with stridor, respiratory distress, and worsening ventilation due to airway narrowing, tumor extension, and bilateral vocal cord palsy.[7]

This is commonly seen in tracheal, laryngeal, esophageal tumors, lung cancer, thyroid carcinomas, metastatic lesions directly to bronchial tree and lymph nodes, and rarely obstructive lymphedema. Often, patients can be asymptomatic, but may worsen with gradual progression of symptoms or may rapidly deteriorate rapidly deteriorate due to lack of respiratory reserve and an already compromised airway.

A thorough clinical history and comprehensive airway assessment are crucial for diagnosis, urgency determination, and effective management planning.

It is important to elicit location of the lesion, degree of compromised airway, patient's work of breathing and accompanying hypoxemia, alerting urgency, and challenges associated with providing ventilation and securing the airway.

Nasoendoscopy can provide comprehensive information about airway and structures, however, CT scan is a useful modality to swiftly and accurately assess airway structures, in an elective setting.

Objectives of Safe Airway Management

These are mainly the following: Timely airway protection, maintenance of oxygenation, and ensuring effective ventilation (to eliminate CO_2). One must remember that *it not failure to intubate that harms/kills the patient, but the failure to oxygenate.*

High-flow nasal oxygen use has shown to improve and maintain oxygenation and airway patency through low-level positive pressure ventilation with decrease in work of breathing.

Steroid therapy may be used in inflammation or edema of airway.

Continuous positive airway pressure or noninvasive ventilation (NIV) can be beneficial as an adjunct during airway obstruction and treatment of pulmonary edema that is associated with postobstruction re-expansion of lungs.

Approach to an Obstructed Airway

It is important to have a contingency back up plans if initial plan fails. Smaller-sized endotracheal tubes and supraglottic airway (SGA) should be kept ready. It is better to avoid long-acting sedatives and muscle relaxants. Airway plans should involve awake techniques, and preparation of invasive rescue measures such as tracheostomy or cricothyrotomy if airway cannot be secured.

Awake Fiberoptic intubation can be done in anticipated difficult face-mask ventilation. Sometimes awake tracheostomy—in case of significant upper airway supraglottic or glottic obstruction with difficult or impossible mask ventilation or intubation may be preferred.

Mediastinal Mass

Patients may present to ICU with superior vena cava syndrome.

It is necessary to maintain high degree of suspicion in patients presenting with acute airway obstruction and respiratory distress. Symptoms severity can differ according to the location and extent of tumor in the mediastinum-anterior mediastinum; superior mediastinum; middle or visceral mediastinum; and posterior or paravertebral mediastinum.[8]

Patients may be unable to lie supine due to the tumor causing difficulty in getting diagnostic imaging. They may present with facial edema, acute breathlessness, cough dyspnea on mild exertion or sometimes at rest, change in voice, noisy breathing, intractable cough, and chest discomfort. Some paraneoplastic tumors can present with symptoms due to release of hormones and cytokines, compression of vascular structures such as pulmonary artery compression can cause profound hypoxia. Pleural and pericardial effusion can contribute to breathlessness and hemodynamic instability. It must be remembered that increased intrathoracic pressure with invasive positive pressure ventilation (IPPV) can increases compression.

Preparation for emergency surgical airway, rigid bronchoscopy and possible extracorporeal membrane oxygenation (ECMO) may have to be considered as rescue.

Commonly, tumors present with airway compression through direct invasion or external compression of airway. If >50% occlusion occurs either at the trachea, carina, or main-stem bronchi, there is risk of acute decompensation of already compromised airway.

This is commonly seen in patients with advanced primary lung cancers, metastatic disease in thorax, endoluminal, metastatic, lymph nodes, and mediastinal disease.

Acute onset may be catastrophic with significant obstruction causing enough narrowing to disrupt airflow and cause dyspnea. Almost complete occlusion occurs in severely narrowed airways with mucous plugging.

Airway stenting may be lifesaving in these patients. Silicone stenting maintains airway patency after an initial ablative procedure. Combined silicone and metal stents (hybrid stents) are frequently used. Complications during these procedures include pneumothorax, airway trauma, infection, stent migration, respiratory compromise, and mortality.

Intraoral Lesions

Intraoral lesions can commonly present with difficult airway, awake intubation by fiberoptic bronchoscope may be considered in extremely difficult airways.

These patents commonly present with postoperative airway emergencies.

In the postoperative period, head and neck cancer patients are considered difficult airway owing to dissection, reconstruction and bulky flaps causing compromised airways. Thus, nasal endotracheal tube is usually kept for a longer time or intraoperative tracheostomy is done if indicated. But if loss of airway happens in such patients after extubation, then an awake tracheostomy/cricothyrotomy is performed if patient is unable to maintain patent airway and desaturates. Usually, difficult airway extubations should be an elective procedure and in certain cases done over tube exchanger and bronchoscope.

Postoperative neck hematoma can be another life-threating emergency. Following thyroid and parathyroid surgery, patients may arrive to the ICU with neck hematomas **(Flowchart 1)**. If signs of airway compromise present evacuate hematoma. If small and not causing airway compromise, can be decompressed through aspiration, for larger hematomas, release of surgical staples for surgical evacuation is required.

EQUIPMENT FOR DIFFICULT AIRWAY TROLLEY DURING DIFFICULT AIRWAY MANAGEMENT IN ICU

Every ICU should have an immediately available difficult airway trolley which should undergo regular checks and restocking of the trolley.

Contents include:

- Supraglottic airways such as laryngeal mask airways (LMAs), i-gels, ProSeal
- Variety of laryngoscopes, blades
- Airways and airway conduits (including airway intubating catheters and airway exchange catheters)
- Equipment for front of neck access (needle cricothyroidotomy and surgical cricothyrotomy)
- Videolaryngoscopes improve glottic view and allow for expert supervision during intubation; should be available in ICUs to rescue difficult intubation or unsuccessful first-pass laryngoscopy, especially in expert hands. However, randomized controlled trials suggest that the systematic use of videolaryngoscopes for every intubation cannot yet be recommended, especially in nonexpert hands.
- Intubating bronchoscope
- Cricothyroidotomy equipment—NAP4 findings suggest that 60% of attempted needle cricothyroidotomies in ICU were unsuccessful while all surgical cricothyroidotomies achieved access to the trachea.
- Capnography for all airway interventions according to NAP4 report
- ICU staff should be trained in the use of this equipment and be familiar with difficult airway management algorithms.

Jaber et al., have suggested that the use ICU intubation bundle, which has 3 components, i.e., preintubation, during, and after intubation, is helpful to improve patient outcomes by preventing hypoxia and minimizing chances of cardiovascular collapse.[9]

Intubation Bundle Components

1. *Preintubation:*
   i. Presence of two operators
   ii. Fluid loading (isotonic saline 500 mL or starch 250 mL) in absence of cardiogenic pulmonary edema
   iii. Preparation of long-term sedation
   iv. Preoxygenation for 3 minutes with noninvasive positive pressure ventilation (NIPPV) in case of acute respiratory failure [fraction of inspired oxygen (FiO_2) 1.0, pressure support ventilation level between 5 and 15 cmH_2O to obtain an expiratory tidal volume between 6 and 8 mL/kg and positive end-expiratory pressure (PEEP) 5 cmH_2O]
2. *During intubation:*
   i. *Rapid sequence induction (RSI) and intubation:* Etomidate 0.2–0.3 mg/kg or ketamine 1.5–3 mg/kg combined with succinylcholine 1–1.5 mg/kg (in absence of allergy, hyperkalemia, severe acidosis, acute or chronic neuromuscular disease, burn patient for >48 hours)
   ii. Sellick maneuver
3. *Postintubation:*
   i. Immediate confirmation of tube placement by capnography
   ii. Norepinephrine if diastolic blood pressure <35 mm Hg

Flowchart 1: Management of suspected hematoma thyroid surgery.

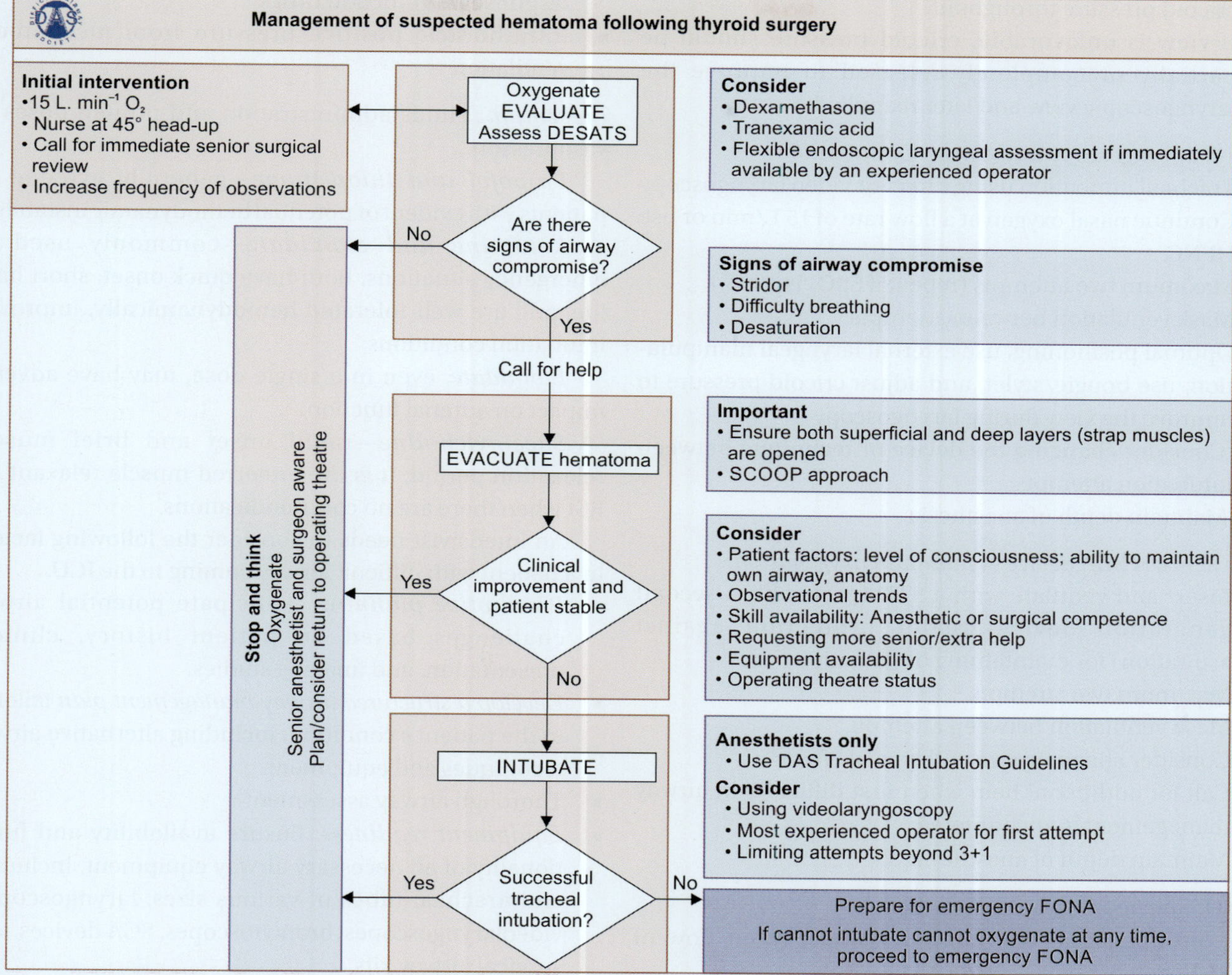

(DAS: Difficult Airway Society; DESATS: difficulty in swallowing/discomfort, EWS, swelling, anxiety, tachypnea, stridor; SCOOP: skin exposure, cut sutures, open skin, open muscles, pack wound; FONA: front-of-neck airway)

iii. Initiate long-term sedation
iv. *Initial "protective ventilation":* Tidal volume 6–8 mL/kg of ideal body weight, PEEP <5 cmH_2O and respiratory rate between 10 and 20 cycles/min, and FiO_2 1.0 for a plateau pressure <30 cmH_2O

Always confirm tracheal placement of endotracheal tube using capnography.

ALL INDIA DIFFICULT AIRWAY ASSOCIATION GUIDELINES ALGORITHM FOR INTUBATION IN THE ICU

Step 1: Preoxygenation and induction of anesthesia:

- Two persons (one experienced)
- Optimize preoxygenation—NIV with a pressure support ventilation 5–15 cmH_2O to obtain an expiratory tidal volume between 6 and 8 mL/kg and PEEP 5 cmH_2O.
- Nasal cannula with O_2 flow of 15 L/min-prolong the duration of safe apnea in addition when there is a mask leak or high-flow nasal cannula (HFNC) with 70 L/min of oxygen flow during intubation and leads to decrease desaturation and higher first attempt success without hypoxemia.
- Induction—ketamine or etomidate and paralysis with succinylcholine or rocuronium
- Use cricoid pressure
- IPPV using bag-valve mask with reservoir bag using external PEEP valve set to 5–10 cmH_2O PEEP if

available or IPPV using the ventilator maintaining a cricoid pressure throughout.
- If view is unfavorable, cricoid pressure should be partially or completely released to improve the laryngoscopic view and later reapplied.

Step 2: Laryngoscopy and tracheal intubation:
- Tracheal intubation using direct or video laryngoscopy
- Continue nasal oxygen at a flow rate of 15 L/min or use HFNC
- Maximum two attempts (repeat if SpO_2 is ≥95%)
- Mask ventilation between attempts
- Optimal positioning, use external laryngeal manipulation, use bougie/stylet, and adjust cricoid pressure to improve the view during laryngoscopy
- Consider changing the device or technique between intubation attempts
- Maintain depth of anesthesia

Step 3: Insert SGA device to maintain oxygenation:
- Insert and ventilate with a SAD (preferably a second generation device-greater protection against aspiration) for maintaining oxygenation
- Maximum two attempts
- Mask ventilation between attempts
- Consider changing size and type of SAD
- Call for additional help when first difficulty in airway management is encountered
- Maintain depth of anesthesia

Step 4: Rescue face mask ventilation:
- Continue nasal oxygenation using oxygen flow of 15 L/min or HFNC
- Ensure complete neuromuscular blockade
- Additional help when the final attempt at rescue mask ventilation fails
- One final attempt at face mask ventilation using optimal technique and adjuncts

Step 5: Emergency cricothyroidotomy:
- Continue nasal oxygenation using oxygen flow at 15 L/min or HFNC oxygen and call for additional help
- Either needle or surgical cricothyroidotomy

PHARMACOLOGICAL CONSIDERATIONS[10]

An intubation in a critically ill patient may be followed by cardiovascular collapse within few minutes due to:
- Drug-induced vasodilation and myocardial depression
- Hypovolemia
- Suppression of the body's natural sympathetic response by induction drugs
- Intrathoracic positive pressure from mechanical ventilation

Prevention: Fluids administration and titrated doses of vasopressors.

Propofol and thiopentone—generally avoided in patients with evident or potential hemodynamic instability.

Ketamine and etomidate—commonly used in emergency situations, both have quick onset, short half-life, and are well-tolerated hemodynamically, improved intubation conditions.

Etomidate, even in a single dose, may have adverse impact on adrenal function.

Succinylcholine—rapid onset and brief muscle relaxation period, it is the preferred muscle relaxant for RSI when there are no contraindications.

An intensivist needs to consider the following factors in a patient with difficult airway coming to the ICU.
- *Preemptive planning:* Anticipate potential airway challenges based on patient history, clinical presentation, and imaging studies.
- *Develop a structured airway management plan* tailored to the patient's condition, including alternative airway techniques and equipment.
- Thorough airway assessment
- *Equipment readiness:* Ensure availability and functionality of all necessary airway equipment, including endotracheal tubes of various sizes, laryngoscopes, videolaryngoscopes, bronchoscopes, SGA devices, and surgical airway kits.
- *Alternative Airways:* Have a contingency plan for difficult airway scenarios, including availability of alternative airway devices and techniques.
- *Monitoring:* Continuous monitoring of oxygenation, ventilation, and hemodynamics. Monitor vital signs, SaO_2, and end-tidal carbon dioxide continuously.
- *Resuscitation readiness:* Ensure readiness for immediate resuscitation in case of airway-related complications, with appropriate equipment and readily available medications.
- *Adjuncts and techniques:* Utilize NIV techniques such as HFNC or continuous positive airway pressure to support oxygenation and ventilation in selected patients.
- *Consider awake fiberoptic intubation or bronchoscopy-*guided intubation patients with anticipated difficult

airways or compromised respiratory function. Employ advanced airway techniques including video laryngoscopy or bronchoscopy, SGA devices, and percutaneous tracheostomy when appropriate.

- *Pharmacological considerations:* Select sedative and induction agents carefully, considering hemodynamic stability, respiratory status, and potential drug interactions. Titrate medications cautiously to achieve adequate sedation and minimize the risk of respiratory depression.
- *Complication management:* Prompt and effective management of potential airway complications—desaturation, hypotension, laryngospasm, or aspiration. Ensure adequate training and resources for managing difficult airway scenarios, including difficult airway algorithm implementation and simulation exercises.

CONCLUSION

Airway management in the oncological ICU requires a tailored and multidisciplinary approach to address the unique challenges posed by critically ill cancer patients. Prioritizing preemptive planning, comprehensive airway assessment, and utilization of appropriate techniques and equipment are essential for optimizing patient outcomes and minimizing complications. Collaborative teamwork and ongoing education are key to ensuring safe and effective airway management in this complex patient population.

REFERENCES

1. Azoulay E, Soares M, Darmon M, et al. Intensive care of the cancer patient: recent achievements and remaining challenges. Ann. Ann Intensive Care. 2011;1(1):5.
2. Cook TM, Woodall N, Frerk C; Fourth National Audit Project. Major complications of airway management in the UK: Results of the fourth national audit project of the Royal College of Anaesthetists and the difficult airway society. Part 1: Anaesthesia. Br J Anaesth. 2011;106:617-31.
3. De Jong A, Molinari N, Terzi N, Mongardon N, Arnal JM, Guitton C, et al. Early identification of patients at risk for difficult intubation in the Intensive Care Unit: Development and validation of the MACOCHA score in a multicenter cohort study. Am J Respir Crit Care Med. 2013;187:832-9.
4. Crawley SM, Dalton AJ. Predicting the difficult airway. Bja Education. 2015;15(5):253-7.
5. Jain K, Gupta N, Yadav M, Thulkar S, Bhatnagar S. Radiological evaluation of airway - What an anaesthesiologist needs to know! Indian J Anaesth. 2019;63(4):257-64.
6. Kundra P, Mishra SK, Ramesh A. Ultrasound of the airway. Indian J Anaesth. 2011;55(5):456-62.
7. Lynch J, Crawley SM. Management of airway obstruction. BJA Educ. 2018;18(2):46-51.
8. Hariharan U. Mediastinal masses and emergency management challenges-the great mimic. Emerg Med Inves. 2017;127.
9. Jaber S, Jung B, Corne P, Sebbane M, Muller L, Chanques G, et al. An intervention to decrease complications related to endotracheal intubation in the intensive care unit: A prospective, multiple-center study. Intensive Care Med. 2010;36:248-55.
10. Divatia JV, Khan PU, Myatra SN. Tracheal intubation in the ICU: Lifesaving- or life threatening? Indian J Anaesth. 2011;55(5):470-5.

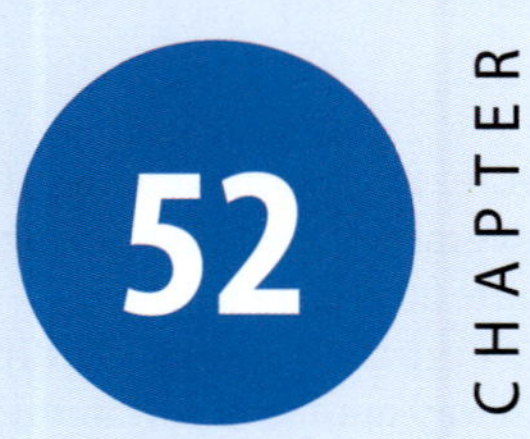

Disorders of Calcium, Sodium, Phosphate, and Potassium Equilibrium

Satish Vishnu Sarode, Suhail Sarwar Siddiqui

CALCIUM HOMEOSTASIS AND DISORDERS OF CALCIUM IMBALANCE

INTRODUCTION

Calcium is an essential macronutrient with a recommended dietary allowance (RDA) of 1,000–2,000 mg/day. About 1–2% of adult body weight is made up of calcium, 99% of which is stored in the bone as hydroxyapatite and serves an important role in skeletal mineralization. Calcium plays an important structural role in the mineralization of teeth and bones. It also plays a crucial physiological role at the cellular level. It acts as a clotting factor, intra and extracellular messenger, skeletal muscle contraction through coupling and decoupling, smooth muscle contractions and relaxations, to maintain vascular tone, nerve conduction, release of various hormones, as a catalyst in various metabolic processes.

Despite being stored in bones in large quantities, its serum and cellular levels are tightly controlled in a narrow range of 8.8–10.3 mg/dL by positive and negative feedback systems through the interplay of parathyroid hormone (PTH), and calcitriol and calcitonin levels. Any prolonged imbalance between them may lead to structural abnormalities due to altered bone mineralization. However, this topic is intended to discuss acute changes in calcium homeostasis and its physiological effects.

CALCIUM HOMEOSTASIS

As mentioned, serum calcium levels are tightly controlled in the narrow range of 8.8–10.3 mg/dL (2.2–2.6 mmol/L) by increased or reduced levels of PTH or calcitonin through positive or negative feedback mechanisms.

In serum, calcium exists in three forms in blood, i.e., albumin bound, ionized, and chelated.[1] Details of physiological forms of calcium are summarized in **Table 1**.

TABLE 1: Calcium in various forms.

S. No.	*Forms of calcium*	*Fraction of total calcium*	*Comments*
1.	Protein bound	45%	It is in equilibrium with ionized form and works as an immediate source of ionized calcium for the body
2.	Ionized	45%	Physiologically active form
3.	Chelated	9–10%	Calcium is chelated with anions like citrate, carbonate, and phosphate

REGULATION OF CALCIUM

Calcium homeostasis is a crucial physiological process that maintains optimal calcium levels in the body. Three key hormones play pivotal roles in regulating calcium balance: PTH, calcitriol, and calcitonin.

1. *Role of PTH:* The parathyroid glands release PTH in response to a decrease in serum-ionized calcium. Raised PTH increases serum-ionized calcium and reduces serum phosphate levels by:[2]
   - Increased calcium reabsorption in the ascending loop of Henle, the distal convoluted tubule (DCT), and the collecting duct in kidneys.
   - Inhibiting the reabsorption of phosphate, which competes with calcium for absorption.
   - The kidney also responds to PTH by increasing the secretion of vitamin D_3, which in turn stimulates calcium absorption through the gut.
   - It acts on the bones to stimulate osteoclasts involved in bone reabsorption and the release of free calcium.
2. *Role of calcitonin:* Calcitonin is released by the thyroid parafollicular cells (C-cells) in response to an increase in serum-ionized calcium.

- Calcitonin stimulates osteoblasts in bone leading to calcium deposition.
- Calcitonin inhibits renal reabsorption of calcium.
- It also acts by calcium absorption in the intestines.

These processes lead to decreased serum calcium and increased phosphate levels.

3. *Role of calcitriol (vitamin D_3)*: Renal synthesis of calcitriol is enhanced in response to raised PTH levels, which are elevated in response to hypocalcemia. Calcitriol plays a pivotal role in raising serum calcium levels by:
   - Enhancing absorption of calcium and phosphate from the intestines by increasing the expression of calcium transporters.
   - Promoting the reabsorption of calcium in the proximal tubules of the kidneys.
   - Parathyroid hormone-dependent calcitriol activation promotes bone osteoclastogenesis and reabsorption, raising serum calcium and phosphate levels.

Together, these hormones work in a delicate balance to maintain calcium homeostasis. PTH and calcitriol raise blood calcium levels, while calcitonin lowers it. Dysregulation of these hormones can lead to conditions such as hypercalcemia or hypocalcemia.

HYPOCALCEMIA

Hypocalcemia is one of the common electrolyte imbalances observed in the intensive care unit (ICU) and perioperative care and is labeled when the corrected serum calcium level falls <8.4 mg/dL or ionized calcium is <4.2 mg/dL. Hypocalcemia occurs due to failure to release PTH from the parathyroid gland due to various causes, i.e., hypoparathyroidism. Here serum PTH levels are reduced. A normal parathyroid gland responds to hypocalcemia of any cause by increased secretion of PTH. Hence, etiology of hypocalcemia is broadly categorized into two groups:

1. Hypocalcemia with low PTH
2. Hypocalcemia with raised PTH

The causes of hypocalcemia are enumerated in **Table 2**.

TABLE 2: Causes of hypocalcemia.

A	Low PTH	• Postsurgical-post-thyroidectomy, postparathyroidectomy • Autoimmune destruction of parathyroid gland • Abnormal parathyroid gland development
B	High PTH	• Vitamin D deficiency • Chronic kidney disease (CKD) • Pseudohypoparathyroidism (PHP)
C	Miscellaneous	• Respiratory alkalosis • Acute pancreatitis • Massive blood transfusion • Tumor lysis syndrome • Sepsis • Hypomagnesemia • Acute hyperphosphatemia • Osteoblastic metastasis • *Drugs:* Bisphosphonates, denosumab, cinacalcet, cisplatin, and foscarnet

(PTH: parathyroid hormone)

Hypocalcemia with Low Parathyroid Hormone

Monitoring for serum calcium levels and symptoms of hypocalcemia should be performed meticulously in postoperative cases of thyroid, parathyroid, and other radical neck surgeries.[3] In these patients, hypocalcemia can be permanent due to loss of the parathyroid gland or transient due to manipulation of blood supply to the parathyroid gland.[3]

Autoimmune destruction of the parathyroid gland is one of the most common causes of acquired hypoparathyroidism, which is frequently associated with polyglandular autoimmune syndrome type I. This is a familial disorder, typically presenting in childhood with candidiasis, followed by several years later by hypoparathyroidism, and then adrenal insufficiency during adolescence. Rare causes of parathyroid gland destruction include irradiation, hemochromatosis, and Wilson's disease.

Inherited causes of hypothyroidism and hypocalcemia are related to abnormal development of the parathyroid gland and altered regulation of PTH secretion.

Hypocalcemia with High Parathyroid Hormone

When the structure and function of the parathyroid gland are preserved, PTH is released in response to low serum calcium levels. If reduced calcium levels are marginal and transient, elevated PTH succeeds to normalize calcium level producing a subclinical state without any sign or symptoms of hypocalcemia. But if hypocalcemia is severe or its etiology is not reversed early, PTH fails to normalize serum calcium despite being elevated beyond the normal range. Common causes are discussed below.

- *Chronic kidney disease (CKD):* Reduced production of calcitriol in CKD patients results in chronic hypocalcemia requiring daily calcium and vitamin D_3 supplements, calcium chelation due to hyperphosphatemia in CKD is another mechanism that aggravates hypocalcemia. PTH levels are elevated in response to low calcium levels.
- *Vitamin D_3 deficiency:* Dietary deficiency of vitamin D_3 can cause hypocalcemia with raised PTH. In contrast to CKD patients, phosphate levels are low due to its enhanced urinary loss.
- *Pseudohypoparathyroidism:* It occurs due to resistance of PTH action on its target organs, i.e., gut, kidney, and bones. It is characterized by hypocalcemia and hypophosphatemia with elevated PTH levels. Severe hypomagnesemia may lead to PTH resistance and hypocalcemia.
- *Calcium chelation:* Chelation of calcium is one of the common factors causing acute symptomatic hypocalcemia in critically ill patients. Calcium may get chelated with phosphate, citrate, or drugs. As discussed, hyperphosphatemia in CKD is one of the contributing factors for the development of chronic hypocalcemia.

In case of rhabdomyolysis and tumor lysis syndrome,[4] large quantities of phosphate are released into the bloodstream, producing hyperphosphatemia. It forms calcium phosphate crystals leading to acute hypocalcemia.

Those patients who receive large quantities of blood products develop hypocalcemia as it gets chelated with citrate, which is used as an anticoagulant in blood components. Intravenous (IV) calcium supplements must be provided to patients requiring massive blood transfusions.

In acute pancreatitis, calcium levels need to be monitored at regular intervals as these patients are prone to develop hypocalcemia. Calcium soaps are formed in the abdominal cavity. The exact mechanism is unknown behind chelation of calcium in acute pancreatitis.

In severe sepsis, hypocalcemia is multifactorial. Sepsis may lead to reduced PTH secretion and reduced calcitriol synthesis leading to hypocalcemia.

Respiratory alkalosis due to hyperventilation increases calcium binding to albumin. It results in a transient reduction of ionized calcium levels with normal total calcium levels.

Clinical Features

Clinical manifestations of hypocalcemia vary from asymptomatic at mild deficiency to life-threatening symptoms like seizures, heart failure, or laryngospasm if severe. Also, the clinical symptoms depend on the rate of onset and chronicity of hypocalcemia.

- *Paresthesia:* Circumoral and distal extremity tingling or numbness generally occurs.
- *Tetany:* Generally, it occurs due to a rapid decrease in serum-ionized calcium. Acute hypocalcemia increases the excitability of neurons generating repetitive discharges to a single stimulus. Though any muscle can undergo spasmodic contractions, spasm of carpopedal muscles is classical and can easily be triggered.[5]
  - *Trousseau's sign or carpopedal spasm:* When a blood pressure (BP) cuff is applied on the arm and inflated above systolic BP for 3–5 minutes, a carpopedal spasm sets in. It is also called Trousseau's sign. Components of this sign are flexion of the thumb, wrist, and metacarpophalangeal joints with extension of the fingers.[6]
  - *Chvostek's sign:* When the facial nerve is stimulated by tapping it in front of the tragus, it will result in ipsilateral contraction of the facial muscles. It is named Chvostek's sign.[6]
  - *Laryngospasm* due to hyperexcitability of laryngeal muscles could turn fatal if not detected early.
- *Cardiovascular manifestations:* Calcium is essential for excitation–contraction coupling of cardiac muscles, the deficiency of which may precipitate hypotension and congestive heart failure.
  - Hypocalcemia prolongs phase 2 of myocardial action potential, which leads to QTc prolongation. Although rare, severe hypocalcemia may precipitate ventricular tachyarrhythmia.
- Severe hypocalcemia may cause seizures, and it may be the sole presenting symptom. Evaluation of new onset seizures is incomplete without assessment of serum calcium levels.
- Psychiatric manifestations such as anxiety, depression, and emotional liability are frequent and reversible with treatment. Hallucinations and acute psychosis are rare symptoms.

Diagnosis

When hypocalcemia is suspected, evaluation should be directed to confirm hypocalcemia and find its etiology.

- *Hypocalcemia confirmation:* When hypocalcemia is identified as a low serum total calcium, the patient should be further evaluated with serum-ionized calcium levels. Serum total calcium level is less specific than ionized calcium and is affected by serum albumin levels and factors affecting its binding to calcium. If a facility to test ionized calcium is not available, hypocalcemia should be defined based on corrected total calcium levels where measured calcium levels are corrected to hypo or hyperalbuminemia. For 1 g/dL increase or decrease in albumin level below 4 g/dL, 0.8 mg/dL should be subtracted or added respectively to the total serum calcium level. The corrected calcium formula is mentioned below:

  Corrected total calcium = measured total calcium + [0.8 × (4.0 – Albumin)]
- *Etiological diagnosis of hypocalcemia:* Most of the time hypocalcemia is associated with obvious clinical scenarios, such as CKD, post-thyroidectomy, parathyroidectomy, and massive blood transfusion during hemorrhagic shock management. Further testing may be needed to confirm the etiological diagnosis or if an obvious cause of hypocalcemia cannot be identified on clinical history.

  The investigation required for the further etiological diagnosis of hypocalcemia is serum HCO_3, serum creatinine, serum albumin, serum magnesium, serum phosphate, and intact PTH, serum vitamin D_3 levels.

Once the hypocalcemia is identified, the next step is to see serum PTH, phosphate, and vitamin D_3 levels. Hypoparathyroidism is characterized by low serum calcium, low PTH, and elevated PO_4 levels. Pseudohypoparathyroidism (PHP) and CKD are associated with PTH and PO_4 levels that are elevated along with low calcium. Patients with vitamin D_3 deficiency will show reduced calcium and PO_4 and elevated PTH levels.

The correlation of serum calcium, PTH, and PO_4 in different disorders is summarized in **Table 3**.

TABLE 3: Correlation of PTH, PO_4, calcium, and vitamin D in various disorders.

Disease	*Calcium*	*PTH*	*PO_4*	*Vitamin D*
Hypoparathyroidism	Low	Low	Elevated	Normal
Pseudohypoparathyroidism	Low	Elevated	Elevated	Normal
Chronic kidney disease	Low	Elevated	Elevated	Normal
Vitamin D deficiency	Low	Elevated	Low	Low

Treatment

Hypocalcemia treatment mainly depends on the severity of symptoms, acuity of hypocalcemia, and its etiology. Recommendations of hypocalcemia correction are widely based on accepted clinical practice and experience as limited studies are available on the optimal treatment of hypocalcemia.

Asymptomatic patients and patients with mild symptoms with gradual onset of hypocalcemia are managed with oral calcium supplements along with treatment of etiology.

However, those patients having severe symptoms or mild symptoms but rapid drop in calcium levels require IV calcium supplementations. Patients with the following symptoms are suggested to be treated with IV calcium supplements.[7]

- Seizures, behavioral changes
- Coagulopathy
- Congestive cardiac failure or hypotension
- Electrocardiogram (ECG) changes with QTc prolongation or arrhythmias
- Laryngospasm
- Carpopedal spasm

Intravenous calcium supplements are available as calcium gluconate or calcium chloride. Calcium gluconate is preferred over calcium chloride as the latter has more tendency to cause tissue necrosis if extravasated. A 10% calcium gluconate contains 90 mg of elemental calcium/10 mL, and usually 1–2 ampules (180 mg of elemental calcium) diluted in 50–100 mL of 5% dextrose (5% D) is infused slowly over 10–20 minutes.[7] In severe hypocalcemia infusion of 60 mL of calcium gluconate in 500 mL of 5% D is prepared and given at an infusion rate of 0.5–2.0 mg/kg/h. IV calcium supplements are continued till symptoms reversed and oral calcium supplements are started. Concurrent hypomagnesemia should be treated if present.

Disease-specific treatment modifications are required based on the etiology of hypocalcemia. Patients with hypoparathyroidism require lifelong calcium supplementation along with calcitriol. Despite oral calcium supplements, the patient may develop intermittent hypocalcemia attacks.

HYPERCALCEMIA

Introduction

Though hypercalcemia in ICU is less frequent, it requires immediate attention and treatment, if severe. It may cause life-threatening complications if remains undetected. Hypercalcemia is labeled when serum total calcium levels are >10.8 mg/dL. It occurs due to reduced urinary excretion of calcium, increased absorption or dietary intake of calcium, or increased calcium release from bones. Mild-to-moderate hypercalcemia is generally well tolerated if the serum calcium rise is gradual. Even mild hypercalcemia may produce symptoms if the rise in serum calcium is acute.

Etiology

Causes of hypercalcemia are broadly classified into two categories, i.e., parathyroid-mediated and nonparathyroid-mediated. Among all causes, primary hyperparathyroidism and malignancy are the most common contributors, accounting for over 90%.

Parathyroid-Mediated

- *Primary hyperparathyroidism:* Increased PTH secretion due to parathyroid adenoma or hyperplasia leads to hypercalcemia and hypophosphatemia.[8] Increase in serum calcium levels is usually gradual. Parathyroid hyperplasia is also associated with multiple endocrine neoplasia (MEN) syndromes: MEN type 1 and MEN type 2A.
- *Tertiary hyperparathyroidism:* CKD patients usually develop secondary hyperparathyroidism, i.e., increased PTH and PO_4 but low calcium levels. Few long-standing CKD patients may develop parathyroid hyperplasia releasing inappropriately high PTH levels which leads to hypercalcemia.
- Familial hypocalciuric hypercalcemia is an autosomal dominant condition associated with reduced urinary calcium excretion due to increased calcium absorption through renal tubules.[9] It leads to hypercalcemia. Serum PTH levels are normal or marginally raised.

Nonparathyroid-Mediated

- *Malignancy:* Hypercalcemia due to malignancy is often acute and severe and usually symptomatic. The following mechanisms are responsible for hypercalcemia in malignancy:[10]
  - *Metastatic bone resorption:* Bone metastasis increases bone resorption by stimulating osteoclast growth and differentiation through the local release of cytokines. Metastatic breast cancer, renal cell carcinoma, and multiple myeloma are common examples.[10]
  - *Release of parathyroid hormone-related peptide (PTHrP):* PTHrP acts similarly to PTH on PTH-1 receptors. Hence, when produced in an uncontrolled manner, it leads to hypercalcemia through its action on bone, kidney, and gut. The PTHrP-related hypercalcemia is the most common cause of hypercalcemia in malignancy, also called humoral hypercalcemia of malignancy. It has a common association with squamous cell carcinoma of the lung and the head and neck region. It is also seen with carcinoma of the breast, ovaries, kidney, and bladder. The PTHrP is often produced when the disease is advanced and is a marker of poor prognosis.[11]
  - *Increased production of calcitriol:* In lymphoma, there is extrarenal production of calcitriol from calcidiol by lymphocytes and macrophages. This calcitriol production is independent of PTH. As it is independent of PTH, its production will not get suppressed with normal calcium levels.[10] And hence, continuous increased production of calcitriol leads to hypercalcemia. It is commonly seen in Hodgkin's and non-Hodgkin's lymphoma.
- *Hypervitaminosis D:* Increased either calcidiol or calcitriol levels will increase bone resorption and calcium absorption from the gut causing hypercalcemia. Hypervitaminosis D is observed in patients for whom vitamin D is prescribed for a longer duration, such as CKD and osteoporosis. It can also be seen with excessive intrinsic production of calcitriol, which is observed in malignant lymphomas and chronic granulomatous condition.[12]
- *Miscellaneous causes:* These are rare but important causes of hypercalcemia.
  - Endocrine causes: Thyrotoxicosis, pheochromocytomas, and adrenal insufficiency.
  - High bone turnover due to prolonged immobilization.
  - *Milk alkali syndrome:* It is a triad of hypercalcemia, alkalosis, and acute kidney injury.
  - Drug induced: Thiazide diuretics, lithium, calcium, vitamin D supplements, and vitamin A supplements.

Clinical features: There are no hallmark clinical signs and symptoms of hypercalcemia and mostly its presentation is vague and nonspecific. Though symptoms increase with the severity of hypercalcemia, it is not linearly related to its serum levels. Symptoms are prominent if the rise in serum calcium is acute even with mild to moderate hypercalcemia.[13]

Hypercalcemia is classified into three severity grades based on serum calcium levels in **Table 4.**[13]

Mild hypercalcemia is usually asymptomatic. Patients may have nonspecific symptoms of generalized weakness, fatigue, and constipation in acute mild hypercalcemia or gradual onset moderate hypercalcemia.

In cases of severe hypercalcemia or acute onset moderate hypercalcemia, symptoms are profound including nausea, vomiting, anorexia, polydipsia, polyuria, neuromuscular weakness, irritability, and confusion. These symptoms may progress to drowsiness, stupor, coma, seizure, anuria due to acute kidney injury, hemodynamic instability due to life-threatening arrhythmias.[13,14]

Hypercalcemia should always be ruled out in patients presenting with acute pancreatitis, peptic ulcer disease, nephrolithiasis, and CKDs.[15]

Diagnosis: Acute onset moderate-to-severe hypercalcemia can turn fatal, hence rapid and accurate diagnosis and treatment is essential to improve overall outcomes. It is also essential to find the underlying cause of hypercalcemia to prevent its recurrence and other complications. Detailed history and physical examination along with investigation is the main stay of diagnosis.

TABLE 4: Severity of hypercalcemia.

S. No.	Severity of hypercalcemia	Serum calcium levels (mg/dL)
1.	Mild hypercalcemia	10.8–12
2.	Moderate hypercalcemia	12.1–14
3.	Severe hypercalcemia	>14

Confirmation of hypercalcemia: When suspected, hypercalcemia should be confirmed with serum total calcium and ionized levels. As discussed in the hypocalcemia section of this chapter, serum total calcium levels are affected by many factors like serum albumin levels and acid–base balance.[1] If testing of ionized calcium testing facilities is not available, the diagnosis should be made based on corrected total calcium levels with the help of the following formula:

Corrected total calcium = measured total calcium + [0.8 × (4.0 – albumin)]

Once the hypercalcemia is confirmed, further evaluation is done to diagnose the underlying cause. Further testing includes serum PTH, PTHrP, calcitonin, vitamin D, phosphorus, magnesium, alkaline phosphatase levels, serum creatinine and urinary calcium–creatinine ratio, serum protein electrophoresis (SPEP,) and appropriate tumor markers and imaging to detect malignancy, parathyroid adenoma, or hypertrophy. **Flowchart 1** gives the diagnostic approach to reach the etiological diagnosis and should be interpreted with the patient's clinical scenario.

Treatment

Measures to treat hypercalcemia are broadly divided into two categories:

Flowchart 1: Diagnostic approach to hypercalcemia.

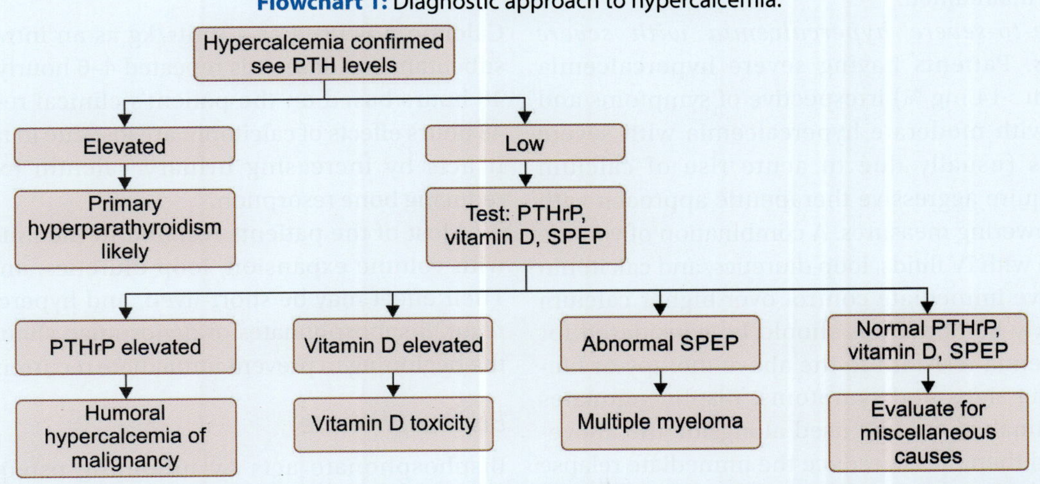

(PTH: parathyroid hormone; PTHrP: parathyroid hormone-related protein; SPEP: serum protein electrophoresis)

1. Measures to reduce serum calcium levels
2. Treatment of the underlying cause of hypercalcemia to prevent recurrence

Measures to reduce serum calcium levels: Serum calcium levels can be reduced by the following measures:[13,16]

- *Increase calcium elimination from the extracellular fluid (ECF):* Volume expansion by IV fluids, loop diuretics, and hemodialysis
- *Inhibition of gastrointestinal (GI) absorption:* Glucocorticoids and oral phosphate
- *Inhibition of bone resorption:* Bisphosphonate, calcitonin, and denosumab

The therapeutic approach to control calcium levels includes a combination of the above therapeutic measures. The choice of the therapy depends upon its rapid onset of action and its duration of action. It also depends upon the acuity of calcium rise, the severity of symptoms, serum calcium levels, and the etiology of hypercalcemia. The therapeutic approach to treat hypercalcemia is broadly divided into two categories: (1) Mild-to-moderate asymptomatic or mild symptomatic hypercalcemia and (2) moderate-to-severe hypercalcemia with severe symptoms.

1. *Mild-to-moderate asymptomatic or mild symptomatic hypercalcemia:* Patients with mild-to-moderate hypercalcemia in whom calcium rise is gradual manifest no symptoms or mild symptoms. These patients do not require immediate therapy. Treatment is targeted toward the etiology of hypercalcemia. Factors that influence calcium excretion should be avoided such as dehydration, thiazide diuretics, lithium, calcium, and vitamin D supplements. Adequate oral hydration should be maintained.
2. *Moderate-to-severe hypercalcemia with severe symptoms:* Patients having severe hypercalcemia (s. calcium >14 mg %) irrespective of symptoms and patients with moderate hypercalcemia with severe symptoms (usually due to acute rise of calcium levels) require aggressive therapeutic approach with calcium lowering measures. A combination of volume expansion with IV fluids, loop diuretics, and calcitonin will achieve immediate control over higher calcium levels. Early hemodialysis should be considered for hypercalcemia resistant to the above therapy or life-threatening signs and symptoms. Bisphosphonates or denosumab should be used alongside the above-mentioned therapies to reduce the immediate relapse rate of hypercalcemia.

Volume Expansion

Patients with hypercalcemia usually have severe dehydration. Dehydration itself reduces urinary excretion of calcium. Volume expansion should be given for an initial 48 hours with isotonic saline as a preferred crystalloid.[17] Rate of fluid administration should be individualized and done with caution in patients with poor cardiac reserve. For those with good cardiac reserve, the initial rate of fluid infusion should be 200–300 mL/h for the first 4–6 hours targeting 100–150 mL/h urine output.

Loop Diuretics

Loop diuretics can be added with IV fluids once dehydration is corrected. One must make a note that loop diuretics should not be used if volume expansion is not achieved as it may worsen dehydration and hypercalcemia. Additionally, it is important to note that, thiazide diuretics are contraindicated in hypercalcemia as it reduces calcium excretion through the kidneys which leads to further worsening of hypercalcemia.

Hemodialysis

Hemodialysis as a first line of therapy in hypercalcemia should be reserved for patients with poor renal functions as these patients are unlikely to respond to volume expansion and loop diuretic and those with very poor cardiac reserve. Hemodialysis should be done as a first line of therapy for those presenting with life-threatening complications of hypercalcemia. It is used as a rescue measure if hypercalcemia is resistant to initial management with volume expansion, loop diuretics, and calcitonin.

Calcitonin

Calcitonin is used as 4 units/kg as an intramuscular or subcutaneous dose. It is repeated 4–6 hourly for an initial 48 hours based on the patient's clinical response. After 48 hours effects of calcitonin are lost due to tachyphylaxis. It acts by increasing urinary calcium excretion and reducing bone resorption.[18]

Most of the patients respond to the initial treatment with volume expansion, loop diuretics, and calcitonin. Their effect may be short-lived, and hypercalcemia may recur. Bisphosphonates or denosumab should be used in the beginning to prevent immediate recurrence.

Bisphosphonate

Bisphosphonate acts by inhibiting osteoclastic bone resorption. Their effect starts after 24–36 hours after initiation of therapy and lasts for about 7 days. Zoledronic acid is given as a 4 mg IV over 15 minutes.[19] It is repeated after every 7 days in cases of malignancy-induced hypercalcemia. Bisphosphonates are preferred over denosumab as the risk of iatrogenic hypocalcemia is lower with them. However, Endocrine Society Clinical Practice Guidelines suggest the use of denosumab over bisphosphonates for initial therapy of hypercalcemia of malignancy.[20] Bisphosphonates are associated with significant side effects. Oral bisphosphonates can cause severe esophagitis and hence contraindicated in cases of reflux disease, esophageal stricture, and Barrett's esophagus. IV bisphosphonate therapy may cause flu-like symptoms lasting for 24–48 hours. Precipitous hypocalcemia is observed in few cases treated with oral or IV bisphosphonates.

Denosumab

Denosumab is a monoclonal antibody, used to treat hypercalcemia in patients with CKD where bisphosphonates are contraindicated; it is also used when hypercalcemia is resistant to initial therapy with bisphosphonates. It is administered as a 60–120 mg single dose subcutaneously. It can be repeated after 5–7 days based on clinical response. Daily calcium monitoring is recommended for early detection hypocalcemia.[20]

Etiology-specific Treatment

Once the calcium levels are controlled, surgical removal of parathyroid adenoma/gland should be performed. Humoral hypercalcemia of malignancy usually occurs in the advanced stage with limited therapeutic options. Detailed discussion on etiology-specific treatment is beyond the scope of this chapter.

Conclusion

Hypercalcemia presents as a multifaceted clinical challenge, demanding a comprehensive understanding of its etiology, diagnosis, and management. While primary hyperparathyroidism remains a leading cause, the differential diagnosis must encompass a spectrum of conditions, from malignancies to medication-induced effects. Timely recognition and appropriate intervention are imperative to mitigate potential complications, ranging from renal impairment to cardiovascular events. Despite advancements in diagnostic modalities and therapeutic strategies, ongoing research is needed to refine our approach and improve patient outcomes. Through interdisciplinary collaboration and continued vigilance, healthcare professionals can effectively navigate the complexities of hypercalcemia, ultimately enhancing patient care and quality of life.

SODIUM HOMEOSTASIS AND DISORDERS OF SODIUM IMBALANCE

SODIUM HOMEOSTASIS

Sodium serves as the primary extracellular cation, contributing to around 88% of ECF osmolality. It is an essential electrolyte and plays a crucial role in maintaining homeostasis and supporting various physiological processes within the human body. Its function encompasses fluid balance, nerve transmission, and muscle contraction, among others. Understanding the intricate physiology of sodium is paramount for comprehending its profound impact on human health and well-being.

Distribution and Concentration of Sodium

Sodium is distributed throughout the body, primarily in ECF compartments such as the blood plasma and interstitial fluid. The concentration of sodium in these compartments is tightly regulated to ensure optimal cellular function. The movement of sodium across cell membranes is facilitated by various transport proteins, including sodium–potassium pumps and sodium channels.[21]

Extracellular Sodium Concentration

Sodium is found in the ECF at a concentration of approximately 145 mEq/L. Unlike calcium or magnesium, sodium is not bound to protein. Strong electrolytes, such as NaCl, behave as independent Na^+ and Cl^- ions in aqueous solutions when sufficiently diluted. However, in physiological concentrations, this is mostly true, except in the renal medulla where concentrations are significantly higher than in the ECF.

Intracellular Sodium Concentration

The intracellular sodium concentration is typically lower than the extracellular concentration, maintained by the action of sodium–potassium pumps. These pumps actively transport sodium out of the cell while simultaneously moving potassium into the cell. This process is crucial for maintaining the electrochemical gradient across the cell membrane.

Sodium Regulation

Water primarily follows osmotic gradients across membranes. The sodium pump plays a crucial role in maintaining ECF volume by confining sodium to the ECF, acting as the osmotic framework. Changes in sodium balance predominantly affect ECF volume rather than plasma sodium concentration, contrary to the common misconception. The regulation of plasma sodium concentration is governed by mechanisms that control water balance, including thirst, the secretion of antidiuretic hormone (ADH), and the renal response to it.

The main stimulus for thirst and ADH secretion is an increase in plasma sodium concentration, which elevates the concentration of the interstitial fluid surrounding the osmoreceptors responsible for thirst and ADH release. Both groups of osmoreceptors are located within the hypothalamus. ADH is synthesized in other hypothalamic neurons before being stored in the posterior pituitary gland.[22]

When the water loss from ECF occurs, serum sodium concentration will increase which leads to increased serum osmolality. It stimulates osmoreceptors which stimulate thirst and releases ADH. The ADH will act on kidneys to reabsorb free water producing concentrated urine. Any imbalance in the distribution and concentration of sodium can have detrimental effects on cellular function and overall health. Hyponatremia, a condition characterized by low sodium levels in the blood, can lead to symptoms such as lethargy, confusion, seizures, and even coma. On the other hand, hypernatremia, an elevated sodium level in the blood, can cause symptoms such as thirst, dehydration, and neurological abnormalities. These imbalances can occur due to various factors, including kidney dysfunction, hormonal imbalances, excessive sweating, or inadequate sodium intake.

Laboratory testing of sodium is done by direct and indirect ion-selective electrode (ISE) methods. Indirect ISE is the most commonly utilized method in clinical laboratories to measure sodium levels. In the indirect ISE method, sodium is tested on separated serum or plasma. Hence, it measures sodium activity in an aqueous solution. In case of hyperlipidemia or hyperproteinemia, the measured sodium value would be lower due to the dilutional effect of lipids or proteins. However, direct ISE overcomes this drawback as sodium measurement is done directly on whole blood.

HYPONATREMIA

Definition

Hyponatremia is when the level of sodium in the blood drops <135 mEq/L.[23] This condition can be linked to low, normal, or high tonicity. Effective osmolality or tonicity refers to the contribution to osmolality of solutes, like sodium and glucose, that cannot freely move across cell membranes, leading to shifts in water within cells. The most common type of hyponatremia is dilutional hyponatremia, which occurs due to water retention. If the kidneys cannot eliminate water as quickly as it is consumed, it dilutes the body's solutes, resulting in lower osmolality and hypotonicity.

The duration of hyponatremia is classified based on its onset:

- *Acute:* Hyponatremia is considered acute if it develops over a period of *fewer than 48* hours.
- *Chronic:* Hyponatremia is termed chronic if it has been present for *48 hours or more.*

The acuity of hyponatremia influences the risk of complications, such as cerebral edema and seizures, and determines the need for aggressive therapy. Acute hyponatremia poses a higher risk of complications and requires more aggressive treatment. Conversely, chronic hyponatremia, particularly with lower serum sodium concentrations, carries a risk of complications from overly aggressive therapy. Therefore, careful monitoring of serum levels is crucial to prevent overcorrection.

Severity of Hyponatremia

Hyponatremia severity is categorized as follows:

- *Severe hyponatremia:* Serum sodium concentration <120 mEq/L is classified as severe hyponatremia.
- *Moderate hyponatremia:* Serum sodium concentration ranging from 120 to 129 mEq/L is considered moderate hyponatremia.
- *Mild hyponatremia:* Serum sodium concentration between 130 and 134 mEq/L falls under mild hyponatremia.

These classifications help guide the management and treatment of hyponatremia, with more severe cases requiring closer monitoring and potentially more aggressive interventions to avoid complications.

Hyponatremia can be further classified into different subtypes based on its underlying causes and characteristics **(Flowchart 2)**.[24]

- *Pseudo (normo-osmolal) or isotonic hyponatremia:* This type of hyponatremia occurs due to conditions such as hypertriglyceridemia or increased plasma proteins, as seen in multiple myeloma. In pseudohyponatremia, although the sodium concentration and plasma osmolality remain unchanged, the measured sodium concentration appears low because the specimen contains less plasma water. This condition can occur when the plasma water fraction falls below 80%, as seen in marked hyperlipidemia or hyperproteinemia (paraproteinemia).
- *Translocational (hyperosmolal) or hypertonic or redistributive hyponatremia:* This type of hyponatremia results from the presence of osmotically active solutes in the serum, such as mannitol or glucose. When significant amounts of unmeasured solutes are present in the plasma, accurate calculation of plasma osmolality becomes challenging and requires direct measurement.
- *True (hypoosmolal) hyponatremia:* True hyponatremia is characterized by a reduction in serum osmolality and is further classified based on volume status in **Table 5**.

Hypovolemic Hyponatremia

This condition is associated with low plasma volume; as mentioned above, the causes of this condition can be either due to renal sodium loss or extra-renal sodium loss.

- *Cerebral salt wasting (CSW):* It is a condition that shares similarities with the syndrome of inappropriate antidiuretic hormone (SIADH) secretion, but with distinct differences. In CSW, the primary defect lies in renal salt wasting and volume depletion, leading to a secondary increase in ADH levels. On the other hand, patients with SIADH experience a high level of arginine vasopressin (AVP) as the main etiologic event.

Flowchart 2: Types of hyponatremia.

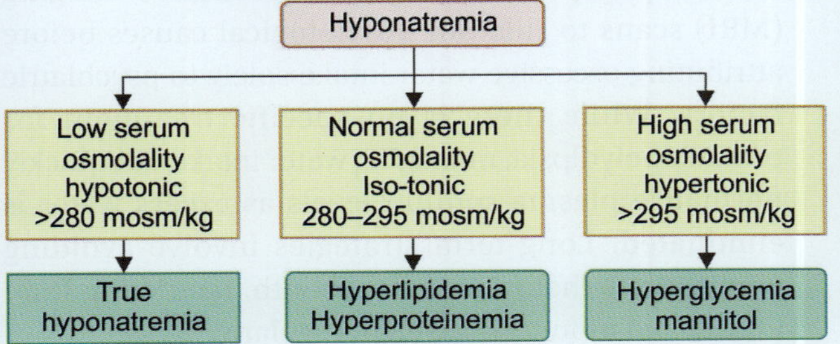

- *Diuretic-induced hyponatremia:* It is a well-documented phenomenon, particularly prevalent with the use of thiazides. This condition typically manifests *shortly after the initiation* of thiazide therapy and is frequently observed in elderly female patients. Notably, the concentration of sodium and potassium in urine surpasses that in the plasma, leading to a direct reduction in plasma sodium levels. In contrast,

TABLE 5: Subtypes of hypoosmolal hyponatremia.

Sr. no.	*Type of hyponatremia*	*Causes*	
1.	Euvolemic hyponatremia	• Thiazide diuretics • Hypothyroidism • Adrenal insufficiency • Syndrome of inappropriate secretion of antidiuretic hormone • Excessive water intake • Primary polydipsia • Decreased intake of solutes • Beer potomania • "Tea-and-toast" syndrome	
2.	Hypervolemic hyponatremia	• Congestive heart failure • Cirrhosis • Nephrotic syndrome • Renal failure (acute or chronic) • Pregnancy	
3.	Hypovolemic hyponatremia	Renal sodium loss	• Diuretic agents • Osmotic diuresis (glucose, urea, mannitol) • Adrenal insufficiency • Salt-wasting nephropathy • Bicarbonaturia (renal tubular acidosis, disequilibrium stage of vomiting) • Ketonuria
		Extrarenal sodium loss	• Diarrhea • Vomiting • Blood loss • Excessive sweating (e.g., in marathon runners) • Fluid sequestration in "third space" – Bowel obstruction – Peritonitis – Pancreatitis – Muscle trauma – Burns

hyponatremia is less commonly associated with loop diuretics. Furosemide-related hyponatremia, on the other hand, tends to manifest *after prolonged treatment periods*, often coinciding with the onset of concurrent illnesses.

- *Extrarenal sodium losses* can occur in various medical conditions such as excessive sweating, pancreatitis, small bowel obstruction, vomiting, and diarrhea. If these losses are not replenished, they can lead to a decrease in effective circulating volume and a nonosmotic release of AVP. Hypovolemic hyponatremia, caused by conditions like diarrhea or third space loss, can result in low urine sodium levels due to increased renal sodium reabsorption. Hypovolemia from gastric losses of hydrochloric acid can lead to low urine chloride levels due to increased renal chloride reabsorption, although urine sodium levels may not necessarily be low due to metabolic alkalosis and resulting bicarbonaturia.
- *Mineralocorticoid deficiency* is a rare but another significant factor contributing to hypovolemic hyponatremia. Primary adrenal insufficiency, also known as Addison's disease, is characterized by mineralocorticoids and glucocorticoid deficiency. This condition leads to renal sodium wasting and subsequent volume depletion, triggering the nonosmotic release of AVP. The lack of cortisol further increases AVP release. Patients with Addison's disease typically present with symptoms such as hypovolemia, hyponatremia, hyperkalemia, decreased bicarbonate, and increased urine sodium. However, it is important to note that not all individuals with primary adrenal insufficiency will exhibit this classic presentation.

Euvolemic Hyponatremia

Euvolemic hyponatremia is a condition characterized by normal or slightly decreased total body sodium content alongside an increase in total body water. This imbalance can be caused by various factors such as SIADH, diuretic use, CKD, decreased solute intake, primary polydipsia, glucocorticoid and thyroid deficiency, and reset osmostat.

- *SIADH:* Syndrome of inappropriate antidiuretic hormone is the most common cause of euvolemic hyponatremia and accounts for almost 60% of the cases of hyponatremia. It occurs due to disturbed regulation of ADH hormone. ADH is secreted inappropriately irrespective of serum osmolality.

  Syndrome of inappropriate antidiuretic hormone is commonly seen in the following conditions:
  - *Central nervous system (CNS) disorders:* Intracranial hemorrhage, stroke, trauma, and meningitis
  - *Malignancies:* As part of par neoplastic syndrome in pulmonary and extrapulmonary small cell carcinoma, head and neck malignancies, and neuroblastomas
  - *Drugs:* Carbamazepine, chlorpropamide, haloperidol, and cyclophosphamide are commonly associated with SIADH.
  - *Miscellaneous:* Postpituitary surgery, pulmonary infections, and human immunodeficiency virus (HIV)

  Syndrome of inappropriate antidiuretic hormone is characterized by:
  - Euvolemia with decreased measured serum osmolality (100 mOsm/kg H_2O)
  - Urinary osmolality (>100 mOsm/kg H_2O)
  - Urinary [Na^+] >40 mmol/L
  - Fractional sodium excretion >1%; fractional urea excretion >55%
  - Failure to improve or worsening of hyponatremia after 0.9% saline infusion
  - Improvement of hyponatremia with fluid restriction (FR)
- *Exercise-related hyponatremia:* This condition can occur in marathon runners, excessive water intake can be associated with persistent ADH secretion.
- *Primary polydipsia:* Primary polydipsia is usually associated with a psychiatric condition, characterized by excessive intake of water. Patients of primary polydipsia can produce over 400–600 mL of dilute urine per hour. when ADH is suppressed, with a minimum urine osmolality of 40 mOsm/kg. Although these individuals typically maintain normal or slightly reduced serum sodium levels and may exhibit symptoms such as polydipsia and polyuria, they struggle to excrete excessive water loads, which can lead to fatal hyponatremia. Patients with polydipsia should undergo brain imaging tests like computed tomography (CT) or magnetic resonance imaging (MRI) scans to rule out physiological causes before attributing excessive water intake solely to psychiatric factors. While there is no specific treatment for primary polydipsia, managing water intake can quickly normalize plasma sodium levels as excess water is eliminated. Long-term strategies involve avoiding medications that induce dry mouth, restricting fluid intake, and monitoring weight regularly.

Hypervolemic Hyponatremia

This type of hyponatremia is a common occurrence in various conditions such as congestive heart failure, cirrhosis of the liver, nephrotic syndrome, and CKD. Despite the increase in plasma and extracellular volumes in heart failure and cirrhosis, there is still stimulation of ADH as part of the pathogenesis. The presence of hyponatremia is often indicative of a poor prognosis. In cases of acute and chronic renal failure, hyponatremia is frequently seen due to the kidneys' inability to effectively excrete excess water. However, hyponatremia is not as prevalent in nephrotic syndrome unless there is a significant decrease in glomerular filtration rate (GFR). In instances of severe hypoalbuminemia (<2 g/dL), intravascular hypovolemia may occur, triggering the nonosmotic release of AVP and subsequent retention of hypotonic fluids.

Clinical Features

Mainly the clinical picture of hyponatremia depends on the severity of hyponatremia and the rate at which it develops. Symptoms generally occur when serum sodium concentration <125 mEq/L. Elderly patients are usually more symptomatic. Early symptoms of hyponatremia are nonspecific and often missed. The patient may have muscle cramps, generalized weakness, anorexia, increased sleepiness, nausea, and vomiting. Patients with severe hyponatremia or acute mild to moderate hyponatremic patients may have early severe symptoms like drowsiness, seizures, or even coma.[25]

Diagnosis Approach of Hyponatremic Patient

When diagnosing hyponatremia, it is crucial to determine the patient's volume status, such as dehydration, edema, or ascites. Clinical signs of volume depletion, like orthostatic changes in BP and pulse rate, dry mucus membranes, and decreased skin turgor, indicate hypovolemia. Direct hemodynamic measurements can further support the clinical assessment. Signs of hypothyroidism or adrenal insufficiency should be noted, and a thorough examination should be conducted to identify any CNS or lung lesions.

Investigations

Measurement of Serum Sodium Levels

Serum sodium measurement is a critical step in assessing electrolyte balance, with the ideal method being an ion-specific electrode (ISE) using direct potentiometry to avoid pseudohyponatremia.

Measurement of Serum Osmolality

Differentiating true, pseudo, or translocational hyponatremia involves measuring serum osmolality, ideally using an osmometer. In the absence of an osmometer, assessing blood sugar, serum triglyceride, and serum protein levels can aid in distinguishing between the three types.

Serum osmolality is calculated using the following formula:

$$\text{Serum osmolality } (mOsm/kg\ H_2O) = 2 \times \text{Serum } [Na^+]\ (mEq/L) + \text{Glucose } (mg/dL)/18 + \text{BUN } (mg/dL)/2.8$$

Measurement of Urine Osmolality

Urine osmolality serves as a valuable indicator to differentiate between impaired water excretion and hyponatremia with normal water excretion. When urine osmolality exceeds 100 mOsm/kg, it suggests impaired water excretion. In cases of hyponatremia with normal water excretion, the typical response involves a significant reduction in ADH secretion, leading to the excretion of highly diluted urine with an osmolality below 100 mOsm/kg and a specific gravity of ≤1.003. Elevated values above this threshold indicate an inability to effectively excrete free water, often due to the persistent secretion of ADH.

Measurement of Urinary Sodium Levels

Measuring urinary sodium losses can help differentiate whether the sodium loss is renal or nonrenal. In cases of inappropriate urine concentration, analyzing urine sodium and chloride concentrations can help differentiate between hypovolemic and euvolemic hyponatremia. Patients with hypovolemic hyponatremia are associated with metabolic alkalosis due to vomiting, a urine sodium concentration >20 mEq/L, and a low urine chloride concentration (<20 mEq/L) may indicate the cause of sodium loss.

Fractional Excretion of Sodium (Flowchart 3)

Fractional excretion of sodium (FENa) is a valuable tool for assessing volume status, as it takes into account variations in urine volume that can affect urine sodium levels. In patients with normal renal function and hyponatremia, a FENa cut-off of <1% indicates hypovolemic hyponatremia, while a FENa >1% suggests hypervolemic or normovolemic hyponatremia.

Flowchart 3: Interpretation of fractional excretion of sodium (FENa)

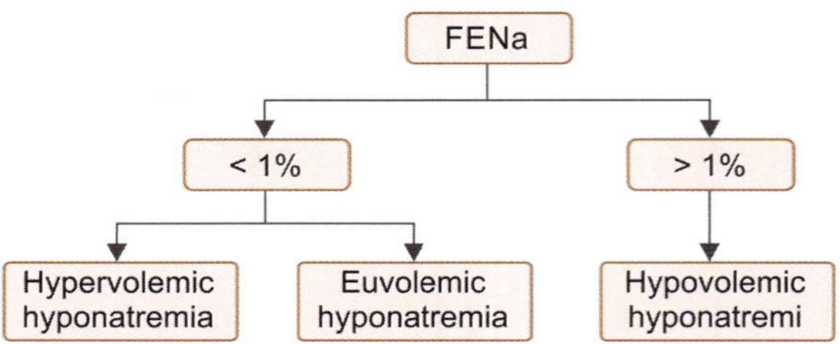

Management of Hyponatremia

The management of hyponatremia mainly depends on etiology, degree of hyponatremia, duration of hyponatremia (acute or chronic), severity of symptoms (severe or mild), and volume status. The rate of correction depends on the acuity with which it develops and also on the degree of symptoms present in the patients. The goal of therapy in hyponatremia is to correct plasma sodium concentration at a safe rate, replace both sodium and potassium deficit, and also treat the underlying etiology.

Rate of Correction

In patients with acute hyponatremia or severely symptomatic chronic hyponatremia, characterized by altered mental status, seizures, and frequent vomiting, it is crucial to swiftly reverse cerebral edema by elevating plasma sodium levels by 5 mEq/L.[23] Conversely, for individuals with chronic hyponatremia, caution must be exercised to ensure that plasma sodium levels are not increased by >10 mEq/L within 24 hours.[23,25,26]

The equation used to estimate the efficacy of initial therapy in hyponatremia patients involves the AdroguéMadias formula which gives an increase in serum sodium by administration of 1 L of infusate. Based on the amount of infusate required to achieve the desired change in sodium is calculated. The infusion rate is decided based on the desired rate of sodium correction.

$$\text{Increase in S. Na} = (\text{Infusate } [\text{Na} + \text{k}] - \text{S. Na}) \div (\text{TBW} + 1)$$

TBW is the estimated total body water (lean body weight times 0.5 for women and 0.6 for men).

Total infusate required to achieve target sodium = Increase in Na by 1 L of infusate/desired increase in Na targeted

It is important to note that this formula should not be the sole basis of therapy decisions, as regular monitoring of serum sodium levels is crucial.

Potassium added to the solution should be included in the formula (i.e., "Infusate [Na + K]" rather than "Infusate [Na]") as potassium administration for concurrent hypokalemia can raise the serum sodium concentration.

However, these formulas have limitations and may not accurately predict changes in serum sodium, necessitating frequent measurements.

Fluid Restriction

Fluid restriction below the level of urine output is recommended for the treatment of symptomatic or severe hyponatremia in conditions such as heart failure, cirrhosis, SIADH, and advanced kidney function impairment. A restriction to 50–60% of daily fluid requirements may be necessary to achieve the desired negative water balance. It is advised to keep fluid intake <800 mL/day.[27] In cases where urine is highly concentrated (500 mOsm/kg or higher), FR alone may not be enough to correct hyponatremia. It is also useful in hyponatremia patients with primary polydipsia. The urine-to-serum cation ratio, which compares the concentrations of urine cations (sodium and potassium) to serum sodium, can help predict the effectiveness of FR. A ratio of <0.5 suggests that serum sodium will increase with FR, while a ratio >1 indicates it will not.

Loop Diuretics

In patients with SIADH exhibiting a urine-to-serum cation ratio exceeding 1, the concurrent use of a loop diuretic like furosemide may prove beneficial. Thiazides should not be used.

Demeclocycline

Demeclocycline induces a nephrogenic form of diabetes insipidus (DI), leading to reduced urine concentration despite elevated plasma AVP levels. The recommended dosage of demeclocycline typically falls between 600 and 1,200 mg/day, divided into multiple doses.

Vaptans

Vasopressin receptor antagonists, known as vaptans, target various vasopressin receptors such as V1a, V1b, and V2. While V2 receptors promote antidiuresis, V1a and V1b receptors trigger vasoconstriction and adrenocorticotropic hormone (ACTH) release, respectively. By inducing aquaresis, vaptans facilitate water loss without impacting sodium and potassium excretion.[28] This makes them a preferred method for addressing hyponatremia, as they maintain electrolyte balance and eliminate the need for FR. Importantly, vaptans operate without stimulating the neurohormonal system or causing renal impairment. The efficacy of oral tolvaptan was studied in multicenter trials (SALT-1 and SALT-2) with hyponatremia caused by SIADH. Tolvaptan showed a significant increase in serum sodium concentration and led to improvements in mental scores, although the clinical significance of these effects was uncertain due to the short 30-day follow-up period.[29] The starting dose of tolvaptan is 15 mg on the first day and the dose can be titrated to 30 and 60 mg at 24-hour intervals if the serum Na remains <135 mmol/L or the increase in serum Na is <5 mmol/L in the previous 24 hours.

Treatment of Hypovolemic Hyponatremia

In the treatment of hypovolemic hyponatremia, the presentation can vary between acute and chronic cases. Chronic cases often require the administration of sodium chloride, typically in the form of 0.9% NaCl, to correct the volume deficit. It is important to note that 3% normal saline is not recommended for this condition. Sodium chloride corrects hyponatremia through two mechanisms: (1) By slowly increasing serum sodium levels and (2) by addressing hypovolemia, thus reducing the stimulus for ADH release. In cases of GI losses, both potassium and bicarbonate deficits should be corrected alongside volume correction. Thiazide-induced hyponatremia, often chronic, should be corrected gradually due to the high risk of osmotic demyelination syndrome (ODS). Patients with this condition should not be rechallenged with thiazides. Mineralocorticoid deficiency-associated hyponatremia typically responds well to 0.9% NaCl, with long-term treatment possibly requiring fludrocortisone. Increasing dietary salt intake is preferred for chronic hyponatremia, while vaptans are not recommended for hypovolemic cases.

Hypervolemic Hyponatremia Treatment

Hypervolemic hyponatremia is a common occurrence in conditions such as congestive heart failure (CHF) and cirrhosis. When managing edematous patients, it is important to note that salt administration or 3% NaCl is typically not recommended for chronic hyponatremia except in cases of acute symptomatic hyponatremia. Water restriction is essential for treatment, with cirrhotic patients sometimes requiring severe limitations (<750 mL/d), albeit challenging to implement. Loop diuretics play a pivotal role in addressing hypervolemic hyponatremia, while additional therapies for CHF may involve neurohormonal blockade, angiotensin-converting enzyme (ACE) inhibitors, and β-adrenergic antagonists. Terlipressin, a V1a receptor agonist, is utilized in the treatment of hepatorenal syndrome.

Vaptans are a potential treatment option for managing fluid overload and/or hyponatremia in patients with CHF when water restriction and diuretics have been ineffective. Correcting hyponatremia in CHF is essential for normalizing serum sodium levels and alleviating symptoms, ultimately optimizing diuretic therapy.[29,30] Research suggests that hyponatremia in CHF may be linked to higher mortality rates and increased re-hospitalization rates in patients with acute heart failure. On the other hand, tolvaptan has been associated with hepatotoxicity, leading the United States Food and Drug Administration (USFDA) to restrict its use to hyponatremic patients with end-stage liver disease awaiting imminent liver transplantation. While earlier studies showed improved serum sodium levels with vaptans in cirrhotic patients, there was no significant difference in outcomes such as mortality, variceal bleeding, hepatic encephalopathy, or renal failure compared to control groups.

CONCLUSION

Hyponatremia stands as a prevalent electrolyte disorder in hospital settings, linked to significant short- and long-term health implications. While the precise causal relationship awaits further exploration in upcoming trials, SIADH secretion emerges as a common underlying factor necessitating meticulous diagnostic evaluation. Notably, nearly half of SIADH cases do not respond to initial frontline treatments like FR. In the absence of robust evidence guiding secondary interventions for hypotonic hyponatremia, recent insights highlight tolvaptan and urea as promising options post-FR failure. Vigilant monitoring and proactive measures to prevent sodium overcorrection are paramount considerations when utilizing these therapies, emphasizing the importance of tailored patient care for optimal outcomes.

HYPERNATREMIA

INTRODUCTION

As discussed, sodium balance is maintained in tight a narrow range by maintaining water balance. Hypernatremia is defined as serum plasma concentration

>145 mEq/L Hypernatremia mainly occurs due to water loss in excess of sodium or sodium intake in excess of water. It results in increased sodium levels and serum osmolality which stimulates osmoreceptors in the hypothalamus to release ADH from the pituitary. ADH mainly acts by two mechanisms: (1) By increasing thirst and (2) by increasing water reabsorption via the collecting duct in the kidney. Failure to increase free water intake or reabsorption precipitates hypernatremia. And causes of hypernatremia are broadly divided into the following two categories, i.e., (1) excess free water loss and (2) excess sodium gain.

ETIOLOGY OF HYPERNATREMIA

Excess Free Water Loss

One must understand that when water is lost from the body through the skin, gut, or kidney along with sodium with a concentration similar to plasma, the patient develops dehydration without a change in serum sodium levels. However, if water is lost with a lower concentration of sodium compared to serum, hypernatremia sets in.[31]

- *Renal causes:*
  - *Central diabetic insipidus* occurs due to inadequate production of ADH. It occurs in patients when the hypothalamus-pituitary axis is disrupted due to cranial surgery, head injury, lesion in the hypothalamus, and the pituitary region or brainstem herniation.[32]
  - *Nephrogenic diabetic insipidus* occurs due to tubular unresponsiveness to the action of ADH—defect in the V2 receptor.
  - *Diuretics induced:*
    - Osmotic diuretics: For example, mannitol and urea.
    - Loop diuretics—furosemide and mannitol, in the initial phase may produce hyponatremia as it drags water out of the intracellular compartment. In the later stage, mannitol gets excreted through the kidneys which drags water due to the osmotic effect. And this free water loss leads to hypernatremia.

  Loop diuretics have a tendency of free water loss and development of hypernatremia. However, thiazide diuretics cause excess sodium loss along with water which may lead to the development of hyponatremia.
  - *Miscellaneous causes:* Uncontrolled diabetes mellitus, lithium toxicity, and hypercalcemia.
- *Gastrointestinal tract water loss:* GI secretions have a low concentration of sodium compared to serum, and hence, excessive GI secretions will result in hypernatremia. Examples are:
  - Vomiting
  - Diarrhea—osmotic diarrhea
  - Prolonged nasogastric drainage
- *Insensible loss through the skin:* Similar to the GI tract, water lost through the skin has less sodium concentration. Hence, excessive water loss through the skin due to severe burns and excessive sweating in fever, heat exposure, and exercise leads to hypernatremia.

TABLE 6: Causes of hypernatremia.

Excess free water loss	
Renal loss of water	***Extrarenal loss of water***
• Central diabetes insipidus • Nephrogenic diabetes insipidus • *Diuretics:* Osmotic diuresis, loop diuretics • *Miscellaneous:* Lithium toxicity, hyperglycemia, and hypercalcemia	• *Gastrointestinal tract (GI) water loss:* Vomiting, diarrhea, and prolonged nasogastric drainage • *Skin loss:* Burns, fever, heat exposure, and excessive sweating
Sodium gain	
• Hypertonic saline infusion • Excessive 0.9% saline infusion • Salt water drowning • Sodium toxicity	

Sodium Gain

Except few rare reasons like salt water drowning, hypernatremia due to sodium gain is commonly due to iatrogenic infusion of hypertonic saline or large quantities of isotonic saline. Infusion of 3% saline at a higher rate for hyponatremia correction may lead to hypernatremia. Patients who receive large quantities of 0.9% saline also develop hypernatremia. It usually occurs in patients undergoing major surgeries, especially in oncosurgical cases, critically ill patients, and patients with trauma with hemorrhagic shock.[33] Causes of hypernatremia are enumerated in **Table 6**.

CLINICAL FEATURES

Clinical features mainly depend on the duration of onset and magnitude of hypernatremia. Patients with acute hypernatremia, i.e., within 24 hours will present with complaints of thirst, generalized weakness, irritability, lethargy, and confusion. Symptoms may rapidly progress to stupor, coma, and seizures. Shrinkage of cerebral cells may cause traction of cerebral sinuses and arteries, which leads to bleeding and subarachnoid hemorrhage (SAH). The rapid increase in sodium levels may cause ODS. The severity of symptoms is less when hypernatremia is chronic and gradual. Also, symptoms occur at higher magnitude of sodium levels compared to the acute state. SAH and osmotic demyelination are usually not seen in chronic hypernatremia.

DIAGNOSTIC APPROACH

In the majority of the cases, the etiology of hypernatremia is easily identified on detailed history and clinical examination. However, few cases require further laboratory workup.

Patients with serum sodium levels >145 mEq/L are further evaluated with serum osmolality, urinary sodium and osmolality, blood sugar levels (BSLs), and renal function tests. Hypernatremic patients have raised serum osmolality >295 mOsm/L.

If the urine osmolality is <300 mOsm/L, hypernatremia is either due to decreased production of AVP, i.e., central DI or its resistance, i.e., nephrogenic DI. If AVP is administered, urine osmolality will be increased in patients with AVP deficiency but not in AVP resistance. When the urine osmolality is between 300 and 600 mOsm/L, then hypernatremia is likely due to osmotic diuresis.

Urine osmolality >600 mOsm/L indicates adequate AVP production and its action on kidneys in response to hypernatremia. Hence increased urine osmolality will be observed in extrarenal losses of water through skin and gut or due to sodium gain caused by iatrogenic infusion of 0.9% or hypertonic saline. These two conditions can be differentiated based on urinary sodium levels. Urinary sodium levels <20 mEq/L are seen in extrarenal water loss and >100 mEq/L are seen in sodium gain. The diagnostic approach to hypernatremia is summarized in **Flowchart 4**.

TREATMENT

The treatment approach to a hypernatremic patient depends upon the duration of hypernatremia and the severity of symptoms. The mainstay of treatment is to correct water deficit and stop ongoing fluid loss by various means.

Correction of free water deficit: Hypernatremic patients are dehydrated and require replacement of free water devoid of sodium. Assessment and calculation of total water deficit and deciding the rate of fluid replacement is the single most important factor in the treatment of hypernatremia. Free water deficit is calculated by the following formula:

Free water deficit in male

$$= (0.6 \times \text{weight in kg}) \times \frac{(\text{serum Na} - 140)}{140}$$

Free water deficit in female

$$= (0.5 \times \text{weight in kg}) \times \frac{(\text{serum Na} - 140)}{140}$$

Once the free water deficit is calculated, its rate of replacement is decided based on the duration and severity of hypernatremia.

Flowchart 4: Diagnostic approach to hypernatremia.

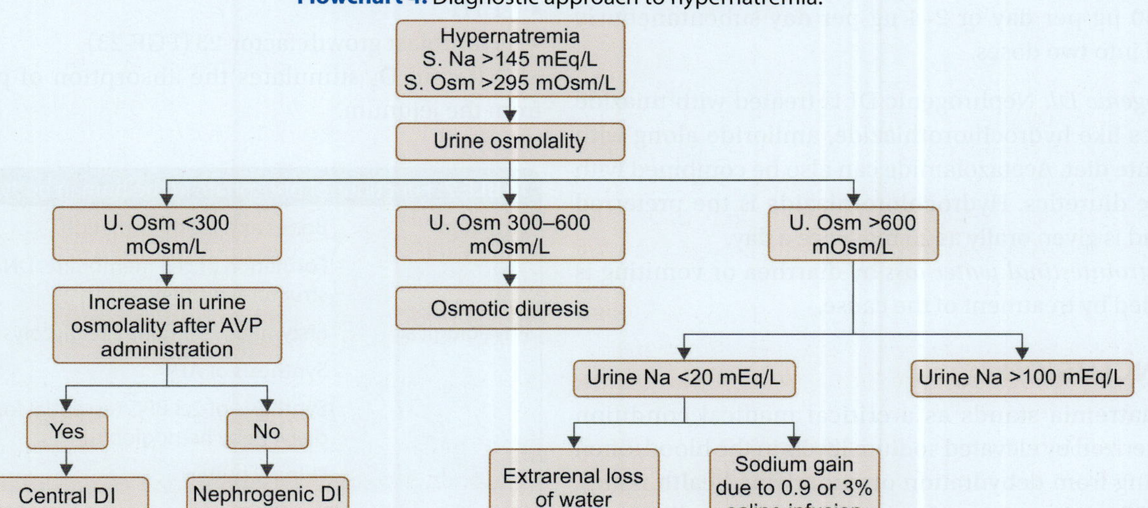

(AVP: arginine vasopressin; DI: diabetes insipidus; S. Na: serum sodium; S. Osm: serum osmolality; U. Osm: urine osmolality)

RATE OF FREE WATER REPLACEMENT

Acute hypernatremia with onset within 48 hours, total free water replacement can be done within the next 24 hours without increasing the risk of cerebral edema. Usually, 5% D is used as a fluid to replace free water intravenously. The rate of 5% D is calculated by the following formula:

Free water infusion rate in acute hypernatremia in mL/h = Total water deficit in mL/24 h

In chronic hypernatremia, due to the shrinkage of brain cells, rapid hypernatremia correction can cause cerebral edema and neurological worsening. Though no randomized controlled trials (RCTs) are available to define a safer rate of sodium correction, it is recommended to limit the sodium correction rate to 10 mEq/L for the first 24 hours. During the hypernatremia correction, the rate of correction should not be faster than 1 mEq/L/h during any hour. 5% D infusion rate to achieve this correction rate is calculated by the following formula:[34]

Free water infusion rate in chronic hypernatremia in mL/h = 3 × body weight in kg × 10

Patients should be monitored carefully for the rate of correction, urine output, and ongoing losses.

Control ongoing water loss: Control of ongoing loss needs treatment of cause, which should be initiated simultaneously with free water replacement. Ongoing water loss should be monitored closely and treated to avoid recurrence of hypernatremia.

Central DI: Patients with central DI are treated with desmopressin (DDAVP). It is given as an intranasal spray of 10–40 µg per day or 2–4 µg per day subcutaneously divided into two doses.

Nephrogenic DI: Nephrogenic DI is treated with thiazide diuretics like hydrochlorothiazide, amiloride along with low solute diet. Acetazolamide can also be combined with thiazide diuretics. Hydrochlorothiazide is the preferred drug and is given orally as 25 mg twice a day.

Gastrointestinal water loss by diarrhea or vomiting is controlled by treatment of the cause.

CONCLUSION

Hypernatremia stands as a critical medical condition characterized by elevated sodium levels in the blood, often stemming from dehydration or underlying health issues. Its manifestations range from mild symptoms like thirst and restlessness to severe neurological impairments and life-threatening complications. Timely diagnosis, coupled with appropriate treatment focusing on fluid repletion and addressing the underlying cause, is essential in managing hypernatremia effectively.

PHOSPHATE HOMEOSTASIS

INTRODUCTION

Like calcium, in the body, phosphate is also available in abundant quantity comprising 1% of body weight. It plays a major role both in cytoskeletal formation and physiological functions at the cellular level. Functions of phosphate in the body are enumerated in **Table 7**.[35,36]

REGULATION OF PHOSPHATE METABOLISM

Despite phosphate being present in large quantities in the body, only 1% is present in ECF. Around 85% of phosphate is stored in bones and teeth, and the remaining 14% is present in cellular and intracellular structures. The normal serum concentration of phosphate is 2.5–4.5 mg/dL. Serum phosphate levels are tightly regulated in this narrow range by the following mechanisms:

- Regulation of phosphate absorption through the jejunum
- Excretion and reabsorption of phosphate through the kidney
- Movement of phosphate from bone and intracellular fluid to ECF or vice versa

This regulation is achieved by actions of:

- Vitamin D_3
- PTH
- Fibroblast growth factor-23 (FGF-23)

Vitamin D_3 stimulates the absorption of phosphate from the jejunum.

TABLE 7: Functions of phosphate in the human body.

Structural	Bones and teeth formation
	Formation of cell membrane, DNA, RNA, structural proteins
Physiological	Enzymatic reactions like glycolysis.
	Synthesis of ATP
	Synthesis of 2,3 BPG (essential for O_2 delivery by hemoglobin)
	Urinary buffer

(ATP: adenotriphosphate; BPG: bisphosphoglycerate; DNA: deoxyribonucleic acid; RNA: ribonucleic acid)

Parathyroid hormone, which is released in response to hypocalcemia, indirectly acts on the jejunum to increase the absorption of phosphate. It acts by activation of vitamin D. However, PTH directly acts on kidneys (proximal convoluted tubules) causing reduced phosphate reabsorption resulting in hypophosphatemia and phosphaturia.[36]

Fibroblast growth factor-23 which is released by osteoblasts and osteocytes in response to hyperphosphatemia, acts directly on the jejunum to reduce phosphate absorption. It also acts on proximal convoluted tubules (PCTs) in kidneys to inhibit its absorption causing phosphaturia.[35]

Any acute change in phosphate regulation leads to hypo or hyperphosphatemia affecting phosphate-dependent physiological functions without any skeletal abnormalities. Discussion on the chronic effects of hypo and hyperphosphatemia on skeletal abnormalities is beyond the scope of this topic.

HYPOPHOSPHATEMIA

Hypophosphatemia is relatively less prevalent in ICU and is labeled when serum phosphate falls <2.5 mg/dL. Based on serum phosphate levels, the severity of hypophosphatemia is classified into three categories, i.e., mild, moderate, and severe **(Table 8)**.

Mild to moderate hypophosphatemia is usually asymptomatic and often remains undetected in the ICU. Severe hypophosphatemia is often associated with other electrolyte abnormalities, which may lead to severe symptoms such as arrhythmias, heart failure, or metabolic encephalopathy.

CAUSES OF HYPOPHOSPHATEMIA

Based on mechanisms, causes of hypophosphatemia are broadly divided into the following three categories.

1. Reduced intestinal absorption
2. Phosphate loss through kidneys or by renal replacement therapies
3. Intracellular phosphate shift

The causes of hypophosphatemia are enumerated in **Table 9**.

TABLE 8: Severity classification of hypophosphatemia.

Sr. no.	*Severity class*	*Serum phosphate levels*
1.	Mild	2–2.49 mg/dL
2.	Moderate	1–1.99 mg/dL
3.	Severe	<1 mg/dL

TABLE 9: Causes of hypophosphatemia.

Sr. no.	*Mechanism of hypophosphatemia*	*Causes*
1.	Reduced intestinal absorption of phosphate	Vitamin D deficiency
		Chronic diarrhea
		Chronic alcoholism (reduced intake and malabsorption)
		Drugs: Chronic antacid use, overtreatment with phosphate binders in CKD
2.	Phosphate loss through kidneys or by renal replacement therapies	Primary hyperparathyroidism
		Secondary hyperparathyroidism due to vitamin D deficiency or resistance
		Fanconi syndrome
		Genetic disorders: Hypophosphatemic rickets (X-linked, autosomal dominant, autosomal recessive)
		Postrenal transplant urinary phosphate loss
		Diabetic ketoacidosis
		• *Drugs:* Diuretics: Acetazolamide and metolazone • *Chemotherapeutic agents:* Sorafenib and imatinib
		Renal replacement therapy, especially CRRT
3.	Intracellular phosphate shift	Refeeding syndrome
		Acute respiratory alkalosis

(CKD: chronic kidney disease; CRRT: continuous renal replacement therapy)

Reduced Intestinal Absorption of Phosphate

The daily phosphate requirement (RDA) of adults is around 800–1,500 mg/dL. Almost all natural foods contain adequate phosphate; hence, the RDA is easily matched unless the patient is having chronic malnutrition, such as chronic alcoholics, or absorption of phosphate is affected. Chronic diarrhea may lead to poor phosphate absorption, causing hypophosphatemia.

Secondary hyperparathyroidism due to vitamin D deficiency or resistance impairs phosphate absorption despite adequate intake. Indirectly, it also leads to increased urinary loss of phosphate which is mediated by raised PTH levels.

Antacids containing magnesium and aluminum salts bind with phosphate making it unavailable for absorption. Prolonged use of these antacids may precipitate hypophosphatemia. Overzealous treatment of CKD patients with phosphate binders can also lead to hypophosphatemia.

Phosphate Loss Through Kidneys or by Renal Replacement Therapies

Almost 70% of the filtered phosphate is absorbed in proximal convoluted tubules through sodium-phosphate cotransporters. The function of these cotransporters is inhibited by PTH and FGF-23. Any conditions that lead to elevated PTH or FGF-23 will cause urinary phosphate loss and hypophosphatemia.

Primary hypoparathyroidism is associated with increased secretion of PTH from the parathyroid gland causing hypercalcemia. Serum phosphate levels are usually normal or in the range of mild hypophosphatemia, which is often asymptomatic. Secondary elevated PTH levels due to vitamin D deficiency or resistance often produce hypophosphatemia through two mechanisms: (1) Reduced absorption from the intestine (direct action of vitamin D3) and (2) Urinary phosphate loss due to secondary elevated PTH levels.

Fanconi syndrome is associated with generalized impairment of proximal tubular function of the kidney, which leads to hypophosphatemia. It is associated with proximal renal tubular acidosis, glycosuria, aminoaciduria, and hypouricemia.[37]

Hereditary causes of hypophosphatemic rickets are associated with X-linked or autosomal mutations causing urinary phosphate losses.

In postrenal transplant patients, urinary loss of phosphate is due to multiple effects, i.e., inadequate reabsorption of phosphate through the transplanted kidney, excessive diuretic use, and elevated FGF-23 in post-transplant patients.

Intracellular Phosphate Shift

During the process of glycolysis inorganic phosphate is utilized in large quantities for ATP production. During the process of glycolysis, phosphate is shifted from extracellular to intracellular compartment causing marginal reduction in serum phosphate levels in healthy individuals. This effect is mediated by insulin.

Refeeding Syndrome

This effect of intracellular shift of phosphate is augmented in a particular subset of patients causing a rapid and severe drop in serum phosphate levels. When chronic alcoholic patients with poor nutritional status and patients with prolonged fasting receive enteral or parenteral carbohydrate loading, a rapid intracellular shift of phosphate and potassium occurs, leading to severe life-threatening hypophosphatemia and hypokalemia.

Acute Respiratory Alkalosis

An increase in intracellular pH in acute respiratory acidosis stimulates glycolysis, leading to intracellular phosphate shift and hypophosphatemia.

CLINICAL MANIFESTATIONS

As mentioned earlier, hypophosphatemia remains asymptomatic unless the serum phosphate level falls <1 mg/dL.

Manifestations of hypophosphatemia are due to impaired tissue oxygenation due to reduced 2,3-DPG levels and reduced tissue energy supply due to impaired ATP synthesis.

In critically ill patients, hypophosphatemia should be suspected and evaluated in the following scenarios.

Persistent Hypokalemia or Hypomagnesemia Despite Aggressive Electrolyte Corrections

Hypophosphatemia impairs renal reabsorption of calcium, magnesium, and potassium, which can cause other electrolyte abnormalities such as hypocalcemia, hypokalemia, and hypomagnesemia. These electrolyte abnormalities are resistant to corrections unless phosphate is replaced.

Unexplained Heart Failure or Arrhythmias

Depletion of ATP impairs myocardial contractility resulting in heart failure. Hence, malnourished patients with unexplained heart failure should be evaluated for hypophosphatemia. Ventricular arrhythmias are also common among hypophosphatemic patients.[38]

Unexplained Metabolic Encephalopathy

Severe hypophosphatemia may present with neurological symptoms such as paresthesia, irritability, confusion, or coma. Hypophosphatemia can also precipitate generalized seizures.

Critical Illness Neuromyopathy with or without Ventilatory Weaning Failure

Severe hypophosphatemia causes proximal muscle weakness. Respiratory muscles also get involved, leading to ventilatory weaning failure.[39]

EVALUATION OF HYPOPHOSPHATEMIA

- *Serum phosphate levels:* Patients with suspected hypophosphatemia should be tested for serum phosphate levels.
- *Evaluate for associated electrolyte abnormalities:* Once hypophosphatemia is detected, serum calcium, magnesium, and potassium levels should be assessed to find out any abnormality.

Most common causes of hypophosphatemia, i.e., malnutrition or prolonged fasting are easily identified with clinical history, hence further workup is not required. Those patients with unexplained hypophosphatemia should be evaluated further to ascertain its cause.

The first step toward finding the cause of hypophosphatemia is to identify whether the kidneys are conserving phosphate through increased absorption or not. A 24-hour urine phosphate level of >100 mg or a fractional excretion of phosphate (FEPO4) >5% indicates inappropriate urinary phosphate loss. It is associated with hyperparathyroidism, Fanconi syndrome, hypophosphatemic rickets, diabetic ketoacidosis, or the use of diuretics.

Fractional excretion of phosphate is calculated by the following formula:

$$FEPO_4 = \frac{UPO_4 \times S.\ Cr \times 100}{SPO_4 \times U.\ Cr}$$

$FEPO_4$ = Fractional excretion of phosphate

S. Cr = Serum creatinine levels

U. Cr = Urine creatinine levels

UPO_4 = Urine phosphate levels

24-hour urine phosphate levels are 600–1,200 mg and FEPO4 ranges between 5 and 20% in normal individuals.

Elevated PTH levels with hypercalcemia indicate primary hyperparathyroidism. Elevated PTH with hypocalcemia is associated with secondary hyperparathyroidism likely due to vitamin D deficiency which is confirmed by measuring vitamin D3 levels.

Urinary phosphate loss is also associated with hypophosphatemic rickets where PTH, vitamin D3, and calcium levels are normal. These patients may show elevated FGF-23 levels.

Diuretics are associated with hypophosphatemia due to urinary loss of phosphate. These patients may have associated other electrolyte abnormalities.

Patients with Fanconi syndrome show elevated urine phosphate excretion along with glycosuria, aminoaciduria, low serum bicarbonate, and uric acid levels.

24-hour urine phosphate <100 mg or $FEPO_4$ <5% suggests phosphate conservation by kidneys in response to reduced serum phosphate levels. It is seen in conditions of intracellular phosphate shifts or malabsorption.

Stepwise evaluation and its interpretation are summarized in **Flowchart 5.**

TREATMENT

Most of the patients with mild to moderate hypophosphatemia are asymptomatic and do not require phosphate supplements. Once the cause is reversed, phosphate levels are rapidly restored to normal range. Such as hypophosphatemia in diabetic ketoacidosis is rapidly reversed without phosphate supplements once oral intake is reestablished.

Those patients who are symptomatic or have severe phosphate deficiency should be supplemented with either oral or IV phosphate. Oral phosphate therapy is preferred unless the patient is having severe life-threatening complications such as arrhythmias, heart failure, metabolic encephalopathy, and seizures.

Oral Phosphate Therapy

Asymptomatic hypophosphatemic patients with serum phosphate levels >1.5 mg/dL and good oral intake should be treated with oral phosphate supplements. 30–90 mmol of oral phosphate (1–1.5 mmol/kg) should be given daily in

Flowchart 5: Evaluation of hypophosphatemia.

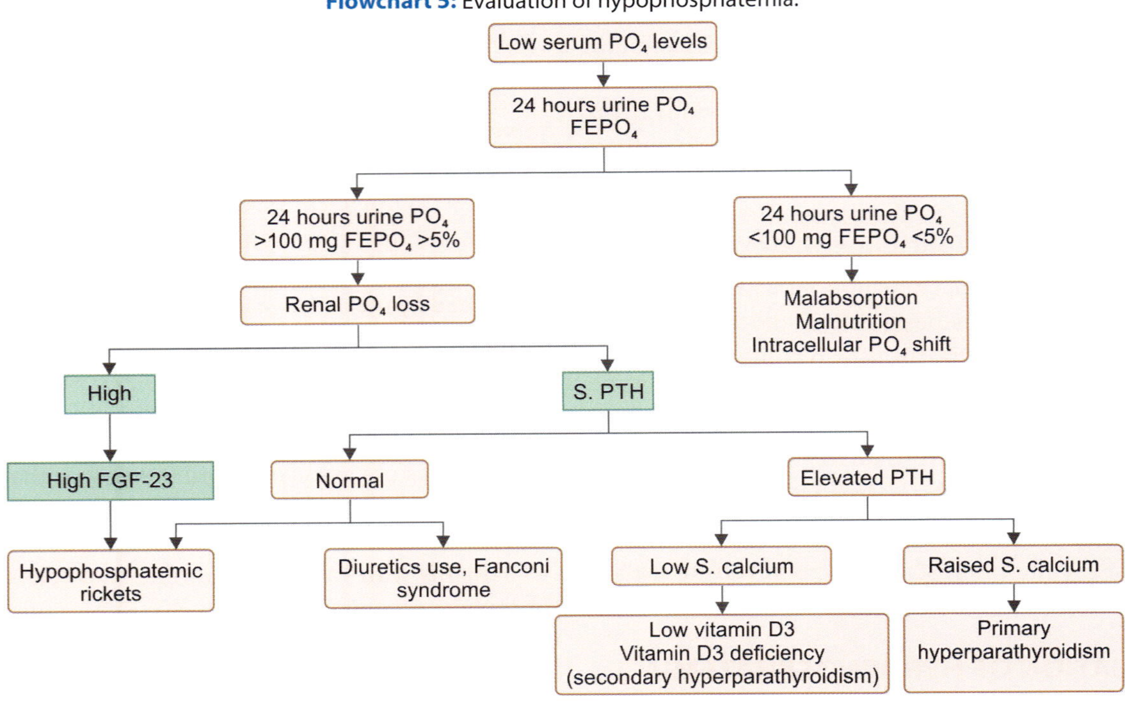

(FGF-23: fibroblast growth factor-23; $FEPO_4$: fractional excretion of phosphate; PTH: parathyroid hormone)

2–3 divided doses. Duration of therapy should be decided based on daily phosphate monitoring.

Intravenous Phosphate Therapy

Intravenous phosphate therapy is recommended for those having symptoms or phosphate levels <1.5 mg/dL. The IV phosphate preparations are available in two forms, i.e., potassium phosphate and sodium phosphate. When hypophosphatemia has associated hypokalemia, potassium phosphate preparation is preferred over sodium phosphate. 1 mL of potassium phosphate contains 4.5 mmol of potassium and 3 mmol of phosphate. Hence, potassium phosphate should be appropriately diluted with normal saline and given in IV infusion form. The recommended dose of phosphate replacement is 0.2–04 mmol/kg over 4–6 hours slowly via infusion. Repeat dosing is decided by 6 hourly phosphate monitoring.

Remember that IV phosphate therapy has its own risk profile and hence should be given cautiously only when indicated. An IV phosphate therapy may lead to the chelation of serum calcium and cause life-threatening hypocalcemia-induced arrhythmias. Caution should be taken for speed of potassium phosphate infusion as it contains potassium at high concentration which may lead to life-threatening arrhythmias if given at a faster rate.

CONCLUSION

Phosphate plays a very crucial role in the body's structural makeup as well as physiological functions at a cellular level. It is a component of the fuel of the body, i.e., ATP. Though the incidence of hypophosphatemia is less as it is available in all natural foods, critically ill patients may develop severe life-threatening hypophosphatemia due to various reasons. Early detection and replacement of phosphate improves overall clinical outcomes.

HYPERPHOSPHATEMIA

INTRODUCTION

Serum phosphate levels >4.5 mg/dL are labeled as hyperphosphatemia. Hyperphosphatemia is uncommon in critical care settings as serum phosphate levels are well regulated by vitamin D, PTH, and FGF-23 levels through their action on gut, kidneys, and bone. Though the average daily consumption of phosphate is 800–1,500 mg/day, kidneys are capable of excreting excess phosphate even if the daily intake is as high as 4,000 mg/day without causing hyperphosphatemia. Despite this, hyperphosphatemia is caused due to several conditions, which may precipitate severe hypocalcemia and life-threatening arrhythmias.

CAUSES OF HYPERPHOSPHATEMIA

Hyperphosphatemia ensues when daily intake exceeds beyond the filtration ability of the kidneys due to reduced kidney functions or excessive dietary intake >4,000 mg/day or a combination of both. Acute release of intracellular phosphate also leads to hyperphosphatemia. Hence, the causes of hyperphosphatemia are broadly divided into three categories:

1. Excessive phosphate intake: Dietary/iatrogenic
2. Increased renal excretion or reduced reabsorption: Acute or chronic renal dysfunction and hypoparathyroidism
3. Release of intracellular phosphate into ECF: Transcellular shift or cell breakdown

Excessive Phosphate Intake: Dietary/Iatrogenic

Hyperphosphatemia due to excessive intake is rare, though it can occur due to the following conditions:

- Excessive dietary intake with reduced renal functions
- Milk alkali syndrome
- Excessive phosphate-containing laxatives or enema use
- Excessive parenteral supplementation of phosphate
- Vitamin D intoxication causing excessive phosphate absorption and reduced renal excretion

Reduced Renal Excretion or Increased Reabsorption of Phosphate

Almost 80–85% of the filtered phosphate load is reabsorbed in the proximal convoluted tubule. This reabsorption is inhibited by both PTH and FGF-23. Renal handling of phosphate is altered leading to hyperphosphatemia by following mechanisms:

1. *Renal dysfunction:* Among all, chronic renal failure is the most common cause of hyperphosphatemia. Acute or chronic renal dysfunction reduces the kidney's capacity of phosphate filtration leading to its accumulation and hyperphosphatemia. In early phases of renal dysfunction, serum levels of phosphate are maintained in the normal range by increased excretion of phosphate. This is achieved by increased secretion of PTH and FGF-23, which acts on PCT to inhibit phosphate reabsorption. Once the GFR drops below 25%, this compensation fails leading to hyperphosphatemia.
2. *Hypoparathyroidism:* Reduced PTH release, i.e., primary hypoparathyroidism due to any cause (see causes of hypocalcemia) will lead to increased reabsorption of phosphate and hyperphosphatemia. PTH resistance in severe hypomagnesemia and PHP also shows a similar picture.
3. *Tumoral calcinosis:* It is an autosomal recessive condition caused due to either reduced secretion of FGF-23 or its resistance. It causes excessive phosphate absorption and hypophosphatemia, which is often associated with elevated vitamin D levels.
4. *Drug induced*
   a. *Vitamin D toxicity:* Excessive prolonged vitamin D intake leads to hyperphosphatemia directly by increasing phosphate absorption through the gut and indirectly by inhibition of PTH release resulting in increased renal phosphate reabsorption.
   b. Bisphosphonates may cause mild hyperphosphatemia.
   c. *FGF receptor inhibitors:* Cancer patients receiving immunotherapy with fibroblast growth factor receptor (FGFR) inhibitors such as pemigatinib, infigratinib, and erdafitinib are at risk of developing hyperphosphatemia. This drug acts by inhibiting FGF receptors, which causes a loss of inhibitory effect of FGF-23 on phosphate reabsorption causing hyperphosphatemia.

Release of Intracellular Phosphate into Extracellular Fluid

In case of tumor lysis syndrome and rhabdomyolysis, it causes rapid cellular breakdown and release intracellular contents into ECF. Potassium and phosphate are predominantly intracellular ions that are spilled out into ECF resulting in acute severe hypercalcemia and hyperphosphatemia.

Tumor lysis syndrome occurs due to rapid lysis of tumor cells either due to spontaneous breakdown of cancer cells or due to cellular death in response to chemotherapy. It is commonly observed with hematological malignancies such as lymphomas and leukemia. However, it can also occur in solid organ malignancies. Tumor lysis syndrome is characterized by hyperkalemia, hyperphosphatemia, hyperuricemia, and hypocalcemia. Hypocalcemia is a secondary electrolyte abnormality that occurs due chelation of calcium with excessively released phosphate in bloodstream. Electrolyte abnormalities in tumor lysis syndrome are acute and severe. If not detected and treated early, can lead to life-threatening arrhythmias and death.[40] Rhabdomyolysis is seen in patients of burns, compartment syndromes, severe hypokalemia, and hypophosphatemia-induced muscle lysis. It depicts a similar metabolic picture of tumor lysis syndrome but also associated with myoglobinuria which precipitates acute kidney injury. This acute kidney injury can further worsen hyperkalemia and hyperphosphatemia.[41]

Rarely, acute hemolysis due to various causes can mimic a similar picture.

Acute extracellular shift of phosphate can be observed in metabolic acidosis. However, the effect on serum phosphate level is mild and clinically insignificant.

CLINICAL FEATURES

Hyperphosphatemia is usually asymptomatic; however, in severe form, it presents with symptoms of hypocalcemia, i.e., tingling, numbness, muscle cramps, tetany, or even seizures, and encephalopathy (refer to symptoms of hypocalcemia) due to chelation of calcium with excessive phosphate. It is associated with a positive Trousseau's or Chvostek's sign. Conditions that lead to acute severe hyperphosphatemia such as tumor lysis syndrome and rhabdomyolysis are associated with other electrolyte abnormalities, i.e., hyperkalemia which can be fatal due to life-threatening arrhythmias.

Chronic hyperphosphatemia often seen with CKD patients is associated with cardiovascular abnormalities, which is likely due to endovascular calcium phosphate deposition. Chronic hyperphosphatemia is associated with skeletal abnormalities and soft tissue calcifications.

DIAGNOSIS

If hyperphosphatemia is suspected based on history and clinical findings, it should be further evaluated to confirm the diagnosis and to reach out the cause.

- Serum phosphate levels—to confirm hyperphosphatemia and assess for severity
- Serum ionized and total calcium levels—to assess the impact of hyperphosphatemia on serum calcium levels.
- Associated other electrolyte abnormalities: Serum potassium levels and serum magnesium
- *Assessment of renal functions:* Serum urea, creatinine, and serum uric acid levels
- Serum PTH, S. FGF-23 levels
- S. vitamin D3 levels
- ECG to look for arrhythmias
- Abdominal ultrasound to find out the cause of renal dysfunction if present.

Once hyperphosphatemia is detected, $FEPO_4$ should be calculated. $FEPO_4$ <5% suggests impaired renal excretion of phosphate due to renal dysfunction or hypoparathyroidism. $FEPO_4$ >20% suggests an intact response of kidney to hyperphosphatemia in the form of excessive phosphate excretion. It is observed in excessive phosphate ingestion and phosphate release due to cellular lysis.

TREATMENT

Treatment strategy for hyperphosphatemia depends upon several factors such as:

- Acute or chronic nature of hyperphosphatemia
- Associated hypocalcemia
- Severity of symptoms
- Cause of hyperphosphatemia
- Underlying renal functions

Patients with acute severe hyperphosphatemia due to cellular lysis, usually seen in tumor lysis syndrome and rhabdomyolysis, are associated with severe hypocalcemia and hyperkalemia. The treatment strategy includes:

- It requires IV calcium supplement based on severity (refer to treatment of hypocalcemia) and rapid correction of hyperkalemia.
- Treatment of hyperphosphatemia:
  - *Volume expansion:* If underlying kidney functions are normal, intravascular volume expansion with IV crystalloids is recommended. It improves renal phosphate clearance. However, crystalloids can dilute calcium and symptoms may worsen. Hence concomitant calcium replacement should be achieved.
  - *Diuretics:* Forced diuresis along with volume expansion in patients with normal kidney functions can normalize hyperphosphatemia within 6–12 hours. Loop diuretics are recommended.
  - *Dialysis:* Patients who develop acute kidney injury, especially in cases of rhabdomyolysis, may not respond to fluid therapy and diuretics, and hence dialysis is recommended.

TREATMENT OF CHRONIC HYPERPHOSPHATEMIA

Patients with CKD with GFR <25 mL/min are at high risk of developing hyperphosphatemia. Those who are on dialysis also remain hyperphosphatemic as only 400–500 mg of phosphate is removed with each session of dialysis. Hence, these patients require a strategic approach to control serum phosphate levels as prolonged hyperphosphatemia is associated with poor cardiovascular outcomes.

Treatment strategies include:

- *Diet:* Dietary modifications with a low phosphate diet are recommended. However, natural food is rich in phosphate; hence, dietary modifications alone barely control hyperphosphatemia.
- *Use of phosphate binders:* Based on serum phosphate levels, CKD patients are advised to take phosphate binders along with food.[42]
    - Calcium-based phosphate binders: Calcium citrate and calcium carbonate.
    - Hyperphosphatemic CKD patients with associated hypocalcemia are treated with calcium-based phosphate binders. These are associated with the risk of hypercalcemia.
    - Aluminum-based phosphate binders are barely used nowadays due to the risk of aluminum toxicity.
    - Noncalcium, nonaluminum-based phosphate binders: Sevelamer, ferric citrate, sucroferric oxyhydroxide, and lanthanum carbonate.

  Sevelamer is used as a first line of phosphate binder or in combination with calcium-based therapy.
- *Sodium-hydrogen exchanger 3 (NHE3) inhibitors:* Tenapanor NHE3 inhibitor inhibits sodium and phosphate absorption from gut. It is approved to use as a first line of therapy or in combination with phosphate binders to control hyperphosphatemia.

CONCLUSION

Hyperphosphatemia due to tumor lysis syndrome and rhabdomyolysis is rapid and severe. It is associated with several other electrolyte abnormalities and can lead to death if not treated. Hence, early detection and prompt treatment are necessary to improve outcomes and avoid life-threatening arrhythmias.

Chronic hyperphosphatemia due to CKD, if not controlled, is associated with poor cardiovascular outcomes.

DISORDERS OF POTASSIUM HOMEOSTASIS

PHYSIOLOGY OF POTASSIUM BALANCE

Potassium is the most abundant cation in the human body (50–75 mmol/kg body weight), and 98% of K^+ is found in intracellular space, while only a small fraction (2%) is found in the extracellular space. This substantial K^+ gradient between intracellular and extracellular compartments plays a crucial role in maintaining cell membrane potential, cellular excitability, nerve impulse conduction, muscle contraction (skeletal, cardiac, and smooth), GI motility, osmolality regulation, acid–base balance, hormone secretion, mineralocorticoid function, renal concentrating ability, and overall fluid and electrolyte equilibrium.

REGULATION OF POTASSIUM

Maintaining optimal K^+ levels in the blood is a critical physiological process that relies on a complex interplay of regulatory mechanisms. The normal range of blood K^+ levels is tightly controlled between 3.5 and 5.0 mmol/L. The daily intake of dietary K^+ (typically 70–100 mEq) is efficiently absorbed in the GI tract, and this influx is matched by an equivalent increase in K^+ excretion, with approximately 90% excreted in the urine and the remaining 10% in the feces. As a result, alterations in renal K^+ secretion have a significant impact on overall K^+ balance.

Potassium regulation is via two main mechanisms:

1. Regulation of potassium by balancing total body potassium concentration via renal potassium handling
2. Transferring potassium between intracellular and extracellular compartments[43]

Renal Handling of Potassium

The kidney plays a central role in the maintenance of K^+ homeostasis. Potassium is filtered by the glomerulus and then reabsorbed in the proximal tubule (65%) and the Henle's loop (20%), with the final regulation occurring in the distal tubule and collecting duct cells, where the aldosterone receptors are present. The final urine potassium concentration is determined by modifying the amount of tubular secretion. An increasing serum potassium concentration, an increased aldosterone level, a high potassium diet, and higher tubular sodium content increase potassium secretion. Angiotensin II and a low-potassium diet inhibit potassium secretion. Healthy kidneys can maximally conserve potassium when the total body potassium level is low and can excrete excess potassium when the total body potassium level is high.

Cellular Shift

When the body experiences a decline in potassium intake or an increase in renal or GI losses, there is an upregulation of the Na^+/ K^+ ATPase activity in the skeletal muscle and liver, which facilitates a net shift of potassium from the intracellular fluid to the plasma. A similar shift is induced by acidosis, hyperosmolarity, alpha-adrenergic agonists, or strenuous exercise. Furthermore, in an attempt to maintain normal potassium levels, hypokalemia results in insulin resistance which reduces K^+ uptake into muscle cells, increases the reabsorption of K^+ (via the increased activity of H^+- K^+ ATPase), and decreases aldosterone secretion leading to an increase in the reabsorption and a decrease in the tubular excretion of K^+.

HYPOKALEMIA

Hypokalemia, defined as a serum or plasma K^+ <3.5 mmol/L, is a common electrolyte disorder that may develop due to decreased K^+ intake, increased shift from the extracellular to the intracellular space, or increased K^+ losses in the urine or through the GI tract.

Hypokalemia can be classified as mild (serum K^+ 3.0–3.4 mmol/L), moderate (serum K^+ 2.5–2.9 mmol/L), or severe (serum K^+ < 2.5 mmol/L).

NONRENAL LOSS OF POTASSIUM

The loss of potassium (K^+) in sweat is usually minimal, except during extreme physical activity. Direct gastric losses of K^+ due to vomiting or nasogastric suction are also small; however, the resulting hypochloremia alkalosis leads to ongoing kaliuresis because of secondary hyperaldosteronism and bicarbonaturia, meaning a renal loss of K^+. Diarrhea is a global cause of hypokalemia due to the prevalence of infectious diarrheal diseases. Noninfectious GI conditions such as celiac disease, ileostomy, villous adenomas, inflammatory bowel disease, colonic pseudo-obstruction (Ogilvie's syndrome), VIPoma's, and chronic laxative misuse can also lead to notable hypokalemia. In many of these disorders, an increased intestinal secretion of potassium through upregulated colonic BK channels has been implicated in the development of hypokalemia.

RENAL LOSS OF POTASSIUM

The investigation of renal loss of potassium (K^+) requires considering several key factors, such as increased mineralocorticoid receptor stimulation, elevated distal nephron delivery of sodium (Na^+), fluid, and the presence of a nonreabsorbable anion or low intratubular chloride (Cl^-) concentration.

The balance between mineralocorticoid activity and distal nephron Na^+ and fluid delivery explains why acute volume changes do not typically affect renal K^+ excretion and why hyperkalemia is less common in nonoliguric, as opposed to oliguric, glomerulonephritis, and acute kidney injury.

DRUG-INDUCED RENAL LOSS OF POTASSIUM

Diuretics that act upstream of the connecting tubule and collecting duct, such as loop diuretics (e.g., furosemide) and thiazide diuretics, can increase Na^+ and fluid delivery to these sites, thereby promoting K^+ secretion. Loop diuretics reduce medullary osmolality, increasing fluid delivery from the loop of Henle to the distal tubule, and may directly inhibit K^+ reabsorption in the thick ascending limb. Thiazide diuretics inhibit Na^+- Cl^- cotransport in the DCT, leading to increased Na^+ delivery to the collecting duct, which stimulates K^+ secretion. The causes of hypokalemia are enumerated in **Table 10**.

Additionally, drugs that inhibit carbonic anhydrase, such as acetazolamide, act on the proximal tubule to increase distal delivery of Na^+ and bicarbonate, a situation also observed in proximal renal tubular acidosis and Fanconi syndrome. Nonreabsorbable anions, including certain penicillin, ketoacids, and organic anions, can directly stimulate K^+ secretion by reducing intratubular Cl^- concentration and enhancing electroneutral K^+- Cl^- cotransport, independent of Na^+ delivery.

Mineral Corticoid Excess

Aldosterone plays a pivotal role in the activation of the epithelial sodium channel (ENaC) within the principal cells of the kidney. Aldosterone increases the driving force for potassium (K^+) excretion, ultimately leading to hypokalemia.

Hyperaldosteronism, either primary or secondary, can contribute to this phenomenon. Primary hyperaldosteronism can be genetic or acquired, with familial hyperaldosteronism types I, II, and III (FH-I, FH-II, and FH-III) representing the major genetic forms. FH-I, also known as glucocorticoid-remediable hyperaldosteronism (GRA), is caused by a chimeric gene duplication that places

TABLE 10: Causes of hypokalemia.

Decreased intake:
- Starvation
- Clay ingestion

Redistribution into cells:
- Acid–base:
  - Metabolic alkalosis
- *Hormonal:*
  - Insulin
  - Increased β_2-adrenergic sympathetic activity: Postmyocardial infarction and head injury
  - β_2-Adrenergic agonists—bronchodilators and tocolytics
  - α-Adrenergic antagonists
  - Thyrotoxic periodic paralysis
  - Downstream stimulation of Na^+/ K^+ -ATPase: Theophylline and caffeine
- Anabolic state:
  - Vitamin B_{12} or folic acid administration (red blood cell production)
  - Granulocyte-macrophage colony-stimulating factor (white blood cell production)
  - Total parenteral nutrition
- Other:
  - Pseudohypokalemia
  - Hypothermia
  - Familial hypokalemia periodic paralysis
  - Barium toxicity: Systemic inhibition of "leak" K^+ channels

Increased loss:
- Nonrenal:
  - Gastrointestinal loss (diarrhea)
  - Integumentary loss (sweat)
- Renal:
  - Increased distal flow and distal Na^+ delivery: Diuretics, osmotic diuresis, and salt-wasting nephropathies
  - Increased secretion of potassium:
    - Mineralocorticoid excess: Primary hyperaldosteronism (aldosterone-producing adenomas, primary or unilateral adrenal hyperplasia, idiopathic hyperaldosteronism due to bilateral adrenal hyperplasia, and adrenal carcinoma), genetic hyperaldosteronism (familial hyperaldosteronism types I/II/III, congenital adrenal hyperplasia), secondary hyperaldosteronism (malignant hypertension, renin-secreting tumors, renal artery stenosis, hypovolemia), Cushing's syndrome, Bartter's syndrome, and Gitelman's syndrome
    - Apparent mineralocorticoid excess: Genetic deficiency of 11β-dehydrogenase-2 (syndrome of apparent mineralocorticoid excess), inhibition of 11β-dehydrogenase-2 (glycyrrhetinic/glycyrrhizinic acid and/or carbenoxolone; licorice, food products, drugs), and Liddle's syndrome (genetic activation of epithelial Na^+ channels)
    - Distal delivery of nonreabsorbed anions: Vomiting, nasogastric suction, proximal renal tubular acidosis, diabetic ketoacidosis, glue-sniffing (toluene abuse), penicillin derivatives (penicillin, nafcillin, dicloxacillin, ticarcillin, oxacillin, and carbenicillin)
  - Magnesium deficiency

the aldosterone synthase (CYP11B2) under the control of the ACTH-responsive 11β-hydroxylase (CYP11B1) promoter, rendering it sensitive to glucocorticoid regulation. In contrast, FH-III is associated with mutations in the *KCNJ5* gene, leading to altered sodium permeability and calcium influx in adrenal glomerulosa cells, thereby stimulating aldosterone secretion and cell proliferation.

Acquired causes of primary hyperaldosteronism include aldosterone-producing adenomas (APAs), primary or unilateral adrenal hyperplasia (PAH), and idiopathic hyperaldosteronism (IHA) due to bilateral adrenal hyperplasia. Somatic mutations in KCNJ5, as well as less frequently in the *ATP1A1* and *ATP2B3* genes, have been detected in APAs, further contributing to the dysregulation of aldosterone production.

Hypokalemia may also occur in conditions leading to systemic increase in glucocorticoids, such as Cushing's syndrome.

Defects in multiple renal tubular transport pathways are associated with hypokalemia, for example, loss-of-function mutations in the subunits of the acidifying H+-ATPase in alpha-intercalated cells can lead to hypokalemia distal renal tubular acidosis, as can various acquired disorders of the distal nephron.

Liddle's syndrome is caused by autosomal dominant gain-in-function mutations of ENaC subunits, resulting in increased expression of activated ENaC channels in the plasma membrane of principal cells. This typically manifests as severe hypertension with hypokalemia.

Loss of transport functions in the thick ascending limb of the loop of Henle (TALH) and DCT nephron segments can cause hereditary hypokalemic alkalosis, known as Bartter's syndrome (BS) and Gitelman's syndrome (GS), respectively. Patients with classic BS often experience polyuria, polydipsia, and hypercalciuria, along with marked activation of the renin-angiotensin-aldosterone axis. In contrast, GS is genetically homogeneous, caused primarily by loss-of-function mutations in the thiazide-sensitive Na^{+}- Cl^{-} cotransporter of the DCT, and is characterized by hypomagnesemia and hypercalciuria. While GS is generally a milder phenotype than BS, it can still be associated with chondrocalcinosis, an abnormal deposition of calcium pyrophosphate dihydrate in joint cartilage.

MAGNESIUM DEFICIENCY AND HYPOKALEMIA

Magnesium depletion has a significant impact on the regulation of muscle Na^{+}/ K^{+} -ATPase activity, leading to a reduction in potassium influx into muscle cells and leading to kaliuresis, or excessive excretion of potassium. Furthermore, magnesium deficiency can exacerbate potassium secretion by the distal nephron, an effect attributed to a diminished magnesium-dependent, intracellular blockade of potassium efflux through the secretory potassium channels in principal cells. As a result, patients with hypomagnesemia often exhibit clinical refractoriness to potassium replacement therapy unless the underlying magnesium deficiency is addressed.

CONSEQUENCES OF HYPOKALEMIA

Due to hypokalemia, the cell membrane becomes hyperpolarized, impairing the ability of the myocytes to contract.

Effect on Cardiac Muscles

Hyperpolarization of the cardiac cells can disrupt cardiac conduction, causing characteristic changes on ECG. These alterations include ST depression, decreased amplitude of T waves, increased amplitude of U waves, and prolongation of the PR and QT intervals. The subsequent manifestation of these ECG changes can lead to a variety of arrhythmias, ranging from premature atrial and ventricular beats to more severe conditions such as bradycardia, tachycardia, atrioventricular (AV) block, and even ventricular tachycardia or fibrillation.

Effect on Other Muscles

Profound potassium depletion can have consequences on skeletal muscle function. This depletion may manifest as muscle weakness and diminished reflexes. Accompanying hypophosphatemia is common, as a consequence of renal tubular phosphate wasting, which further exacerbates the situation. Additionally, impaired gut motility may lead to the development of paralytic ileus, while vascular smooth muscle contractility may be reduced, resulting in diminished pressor responses to catecholamines and angiotensin.

Renal Effects

Hypokalemia can lead to a state resembling DI, primarily due to the reduced concentration of solutes in the renal medulla. Additionally, there is a well-established association between potassium depletion and metabolic alkalosis, particularly in patients with hypovolemia. This relationship is at least partially attributed to the shift of hydrogen ions into the cells, but it may also reflect an increase in renal sodium and bicarbonate retention, further contributing to the development of metabolic alkalosis.

Approach Toward Hypokalemia

Identifying the underlying cause of hypokalemia is a critical step in clinical management. A thorough history, physical examination, and basic laboratory tests can often provide valuable clues. The history should focus on potential contributing factors, such as medication use (e.g., laxatives, diuretics, antibiotics), dietary habits (e.g., excessive licorice consumption), and symptoms that may suggest a specific etiology (e.g., periodic weakness, diarrhea). Renal K^{+} excretion can be assessed with a 24-hour urine collection; a 24-hour K^{+} excretion of <15 mmol is indicative of extrarenal loss of potassium.[44]

The transtubular potassium gradient (TTKG) has been proposed as a useful tool to assess renal potassium handling because the equation takes into consideration the effect of renal water handling on urine potassium concentration. However, no data supported its usefulness

Flowchart 6: Approach toward hypokalemia.

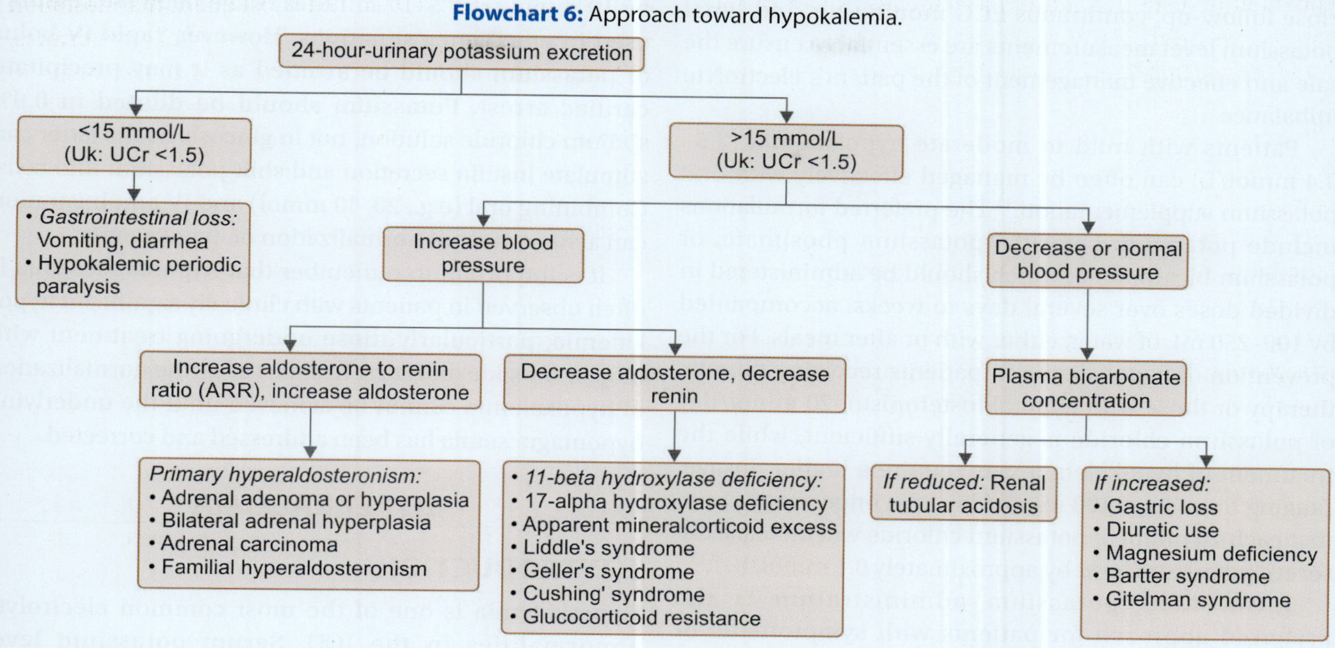

to identify urinary loss of potassium, and hence its use is not recommended by many experts:

TTKG = (Urine K × Serum Osmolality) ÷ (Serum K × Urine Osmolality)

In an otherwise healthy individual ingesting a typical Western diet, TTKG ranges from 8 to 9 and will increase to >11 with increased potassium intake. In patients with hypokalemia caused by extrarenal potassium losses, TTKG should decrease to <3. Although the TTKG is of interest, in most settings, a spot urine potassium concentration and the clinical setting will be sufficient to determine the cause of potassium disturbances. Calculation of the TTKG may prove useful in patients in whom the cause of dyskalemia remains in doubt.

Alternatively, a urinary K^+-to-creatinine ratio of >13 mmol/g creatinine (>1.5 mmol/mmol creatinine) is compatible with excessive renal K^+ excretion. Urine Cl^- is usually decreased in patients with hypokalemia from a nonabsorbable anion, such as antibiotics or HCO_3^-. The most common causes of chronic hypokalemia alkalosis are surreptitious vomiting, diuretic abuse, and GS; these can be distinguished by the pattern of urinary electrolytes. Other tests, such as urinary Ca^{2+}, thyroid function tests, and/or plasma renin activity (PRA) and aldosterone levels, may also be appropriate in specific cases.

Diagnostic approach to hypokalemia is summarized in **Flowchart 6**.

TREATMENT

The management of hypokalemia requires a comprehensive approach focused on addressing the underlying causes and restoring the patient's potassium balance. The primary objectives of the treatment are to reduce ongoing potassium losses, replenish the depleted potassium stores, evaluate and mitigate potential complications, and determine the underlying etiology to prevent future episodes. Key strategies include discontinuing the use of laxatives, selecting potassium-neutral or potassium-sparing diuretics when diuretic therapy is necessary (as in heart failure), treating diarrhea or vomiting, utilizing H2 blockers for patients with nasogastric suction, and effectively managing hyperglycemia in the presence of glycosuria.

The decision to administer oral or IV potassium should be based on the severity of the patient's hypokalemia. While the general guideline suggests that a 1 mEq/L decrease in serum potassium corresponds to a potassium deficit of approximately 200–400 mEq, this calculation may not always accurately reflect the true potassium deficit. Patients with mild to moderate hypokalemia, defined as potassium levels between 2.5 and 3.5 mEq/L, may be adequately treated with oral potassium replacement. However, for patients with potassium levels <2.5 mEq/L, representing severe hypokalemia, IV potassium administration is recommended. In such cases, close follow-up, continuous ECG monitoring, and serial potassium level measurements are essential to ensure the safe and effective management of the patient's electrolyte imbalance.

Patients with mild to moderate hypokalemia (2.5–3.4 mmol/L) can often be managed effectively with oral potassium supplementation.[45] The preferred formulations include potassium chloride, potassium phosphate, or potassium bicarbonate, which should be administered in divided doses over several days to weeks, accompanied by 100–250 mL of water, either with or after meals. For the prevention of hypokalemia in patients receiving diuretic therapy or those with hyperaldosteronism, 20 mmol/day of potassium chloride is generally sufficient, while the treatment of hypokalemia may require a higher dosage, ranging from 40 to 100 mmol/day. It is important to note that each 10 mmol of potassium chloride will increase the serum potassium level by approximately 0.1 mmol/L.[45,46]

Intravenous potassium administration is the preferred approach for patients with symptomatic or severe hypokalemia (<2.5 mmol/L) or life-threatening arrhythmias or neuromuscular dysfunction. Continuous ECG monitoring and serial potassium level measurements are essential to avoid overcorrection and the development of hyperkalemia.

For asymptomatic patients without severe heart disease, potassium can be gradually replaced at a rate of 10 mmol/h.[45] The maximum recommended IV dose is 20 mmol/h, but higher rates using central venous catheters (up to 40 mmol/h or 2 mmol/min for 10 minutes, followed by 10 mmol over 5–10 minutes) have been successfully used in emergency situations. However, rapid IV bolus of potassium should be avoided as it may precipitate cardiac arrest. Potassium should be diluted in 0.9% sodium chloride solution, not in glucose, as the latter can stimulate insulin secretion and shift potassium into cells. Combining oral (e.g., 20–40 mmol) and IV administration can achieve a rapid normalization of hypokalemia.

It is important to remember that hypomagnesemia is often observed in patients with clinically significant hypokalemia, particularly those undergoing treatment with loop or thiazide diuretics. In such cases, the normalization of hypokalemia cannot be achieved until the underlying hypomagnesemia has been addressed and corrected.

HYPERKALEMIA

INTRODUCTION

Hyperkalemia is one of the most common electrolyte abnormalities in the ICU. Serum potassium level >5.5 mEq/L is labeled as hyperkalemia. It is a part of several crystalloids, which are routinely used for maintenance or resuscitation in the ICU. Several patients in ICU either have acid–base imbalance, which can cause a transcellular shift of potassium, or they may have renal dysfunction which reduces potassium excretion. All these conditions make ICU patients prone to the development of hyperkalemia which mandates frequent monitoring. The causes of hyperkalemia are summarized in **Flowchart 7**.

Flowchart 7: Causes of hyperkalemia.

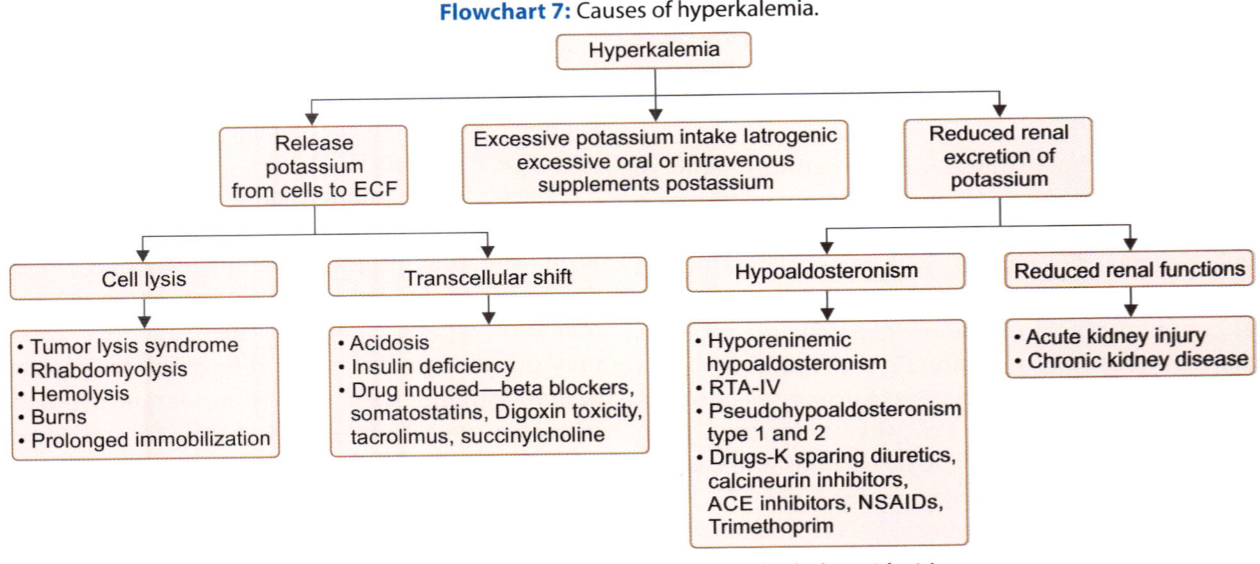

(ECF: extracellular fluid; RTA-IV: type 4 renal tubular acidosis)

CAUSE OF HYPERKALEMIA

Release of Intracellular Potassium to Extracellular Fluid

Cellular Lysis

Tissue breakdown releases intracellular contents into ECF. Potassium is predominantly an intracellular cation. Conditions such as tumor lysis syndrome, rhabdomyolysis, burns, and prolonged immobilization, where rapid tissue lysis occurs, release potassium into ECF in large quantities. It may lead to acute severe hyperkalemia, which can precipitate life-threatening arrhythmias.

Transcellular Shift

- *Acidosis:* In metabolic acidosis, excessive H^+ ions are moved from plasma to intracellular space in exchange for K^+ ions to maintain the equilibrium of pH and electroneutrality.

  This effect is less severe but remains for a prolonged duration in case of respiratory acidosis.[47]

  In diabetic ketoacidosis, movement of potassium from intra to extracellular space is due to multiple effects, i.e., insulin insufficiency, hyperosmolarity, and acidosis.
- *Drug induced:* Beta-blockers, somatostatin analogs, digitalis toxicity, tacrolimus, and nicorandil can cause mild increases in serum potassium levels by transcellular shift. Though the impact on serum potassium concentration by these drugs in healthy individuals is minor, it can produce clinically significant hyperkalemia in patients with acute or CKD.

Succinylcholine, on the other hand, can produce life-threatening hyperkalemia in susceptible individuals, i.e., in patients with burns, neuromuscular disorders, spinal cord injury, prolonged bed rest, and CKD.

Excessive Potassium Intake

Though less common, iatrogenic excessive administration of potassium through oral or IV form can lead to hyperkalemia. Regular monitoring of potassium during hypokalemia correction is recommended.

Dietary intake of food containing higher potassium, such as citrus fruits and coconut water, can also cause hyperkalemia in those with underlying renal dysfunction.

Reduced Renal Excretion of Potassium

Renal dysfunction: Impaired renal function (acute or chronic) beyond the level of maintaining adequate potassium excretion will result in hyperkalemia. Hyperkalemia is a result of resistance to aldosterone. The development of hyperkalemia is one of the absolute indications to initiate dialysis.

Hypoaldosteronism: Reduced levels of aldosterone will reduce kidneys' ability to excrete potassium leading to hyperkalemia.

It is seen in hyporeninemic hypoaldosteronism and distal renal tubular acidosis IV. A similar clinical effect is produced by certain types of drugs, i.e., nonsteroidal anti-inflammatory drugs (NSAIDs), ACE inhibitors, and calcineurin inhibitors, leading to hyperkalemia.

Despite normal aldosterone levels, conditions such as acute kidney injury, CKD, and potassium-sparing diuretics (spironolactone, eplerenone, and amiloride) cause hyperkalemia due to resistance to aldosterone.

Pseudohypoaldosteronism type 1 is an autosomal dominant condition associated with aldosterone resistance and hyperkalemia.

Pseudo-hypoaldosteronism type 2, i.e., Gordon's syndrome, is an inherited condition associated with selective impairment of potassium secretion. It is characterized by hyperkalemia, volume expansion, and hypertension with normal renal functions.

CLINICAL FEATURES OF HYPERKALEMIA

Signs and symptoms of hyperkalemia depend upon the severity and rate of potassium rise. Hyperkalemia reduces neuronal and muscular excitability by altering cellular action potential.

Skeletal Muscle Weakness

Hyperkalemia is associated with proximal muscle weakness. It is usually an ascending type which mimics Guillain–Barré syndrome. Involvement of cranial nerves and sphincters is absent. Respiratory muscles are rarely affected.[48]

CARDIAC MANIFESTATIONS

Patients may present with giddiness, syncope, palpitations due to cardiac arrhythmias, and conduction abnormalities caused by hyperkalemia. Even sudden cardiac death is possible due to ventricular arrhythmias or asystole. However, ECG changes precede any adverse cardiac event.[49]

The progression of ECG changes with hyperkalemia severity is mentioned below in sequence:

- Tall and peak T waves

- Shortened QT interval
- Progressive lengthening of PR interval and QRS duration
- Disappearance of P wave
- Sine wave pattern
- Asystole

Hyperkalemia also produces conduction abnormalities. It causes reduced excitation of the sinus node, AV node, and overall conduction system—sinus bradycardia, junctional rhythm, right bundle and left bundle blocks, and A-V blocks of various severity. Ventricular arrhythmias are a common cause of cardiac arrest.

One must note that the progression of ECG changes does not always correlate with serum potassium levels. Acute rise in potassium may induce more advanced ECG changes at lower serum levels compared to chronic hyperkalemia. Important facts about the correlation between potassium and ECG changes are mentioned below.

- ECG changes are more likely if hyperkalemia is rapid in onset. Chronic hyperkalemia produces similar changes at higher serum potassium levels.
- ECG changes appear early if associated with other electrolyte abnormalities present such as calcium and phosphate abnormalities.
- It is unlikely to have a normal ECG if serum potassium is >9 mEq/L.[50]

EVALUATION

If hyperkalemia is detected, the possibility of pseudohyperkalemia due to sampling error should be ruled out by repeat sampling with a standard technique unless ECG changes are present.

ECG should be done in all patients with hyperkalemia. It assists in the treatment of hyperkalemia.

Renal function tests, i.e., serum urea, serum creatinine, and uric acid levels, should be done to see underlying renal function. Arterial blood gas analysis is done to identify the associated acid–base abnormality.

24-hour urine potassium and TTKG can be calculated to assess urinary excretion of potassium. However, no research data validate its reliability, and hence it is not recommended by many experts.

Serum phosphorus and uric acid levels are raised in tumor lysis syndrome and rhabdomyolysis.

Rhabdomyolysis is also associated with raised creatine phosphokinase (CPK) levels and the presence of myoglobin in urine.

TREATMENT

The approach to hyperkalemia depends on the severity of symptoms, the associated ECG changes, the acuity of potassium rise, and serum potassium levels. Though not a rule, the following category of patients should be treated as a hyperkalemic emergency:

- Patients having any of the ECG changes suggestive of hyperkalemia
- Hyperkalemia-induced muscular weakness
- Serum potassium levels >7 mEq/L with or without ECG changes
- Even if serum potassium is lower than 7 mEq/L, hyperkalemic emergency should be considered if the rate of rise of serum potassium is rapid, patients having underlying renal dysfunction, ongoing cell lysis in rhabdomyolysis or tumor lysis syndrome or GI bleeding causing persistent potassium absorption through gut.[51]

Treatment of hyperkalemia includes the following modalities:

- *Membrane stabilization:* With IV calcium gluconate.
- *Intracellular shift of potassium:* Insulin with or without dextrose, inhalational or systemic beta-agonists, and sodium bicarbonate
- *Removal of potassium from body:* Potassium-binding resins, diuretics, and dialysis

All hyperkalemic emergencies should receive immediate IV calcium and insulin-dextrose in addition to other hyperkalemic measures.

Membrane Stabilization by Intravenous Calcium Supplementation

Hyperkalemia is prone to cardiac arrhythmias by causing depolarization of the cell membrane of cardiac cells. This effect is even more pronounced in the presence of hypocalcemia. This effect is minimized by IV administration of calcium in the form of calcium gluconate of calcium carbonate.[51]

1,000 mg of 10% calcium gluconate (10 mL) or 10% calcium carbonate (3.5 mL) should be administered slowly over 5–10 minutes under continuous ECG monitoring. The effect of calcium starts within minutes and lasts for approximately 30 minutes. Calcium should be repeated after 30 minutes if needed.

Intracellular Shift of Potassium

After membrane stabilization, measures to reduce serum potassium levels must be started immediately. It is either achieved by intracellular shift or by removal of potassium from the body.

Intravenous Insulin

Intravenous insulin bolus is the fastest measure to reduce serum potassium levels. 10 units of insulin bolus along with 25 g of dextrose (either 50 mL of 50% dextrose or 100 mL of 25% dextrose) should be administered as a bolus dose. Dextrose should not be supplemented with insulin if serum glucose levels are >250 mg%. 1 hourly BSL monitoring is performed at least for 4–6 hours.[52]

10 units of insulin bolus reduce serum potassium levels approximately by 1. Its effects last for at least 4–6 hours and hence therapy should be repeated 4–6 hourly if required.

Beta-2 Agonist

Beta-2 receptor stimulation enhances intracellular uptake of potassium. Fastest-acting beta-2 agonists like albuterol are preferred. Nebulization of 10 mg of albuterol with 4–5 mL of saline reduces potassium level by approximately 0.7–1 mEq/L. Peak action of albuterol starts after 15–20 minutes and lasts for 3–4 hours. Hence, it should be repeated after 4 hours. Beta-2 agonists may induce tachycardia or arrhythmias.

Sodium Bicarbonate

Routine use of sodium bicarbonate to reduce serum potassium level is not recommended. Its use is only considered in cases of hyperkalemia associated with severe metabolic acidosis.[53]

Removal of Potassium from Body

Diuretics

Loop diuretics enhance the urinary excretion of potassium. Its use is influenced by underlying kidney function and intravascular volume status.

Use of loop diuretics is recommended with normal or mild to moderately impaired kidney function. If hypovolemia is present, IV hydration with potassium-deficient crystalloids followed by the use of diuretics is suggested. Patients with euvolemia or hypervolemia are treated without IV fluids.

Hemodialysis

Patients having underlying severe renal dysfunction do not respond to diuretics therapy. Patients with hyperkalemic emergency with underlying renal dysfunction and those who do not respond to other potassium-lowering therapies should undergo dialysis.

Potassium-binding Resins

Sodium polystyrene sulfonate (SPS) is a potassium-binding GI resin used at doses of 15–30 g 2–3 times a day. It can reduce potassium levels by 1 mEq/L per day, but its onset of action is gradual. Caution and close monitoring should be done for early detection of SPS-induced bowel necrosis.

The treatment of hyperkalemia is summarized in **Table 11**.

TABLE 11: Antihyperkalemic measures.

	Measures	*Dosing*	*Mechanism of action*	*Onset/duration*	*Effect on potassium decline*
1.	Calcium	1 g of 10% calcium gluconate or calcium chloride infused IV over 2–3 minutes	Raises threshold potential and reestablishes cardiac excitability	Immediate onset, lasting 30–60 minutes	No effect on potassium decline
2.	Insulin	10 units of regular insulin IV, with D25% if no significant hyperglycemia	Increases potassium intracellular uptake	Onset at 15 minutes, lasting 6–8 hour	Approximately 1 mEq/L
3.	Albuterol	10–20 mg given by nebulized inhalation over 15 minutes or 0.5 mg in 100 mL of 5% dextrose infused over 15 minutes	Upregulates cyclic adenosine monophosphate, shifts K^+ into cell	Onset at 10–30 minutes, lasting 3–6 hours	Approximately 1–1.5 mEq/L
4.	Loop ± Thaizide diuretics	Widely variable dose depends on GFR	Renal K^+ excretion	Onset at 30–60 minutes, lasting 4–6 hours) duration prolonged in renal insufficiency)	Depends on the diuretic response, and can vary from patient to patient

Contd...

Contd...

	Measures	Dosing	Mechanism of action	Onset/duration	Effect on potassium decline
5.	Sodium polystyrene sulfonate	25–50 g mixed in 100 mL 20% sorbitol PO or 50 g in 200 mL 30% sorbitol per rectum	Exchanges resin Na^+ for K^+	Onset at 1–2 hours, lasting 4–5 hours	0.5–1.0 mEq/L
6.	Sodium bi-carbonate	2–4 mEq/min in drip (3 ampules $NaHCO_3$ in sterile water or 5% dextrose) until bicarbonate normalized	Shifts potassium into the cell	Onset at 4 hours, lasting >6 hours	0.5–0.75 mEq/L
7.	Hemodialysis	Variable, based on starting potassium	Removal from plasma	Immediate onset, lasting until dialysis completion	Variable based on dialysis duration and dialysate

(GFR: glomerular filtration rate; IV: intravenous)

CONCLUSION

Hyperkalemia is one of the common electrolyte abnormalities, which has potential to cause major adverse cardiac events. It is preventable and easily treatable if detected early.

REFERENCES

1. Maeda Y, Shiigai T. Blood ionized calcium fraction in various serum albumin levels surveyed in non-dialysis patients. Nihon Jinzo Gakkai Shi. 2005;47(7):821-7.
2. Vantour L, Goltzman D. Regulation of calcium homeostasis. In: Bilezikian JP (Ed). Primer on the Metabolic Bone Diseases and Disorders of Mineral Metabolism, 9th edition. Hoboken: Wiley-Blackwell; 2018. p. 163.
3. Fitzpatrick LA, Arnold A. Hypoparathyroidism. In: DeGroot LJ (Ed). Endocrinology, 3rd edition. Philadelphia: Saunders; 1995. p. 1123.
4. Howard SC, Jones DP, Pui CH. The tumor lysis syndrome. N Engl J Med. 2011;364(19):1844-54. Erratum in: N Engl J Med. 2018;379(11):1094.
5. Bilezikian JP. Hypoparathyroidism. J Clin Endocrinol Metab. 2020;105(6):1722-36
6. Cooper MS, Gittoes NJ. Diagnosis and management of hypocalcaemia. BMJ. 2008;336(7656):1298-302. BE. Erratum in: BMJ. 2008;336(7659).
7. Turner J, Gittoes N, Selby P. Society for endocrinology emergency endocrine guidance: emergency management of acute hypocalcaemia in adult patients. Endocr Connect. 2019;8(6):X1.
8. Bilezikian JP, Khan AA, Silverberg SJ, Fuleihan GE, Marcocci C, Minisola S, et al. International Workshop on Primary Hyperparathyroidism. Evaluation and management of primary hyperparathyroidism: summary statement and guidelines from the fifth international workshop. J Bone Miner Res. 2022;37(11):2293-314.
9. Bai M, Pearce SH, Kifor O, Trivedi S, Stauffer UG, Thakker RV, et al. In vivo and in vitro characterization of neonatal hyperparathyroidism resulting from a de novo, heterozygous mutation in the Ca^{2+}-sensing receptor gene: normal maternal calcium homeostasis as a cause of secondary hyperparathyroidism in familial benign hypocalciuric hypercalcemia. J Clin Invest. 1997;99(1):88-96.
10. Clines GA, Guise TA. Hypercalcaemia of malignancy and basic research on mechanisms responsible for osteolytic and osteoblastic metastasis to bone. Endocr Relat Cancer. 2005;12(3):549-83.
11. Pecherstorfer M, Schilling T, Blind E, Zimmer-Roth I, Baumgartner G, Ziegler R, et al. Parathyroid hormone-related protein and life expectancy in hypercalcemic cancer patients. J Clin Endocrinol Metab. 1994;78(5):1268-70.
12. Jacobs TP, Bilezikian JP. Clinical review: rare causes of hypercalcemia. J Clin Endocrinol Metab. 2005;90(11):6316-22.
13. Walker MD, Shane E. Hypercalcemia: a review. JAMA. 2022;328(16):1624-36.
14. Inzucchi SE. Understanding hypercalcemia. Its metabolic basis, signs, and symptoms. Postgrad Med. 2004;115(4):69-70, 73-6.
15. Gardner EC Jr, Hersh T. Primary hyperparathyroidism and the gastrointestinal tract. South Med J. 1981;74(2):197-9.
16. Bilezikian JP. Management of acute hypercalcemia. N Engl J Med. 1992;326(18):1196-203.
17. Hosking DJ, Cowley A, Bucknall CA. Rehydration in the treatment of severe hypercalcaemia. Q J Med. 1981;50(200):473-81.
18. Marte F, Sanchez M, Neel S, Pauly J, Valentine J. Evaluation of a pharmacy-driven calcitonin protocol for treating hypercalcemia in hospitalized patients: a multisite study. J Pharm Pract. 2022;35(6):874-8.
19. Kawada K, Minami H, Okabe K, Watanabe T, Inoue K, Sawamura M, et al. A multicenter and open label clinical

trial of zoledronic acid 4 mg in patients with hypercalcemia of malignancy. Jpn J Clin Oncol. 2005;35(1):28-33.

20. El-Hajj Fuleihan G, Clines GA, Hu MI, Marcocci C, Murad MH, Piggott T, et al. Treatment of hypercalcemia of malignancy in adults: an endocrine society clinical practice guideline. J Clin Endocrinol Metab. 2023;108(3):507-28.
21. Edelman IS, Leibman J, O'meara MP, Birkenfeld LW. Interrelations between serum sodium concentration, serum osmolarity and total exchangeable sodium, total exchangeable potassium and total body water. J Clin Invest. 1958;37(9):1236-56.
22. Robayo-Amortegui H, Quintero-Altare A, Florez-Navas C, Serna-Palacios I, Súarez-Saavedra A, Buitrago-Bernal R, et al. Fluid dynamics of life: exploring the physiology and importance of water in the critical illness. Front Med (Lausanne). 2024;11:1368502.
23. Adrogué HJ, Tucker BM, Madias NE. Diagnosis and management of hyponatremia: a review. JAMA. 2022; 328(3):280-91.
24. Sterns RH. Disorders of plasma sodium—causes, consequences, and correction. N Engl J Med. 2015;372(1):55-65.
25. Sterns RH, Nigwekar SU, Hix JK. The treatment of hyponatremia. Semin Nephrol. 2009;29(3):282-99.
26. Spasovski G, Vanholder R, Allolio B, Annane D, Ball S, Bichet D, et al. Hyponatraemia Guideline Development Group. Clinical practice guideline on diagnosis and treatment of hyponatraemia. Eur J Endocrinol. 2014;170(3):G1-47. Erratum in: Eur J Endocrinol. 2014 Jul;171(1):X1.
27. Adrogué HJ, Madias NE. Hyponatremia. N Engl J Med. 2000;342(21):1581-9.
28. Greenberg A, Verbalis JG. Vasopressin receptor antagonists. Kidney Int. 2006;69(12):2124-30.
29. Schrier RW, Gross P, Gheorghiade M, Berl T, Verbalis JG, Czerwiec FS, et al.; SALT Investigators. Tolvaptan, a selective oral vasopressin V2-receptor antagonist, for hyponatremia. N Engl J Med. 2006;355(20):2099-112.
30. Dasta JF, Chiong JR, Christian R, Lin J. Evaluation of costs associated with tolvaptan-mediated hospital length of stay reduction among US patients with the syndrome of inappropriate antidiuretic hormone secretion, based on SALT-1 and SALT-2 trials. Hosp Pract (1995). 2012;40(1):7-14.
31. Rose BD. New approach to disturbances in the plasma sodium concentration. Am J Med. 1986;81(6):1033-40.
32. Verbalis JG. Acquired forms of central diabetes insipidus: mechanisms of disease. Best Pract Res Clin Endocrinol Metab. 2020;34(5):101449.
33. Lindner G, Kneidinger N, Holzinger U, Druml W, Schwarz C. Tonicity balance in patients with hypernatremia acquired in the intensive care unit. Am J Kidney Dis. 2009;54(4):674-9.
34. Sterns RH. Disorders of plasma sodium—causes, consequences, and correction. N Engl J Med. 2015;372(1):55-65.
35. Gattineni J, Baum M. Regulation of phosphate transport by fibroblast growth factor 23 (FGF23): implications for disorders of phosphate metabolism. Pediatr Nephrol. 2010;25(4):591-601.
36. Murer H. Homer Smith Award. Cellular mechanisms in proximal tubular Pi reabsorption: some answers and more questions. J Am Soc Nephrol. 1992;2(12):1649-65.
37. Taylor HC, Elbadawy EH. Renal tubular acidosis type 2 with Fanconi's syndrome, osteomalacia, osteoporosis, and secondary hyperaldosteronism in an adult consequent to vitamin D and calcium deficiency: effect of vitamin D and calcium citrate therapy. Endocr Pract. 2006;12(5):559-67.
38. Davis SV, Olichwier KK, Chakko SC. Reversible depression of myocardial performance in hypophosphatemia. Am J Med Sci. 1988;295(3):183-7.
39. Ravid M, Robson M. Proximal myopathy caused by latrogenic phosphate depletion. JAMA. 1976;236(12):1380-1.
40. Arrambide K, Toto RD. Tumor lysis syndrome. Semin Nephrol. 1993;13(3):273-80.
41. Llach F, Felsenfeld AJ, Haussler MR. The pathophysiology of altered calcium metabolism in rhabdomyolysis-induced acute renal failure. Interactions of parathyroid hormone, 25-hydroxycholecalciferol, and 1,25-dihydroxycholecalciferol. N Engl J Med. 1981;305(3): 117-23.
42. Ketteler M, Liangos O, Biggar PH. Treating hyperphosphatemia—current and advancing drugs. Expert Opin Pharmacother. 2016;17(14):1873-9.
43. Unwin RJ, Luft FC, Shirley DG. Pathophysiology and management of hypokalaemia: a clinical perspective. Nat. Rev. Nephrol. 2011;7:75-84.
44. Palmer BF. A physiologic-based approach to the evaluation of a patient with hypokalaemia. Am. J. Kidney Dis. 2010;56(6):1184-90.
45. Cohn JN, Kowey PR, Whelton PK, Prisant LM. New guidelines for potassium replacement in clinical practice: a contemporary review by the National Council on Potassium in Clinical Practice. Arch Intern Med. 2000; 160(16):2429-436.
46. Krogager ML, Kragholm K, Thomassen JQ, Søgaard P, Lewis BS, Wassmann S, et al. Update on management of hypokalaemia and goals for the lower potassium level in patients with cardiovascular disease: a review in collaboration with the European Society of Cardiology Working Group on Cardiovascular Pharmacotherapy. Eur Heart J Cardiovasc Pharmacother. 2021;7(6): 557-67.
47. Adrogué HJ, Madias NE. Changes in plasma potassium concentration during acute acid-base disturbances. Am J Med. 1981;71(3):456-67.
48. Finch CA, Sawyer CG, Flynn JM. Clinical syndrome of potassium intoxication. Am J Med. 1946;1:337-52.
49. Durfey N, Lehnhof B, Bergeson A, Durfey SNM, Leytin V, McAteer K, et al. Can the electrocardiogram risk stratify for short-term adverse events? West J Emerg Med. 2017; 18(5):963-71.

50. Szerlip HM, Weiss J, Singer I. Profound hyperkalemia without electrocardiographic manifestations. Am J Kidney Dis. 1986;7(6):461-5.
51. Clase CM, Carrero JJ, Ellison DH, Grams ME, Hemmelgarn BR, Jardine MJ, et al.; Conference Participants. Potassium homeostasis and management of dyskalemia in kidney diseases: conclusions from a Kidney Disease: Improving Global Outcomes (KDIGO) Controversies Conference. Kidney Int. 2020;97(1):42-61.
52. Pergola PE, DeFronzo R. Clinical disorders of hyperkalemia. In: Seldin DW, Giebisch G (Eds). The Kidney: Physiology and Pathophysiology, Volume 2. Lippincott Williams & Wilkins; 2000. p. 1647.
53. Blumberg A, Weidmann P, Shaw S, Gnädinger M. Effect of various therapeutic approaches on plasma potassium and major regulating factors in terminal renal failure. Am J Med. 1988;85(4):507-12.

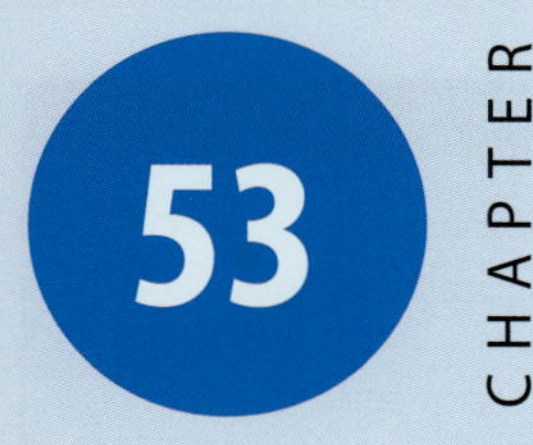

CHAPTER

Managing Children with Hematological Malignancy in ICUs

Sudivya Sharma, Shilpushp J Bhosale

INTRODUCTION

Hematologic malignancies in children account for over 40% of all new cancer diagnoses and majority of these are leukemias representing approximately 28% of cancer diagnosis. Acute lymphoblastic leukemia is the most common type of cancer, while lymphomas account for 9% (third after brain tumors).[1]

The hematological malignancies in children are also characterized by significantly higher illness severity, infection rates, and hospital mortality as compared to those with solid tumors.[2] Additionally, two thirds of pediatric cancer patients require at least one intensive care admission throughout their disease course.

However, amid vast improvements in cancer treatment, the 5-year survival for a child with cancer has improved to around 90%.[3]

Although the mortality in pediatric cancers has improved significantly over the last decades it remains quite high. According to recent meta-analysis by Asperen et al., the pooled weighted pediatric intensive care unit (PICU) mortality was 27.8%. The estimated pooled PICU mortality was even higher i.e., 46.2% among patients with sepsis.[4]

In a tertiary cancer center in India, hospital mortality of critically ill children was 61.5%. Mechanical ventilation [odds ratio (OR), 14.64], inotropes (OR, 9.81) and the presence of coagulopathy (OR, 3.86) were independent predictors of hospital mortality.[5]

EARLY RECOGNITION AND ICU TRANSFER

Pediatric oncology patients are at risk of severe clinical deterioration even while in the hospital. PEWS stands for "Pediatric Early Warning Scores," which are recorded in hospital wards that help in clinical decision-making for timely intensive care unit (ICU) transfers. They include scoring for clinical condition pertaining to respiration, circulation, neurological status, staff concern, and family concern. Worsening PEWS should trigger flagging of these children and escalation for ICU consult or call of rapid response teams **(Table 1)**.

CAUSES OF ADMISSION TO THE ICU

The most common causes of admission to ICU are respiratory failure and septic shock. Other causes are bleeding, neurological deterioration, oncological emergencies, decompensation from treatment, mass effect, organ failure, etc. Children who have undergone hematopoietic stem cell transplant may also need intensive care for early and late complications.

Severity Scores

Various prognostic scores are in clinical use to predict the risk of death in the ICU. Certain outcome scores are used to describe the course of illness in the ICU. PRISM4 (Pediatric Risk of Mortality 4) and PIM4 (Pediatric Index of Mortality 4) are the current scores recorded at an ICU admission to ascertain the risk of mortality in children. These are population-based indices and should not be used to manage individual patients. Other severity descriptive scores that assess the multiorgan dysfunction are pSOFA, PELOD, etc., which help to see the trend of progress in each patient and are helpful in prognostication **(Table 2)**.[6]

There has been a change in our perspective over the years. Traditionally, there had been a reluctance to admit oncology children to the ICU given their poor outcomes, particularly in hematologic malignancy and patients needing invasive mechanical ventilation. However in recent years, children with cancer are proactively admitted to the ICU and outcomes have improved over the years. ICU survivors achieve long-term survival and complete remission rates comparable with those never admitted to the ICU.[7]

TABLE 1: Pediatric early warning scores.

Component	***0***	***1***	***2***	***3***	***Score***
Behavior/ neurologic	• Playing or sleeping appropriately • Alert at patients baseline	Sleepy, somnolent when not disturbed	• Irritable, difficult to console • Increase in patients' baseline seizure activity	• Lethargic, confused, and floppy • Reduced response to pain • Prolonged or frequent seizures • Pupils asymmetric or sluggish	
Cardiovascular	• Skin tone appropriate for patient • Capillary refill <2 s	• Pale • Capillary refill 3–4 s • Mild tachycardia • Intermittent ectopy or irregular heart rhythm (not new)	• Gray • Capillary refill 4–5 s • Moderate tachycardia	• Gray and mottled • Capillary refill >5 s • Severe tachycardia • New-onset bradycardia • New onset/increase in ectopy, irregular heart rhythm, or heart block	
	• Within normal • Parameters • No retractions	• Mild tachypnea • Mild increased WOB (flaring and retracting) • Up to 40% supplemental • O_2 via mask	• Moderate increased • WOB (flaring and retracting, grunting, and use of accessory muscles) • 40–60% O_2 via mask	• Severe tachypnea • Respiratory rate below normal for age • Severe increased WOB (i.e., head bobbing, paradoxical, breathing) • >60% O_2 via mask	
Respiratory		• Up to 1 LNC > patients baseline need • Mild desaturation • Intermittent apnea self-resolving	• 1–2 LNC > patients baseline need • Nebulizations every • 1–2 hours • Moderate desaturation • Apnea requiring repositioning or stimulation	• > 2 LNC > patients baseline need • Nebulizations every 30 minutes to 1 hour • Severe desaturation • Apnea requiring interventions other than repositioning or stimulation	
Staff concern	Not concerned	Concerned			
Family concern	Not concerned	Concerned or absent			
				Total score	

Vital Sign	***Age***	***Mild***	***Moderate***	***Severe***
Respiratory rate and heart rate	Infant	>10% for age	>15% for age	>25 %for age
	Toddler and older >10% for age	>10% for age	>25% for age	>50% for age
Desaturation from patient baseline O_2 saturation	All ages	5% below	10% below	15% below

Source: Adapted from St. Jude's Hospital

Febrile Neutropenia

Fever is defined as an oral temperature of 38.0 °C for at least 1 hour or a single oral temperature of 38.3 °C.

Neutropenia and profound neutropenia are defined as an absolute neutrophil count (ANCs) of $<0.5 \times 10^9$/L and $<0.1 \times 10^9$/L, respectively).[8] With mild neutropenia,

TABLE 2: Severity scoring systems.

Pediatric Risk of Mortality (PRISM)	• SBP, HR, temperature, respiratory rate, GCS, pupillary reaction, pH, CO_2, arterial pO_2, glucose, potassium, creatinine, urea, WBC, PT, PTT, platelets • Age, admission source, CPR within 24 hours, cancer (acute or chronic), low risk systems of primary dysfunction (endocrine, hematologic, musculoskeletal, and renal)	Physiologic variables are measured only in the first 4 hours of PICU care, and laboratory variables are measured in the time period from 2 hours before PICU admission through the first 4 hours
Pediatric Index of Mortality (PIM)	SBP, PaO_2/ FiO_2, pupillary reaction, mechanical ventilation, base excess, reason for admission, low/high/very high risk diagnosis	Clinical and laboratory indices, underlying illnesses or surgical conditions leading to hospital admission, within 1 hour of admission to ICU
Pediatric Sequential organ Failure Assessment (pSOFA)	PaO_2/FiO_2, platelet, bilirubin, mean arterial pressure, GCS, Creatinine, lactate	pSOFA score of 2 or more was associated with increased hospital mortality
Pediatric Logistic Organ Dysfunction (PELOD) Score	HR, MBP, lactate, PAO_2/FiO_2, $PACO_2$, mechanical ventilation, GCS, pupillary reaction, WBC count, platelets, serum creatine	Worst value in 24 hours; predicts death rate

(HR: heart rate; SBP: systolic blood pressure; FiO_2: inspired oxygen fraction; GCS: Glasgow Coma Scale; FiO_2: MBP: milk basic protein; PaO_2: partial pressure of oxygen in arterial blood; PAO_2: partial pressure of oxygen in the alveoli; $PACO_2$: alveolar partial pressure of carbon dioxide; PICU: pediatric intensive care unit; pSOFA: pediatric sequential organ failure assessment; PT: prothrombin time; PTT: partial thromboplastin time; WBC: white blood cell)

stomatitis, gingivitis, and cellulitis may develop. They are at increased risk of infection from endogenous bacterial flora that reside in the mouth, oropharynx, gastrointestinal tract, and skin. Severe infections occur when the ANC is below 500/mm^3, with perirectal abscesses, colitis, pneumonia, and sepsis being common.[9]

Upper respiratory tract was the most common site followed by ear, bloodstream, and gastrointestinal tract infections. These episodes were more common during intensified therapy phases such as remission, induction, and reinduction.[10]

Multiple FN episodes are associated with invasive infections, shock, and mortality.[11] The outcomes may be affected by the severity and duration of neutropenia.

There are certain risk factors for infection-associated mortality in FN patients such as low platelet count <20,000/mm^3, raised C-reactive protein >90 mg/L, low albumin <2.5 mg/dL, monocyte count <100/mm^3, hemoglobin level <7 g/dL, serum lactate >3 mmol/L, and serum bicarbonate <17 mmol/L.[12-14]

The most common causative organisms are gram-negative bacteria such as *Escherichia coli*, *Klebsiella pneumoniae*, nosocomial such as *Pseudomonas aeruginosa*, and *Acinetobacter baumannii*; while children exposed to prolonged antibiotics may grow MDR organisms such as *Stenotrophomonas* and *Burkholderia*. The possibility of gram-positive bacterial infections should be considered in cellulitis, line-related bacteremia, endocarditis, enterocolitis, etc. These include *Staphylococcus aureus*, enterococci, *Streptococcus pneumoniae*, etc.

Among fungal infections, aspergillosis and candida are most common. Risk factors for invasive fungal infections include prolonged neutropenia, prolonged steroids therapy, relapsed malignancy, and bone marrow transplant.[15]

The infection sources can be central lines, pneumonia, enterocolitis, and cellulitis and these can worsen into septic shock. The most common cause is upper respiratory tract infection. Inaba et al. studied the source of infection over various phases of treatment. Bloodstream infection was most prevalent during induction, followed by reinduction phase; the latter period had much less episodes. Pneumonia was most prevalent during the reinduction or delayed intensification phases. Gastrointestinal tract was a common source of sepsis during induction and reinduction phases, with almost similar episodes.[10]

Role of Granulocyte-colony Stimulating Factor in Febrile Neutropenia

Prolonged neutropenic sepsis not responding to antibiotics and antifungals within an expected timeframe; neutropenic patients with extensive cellulitis, necrotizing fasciitis, perianal infections or severe fungal infections; patients who have had severe delays in previous chemotherapy courses due to neutropenia are given a trial of granulocyte-colony stimulating factor (GCSF). GCSF stimulates the release of neutrophils. GCSF is generally given subcutaneously in a dose of 5–10 μg/kg/day; granulocyte-macrophage colony-stimulating factor (GM-CSF) enhances the release of both neutrophils and macrophages. GM-CSF is administered subcutaneously at 250 $\mu g/m^2$/day. These are continued until neutrophil counts have recovered to more than 1,000/mm^3 for 3 consecutive days. Bone pain, myalgia, and a flu-like syndrome are the most reported side effects.

Acute Respiratory Failure

Acute respiratory failure (ARF) in the oncologic children admitted to ICU can be broadly classified as infectious and non-infectious in origin. The latter can further be classified according to disease-related or treatment-related etiologies . The most common pathophysiology is ventilation perfusion mismatch due to pneumonia.

Respiratory support may be provided in the form of oxygen supplementation by low flow oxygen delivery devices such as face mask or nasal prongs or reservoir masks (partial rebreathing or non-rebreathing); or high-flow systems such as venturi masks and high-flow nasal cannula (HFNC). The choice of delivery system is based on the degree of hypoxia, requirement of precision of delivery, patient comfort, and cost.

As per the recent OXY-PICU trial, we target saturations above 88% or pO_2 above 60 mm Hg. [16]

The common factors that increase the risk of ARF are myeloid over lymphoid proliferation, prolonged neutropenia, allogeneic hematopoietic cell transplantation, underlying structural lung disease; and absence of appropriate prophylaxis. Neutropenic children remain at a higher risk of infections caused by *Staphylococcus* species, gram-negative bacilli, and fungi. *Aspergillus* being the most common cause of fungal pneumonia in neutropenic children, followed by *Zygomycetes* and *Fusarium*.

Using the DIRECT approach by Ezoulay et al., we can differentiate and diagnose causes of ARF such as infection, pulmonary edema, leukostasis, leukemic infiltration, pulmonary tumor lysis syndrome, diffuse alveolar hemorrhage, and chemotoxicity. The approach includes history, examination, tests, and imaging. Leukemic infiltrates due to disease per se follow the lymphatic routes along the bronchovascular bundles, interlobular septa, and pleural interstitial tissue.

Management of acute respiratory failure remain rapid identification of cause, appropriate antimicrobial and oxygen therapy. Various non-invasive oxygen strategies have been used in supporting children with acute respiratory failure such as continuous oxygen therapy, noninvasive ventilation (NIV), and HFNC, each with their advantages and disadvantages.

HFNC currently has gained widespread use in clinical practice. Various benefits of HFNC include effective humidification, mild PEEP, and very well tolerated by children.

NIV has been extensively used with different interfaces for continuous positive airway pressure (CPAP) or bilevel positive airway pressure (BIPAP) such as nasal masks, face masks, full face mask, helmets, etc., depending on patient comfort and utility. According to a recent large ABC trial, HFNC is equivalent to CPAP when compared as a step up for the liberation from respiratory support in acutely ill children.[17]

According to the FLORALI-IM study, the mortality rate did not differ between high-flow nasal oxygen (HFNO) alone and NIV alternating with HFNO in critically ill immunocompromised patients with acute respiratory failure.[18]

Pediatric acute respiratory distress syndrome (PARDS) was defined based on Berlin definition with acute onset (<7 days from known clinical insult), partial pressure of arterial oxygen (PaO_2)/FiO_2 ratio <300, PEEP of 5 cmH_2O, and absence of cardiac failure as the cause. Invasive mechanical ventilation in PARDS recommends using standard lung protective ventilatory strategy.

The lung-protective strategy in children includes low tidal volume ventilation (6–8 mL/kg) [ARDS net (Acute Respiratory Distress Syndrome Network) trial, LUNG SAFE (Large observational study to UNderstand the Global impact of Severe Acute respiratory FailurE trial) trial]; optimizing PEEP (according to ARDSnet tables, pressure volume loops, esophageal manometry), and using lowest possible driving pressures.

Use of recruitment maneuvers are currently not routinely recommended, and early use of neuromuscular blockade has not shown to improve mortality like in adults [Prevention and Early Treatment of Acute Lung Injury (PETAL) trial].

Use of prone ventilation is highly recommended as it has shown to improve ventilation homogeneity in children.

Factors associated with mortality in patients with hematological malignancy with ARF at the time of ICU admission are time between hospital and ICU admission, admission to a low volume ICU, severity scores, hypoxemia (PaO_2/FiO_2 <100). During the ICU stay, factors are development of nonrespiratory organ dysfunction, NIV failure, delayed intubation, high driving pressure (in patients with ARDS), low platelet count (in patients receiving ECMO), diagnosis of invasive fungal infection, undetermined ARF etiology, prolonged ICU length of stay, etc.

Hyperleukocytosis

Hyperleukocytosis, defined as white blood cell (WBC) count >100 × 10^9/L, is a serious presenting feature in acute leukemia children, with reported incidences of upto 20% and are found to be associated with higher morbidity and poor outcomes as compared to children without hyperleukocytosis. In hyperleukocytosis of acute leukemias, the raised cell count in circulation leads to hyperviscosity and reduced deformability. This causes sludging of leukemic blasts in capillary vessels leading to diffuse cerebral, pulmonary and renal microcirculatory failure, and therefore tissue hypoxia, infarct or hemorrhage. These children are also at a higher risk of developing tumor lysis syndrome.

The pathophysiology also involves endothelial injury followed by secretion of cytokines and their effects on various organs. Pulmonary manifestations are dyspnea, hypoxia, tachypnea, and respiratory failure. Neurological manifestations include altered mental status, seizures, focal deficits, delirium, and papilledema. Cardiovascular symptoms such as chest pain maybe present. Other features can be acute kidney injury, renal vein thrombosis, acute limb ischemia, bowel infarctions, bleeding, and coagulopathy.[19]

The management entails aggressive hydration to improve regional blood flow. The definitive treatment and prevention of leukostasis is to commence chemotherapy urgently. In situations where chemotherapy cannot be given, cell reduction therapies such as hydroxyurea are beneficial (50–100 mg/kg/day). The evidence is weak, but theoretically leukopharesis is another option to reduce cell counts. Red cell transfusion is avoided due to hyperviscosity and hemoglobin levels as low as 5 g/dL are well accepted. As this condition may be associated with bleeding, platelets should be maintained above 50,000 and administer fresh frozen plasma and cryoprecipitate, if active bleeding is present.

Interestingly, when samples of these patients are sent, they may spuriously have low paO_2 measurements, due to consumption called leukocyte larceny.

Tumor Lysis Syndrome

Tumor lysis syndrome (TLS) is an oncologic emergency that occurs when there is massive breakdown of cancer cells after initiation of chemotherapy or even spontaneously and release their intracellular contents into the bloodstream leading to life-threatening hyperuricemia, hyperkalemia, hyperphosphatemia, and hypocalcemia. These metabolic derangements increase the risk of complications such as acute kidney injury (AKI), cardiac arrhythmias, seizures, and even death. The incidence of TLS in acute myeloid leukemia (AML) is 3.4% compared to 5.2% for acute lymphoblastic leukemia (ALL). Certain malignancies that are aggressive and rapidly proliferating such as Burkitts, or ALL with high leukemic burden or highly chemosensitive are more likely to develop TLS.

The breakdown of proliferating malignant cells leads to accumulation of nucleic acid which lead to high hypoxanthine levels which further gets converted to xanthine and then uric acid. The hyperuricemia induces acute renal injury by intrarenal uric acid crystallization. The concomitant hyperphosphatemia aggravates precipitation of calcium phosphate crystals in the renal tubules causing inflammation, obstruction, and renal tubular damage ultimately manifesting as nephropathy and acute kidney injury. The Corresponding Hypocalcemia and Hyperkalemia may lead to muscle cramps, tetany, seizures, dysrhythmias, and death.

It is diagnosed using the Cairo and Bishop laboratory and clinical criteria.[20] Laboratory parameters may be repeated every 4–6 hours **(Table 3)**.

Management of TLS warrants vigilant assessment and careful monitoring to early recognize and promptly treat the life-threatening complications.

TABLE 3: Cairo and Bishop laboratory and clinical criteria.

Laboratory (2 or more)	*Clinical*
• Hyperuricemia >8 mg/dL • Hyperkalemia >6 mEq/L • Hyperphosphatemia >4.5 mg/dL • Hypocalcemia <7 mg/dL	• Serum Creatinine >1.5 times • Cardiac arrythmias or sudden death • Seizure

The treatment is directed toward facilitation of renal perfusion by hyperhydration and inhibiting uric acid formation by inhibiting xanthine oxidase enzyme or converting uric acid to soluble form by use of rasburicase. Hyperkalemia is managed medically by transporting it to intracellular compartment with glucose insulin infusion, salbutamol nebulization, and sodium bicarbonate. It can be removed by use of potassium binders but occasionally dialysis may be the treatment of choice for life-threatening conditions. Phosphate binds with calcium and deposits in the kidneys, further exacerbating renal injury and reducing the calcium levels. It is lowered by phosphate binders and removal by continuous renal replacement therapy (CRRT). Hypocalcemia corrects itself with removal of phosphate and giving calcium should be avoided as it can precipitate as calcium phosphate in kidneys and be counterproductive **(Table 4)**.

Indications for dialysis are life-threatening dyselectrolytemia and fluid overload. Hemodialysis clears potassium very fast, but CRRT is the preferred modality for hyperphosphatemia as its clearance is time dependent. Peritoneal dialysis is generally not recommended in children with TLS due to its poor uric acid clearance.

Mediastinal Mass/Superior Vena Cava Syndrome

Mediastinal masses are known to cause life-threatening airway and cardiovascular complications in children. The tumors may compresses the trachea and bronchus causing severe hypoxia while superior vena cava (SVC) obstruction and cardiac compression can lead to severe hemodynamic instability and risk of cardiac arrest. Typically, a child with anterior mediastinal mass presents with airway compromise with dyspnea, tachypnea, stridor, orthopnea, wheezing, cough, etc. This is due to the compression on the trachea. The trachea may be slit like and hence, wheezing and stridor are often present. The mass can sometimes (commonly lymphoma) cause obstruction to the superior vena cavae leading to reduced venous return from head, neck and upper limbs. This congestion above the SVC causes facial swelling, dilated neck veins, cerebral edema, presenting as confusion, lethargy, headache, and papilledema.

These cases are extremely challenging as imaging may not be present to delineate the site and extent of mechanical compression to airway and vessels. These children may not tolerate lying supine. HFNC or non-invasive CPAP

TABLE 4: Management of tumor lysis syndrome.

Fluid	*Allopurinol*	*Rasburicase*	*Sevelamer*	*Hyperkalemia*	*Hypocalcemia*
Hydration diuresis 3 L/m^2/d or 200 mL/kg/d if <10 kg	• Prevents formation of uric acid by inhibiting xanthine oxidase • 50–100 mg/m^2/dose PO tds—maximum 300 mg/m^2/d or 10 mg/kg/d • Divided every 8 h—maximum dose 800 mg/d • Can be given IV 200–400 mg/m^2/day IV in 1–3 divided doses—maximum 600 mg/d	• Recombinant urate oxidase degrades existing uric acid to allantoin • Can be excreted in urine • 0.1–0.2 mg/kg in 50 mL • Normal saline over 30 min for 5 days • C/I G6PD deficiency, prior anaphylaxis/hypersensitivity	• Non-calcium phosphate binder • 100 mg/kg/day to 130 mg/kg/day, every 8 hours	• K bind–sodium polystyrene sulfonate • (1 g/kg with 50% sorbitol) • Insulin (0.1 units/kg IV) and glucose infusion (25% dextrose 2 mL/kg) or sodium bicarbonate (1–2 mEq/kg IV push) • Calcium gluconate (100 to 200 mg/kg/dose) • Dialysis	• Treatment of asymptomatic hypocalcemia is not recommended • Symptomatic hypocalcemia causing muscular, cardiovascular, or • neurologic complications, calcium gluconate (50–100 mg/kg IV)

(G6PD: glucose-6-phosphate dehydrogenase; IV: intravenous; PO: per oral; tds: three times a day)

helps the child breath better by splinting ad assisting the airway respectively. For diagnosis, biopsy may have to be taken in upright position with cautious sedation, while preserving spontaneous respiration. Airway compromise should be anticipated, and one must be ready with video laryngoscope, reinforced smaller size tube and lastly, rigid bronchoscope. Intravenous access should be taken in the lower limbs. One should screen for any thrombosis in the neck veins and upper limbs due to stasis. They may be associated with pleural and pericardial effusions. If there are signs of raised intracranial pressure, administer 3 mL/kg of 3% hypertonic saline.

Once the sample is collected for diagnosis, be it peripheral blood for flowcytometry or tissue biopsy, we can administer steroids. In cases of lymphoma, the response to steroids is rapid and within hours of administration. This may not happen with solid tumors such as germ cell. We should monitor for tumor lysis syndrome. Differential diagnosis includes infective pathology, foreign body aspiration, vascular abnormalities of great vessels, asthma, solid mass tumors, duplication cysts, etc. Differentials of neoplasms include lymphoma, leukemia, neurogenic, germ cell tumors, thymoma, etc.

Cardiovascular Emergencies

Children presenting with shortness of breath should also be screened for cardiogenic shock. This can be due to diastolic or systolic heart failure, pericardial effusion, tamponade, arrythmias, and fluid overload. Anthracyclines are cardiotoxic and part of chemotherapy of most leukemias. They may cause myocardial necrosis. The toxicity is progressive and cumulative (doses above 300 mg/m^2). Other cardiotoxic chemotherapeutic agents include busulfan, cyclophosphamide, 5-fluorocil, cytarabine, cisplatin, etc. Radiation injury also causes myocardial necrosis. Infective causes are myocarditis, endocarditis, and indirect infective causes result in septic cardiomyopathy **(Table 5)**.

Cardiac tamponade presents with symptoms such as chest pain and dyspnea. On examination, there is tachycardia, friction rub on auscultation, and narrow pulse pressure. The classic beck triad includes pulsus paradoxus, elevated jugular venous pressure (JVP), and distant heart sounds. Compression of intrathoracic structures may cause hoarseness, hiccups, nausea, etc. Electrocardiogram (ECG) suggests low voltage, PR depression, and electrical alternans. Chest X-ray shows increased/globular cardiac silhouette. Echocardiography is the investigation of choice for diagnosis and treatment. It suggests right atrial collapse for more than one third of cardiac cycle; early diastolic collapse of right ventricle, Inferior vena caval dilatation, etc.

TABLE 5: Spectrum of cardiac dysfunction in children with hematological malignancy.

Disease spectrum	*Anthracycline cardiotoxicity*	*Septic cardiomyopathy*	*Infective myocarditis*
• Pericardial effusion • Serositis, neoplastic, thrombotic microangiopathy	Progressive, cumulative	• Global hypokinesia • Improves within 10 days, once primary sepsis resolves	Tachycardia, raised troponin, EBV, CMV, adenovirus

Neurological Manifestations

Neurological emergencies is a common cause of oncology children admitted to the ICU.[21] Various etiologies can be raised intracranial pressure secondary to brain mass lesions, impaired cerebrospinal fluid drainage, or intracranial inflammation. Presenting symptoms include headaches, vomiting, visual disturbances, altered sensorium or siesures . When a child presents with altered sensorium, assess for airway, breathing and circulation. Check for glucose and calcium. If GCS is 8 or less, airway protection by intubation will be required. Hemodynamic instability will need fluid resuscitation and vasopressors. One should rule out a postictal state, ongoing non convulsive status epilepticus, posterior reversible leukoencephalopathy, stroke or venous thrombosis, intracranial hemorrhage, central nervous system (CNS) infiltration of disease, dyselectrolytemia, and infective pathology such as meningitis and encephalitis.

Hyponatremia, hypernatremia, hypoglycemia, hypocalcemia, acidosis, uremia, and hyperammonemia are easily treatable metabolic causes of seizures.

Certain chemotherapeutic drugs also have neurological manifestations, such as methotrexate, vincristine, and ifosfamide.

Management of super refractory status epilepticus is outlined in **Box 1**.

BOX 1: Management of super refractory status epilepticus.

Management of super refractory status epilepticus:

1. Initial first-line (5–10 minutes) management with first benzodiazepine (injection midazolam 150 µg/kg), then second benzodiazepine (injection midazolam 150 µg/kg),
   - Second-line management (10–30 minutes) with injection levetiracetam (40 mg/kg over 5 minutes)/injection phenytoin (20 mg/kg over 20 minutes)
   - Third-line management (30–60 minutes) is with anesthetic medications (injection midazolam infusion, injection thiopentone (3–5 mg/kg bolus then 3–8 mg/kg/min)/ injection propofol (2 mg/kg bolus, 1–10 mg/kg/h).
     This will need securing of airway by endotracheal intubation
2. After seizure is aborted, we need not always start on midazolam infusion and can assess if the patient can be woken up.
3. If not, midazolam infusion is started at 0.1 mg/kg/h, clinical seizure while on midazolam can lead to either increasing midazolam dose (stepwise, maximum 1 mg/kg/h) or addition of another antiepileptic/going up on dose of existing antiepileptic, e.g., levetiracetam maximum 60 mg/kg/day, phenytoin maximum 5 mg/kg/day, valproate maximum 40 mg/kg/day.
   More than three antiepileptics and still having breakthrough seizures are associated with poor prognosis. Adding lacosamide, topiramate, etc., is the next step but we should also think about withdrawing the antiepileptic which does not seem to be working
4. Seizure-free period of 24 hours can guide us to taper midazolam or third line of drugs. One should taper midazolam either way after 48 hours even if breakthrough seizures are happening, because this indicates midazolam may not be working
5. Fourth-line drugs include thiopentone aiming suppression of seizure activity on electroencephalogram (EEG), ketamine infusion, ketogenic diet, therapeutic hypothermia, immune modulation, intravenous (IV) magnesium, etc.

Posterior Reversible Encephalopathy Syndrome

Posterior reversible encephalopathy syndrome (PRES) is a rare but increasingly reported neurological manifestation in the pediatric oncology population. The true incidence of PRES is difficult to determine because there are no standardized diagnostic criteria (both clinical and radiological).

The etiology is not very well understood but is commonly associated with hypertension, steroids, cytotoxic agents and renal failure. Commonly, the posterior part of the brain is swollen by edema but not limited to posterior part of the brain. The vasogenic edema occurs because of a leaky blood–brain barrier.

Patient commonly presents as headache, altered mental status, seizure, and vision changes with brain MRI white matter changes in the bilateral parieto-occipital lobes. It is supposed to be caused by sudden elevations in blood pressure or medication-induced vascular endothelial damage resulting in capillary leakage and vasogenic edema. It occurs most commonly during induction therapy where high-dose steroids, vincristine, intrathecal methotrexate, cytarabine, and asparaginase are given. The treatment comprises antihypertensive and antiepileptic medications. It usually resolves in around 48 hours with the brain MRI findings resolving over 3–6 months. Similar presentation can also occur due to SIADH (syndrome of inappropriate antidiuretic hormone secretion), CNS leukemia, primary CNS infections, metabolic (uremia, polycythemia, and anemia), toxic (methotrexate, hypervitaminosis), infectious, or vascular (hypertension and thrombosis) causes. It is quite encouraging that most PRES are reversible and have favorable outcomes.

Hemophagocytic Lymphohistiocytosis

Hemophagocytic lymphohistiocytosis (HLH) is a highly fatal condition manifested as severe systemic hyperinflammation. The HLH disorders may be primary (inherited/familial) or secondary such as in response to specific types of infections, malignancies, rheumatologic disorders or immune system-modifying treatments. It is a hyperinflammatory syndrome with significant CD8 T-cell and macrophage activation and severe hypercytokinemia. After a triggering event, such as a viral infection, CD8 T-cells are activated by antigen-presenting cells, which monoclonally expand in the blood and in the tissue. They secrete multiple cytokines including interleukin (IL)-18, IL-10, IL-6, IL-1β, and tumor necrosis factor-alpha (TNF-α), interferon-γ, etc. As the virally infected cells cannot be eliminated due to defective degranulation of CD8 T-cells and NK cells, there is persistent antigenemia and positive feedback loop for further CD8 T-cell activation.

The presentation is similar to sepsis. The characteristic features are high-grade fever, cytopenias, hepatosplenomegaly, and elevated levels of HLH biomarkers. Patients can develop transaminitis with signs

BOX 2: Diagnosis of HLH by HLH 2004 criteria.[22]

Diagnostic criteria for HLH fulfilled (5 of the 8 criteria below):

1. Fever
2. Splenomegaly
3. Cytopenias (affecting ≥2 of 3 lineages in the peripheral blood)
   - Hemoglobin <90 g/L (hemoglobin <100 g/L in infants <4 weeks)
   - Platelets <100 × 10^9/L
   - Neutrophils <1.0 × 10^9/L
4. Hypertriglyceridemia and/or hypofibrinogenemia
   - Fasting triglycerides ≥3.0 mmol/L (i.e., ≥265 mg/dL)
   - Fibrinogen ≤1.5 g/L
5. Hemophagocytosis in bone marrow or spleen or lymph nodes; no evidence of malignancy
6. Low or no NK-cell activity (according to local laboratory reference)
7. Ferritin ≥500 µg/L
8. sCD25 (i.e., soluble IL-2 receptor) ≥2,400 U/mL

fHLH gene mutations

of liver failure, coagulopathy, CNS manifestations and eventually multiorgan failure.

Diagnosis is clinical and can be guided by using the 2004 criteria or the H-score **(Box 2 and Table 6)**.[22,23]

Some distinguishing features are disseminated intravascular coagulation (DIC) with hypofibrinogenemia, hyperferritinemia (particularly >10,000 µg/L), hypertriglyceridemia (secondary to elevated TNF-α levels).

The principle of management is to control hyperinflammation, targeting activated immune cells, and treating infections. This is done by using corticosteroids, etoposide (reverse defective apoptosis, target activated T cells), rarely using combination with vinblastine/etoposide/teniposide/antithymocyte globulin.

Other modalities used are IV immunogloblins, Anakinra, and Rituximab depending on suspected etiology along with other supportive care. Use of Alemtuzumab and Ruxolutinib is still under evaluation.

Long-term approach replacing the defective immune system through a hematopoietic cell transplant (HCT) in familial HLH or refractory secondary HLH.[24]

ISSUES OF ICU SURVIVORS

Prolonged ICU stay can result in delay or modification of oncological treatment. After discharge from ICU, children need further rehabilitation due to physical issues (pulmonary complications, muscle atrophy, weakness, dental problems, and sensory impairments) and mental challenges (diminished quality of life, increased risk of posttraumatic stress disorder, and various psychological and neurocognitive impairments, including memory deficits, attention problems, concentration difficulties, and reduced mental processing speed).[25]

TABLE 6: H score[23] Pediatric cut-off >141 (sensitivity 100%, specificity 88%).

Parameter	*No. of points (criteria for scoring)*
Known underlying immunosuppression*	0 (no) or 18 (yes)
Temperature (°C)	0 (<38.4), 33 (38.4–39.4), or 49 (>39.4)
Organomegaly	0 (no), 23 (hepatomegaly or splenomegaly), or 38 (hepatomegaly and splenomegaly)
No. of cytopenias†	0 (1 lineage), 24 (2 lineages), or 34 (3 lineages)
Ferritin (µg/L)	0 (<2000), 35 (2000-6000), or 50 (>6000)
Triglyceride (mmol/L)	0 (<1.5), 44 (1.5-4), or 64 (>4)
Fibrinogen (g/L)	0 (>2.5) or 30 (≤2.5)
Aspartate aminotransferase (U/L)	0 (<30) or 19 (≥30)
Hemophagocytosis on bone marrow aspirate	0 (no) or 35 (yes)

*Human immunodeficiency virus positive or receiving long-term immunosuppressive therapy (i.e., glucocorticoids, cyclosporine, azathioprine).

†Defined as a hemoglobin level of ≤9.2 g/dL and/or a leukocyte count of ≤5,000/mm³ and/or a platelet count of ≤110,000/mm³.

CONCLUSION

One in five children with hematological malignancy require intensive care. Early recognition, early transfer, safer medications, better diagnostic modalities and treatment options have improved the survival of these children to the order of 80–90%. This is very much achievable in resource limited settings as well. This cohort is unique due to the presence of cytopenias, susceptibility to infections, long course of treatment, tumor and therapy related complications.

REFERENCES

1. Siegel RL, Miller KD, Fuchs HE, Jemal A. Cancer Statistics, 2021. CA Cancer J Clin. 2021;71(1):7-33. Erratum in: CA Cancer J Clin. 2021;71(4):359.
2. Ali AM, Sayed HA, Mohammed MM. The outcome of critically ill pediatric cancer patients admitted to the

pediatric intensive care unit in a tertiary university oncology center in a developing country: a 5-year experience. J Pediatr Hematol Oncol. 2016;38(5):355-9.
3. Inaba H, Greaves M, Mullighan CG. Acute lymphoblastic leukaemia. Lancet. 2013;381(9881):1943-55.
4. Wösten-van Asperen RM, van Gestel JPJ, van Grotel M, Tschiedel E, Dohna-Schwake C, Valla FV, et al; POKER (PICU Oncology Kids in Europe Research group) research consortium. PICU mortality of children with cancer admitted to pediatric intensive care unit a systematic review and meta-analysis. Crit Rev Oncol Hematol. 2019;142:153-63.
5. Bhosale SJ, Joshi M, Patil VP, Kothekar AT, Myatra SN, Divatia JV, et al. Epidemiology and predictors of hospital outcomes of critically ill pediatric oncology patients: a retrospective study. Indian J Crit Care Med. 2021;25(10):1183-8.
6. Jyotsna, Kumar R, Sharan S, Kishore S, Prakash J. The various scoring systems in pediatric intensive care units: a prospective observational study. Cureus. 2023;15(5):e39679.
7. Schellongowski P, Staudinger T, Kundi M, Laczika K, Locker GJ, Bojic A, et al. Prognostic factors for intensive care unit admission, intensive care outcome, and post-intensive care survival in patients with de novo acute myeloid leukemia: a single center experience. Haematologica. 2011; 96(2):231-7.
8. Freifeld AG, Bow EJ, Sepkowitz KA, Boeckh MJ, Ito JI, Mullen CA, et al; Infectious Diseases Society of America. Clinical practice guideline for the use of antimicrobial agents in neutropenic patients with cancer: 2010 update by the Infectious Diseases Society of America. Clin Infect Dis. 2011;52(4):e56-93.
9. Lehrnbecher T, Robinson P, Fisher B, Alexander S, Ammann RA, Beauchemin M, et al. Guideline for the management of fever and neutropenia in children with cancer and hematopoietic stem-cell transplantation recipients: 2017 Update. J Clin Oncol. 2017;35(18):2082-94.
10. Inaba H, Pei D, Wolf J, Howard SC, Hayden RT, Go M, et al. Infection-related complications during treatment for childhood acute lymphoblastic leukemia. Ann Oncol. 2017;28(2):386-92.
11. Bothra M, Seth R, Kapil A, Dwivedi SN, Bhatnagar S, Xess I. Evaluation of predictors of adverse outcome in febrile neutropenic episodes in pediatric oncology patients. Indian J Pediatr. 2013;80(4):297-302.
12. Das A, Trehan A, Bansal D. Risk factors for microbiologically-documented infections, mortality and prolonged hospital stay in children with febrile neutropenia. Indian Pediatr. 2018;55: 859-64.
13. Phillips RS, Sung L, Ammann RA, Riley RD, Castagnola E, Haeusler GM, et al. Predicting microbiologically defined infection in febrile neutropenic episodes in children: Global individual participant data multivariable meta-analysis. Br. J. Cancer. 2016;114:623-30.
14. Rondinelli PI, Ribeiro Kde C, de Camargo B. A proposed score for predicting severe infection complications in children with chemotherapy-induced febrile neutropenia. J Pediatr Hematol. Oncol. 2006;28:665-70.
15. Lai H-P, Chen Y-C, Chang L-Y, Lu C-Y, Lee C-Y, Lin K-H, et al. Invasive fungal infection in children with persistent febrile neutropenia. J Formos Med Assoc. 2005;104:174-9.
16. Peters MJ, Gould DW, Ray S, Thomas K, Chang I, Orzol M, et al; Oxy-PICU Investigators of the Pediatric Critical Care Society Study Group (PCCS-SG). Conservative versus liberal oxygenation targets in critically ill children (Oxy-PICU): A UK multicentre, open, parallel-group, randomised clinical trial. Lancet. 2024;403(10424):355-64. Erratum in: Lancet. 2024;403(10424):354.
17. Ramnarayan P, Richards-Belle A, Drikite L, Saull M, Orzechowska I, Darnell R, et al; FIRST-ABC Step-Up RCT Investigators and the Pediatric Critical Care Society Study Group. Effect of high-flow nasal cannula therapy vs continuous positive airway pressure therapy on liberation from respiratory support in acutely ill children admitted to pediatric critical care units: a randomized clinical trial. JAMA. 2022;328(2):162-72.
18. Coudroy R, Frat JP, Ehrmann S, Pène F, Decavèle M, Terzi N, et al; FLORALI-IM study group and the REVA Research Network. High-flow nasal oxygen alone or alternating with non-invasive ventilation in critically ill immunocompromised patients with acute respiratory failure: a randomised controlled trial. Lancet Respir Med. 2022;10(7):641-9.
19. Yuan S, Yarmis SJ, Hu KM. Hyperleukocytosis and leukostasis. In: Todd KH, Thomas Jr CR, Alagappan K, (Eds). Oncologic Emergency Medicine. Cham: Springer; 2021.
20. Cairo MS, Bishop M. Tumour lysis syndrome: New therapeutic strategies and classification. Br J Haematol. 2004;127(1):3-11.
21. Faraci M, Bagnasco F, Giardino S, Conte M, Micalizzi C, Castagnola E, et al. Intensive care unit admission in children with malignant or nonmalignant disease: incidence, outcome, and prognostic factors: a single-center experience. J Pediatr Hematol Oncol. 2014;36(7):e403-9.
22. Henter JI, Horne A, Aricó M, Egeler RM, Filipovich AH, Imashuku S, et al. HLH-2004: Diagnostic and therapeutic guidelines for hemophagocytic lymphohistiocytosis. Pediatr Blood Cancer. 2007;48(2):124-31.
23. Fardet L, Galicier L, Lambotte O, Marzac C, Aumont C, Chahwan D, et al. Development and validation of the HScore, a score for the diagnosis of reactive hemophagocytic syndrome. Arthritis Rheumatol. 2014;66(9):2613-20.
24. La Rosée P, Horne A, Hines M, von Bahr Greenwood T, Machowicz R, Berliner N, et al. Recommendations for the management of hemophagocytic lymphohistiocytosis in adults. Blood. 2019;133(23):2465-77.
25. Herridge MS, Azoulay E. Outcomes after critical illness. N Engl J Med. 2023;388(10): 913-24.

54

CHAPTER

Sepsis in Cancer

Sudipta Mukherjee, Pralay Shankar Ghosh

INTRODUCTION

Sepsis with multidrug resistant (MDR) organisms and malignancy are two most important burdens on present healthcare system and two most important leading causes of death. Incidence of cancer is increasing and also its treatment options. As a result, a large number of cancer patients are currently present in the community and seeking healthcare services due to varied medical aids. Malignancy has become a kind of comorbidity. They form a unique cohort of immunocompromised patients—immunosuppression is either due to underlying malignancy or related to its treatment. This cohort of patients are prone to develop varied kinds of infection depending on types of adaptive immune dysfunction.[1] Besides, postintensive care syndrome (PICS) after discharge can cause significant physical and psychological morbidity, even mortality. Sepsis leading to residual organ dysfunction may curtail further cancer therapy and leads to progression of the disease process. So, there can be a vicious cycle formed by these two disease processes, complicating the medical journey of cancer patient population.

CANCER AND IMMUNOMODULATION

Sepsis, by definition, is a state of dysregulated immune response of the body against invasion of microbes.[2] There have to be a suspected or proven infection, leading to triggering of different immunological cascades such as inflammatory pathway, complement activation pathway, and coagulation pathway. All these pathways have significant overlapment in terms of involved immune cells, cytokines, and chemokines. Different changes at the cellular level (apoptosis, necroptosis, and mitochondrial dysfunction) will also alter internal metabolic and endocrine milieu. These all lead to endothelial activation, microvascular pathology, and microbial dysgenesis. Both proinflammatory and anti-inflammatory pathway can work together and decide the clinical course of the host.[3] Both the pathways can continue together in the same or different compartments of the body. Hyperimmune response leads to cytokine storm, severe systemic inflammatory response syndrome (SIRS), shock, and end organ damage. On the other hand, anti-inflammatory pathway leads to poor immune response to invading micro-organisms, leading to recurrent sepsis. Septic shock is more progressive clinical stage and characterized by profound circulatory, cellular, and metabolic abnormalities with significantly higher mortality (40%, compared to sepsis, i.e., 10%). So, the key point of sepsis prognostication is new onset or worsening organ failure.

Malignant cells can hide themselves from the immune response of the host, and they create a conducive microenvironment suitable for cell multiplication and survival. Due to altered cytokine signaling in the tumor microenvironment, proinflammatory activities of the macrophages can be limited like decreased chemotaxis, phagocytosis, and dendritic cells/T cells activation; but profibroblastic activity and angiogenesis may work in favor of cancer cells. Natural killer (NK) cells and T-cell dysfunction, exhaustion, and senescence promote tumor cell proliferation. All these immune modifications can be done by cancer itself or by its therapy (chemotherapy and radiotherapy), leading to frequent infective episodes in oncology patients along with hospital and ICU admission. Besides, some cancer patients have genetic preponderance for development of sepsis. Transcriptomic studies of tumor and peritumor tissues have shown distinct sepsis signature pattern among certain ethnic population while having colorectal malignancy.[4] Cellular changes like epithelial junctional remodeling and impaired expulsion of virus have been well documented.

Different overlapping immunomodulations have been reported in sepsis and cancer. Downregulation of different innate and adaptive immune regulatory pathways plays a key role in both the disease processes. Checkpoint inhibitors are an evolving area of interest. Their role in cancer therapy is well established (PD-1 and PD-L1) along with some positive result in preclinical sepsis studies.[5] Their effect can be more prominent on different immune cell lineage. For example, sepsis has more influence on $CD4^+$ T-cell transcription, but cancer has more effect on $CD8^+$ T-cell transcription. All these can affect cytokine production (both pro- and anti-inflammatory) during the disease process. But checkpoint inhibitors have failed to show outcome benefit (e.g., survival) in sepsis even in animal models. This may be due to decrease in PD-1 responder cells and $CD8^+$ T cells (changes in receptor expression) or upregulation of some checkpoint regulators in cancer cells.

Animal Models

Interaction between cancer and sepsis biology at cellular level has been explored in animal model for better understanding. A chronic dysregulated host response due to cancer, when intervened with acute dysregulated host response by sepsis, can generate a heterogenous outcome. To some extent, it depends on the type of cancer and site of sepsis. There are evidence in favor of increased bacteremia, increased gut epithelial apoptosis, decreased intestinal proliferation, increased local infection, and worsening renal function.[6] Immunological responses of lymphocytes are very variable as per animal model. Whereas splenic CD4 T lymphocytes had shown apoptosis;[7] gut CD4 and CD8 T and B lymphocytes had shown opposite response—decrease apoptosis and increase cell proliferation. Depending on CD8 T-cell expression (activation or suppression), tumor growth has been shown to be modified accordingly.[8] Immunological response of cancer and sepsis needs to be explored more in practical aspect to draw any conclusion.

Role of tumor-induced immunomodulation on clinical course of sepsis has also been evaluated. Depletion of tumor-specific CD8 T cells in animal models shown to improve survival.[9] It has been shown in different animal models with different cancer types. Tumor-specific T cells cause activation of endogenous T cells, but during sepsis they stimulate apoptosis of the same cell lineage along with impaired interferon γ (IFN-γ) production. Role of NK cells has also been evaluated for immunomodulator. Toll-like receptors (TLRs), especially TLR-2 and 4, have antitumor signaling,[10] and NK cells can have some impact in that alone with increased production of IFN-γ and intracellular degranulation.

In vitro association between sepsis and malignancy has also been explored. Some infections can influence tumor growth to some extent. Historically, *Streptococcus pyogenes* (bacteria and its products) had been injected in inoperable cancer patients of more than 1,000 in number; this "Coley's toxin"[11] had shown tumor remission. In different animal models, intratumor injection of attenuated strain of *Clostridium novyi*[12] has caused tumor regression. Recent human trial in patients with refractory solid tumor has also shown disease regression in 40% cases[13] with occasional development of gas gangrene. Sepsis also influences the development of future cancer, and it has been evaluated in a large database of 4 lac adult population. Risk of carcinoma of colon, liver, cervix, rectum, and lung with acute and chronic myeloid leukemia and myelodysplastic syndrome has shown to be increased after sepsis. Besides, there is association with cancer risk reduction for carcinoma breast, thyroid, kidney, and prostrate with melanoma, follicular, and B cell lymphoma.[14]

Cellular targets for sepsis management may respond differently in presence of cancer. CXCR 4 (chemokine receptor) expressed by T cells and cellular apoptosis of lymphocyte and gut epithelium have shown significant impact on sepsis outcome. Blockage of CXCR4 receptor has shown to improve survival in animal model. Prevention of lymphocyte and gut epithelium apoptosis leads to improved survival in pneumonia and intra-abdominal sepsis of mono- and polymicrobial etiology.[15] But this result could not be replicated in the background of malignancy. Besides, due to different immune pathway activation, similar interventions have shown to have increased mortality in cancer animal models.[16,17]

TYPES OF CANCER AND SEPSIS OUTCOME

Sepsis is one of the biggest challenges related to cancer treatment. Cancer patients are at significantly higher risk of sepsis (as high as 10 times), with three times higher risk of death compared to general population.[18] Sepsis can contribute up to 30% of death in cancer subgroup.[19] Compared to noncancer population, mortality in cancer patients is significantly higher due to sepsis. It has been shown among all subgroup categories like age, infection site, severity of sepsis and organ failure, and sepsis recurrence.[20] Regarding the hospital admission, solid organ malignancy predominates (≈60–80%) compared to hematological malignancy, but mortality is higher in hematology group.[21] Overall mortality trend due to sepsis is decreasing in cancer patients over last two decades, probably due to early identification, aggressive initial resuscitation, optimal "ICU trial," and selective organ support.

Hematological Malignancy

Hematological patients are at high risk of sepsis even in the absence of neutropenia due to multiple reasons. Neutropenia (total leukocyte count <1,000/cm^3) can be seen up to 30% patients during intensive care unit (ICU) shift. Functional neutropenia is common when neutrophils are immature [after granulocyte colony-stimulating factor (G-CSF)] or pathological, i.e., unable to generate adequate oxygen burst to kill microbes. This commonly occurs after chemotherapy or radiation-induced bone marrow toxicity, or direct infiltration of primary malignancy to bone marrow. It can cause significant immunosuppression depending on severity and duration of neutropenia and associated monocyte dysfunction. There can also be lymphocyte abnormality, leading to both cellular and humoral immune dysfunction. B-cell pathology leads to inappropriate antibody production due to dysfunctional immunoglobulin [immunoglobulin (Ig) G, Ig M, and Ig A in combination]. T-cell abnormality can lead to cell-mediated immune dysfunction, making the person more prone to viral [herpes simplex virus (HSV), varicella zoster virus, and cytomegalovirus] and pneumocystis infection. Patients with acute leukemia have the highest risk of infection, and sepsis is one of the presenting symptoms for the disease. Mortality can be significantly high in ICU stay. Even if the patients come out of the initial crisis, 30-day and 90-day mortality remain very high[22] (33% and 49%, respectively), mostly due to recurrent sepsis and inadequate scope for treatment of primary malignancy, eventually leading to multiorgan failure. Most common types of sepsis are pneumonia and catheter-associated bloodstream infection, each contributing one-third of the total load. Resistant gram-negative bacteria (GNB) (Enterobacteriaceae, *Pseudomonas,* and *Acinetobacter*) are the main causative agents. Due to MDR and carbapenem resistance, the treatment options are very limited. Progressive organ failure (e.g., mechanical ventilation, shock, hepatic failure, and delirium) along with persistent cytopenias is important causes of poor clinical outcome, including mortality.[23,24]

Solid Organ Malignancy

Solid organ malignancies also have some overlapping risk factors for poor clinical outcome (e.g., organ failure) like hematological malignancy. Neutropenia postchemotherapy is usually less profound and of short duration because of apparently normal bone marrow responding well with G-CSF. Neutropenia due to metastatic disease or sepsis induced, has poor prognosis. Locally progressive tumor can cause significant distortion of organ anatomy, leading to high risk of sepsis and challenging source control. Poor general condition may not allow high-risk interventions. On the other hand, patients with cancer remission may behave like noncancer patients during their sepsis journey. These lead to a spectrum of heterogenous prognosis among solid organ malignancy patients. Clinically applicable prediction model using machine learning principle has been explored to identify different risk factors for sepsis-associated mortality in solid organ malignancy patients.[25] It was shown that emergent ICU admission, baseline comorbidities and disease severity, organ failure (e.g., respiratory failure, shock, and acute kidney injury) requiring organ support (e.g., mechanical ventilation, vasopressor support, and hemodialysis), and metastatic cancer are the risk factors for ICU mortality.

Effect of Chemotherapeutic Agents

Anticancer therapy can affect different aspects of body immunity. Corticosteroids and tyrosine kinase inhibitors (TKI) can hinder phagocytosis, causing increased risk for bacterial and fungal infection. After prolong usage, it can affect cell-mediated immunity (CMI) too. Cytotoxic anticancer drugs mostly damage other rapidly dividing cells outside malignant cells, like gastrointestinal mucosal cells and bone marrow cells. This can compromise gut mucosal integrity and may lead to bacterial transmigration from bowel. Similar effects are seen with antimetabolites like methotrexate and fluorouracil. Along with alkylating agents (cyclophosphamide) and anthracyclines (doxorubicin), they can cause significant neutropenia. T-cell abnormality caused by purine analogs (fludarabine) leads to higher risk for viral and pneumocystis infection. Antilymphocyte monoclonal antibody (rituximab), mycophenolate, calcineurin inhibitors (cyclosporin and tacrolimus), and alemtuzumab cause B- and/or T-type lymphocytopenia. Besides, endothelial injury caused by chemotherapeutic agents can lead to potential vasopressor refractoriness, without much clinical evidence.

Overall effect of immunosuppression on clinical outcome is not well understood. Multicentric retrospective study on noncancer patients on long-term immunosuppression did not show poor outcome in terms of ICU and 30-day mortality.[26] This may be due to similar inflammatory marker profile between these two groups, except interleukin 2 and 10. There is a lack of hemodynamic adverse effect in the immunosuppression group shown in the animal model.[27]

EPIDEMIOLOGY

Acquired immunosuppression is the main etiology of sepsis in cancer patients. Western data suggests that around 6.6% of the whole population of United States (US) are on some kind of immunosuppression.[28] Along with rheumatological disease and postorgan transplant scenario, cancer patients are one of the main contributors in this population. The incidence of cancer is increasing in our society. On the other hand, due to effective cancer screening protocol, early diagnosis, lifestyle modification, and availability of novel anticancer therapies, there is a decrease in attributable mortality related to oncology (up to 33%).[29] Because of that, currently we have an increasing population of patients at high risk of infection. We have robust western data in this scenario compared to Indian perspective.[30] Oncology patients have a significantly higher rate of sepsis, cardiorespiratory failure, and hospital admission after their emergency department (ED) visit compared to nononcology patients. Co-occurrence of cancer and sepsis is very common during hospital admission. A large US database of more than 270 lakh hospital admission patients had shown that 5.75% had both sepsis and cancer. In EPISEPSIS study,[31] conducted in 206 French ICUs, 12.8% of septic patients have underlying malignancy—hematological (5.3%) or metastatic solid organ (7.5%) cancer. But EPIC 2 study[32] involving 13,796 ICU patients had shown only 2% hematological malignancy (solid organ malignancy was 15.1%), while 51% have infection-related challenges. Similar observation was found in EPIC 3 study[33] involving 15,202 ICU patients (cancer = 16.7%, hemato-oncology = 2.8% with sepsis in 50–75% cases). It shows that there may be hindrance of shifting septic hemato-oncology patients to ICU in certain institutes/regions. But the septic complications have been showing increasing trend over last two decades involving gram-negative and gram-positive bacteria, anaerobes, and fungus.

Common infections causing hospital admission in this population are pneumonia (most common), intra-abdominal sepsis, urinary tract infection, skin and soft tissue infection, and catheter-associated infection.

DIAGNOSTIC CHALLENGES

Differentiating infection from inflammatory response/immune reconstitution can be very challenging in cancer patients. Due to immunosuppressed state (neutropenia and lymphopenia), inflammatory response of infection may not be present. Lack of local inflammatory response like calor, dolor, rubor, and tumor can make identification of source very difficult.[34] Corticosteroid can suppress febrile response of infection. On the other hand, resolution of neutropenia can give a clinical picture like immune reconstitution syndrome, leading to fever and organ failure (e.g., hypoxemia due to acute respiratory distress syndrome). Chemotherapy (cytosine, dacarbazine, and cyclophosphamide) induced febrile episodes are also not uncommon. There are other sepsis mimickers in oncology practice due to hyperimmune response of the body such as neutropenic enterocolitis, tumor lysis syndrome, cytokine release syndrome after immune check point inhibitors or CAR-T therapy, engraftment syndrome, differentiation syndrome, hemophagocytic lymphohistiocytosis, and engraftment syndrome after bone marrow transplant (BMT). Some of them need empirical antibiotics, but conservative medical management with organ support is the key treatment needed.

Routine infection markers like total leukocyte count can be really misleading—low in postchemotherapy and high in post G-CSF scenario. Serial biomarkers like procalcitonin can be helpful, but definitive cut offs of procalcitonin this cancer patients with/without neutropenia are lacking. Baseline value can be higher in oncology patients, especially with mucositis, postchemotherapy, graft-vs-host disease (GVHD), or by malignancy itself (thyroid medullary carcinoma, hepatocellular carcinoma, and lung carcinoma). Hematological malignancy has higher baseline procalcitonin value compared to solid organ malignancy.[35] C-reactive protein, due to its slow pharmacokinetics, is used less frequently in critical care. Its value depends on underlying inflammation rather than infection. So, variable results have been reported for CRP in oncology subgroup.[36] Thorough clinical assessment to identify organ failure and its course can help to understand patient's condition and guide about further therapy. Disease severity scores such as Acute Physiology and

Chronic Health Evaluation (APACHE) 4 and Sequential Organ Failure Assessment (SOFA) can be helpful to assess and predict clinical course. Combining these clinical scores with trends of biomarkers can be helpful in sepsis management, especially to understand clinical response and prognostication.[37] New biomarkers like pro-adrenomedullin and presepsin are showing promising outcome in the initial evaluation. For identifying fungal infection, fungal specific biomarkers (e.g., beta d glucan, galactomannan, and mannan) or polymerase chain reaction (PCR)-based test [e.g., *Candida* PCR, *Aspergillus* PCR, *Pneumocystis jirovecii* (PCP) PCR] can be considered to rationalize antifungal usage.

TREATMENT

Early diagnosis and appropriate treatment are the keys for good clinical outcome. The basic principles of sepsis management do not differ between oncology and nononcology patient populations. Because of advance in cancer therapies, overall survival with good quality of life has increased significantly in cancer patients over last few decades. So, acute medical management including ICU transfer and organ support (e.g., mechanical ventilation) should be offered judiciously and preferably in a time-bound manner. Oncology patients are usually sicker with less margin of safety. Overall outcome of this subgroup with sepsis and septic shock is poor compared to general population. This is mostly due to elderly population, multiple comorbidities, frailty, advanced metastatic malignancy, treatment-associated toxicity, immunosuppression, poor nutritional status, dyselectrolytemia, and MDR bacterial colonization due to repeated healthcare exposure.[20] In Indian and southeast Asian scenario, infection with resistant GNB is most common **(Table 1)**.

TABLE 1: Susceptibility pattern of bloodstream infections by gram-positive and gram-negative bacteria in tertiary care oncology center over 5 years' time period.[53]

	2020	*2019*	*2018*	*2017*	*2016*
Total blood culture done (n)	5,445	5,398	4,656	4,582	4,360
Positivity rate (%)	12.49	12.7	12.2	13.2	13.5
Third generation cephalosporin sensitivity (%)					
Escherichia coli	34.83	34	42.97	34.07	26.56
Klebsiella spp.	33.08	33.12	36.13	28.94	31.25
Meropenem sensitivity (%)					
E. coli	84.83	76	84	79.25	67.18
Klebsiella spp.	47.79	51.53	49.57	42.1	44.53
Pseudomonas	85.71	88.88	80.95	79.03	77.04
Acinetobacter	55.17	66.67	41.93	50	32.72
Colistin/polymyxin sensitivity (%)					
E. coli	100	99.33	100	100	100
Klebsiella spp.	91.17	93.86	87.39	96.05	95.31
Pseudomonas	100	100	100	100	100
Acinetobacter	96.55	90.90	96.77	90.62	87.27
Methicillin resistance (%)					
Staphylococcus aureus	20.59	0	0	32.15	27.59
Glycopeptide resistance					
Enterococcus	36.37	11.77	22.59	21.74	6.67

Early Diagnosis

High index of suspicion is one of the key factors for early diagnosis of sepsis in cancer patients. There are different scoring systems available to decide regarding the need for hospital admission in patients with neutropenic fever/neutropenic sepsis. Multinational Association for Supportive Care in Cancer (MASCC[38]) and Clinical Index of stable febrile neutropenia (CISNE[39]) models have been explored without significant clinical benefit. Combining both scoring systems may be beneficial for the emergency doctors to decide about treatment plan in neutropenic patients. In a systematic review and meta-analysis, Zheng et al.[40] have shown that CISNE may be more sensitive compared to MASCC to identify acute conditions. But, there is no definite scoring system for non-neutropenic oncology patient population. Different early warning scoring systems such as SIRS, National Early Warning Score (NEWS), Modified Early Warning Score (MEWS), or quick Sequential Organ Failure Assessment (q-SOFA) score have been explored in oncology patients with variable success. MEWS has the most robust data in oncology and has been shown to predict need for ICU admission in septic oncology patients.[41] Besides, different advanced technologies have been tried to pick up early deterioration of clinical conditions such as smartwatches, fitness trackers, and patched medical devices. There are different protocol-based approaches/decision trees,[25] machine learning,[42] artificial neural network, and artificial intelligence-based approach explored in sick oncology patients for early diagnosis; we need more experience to understand their clinical role.

Intensive Care Unit Admission

There is significant clinical dilemma regarding transfer of septic cancer patients to ICU. In one hand, early diagnosis and resuscitation of sepsis/septic shock can result in better clinical outcome; on the other hand, there will be risk of unnecessary utilization of health resources in advance cancer patients without much clinical outcome. So, decision to shift to ICU depends on factors associated with long-term prognosis such as general condition and quality of life of the patient, cancer under remission/realistic treatment plan available in future, reversible current pathology, cancer in remission/no active therapy required immediately, patient and family members understand the clinical journey, etc.; so, a clear escalation plan should be made a priori to get best possible clinical outcome. In a resource-limited setting, a prioritization model[43] can be really helpful for best possible utilization of resources, like ICU bed. It is also advisable that critically ill patients with advanced/metastatic malignancy should be reviewed regularly in terms of the need of aggressive therapy and should be discussed with family members and/or legal aids.[44] The concept of "ICU trial"[45] is evolving in practice, where full escalation of therapy will be done for first 48–72 hours of ICU admission and after that, further clinical course will be decided depending on clinical response of the patient along with detailed discussion with family members and treating oncologists.

Management

Management of septic oncology patients can be guided by standard surviving sepsis guideline[46] including initial resuscitation, appropriate microbiology sampling, broad-spectrum antibiotics, and organ support. But due to varied immunosuppression, source of infection, anticipated microbes, and empirical antimicrobials may vary in oncology patients. Atypical microbial profile, clinical sample, and the choice of empirical antimicrobials will vary from patient to patient.

Early initiation of appropriate broad-spectrum antibiotics with appropriate source control is strongly recommended. The choice of empiric antibiotics will depend on type and duration of immunosuppressive therapy/anticancer therapy, antimicrobial prophylaxis received, colonization profile with drug-resistant bacteria/fungus, organ involved in sepsis, and local and institutional antibiogram. Delay in appropriate antibiotic can increase mortality risk by manyfold.[47,48] ICU-associated MDRO infection varies among institutes and depends on infection control and antimicrobial stewardship policy. Some studies have reported no such increase in oncology ICU (e.g., CIMDREA trial[49]). Choice of empirical antibiotics is usually an antipseudomonal cephalosporin or piperacillin–tazobactam (+/– aminoglycosides) or a carbapenem (e.g., meropenem). Additional gram-positive bacterial coverage is needed in case of lobar pneumonia, septic shock, skin and soft tissue infection, central line-associated bloodstream infection, positive blood culture with gram-positive bacteria, and colonization with resistant *Staphylococcus* or *Enterococcus* strain. Similarly, empirical antifungal therapy (against candida or mold) may also be needed depending on clinical condition, level of immunosuppression, and underlying risk factors.

Antimicrobial prophylaxis is recommended in certain oncology patients with high risk. Antibiotic prophylaxis is used in oncosurgical patients targeting to prevent surgical site infection, and mostly the antibiotic is targeting skin organisms such as *Streptococcus* and *Staphylococcus*. Usually, one dose of antibiotic is enough given 30 minutes before surgery; antibiotic needs to be repeated for prolong surgery (>3 hours). For contaminated or clean contaminated surgery, probably a longer duration of antibiotics is required depending on severity of sepsis and extent of source control.

Hemato-oncology patients with neutropenia may receive antifungal prophylaxis to cover against candida and/or aspergillus, depending on the severity of immunosuppression. Patients having T lymphocyte disease (acute lymphoid leukemia or lymphoma) or receiving T lymphocyte-depleting chemotherapy, may need prophylaxis against *Pneumocystis jirovecii* (PCP) and HSV. Antibiotic prophylaxis in hemato-oncology subgroup of patients with neutropenic is debatable. There are some evidences of using ciprofloxacin or levofloxacin in mucositis to prevent *Streptococcus viridans*. But, this is not a standard practice due to risk of selection pressure to develop drug-resistant bacteria.

OUTCOME

Morbidity and mortality in patients with sepsis with cancer are significantly higher compared to nononcology patients. Hensley et al.[20] in his study had found that hospital mortality due to sepsis was nearly 50% higher in oncology patients (27.9%) compared to nononcology patients (19.5%). It also varies from hospital to hospital depending on internal policy regarding ICU shifting and therapy escalation. There is a tendency to delay ICU shift and presumptively that may also contribute to very high mortality in some studies[50] (up to 60%). Long-term outcome is also unsatisfactory in this population, especially if the primary disease is not in remission and general condition of the patient is poor during ICU discharge for receiving further anticancer treatment. Data from more than 3 lakh septic oncology patients over 9 years had shown significantly high 30-day and 1-year mortality[51] (52% and 81.2%, respectively). Hematological malignancy usually has a poorer outcome compared to solid organ malignancy, in terms of higher short-term and long-term mortality. Some studies had reported similar outcome data too.[52] Predictors of poor ICU survival include poor general condition [Eastern Cooperative Oncology Group (ECOG) score 3 or 4], metastatic cancer, respiratory failure requiring invasive ventilation, severity of the disease (high SOFA score) on admission and during ICU stay, high lactate, positive microbiological culture, and worsening organ function like thrombocytopenia and hyperbilirubinemia.

CONCLUSION

Sepsis in oncology patients creates a unique high-risk population. Due to underlying immunosuppression and cancer-related challenges, a wide range of microbes including bacteria, fungus, and virus can cause sepsis in this vulnerable population. Empirical antibiotics have to be modified according to local antibiogram and may vary from general medical surgical ICU protocol. Conventional clinical and laboratory findings of sepsis may be absent and as a result, a high index of suspicion for sepsis as the cause of new onset organ failure should be kept in mind. Delay in resuscitation in septic patients leads to poor outcome. So, patients with anticipated good long-term outcome should be shifted to ICU early during their acute clinical condition to have better outcome. In case of poor clinical response to initial therapy or with anticipated long-term poor outcome from cancer perspective, palliative care team should be involved early during ICU stay after initial "ICU trail" of therapy.

REFERENCES

1. Williams JC, Ford ML, Coopersmith CM. Cancer and sepsis. Clin Sci (Lond). 2023;137(11):881-93.
2. Singer M, Deutschman CS, Seymour CW, Shankar-Hari M, Annane D, Bauer M, et al. The Third International Consensus Definitions for Sepsis and Septic Shock (Sepsis-3). JAMA. 2016;315(8):801-10.
3. Wiersinga WJ, van der Poll T. Immuno-pathophysiology of human sepsis. E Bio Med. 2022;86:104363.
4. Glibetic N, Shvetsov YB, Aan FJ, Peplowska K, Hernandez BY, Matter ML. Transcriptome profiling of colorectal tumors from patients with sepsis reveals an ethnic basis for viral infection risk and sepsis progression. Sci Rep. 2022;12(1):20646.
5. Chen CW, Xue M, Zhang W, Xie J, Coopersmith CM, Ford ML. 2B4 but not PD-1 blockade improves mortality in septic animals with preexisting malignancy. JCI Insight. 2019;4(22):e127867.
6. Fox AC, Robertson CM, Belt B, Clark AT, Chang KC, Leathersich AM, et al. Cancer causes increased mortality and is associated with altered apoptosis in murine sepsis. Crit Care Med. 2010;38(3):886-93.
7. Lyons JD, Mittal R, Fay KT, Chen CW, Liang Z, Margoles LM, et al. Murine Lung Cancer Increases CD4+ T Cell Apoptosis and Decreases Gut Proliferative Capacity in Sepsis. PloS One. 2016;11(3):e0149069.
8. Cavassani KA, Carson WF 4th, Moreira AP, Wen H, Schaller MA, Ishii M, et al. The post sepsis-induced expansion and enhanced function of regulatory T cells create an environment to potentiate tumor growth. Blood. 2010;115(22):4403-11.
9. Chen CW, Bennion KB, Swift DA, Morrow KN, Zhang W, Oami T, et al. Tumor-Specific T Cells Exacerbate Mortality and Immune Dysregulation during Sepsis. J Immunol. 2021;206(10):2412-9.
10. Vigneron C, Mirouse A, Merdji H, Rousseau C, Cousin C, Alby-Laurent F, et al. Sepsis inhibits tumor growth in mice with cancer through Toll-like receptor 4-associated enhanced Natural Killer cell activity. Oncoimmunology. 2019;8(11):e1641391.
11. McCarthy EF. The toxins of William B. Coley and the treatment of bone and soft-tissue sarcomas. Iowa Orthop J. 2006;26:154-8.
12. Roberts NJ, Zhang L, Janku F, Collins A, Bai RY, Staedtke V, et al. Intratumoral injection of Clostridium novyi-NT spores induces antitumor responses. Sci Transl Med. 2014;6(249):249ra111.
13. Janku F, Zhang HH, Pezeshki A, Goel S, Murthy R, Wang-Gillam A, et al. Intratumoral Injection of Clostridium novyi-NT Spores in Patients with Treatment-refractory Advanced Solid Tumors. Clin Cancer Res. 2021;27(1):96-106.
14. Liu Z, Mahale P, Engels EA. Sepsis and Risk of Cancer Among Elderly Adults in the United States. Clin Infect Dis. 2019;68(5):717-24.
15. Hotchkiss RS, Osmon SB, Chang KC, Wagner TH, Coopersmith CM, Karl IE. Accelerated lymphocyte death in sepsis occurs by both the death receptor and mitochondrial pathways. J Immunol. 2005;174(8):5110-8.

16. Coopersmith CM, Stromberg PE, Dunne WM, Davis CG, Amiot DM 2nd, Buchman TG, et al. Inhibition of intestinal epithelial apoptosis and survival in a murine model of pneumonia-induced sepsis. JAMA. 2002;287(13):1716-21.
17. Zhang W, Chihade DB, Xie J, Chen CW, Ramonell KM, Liang Z, et al. Preexisting malignancy abrogates the beneficial effects of CXCR4 blockade during sepsis. J Leukoc Biol. 2020;107(3):485-95.
18. Danai PA, Moss M, Mannino DM, Martin GS. The epidemiology of sepsis in patients with malignancy. Chest. 2006;129(6):1432-40.
19. Rosolem MM, Rabello LS, Lisboa T, Caruso P, Costa RT, Leal JV, et al. Critically ill patients with cancer and sepsis: clinical course and prognostic factors. J Crit Care. 2012;27(3):301-7.
20. Hensley MK, Donnelly JP, Carlton EF, Prescott HC. Epidemiology and Outcomes of Cancer-Related Versus Non-Cancer-Related Sepsis Hospitalizations. Crit Care Med. 2019;47(10):1310-6.
21. Sharma A, Nguyen P, Taha M, Soubani AO. Sepsis Hospitalizations With Versus Without Cancer: Epidemiology, Outcomes, and Trends in Nationwide Analysis From 2008 to 2017. Am J Clin Oncol. 2021;44(10):505-11.
22. Silva LLe, Ferreira DB, Goto JM, Becker OM, Tuma P, MedEoros EAS. Sepsis and shock septic among patients with hematological malignancies: Factors associated with mortality. Research Square. 2023.
23. Lemiale V, Pons S, Mirouse A, Tudesq JJ, Hourmant Y, Mokart D, et al. Sepsis and Septic Shock in Patients With Malignancies: A Groupe de Recherche Respiratoire en Réanimation Onco-Hématologique Study. Crit Care Med. 2020;48(6):822-9.
24. Tao J, Seier K, Marasigan-Stone CB, Simondac JS, Pascual AV, Kostelecky NT, et al. Delirium as a Risk Factor for Mortality in Critically Ill Patients With Cancer. JCO Oncol Pract. 2023;19(6):e838-e847.
25. Ma C, Sun G, Yang X, Yang S. A clinically applicable prediction model for the risk of in-hospital mortality in solid cancer patients admitted to intensive care units with sepsis. J Cancer Res Clin Oncol. 2023;149(10):7175-85.
26. Vaidie J, Peju E, Jandeaux LM, Lesouhaitier M, Lacherade JC, Guillon A, et al. Long-term immunosuppressive treatment is not associated with worse outcome in patients hospitalized in the intensive care unit for septic shock: the PACIFIC study. Crit Care. 2023;27(1):340.
27. Kieslichova E, Rocen M, Merta D, Kudla M, Splichal I, Cap J, et al. The effect of immunosuppression on manifestations of sepsis in an animal model of cecal ligation and puncture. Transplant Proc. 2013;45(2):770-7.
28. Martinson ML, Lapham J. Prevalence of Immunosuppression Among US Adults. JAMA. 2024;331(10):880-2.
29. Siegel RL, Miller KD, Wagle NS, Jemal A. Cancer statistics, 2023. CA Cancer J Clin. 2023;73(1):17-48.
30. Rivera DR, Gallicchio L, Brown J, Liu B, Kyriacou DN, Shelburne N. Trends in Adult Cancer-Related Emergency Department Utilization: An Analysis of Data From the Nationwide Emergency Department Sample. JAMA Oncol. 2017;3(10):e172450.
31. Brun-Buisson C, Meshaka P, Pinton P, Vallet B; EPISEPSIS Study Group. EPISEPSIS: a reappraisal of the epidemiology and outcome of severe sepsis in French intensive care units. Intensive Care Med. 2004;30(4):580-8.
32. Vincent JL, Rello J, Marshall J, Silva E, Anzueto A, Martin CD, et al.; EPIC II Group of Investigators. International study of the prevalence and outcomes of infection in intensive care units. JAMA. 2009;302(21):2323-9.
33. Vincent JL, Sakr Y, Singer M, Martin-Loeches I, Machado FR, Marshall JC, et al.; EPIC III Investigators. Prevalence and Outcomes of Infection Among Patients in Intensive Care Units in 2017. JAMA. 2020;323(15):1478-87.
34. Guarana M, Nucci M, Nouér SA. Shock and Early Death in Hematologic Patients with Febrile Neutropenia. Antimicrob Agents Chemother. 2019;63(11):e01250-19.
35. El Haddad H, Chaftari AM, Hachem R, Chaftari P, Raad II. Biomarkers of Sepsis and Bloodstream Infections: The Role of Procalcitonin and Proadrenomedullin With Emphasis in Patients With Cancer. Clin Infect Dis. 2018;67(6):971-7.
36. Gradel KO, Póvoa P, Garvik OS, Vinholt PJ, Nielsen SL, Jensen TG, et al. Longitudinal trajectory patterns of plasma albumin and C-reactive protein levels around diagnosis, relapse, bacteraemia, and death of acute myeloid leukaemia patients. BMC Cancer. 2020;20(1):249.
37. Sakr Y, Sponholz C, Tuche F, Brunkhorst F, Reinhart K. The role of procalcitonin in febrile neutropenic patients: review of the literature. Infection. 2008;36:396-407.
38. Bhardwaj PV, Emmich M, Knee A, Ali F, Walia R, Roychowdhury P, et al. Use of MASCC score in the inpatient management of febrile neutropenia: a single-center retrospective study. Support Care Cancer. 2021; 29(10):5905-14.
39. Moon H, Choi YJ, Sim SH. Validation of the Clinical Index of Stable Febrile Neutropenia (CISNE) model in febrile neutropenia patients visiting the emergency department. Can it guide emergency physicians to a reasonable decision on outpatient vs. inpatient treatment? PLoS One. 2018;13(12):e0210019.
40. Zheng B, Toarta C, Cheng W, Taljaard M, Reaume N, Perry JJ. Accuracy of the Multinational Association of Supportive Care in Cancer (MASCC) and Clinical Index of Stable Febrile Neutropenia (CISNE) scores for predicting serious complications in adult patients with febrile neutropenia: A systematic review and meta-analysis. Crit Rev Oncol Hematol. 2020;149:102922.
41. Allarakia J, Felemban T, Alghamdi A, Ashi A, Al Talhi YM, Alsahafi A, et al. Modified Early Warning Score (MEWS) as a predictor of intensive care unit admission in cancer patient on chemotherapy with positive blood culture:

A retrospective cohort study. J Infect Public Health. 2023;16(6):865-9.

42. Ocampo-Quintero N, Vidal-Cortés P, Del Río Carbajo L, Fdez-Riverola F, Reboiro-Jato M, Glez-Peña D. Enhancing sepsis management through machine learning techniques: A review. Med Intensiva (Engl Ed). 2022;46(3):140-56.
43. Guidelines for intensive care unit admission, discharge, and triage. Task Force of the American College of Critical Care Medicine, Society of Critical Care Medicine. Crit Care Med. 1999;27(3):633-8.
44. Nates JL, Nunnally M, Kleinpell R, Blosser S, Goldner J, Birriel B, et al. ICU Admission, Discharge, and Triage Guidelines: A Framework to Enhance Clinical Operations, Development of Institutional Policies, and Further Research. Crit Care Med. 2016;44(8):1553-602.
45. Lecuyer L, Chevret S, Thiery G, Darmon M, Schlemmer B, Azoulay E. The ICU trial: a new admission policy for cancer patients requiring mechanical ventilation. Crit Care Med. 2007;35(3):808-14.
46. Evans L, Rhodes A, Alhazzani W, Antonelli M, Coopersmith CM, French C, et al. Surviving sepsis campaign: international guidelines for management of sepsis and septic shock 2021. Intensive Care Med. 2021;47(11):1181-247.
47. Mokart D, Saillard C, Sannini A, Chow-Chine L, Brun JP, Faucher M, et al. Neutropenic cancer patients with severe sepsis: need for antibiotics in the first hour. Intensive Care Med. 2014;40(8):1173-4.
48. Hechtman RK, Kipnis P, Cano J, Seelye S, Liu VX, Prescott HC. Heterogeneity of Benefit from Earlier Time-to-Antibiotics for Sepsis. Am J Respir Crit Care Med. 2024;209(7):852-60.
49. Kreitmann L, Vasseur M, Jermoumi S, Perche J, Richard JC, Wallet F, et al. Relationship between immunosuppression and intensive care unit-acquired colonization and infection related to multidrug-resistant bacteria: a prospective multicenter cohort study. Intensive Care Med. 2023;49(2):154-65.
50. Nazer L, Lopez-Olivo MA, Cuenca JA, Awad W, Brown AR, Abusara A, et al. All-cause mortality in cancer patients treated for sepsis in intensive care units: a systematic review and meta-analysis. Support Care Cancer. 2022;30(12):10099-109.
51. Kim YJ, Kim MJ, Kim YJ, Kim WY. Short and Long-Term Mortality Trends for Cancer Patients with Septic Shock Stratified by Cancer Type from 2009 to 2017: A Population-Based Cohort Study. Cancers (Basel). 2021;13(4):657.
52. Le Borgne P, Feuillassier L, Schenck M, Herbrecht JE, Janssen-Langenstein R, Simand C, et al. Comparison of Short- and Long-Term Mortality in Patients with or without Cancer Admitted to the ICU for Septic Shock: A Retrospective Observational Study. Cancers (Basel). 2022;14(13):3196.
53. Mukherjee S, De MS, Goel G, Bhattacharyya A, Mallick I, Dabkara D, et al. Multi-drug resistant (MDR) and extensively drug-resistant (XDR) bacteraemia rates among cancer patients in an oncology hospital in eastern India: an 11-year retrospective observational study. Infect Prev Pract. 2023;5(2):100275.

CHAPTER 55

Nutrition in Oncocritical Care Setting

Snany Surendran A, Deepa Chandramohan

INTRODUCTION

Providing nutritional support is one of the most fundamental aspects of any care pathway dealing with any critically ill patient. Critical illnesses are associated with excessive loss of muscle mass, and hence, critically ill patients are at high risk of malnutrition. Proteolysis-related muscle loss can be prevented by initiating a nutrition care plan from the day of admission to the intensive care unit (ICU). It is recommended that any critically ill patient who is expected to stay >72 hours in the ICU should undergo a complete nutritional assessment for an individualized or "personalized" nutritional management. This includes five steps, namely: (1) Assessment of nutrition risk through screening, (2) assessment of nutritional status through nutritional assessment techniques, (3) calculation of protein and energy requirements, (4) provision of the individualized nutritional requirements, and (5) monitoring and evaluation.

Malnutrition, anorexia, and weight loss are common in cancer patients right from their first visit to a cancer care hospital. The prevalence of malnutrition among oncological patients is as high as 40–80%. The prevalence of malnutrition is the highest in the oncological population compared to all other specialties.[1] As nutritional status is a significant parameter that affects treatment outcome, malnutrition is to be addressed with utmost care in all phases of oncological management **(Flowchart 1)**. Medical nutrition therapy is a vital component in oncocritical care as it reduces complication rates, shortens hospital stay, improves treatment outcomes, and enhances the quality of life.

NUTRITIONAL SCREENING

There are various nutritional screening tools that can be validated for oncological patients. These help to identify the risk of malnutrition in ICU patients. Nutritional risk screening (NRS) 2002[3] and NUTRIC score[4] are commonly used and recommended tools as per American Society for Parenteral and Enteral Nutrition (ASPEN) and ESPEN guidelines. The NUTRIC score ≤5 is not at nutritional risk,

Flowchart 1: Structure of the ESPEN practical guideline: "Clinical nutrition in cancer."[2]

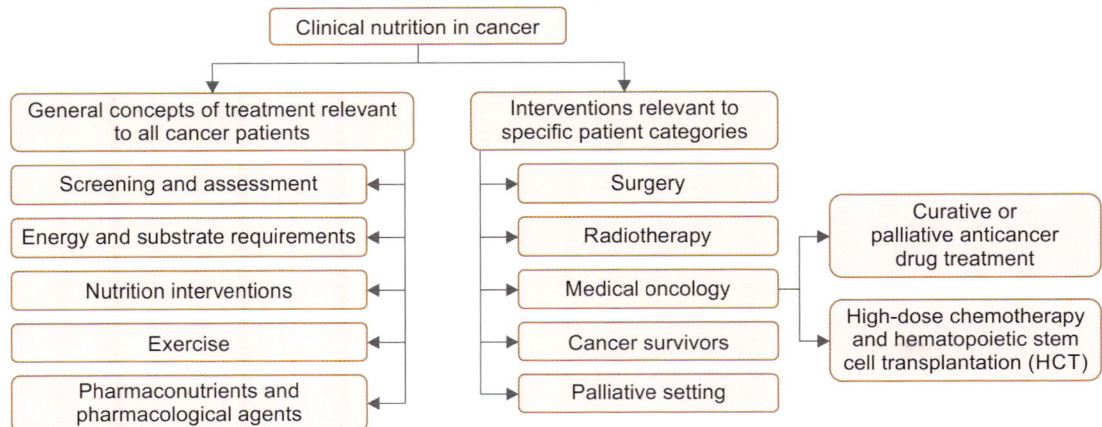

(ESPEN: European Society for Clinical Nutrition and Metabolism)

but others need a comprehensive nutritional assessment of nutritional intake, nutrition impact symptoms, muscle mass, physical performance, etc. An NRS-2002 score >3 must need specialized nutrition therapy from day 1 of the ICU stay.[5] The Nutritional Risk Index (NRI)[6] is a tool used to assess the nutritional status of patients, particularly to identify malnutrition and predict potential complications related to nutrition in clinical settings. It helps healthcare professionals determine the need for nutritional support, particularly in surgical or chronically ill patients. The NRI is calculated using the following formula: NRI = (1.519 × serum albumin level, g/dL) + [41.7 × (current weight/usual weight)]. This index is particularly useful for identifying at-risk individuals who may not appear undernourished but still face nutritional challenges that could affect their health outcomes.

ASSESSMENT OF NUTRITIONAL STATUS

The assessment of nutritional status is essential for providing adequate medical nutrition therapy to ICU patients.[5]

- *Anthropometric assessment:* Height, weight, body mass index (BMI), skin fold thickness, midupper arm circumference, etc., are the various parameters in the anthropometric assessment. But if the patient is not conscious or if the patient has generalized edema, these parameters will be of a limited value.
- *Biochemical values:* S. albumin is not the only marker that helps to know the severity of the condition as its levels can fluctuate, being an acute phase reactant. Hemoglobin values, transferrin, lymphocyte count, serum electrolyte values, C-reactive protein (CRP), visceral proteins, etc., are useful in assessing the inflammation and disease status, but it can be influenced by various factors of patients such as hydration status, internal or external bleeding, etc.
- *Clinical findings:* Pedal edema, ascites, temporal wasting, sarcopenia, signs of micronutrient deficiencies, nonhealing ulcers, etc., are the clinical findings that help to assess the nutritional status of the patients.
- *Dietary recall:* Diet history of a self-defined period gives the data of the feeding pattern and expected nutrient deficiency of the patient.
- *Other measures:* If the patient is conscious, the muscle function can be assessed using a handgrip dynamometer. Biomedical impedance, muscle function studies, body composition, etc., can be done to assess muscle mass and strength.

A subjective global assessment (SGA)[7] is a simple, inexpensive, and reliable assessment tool for ICU patients. The SGA allows a more concise and simple way of collecting a large part of patient history and nutritional risk. The early diagnosis of malnutrition or risk of malnutrition allows the establishment of adequate diet therapy, which in turn contributes to better treatment outcomes. The ultrasound scan and computed tomography (CT) scan assess the muscle distribution and tissue deposit in the body which can indirectly give the knowledge of patients energy storage.

PROTEIN AND ENERGY REQUIREMENTS

The body gets energy from macronutrients and micronutrients. Adequate nutritional requirement is to be met in ICU patients to prevent undernutrition as well as overnutrition. Improper nutritional management will lead to refeeding syndrome also.[8] Due to the catabolic nature of critical illnesses, high calories/proteins are required in most cases. Indirect calorimetry is a standard in determining energy expenditure and calorie needs. In the absence of an indirect calorimeter, validated equations like Harris-Benedict equation[9] can be used.

Guidelines[8] recommend giving 25–30 kcal/kg of calories in critically ill cancer patients. In the acute phase of critical illness, 20–25 kcal/kg and in recovery 25–30 kcal/kg of energy is needed. In critically ill oncology patients, guidelines recommend 1.2–2.0 g/kg of protein per day and try to attain 100% of protein targets within 48–72 hours to prevent muscle loss during the ICU stay.[8] In mechanically ventilated patients, the caloric needs should be estimated with the Penn State equation.[10] Carbohydrate intake should not exceed 4 g/kg/day and blood glucose levels should remain below 180 mg/dL. The recommended lipid supply is 0.7–1.5 g/kg/day, and the use of lipid emulsions with a high omega-6 fatty acid content should be avoided in critically ill patients. The supply of amino acids must be adjusted to 1–1.8 g/kg/day, depending on the level of metabolic stress.

The requirement of micronutrients should be managed if the requirement of macronutrients is addressed in healthy people. In the case of critically ill patients, micronutrients like zinc, selenium, copper, vitamins, other trace elements, etc., get deficient due to loss through drains or malabsorption. As per the recommended dietary allowance, the micronutrient requirement should be managed orally/enterally/parenterally.

ADMINISTRATION OF NUTRIENTS

Routes of administration of nutrients: The effect of nutrition intervention depends on the route of delivering the nutrients into the body, i.e., oral, enteral, or parenteral.[8] If the patient is conscious with a functional gastrointestinal (GI) tract, the oral route is preferable. If the patient is unconscious or has difficulty in swallowing but with a functional GI tract, enteral routes like nasogastric (NG)/nasojejunal (NJ), oral tubes, percutaneous endoscopic gastrostomy (PEG), and percutaneous endoscopic jejunostomy (PEJ) can be considered. If the patient needs parenteral nutrition (PN), peripheral IV lines or central venous lines can be used, depending upon the osmolarity of the PN preparation.

A. Enteral Nutrition[11-13]

Enteral nutrition (EN) is crucial in critical care, particularly in patients who are unable to consume food orally but have a functioning GI tract. An enteral route is preferred to parenteral due to the following reasons:

- *Maintains gut integrity:* Enteral feeding stimulates the gut and maintains the structural and functional integrity of the intestinal mucosa, reducing the risk of atrophy and bacterial translocation, which can lead to infections. A functioning gut plays a role in the immune response, helping prevent systemic infections and reducing the risk of sepsis.
- *Reduces infection risk:* Compared to PN, EN is associated with a lower risk of infectious complications, as it helps maintain gut flora and reduces bacterial overgrowth in the gut.
- *Cost-effective:* EN is generally more cost-effective compared to PN, as it avoids the high costs and risks associated with intravenous feeding.
- *Fewer metabolic complications:* EN is associated with fewer metabolic complications (such as hyperglycemia or electrolyte imbalances) than PN. This is because nutrients are delivered more physiologically through the GI tract, allowing for better nutrient absorption and utilization.
- *Improved GI function:* Continuous enteral feeding promotes gut motility, preventing ileus (intestinal obstruction) and reducing the risk of GI complications such as constipation or diarrhea.

Enteral Feeding Composition[8]

Enteral nutrition formulas can be categorized as standard polymeric, oligomeric, immune modulating, and disease-specific.

- *Standard polymeric:* Critically ill patients with normal GI tracts benefit from oligomeric formulas. They have intact nutrients, usually with carbohydrates in the form of maltodextrin and corn syrup solids, protein as soy protein isolate or caseinates, and fats such as safflower, canola, or soybean oil. They are available in different concentrations, from 1 to 2 kcal/mL. The ASPEN/Society of Critical Care Medicine (SCCM) guidelines for nutrition support in a critical illness state that a standard formula with or without fiber may be tolerated by most ICU patients. Fiber-containing formulas should be avoided in patients who are hemodynamically unstable and at risk for bowel ischemia.[5]
- *Oligomeric-based/elemental/semielemental formula:* Oligomeric formulas are predigested and are formulated to require minimal digestion by the GI tract. Peptide-based formulas may be used in patients with malabsorption or who have demonstrated GI intolerance of standard formulas. These formulas are easier to digest as protein is hydrolyzed into small-chain peptides, and fat sources include medium-chain triglycerides and/or fish oil structured lipids. They are beneficial in critically ill patients, especially in those receiving additional calories from IV solutions which necessitates a lower EN rate to avoid overfeeding. Many peptide-based formulas also contain higher amounts of antioxidant micronutrients, such as vitamins C, D, E, and selenium, and the omega-3 fatty acids eicosapentaentoic acid (EPA) and docosahexaenoic acid (DHA).
- *Immune modulating:* The ASPEN/SCCM nutrition support guidelines in critical care recommend the consideration of immune-modulating formulas in postoperative patients (containing arginine, glutamine, etc.), but not recommended in medical ICU and septic patients.[8]
- *Disease-specific:* The ASPEN/SCCM nutrition support in the critical illness guidelines does not recommend the routine use of disease-specific formulas in medical and surgical ICU (SICU) patients.[8] However, their use in some subsets of patients may be of benefit. The ESPEN guidelines do not specifically address disease-specific formulas.

Complications of Enteral Nutrition[14,15]

Enteral feeding, while beneficial in critical care, is not without risks. EN is associated with GI, mechanical, metabolic, and infectious complications which have been listed in **Box 1**.

Enteral Feeding Methods[16]

Enteral feeding can be administered in various ways, depending on the patient's needs and GI function. These methods include bolus, intermittent, continuous, and trophic feeding.

- *Bolus feeding:* It involves delivering a specific volume of formula (usually 200–400 mL) over a short period, typically 15–30 minutes, 3–6 times a day. It mimics regular eating patterns. It is suitable for patients with normal gastric function, a functioning stomach, and those with gastrostomy tubes (G-tube). It is often used for home EN and is not a preferred method in critically ill patients.
- *Intermittent feeding:* Similar to bolus feeding, intermittent feeding involves administering a set volume of formula over a longer period (30–60 minutes), 4–6 times a day, using gravity or a feeding pump. It is used when bolus feeding is not well-tolerated but the patient still has good gastric function. It can also be used in patients with NG, NJ, or gastrostomy tubes.

BOX 1: Complications of enteral nutrition.

- Gastrointestinal complications
  - Aspiration pneumonitis
  - Diarrhea
  - Constipation
  - Nausea and vomiting
  - Bloating and abdominal distension
  - Gastrointestinal ischemia or necrosis
- Mechanical complications
  - Feeding tube displacement or dislodgment
  - Tube occlusion
  - Sinusitis or nasopharyngeal ulceration
- Metabolic complications
  - Refeeding syndrome
  - Electrolyte imbalances
  - Hyperglycemia
  - Dehydration or fluid overload
- Infectious complications
  - Aspiration pneumonia
  - Contamination of feeding formula leading to infections like gastroenteritis
  - Sinusitis
- Psychological and patient comfort issues

- *Continuous feeding:* It involves delivering the feed at a slow and steady rate over 16–24 hours using a feeding pump. It is often used in critically ill patients or those with feeding intolerance. It is ideal for patients with a high risk of aspiration, delayed gastric emptying, or those requiring feeding directly into the small intestine (e.g., jejunostomy tubes). It is commonly used in ICUs.
- *Trophic feeding (minimal EN):* Trophic feeding, also called "gut-priming" or "trickle feeding," involves giving a very small volume of formula (typically 10–30 mL/h) to stimulate the GI tract without providing full caloric needs. This method is typically used in postoperative patients, and IN critically ill patients, especially in those with hemodynamic instability. It is used in patients who are not ready for full enteral feeding but need to maintain gut integrity and prevent atrophy of the intestinal mucosa. As it does not meet the patient's full nutritional needs, it is often combined with PN.

B. Parenteral Nutrition[17,18]

Parenteral nutrition is particularly important in critical care when patients are unable to tolerate or use EN due to conditions such as intestinal obstruction, severe malabsorption, or prolonged ileus. PN provides essential nutrients including carbohydrates, proteins, fats, vitamins, and minerals to meet the metabolic needs of critically ill patients. The chief indications include (1) nonfunctional or inaccessible GI tract—short bowel syndrome, severe pancreatitis, bowel ischemia, or bowel obstruction; (2) EN intolerance—severe diarrhea, vomiting, or high-output fistulas; (3) delayed or failed enteral feeding—critically ill patients where EN is not possible within the first 5–7 days of hospitalization; and (4) severe malnutrition—as a supplement to EN.

Types of Parenteral Nutrition

Depending on the route of administration and the duration of therapy, PN is of two main types, namely total parenteral nutrition (TPN) and peripheral parenteral nutrition (PPN). TPN provides all daily nutritional requirements (carbohydrates, proteins, fats, electrolytes, vitamins, and trace elements) via a central venous catheter (CVC) inserted into a large vein, such as the subclavian or jugular vein. Patients with a nonfunctioning GI tract such as in bowel obstruction, severe pancreatitis, or short bowel syndrome can be benefitted with high-calorie formulas to provide complete nutrition, meeting all caloric and micronutrient needs over a long duration (>7 days). PPN is administered through a peripheral vein and provides partial nutritional support. It is generally used for short-term or lower-calorie needs. Mildly ill patients or those with temporary GI issues benefit from PPN. It cannot provide full nutritional needs for critically ill patients.

Complications of Parenteral Nutrition[18]

Parenteral nutrition is associated with infectious, metabolic, hepatic, mechanical, and nutritional complications which have been listed in **Box 2**.

NUTRITIONAL STRATEGIES IN AN INTENSIVE CARE UNIT[18-22]

Nutritional strategies in the ICU are vital for the recovery and survival of critically ill oncology patients. These strategies aim to provide adequate calories and nutrients to prevent malnutrition, support immune function, and reduce the risk of complications in nonsurgical patients, surgical patients, and those on palliative care **(Flowchart 2)**.

BOX 2: Complications of parenteral nutrition.

- Infectious complications
  - Catheter-related bloodstream infections (CRBSIs)
  - Sepsis
  - Contaminated PN solutions
- Metabolic complications
  - Hyperglycemia
  - Refeeding syndrome
  - Electrolyte imbalances
  - Hypertriglyceridemia
  - Metabolic acidosis or alkalosis
  - Fluid overload
  - Dehydration
  - Osteoporosis and osteomalacia
- Hepatic complications
  - Parenteral nutrition-associated liver disease (PNALD)
  - Cholestasis
  - Cholelithiasis and cholecystitis
- Mechanical complications
  - Catheter occlusion
  - Catheter malposition
  - Venous thrombosis, deep vein thrombosis and pulmonary embolism
- Nutritional deficiencies and toxicities
  - Vitamin deficiencies
  - Trace element imbalances
  - Aluminum toxicity—particularly in pediatric patients

Flowchart 2: Nutritional strategies in intensive care unit (ICU).[18]

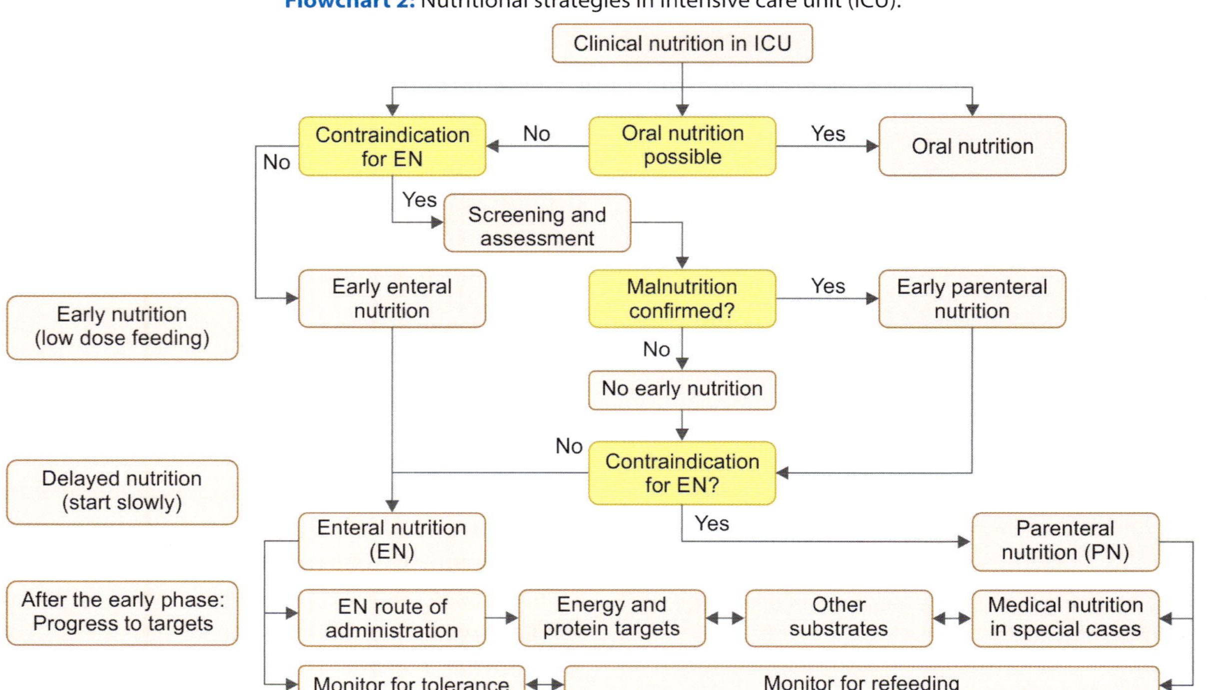

In Surgical Patients Following Major Cancer Surgeries[24]

Nutritional strategies in surgical patients following cancer surgeries are critical for promoting recovery, reducing complications, and improving long-term outcomes. Cancer surgery, especially when it involves the GI tract, can significantly impact the patient's nutritional status due to pre-existing malnutrition, postoperative stress, and changes in digestive function.

The nutritional assessment before surgery is essential, as many cancer patients are at risk of malnutrition due to the cancer itself, treatments, or reduced oral intake. Tools such as the SGA, the Malnutrition Universal Screening Tool (MUST), or NRS-2002 can help identify malnourished patients early. If malnutrition is present, initiate nutritional support (oral supplements, enteral, or PN) prior to surgery to improve nutritional reserves and wound healing capacity. Supplementing with specific nutrients such as arginine, omega-3 fatty acids, and nucleotides 5–7 days before surgery has been shown to improve immune function, reduce postoperative infections, and enhance recovery in GI cancer patients.

Early initiation of EN (within 24–48 hours postsurgery) is recommended,[25] as it helps to preserve gut function, reduce the risk of infections, and support wound healing. For patients who are unable to tolerate EN, such as those with severe postoperative ileus, anastomotic leaks, or short bowel syndrome, PN may be required to meet their nutritional needs. However, PN is associated with higher risks of infections and metabolic complications. When used, it is critical to transition to EN as soon as feasible.

Postoperative patients generally have increased metabolic demands due to the surgical stress response. A typical target for calorie intake is 25–30 kcal/kg/day. Higher energy requirements may be needed for patients with complications, sepsis, or extensive resections. Protein needs are elevated to support tissue repair, wound healing, and immune function. Aim for 1.5–2.0 g/kg/day of protein, especially in patients with significant tissue loss or catabolism due to surgery, is suggested. Vitamins and minerals play a key role in recovery, especially in cancer patients who are often deficient in micronutrients. Supplementation of vitamins (such as A, C, and D) and minerals (such as zinc and selenium) is important for immune support, wound healing, and prevention of deficiencies postsurgery.

Tailored Nutrition Based on the Type of Surgery

- *Head and neck surgeries:*[26] The nutritional management in surgical patients following head and neck cancer surgeries is challenging due to factors such as dysphagia, mucositis, trismus, and loss of appetite, all of which impact their ability to consume adequate nutrition orally. Many patients experience dysphagia due to surgical alterations, nerve damage, or postoperative edema. If oral intake is possible, texture-modified diets (soft or pureed) based on swallowing assessments by a speech-language pathologist (SLP) are advised. Oral nutritional supplements (ONS) like high-protein and high-calorie liquid formulas can bridge the gap between inadequate oral intake and nutritional needs. For patients with severe dysphagia or those unable to meet nutritional needs orally, enteral feeding or NG tube feeding is considered. If oral intake is significantly delayed or not possible for several weeks or months (common in patients with extensive resections or postradiation therapy), PEG feeding is advisable.
- *Gastrointestinal and major abdominal surgeries:*[27] The nutritional management in surgical patients who have undergone major resections (e.g., gastrectomy, esophagectomy, pancreatectomy, or colorectal surgery) often face challenges such as altered GI function, malabsorption, and an increased risk of malnutrition. The key to a successful nutritional strategy involves early identification of nutritional needs, maintaining gut integrity, minimizing the risk of postoperative complications like ileus and infections, and ensuring adequate calorie, protein, and micronutrient intake. For patients undergoing surgeries like esophagectomy, gastrectomy, or colorectal resections, EN can be administered via an NJ tube or jejunostomy to bypass any surgical sites. Small, frequent meals or liquid diets may be introduced later. In colorectal cancer surgery, postoperative ileus is common, so early mobilization and gradual introduction of nutrition, either orally or via enteral routes, are essential. If an anastomotic leak or fistula develops postoperatively, EN may be contraindicated, depending on the location and severity of the leak or fistula. In those cases, PN may be required until the leak is resolved or is surgically repaired. Cancer patients, especially those undergoing gastric or esophageal surgery, may develop feeding intolerance, characterized by delayed gastric emptying,

nausea, and vomiting. Gradual feeding with small, frequent meals and the use of prokinetic agents may help manage this.

- *Superficial/limb surgeries:*[28] In surgical patients following superficial or limb cancer surgeries (e.g., sarcoma resection, melanoma excision, or soft tissue tumor removal), the primary goals of nutrition management are to support wound healing, minimize infection risk, and maintain muscle mass, while promoting functional recovery. These patients may not face the same GI challenges as those who undergo abdominal surgeries, but they still have significant metabolic and nutritional needs, especially if they are critically ill in the SICU. Most patients undergoing superficial or limb cancer surgeries retain GI function and may be able to tolerate oral feeding postoperatively. Oral intake should be encouraged as soon as it is safe. Postoperative hyperglycemia is common, especially in critically ill patients, and can impair wound healing and increase infection risk. Tight glycemic control (target 140–180 mg/dL) is important in reducing the risk of complications.

In Critically Ill Nonsurgical Oncology Patients[18,19]

Nutrition strategies for nonsurgical oncology patients in the ICU need to be carefully managed, considering their unique metabolic and immune challenges, treatment effects (chemotherapy, radiation), and the overall critical nature of their illness. Nutrition intervention aims to minimize malnutrition, manage inflammation, and optimize recovery while balancing calorie and protein intake.

Early screening within 24–48 hours of ICU admission to assess nutritional status, severity of illness, and the risk of malnutrition is recommended in these patients. Biochemical markers such as albumin, prealbumin, and CRP may help in assessing the inflammatory state, though they are not direct indicators of the nutritional status.

Cancer patients may have increased metabolic demands, so energy requirements need to be individualized. The general recommendation is 25–30 kcal/kg/day, adjusted based on metabolic demands, underlying cancer, and ICU status. If the patient is hypermetabolic or undergoing treatment that alters the metabolic rate, indirect calorimetry can be considered. Adequate protein intake is essential to counteract muscle wasting (from both critical illness and cancer cachexia) and to improve immune function. Oncology patients in the ICU typically require 1.2–2.0 g/kg/day of protein, depending on the degree of stress, muscle wasting, and renal function.

Enteral nutrition is recommended within 24–48 hours if the GI tract is functional. Trophic or low-volume feeding (10–20 mL/h) can be initiated to maintain gut integrity, with the goal of gradually advancing to full nutrition as tolerated. Standard formulas are used typically, but specific oncology or immune-modulating formulas can be considered for patients with cachexia or severe inflammation. PN is to be considered if EN is contraindicated or insufficient (e.g., bowel obstruction, severe mucositis from chemotherapy). Aim to start PN only if EN is not possible after 5–7 days.

Oncology patients often have a high inflammatory burden, which may be further exacerbated by critical illness. Immune-modulating formulas contain omega-3 fatty acids, glutamine, arginine, and nucleotides, which may help modulate inflammation and enhance immune function, particularly in patients with significant cachexia or sepsis. Omega-3 fatty acids have been shown to reduce inflammation and may be beneficial in critically ill cancer patients with high inflammatory markers. Micronutrient supplementation needs to be considered in cancer patients as they are often deficient in vitamins (thiamine, vitamins A, C, D, and E) and trace elements (zinc, selenium) due to the disease, treatments, and critical illness.

Cancer treatments and critical illness often lead to electrolyte imbalances, particularly potassium, magnesium, calcium, and phosphorus, which require regular monitoring and correction. Hyperglycemia is a common issue in critically ill patients, especially those receiving steroids or chemotherapy. Maintain blood glucose levels between 140 and 180 mg/dL to reduce the risk of infections and complications to avoid adverse effects associated with both hyperglycemia and hypoglycemia.

Specific Considerations

- *Hemodynamically unstable:*[20] In patients with hemodynamic instability (e.g., hypotension, ongoing vasopressor use, or shock), the primary focus is to stabilize the cardiovascular system before aggressively initiating nutrition. Nutrition is generally not prioritized until the patient is more stable. Begin with trophic feeds until hemodynamics improve, to prevent ischemic complications. Start with 10–15 kcal/kg/day (or 50–70% of estimated needs), increasing as the patient stabilizes and gradually increase to 25–30 kcal/kg/day as the patient becomes hemodynamically stable.

- *Multiorgan dysfunction:*[21] In critically ill oncology patients with multiorgan dysfunction syndrome (MODS), nutritional strategies must be highly individualized and cautious due to the complexity of the metabolic and physiological disturbances present.
  - *Renal dysfunction:* If acute kidney insufficiency (AKI) or chronic kidney disease (CKD) is present, electrolyte levels, particularly potassium, magnesium, and phosphate should be closely monitored. Protein intake should be adjusted depending on whether the patient is on renal replacement therapy (RRT).
  - *In AKI without dialysis:* Protein may need to be reduced to 0.8–1.0 g/kg/day to prevent nitrogen accumulation.
  - *On RRT:* Protein requirements increase to 1.5–2.0 g/kg/day due to losses during dialysis.

Fluid restriction is advisable if the patient is oliguric or anuric. Sodium and potassium intake should be monitored closely.

  - *Hepatic dysfunction:* In patients with liver failure or hepatic encephalopathy, protein intake should be moderated to 0.8–1.2 g/kg/day, depending on the severity of hepatic dysfunction. Branched-chain amino acids can be considered to improve tolerance to protein and manage encephalopathy. The intake of carbohydrates and fats is limited as it can exacerbate hepatic steatosis or hyperglycemia.
  - *Respiratory dysfunction:* In patients with respiratory failure or on mechanical ventilation, avoid overfeeding as it can increase carbon dioxide production, complicating weaning from the ventilator. Carbohydrates should be provided in moderate amounts to prevent excessive CO_2 production. Fat-based nutrition (e.g., higher lipid formulas) can be considered if needed. For patients with specific conditions like acute respiratory distress syndrome (ARDS), high-protein and low-carbohydrate formulas can reduce the carbon dioxide burden and support lung function.
  - *Cardiovascular dysfunction:* Patients with cardiovascular instability or heart failure may require fluid-restricted feeds to prevent volume overload, particularly if they have third-spacing or are receiving vasopressors.
- *Neutropenic colitis and diarrhea:*[23] In critically ill oncology patients with neutropenic colitis (also known as typhlitis) and diarrhea, the nutritional management is highly complex due to their compromised immune system, high risk of infections, GI inflammation, and potential malabsorption. The primary goals of nutrition in this context are to maintain gut integrity, prevent malnutrition, and minimize the risk of infections while addressing the challenges posed by neutropenia, colitis, and diarrhea. The following points should be considered:
  - Begin with trophic or minimal enteral feeding (e.g., 10–20 mL/h) to stimulate the gut and prevent atrophy. This can be beneficial even if the patient has diarrhea, provided there are no signs of severe GI intolerance.
  - Consider using elemental or semielemental formulas, which are easier to digest and absorb, particularly if the patient has severe diarrhea and malabsorption.
  - Watch for signs of feeding intolerance (e.g., worsening diarrhea, abdominal pain, distension, and high gastric residual volumes) and adjust feeding as needed. In cases of neutropenic colitis, the bowel can be significantly compromised, so feeds should be advanced cautiously.
  - Use a low-residue or low-fiber enteral formula to minimize bowel stimulation and reduce the risk of exacerbating diarrhea.
  - Avoid probiotics in neutropenic patients, as they carry a risk of bacterial or fungal translocation leading to bloodstream infections.
  - Consider implementing a neutropenic diet, which limits exposure to raw foods, unpasteurized products, and certain bacteria that could pose a risk for infections. The diet focuses on cooked and sterilized foods to minimize the risk of infection in neutropenic patients.
  - If the patient is extremely ill with bowel rest, PN can be considered.

In Oncology Patients on Palliative Care[29]

Nutrition in the ICU for palliative cancer patients must be approached with sensitivity, considering the patient's overall prognosis, quality of life, and comfort rather than focusing solely on nutritional optimization or life extension.

The primary goal is to enhance patient comfort and reduce suffering. Since cancer treatments can alter taste and offer foods that are appealing and enjoyable, even if they are not nutritionally optimal unlike in curative settings, aggressive nutrition interventions might not be appropriate. Artificial nutrition or hydration should be carefully evaluated in cases where life extension is not a goal.

If the patient can still eat, offering small, easily digestible meals is ideal. Focus on the patient's preferences to maximize satisfaction and comfort. Open discussions with the patient and their family about the benefits and burdens of feeding and hydration are essential. The ethical principle of "do no harm" should guide decisions, balancing the need for nutrition with the potential distress caused by interventions. If the patient is unable to eat but still has a functioning GI tract, EN can be considered. However, in the palliative setting, the focus should be on noninvasive options that enhance comfort.

In many cases, it may be appropriate to withhold or withdraw artificial nutrition if it no longer provides comfort or increases suffering. In terminal stages, aggressive hydration may cause fluid overload, discomfort, or respiratory distress. Oral sips or small amounts of water may be offered to alleviate thirst, but IV fluids are typically minimized.

MONITORING AND EVALUATION[30,31]

Enteral nutrition: Monitoring EN in critically ill patients is essential to ensure adequate nutrient delivery, avoid complications, and adjust feeding protocols as needed. The frequency of monitoring can vary based on the patient's condition and the phase of their critical illness **(Box 3)**.

Parenteral nutrition: Monitoring patients receiving PN is critical to ensure nutrient adequacy, prevent complications, and make necessary adjustments to the PN regimen. The frequency of monitoring varies depending on whether the patient is in the initiation phase, stabilization phase, or long-term use of PN **(Table 1)**.

Refeeding Syndrome[32]

Refeeding syndrome is a potentially life-threatening condition that occurs when initiating EN or PN in severely malnourished patients. It occurs when nutritional support, particularly carbohydrates, is introduced too rapidly to severely malnourished individuals. It is characterized by shifts in fluids and electrolytes, especially phosphate, magnesium, and potassium, leading to significant metabolic complications. It results in a rapid drop in serum phosphate, potassium, and magnesium levels as the body shifts from a catabolic to an anabolic state. It can lead to serious complications like heart failure, arrhythmias, respiratory failure, and muscle weakness. Slow initiation of PN with careful monitoring and correction of electrolyte imbalances prevents refeeding incidences.

BOX 3: Parameters to be monitored during EN.

- *Gastric residual volume (GRV):* Check GRV every 4–6 hours in the initial phase (for the first 48 hours), then adjust based on tolerance. GRV measurements are controversial. Some guidelines suggest reducing reliance on routine GRV checks unless there are signs of intolerance (vomiting and abdominal distention). GRV < 500 mL should not automatically stop feeding in the absence of other symptoms
- *GI intolerance:* GI intolerances such as vomiting, bloating, diarrhea, and abdominal distention should be assessed every 8 hours or more frequently if the patient is unstable or showing symptoms
- *Bowel movements:* These should be checked daily to rule out signs of ileus
- *Hydration and fluid balance:* For assuring fluid balance and proper hydration track input (EN, intravenous fluids, and oral sources)/output(urine, drains, and ostomies) chart on a daily basis. In the acute phase of critical illness, body weight helps to assess fluid retention or dehydration
- *Electrolytes, glucose, and laboratory values:* Electrolytes (sodium, potassium, calcium, magnesium, and phosphate) are to be checked during the initiation of EN and then every 2–3 days once stable. More frequent monitoring is necessary in patients with renal dysfunction, those on diuretics, or those at risk of refeeding syndrome
- Blood glucose should be monitored daily for stable patients and every 6 hours in patients with hyperglycemia
- Liver and renal function tests (bilirubin, AST, ALT, creatinine, and BUN) should be checked weekly unless abnormalities arise. More frequent monitoring in patients with liver or renal dysfunction
- Prealbumin, albumin, and other markers can be checked weekly or as clinically indicated. These markers help assess a long-term nutritional status but may be affected by inflammation or acute illness
- Phosphate, potassium, and magnesium should be checked in severely malnourished patients while initiating EN to rule out the possibility of refeeding syndrome. Rapid electrolyte shifts associated with refeeding syndrome, particularly in the first few days after initiation of EN should be monitored

(AST: aspartate aminotransferase; ALT: alanine aminotransferase; BUN: blood urea nitrogen; EN: enteral nutrition; GI: gastrointestinal)

TABLE 1: Monitoring frequency of parenteral nutrition.

Parameter	Frequency (initiation)	Frequency (stable/ long-term)
Electrolytes	Daily	2–3 days/weekly
Blood glucose	Every 4–6 hours	Daily
Liver function tests	Weekly	Weekly
Renal function (BUN, Cr)	Daily	2–3 days/weekly
Serum triglycerides	Baseline, then weekly	Weekly
Prealbumin, albumin	Weekly	Weekly
Fluid balance/intake-output	Every 4–6 hours	Daily
Body weight	Daily	Weekly
Acid–base balance (ABG)	Daily	2–3 days
Complete blood count	Weekly	Weekly
Micronutrients/vitamins	Baseline, every 1–3 months	Every 1–3 months
Catheter site	Daily	Daily
Refeeding syndrome (electrolytes)	Every 6–12 hours during risk	Daily until stable

(BUN: blood urea nitrogen)

Prevention: The best approach to refeeding syndrome is prevention through careful nutritional planning and monitoring, especially in high-risk patients.

- *Identify high-risk patients*: Assess malnutrition risk by using criteria such as BMI <16 kg/m^2, unintentional weight loss >15% in the last 3–6 months, or negligible food intake for >5 days.
- *Start nutrition slowly:* Energy intake—Begin at 10–20 kcal/kg/day (approximately 50% of calculated energy needs) and increase slowly over 4–7 days. For high-risk patients, start as low as 5–10 kcal/kg/day. Limit carbohydrate intake initially to prevent a surge in insulin production. Provide 100–150 g/day initially.
- *Electrolyte supplementation:* Ensure adequate replacement of phosphate, potassium, and magnesium before starting nutritional support and continue supplementation as needed.
- *Vitamin supplementation:* Administer thiamine (100–300 mg/day) before and during refeeding to prevent Wernicke's encephalopathy. Provide a general multivitamin daily, including other B-complex vitamins.
- *Monitor electrolytes closely:* Check serum phosphate, potassium, magnesium, and glucose before starting nutrition, then daily for the first 5–7 days. Continue monitoring until it becomes stable.

CONCLUSION

There is a high risk of malnutrition among cancer patients due to the disease itself and also due to the different modalities of treatment faced by them. Medical nutrition therapy via a systematic approach is indispensable during all the phases of cancer therapy. Nutrition therapy starts from the time of admission to the hospital and continues through the critical phase to recovery and rehabilitation phases. Proper nutrition monitoring and evaluation help the cancer patients to improve their quality of life even after ICU discharge.

KEY POINTS

- Prevalence of malnutrition among oncological patients is high as 40–80%.
- Any critically ill patient who is expected to stay >72 hours in the ICU should undergo a complete nutritional assessment for an individualized or "personalized" nutritional management.
- Guidelines recommend 25–30 kcal/kg of calories and 1.2–2.0 g/kg of protein per day in critically ill cancer patients. Try to attain 100% of protein targets within 48–72 hours to prevent muscle loss during the ICU stay.
- If the patient is conscious with a functional GI tract, the oral route is preferable. If the patient is unconscious or has difficulty in swallowing but with a functional GI tract, EN routes such as NG/NJ tubes, oral tubes, PEG, and PEJ can be considered.
- PN is particularly important in critical care when patients are unable to tolerate or use EN, i.e., those with nonfunctional or inaccessible GI tract, EN intolerance, delayed or failed enteral feeding, and severe malnutrition.
- Trophic feeding, combined with PN, is typically used in postoperative patients, and in critically ill patients, especially in those with hemodynamic instability, who are not ready for full enteral feeding but need to maintain gut integrity and prevent atrophy of the intestinal mucosa.
- The goal in nonsurgical oncology patients in the ICU is to deliver personalized nutrition that prevents

malnutrition, supports immune function, and promotes recovery, while carefully monitoring for complications related to both critical illness and cancer.

- A combination of early EN, individualized caloric and protein support, and monitoring for specific micronutrient deficiencies is key for postoperative nutritional management in cancer surgery patients.
- By closely monitoring various parameters at appropriate intervals and timely adjustments, healthcare teams can optimize EN and PN and minimize potential complications in critically ill patients.
- Refeeding syndrome is a serious complication in oncocritical care which can be prevented by careful monitoring of electrolytes, gradual introduction of nutrition, and supplementation of vitamins and electrolytes.

REFERENCES

1. Hébuterne X, Lemarié E, Michallet M, de Montreuil CB, Schneider SM, Goldwasser F. Prevalence of malnutrition and current use of nutrition support in patients with cancer. JPEN J Parenter Enteral Nutr. 2014;38(2):196-204.
2. Muscaritoli M, Arends J, Bachmann P, Baracos V, Barthelemy N, Bertz H, et al. ESPEN practical guideline: clinical nutrition in cancer. Clin Nutr. 2021;40(5):2898-913.
3. Reber E, Gomes F, Vasiloglou MF, Schuetz P, Stanga Z. Nutritional risk screening and assessment. J Clin Med. 2019;8(7):1065.
4. Wełna M, Adamik B, Kübler A, Goździk W. The NUTRIC score as a tool to predict mortality and increased resource utilization in intensive care patients with sepsis. Nutrients. 2023;15(7):1648.
5. Castillo-Martínez L, Castro-Eguiluz D, Copca-Mendoza ET, Pérez-Camargo DA, Reyes-Torres CA, Ávila EA, et al. Nutritional assessment tools for the identification of malnutrition and nutritional risk associated with cancer treatment. Rev Invest Clin. 2018;70(3):121-5.
6. Prasad N, Sinha A, Gupta A, Bhadauria D, Manjunath R, Kaul A, et al. Validity of nutrition risk index as a malnutrition screening tool compared with subjective global assessment in end-stage renal disease patients on peritoneal dialysis. Indian J Nephrol. 2016;26(1):27-32.
7. Surendran S, Sankar UV, Nochikkattil S, Cheekapravan R, Warrier N, Babu S, et al. Subjective global assessment as a pre-operative nutrition status screening tool for head and neck cancer patients of a tertiary health care setting. J Canc Therapy. 2022;13(8).
8. McClave SA, Taylor BE, Martindale RG, Warren MM, Johnson DR, Braunschweig C, et al. Guidelines for the provision and assessment of nutrition support therapy in the adult critically ill patient. Society of Critical care Medicine (SCCM) and American Society for Parenteral and Enteral Nutrition (A.S.P.E.N.). J Parenter Enteral Nutr. 2016;40:159-211.
9. Pavlidou E, Papadopoulou SK, Seroglou K, Giaginis C. Revised Harris-Benedict equation: new human resting metabolic rate equation. Metabolites. 2023;13(2):189.
10. Wu S, Iqbal S, Giroux M, Alam N, Campisi J, Razek T, et al. Penn State equation versus indirect calorimetry for nutritional assessment in patients with traumatic brain injury. Can J Surg. 2022;65(3):E320-5.
11. Nutrition Support for Adults: Oral Nutrition Support, Enteral tube Feeding and Parenteral Nutrition NICE Clinical Guidelines, No 32 National Collaborating Centre for Acute Care (UK) 2006. [online] Available from https://www.nice.org.uk/guidance/cg32. [Last accessed March, 2025].
12. Kreymann KG, Berger MM, Deutz NEP, Hiesmayr M, Jolliet P, Kazandjiev G, et al. DGEM (German Society for Nutritional Medicine); ESPEN (European Society for Parenteral and Enteral Nutrition). ESPEN guidelines on enteral nutrition: intensive. 2006;25(2):210-23.
13. Tannuri U, et al. ASPEN Nutrition Support Manual, 2nd edition. Intensive Care Med; 1998. pp. 848-59.
14. Wanden-Berghe C, Patino-Alonso MC, Galindo-Villardón P, Sanz-Valero J. Complications associated with enteral nutrition: CAFANE study. 2019;11(9):2041.
15. Boullata JI, Carrera AL, Harvey L, Escuro AA, Hudson L, Mays A, et al. ASPEN Safe Practices for Enteral Nutrition Therapy. J Parenter Enteral Nutr. 2017;41(1):15-103.
16. Ichimaru S. Methods of enteral nutrition administration in critically ill patients: continuous, cyclic, intermittent, and bolus feeding. 2018;33(6):790-5.
17. Cotogni P. Management of parenteral nutrition in critically ill patients. World J Crit Care Med. 2017;6(1):13.
18. Singer P, Blaser AR, Berger MM, Szczeklik W, van Zanten ARH, Bischoff SC, et al. ESPEN practical and partially revised guideline: Clinical nutrition in the intensive care unit. Clinical Nutrition. 2023;42(9):1671-89.
19. Muscaritoli M, Arends J, Aapro M. From guidelines to clinical practice: a roadmap for oncologists for nutrition therapy for cancer patients. Ther Adv Med Oncol. 2019;11:1758835919880084.
20. Singer P, Blaser AR, Berger MM, Alhazzani W, Calder PC, Casaer MP, et al. ESPEN guideline on clinical nutrition in the intensive care unit. Clin Nutr. 2019;38(1):48-79.
21. Heyland DK, Dhaliwal R, Drover JW, Gramlich L, Dodek P, Canadian Critical Care Clinical Practice Guidelines Committee. Canadian clinical practice guidelines for nutrition support in mechanically ventilated, critically ill adult patients. J Parenter Enteral Nutr. 2003;27(5):355-73.
22. Desai SV, McClave SA, Rice TW. Nutrition in the ICU: an evidence-based approach.Chest. 2014;145(5):1148-57.
23. Babakhanlou R, Ravandi-Kashani F, Kontoyiannis DP. Neutropenic enterocolitis: an uncommon, but fearsome complication of leukemia. J Hematol. 2023;12(2):59-65.

24. Baji DB, Patel JP, Konanur Srinivasa NK, Gande A, Anusha M, Dar H. Nutrition care in cancer surgery patients: a narrative review of nutritional screening and assessment methods and nutritional considerations. Cureus. 2022;14(12):e33094.
25. Kim JY, Wie GA, Cho YA, Kim SY, Sohn DK, Kim SK, et al. Diet modification based on the enhanced recovery after surgery program (ERAS) in patients undergoing laparoscopic colorectal resection. Clin Nutr Res. 2018;7(4):297-302.
26. Talwar B, Donnelly R, Skelly R, Donaldson M. Nutritional management in head and neck cancer: United Kingdom National Multidisciplinary Guidelines. J Laryngol Otol. 2016;130(Suppl 2):S32-40.
27. Cencioni C, Trestini I, Piro G, Bria E, Tortora G, Carbone C, et al. Gastrointestinal cancer patient nutritional management: from specific needs to novel epigenetic dietary approaches. Nutrients. 2022;14(8):1542.
28. Baji DB, Patel JP, Konanur Srinivasa NK, Gande A, Anusha M, Dar H. Nutrition care in cancer surgery patients: a narrative review of nutritional screening and assessment methods and nutritional considerations. Cureus. 2022;14(12):e33094.
29. Cotogni P, Stragliotto S, Ossola M, Collo A, Riso S, On Behalf Of The Intersociety Italian Working Group For Nutritional Support In Cancer. The role of nutritional support for cancer patients in palliative care. Nutrients. 2021;13(2):306.
30. Gostyńska A, Stawny M, Dettlaff K, Jelińska A. Clinical nutrition of critically ill patients in the context of the latest ESPEN guidelines. Medicina (Kaunas). 2019;55(12):770.
31. Akbulut G. New perspective for nutritional support of cancer patients: enteral/parenteral nutrition. Exp Ther Med. 2011;2(4):675-84.
32. Stanga et al. Nutrition in clinical practice—the refeeding syndrome: illustrative cases and guidelines for prevention and treatment. Eur J Clin Nutr. 2008;62(6):687-94.

Cancer Pain Management

56 CHAPTER

Acute Pain Management after Oncosurgeries

Sheetal Gaikwad, Sumitra Bakshi

INTRODUCTION

With better understanding of the cancer biology, newer treatment options for cancer have surfaced in the past few decades. However, surgery still remains the primary modality for treatment of solid tumors.[1] Aggressive treatments such as hyperthermic intraperitoneal chemotherapy (HIPEC), are now more frequently utilized for locally advanced cancers. Patients frequently experience significant acute pain in the postoperative period. Effective acute pain management is crucial in the postoperative period, as pain from tissue manipulation and dissection is unavoidable during surgery. Poorly managed postoperative pain can lead to complications, including reduced mobility, compromised pulmonary function due to inadequate chest rehabilitation, the increased risk of respiratory complications, sleep disturbances, and prolonged hospitalization. The sympathetic and psychological impacts of unrelieved pain are considerable, and untreated acute pain is a known precursor to chronic pain syndromes.

Inadequate analgesia following major cancer surgery has been linked to persistent pain syndromes and prolonged opioid use, both of which increase patient suffering and can contribute to poorer outcomes.[2] This ongoing pain often leads to emotional and social distress, contributing to psychological conditions such as depression, anxiety, and sleep disturbances. Such conditions can further exacerbate the pain, creating a cycle of persistent suffering. The burden of chronic pain may foster isolation and dependency, amplifying patient distress and hindering recovery. Predictors of persistent pain include factors such as the type and invasiveness of the tumor, the specific treatment regimens used, the time elapsed since treatment, and the adequacy of initial pain management.

Globally, of the 310 million major surgeries performed each year, up to one-third of patients report persistent postsurgical pain (PPSP): pain one year after surgery.[3,4] In the case of cancer surgeries, this risk is heightened, making acute pain management an essential element in the perioperative care of oncology patients.

Furthermore, experimental studies suggest that the elevated catecholamine levels and inflammatory markers associated with surgical pain may facilitate the seeding of circulating cancer cells in distant organs and support the growth of dormant tumors and micrometastases, collectively known as minimal residual disease (MRD).[2] Thus, treating pain effectively may not only improve postoperative recovery but may also be critical for the long-term survival of cancer patients.

CHALLENGES OF TREATING ACUTE PAIN IN ONCOSURGERIES

Recent studies indicate a high incidence of moderate-to-severe postoperative pain following oncosurgeries, with rates of 41–61% in developed countries and 60–80% in developing countries. According to the American Pain Society, this prevalence has remained persistently high, affecting over 80% of postoperative cancer patients.[5-7] The likelihood of acute pain after oncologic surgeries is heightened by several factors:

Preoperative Pain

- *Chemotherapy and radiotherapy:* Cancer patients often require neoadjuvant therapies such as chemotherapy and radiotherapy before surgery, which can cause peripheral neuropathy, mucositis, and other painful conditions. Chemotherapy and radiation-induced sensitization create central and peripheral hyperalgesia, increasing postoperative pain severity. As a result, many patients require multianalgesic regimens, including opioids, even before surgery. Furthermore, therapies such as immunotherapy and aromatase inhibitors can contribute to musculoskeletal pain.[8]

- *Primary tumor-related pain:* Many cancer patients enter surgery already on opioid therapy due to inflammatory mediators released from the tumor or from previous treatments. Chronic conditions such as radiation-induced proctitis, colitis, plexopathies, and even fractures further complicate the management of postoperative pain.

Surgical Factors

- *Complexity of oncosurgeries:* Cancer surgeries are typically lengthy and complex, often involving extensive dissection of tissues and lymph nodes to ensure complete disease clearance. These procedures are frequently performed using an open surgical approach, requiring significant tissue retraction and manipulation, which can lead to iatrogenic nerve damage and increased postoperative pain.
- *Use of drains and invasive measures:* Due to the need for effective drainage and postoperative care, drains are commonly placed, adding another source of discomfort for patients.
- *Higher pain levels:* Postoperative pain following oncosurgeries is often moderate to severe, requiring intensive pain management strategies.

Anxiety and Psychological Aspects

Cancer is an inherently distressing diagnosis, associated with a substantial physical, emotional, financial, and social burden. The cumulative stress of navigating a cancer diagnosis, treatment side effects, and financial strain exacerbates postoperative pain perception. The psychological toll amplifies physical pain, further complicating pain management in the post-surgical period.

In summary, managing acute postoperative pain in cancer patients is highly complex due to these multifactorial challenges. Each of these factors—preexisting pain, surgical complexity, and psychological stressors—demands a comprehensive, multimodal approach to adequately address pain and improve patient outcomes.

PRINCIPLES OF MANAGEMENT OF POSTOPERATIVE PAIN FOLLOWING ONCOSURGERIES

The need for aggressive postoperative pain management following oncosurgeries cannot be over emphasized. Opioids are the most effective and oldest known pain killers to mankind. Opioids have played a critical role in advancing perioperative pain management, helping to reduce patient distress and improve surgical outcomes. However, the widespread use of high-dose opioids has exposed significant limitations. While effective for baseline pain control, opioids often fall short in managing pain during movement, a critical aspect for postoperative mobility and rehabilitation.[9] Furthermore, dose-dependent side effects—including postoperative ileus, urinary retention, nausea, vomiting, and opioid-induced ventilatory impairment (OIVI)—can be highly disabling and delay recovery.[10]

An additional challenge is opioid-induced hyperalgesia (OIH), where opioid use paradoxically increases pain sensitivity, leading to both acute and chronic pain that complicates effective pain management. OIH, observed with agents such as remifentanil and fentanyl, can present as heightened pain, pain spread beyond the initial site, or increased sensitivity to stimuli, often requiring higher postoperative opioid doses.[10] This paradoxical response, coupled with opioid tolerance, where escalating doses are needed to maintain analgesic effects, underscores the need for a rational, balanced approach to perioperative opioid prescribing. Integrating alternative analgesic strategies alongside careful opioid use can optimize pain relief, minimize side effects, and support faster rehabilitation.

Opioids and Cancer Recurrence

The effect of opioids on tumor growth and progression remains a complex and debated issue. Studies suggest a dual nature of opioid impact on cancer cells, with both inhibitory and stimulatory effects observed depending on dosage, timing, and specific opioid used. In high concentrations (>10 μM), morphine has been shown to significantly reduce cell proliferation and inhibit tumor growth in cancers such as breast and colon cancer.[11,12] Additionally, morphine demonstrates antiangiogenic properties, meaning it can inhibit the formation of new blood vessels needed by tumors for growth, as well as antiapoptotic effects, potentially protecting healthy cells during stressful treatments such as chemotherapy.[13]

These properties highlight a possible role for opioids in limiting cancer cell growth under certain conditions.

Contrastingly, other preclinical animal and retrospective clinical studies indicate that opioids may encourage tumor growth and spread by modulating the immune system and potentially enhancing cancer cell proliferation. Opioids can exert immunosuppressive effects, which may compromise the body's ability to identify and destroy cancer cells, and there is evidence to suggest that some opioids could potentially facilitate tumor-promoting pathways. This contradiction is observed in various studies where opioid use has been linked to both tumor inhibition and growth depending on several factors, including the type of cancer, type and dose of opioid, and duration of use.

A recent meta-analysis has added further nuance to this conversation. It concluded that intraoperative opioid administration during cancer surgery does not significantly impact progression-free survival (PFS) or overall survival (OS), which are commonly used metrics to assess cancer prognosis.[14] However, high doses of opioids administered postoperatively were found to have a negative impact on PFS, suggesting that while opioids may be safe in surgical doses during the operation, higher postoperative doses could potentially influence cancer outcomes unfavorably.[14]

Given these conflicting findings, it is increasingly recommended to approach opioid use in cancer surgeries with caution. A balanced, multimodal analgesic strategy that minimizes opioid use—often referred to as opioid-sparing analgesia—is encouraged during the perioperative period. Multimodal opioid-sparing analgesia combines various non-opioid medications (such as NSAIDs, acetaminophen, and local anesthetics) with nonpharmacologic techniques (such as regional anesthesia or nerve blocks) to provide effective pain relief while reducing reliance on opioids.

This opioid-sparing approach offers several benefits. First, it reduces potential opioid-induced side effects, such as respiratory depression, sedation, nausea, and vomiting, which can complicate recovery and delay mobilization. By lowering opioid doses, this strategy may also help mitigate potential tumor-promoting risks associated with opioid-induced immunosuppression or other biological pathways potentially favorable to cancer growth. Additionally, nonopioid analgesic components have their own unique benefits, including anti-inflammatory properties, which may further support an environment less conducive to tumor growth.

Ultimately, the prudent approach for managing pain in cancer patients undergoing surgery is to individualize analgesia plans that balance effective pain control with minimized opioid exposure. This balanced approach is especially important in cancer surgery, where pain management needs must be weighed against the broader goals of reducing perioperative stress, minimizing immunosuppression, and supporting a prompt and smooth recovery.

Regional Anesthesia

Regional anesthesia is increasingly recognized for its role in reducing perioperative morbidity in patients undergoing major cancer surgeries. By mitigating the risk of complications such as myocardial infarction, pneumonia, and venous thromboembolism, regional anesthesia contributes to safer recovery in patients undergoing high-risk procedures, such as major abdominal surgery for cancer.[15,16] Although some retrospective studies have shown no clear association between regional anesthesia and improved long-term cancer outcomes, a reduction in perioperative morbidity is often observed in regional anesthesia groups.[17] These groups experience benefits such as reduced opioid consumption, decreased postoperative ICU stays, and lower rates of complications such as pneumonia and anastomotic leaks, particularly in complex surgeries such as esophagectomy.[18] While not definitively linked to decreased cancer recurrence, regional anesthesia has become a cornerstone in oncoanesthesia, allowing individualized perioperative planning to lower stress responses, expedite recovery, and support timely progression to subsequent cancer therapies.

In practice, the decision to use regional anesthesia is best tailored to individual patient characteristics and the nature of the surgical procedure rather than the goal of reducing cancer recurrence. Regional anesthesia's value lies in its ability to reduce overall surgical stress and perioperative morbidity while improving pain management. It serves an especially useful function in oncoanesthesia, where enhancing recovery and minimizing stress responses are the key to managing the multimodal needs of cancer patients.

Epidural Anesthesia/Analgesia

Thoracic epidural analgesia (TEA) forms the backbone of pain management in multimodal opioid-sparing pain management technique. The initial bundle of interventions introduced to enhance recovery after surgery enhanced recovery after surgery (ERAS) protocols emphasize on the use of epidural analgesia after major open abdominal and thoracic oncosurgeries.[19,20] Thoracic epidural analgesia offers complete pain relief, which includes both the somatic and visceral pain following surgery. However, performance of these blocks will require expertise and has a significant learning curve for the novices. TEA also warrants meticulous monitoring in the postoperative period and can be associated with serious complications.

For patients who cannot receive neuraxial techniques such as epidural anesthesia—due to contraindications such as thrombocytopenia, neutropenia, difficult anatomy, or coagulation disorders—fascial plane blocks (FPBs) offer a viable alternative within a multimodal, opioid-sparing approach.[21-23] Although FPBs lack the visceral pain coverage provided by TEA, they have been found to offer comparable analgesic benefits, which can help support recovery. FPBs come with notable advantages over TEA, such as a lower incidence of hypotension, reduced need for ICU monitoring, and the potential for earlier mobilization. FPB are now considered as effective as epidural analgesia in the ERAS protocol. Furthermore, FPBs may prove to be more cost effective and can be performed with greater accessibility, particularly when ultrasound-guided techniques are available.

Fascial plane blocks are well-suited for surgeries where neuraxial techniques may be inaccessible or unsuitable, such as clavicular or lower limb orthopedic procedures where motor-sparing analgesia is desired. Their superficial nature, ease of application with ultrasound, fewer contraindications, and low rates of significant hemodynamic and neurological complications have increased their adoption in practice, making them a useful option alongside or as an alternative to TEA and peripheral nerve blocks.

Beyond immediate postoperative benefits, regional anesthesia has gained attention for its potential to modulate surgical inflammatory and immune responses. Theories suggest these modulations could reduce cancer recurrence risk, as inflammation and immune responses are closely linked to cancer progression. While intriguing, these hypotheses remain unproven.[2] A recent consensus from the American and European Societies for Regional Anesthesia emphasized that evidence does not currently support the routine use of regional anesthesia to prevent cancer recurrence.[2] Therefore, the primary indication for regional anesthesia in cancer surgeries should be based on patient-centered considerations, specific to the surgical procedure and intended to improve perioperative morbidity, pain management, and recovery outcomes rather than on unproven oncological benefits.

Ultimately, regional anesthesia's place within onco-anesthesia is solidified by its demonstrated ability to reduce perioperative opioid and general anesthetic use, limit complications, and facilitate early mobilization and enhanced recovery. By combining these effects with a patient-centered approach, regional anesthesia continues to play a fundamental role in comprehensive cancer care and in enabling patients to resume their oncological treatments as quickly and safely as possible.

Coanalgesics

The role of various non-opioid analgesics in multimodal pain management is crucial in reducing opioid consumption and associated side effects, but each class comes with its own benefits, risks, and limitations that must be considered in perioperative and long-term pain management.

Nonsteroidal Anti-inflammatory Drugs

Non-steroidal anti-inflammatory drugs (NSAIDs) work primarily by inhibiting cyclooxygenase (COX) enzymes, which play a key role in the synthesis of prostaglandins, the molecules responsible for sensitizing peripheral nerves and amplifying pain signals (hyperalgesia).[24] This inhibition provides effective analgesia, particularly for inflammatory pain, and can reduce opioid requirements. NSAIDs also act on spinal COX enzymes, contributing to their central analgesic effects.

However, there are significant concerns surrounding NSAID use in the perioperative setting due to their potential side effects, such as acute kidney injury and anastomotic leaks—complications particularly relevant in abdominal surgery where NSAIDs have been associated, albeit inconclusively, with higher leak rates.[25-27] The recent reviews, including a Cochrane review, highlight uncertainties about the renal safety of perioperative NSAIDs. Given these risks, the recommendationis often to evaluate NSAID use on an individual basis, considering potential thromboembolic events, gastrointestinal bleeding, and heart failure exacerbation, especially in vulnerable populations.

Paracetamol (Acetaminophen)

In multimodal analgesic strategies, paracetamol is widely favored due to its opioid-sparing effects, particularly when administered intravenously in a prophylactic manner. This can reduce postoperative nausea and vomiting by enabling better pain control with fewer opioids. Unlike NSAIDs, paracetamol carries a lower risk of renal and gastrointestinal complications, although hepatotoxicity remains a concern at high doses.[28,29] In the perioperative setting, therapeutic doses are generally considered safe, making paracetamol a valuable component of multimodal regimens for enhancing pain control and minimizing opioid use.

Gabapentinoids (Gabapentin and Pregabalin)

Gabapentin and pregabalin, traditionally antiepileptic drugs, are also employed for neuropathic pain due to their effects on neuronal excitability, mediated by their interaction with the $\alpha 2\delta$ subunit of calcium channels. This interaction is thought to reduce excitatory neurotransmission and alter the affective component of pain by enhancing descending pain inhibition pathways. However, their use in perioperative pain management is increasingly questioned due to their adverse effects, which include dizziness and visual disturbances.

Recent systematic reviews and meta-analyses indicate that gabapentinoids offer no significant analgesic benefit for perioperative pain and do not effectively prevent chronic postoperative pain, while carrying a risk of adverse events.[30] Consequently, the routine use of gabapentinoids for postoperative pain is generally not recommended, and their use should be individualized. Many cancer patients experience neuropathic pain due to tumor invasion, chemotherapy, or radiotherapy, leading to preoperative gabapentinoid use. However, once the primary tumor is excised, the underlying cause of neuropathic pain may be alleviated, potentially justifying gabapentinoid discontinuation. Conversely, patients with neuropathic pain related to chemo- or radiotherapy, or from surgical procedures like thoracotomy and mastectomy, may benefit from long-term gabapentinoid therapy. The decision to continue or discontinue gabapentinoids postoperatively should, therefore, be based on individual needs and ongoing symptoms.

Ketamine

Ketamine, an N-methyl-D-aspartate (NMDA) receptor antagonist, is valuable in multimodal analgesia for its opioid-sparing properties, particularly in patients with escalating opioid requirements. However, ketamine is associated with a range of dose-dependent adverse effects, such as hypersalivation, nausea, vomiting, and central nervous system (CNS) effects, including hallucinations, vivid dreams, blurred vision, and delirium. While these psychotomimetic effects can limit its routine use in ERAS protocols, ketamine may be effective in carefully selected cases requiring intense, multimodal pain control.

For patients with chronic or difficult-to-manage pain, such as those with high opioid tolerance or cancer-related pain, ketamine can serve as a valuable adjunct when traditional analgesics provide insufficient relief. The addition of ketamine can potentially minimize the need for higher opioid doses, thus reducing opioid-related side effects and improving pain control in these complex cases. However, due to its CNS side effects, ketamine should generally be used at the lowest effective dose and tailored to each patient's needs. Routine use of ketamine remains controversial, and its role is often reserved for specific clinical contexts where other analgesic options prove inadequate.

Alpha-2 Receptor Agonists

Alpha-2 (α-2) receptor agonists, such as clonidine and dexmedetomidine, are increasingly used in perioperative care for their opioid-sparing effects and ability to prolong the duration of nerve blocks. By activating α-2 adrenergic receptors, these agents provide analgesia and sedation, reducing the overall need for opioids. However, their benefits come with potential side effects, as even a single dose may cause sedation and hypotension, limiting their routine use. The common routes of administration include oral, intravenous, perineural, and field blocks, allowing for flexibility in tailoring them to patient needs and surgical procedures.

Intravenous Lignocaine

Intravenous lignocaine (lidocaine), particularly in preservative-free form, has shown promise as a perioperative analgesic, effectively reducing postoperative pain and opioid requirements. Its precise mechanisms are under investigation, though it is believed to modulate inflammatory responses to surgery, potentially influencing pain pathways and immune response. Beyond pain relief, low-dose lidocaine infusions are associated with a reduction in postoperative nausea and vomiting, shorter duration of postoperative ileus, and reduced hospital stays, making it a valuable addition to multimodal analgesia. Its anti-inflammatory effects and opioid-sparing benefits contribute to faster recovery, particularly in procedures where pain and inflammation are significant.

Overall, these analgesics, each contribute uniquely to opioid-sparing strategies in perioperative and cancer pain management. Multimodal regimens that combine these agents, while carefully balancing their risks and benefits, allow for a more individualized approach to pain control, potentially enhancing patient recovery while minimizing adverse effects.

Acute Pain Service

For years, acute postoperative pain has been underemphasized in patient care, despite evidence showing that a significant percentage of patients endure moderate-to-severe pain following surgery. Effective pain management requires a specialized team that can assess pain levels, consider each patient's comorbidities, and navigate the side effects of various analgesics. This need led to the development of the Acute Pain Services (APS), a multidisciplinary team ideally comprising anesthesiologists, surgeons, and nurses, with anesthesiologists playing a central role due to their expertise in regional anesthesia and pharmacotherapy.

The APS pathway begins with a preoperative assessment to establish a personalized pain management plan. This collaborative, patient-centered approach allows the APS team and surgeons to work together, placing patients at the center of care. By identifying factors such as anxiety, chronic pain, or prior opioid use early, the team can tailor pain strategies to individual needs, promote nonopioid options, and set realistic expectations. This proactive engagement helps patients and families take an active role in their care, enhancing recovery and supporting effective pain management throughout the surgical process. It then extends through the postoperative period; the APS team does consistent pain assessment and side effect monitoring. Standardized tools, such as the Numeric Rating Scale, Visual Analogue Scale, Wong Baker Scale, and FLACC (Face, Legs, Activity, Cry, Consolability) scale, are crucial for this evaluation, providing reliable feedback for pain interventions.

Persistent Postsurgical Pain

Chronic pain is a known complication following nearly all types of surgery, with a particularly high prevalence (>20%) in areas that are frequently operated on in oncology, such as the breast, thorax, and spine.[8,31] The high rates of persistent pain after cancer surgery are often attributed to iatrogenic nerve injury, though other factors—including central sensitization and preexisting pain in the operated area—also play significant roles in its development.

The pathophysiology of persistent postsurgical pain (PPSP) is complex, with multiple contributing factors, making it challenging to establish definitive preventive strategies. The current research is limited by small sample sizes and methodological inconsistencies, and recent meta-analyses have not been able to draw conclusive recommendations.[32] Nevertheless, PPSP presents an opportunity for perioperative intervention. For anesthetists and pain specialists, targeting identifiable risk factors during the acute perioperative period (preoperative, intraoperative, and immediate postoperative phases) is essential to minimizing the incidence and impact of PPSP.

The recognition of PPSP as a distinct diagnosis in the International Classification of Diseases 11th Revision (ICD-11) highlights the significant clinical challenge it poses.[33,34] Effective management requires a multidisciplinary, holistic approach that integrates pharmacotherapy, targeted pain or surgical interventions, and psychological support. Addressing PPSP through such a comprehensive strategy has the potential to mitigate its biopsychosocial impacts, improving quality of life and long-term outcomes for cancer surgery patients.

Transitional Pain Service

The concept of the Transitional Pain Service (TPS), developed in 2014, emerged to address PPSP by providing a structured, interdisciplinary approach to pain management that extends beyond the immediate postoperative phase.[35] The TPS has three primary goals: (1) To proactively manage pain for patients at risk of CPSP or pain-related disability; (2) to oversee opioid management, especially for medically complex patients after discharge; and (3) to support patient coping and overall quality of life through improved functioning. TPS bridges the perioperative continuum, offering continued support to patients for up to 6 months post-discharge, facilitating a smoother transition from acute to long-term pain management, while also focusing on personalized opioid-tapering plans.

A typical TPS team includes a diverse set of professionals such as anesthesiologists, pain specialists, pain nurse practitioners, psychologists, physiotherapists, and care coordinators. This team provides three core interventions: (1) Acute postoperative pain control with multimodal analgesia and careful opioid use, aimed at reducing long-term dependence; (2) nonpharmacological therapies such as physiotherapy and yoga to support recovery; and (3) psychological interventions, including patient education and cognitive behavioral therapy based on the acceptance and commitment model, to help patients cope with pain and stress.

The TPS model aims to close the traditional gaps in postoperative pain management, where the responsibility often shifts among various providers—surgeons, anesthesiologists, pain nurses, and primary care physicians. By identifying at-risk patients, such as those with high preoperative opioid use, substance abuse history, uncontrolled postoperative pain, or psychological risk factors such as anxiety, depression, and pain catastrophizing, TPS works to prevent acute pain from progressing to CPSP. Ideally, vulnerable patients are referred to the TPS preoperatively by surgeons or anesthesiologists, but pathways also exist for referrals postoperatively, especially if unanticipated pain complications arise or chronic pain trajectories develop.

The impact of TPS has shown promising results in reducing postoperative opioid consumption and improving functional outcomes, although definitive evidence on reducing CPSP incidence remains limited. Future expansion of TPS, particularly through e-health and digital applications, could enhance accessibility and cost-effectiveness, making it a sustainable and far-reaching solution in managing transitional pain effectively.

CONCLUSION

In summary, modern perioperative pain management prioritizes a patient-centered, multidisciplinary approach that addresses both immediate and long-term pain relief needs. The APS streamline pain care in the immediate postoperative period, ensuring tailored, effective analgesia, while TPS provide extended support for high-risk patients to prevent chronic postsurgical pain. Through multimodal analgesia and nonpharmacological strategies, these frameworks help reduce opioid use and improve recovery outcomes. Ongoing research and technological advancements, such as digital health integration, are essential to further enhance these services, ultimately supporting better patient outcomes and quality of life in perioperative care.

REFERENCES

1. Karakousis CP. Refinements of surgical technique in oncologic surgery. J Surg Oncol. 2010;101(8):647-8.
2. Cata JP, Corrales G, Speer B, Owusu-Agyemang P. Postoperative acute pain challenges in patients with cancer. Best Pract Res Clin Anaesthesiol. 2019;33(3).
3. Bruce J, Quinlan J. Chronic Post Surgical Pain. Rev Pain. 2011;5(3):23-9.
4. Dobson GP. Trauma of major surgery: A global problem that is not going away. Int J Surg. 2020;81:47-54.
5. Gan TJ. Poorly controlled postoperative pain: prevalence, consequences, and prevention. J Pain Res. 2017;10:2287-98.
6. Apfelbaum JL, Chen C, Mehta SS, Gan TJ. Postoperative pain experience: results from a national survey suggest postoperative pain continues to be undermanaged. Anesthesia Anal. 2003;97:534-40.
7. Chou R, Gordon DB, de Leon-Casasola OA, Rosenberg JM, Bickler S, Brennan T, et al. Management of postoperative pain: A clinical practice guideline from the American pain society, the American Society of Regional Anesthesia and Pain Medicine, and the American Society of Anesthesiologists' committee on regional anesthesia, executive committee, and administrative council. J Pain. 2016;17:131-57.
8. Glare P, Aubrey K, Gulati A, Lee YC, Moryl N, Overton S. Pharmacologic Management of Persistent Pain in Cancer Survivors. Drugs. 2022;82(3):275-91.
9. Beloeil H. Opioid-free anesthesia. Best Pract Res Clin Anaesthesiol. 2019;33(3):353-60.
10. Adams TJ, Dalia Mohammed Aljohani, Forget P. Perioperative opioids: A narrative review contextualising new avenues to improve prescribing. Br J Anaesth.2023;130(6):709-18.
11. Tegeder I, Grösch S, Schmidtko A, Häussler A, Schmidt H, Niederberger E, et al. G protein-independent G1 cell cycle block and apoptosis with morphine in adenocarcinoma cells: involvement of p53 phosphorylation. Cancer Res. 2003;63(8):1846-52.
12. Yeager MP, Colacchio TA. Effect of morphine on growth of metastatic colon cancer in vivo. Arch Surg. 1991; 126(4):454-6.
13. Gach K, Wyrębska A, Fichna J, Janecka A. The role of morphine in regulation of cancer cell growth. Naunyn Schmiedebergs Arch Pharmacol. 2011;384(3):221-30.
14. Zheng J, He J, Wang W, Zhou H, Cai S, Zhu L, et al. The impact of pain and opioids use on survival in cancer patients: results from a population-based cohort study and a meta-analysis. Medicine. 2020;99(9):e19306.
15. Dockrell L, Buggy DJ. The role of regional anaesthesia in the emerging subspecialty of onco-anaesthesia: a state-of-the-art review. Anaesthesia. 2021;76(S1):148-59.
16. Myles PS, Peyton P, Silbert B, Hunt J, Rigg JRA, Sessler DI; ANZCA Trials Group Investigators. Perioperative epidural analgesia for major abdominal surgery for cancer and recurrence-free survival: Randomised trial. Br Med J. 2011; 342: d1491.

17. Heinrich S, Janitz K, Merkel S, Klein P, Schmidt J. Short- and long term effects of epidural analgesia on morbidity and mortality of esophageal cancer surgery. Langenbeck's Arch Surg. 2015;400:19-26.
18. Li W, Li Y, Huang Q, Ye S, Rong T. Short and long-term outcomes of epidural or intravenous analgesia after esophagectomy: a propensity-matched cohort study. PLoS One. 2016;11:e0154380.
19. Felling DR, Jackson MW, Ferraro J, Battaglia MA, Albright JJ, Wu J, et al. Liposomal bupivacaine transversus abdominis plane block versus epidural analgesia in a colon and rectal surgery enhanced recovery pathway: A randomized clinical trial. Dis Colon Rectum. 2018;61(10):1196-204.
20. Holtz M, Liao N, Lin JH, Asche CV. Economic outcomes and incidence of postsurgical hypotension with liposomal bupivacaine vs epidural analgesia in abdominal surgeries. J Health Econ Outcomes Res. 2019;9(2):86-94.
21. Marciniak D, Kelava M, Hargrave J. Fascial plane blocks in thoracic surgery: a new era or plain painful? Curr Opin Anaesthesiol. 2020;33(1):1-9.
22. Carver A, Wou F, Pawa A. Do outcomes differ between thoracic epidurals and continuous fascial plane blocks in adults undergoing major abdominal surgery? Curr Anesthesiol Rep. 2024;14:25-41.
23. Parab SY, Gaikwad S. Unlocking precision pain relief: The rise of fascial plane blocks in perioperative care: A commentary. Indian J Anaesth. 2024;68(9):828-31.
24. Khatib S, Razvi SSN, Shaikh MM, Khan MM. In: Ng-Pellegrino A, Stawicki SP. Acute post-operative pain management. Updates in Anesthesia—The Operating Room and Beyond. USA: Intechopen.com; 2023.
25. Small C, Laycock H. Acute postoperative pain management. Br J Surg. 2020;107(2):70-80.
26. Lydrup M-L, Rutegård J, Matthiessen P, Rutegård M. Nonsteroidal anti-inflammatory drugs and the risk of anastomotic leakage after anterior resection for rectal cancer. Eur J Surg Oncol. 2017;43:1908-14.
27. Huang Y, Tang SR, Young CJ. Nonsteroidal anti-inflammatory drugs and anastomotic dehiscence after colorectal surgery: a meta-analysis. ANZ J Surg. 2018;88:959-65.
28. Apfel CC, Turan A, Souza K, Pergolizzi J, Hornuss C. Intravenous acetaminophen reduces postoperative nausea and vomiting: a systematic review and meta-analysis. Pain. 2013;154:677-89.
29. Dart RC, Bailey E. Does therapeutic use of acetaminophen cause acute liver failure? Pharmacotherapy. 2007;27:1219-30.
30. Verret M, Lauzier F, Zarychanski R, Perron C, Savard X, Pinard AM; the Canadian Perioperative Anesthesia Clinical Trials (PACT) Group. Perioperative Use of gabapentinoids for the management of postoperative acute pain: A systematic review and meta-analysis. Anesthesiology. 2020;:265-79.
31. Denk F, McMahon SB, Tracey I. Pain vulnerability: A neurobiological perspective. Nat Neurosci. 2014; 17(2):192-200.
32. Carley ME, Chaparro LE, Choinière M, Kehlet H, Moore RA, Kerkhof EVD, et al. Pharmacotherapy for the prevention of chronic pain after surgery in adults: an updated systematic review and meta-analysis. Anesthesiology. 2021;135:304e25.
33. Treede RD, Rief W, Barke A, Aziz Q, Bennett MI, Benoliel R, et al. Chronic pain as a symptom or a disease: the IASP Classification of Chronic Pain for the International Classification of Diseases (ICD-11). Pain. 2019;160(1):19-27.
34. Schug SA, Lavand'Homme P, Barke A, Korwisi B, Rief W, Treede RD, et al. The IASP classification of chronic pain for ICD-11: Chronic postsurgical or post traumatic pain. Pain. 2019;160:45-52.
35. Klimke R, Ott A, Romero CS, Berendes A, Urman RD, Luedi MM, et al. Transitional pain service: An update. Curr Pain Headache Rep. 2024;28:457-64.

57 CHAPTER

Assessment Tools for Cancer Pain

Mohd Shazrul M Ramly, Donal J Buggy

INTRODUCTION

Epidemiology of Cancer Pain

More than 50% of patients with cancer will experience pain at any stage during their diagnosis. The majority of these patients are undergoing active treatment for their disease. A higher percentage of these patients with pain have metastatic or advanced disease.

There is a spectrum of severity of pain in this population. Moderate or severe pain occurs in approximately 35% of patients with cancer diagnoses but can be as high as 80% in patients with advanced cancer diagnoses. The severity of pain can, and will, affect their ability to function—whether basic tasks as activity of daily living or their ability to enjoy those activities.

The study showed that 66% of patients with cancer diagnosis present to the emergency department with pain as their primary problem.[1] When presenting to palliative care, 68% of patients with advanced cancer reported pain as the primary complaint.

Thus, pain in cancer is a huge financial, psychological, and medical burden to the healthcare system and globally. The World Health Organization (WHO) and the International Agency for Research on Cancer (IARC) estimated 20 million new cancer cases and 9.7 million deaths worldwide in 2022. By 2050, it is predicted that 35 million new cancer cases will be diagnosed, an increase of 77% from 2022 estimation.[2]

The challenge with cancer pain is with the diagnosis, evaluation and assessment tools, and the treatment modality options available to patients. To date, there is no universally accepted pain assessment tool for cancer pain, reflecting the complexity of pain, added by the heterogeneity of cancer types and thus the difficulty of having one tool that fits all. In this chapter, we will first explore the neurophysiology of pain and cancer pain syndromes, followed by the assessment tools and the challenges in assessing cancer pain and pain syndromes.

Cancer Pain Definition and Etiology

In 1986, the first WHO analgesic ladder (or pain ladder) was published for the management of cancer pain. Now, the analgesic ladder is being used worldwide among medical practitioners to guide pain management in all areas of medicine. As the specialty of pain and oncology evolves with the advancement in medical science, so does the understanding of pathophysiology and options for therapeutic interventions.

In 1975, the International Association for the Study of Pain (IASP) subcommittee on taxonomy achieved a consensus on the classification of chronic pain syndromes, for both malignant and nonmalignant diseases. Chronic pain syndrome is assigned a code based on five domains: Anatomical site, organ systems whose abnormal function produces the pain, temporal characteristics, pain intensity and time since onset of pain, and pain etiology. This classification is a physician-based assessment, consisting of patient's medical history, physical examination, and appropriate, relevant investigations.[3]

The International Classification of Diseases-11 (ICD-11) is an update from ICD-10 with regard to the chronic pain classification. In the new classification, chronic cancer-related pain, along with several other chronic pain syndromes, is categorized as chronic secondary pain.[4] Chronic pain is defined as the pain that persists or recurs for >3 months. The associated disease burden from chronic pain includes functional impairment and disability, emotional distress, and direct and indirect societal and financial costs. Chronic cancer pain is defined as the chronic pain caused by the primary cancer itself or metastases (chronic cancer pain) or its treatment (chronic postcancer treatment pain).[4] There is not necessarily a correlation between the severity of pain and the severity of the disease.

The update is partly due to the fact that chronic cancer-related pain was not represented in ICD-10.

The chronic pain classification in ICD-10 did not reflect the biopsychosocial model of pain, plus chronic cancer-related pain, chronic neuropathic pain, and chronic pain after surgery or trauma were all consolidated into one category. Giving the different chronic pain their own classification will help improve the understanding of chronic pain and its global burden.

Prior to 2020, the IASP definition of *pain* was using the recommendation by the Subcommittee on Taxonomy and adopted by the IASP Council in 1979. In 2018, the IASP formed a Presidential Task Force to evaluate the current definition of *pain* and ultimately recommended the *pain* definition to be revised. The new definition and accompanying notes were accepted by the IASP Council in 2020.

Pain is defined as "an unpleasant sensory and emotional experience associated with, or resembling that associated with, actual or potential tissue damage".[5] The above definition recommended by the IASP is expanded upon six keynotes and the etymology of the word *pain* to provide context.

- Pain is a personal experience that is influenced to varying degrees by biological, psychosocial, and social factors.
- Pain and nociception are different phenomena; thus, pain cannot be inferred solely from the activities in sensory neurons.
- Individuals learn the concept of pain through personal life experiences.
- A person's report of pain experience should be respected.
- Pain usually serves as an adaptive role, but it may have adverse effects on function, social, and psychological well-being.
- Verbal description is only one of the several behaviors to express pain; as such, the inability to communicate does not negate the possibility of pain experience.

Cancer pain can be nociceptive (arising from visceral or somatic) or neuropathic. More commonly, pain experienced in patients with cancer is mixed in nature. Cancer pain can be intermittent or continuous.

There are multiple etiologies for cancer pain:[6]

- *Pain from local mass effect:* Cancer growth can produce local inflammation, compression, edema, and ischemia of surrounding tissues. These can affect neural and nonneural tissue, including bone. Cancer cells release inflammatory mediators including interleukins, leukotrienes, prostaglandins, histamine, bradykinins, and tumor necrosis factor (TNF)-alpha. These mediators also act as pain-producing substances toward local tissues. Local swelling will impede blood oxygen and nutrient supply, thus causing ischemic pain of the affected tissue.
- *Pain as a result of treatment:* These include chronic postsurgical pain, radiation-induced neuritis, plexopathy, and peripheral neuropathy from chemotherapeutic agents.
- *Paraneoplastic phenomena:* Peripheral neuropathy or poly-/mononeuritis from the production of anti-Hu and anti-Yo neuronal antibodies, anti-CV2, and antiamphiphysin antibodies[7]. Subacute sensory neuronopathy associated with the anti-Hu antibody is the most frequently seen peripheral neuropathy.[8] Peripheral nerve involvement can be in the form of sensory neuronopathy, sensory neuropathy, polyradiculopathy, and neuromyotonia.
- *Pain from associated conditions:* Pain from infection, immunosuppression-induced herpetic reactivation, hypercalcemia and bone pain, osteoporosis and pathological fracture bone pain, and pain from prolonged immobility.

Patients with cancer also may suffer from pre-existing pain conditions, for example, chronic lower back pain, fibromyalgia, and diabetic neuropathy. These pain conditions are beyond the scope of this chapter; however, it is pertinent to approach cancer pain in a holistic manner that includes and considers pre-existing conditions to better evaluate and manage pain in cancer patients.

CANCER PAIN SYNDROMES

The constellation of symptoms and signs may suggest a specific cancer pain syndrome. The identification of these syndromes may aid in determining the etiology of the pain experienced, help direct diagnostic evaluation, and then further clarify prognosis of the pain or even the disease itself, and thus guide therapeutic management and intervention.

Broadly, cancer pain syndromes can be categorized as acute and chronic.[9]

Acute Cancer Pain Syndrome

Acute pain syndromes in cancer are related to either the diagnostic or therapeutic intervention for the cancer (iatrogenic), or due to the disease itself.

These include (but not limited to):

- *Acute postoperative pain:* Laparoscopic shoulder tip pain, laparotomy pain
- *Acute postdiagnostic intervention pain:* Postlumbar puncture back pain and dural puncture headache and pain from bone marrow biopsy
- *Acute post-therapeutic procedural pain:* Pleurodesis pain, tumor embolization, and nephrostomy/chest drain/percutaneous cholecystostomy pain
- *Acute pain from cancer treatment:*
  - Acute pain from chemotherapeutic agent infusion
  - Chemotherapy toxicity: Mucositis, arthralgia, peripheral neuropathy, and headache
- Acute pain associated with opportunistic infection, such as herpetic neuralgia
- *Acute pain from vascular events:* Limb pain from deep venous thrombosis and pleuritic chest pain from pulmonary embolism
- *Pain from pathological bone fracture:* Femoral fracture, vertebral compression fracture, rib fracture, and avascular necrosis of femoral head.

Chronic Cancer Pain Syndrome

Chronic cancer pain syndromes can be related to the cancer itself or secondary to the cancer therapy.

These include (but not limited to):

- Cancer-related multifocal or generalized bone pain from metastases or marrow infiltration and expansion
- Facial neuralgia and headache from intracerebral tumor, leptomeningeal involvement and metastases, and trigeminal neuralgia
- Cancer involvement of the peripheral nervous system causing radiculopathy and plexopathy, postherpetic neuralgia, mononeuropathy, and sensorimotor peripheral neuropathy
- Pain syndrome from visceral involvement causing chronic intestinal obstruction, liver distension, pain from peritoneal carcinomatosis, and ureteric obstruction
- Pain syndromes secondary to cancer therapy, such as chronic peripheral neuropathy, femoral and humeral head avascular necrosis, gynecomastia pain from prostate cancer hormonal therapy, postmastectomy pain, postneck dissection pain, post-thoracotomy pain, phantom limb pain, and amputation stump pain
- Pain syndrome after radiation treatment, such as radiation-induced plexopathy, peripheral neuropathy, radiation enteritis and proctitis, and osteoradionecrosis.

PAIN ASSESSMENT TOOLS

General Pain Assessment Tools

The pain assessment starts with a comprehensive pain history and relevant clinical examination. A thorough history and examination are essential in characterizing pain and identifying the underlying pain mechanism. This will then facilitate the decision-making process regarding medical treatment or interventional approach.

The *SOCRATES* mnemonic is useful in the clinical setting and provides a systematic approach to assessing pain characteristics (Site, Onset, Character, Radiation, Associated factors, Timing, Exacerbating/relieving factors, and Severity). Among the eight characteristics in the mnemonic, it is worth further exploring three of them in more detail.

Pain intensity—exploring pain intensity provides a guide as to the severity of the pain and often aids treatment option decisions. The most frequent scale used to measure pain intensity is the numeric rating scale (NRS). Generally, pain severity is categorized into mild (NRS 1–4), moderate (5–6), and severe (7–10). Changes in the NRS score help evaluate response to treatment and changes in the patient clinical status from intervention.

Pain site—it is not uncommon that patients with cancer present with more than one pain site, especially in advanced disease. Anatomical location can guide which of the pain sites is the most debilitating to patient's function. Using a body map to document the multiple pain sites (and pain intensity) can help evaluate response to treatment.

Timing and temporal variation—pain can be continuous (or background pain) or intermittent. Transient pain occurring on stable background pain is known now as *transient cancer pain exacerbation* (previously termed *breakthrough pain*).[10] Frequent transient cancer pain exacerbation can be a sign of a new or progression of disease.

Investigations for Pain Assessment

Laboratory Investigations

- Platelet count is important as thrombocytopenia will limit interventional procedures available for patients
- Renal, liver profile for medication dosing adjustments and clearance

Radiological and Neurophysiological Investigations

- Bone X-rays to diagnose acute pathological fractures
- Computed tomography (CT) and magnetic resonance imaging (MRI) for local cancer progression, invasion into surrounding tissues, and evidence of bone metastases
- Nuclear medicine bone scan to assess the extent of metastatic involvement of cancer
- Electromyography (EMG) and nerve conduction study (NCS) for evaluating muscle and nerve involvements and distinguishing between muscular or neurogenic pain

UNIDIMENSIONAL PAIN ASSESSMENT TOOL

Unidimensional pain tools mainly assess the intensity of pain and the effect of treatment following an intervention. Unidimensional tools are easy and quick to use, and they are widely used on a daily basis.[11]

- *Visual Analog Scale (VAS):* This was first used by Hayes and Patterson in 1921.[12] It is a self-reported measure of pain intensity. This is the most common pain scale quantification tool, and it is widely used. It is considered to be the best tool to measure the intensity of acute pain.[13]

  It contains a 10-cm line, with two endpoints representing 0 (no pain) and 10 (worst possible pain). The patient is asked to place a mark on the line of their current pain level. The distance from the "no pain" end to the current patient's mark represents the intensity score of pain.

  Example: 6 cm from "no pain" mark represents 6/10 pain.

  The use of this scale has been studied in cancer patients.[14]
- *Numeric rating scale and verbal rating scale (VRS):* The NRS is another unidimensional, patient self-reporting pain tool.

  It is an 11-point scale, with "0" representing "no pain" and "10" representing "severe, disabling pain".

  The NRS is almost similar to the VAS, in which it is a unidimensional scale, bounded on the left of the scale with "no pain" and on the right of the scale with "worst imaginable pain". The difference with the VAS is that, instead of an unmarked straight line, the NRS is marked with numbers 0–10, spread evenly across the line.

  Patients are instructed to circle (or mark) the number that represents their pain at the time of evaluation. A variation of the NRS, the VRS, is when the tool is used verbally—when patients are asked to state their pain intensity on a scale of 0–10. The reported number represents the pain intensity.

  This tool has been studied in cancer patients.[15]

MULTIDIMENSIONAL PAIN ASSESSMENT TOOL

Multidimensional assessment scales evaluate and assess the complexity of pain sensation, not just the severity or intensity of pain at the time of assessment. These scales take into consideration of the intensity of the pain, location, sensory qualities, and the psychological or physical effects on the patient's activities.[11]

- *Edmonton Symptom Assessment Scale (ESAS):* This was developed in 1991 and has now been validated in over 20 languages worldwide. The ESAS has been used in clinical inpatient and outpatient practice and in research areas of pain, palliative medicine, and oncology. It can be reported by the patient or by their caregiver. The use of ESAS provides a longitudinal symptom monitoring tool and provides insight into the progression and trajectory of disease in cancer patients.[16] The ESAS has been used as a predictive model for emergency department visits, determining symptoms associated with decreased quality of life and thus potentially improving symptom management and preventing overtreatment for patients nearing their end of life from the disease.[17]

  The ESAS tool assesses not only pain but also physical activity, nausea, depression, anxiety, drowsiness, appetite, sensation of well-being, and dyspnea in a cancer patient. The ESAS assesses these eight domains and on a VAS, ranging from 0 to 10 (0—absence of symptoms and 10—worse possible severity). The tool also consists of the front and back of a human figure where the patient can mark the area they feel most discomfort. This will also aid in localizing the pain and subsequently focusing the pain management toward the affected area.

- *MD Anderson Symptom Inventory (MDASI):* This is a multisymptom patient-reported outcome questionnaire. The MDASI evaluates 13 core items which include symptoms most found or severe in patients with different cancer and treatment types.[18] These 13 core items are pain, fatigue (tiredness), nausea, disturbed sleep, distress/feeling upset, shortness of breath, difficulty remembering, lack of appetite, drowsiness, dry mouth, sadness, vomiting and sensation of numbness or tingling. The interference items assess how those symptoms interfere with six aspects of patient's daily functioning: daily activity, mood, work, relationship with others, walking, and enjoyment of life.[19] The MDASI assesses the severity of symptoms and the interfering effects of those symptoms toward patient's activity of daily living. The MDASI has been used to evaluate pain and other associated symptoms over a range of cancer diagnoses. Like most assessment tools, the MDASI uses a scale of 0–10 to assess the severity of each symptom (0—not present and 10—worse possible severity), and a scale of 0–10 to assess the interference (0—did not interfere and 10—interfered completely). The MDASI has been translated and validated to multiple languages.
- *Memorial Symptom Assessment Scale (MSAS):* This is another multidimensional tool to assess pain in cancer patients. The MSAS was first introduced as a tool to assess pain and other symptoms in cancer patients in 1994.[20] This scale has been translated and validated to multiple different languages worldwide. A short version of the MSAS (MSAS-SF) measures only the severity and frequency of the symptoms.[21]

  A total of 24 symptoms are listed, and the patient can self-report or symptoms can be reported by their caregiver by filling in the proforma. The symptoms assessed are ones that have occurred during the previous week, including how those symptoms have interfered with their activities.

  The questions focus on the severity and frequency of the symptoms and how much those symptoms distress or bother the patients in the last week prior to the assessment. This tool comprises three major symptom groups: Psychological symptoms, high-prevalence physical symptoms, and low-prevalence physical symptoms.

  For each symptom, the patient marks between 0 and 4 for the severity and frequency (0—no symptoms and 4—very much).
- *Edmonton Classification System for Cancer Pain (ECS-CP):* This assessment instrument has been validated to be used for cancer pain assessment.[22]

  This tool consists of five features: Mechanism of pain, incident pain, psychological distress, addictive behavior, and cognitive function **(Table 1)**.[23]

  The ECS-CP is a physician-rated assessment, based on clinical findings from history, physical examination, patient reports of symptoms, medical records, available diagnostic radiological information, and collateral history from caregivers and family members.

  The ECS-CP scoring is different than most assessment tools, where the completed ECS-CP profile will give a sense of the pain and the effect of the pain on patient's psychosocial domain. There are many possible combinations of the ECS-CP profile.

  Example of an ECS-CP profile: NcIiPoAaCo—nociceptive pain, incident pain present, no psychological distress, addictive behavior present, and normal cognition.[24]
- *Cancer Pain Prognostic Scale (CPPS):* This scale was developed as a prognostic tool for the prediction of pain relief in cancer patients.[3,25] There are four domains, all mainly through self-reporting by patients. It includes an 11-point severity scale (0—no pain and

TABLE 1: Edmonton classification system for cancer pain.

Mechanism of pain	• No • Nc • Ne • Nx	• No pain syndrome • Any nociceptive pain • Neuropathic pain syndrome • Insufficient information to classify
Incident pain	• Io • Ii • Ix	• No incident pain • Incident pain present • Insufficient information to classify
Psychological distress	• Po • Pp • Px	• No psychological distress • Psychological distress present • Insufficient information to classify
Addictive behavior	• Ao • Aa • Ax	• No addictive behavior • Addictive behavior present • Insufficient information to classify
Cognitive function	• Co • Ci • Cu • Cx	• No impairment. Able to provide accurate present and pass pain history • Partial impairment, affecting patient's ability to provide accurate present/past pain history • Total impairment—patient demented, delirious, or unresponsive • Insufficient information to classify

10—worse pain) for pain, emotional well-being from the functional assessment for cancer therapy (FACT-G), daily opioid dose of >60 mg, and the presence of mixed pain. The scale is graded numerically from 0 to 17, with a higher score corresponding to a higher probability of pain relief within 2 weeks for moderate to severe pain.

There has been only one study that adopted this tool.

- *Edinburgh Pain Assessment and Management Tool (EPAT):* The EPAT was developed by Fallon et al. in 2018 as a clinician-delivered bedside assessment tool for cancer patients.[26,27] The EPAT is incorporated into the vital signs chart of the patient.

  The proforma is divided into four main sections: Managing cancer pain, managing breakthrough cancer pain, managing cancer-induced bone pain, and managing cancer neuropathic pain. The EPAT tool also consists of a treatment review chart to document the effects of intervention, including a section on opioid toxicity; a dose titration guide for opioids; a guide for As required (PRN) administration guide for opioids; and a guide for starting amitriptyline or gabapentin for neuropathic pain.

  The use of this tool has shown improvements in the pain outcome in cancer patients with moderate to severe pain. The use of EPAT did not increase opioid-related adverse effects.
- *Brief Pain Inventory (BPI):* This is a questionnaire used to evaluate pain, specifically developed by the Pain Research Group of the WHO Collaborating Centre for Symptom Evaluation in Cancer Care. Although initially developed as an assessment tool for cancer pain, it is now used widely even for noncancer pain conditions.[28]

  The questionnaire is divided into two dimensions: Pain intensity and pain interference. In the pain intensity section, pain is further assessed into four categories: Worst, least, on average, and currently. In the pain interference section, pain is assessed into two further dimensions: Activity interference (general physical aspect of activity) and affective interference (emotional aspect of pain). Pain interference is measured in seven categories: Mood, work, general activity, walking, relationship, enjoyment of life, and sleep.

  Patients are asked to rate their pain on a scale of 0–10 for pain intensity and pain interference (0—no pain/no interference and 10—worse pain/maximum interference). The front and back of a human figure are also incorporated into the form for patients to shade areas representing where they feel pain, and for patients to mark "X" at the area of most pain.

  The BPI has been validated in several different languages for the assessment of pain. A short version (short form) of the Brief Pain Inventory is also available (BPI-SF).
- *McGill Pain Questionnaire (McGill Pain Index):* This scale was developed in 1975 by Ronald Melzack and Warren Torgerson. It is a self-report questionnaire for patients to describe the quality and intensity of their pain.[29] A list of 78 descriptor words related to pain is presented in 20 sections. The sections signify different components of pain: Sensory, affective, evaluative, and miscellaneous. The score is the sum of all the values associated with each word. Scores range from 0 to 78 (representing severe pain).

  Patients circle the best word that describes their pain in each category.

  A short-form version of the questionnaire (SF-MPQ) is also available and commonly used.
- *Total Pain Scale (TPS)*: This new scale was developed and introduced to be used in India in 2023 by Singh.[30] It contains 18 items sectioned into four domains (physical: four items, social: five items, spiritual: four items, and psychological: five items). It was first developed in Hindi language. The questionnaire takes 5 minutes to complete. All the items are scored between 0 and 10 (0—no symptom and 10—worse level of symptom).

BIOPSYCHOSOCIAL ASSESSMENT OF CANCER PAIN

The assessment of pain and cancer pain has evolved significantly over the years. The introduction of the biopsychosocial pain model has improved the way pain is understood and assessed, especially in chronic settings. The biopsychosocial model incorporates the interconnection between pain biology, psychology, and socioenvironmental factors affecting pain perception.[31]

The term *biopsychosocial* was first coined in 1977 by George Engel. The biopsychosocial approach of pain management is to relieve physical pain, increase movement, and improve function. This will include interdisciplinary work including psychiatry, psychology, physiotherapy, occupational therapy, and pain management team. The treatment plan is individualized and tailored to suit each patient, based on their physical, psychological, and social circumstances and needs.

Domains such as anxiety and depression, fatigue, and substance use may affect how pain is perceived, how well the pain is controlled, and how the patient's social and mental health are disturbed due to pain. By assessing these domains, clinicians and pain specialists will be able to gauge the level of how much each domain plays a significant factor in pain experience. Pain experienced by someone who is optimistic and has a strong social support will differ from that experienced by someone who has undergone psychological trauma and is living in poor socioeconomic circumstances.

The tools available may also aid in managing expectations of pain control and agreeing upon a common goal for management and accepted therapy results.

Examples of questionnaires related to pain which have been used to assess domains other than pain, following the biopsychosocial pain model approach, are mentioned in **Table 2**.

TABLE 2: Overview of assessment tools for various domains.

Tool	*Domain assessed*	*Description of tool*
PEG[32]	Pain intensity and pain interference	This is a three-item instrument assessing pain and the effect of pain on patient's enjoyment and general activity
Generalized anxiety disorder 2-item (GAD-2)[33]	Anxiety	This tool is to screen and assess patient's frequency and anxiety and worry
Patient Health Questionnaire 2-item (PHQ-2)[33]	Depression	This tool assesses patient's feeling of depression and anhedonia
Visual Analog Fatigue Scale	Fatigue	This tool assesses the severity of patient's fatigue on an 11-point scale (0–10)
Tobacco, alcohol, prescription medication, and other substance use tool (TAPS)	Substance use	This is a screening questionnaire tool, assessing the frequency of substance use, and experience with substance use (flagging potential concerns)

(PEG: pain, enjoyment, and general activity)

CONCLUSION

Since the introduction of the WHO Pain Ladder in 1986, there has been an increase in the development of pain assessment tools, for cancer and noncancer conditions alike. Many of these assessment tools have been updated to align with medical and technological advancements in pain medicine and pain service.

More and more assessment tools have been developed for cancer pain, although the utility of these tools depends on the institutions and physicians' preferences. Furthermore, the trend is moving toward multidimensional assessment tools, incorporating psychosocial assessment, and not only concentrating on pain, but also the psychological and physical burden pain exerts on the quality of life of cancer patients. There is no tool universally preferred to be used in cancer patients. This reflects the complexity of the disease, the heterogeneity of patient cohort and cancer disease, and the vast area of therapeutic approaches and interventions available for cancer patients.

REFERENCES

1. Fleshner L, Lagree A, Shiner A, Alera MA, Bielecki M, Grant R, et al. Drivers of emergency department use among oncology patients in the era of novel cancer therapeutics: a systematic review. Oncologist. 2023;28(12):1020-33.
2. Bray F, Laversanne M, Sung H, Ferlay J, Siegel RL, Soerjomataram I, et al. Global cancer statistics 2022: GLOBOCAN estimates of incidence and mortality worldwide for 36 cancers in 185 countries. CA Cancer J Clin. 2024;74(3):229-63.
3. Situ D, Wang J, Shao W, Zhu ZH. Assessment and treatment of cancer pain: from Western to Eastern. Ann Palliat Med. 2012;1(1):32-44.
4. Bennett MI, Kaasa S, Barke A, Korwisi B, Rief W, Treede RD, et al. The IASP classification of chronic pain for ICD-11: chronic cancer-related pain. Pain. 2019;160(1):38-44.
5. Raja SN, Carr DB, Cohen M, Finnerup NB, Flor H, Gibson S, et al. The revised International Association for the Study of Pain definition of pain: concepts, challenges, and compromises. Pain. 2020;161(9):1976-82.
6. Scott-Warren JB A. Cancer pain management-part i: general principles. Continuing Education in Anaesthesia, Critical Care & Pain. 2014;14:278-84.
7. Camdessanche JP, Antoine JC, Honnorat J, Vial C, Petiot P, Convers P, et al. Paraneoplastic peripheral neuropathy associated with anti-Hu antibodies. A clinical and electrophysiological study of 20 patients. Brain. 2002; 125(Pt 1):166-75.
8. Zoccarato M, Grisold W, Grisold A, Poretto V, Boso F, Giometto B. Paraneoplastic neuropathies: what's new since

the 2004 recommended diagnostic criteria. Front Neurol. 2021;12:706169.
9. Kocoglu H, Pirbudak L, Pence S, Balat O. Cancer pain, pathophysiology, characteristics and syndromes. Eur J Gynaecol Oncol. 2002;23(6):527-32.
10. Caraceni A, Shkodra M. Cancer pain assessment and classification. Cancers (Basel). 2019;11(4):510.
11. Crisman E, Appenzeller-Herzog C, Tabakovic S, Nickel CH, Minotti B. Multidimensional versus unidimensional pain scales for the assessment of analgesic requirement in the emergency department: a systematic review. Intern Emerg Med. 2024;19(5):1463-71.
12. Delgado DA, Lambert BS, Boutris N, McCulloch PC, Robbins AB, Moreno MR, et al. Validation of digital visual analog scale pain scoring with a traditional paper-based visual analog scale in adults. J Am Acad Orthop Surg Glob Res Rev. 2018;2(3):e088.
13. Breivik H. Fifty years on the Visual Analogue Scale (VAS) for pain-intensity is still good for acute pain. But multidimensional assessment is needed for chronic pain. Scand J Pain. 2016;11:150-2.
14. Hjermstad MJ, Fayers PM, Haugen DF, Caraceni A, Hanks GW, Loge JH, et al. Studies comparing Numerical Rating Scales, Verbal Rating Scales, and Visual Analogue Scales for assessment of pain intensity in adults: a systematic literature review. J Pain Symptom Manage. 2011;41(6):1073-93.
15. Kim HJ, Jung SO. Comparative evaluations of single-item pain-intensity measures in cancer patients: numeric rating scale vs. verbal rating scale. J Clin Nurs. 2020;29(15-16):2945-52.
16. Hui D, Bruera E. The Edmonton Symptom Assessment System 25 years later: past, present, and future developments. J Pain Symptom Manage. 2017;53(3):630-43.
17. Milton L, Behroozian T, Coburn N, Trudeau M, Razvi Y, McKenzie E, et al. Prediction of breast cancer-related outcomes with the Edmonton Symptom Assessment Scale: a literature review. Support Care Cancer. 2021;29(2):595-603.
18. Cleeland CS, Mendoza TR, Wang XS, Chou C, Harle MT, Morrissey M, et al. Assessing symptom distress in cancer patients: the M.D. Anderson Symptom Inventory. Cancer 2000;89:1634-46.
19. Sailors MH, Bodurka DC, Gning I, Ramondetta LM, Williams LA, Mendoza TR, et al. Validating the M. D. Anderson Symptom Inventory (MDASI) for use in patients with ovarian cancer. Gynecol Oncol. 2013;130(2):323-8.
20. Portenoy RK, Thaler HT, Kornblith AB, Lepore JM, Friedlander-Klar H, Kiyasu E, et al. The Memorial Symptom Assessment Scale: an instrument for the evaluation of symptom prevalence, characteristics and distress. Eur J Cancer. 1994;30A(9):1326-36.
21. Chang VT, Hwang SS, Feuerman M, Kasimis BS, Thaler HT. The memorial symptom assessment scale short form (MSAS-SF). Cancer. 2000;89(5):1162-71.
22. Nekolaichuk CL, Fainsinger RL, Aass N, Hjermstad MJ, Knudsen AK, Klepstad P, et al. The Edmonton Classification System for Cancer Pain: comparison of pain classification features and pain intensity across diverse palliative care settings in eight countries. J Palliat Med. 2013;16(5):516-23.
23. Fainsinger RL, Nekolaichuk CL. A "TNM" classification system for cancer pain: the Edmonton Classification System for Cancer Pain (ECS-CP). Support Care Cancer. 2008;16(6):547-55.
24. Fainsinger R, Nekolaichuk C. Edmonton Classification System for Cancer Pain (ECS-CP) Administration Manual. 2019
25. Hwang SS, Chang VT, Fairclough DL, Kasimis B. Development of a cancer pain prognostic scale. J Pain Symptom Manage. 2002;24(4):366-78.
26. Diernberger K, Clausen E, Murray G, Wee B, Kaasa S, Hall P, et al. Cancer pain assessment and management: does an institutional approach individualise and reduce cost of care? BMJ Support Palliat Care. 2024;13(e3):e1258-64.
27. Fallon M, Walker J, Colvin L, Rodriguez A, Murray G, Sharpe M, et al. Pain management in cancer center inpatients: a cluster randomized trial to evaluate a systematic integrated approach-The Edinburgh Pain Assessment and Management Tool. J Clin Oncol. 2018;36(13):1284-90.
28. Cleeland CS, Ryan KM. Pain assessment: global use of the Brief Pain Inventory. Ann Acad Med Singap. 1994; 23(2):129-38.
29. Melzack R. The McGill pain questionnaire: from description to measurement. Anesthesiology. 2005;103(1):199-202.
30. Singh SP, Aggarwal R, Malhotra RK, Shekhar V, Singh VP, Bhatnagar S. Development and Validation of Total Pain Scale for Evaluation of Total Pain in Cancer Patients. Indian J Palliat Care. 2023;29(3):312-23.
31. Meints SM, Edwards RR. Evaluating psychosocial contributions to chronic pain outcomes. Prog Neuropsychopharmacol Biol Psychiatry. 2018;87(Pt B): 168-82.
32. Krebs EE, Lorenz KA, Bair MJ, Damush TM, Wu J, Sutherland JM, et al. Development and initial validation of the PEG, a three-item scale assessing pain intensity and interference. J Gen Intern Med. 2009;24(6):733-8.
33. Bisby MA, Karin E, Scott AJ, Dudeney J, Fisher A, Gandy M, et al. Examining the psychometric properties of brief screening measures of depression and anxiety in chronic pain: the Patient Health Questionnaire 2-item and Generalized Anxiety Disorder 2-item. Pain Pract. 2022;22(4):478-86.

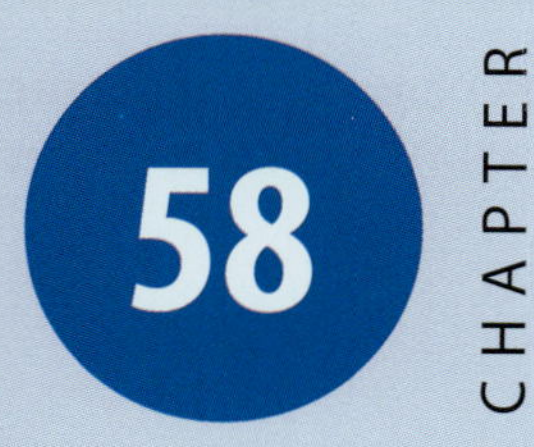

CHAPTER

Pharmacological Management of Chronic Cancer Pain

Nitika Goel, Babita Ghai

INTRODUCTION

Chronic cancer pain is a significant and pervasive issue affecting millions of cancer patients worldwide. It can severely impact quality of life, functional status, and overall well-being. Effective pain management is crucial in oncology care, and pharmacological interventions play a central role in alleviating cancer-related pain. This chapter provides a comprehensive overview of the pharmacological management of chronic cancer pain, including assessment strategies, treatment options, and considerations for special populations.

PAIN ASSESSMENT IN CANCER PATIENTS

Before initiating any pharmacological intervention, a thorough pain assessment is essential. The assessment should include:

- Pain characteristics: Intensity, location, quality, and temporal patterns
- Impact on daily activities and quality of life
- Psychosocial factors influencing pain perception
- Previous pain management strategies and their effectiveness

Several validated pain assessment tools can be used, such as:

- Numerical Rating Scale (NRS)
- Visual Analog Scale (VAS)
- Brief Pain Inventory (BPI)
- McGill Pain Questionnaire (MPQ)

Recent studies have emphasized the importance of patient-reported outcomes in pain assessment. For instance, Bico et al. demonstrated that incorporating patient-reported outcomes into routine cancer pain assessment led to improved pain management and patient satisfaction.[1]

PRINCIPLES OF PAIN MANAGEMENT

The aim is prompt treatment of pain and to prevent its recurrence. It is important to achieve realistic goals of pain relief. Example: If complete relief is not possible without precipitating side effects, at least enough relief to give a comfortable sleep at night should be aimed for. While treating a patient with cancer pain, the following principles should be taken into account:

- *By the mouth*—simple, effective, convenient, and can be taken at home
- *By the clock*—for continuous pain relief, give continuous analgesia to prevent the return of pain. Prescribing "only when needed" for a pain that is continuous is irrational, and the patient will continue to suffer.
- *By the ladder*—the three-step analgesic ladder formulated by the World Health Organization (WHO) in 1986 is a useful guideline: Stronger analgesics for increasing pain is the principle.
- *By the individual*—prescribe according to the patient's comfort and medical condition. Example: Less frequent or reduced dose in renal or hepatic dysfunction.
- *Adjuvant drugs* should be prescribed when required.

WORLD HEALTH ORGANIZATION PAIN LADDER

The WHO Pain Ladder, first introduced in 1986, remains a cornerstone in cancer pain management. The WHO ladder gives a structured, yet flexible, approach to the management of cancer pain. The steps of the ladder indicate that the process of selecting analgesics is based on the assessment of the intensity of pain experienced by the patient, rather than the etiology of the pain **(Fig. 1)**. It is also applicable in nonmalignant chronic pain situations. The analgesic ladder has subsequently been modified over time, with Vargas-Schaffer suggesting the

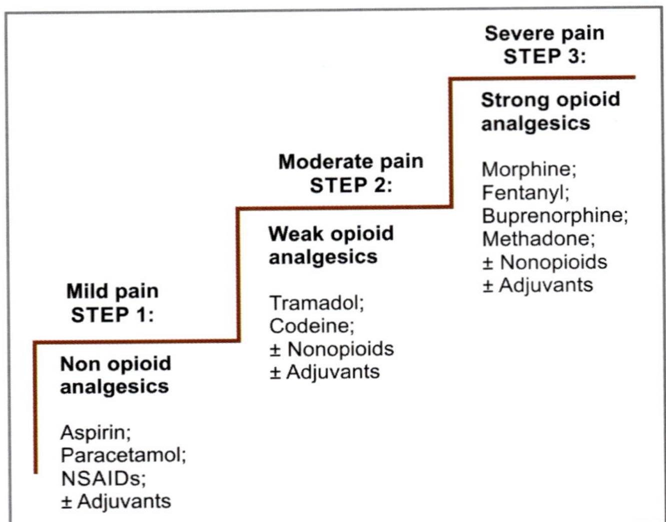

Fig. 1: WHO analgesic ladder for treating chronic cancer pain. (NSAIDs: nonsteroidal anti-inflammatory drugs; WHO: World Health Organization)

inclusion of a fourth step, which added invasive techniques to the pain management armament. Each patient should be regularly reassessed to determine response to treatment, ensure maximum benefit with as few adverse effects as possible, and maintain continuity of care. Anekar et al. documented that tailoring pain management strategies to specific cancer types and patient characteristics led to better outcomes compared to strict adherence to the WHO ladder.[2]

Notes:
- After the assessment of pain, the step necessary for the given intensity of pain can be chosen directly, without necessarily starting from the first step. Example: When pain is severe, start with step 3 (skipping the first two steps).
- Do not give two drugs from the same step. For example, do not give two different nonsteroidal anti-inflammatory drugs (NSAIDs) or two different opioids. If pain persists, move up the ladder or add appropriate adjuvants.

Step 1 Drugs

Nonsteroidal Anti-inflammatory Drugs

Nonsteroidal anti-inflammatory drugs (NSAIDs) are effective in managing mild to moderate cancer pain, particularly bone pain and inflammatory pain. They work by inhibiting cyclooxygenase (COX) enzymes, reducing prostaglandin synthesis. Common NSAIDs used in cancer pain management include:
- Ibuprofen
- Naproxen
- Diclofenac
- Celecoxib (COX-2 selective inhibitor)

Recent research has focused on the potential anticancer effects of NSAIDs. Wang et al. suggested that long-term use of NSAIDs may reduce the risk of certain cancers, particularly colorectal cancer.[3]

Acetaminophen (Paracetamol)

Acetaminophen is widely used for mild to moderate cancer pain. It has a good safety profile and can be combined with other analgesics. The exact mechanism of action is not fully understood, but it is thought to involve central inhibition of prostaglandin synthesis. A recent review demonstrated that combining acetaminophen with low-dose opioids provided effective pain relief while reducing opioid-related side effects in cancer patients.[4]

Step 2 Drugs

Opioid Analgesics

Opioids are the mainstay of moderate-to-severe cancer pain management. They act on opioid receptors in the central nervous system to modulate pain perception. Weak opioids are used for moderate pain or as an intermediate step between nonopioids and strong opioids. Recent research has focused on the genetic variations affecting codeine metabolism. Dean et al. documented that pharmacogenomic testing for CYP2D6 polymorphisms could help predict codeine efficacy and guide dosing decisions.[5]

Common weak opioids include:
- Codeine
- Tramadol
- Dihydroxycodiene

Tramadol has additional pharmacological actions to its opioid effects. It is a synthetic analog of codeine that binds to mu-opioid receptors and also inhibits norepinephrine and serotonin reuptake at the neuromuscular junction. It is rapidly absorbed after oral doses and is metabolized in the liver. It is not classed as a "controlled drug," which has some practical prescribing advantages.

Step 3 Drugs

Strong opioids are used for moderate to severe cancer pain. Recent advances in opioid formulations have led to improved pain control and reduced side effects. Abdel Shaheed et al. demonstrated that a novel extended-release hydromorphone formulation provided better around-the-clock pain control compared to immediate-release formulations, with fewer breakthrough pain episodes.[6]

Common strong opioids include:

- Morphine
- Oxycodone
- Hydromorphone
- Fentanyl
- Methadone

Morphine has been considered the gold standard for treating moderate-to-severe pain. It is the drug of choice at whatever stage of the disease the patient experiences severe pain; NOT reserved only for the terminal stage!

Example: It should be given even when a patient experiences such pain during anticancer treatment (during which time it can be tapered down and stopped as the pain gets relieved with disease control).

Pharmacology:

- Morphine is the principal medical alkaloid of opium derived from the poppy plant.
- Pure agonist. Acts at the opioid receptors in the central nervous system (brain and spinal cord).
- Oral preparation is only one third bioavailable.
- Metabolized mainly in the liver into morphine-3-glucuronide (M3G) and morphine-6-glucuronide (M6G), which are excreted in the urine. M3G does not have a role in analgesia. M6G has analgesic action and is more potent than morphine; hence, caution is needed in prescribing to those with renal dysfunction. It may be necessary to decrease the dose or increase the time interval between doses. Route of choice: Oral—simple, effective, convenient, and acceptable. Other routes: Subcutaneous, intravenous (IV), intramuscular (IM), rectal, subarachnoid, epidural, and topical.

When prescribing morphine:

- Start with: 5–10 mg PO 4th hourly: Waking up dose (say 6 am) 10 am, 2 pm, 6 pm, and bedtime (10 pm). It is not necessary to wake the patient for the 2 am dose. Instead, a double of the 4th hourly dose can be prescribed at bedtime. Provide for "breakthrough" pain—same as the 4th hourly dose between the regular doses.

TABLE 1: Types of pain and their management.

Types of pain	*Management*
Muscular pain	Muscle relaxants/trigger point injections (TPI)
Colicky pain	Antispasmodics
Bone pain	Opioids + NSAIDs ± Corticosteroids
Pain due to constipation	Laxatives
Neuropathic pain	Opioids +/– tricyclic antidepressants (TCA)/*N*-methyl-*D*-aspartate (NMDA) receptor antagonist/invasive techniques
Cutaneous hyperalgesia	Topical agents

- 4th hourly dose to be increased by 50% every 24 hours till pain relief is adequate or an increase in dosage can be made depending upon the number of rescue doses of morphine needed.
- There is no standard dose for oral morphine. The dose is increased to the point at which pain is controlled with tolerable side effects.
- Can continue step 1 analgesics.
- Always prescribe a laxative to prevent constipation (refer to the topic "constipation").
- Prescribe for nausea and vomiting for the initial 3–5 days as a preventive measure.
- Never start on sustained release (SR) preparations of morphine. Effects are not controllable.

Opioid rotation

Opioid rotation involves switching from one opioid to another to improve pain control or reduce side effects. This strategy is based on incomplete cross-tolerance between different opioids. Carver et al. found that opioid rotation improved pain control in 70–80% of cancer patients experiencing inadequate analgesia or intolerable side effects with their current opioid regimen.[7]

Types of pain where oral morphine may not be effective and adjuvant analgesics need to be given **(Table 1)**.

ADJUVANT MEDICATIONS

Adjuvant medications are drugs that are not primarily analgesics but can enhance pain control when used in combination with traditional analgesics.

Antidepressants

Tricyclic antidepressants (TCAs) and serotonin-norepinephrine reuptake inhibitors (SNRIs) are commonly used for neuropathic cancer pain. Wickham documented that duloxetine was particularly effective in managing chemotherapy-induced peripheral neuropathy, with improvements in both pain scores and quality of life measures.[8] Examples include:

- Amitriptyline (TCA)
- Nortriptyline (TCA)
- Duloxetine (SNRI)
- Venlafaxine (SNRI)

Anticonvulsants

Anticonvulsants, particularly gabapentinoids, are effective in managing neuropathic cancer pain. A systematic review by Davari et al. concluded that gabapentin and pregabalin were equally effective in managing cancer-related neuropathic pain, with pregabalin showing a slightly better side effect profile.[9] Common anticonvulsants used include:

- Gabapentin
- Pregabalin
- Corticosteroids

Corticosteroids can help manage cancer pain, particularly in cases of bone metastases, spinal cord compression, or increased intracranial pressure. A recent study by van der Linden et al. demonstrated that a short course of high-dose dexamethasone provided rapid pain relief in patients with bone metastases, with effects lasting up to 4 weeks after treatment cessation.[10] Commonly used corticosteroids include:

- Dexamethasone
- Prednisone

Bisphosphonates and Denosumab

These agents are used to manage bone pain associated with metastatic disease. A comparative study by Stopeck et al. found that denosumab was superior to zoledronic acid in delaying skeletal-related events and reducing bone pain in patients with metastatic breast cancer.[11] Examples include:

- Zoledronic acid (bisphosphonate)
- Denosumab [receptor activator of nuclear factor kappa-B (RANK) ligand inhibitor]

Cannabinoids

The use of cannabinoids in cancer pain management has gained attention in recent years. While evidence is still limited, some studies suggest potential benefits. A randomized controlled trial by Safi et al. found that a standardized cannabis extract containing both tetrahydrocannabinol (THC) and cannabidiol (CBD) provided significant pain relief in patients with advanced cancer, particularly for those with neuropathic pain components.[12]

Topical analgesics

Topical analgesics can be useful for localized pain and may have fewer systemic side effects compared to oral medications. A recent study by Petran et al. demonstrated that a novel high-concentration capsaicin patch provided long-lasting pain relief for patients with localized cancer-related neuropathic pain.[13] Common topical analgesics include:

- Lidocaine patches
- Capsaicin cream
- Nonsteroidal anti-inflammatory drug gels

INTERVENTIONAL PAIN MANAGEMENT TECHNIQUES

While not strictly pharmacological, interventional techniques often involve the administration of medications and can be an important part of comprehensive cancer pain management.

Nerve Blocks

Nerve blocks involve injecting local anesthetics, often combined with corticosteroids, near specific nerves or nerve plexuses to interrupt pain signaling. A prospective study by Chen et al. found that ultrasound-guided celiac plexus neurolysis provided significant pain relief and improved quality of life in patients with pancreatic cancer pain refractory to conventional analgesics.[14]

Intrathecal Drug Delivery

Intrathecal drug delivery systems allow for direct administration of opioids and other analgesics into the cerebrospinal fluid, potentially providing improved pain control with lower systemic doses. A recent systematic review by Mercadante concluded that intrathecal drug delivery was effective for managing refractory cancer pain, with significant improvements in pain scores and reduced systemic opioid requirements.[15]

SPECIAL CONSIDERATIONS IN CANCER PAIN MANAGEMENT

Breakthrough Pain

This refers to pain that "breaks through" a baseline level of analgesia, often seen in patients with cancer pain. The patient generally has good pain relief over 24 hours but experiences episodes of pain in between the 4-hourly doses. An extra dose of oral morphine, the same as the 4th hourly dose, can be given; however, often the patient needs it. A randomized controlled trial by Janknegt et al. demonstrated that a novel sublingual fentanyl formulation provided a faster onset of action and better patient satisfaction compared to oral morphine for managing breakthrough cancer pain.[16]

End-of-dose pain: If pain is experienced before the 4-hourly due dose of immediate-release (IR) morphine, the patient should be given a rescue dose of 100% of the 4-hourly dose. If rescue doses are required more than twice a day on a regular basis, then this is an indication to increase the regular 4-hourly doses.

Incident pain refers to pain caused by an incident such as body movement, cough, or wound dressing. When anticipated, the analgesic can be given half an hour prior to the incident. Management of incident pain with examples: (1) Oral morphine 20–30 minutes prior to wound dressing, (2) NSAID taken prior to movement, when appropriate, and (3) Inj. ketamine (0.25–0.5 mg/kg) taken PO/SL 15 minutes prior to a procedure.

Opioid-induced Constipation

Opioid-induced constipation is a common and distressing side effect of opioid therapy. It is a receptor-binding effect and will stay as long as opioids are given. It is mandatory to prescribe laxatives continuously. A stimulant laxative such as bisacodyl 10 mg HS is increased up to 40 mg/day if required and/or softeners such as docusate can be added, up to 45 mL/day. A recent study by Braun et al. found that the peripherally acting mu-opioid receptor antagonist (PAMORA) naldemedine was effective in managing opioid-induced constipation in cancer patients, with improvements in bowel function and quality of life.[17]

Neuropathic Cancer Pain

Up to 40% of cancer-related pain may have a neuropathic mechanism involved. Neuropathic pain is often challenging to manage and may require a multimodal approach. A recent meta-analysis by Shkodra et al. concluded that a combination of gabapentinoids, SNRIs, and opioids provided the most effective relief for cancer-related neuropathic pain.[18]

Pain in Elderly Cancer Patients

Elderly patients may have altered pharmacokinetics and increased susceptibility to side effects. A personalized approach with careful dose titration is essential. Huang et al. demonstrated that a geriatric-specific pain management protocol, emphasizing lower starting doses and slower titration, led to improved pain control and fewer adverse events in elderly cancer patients.[19]

Cancer Pain in Patients with Substance-use Disorders

Managing cancer pain in patients with a history of substance abuse presents unique challenges. A multidisciplinary approach involving pain specialists, addiction medicine experts, and mental health professionals is often necessary. A recent review by Noreika and Konecny proposed a framework for managing cancer pain in patients with opioid use disorder, emphasizing the use of buprenorphine and close monitoring.[20]

EMERGING THERAPIES AND FUTURE DIRECTIONS

Targeted Drug Delivery Systems

Nanoparticle-based drug delivery systems are being investigated for their potential to improve analgesic efficacy while reducing systemic side effects. A systematic review by Ji et al. demonstrated promising results for a liposomal bupivacaine formulation in managing postsurgical pain in cancer patients, with prolonged analgesia and reduced opioid requirements.[21]

Novel Opioid Receptor Targets

Research is ongoing into developing opioids that selectively activate specific opioid receptor subtypes or biased ligands that preferentially activate analgesic pathways while minimizing side effects. A preclinical study by Piekielna-Ciesielska et al. identified a novel mu-opioid receptor-biased agonist that provided potent analgesia with reduced respiratory depression and constipation in animal models of cancer pain.[22]

Ion Channel Modulators

Drugs targeting specific ion channels involved in pain signaling are under investigation. A review by Pukkanasut et al. showed that a novel selective Na_V1.7 sodium channel blocker provided significant pain relief in patients with chemotherapy-induced peripheral neuropathy.[23]

Immunomodulatory Approaches

Emerging research suggests that modulating the immune system may have analgesic effects in cancer pain. A review by Ciwun et al. found that low-dose naltrexone, thought to act through immunomodulatory mechanisms, provided pain relief and improved quality of life in patients with advanced cancer.[24]

Gene Therapy

Gene therapy approaches are being explored for long-term pain management in cancer patients. These strategies aim to modify gene expression to enhance pain relief or reduce pain sensitivity. A phase I clinical trial by Li et al. demonstrated the safety and potential efficacy of an adeno-associated virus vector delivering the gene for endogenous opioid peptides in patients with intractable cancer pain.[25]

CONCLUSION

The pharmacological management of chronic cancer pain remains a complex and evolving field. While opioids continue to play a central role, a multimodal approach incorporating nonopioid analgesics, adjuvant medications, and interventional techniques is often necessary to achieve optimal pain control. Recent advances in drug formulations, targeted therapies, and personalized medicine approaches have expanded the arsenal of available treatments.

Key points to remember include the following:

- Thorough pain assessment is crucial for effective management.
- The WHO Pain Ladder provides a useful framework, but individualized approaches are often necessary.
- Opioid rotation can be an effective strategy for managing inadequate analgesia or intolerable side effects.
- Adjuvant medications, including antidepressants and anticonvulsants, play an important role in managing neuropathic cancer pain.
- Special considerations are needed for breakthrough pain, opioid-induced constipation, elderly patients, and those with substance use disorders.
- Emerging therapies, including targeted drug delivery systems, novel opioid receptor targets, and immunomodulatory approaches, show promise for future pain management strategies.

As research continues to advance our understanding of cancer pain mechanisms and treatment options, it is crucial for healthcare providers to stay informed about the latest developments in pharmacological pain management. A patient-centered approach, considering individual needs, preferences, and risk factors, remains paramount in providing effective pain relief and improving the quality of life for cancer patients.

Future research directions should focus on:

- Developing more effective and safer analgesics with reduced side effect profiles
- Exploring combination therapies that target multiple pain pathways simultaneously
- Investigating the potential of precision medicine approaches to tailor pain management strategies based on genetic, molecular, and clinical factors
- Evaluating the long-term efficacy and safety of emerging therapies in large-scale clinical trials
- Improving strategies for managing chronic cancer pain in special populations, including pediatric and geriatric patients

By continuing to advance our understanding and treatment of chronic cancer pain, we hope to provide better pain relief, improved quality of life, and enhanced overall care for cancer patients worldwide.

REFERENCES

1. Bico I, Afonso A, Sousa L, Bule MJ, Lopes MJ. Empowering cancer patients with self-care and pain management skills: a quasi-experimental study. Pain Manag Nurs. 2024;25(4):369-76.
2. Anekar AA, Hendrix JM, Cascella M. WHO analgesic ladder. [Updated 2023 Apr 23]. In: StatPearls [Internet]. Treasure Island (FL): StatPearls Publishing; 2024.
3. Wang P, Chen B, Huang Y, Li J, Cao D, Chen Z, et al. The relationship between nonsteroidal anti-inflammatory drugs and cancer incidence: an umbrella review. Heliyon. 2024;10(2):e23203.
4. Kianian S, Bansal J, Lee C, Zhang K, Bergese SD. Perioperative multimodal analgesia: a review of efficacy and safety of the treatment options. Anesthiol Perioper Sci. 2024;2:9.

5. Dean L, Kane M. Codeine therapy and CYP2D6 genotype. 2012 Sep 20 [Updated 2021 Mar 30]. In: Pratt VM, Scott SA, Pirmohamed M, et al., (Eds). Medical Genetics Summaries [Internet]. Bethesda (MD): National Center for Biotechnology Information (US); 2012.
6. Abdel Shaheed C, Hayes C, Maher CG, Ballantyne JC, Underwood M, McLachlan AJ, et al. Opioid analgesics for nociceptive cancer pain: a comprehensive review. CA Cancer J Clin. 2024;74(3):286-313.
7. Carver AC, Foley KM. Therapeutic approaches to cancer pain. In: Kufe DW, Pollock RE, Weichselbaum RR, Bast, Jr RC, Gansler TS, Holland JF, et al. (Eds). Holland-Frei Cancer Medicine, 6th edition. Hamilton, ON: BC Decker; 2003.
8. Wickham R. Review of a study of duloxetine for painful chemotherapy-induced peripheral neuropathy. J Adv Pract Oncol. 2013;4(5):361-8.
9. Davari M, Amani B, Amani B, Khanijahani A, Akbarzadeh A, Shabestan R. Pregabalin and gabapentin in neuropathic pain management after spinal cord injury: a systematic review and meta-analysis. Korean J Pain. 2020;33(1):3-12.
10. van der Linden YM, Westhoff PG, Stellato RK, van Baardwijk A, de Vries K, Ong F, et al. Dexamethasone for the prevention of a pain flare after palliative radiation therapy for painful bone metastases: the multicenter double-blind placebo-controlled 3-armed randomized Dutch DEXA study. Int J Radiat Oncol Biol Phys. 2020;108(3):546-53.
11. Stopeck AT, Lipton A, Body JJ, Steger GG, Tonkin K, de Boer RH, et al. Denosumab compared with zoledronic acid for the treatment of bone metastases in patients with advanced breast cancer: a randomized, double-blind study. J Clin Oncol. 2010;28(35):5132-9.
12. Safi K, Sobieraj J, Błaszkiewicz M, Żyła J, Salata B, Dzierżanowski T. Tetrahydrocannabinol and cannabidiol for pain treatment—an update on the evidence. Biomedicines. 2024;12(2):307.
13. Petran EM, Periferakis A, Troumpata L, Periferakis AT, Scheau AE, Badarau IA, et al. Capsaicin: emerging pharmacological and therapeutic insights. Curr. Issues Mol Biol. 2024;46:7895-943.
14. Chen IW, Sun CK, Chen JY, Chen HT, Lan KM, Hung KC, et al. Comparison of regional vs. general anesthesia on the risk of dementia: a systematic review and meta-analysis. Front Public Health. 2024;12:1362461.
15. Mercadante S. Refractory cancer pain and intrathecal therapy: critical review of a systematic review. Pain Ther. 2023;12(3):645-54.
16. Janknegt R, van den Beuken M, Schiere S, Überall M, Knaggs R, Hanley J, et al. Rapid acting fentanyl formulations in breakthrough pain in cancer. Drug selection by means of the system of objectified judgement analysis. Eur J Hosp Pharm. 2018;25(3):e2.
17. Braun UK, Jackson LK, Garcia MA, Imam SN. A systematic review of naldemedine and naloxegol for the treatment of opioid-induced constipation in cancer patients. Pharmacy (Basel). 2024;12(2):48.
18. Shkodra M, Caraceni A. Treatment of neuropathic pain directly due to cancer: an update. Cancers (Basel). 2022;14(8):1992.
19. Huang L, Zhang T, Wang K, Chang B, Fu D, Chen X. Postoperative multimodal analgesia strategy for enhanced recovery after surgery in elderly colorectal cancer patients. Pain Ther. 2024;13:745-66.
20. Noreika D, Konecny M. The pendulum: the need to develop a safe, effective, and equitable management strategy for opioids in cancer patients. Risk Manag Healthc Policy. 2024;17:1079-82.
21. Ji YD, Harris JA, Gibson LE, McKinley SK, Phitayakorn R. The efficacy of liposomal bupivacaine for opioid and pain reduction: a systematic review of randomized clinical trials. J Surg Res. 2021;264:510-33.
22. Piekielna-Ciesielska J, Malfacini D, Djeujo FM, Marconato C, Wtorek K, Calo G, et al. Functional selectivity of EM-2 analogs at the mu-opioid receptor. Front Pharmacol. 2023; 14:1133961.
23. Pukkanasut P, Jaskula-Sztul R, Gomora JC, Velu SE. Therapeutic targeting of voltage-gated sodium channel $Na_V1.7$ for cancer metastasis. Front Pharmacol. 2024; 15:1416705.
24. Ciwun M, Tankiewicz-Kwedlo A, Pawlak D. Low-dose naltrexone as an adjuvant in combined anticancer therapy. Cancers (Basel). 2024;16(6):1240.
25. Yi-ze Li, Ru-Rong Ji. Gene therapy for chronic pain management. Cell Rep Med. 2024;5(10):101756.

59 CHAPTER

Interventions for Chronic Cancer Pain

Shruti Gairola, Aparna Sanjay Chatterjee

INTRODUCTION

The foundation of interventional therapy is based on a comprehensive understanding of the anatomical structures involved, with particular emphasis on the relevant sensory innervation pathways. The paradigm for managing cancer pain has undergone significant evolution, with accumulating evidence advocating for the early implementation of interventional strategies, rather than considering them merely as options of last resort.

Interventional pain management techniques can be broadly categorized into neuroablative and neuromodulation approaches. Interventional procedures have now been proposed as the fourth step of the ladder.[1] Interventions, such as peripheral nerve and plexus blocks, central neuraxial blocks, sympathetic blocks, neurolytic blocks, intrathecal drug delivery systems, neuromodulation, and neurosurgical procedures could be effective in the management of chronic cancer-related pain. Cancer-related pain interventions are often approached as a last resort due to perceived risks, delaying timely referrals. However, early interventions can effectively control intractable pain, addressing both rest and movement-related discomfort. Also, when pain is inadequately managed with analgesics, interventional pain management techniques provide a viable and effective alternative, offering hope to patients suffering from refractory pain in oncological settings.

The integration of interventional procedures into cancer pain management strategies allows for a multimodal approach, addressing complex pain syndromes and improving the overall care trajectory for patients.

Cornerstones of Cancer Pain Management

- Opioids
- *Adjunctive drugs for cancer pain:* Nonsteroidal anti-inflammatory drugs (NSAIDs), gabapentenoids, antiepileptic, anticonvulsants, local anesthetics, N-methyl-D-aspartate (NMDA) antagonist, ziconotide, bisphosphonates and denosumab, corticosteroids, alpha-adrenergic agonists, Topical capsaicin, acetaminophen, medical cannabis, and some novel and emerging therapies.
- *Interventional procedures:* Destructive neuroablative or nondestructive techniques.
  - *Neuraxial interventional techniques:* Epidural steroid injections, sympathetic blocks.
  - Peripheral nerve blocks and interventions for syndromes, such as:
    - Postmastectomy pain syndrome
    - Brachial plexopathy and brachial plexus pathology
    - Post-thoracotomy pain syndrome
- *Locoregional therapies:*
  - Palliative radiation for cancer
  - *Ablation techniques:* Radiofrequency ablation (RFA), microwave, cryoablation, and high-intensity focused ultrasound (USG).

HISTORY OF INTERVENTIONAL PAIN MANAGEMENT

The field of interventional pain management has evolved over centuries, driven by advances in medical science and innovative techniques targeting specific neural pathways. The development of interventional techniques dates back to the late 1800s with the isolation and naming of cocaine. Chemical neurolysis was first demonstrated in 1863 by Luton, wherein he injected irritant chemicals subcutaneously in patients suffering from sciatic neuralgia.[2] In 1874 Bartholow pioneered the use of subcutaneous injections of chloroform to manage trigeminal neuralgia. Later in 1888, Baccelli introduced subcutaneous phenol injections for neuralgias. Tuffer in

1899 described the use of therapeutic nerve blocks using spinal injections of cocaine to alleviate pain caused by sarcoma of the leg.[3] In 1904 alcohol neurolysis for trigeminal neuralgia was first performed and reported by Schlosser. This technique, which involves the use of alcohol to disrupt neural transmission, gained popularity and became a widely practiced method. In 1919 celiac plexus block was described by Kappis, as a significant milestone in the treatment of visceral pain. This procedure targeted the celiac plexus to provide relief from abdominal pain. Boas in 1978 further refined this technique by distinguishing between retrocrural and transcrural needle placements. This distinction enabled targeted blocking of the splanchnic and celiac plexus nerve fibers, enhancing precision in pain management.[4] Between 1952 and 1953, Robechhi and Capra first described the use of epidural steroid injections for pain relief, which quickly became a standard approach in managing radicular pain.[5] Around the same time, Lievre introduced the transforaminal approach, enabling targeted delivery of steroids and enhancing efficacy.[6]

The application of radiofrequency (RF) techniques for chronic pain management can be traced back to 1931 when Kirscher utilized a direct current of 350 mA with a 10-mm uninsulated needle to treat trigeminal neuralgia. Pulsed radiofrequency (PRF) was introduced in 1998 by Menno Sluijter as a less destructive alternative to conventional radiofrequency (CRF), offering a safer approach to pain management with reduced risk of tissue damage.

INTERVENTIONAL PAIN MANAGEMENT TECHNIQUES IN VARIOUS CANCER PAIN SYNDROMES

Interventional procedures help interrupt the transmission of pain along pathways either temporarily or permanently. Neurolysis is one such interventional procedure that aims to deliberately injure or disrupt the nerve by either physical or chemical means to bring about degenerative changes in the nerve and interrupt the transmission of pain impulses. The nerve injury triggers Wallerian degeneration, characterized by the breakdown of the axon distal to the lesion, facilitating the neurolysis process. This procedure targets and destroys afferent neuronal pathways or associated sympathetic ganglia, thereby interrupting the pain pathway and providing focused pain relief to the patient. Neurolysis can be performed at various points along the pain pathway, ranging from the peripheral nerve transmitting pain signals to the central nervous system.

TABLE 1: Chemical neurolysis—alcohol versus phenol.

Agent	*Alcohol*	*Phenol*
Pain on injection	Yes (can be avoided by preinjection of LA drug)	No
Onset of Block	Immediate	After 15 minutes
Time to full nerve block	3–5 days	1 day
Baricity (water = 1)	0.8	1.1
Concentration used for neurolysis	50–100%	6–10%
Sites of use	Intrathecal, celiac ganglion, lumbar sympathetic chain, cranial nerves, and paravertebral	Epidural, paravertebral, peripheral nerve roots, intrathecal, and cranial nerves

Various techniques for neurolysis include:

- Physical methods
  - RF ablation
  - Cryoablation
- Chemical neurolysis **(Table 1)**
  - Alcohol
  - Phenol
  - Ammonium salts
  - Glycerol

Let us look at the interventions for various cancer-related pain syndromes.

Head and Neck Cancers

Pain is one of the most distressing of symptoms in patients with head and neck cancers even at diagnosis. Managing head and neck cancer pain is particularly challenging due to the dense neural innervation in the region and the functional demands of speech, swallowing, and oral intake, which often exacerbate the pain.[7]

Nerve blocks effectively utilized in the management of head and neck cancer pain include those targeting the trigeminal nerve, glossopharyngeal nerve (GPN), occipital nerve, vagus nerve, sphenopalatine ganglion, and cervical plexus.[8]

When the pain is not relieved adequately with analgesics, the option of pain interventions offers hope. Neuroablation of the trigeminal, glossopharyngeal, occipital, sphenopalatine ganglia and cervical plexus can be performed wherever necessary. Occipital nerve blocks have demonstrated efficacy in alleviating pain and headaches caused by malignancies invading the skull base. This technique can reduce pain intensity and improve the quality of life in patients experiencing secondary headache syndromes due to cancerous spread.

Radiofrequency ablation (RFA) has emerged as a safe and effective modality for managing cancer pain in the head and neck region. It is particularly useful for:

- *Trigeminal neuralgia:* Ablating the trigeminal nerve or its branches can significantly relieve intractable facial pain caused by malignancies or metastatic lesions.
- *Glossopharyngeal neuralgia:* RFA of the GPN can be performed for cancer-related pain localized to the throat or ear, providing sustained relief.
- *Sphenopalatine ganglion ablation:* This procedure is effective for patients with severe facial pain and headache originating from cancer involving the craniofacial region.

By targeting these specific neural pathways, interventional techniques not only alleviate pain but also reduce the reliance on high-dose opioids, minimizing side effects and improving functional outcomes. With advancements in imaging modalities such as fluoroscopy, ultrasound, and computed tomography (CT) guidance, these interventions are performed with increased precision, enhancing both safety and efficacy.

A few interventions for head and neck cancers include:

- Gasserian ganglion block
- Sphenopalatine ganglion block
- Stellate ganglion block (SGB)
- GPN block
- Nerve block for scalp
- Mandibular and maxillary nerve block

Stellate Ganglion Block

Anatomy: Stellate ganglion is a sympathetic ganglion formed by the fusion of the inferior cervical ganglion and the first thoracic ganglion. It is situated on the anterior surface of the longus colli muscle at the level of the C7 and T1 vertebrae. Anatomically, the ganglion is situated anteromedial to the vertebral artery and medial to the common carotid artery and the internal jugular vein as seen below in **Figure 1**. The primary anatomical landmarks for ultrasound-guided SGB include the carotid sheath, the longus colli muscle, and the anterior tubercle of the sixth cervical vertebra.[9]

Position a linear probe over the anterolateral aspect of the neck, aligning it with the anterior border of the sternocleidomastoid muscle at the level of the cricoid cartilage (C6). The C6 vertebral body is recognized by its characteristic "camel hump" anterior tubercle as seen in **Figures 2A and B**. **Figures 3A and B** similar to **Figures 2A and B** shows the cross-sectional CT view and the corresponding sonoanatomy at C7 vertebral level.

The ultrasound probe is positioned at the level of the cricoid cartilage to identify the transverse process of C6, distinguished by its prominent anterior tubercle. To confirm the level of C6, the ultrasound probe is moved caudally to visualize the C7 transverse process, which is characterized by a single (posterior) tubercle. At the C6 level, the typical sonographic landmarks include the transverse process and anterior tubercle of C6, the longus colli muscle (LC), the carotid artery, and the thyroid gland.

At the C7 level, the vertebral artery is visible as a pulsating structure, confirmed by an arterial Doppler signal that can be traced cranially as it enters the foramen transversarium.

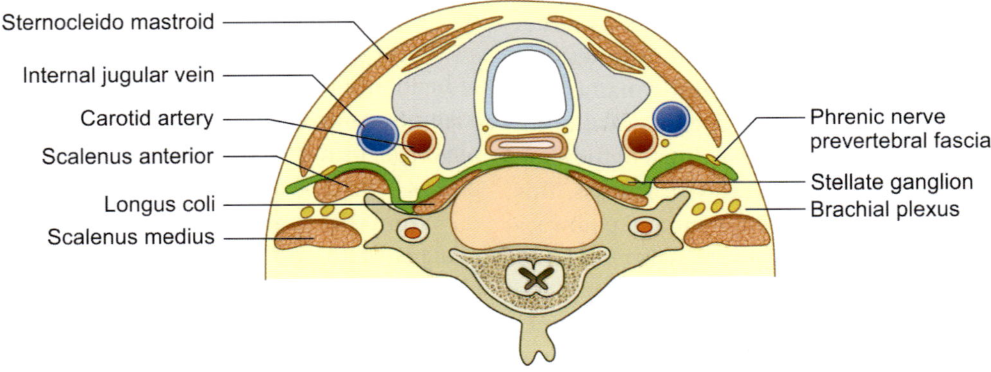

Fig. 1: Cross-section of the neck at C6.

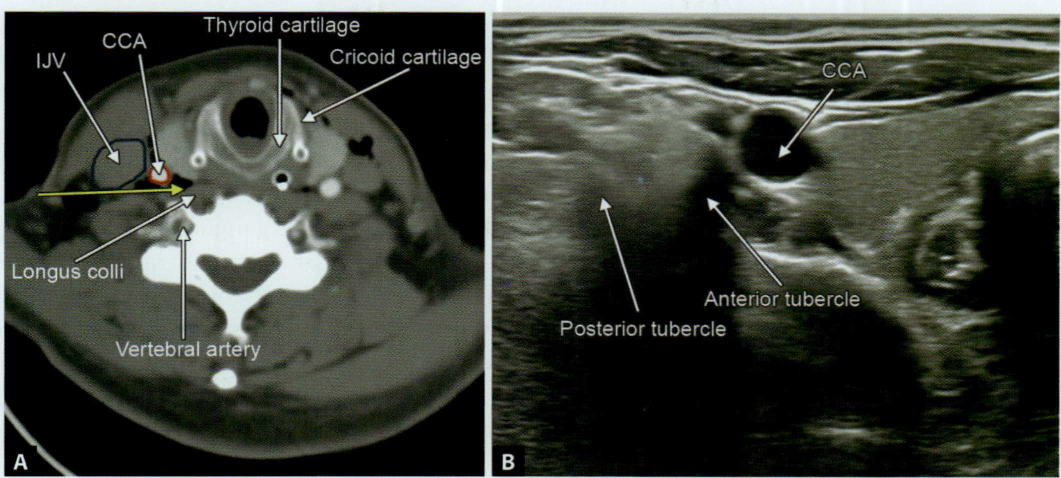

Figs. 2A and B: (A) CT axial view at the level of C6 vertebra; (B) Sonoanatomy at the same level.
Note: The yellow arrow indicates the needle trajectory for the stellate ganglion block.
(CCA: common carotid artery; IJV: internal jugular vein)

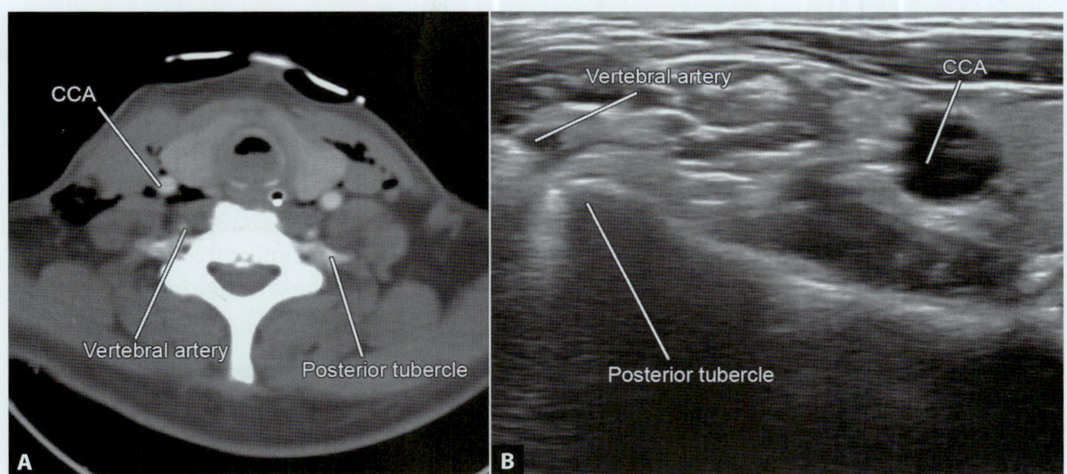

Figs. 3A and B: (A) CT axial view at the level of the C7 vertebra; (B) Sonoanatomy at the same level.
Note: The vertebral artery is exposed at this level.
(CCA: common carotid artery; IJV: internal jugular vein)

For needle insertion, two approaches are commonly used: The 'out-of-plane' anterior approach (similar to the paratracheal approach) and the 'in-plane' lateral approach. With the in-plane approach, the needle is inserted beside the trachea in a lateral-to-medial direction. The needle tip should reach the prevertebral fascia overlying the longus colli muscle, located between the posterior aspect of the carotid artery and the anterior tubercle of C6.[10]

The presence of Horner's syndrome (characterized by symptoms such as ptosis, miosis, anhidrosis, and enophthalmos) serves as a confirmatory sign of a successful SGB. Additional indicators include a warmer, drier extremity and dilated veins on the side where a block is administered. However, due to the presence of Kuntz fibers, which can bypass the stellate ganglion, the absence of an effect in the hand does not necessarily rule out sympathetic involvement.

Arm weakness and/or numbness are typically indicative of a brachial plexus block, which may occur with or without sympathetic blockade. In such cases, it is inconclusive whether the pain is sympathetically mediated.

To ensure the effectiveness of the blockade, it is essential to monitor the ipsilateral arm temperature before and after the procedure, as a temperature increase confirms adequate sympathetic blockade.

Complications of this block include inadvertently injection of the local anesthetic solution into the epidural, subdural, or subarachnoid space which may result in total spinal anesthesia. Other possible complications include pneumothorax, postblock ecchymosis, and hematoma formation.

Trigeminal Nerve Block

Anatomy: The trigeminal nerve, the fifth (V) cranial nerve, is the largest among the twelve cranial nerves and has an extensive area of distribution. It is a mixed cranial nerve with both motor and sensory fibers. The nerve arises from the brainstem (pons) and innervates multiple structures of the head and face.

There are three divisions of the trigeminal nerve: (1) Ophthalmic (V1), (2) maxillary (V2), and (3) mandibular (V3). RFA can either target the Gasserian ganglion of the trigeminal nerve or any of the branches depending on the distribution of pain in the patient.

Gasserian ganglion (trigeminal ganglion) is formed from two roots that exit the ventral surface of the brainstem at the midpontine level. It enters into a recess called "Meckel's cave." The most common method is the intracranial approach to the Gasserian ganglion. Extracranial approaches for targeting specific branches have also been described. **Figure 4A** represents the CT image showing the location of the foramen ovale and a slightly more proximal section as seen in **Figure 4B** which shows the approximate location of Meckel's cave which houses the Gasserian ganglion.

The procedure is performed under fluoroscopic guidance with the patient supine and the head slightly extended. The C-arm is positioned in an oblique submental view to clearly visualize the foramen ovale.[11]

The needle insertion point is 2–3 cm lateral to the commissure of the lips on the affected side as seen in **Figures 5A to D**, aimed at the pupil in the frontal view and 3 cm anterior to the external auditory meatus in the lateral view. After local anesthesia, the needle is advanced coaxially toward the foramen ovale, ensuring the buccal mucosa is intact. The needle's position in Meckel's cavity is verified on lateral fluoroscopy.

The needle is advanced 2–4 mm through the foramen ovale to reach the junction of the petrous ridge and clivus. After removing the stylet, and a negative aspiration which rules out cerebrospinal fluid (CSF) or blood, fluoroscopy after injection of 0.5 mL contrast dye to confirm proper positioning. For RFA a test stimulation at 2 Hz confirms mandibular nerve contact if lower jaw muscle contractions are observed. Once stimulation parameters are optimal,

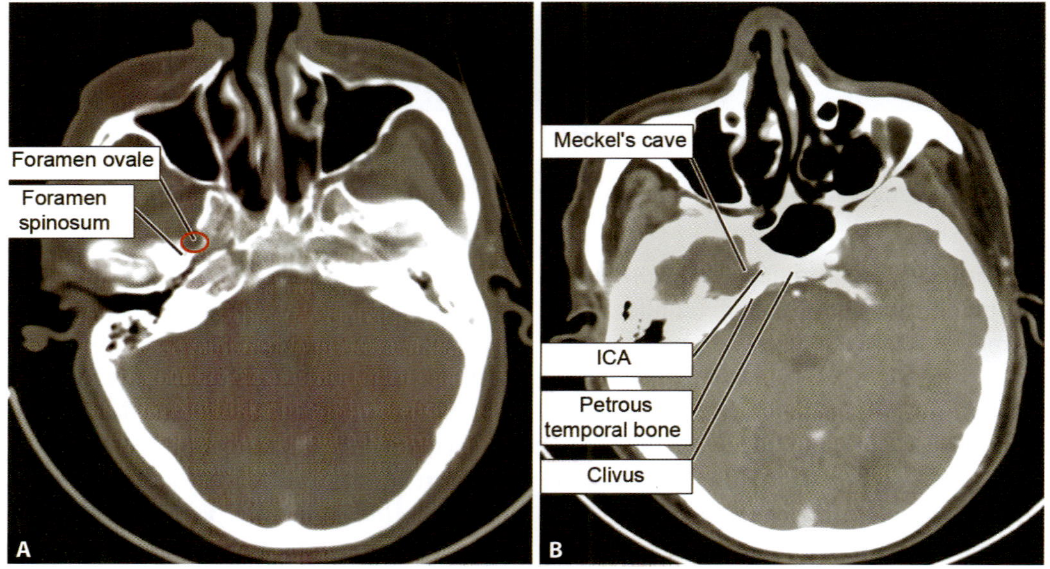

Figs. 4A and B: (A) CT scan axial view showing the anatomy at the location of Gasserian ganglion in the middle cranial fossa; (B) CT scan proximal cut showing the location of Meckel's cave. (CT: computed tomography; ICA: invasive coronary angiography)

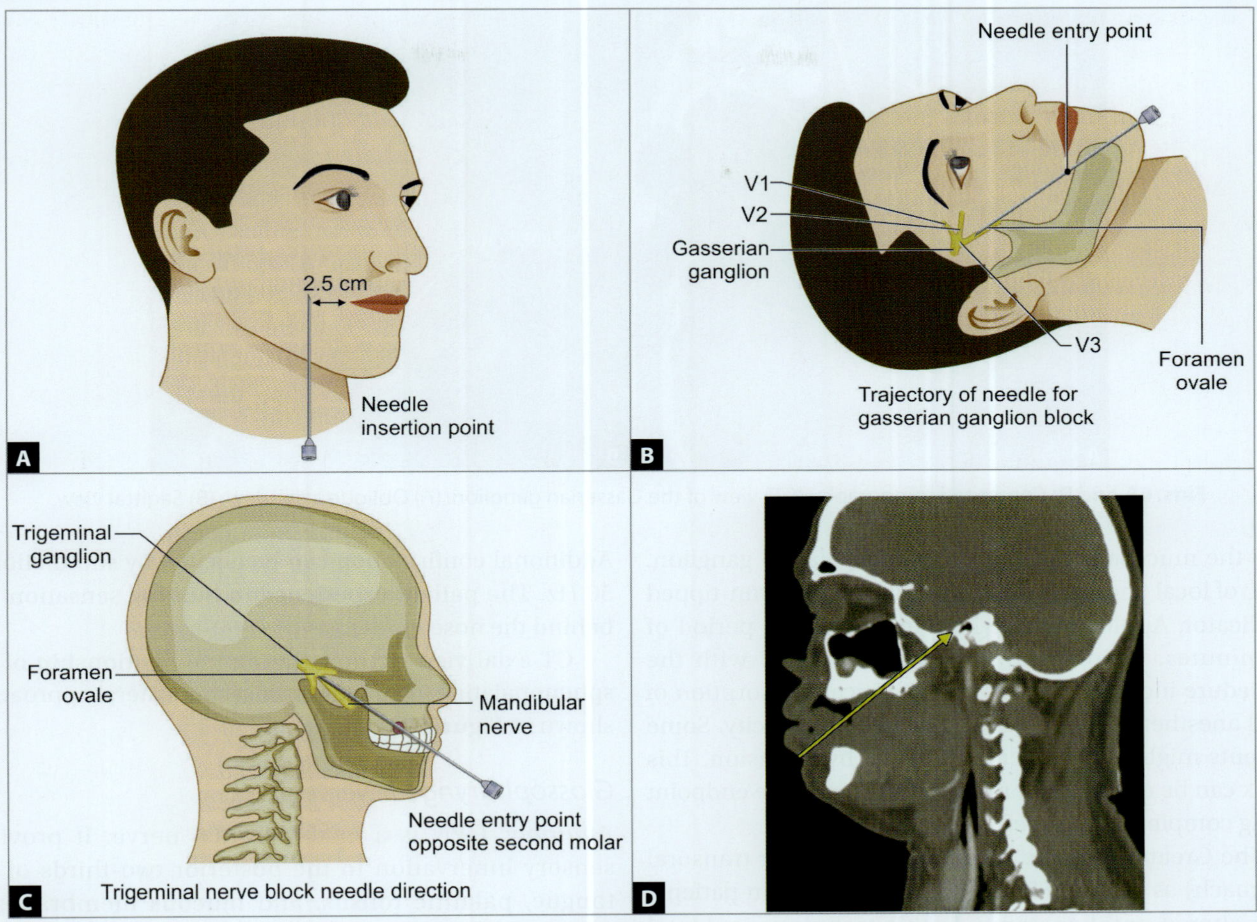

Figs. 5A to D: (A to C) Gasserian ganglion nerve block; (D) Computed tomography (CT) sagittal view showing needle trajectory seen in yellow arrow.

0.5 mL of 0.25% bupivacaine with 40 mg of triamcinolone is injected. After 30 seconds, RFA lesioning is performed at 60°C for 60 seconds, with repositioning as needed for multiple trigeminal branches **(Figs. 6A and B)**.

Complications such as diminished corneal reflex, masseter weakness, dysesthesia, anesthesia dolorosa, keratitis, and transient cranial nerve III or VI paralysis are known.[12]

Sphenopalatine Ganglion Block

It is a large extracranial ganglion located in the pterygopalatine fossa and lies posterior to the middle nasal turbinate. It is covered by a 1–1.5 mm layer of connective tissue and mucous membrane. Because of its superficial location, this block can be achieved with topical anesthesia via the transnasal approach which is a non-invasive and relatively safe technique.

This block can be utilized for the treatment of conditions such as migraine headaches, cluster headaches, facial neuralgias, and intractable orofacial pain syndromes as seen in cancer patients.

Various approaches to block this ganglion include: Transnasal approach, greater palatine foramen approach, and lateral approach.

Transnasal approach: As seen in **Figure 7A** with the patient in a supine position the anterior nares are inspected for any polyps, tumors, and foreign bodies. A small volume of local anesthetic is injected in each nostril and the patient is asked to sniff vigorously to draw local anesthetic posteriorly. Around 10 cm cotton-tipped applicators are soaked in the local anesthetic of choice. The applicator is advanced along the superior border of the middle turbinate of the nostril until the tip comes in contact

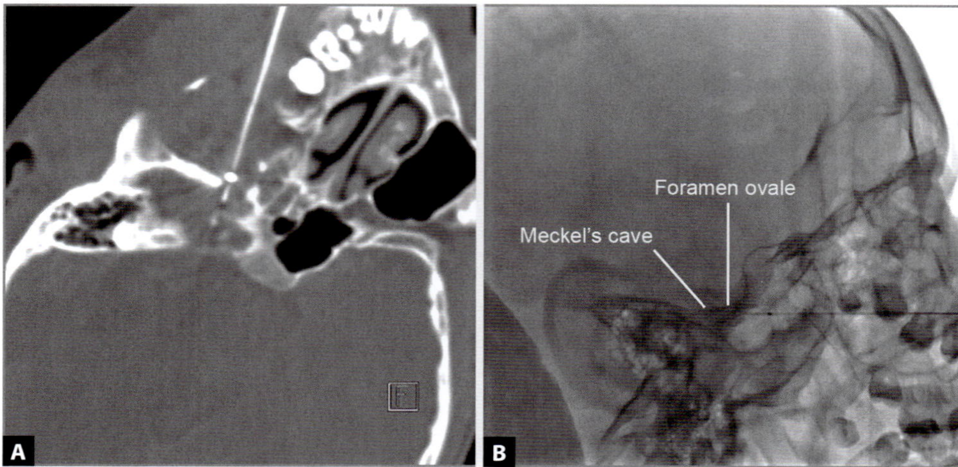

Figs. 6A and B: Computed tomography (CT) view of the Gasserian ganglion. (A) Oblique axial view; (B) Sagittal view.

with the mucosa overlying the sphenopalatine ganglion. 1 mL of local anesthetic is instilled over the cotton-tipped applicator. Applicators are kept in place for a period of 20 minutes. Major complications associated with the procedure include epistaxis and significant absorption of local anesthetic leading to local anesthetic toxicity. Some patients might experience orthostatic hypotension. This block can be carried out on a daily basis with the endpoint being complete pain relief.[13]

The Greater palatine foramen approach (or transoral approach) as seen in **Figure 7B** can be useful in patients with altered nasal anatomy. In this technique, a dental needle with a 120° angle is advanced through the greater palatine foramen, which lies just medial to the gumline of the third molar on the posterior portion of the hard palate. The needle is advanced around 2.5 cm through the foramen in a superior and slightly posterior direction. After negative aspiration, 2 mL of local anesthetic is injected slowly.[14]

Lateral approach: In lateral approach patient is placed supine with the head in the neutral position. The coronoid notch can be located by palpating the area just in front and slightly below the external auditory meatus while the patient opens and closes their mouth. The patient is asked to hold their mouth open in a neutral position. A 3.5″ needle with a stylet is inserted just beneath the zygomatic arch, directly in the middle of the coronoid notch as is seen in **Figure 7C**. The needle is advanced 1.5–2″ perpendicular to the skull until it contacts the lateral pterygoid plate. It is then slightly withdrawn and redirected in a slightly superior and anterior direction. In the fluoroscopic image, the needle tip can be seen to lie just under the lateral nasal mucosa. Additional confirmation can be elicited by stimulation at 50 Hz. The patient experiences a buzzing sensation just behind the nose.

CT axial view demonstrating the relationship of the sphenopalatine fossa in transnasal and lateral approach is shown in **Figure 7D.**

Glossopharyngeal Nerve Block

Anatomy: GPN is a mixed cranial nerve. It provides sensory innervation to the posterior two-thirds of the tongue, palatine tonsils, and mucous membranes of the mouth and pharynx. The landmark for this block is the styloid process of the temporal bone as is seen in **Figures 8A and B**. There are two approaches: (1) Extraoral and (2) intraoral.

Landmark Technique

- *Extraoral approach (peristyloid approach):* A 22G 1.5″ needle is inserted at the midpoint of the line joining the mastoid to the angle of the mandible in a perpendicular plane. The needle should hit the styloid process at a distance of <3 cm. At this point the needle is slightly withdrawn and walked off the styloid process in a posterior direction. Soon after the bony contact is lost after confirmation of negative aspiration of blood or CSF 5–7 mL of local anesthetic is administered. Neurolytic block may be performed using 6.5% aqueous phenol for intractable pain secondary to malignancies.[15]
- *Intraoral approach:* In this approach, the patient is made supine and the tongue is anesthetized with lignocaine. The tongue is retracted downward with

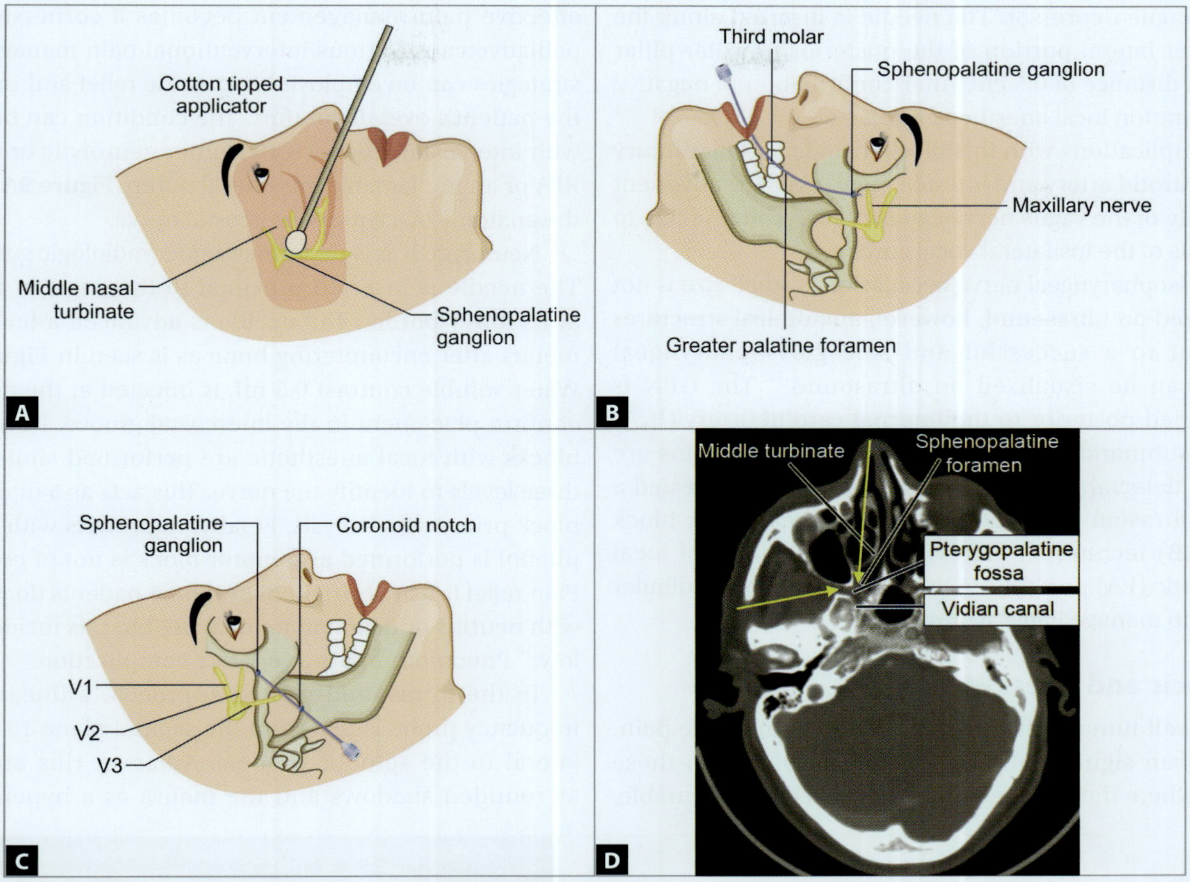

Figs. 7A to D: Different approaches of sphenopalatine block. (A) Transnasal approach; (B) Greater palatine foramen approach; (C) Lateral approach; and (D) CT axial view demonstrating the relationship of the sphenopalatine fossa.
Note: Transnasal and lateral approaches are marked in yellow arrow.
Source: Tashi S, Purohit BS, Becker M. et al. The pterygopalatine fossa: imaging anatomy, communications, and pathology revisited. Insights Imaging 2016;7:589-99. https://doi.org/10.1007/s13244-016-0498-1

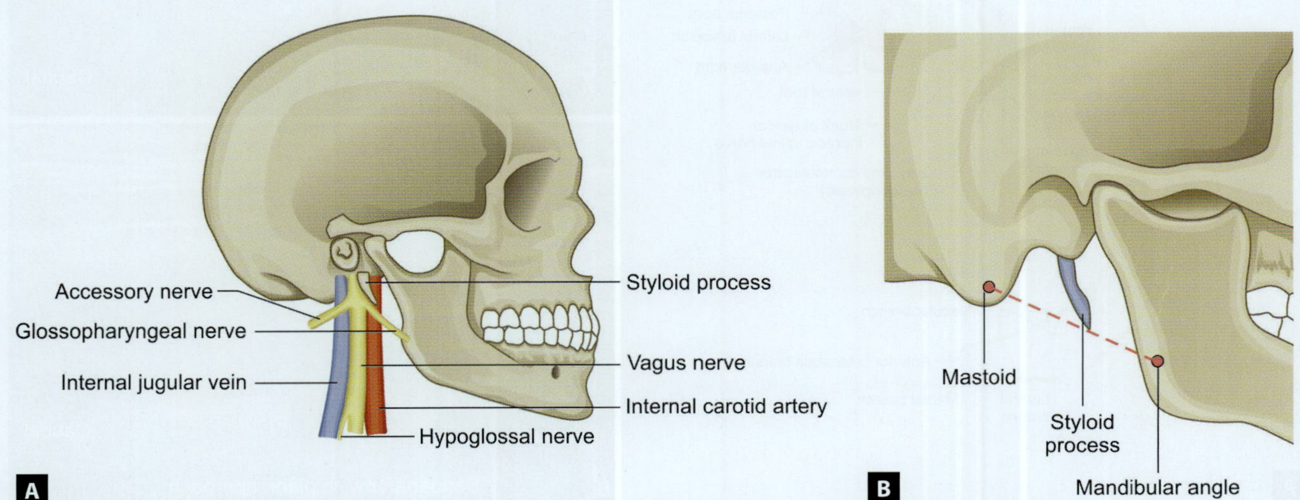

Figs. 8A and B: (A) Relationship of glossopharyngeal nerve to various structures in the neck; (B) Landmark for glossopharyngeal nerve block.

a tongue depressor. The needle is inserted along the lower lateral portion of the posterior tonsillar pillar to a distance of 0.5 cm. After confirmation of negative aspiration local anesthetic is injected.

Complications with this block include vascular injury to the carotid artery and internal jugular vein. Inadvertent blockade of the vagus nerve can lead to dysphonia due to paralysis of the ipsilateral vocal cord.

Glossopharyngeal nerve because of its small size is not visualized on ultrasound, however, anatomical structures relevant to a successful and safe glossopharyngeal block can be visualized on ultrasound.[16] The GPN is positioned posterior to the internal carotid artery (ICA) in the submandibular region. Since ICA pulsations are readily detectable on ultrasound, Punj et al. suggested a novel ultrasound-guided glossopharyngeal nerve block (UGPNB) technique, involving the deposition of local anesthetic (LA) posterior to the ICA in the submandibular region to manage Eagle syndrome.[17]

Thoracic and Chest Wall

Chest wall tumors often lead to severe, intractable pain, which can significantly impair quality of life. In these cases, where the disease is often advanced and incurable, effective pain management becomes a cornerstone of palliative care. Various interventional pain management strategies can be employed to provide relief and improve the patient's overall comfort. The condition can be dealt with intercostal blocks (ICBs) either neurolytic or pulsed RFA or an implantable intrathecal pump. **Figure 9A** shows the anatomy of a typical intercostal nerve.

Neurolytic ICB is performed under radiologic guidance. The needle is inserted proximal to the angle of the rib at its lower border. The needle is advanced a few millimeters after encountering bone as is seen in **Figure 9B**. Water soluble contrast 0.5 mL is injected at the point to confirm placement in the intercostal groove. Diagnostic blocks with local anesthetic are performed similarly at three levels to identify the nerve. This acts as a diagnostic block prior to neurolysis. Finally, neurolysis with 6–10% phenol is performed as a motor block is not of concern. Pain relief is usually immediate. Some patients do present with neuritis or deafferentation pain, but this incidence is low.[18] Pneumothorax is a very rare complication.

In the ultrasound-guided approach, a linear high-frequency probe is placed in the sagittal plane 10–15 cm lateral to the spinous process. Adjacent ribs are seen as rounded shadows and the pleura as a hyperechoic

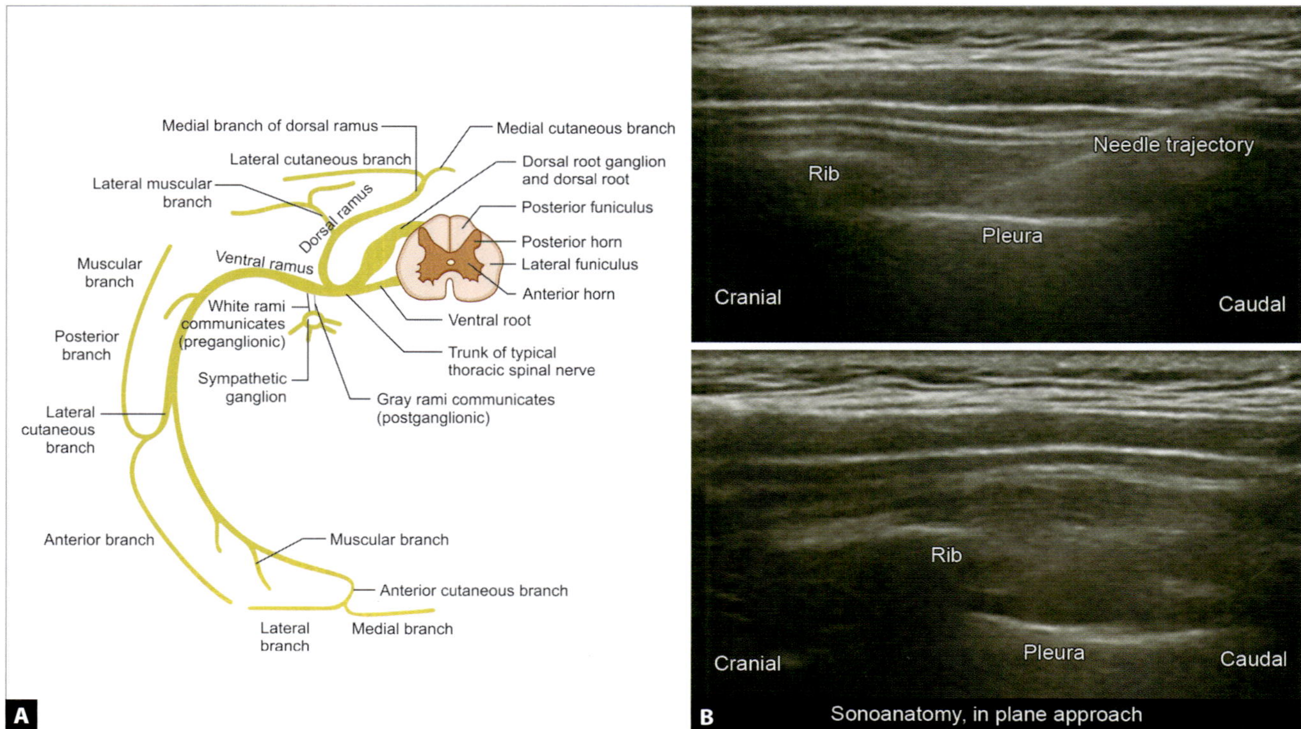

Figs. 9A and B: (A) Anatomy of the intercostal nerve; (B) Sonoanatomy of infraclavicular brachial plexus block (ICB).

line. At this point, the innermost intercostal muscle lies just above the pleura. The neurovascular bundle lies in a triangular space below the superior rib, between the internal and innermost muscles, which is the target site for injection. A 22G, 5 cm needle is placed between the innermost intercostal and pleura.

Abdominal Cancer Pain

Splanchnic and Celiac Plexus Nerve Block

Anatomy: The sympathetic innervation of abdominal organs originates from the anterolateral horn of the spinal cord. The greater (T5–T10), lesser (T10–T11), and least (T11–12) splanchnic nerves provide the major preganglionic contribution to the celiac plexus and transmit most nociceptive information from the viscera. The splanchnic nerves are preganglionic sympathetic fibers that lie retrocrural at the level of the T12 vertebra **(Fig. 10)**.

Celiac ganglia range from 1 to 5 in number with a diameter between 0.5 and 4.5 cm and lie about the level of the L1 vertebra. It lies anterior and anterolateral to the aorta and below the level of the coeliac artery as seen in **Figures 11A to C**. The celiac plexus is formed by the postganglionic fibers, the fibers arising from the preganglionic splanchnic nerves, and the celiac ganglion. It lies anterior to the crura of the diaphragm. The celiac plexus innervates the upper abdominal organs such as the pancreas, liver, spleen, biliary tract, gallbladder, adrenals, kidneys,

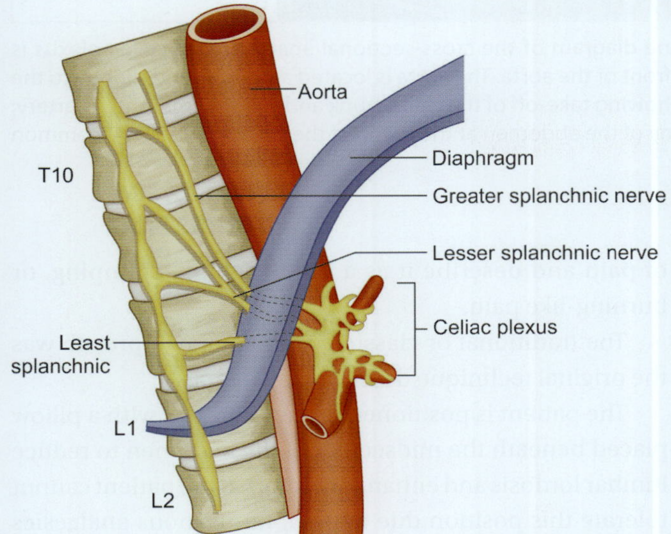

Fig. 10: Relationship of sympathetic ganglia to the splanchnic nerves and celiac plexus.

mesentery, stomach, and bowel till the level of the proximal transverse colon, as well as the blood vessels of the abdomen.[19]

The diagnostic splanchnic block is indicated to rule out whether the upper abdominal pain is sympathetically mediated via the splanchnic nerve. It is reserved for patients with upper abdominal and retroperitoneal pain that fails to respond to coeliac plexus block or in patients with significant preaortic adenopathy, tumor, or postoperative scarring.

The patient is positioned prone with a pillow under the abdomen to flex the thoracolumbar spine. The T12 vertebral body is identified with the help of fluoroscopy by tracing the inferior margin of the 12th rib. At a point 5 cm lateral and inferior to L1 spinous process local is infiltrated. 20G, 13 cm needle with a stylet is inserted at this point and directed at an angle of 45° toward the midline and 35° cephalad under continuous fluoroscopic guidance to ensure contact with the T12 vertebral body. At this point, the needle is withdrawn and redirected in a less medial angle from the midline of around 60 degrees to walk off the lateral surface of the T12 vertebral body. Once the needle walks off the lateral surface of the T12 vertebral body it is advanced around 1.5–2 cm under continuous fluoroscopic guidance so that the tip of the needle lies on just anterior to the lateral border of the vertebral body of T12 and behind the aorta and inferior vena cava in the retrocrural space. After confirming negative aspiration for blood, cerebrospinal fluid or urine a small amount of contrast material is injected through each needle, and the spread of contrast is confirmed radiographically as confined to the midline and concentrated near the T12 vertebral body. For a diagnostic block, 7–10 mL of LA is injected. In the case of neurolysis,10 mL of 50% alcohol is injected but only after a prior diagnostic block is successful. Each needle should be flushed with saline while withdrawing to prevent a tract of neurolytic agent.

Local, intra-abdominal infections, and sepsis are absolute contraindications to this block. Approximately 50% of patients develop postblock diarrhea which could lead to dehydration and electrolyte imbalances. These patients should be rehydrated. The inadvertent intravascular injection can lead to thrombosis of the nutrient vessels in the spinal cord with secondary paraplegia. Too much medial placement of the needle can result in epidural, subdural, or subarachnoid injection. Due to proximity to pleura pneumothorax, it may occur if the needle is placed too cephalad or anterior.

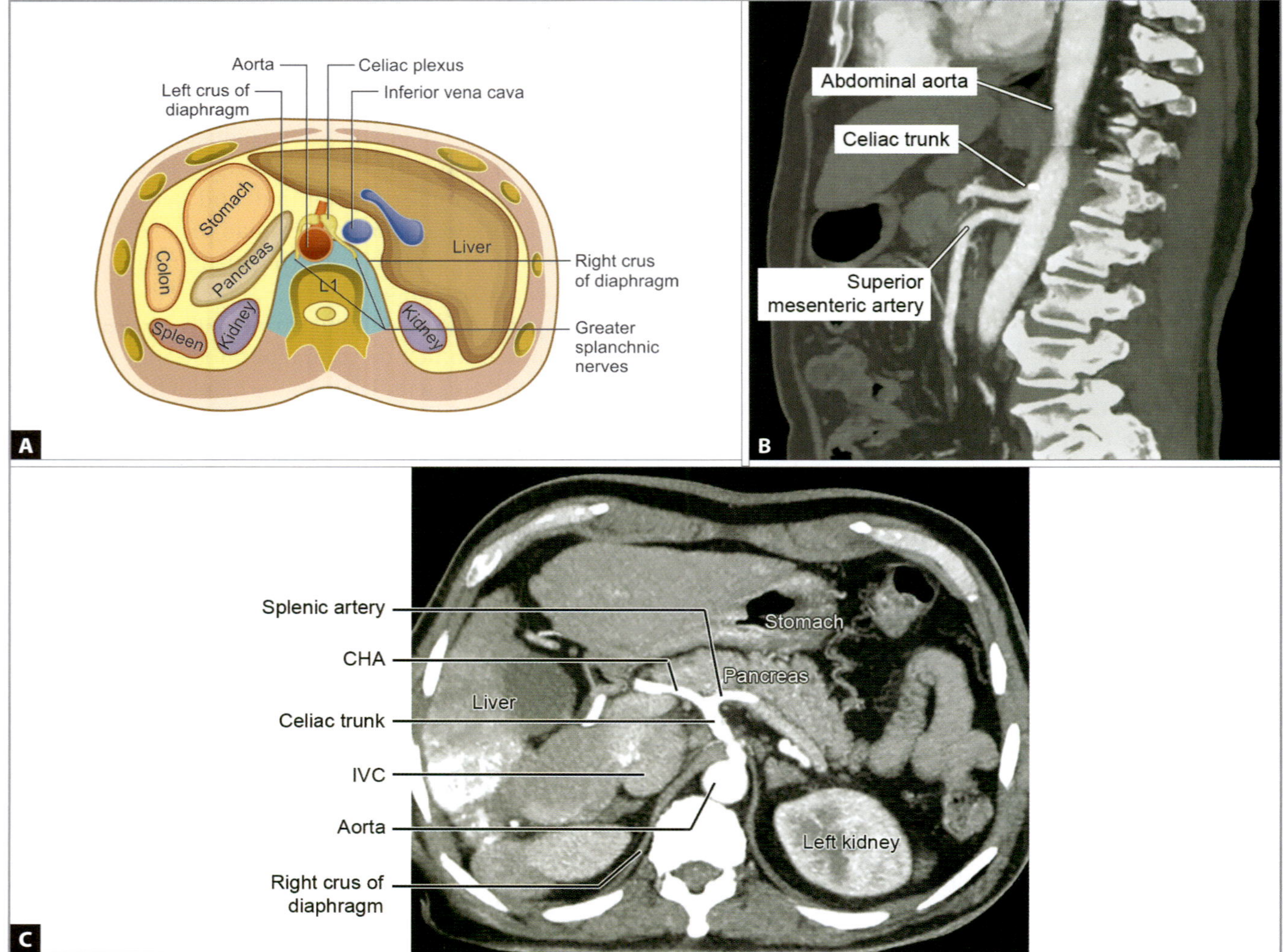

Figs. 11A to C: Cross-sectional anatomy of the celiac trunk. (A) Line diagram of the cross-sectional anatomy. The celiac plexus is positioned in front of the diaphragm's crus, extending around and in front of the aorta. The aorta is located anteriorly and slightly to the left of the anterior margin of the vertebral body; (B) CT sagittal view showing take-off of the celiac trunk and superior mesenteric artery; and (C) CT axial view in arterial phase showing cross-sectional anatomy of the abdomen at the origin of the celiac trunk. (CHA: common hepatic artery; CT: computed tomography; IVC: inferior vena cava)

Coeliac Plexus Block

Important nociceptive triggers in the abdominal cavity include abdominal distension or contraction of hollow organ walls, ischemia of visceral musculature, direct action of chemical substances on the mucosa, formation of allogenic mediators, and traction or compression of ligaments, vessels, or mesentery. This pain from the viscera is transmitted from the nociceptors on the walls of the viscera via the sympathetic and parasympathetic pathways. Patients find it difficult to localize the source of pain and describe it as a vague aching, cramping, or burning-like pain.

The traditional or classic posterolateral approach was the original technique described by Kappis.[20,21]

The patient is positioned prone **(Fig. 12)**, with a pillow placed beneath the midsection of the abdomen to reduce lumbar lordosis and enhance comfort. If the patient cannot tolerate this position due to pain, intravenous analgesics may be administered to assist in positioning. The patient's arms are positioned either under their head or allowed

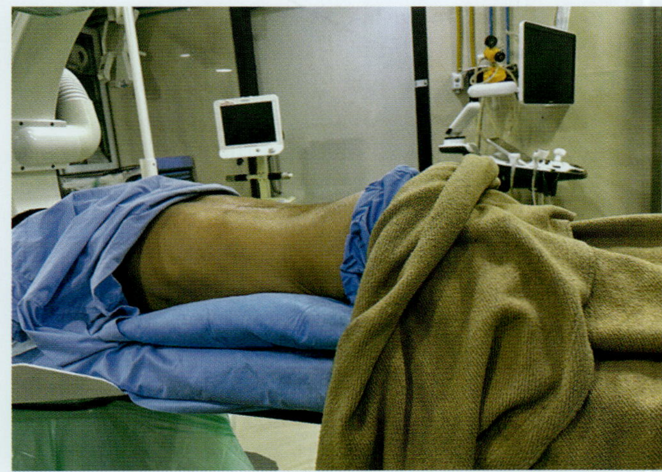

Fig. 12: Patient position for a celiac plexus block (posterior approach).

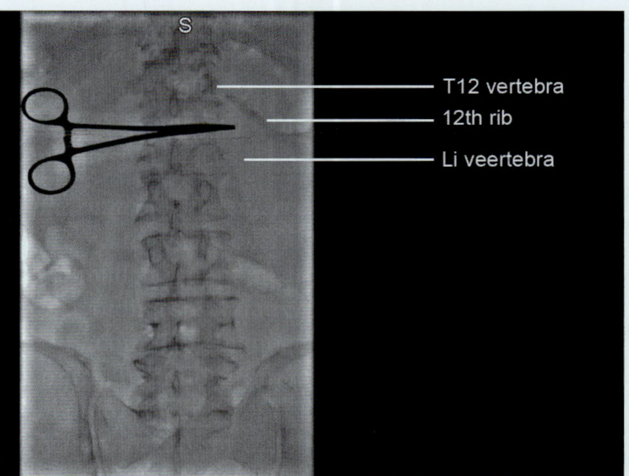

Fig. 13: Locate the L1 vertebra and identify the structures.

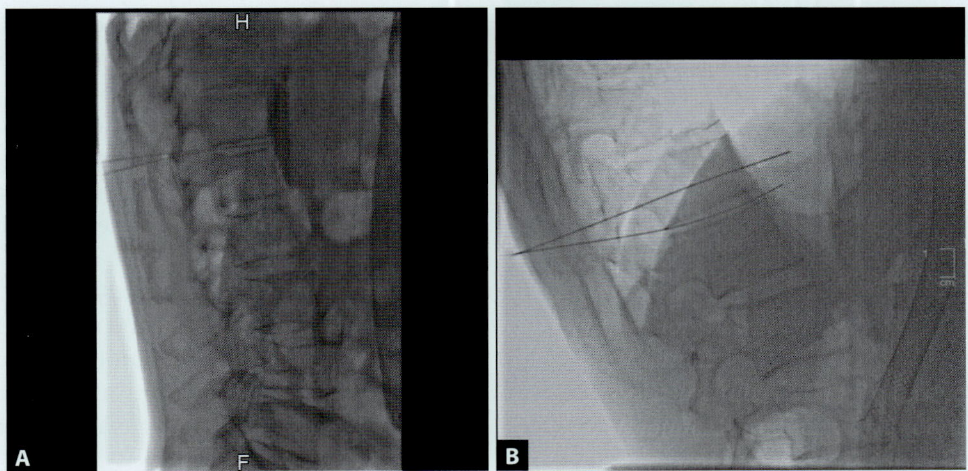

Figs. 14A and B: (A) Lateral Fluoroscopic image showing the spread of the contrast hugging the L1 body (retrocrural); (B) Needles placed antecrural.

to hang off the table. An intravenous line should be secured, and appropriate fluids should be administered. Standard monitoring, including noninvasive blood pressure (NIBP), peripheral capillary oxygen saturation (SpO_2), and electrocardiogram (ECG), must be attached. The classic approach utilizes a two-needle technique and may be performed under fluoroscopic or CT guidance. Key anatomical landmarks include the 12th rib and the T12 and L1 vertebral bodies **(Fig. 13)**. As per Moore, an isosceles triangle is formed by the intersection of the 12th rib and lateral border of paraspinal muscle on both sides and spine if L1 vertebra.

Under strict aseptic precautions, the L1 vertebral body is identified. Local anesthetic is used to raise skin wheals approximately four finger breadths or 6–8 cm from the midline at the L1 vertebral level, typically corresponding to the junction of the paraspinal muscles with the 12th rib. Two 15 cm, 22G spinal or biopsy needles are inserted at the site of the wheals at an angle of 45 degrees to the coronal plane and 15° cephalad, aiming to contact the body of the L1 vertebra. The needle is then slightly withdrawn and redirected an additional 10° until it "walks off" the vertebral body. The final needle position should be 1–1.5 cm anterior to the vertebral body **(Figs. 14A and B)**.

It is recommended that the right needle tip is positioned slightly further forward than the left, as more fibers of the plexus are located on the right. The left needle's proximity to the aorta can be identified by observing its pulsation. After confirming the absence of blood on aspiration, 2–3 mL of water-soluble contrast is injected through each needle **(Fig. 15)**. The dye spread is confirmed on anteroposterior (AP) and lateral views and should remain confined to the T12 and L1 vertebral bodies. This step helps confirm whether the needle placement is retrocrural (1–1.5 cm anterior to the L1 vertebral body), transcrural, or antecrural (an additional 2 cm beyond the retrocrural position). For a transcrural or antecrural approach, the needle tip will be positioned 1–2 cm further anterior compared to the retrocrural location.

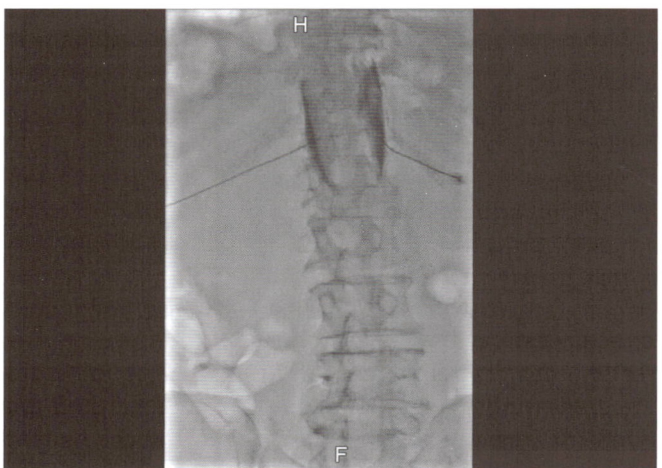

Fig. 15: Spread of contrast in anteroposterior (AP) view.

The contrast gets washed away if in a vessel, if muscle striations are seen, it indicates that the needle is in the diaphragm, and needles should be readjusted and contrast repeated.

Once the needle position is confirmed, 4–5 mL of a local anesthetic (0.25% bupivacaine or 1% lignocaine) is administered through each needle. This serves as a diagnostic block and provides analgesia prior to the injection of the neurolytic agent, as alcohol can cause significant pain upon administration. Subsequently, 15–20 mL of 50% alcohol is injected through each needle, with repeated aspiration to ensure there is no blood return. If the procedure is performed under CT guidance, a smaller volume of the neurolytic agent (8–10 mL) may be used due to the increased precision of needle placement.

Alcohol is the preferred neurolytic agent in this procedure, as it has less affinity for vascular tissue compared to phenol. To prevent the neurolytic agent from remaining in the needle tract and potentially causing skin necrosis, local anesthetic or saline should be injected while withdrawing the needles.

There are several other approaches for the neurolytic celiac plexus block (NCPB) such as the antecrural, retrocrural, transaortic, transdiscal, anterior, and endoscopic. Needle positions and advantages of each are mentioned below **(Figs. 16A and B)**.

- *Transaortic posterolateral approach:*[22] Patient is made to lie in a prone position and a single needle on the left side is used for the technique. The needle is placed just ahead of the anterior wall of the aorta. Hence the position of the needle is as close to the ganglia as is

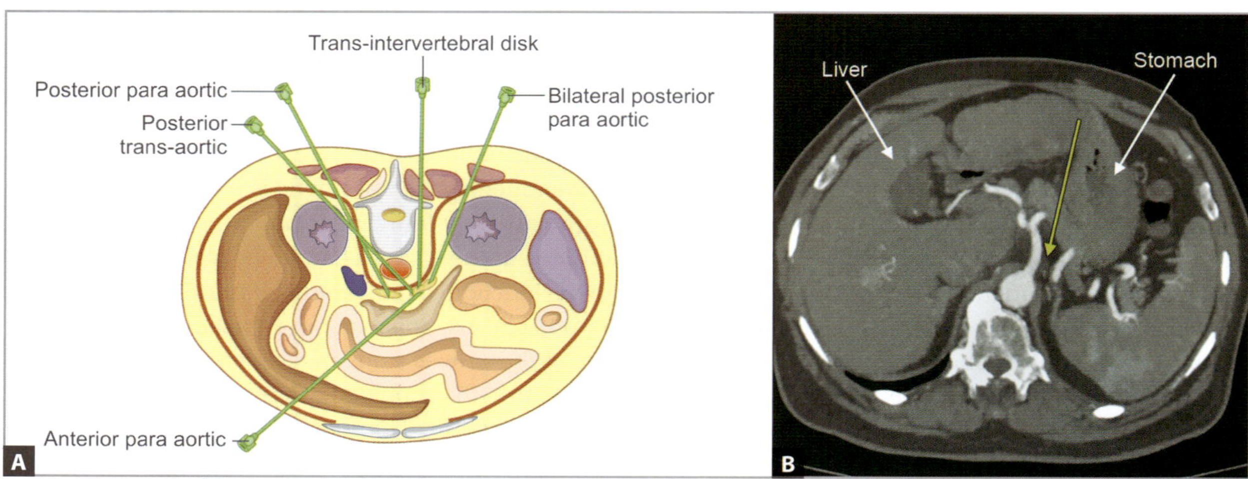

Figs. 16A and B: (A) Approaches to the celiac plexus; (B) CT axial view showing the needle trajectory anterior percutaneous transabdominal approach using USG. (CT: computed tomography; USG: ultrasound)

possible. The neurolytic agent covers the aorta and encircles it. In advanced disease, the tumor is known to invade through all tissues including nerves and the celiac ganglia may be engulfed in tumor mass and thus not reachable. This approach may possibly overcome this problem

- *Transdiscal:*[23] The approach is posterolateral, with the patient positioned prone. The needle is advanced through the T12-L1 intervertebral disc, a technique designed to minimize the risk of organ perforation, particularly in cases of organomegaly. This method also reduces the likelihood of pneumothorax, as its primary target is the splanchnic nerves. However, this approach is not widely utilized. Potential complications include discitis, intervertebral disc degeneration, and other associated risks.
- *Anterior approach:*[24] With the patient in a supine position. A single needle is introduced through the epigastrium till it touches the L1 body and then withdrawn by 1–2 cm. Can be performed under Ultrasound guidance as well as fluoroscopic or CT guidance. Patient comfort is an advantage. Especially useful if the patient cannot lie prone. Also, only a single needle is used
- *Endoscopic approach:*[25,26] The patient is in the left lateral position in the endoscopy suite. The needle is placed anterior to the lateral aspect of the aorta at the level of the celiac trunk. Precision is much improved with Doppler guidance of the interposed vessels. It is an easy technique.

The main adverse events are transient hypotension due to splanchnic vasodilation, diarrhea due to unopposed parasympathetic tone, and needle site pain. Much rarer complications include; paresthesia, paresis, pneumothorax, hematuria, shoulder pain, hemorrhagic gastritis, duodenitis, and rarely death.

The procedure must be performed under imaging either under ultrasound/fluoroscopy/CT for precision and safety. Cardiopulmonary bypass (CPB) is relatively safe and effective and has the best quality of evidence among neurolytic blocks with a reduction in opioid use and better patient satisfaction.[27]

Ultrasound-guided Celiac Plexus

Celiac plexus cannot be visualized clearly by ultrasound and so it is important to be well versed with the sono-anatomy to perform the block safely. An important landmark is the abdominal aorta (AA) which can be seen in the epigastrium as a tubular pulsating anechoic structure. The first artery to arise from the abdominal aorta is the celiac trunk (CT). It is the most important landmark for celiac plexus. At its exit from the aorta, CT presents as a typical ram-horn-like symmetric bifurcation. The second artery to arise from the AA is the superior mesenteric artery.

The origins of the celiac trunk and the superior mesenteric artery are identified using longitudinal ultrasound imaging. Subsequently, the transducer is rotated into a transverse orientation to visualize the origin of the celiac trunk and its bifurcation into the common hepatic artery and splenic artery. The Chiba needle (15 cm, 22G) is used and introduced in plane to the transducer[28] **(Figs. 17A to D)**.

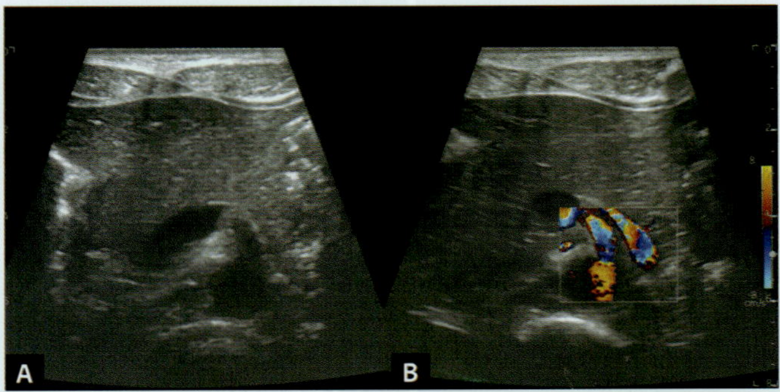

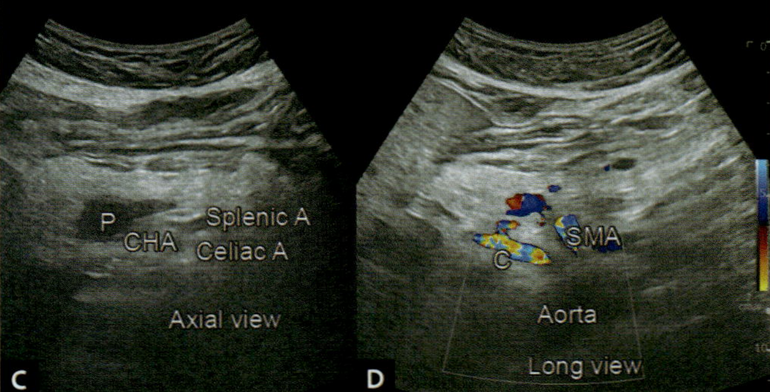

Figs. 17A to D: Ultrasound image of the location of the celiac trunk for anterior percutaneous transabdominal. (A and B) 2D view at the level of origin of the celiac trunk; (C) Axial view; and (D) Sagittal view in color Doppler mode. (C: celiac trunk; CHA: common hepatic artery; P: portal vein; SMA: superior mesenteric artery)

Pelvic Cancer Pain

Superior Hypogastric Plexus Block

The superior hypogastric plexus is a continuation of abdominal aortic plexus and is located bilaterally in the retroperitoneum at the level of L5-S1 vertebral body, anterior to the bifurcation of the aorta, where it

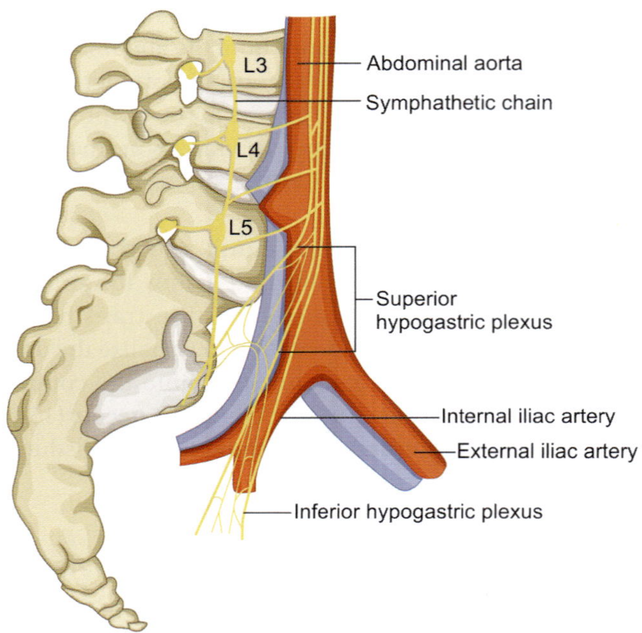

Fig.18: Anatomy of hypogastric plexus (lateral view).

branches into the common iliac vessels **(Fig. 18)**. It then descends into the pelvis as the inferior hypogastric plexus. It innervates various pelvic structures, including the bladder, urethra, vagina, vulva, ovaries, prostate, penis, testicles, uterus, ureter, pelvic floor, descending colon, and rectum.[29] Blocking of this plexus is indicated in the evaluation and management of sympathetically mediated pain from the pelvic viscera.

Superior hypogastric plexus block (SHPB) block was first described in 1990 by Plancarte et al.[30]

Classic Approach

In this fluoroscopy-guided, posterior, two-needle technique patient is placed in a prone position. L4-5 spinous processes are felt and marked. A needle entry point is at L4-5 intervertebral space, 4 finger breadth, or 6–8 cm lateral to the midline. After local infiltration at this point a 22G, 15 cm long blunt tip needle is inserted bilaterally approximately 45° medial and 30° caudal so that its tip is directed toward the anterolateral aspect of the bottom of the L5 vertebral body. Challenges in needle placement include the prominent iliac crest, the L5 transverse process, and the L5 vertebral body. Once the needle contacts the L5 vertebral body, it is redirected off the bone. The goal is to advance the needle approximately 1 cm beyond the vertebral body, where a characteristic "pop" may be felt as the needle pierces the anterior fascia of the psoas muscle. This typically occurs at a depth of 8–12 cm. In the AP fluoroscopic view needle tip should be at the junction of L5-S1 vertebral bodies and in the lateral view needle tip is seen just beyond the anterolateral margin of the vertebral body. The needle tip position is verified by injecting 3–5 mL of a water-soluble contrast medium with the spread of contrast confined to the midline or paramedian region in AP view and as a smooth posterior contour, corresponding to the anterior psoas fascia in the lateral view. This is followed by the injection of 8–10 mL of 0.25% bupivacaine or 1% lignocaine to confirm pain relief. Once confirmed and accepted, 15 mL of 50% alcohol is administered in small increments through each needle, with constant negative aspiration before injection.[31] Gamal et al. described a small randomised control trial of the transdiscal versus classic approach and showed that both methods were safe and effective, though the transdiscal approach was also significantly faster to perform.

Several modifications to the original technique have been introduced, including the transdiscal approach, where the needle is advanced through the L5-S1 disc, and the transarterial approach, where the needle is passed through the iliac artery until blood aspiration ceases. This indicates that the needle is positioned just anterior to the artery, which is retroperitoneal and aligned in the same plane as the superior hypogastric plexus (SHP). These variations were primarily developed to address procedural challenges.[32]

Traditionally performed under fluoroscopic or CT guidance, the use of ultrasound has emerged as a radiation-free, real-time imaging alternative. In the supine position and under aseptic conditions, a low-frequency curved ultrasound probe is placed in the longitudinal axis to identify the aortic bifurcation. The probe is then adjusted to a transverse orientation to visualize the terminal aorta and the bifurcation of the iliac vessels. Also, a sagittal long-axis scan is performed to map the L5/S1 vertebral bodies and intervertebral disc. Local anesthesia is administered with a 1% lidocaine solution, injected 1.0–1.5 inches below the umbilicus. A 15 cm, 22G Chiba needle is inserted using an out-of-plane technique and advanced until contact is made with the L5 vertebral body, carefully avoiding vascular structures. 10 mL of 0.25% bupivacaine is used for diagnostic hypogastric block after confirming a negative aspiration for blood. A 10 mL solution containing 50%

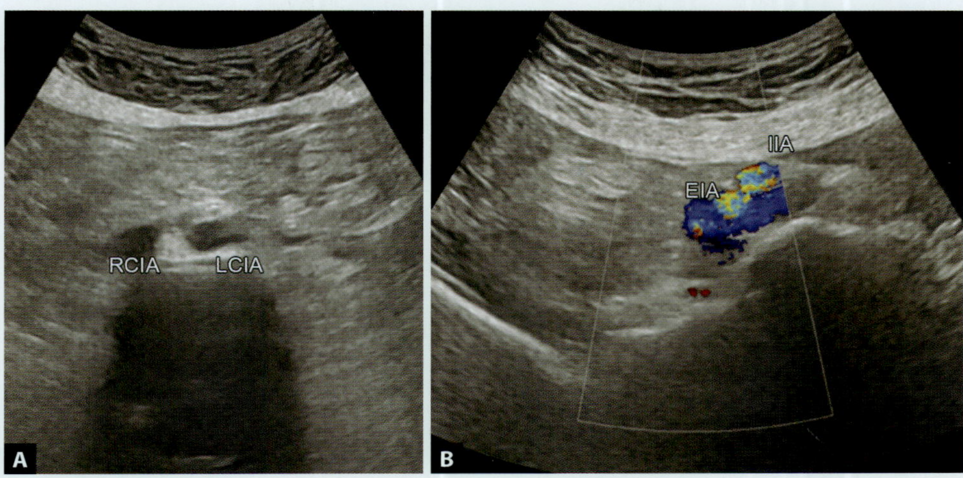

Figs. 19A and B: Ultrasound image. (A) Axial view, aortic bifurcation into right and left common iliac artery (RCIA, LCIA); (B) Sagittal view, division of common iliac into external and internal iliac artery (EIA, IIA).

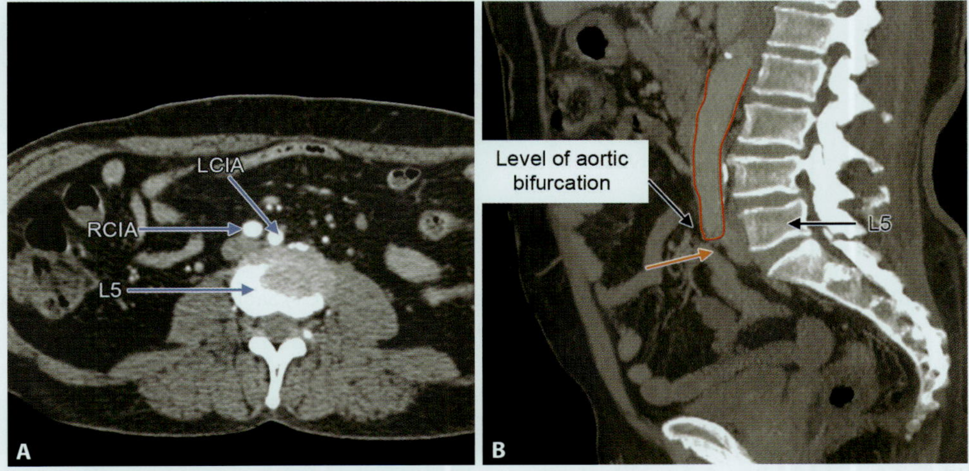

Figs. 20A and B: (A) CT axial view at L5 level; (B) Sagittal view showing aorta in red line. (LCIA: left common iliac artery; RCIA: right common iliac artery)

ethanol is used for neurolysis. The uniform spread of the drug is confirmed with real-time sonography[33] **(Figs. 19 and 20)**.

Ganglion Impar Block

The Ganglion impar is a solitary, unpaired ganglion that represents the fused terminal segment of the paired paravertebral sympathetic chains. It is located in the retroperitoneal space, posterior to the rectum, and situated at the midline or paramedian position near the sacrococcygeal joint (SCJ) or coccyx **(Figs. 21A to C)**. This ganglion provides sympathetic innervation to the perineum, coccyx, anus, distal rectum, vulva, scrotum, urethra, and vagina.

Chronic perineal pain (CPP) is a pain syndrome that may involve either a somatic or sympathetic component. A thorough history and a detailed physical examination are both invaluable for distinguishing between the sympathetic and somatic aspects of CPP. *Sympathetically mediated perineal pain (SMPP)* is characterized by poorly localized discomfort, often described as burning and accompanied by a sense of urgency in the perineal area.[34]

The ganglion impar block is utilized for the management of intractable neoplastic perineal pain of sympathetic origin. This type of pain is typically vague, poorly

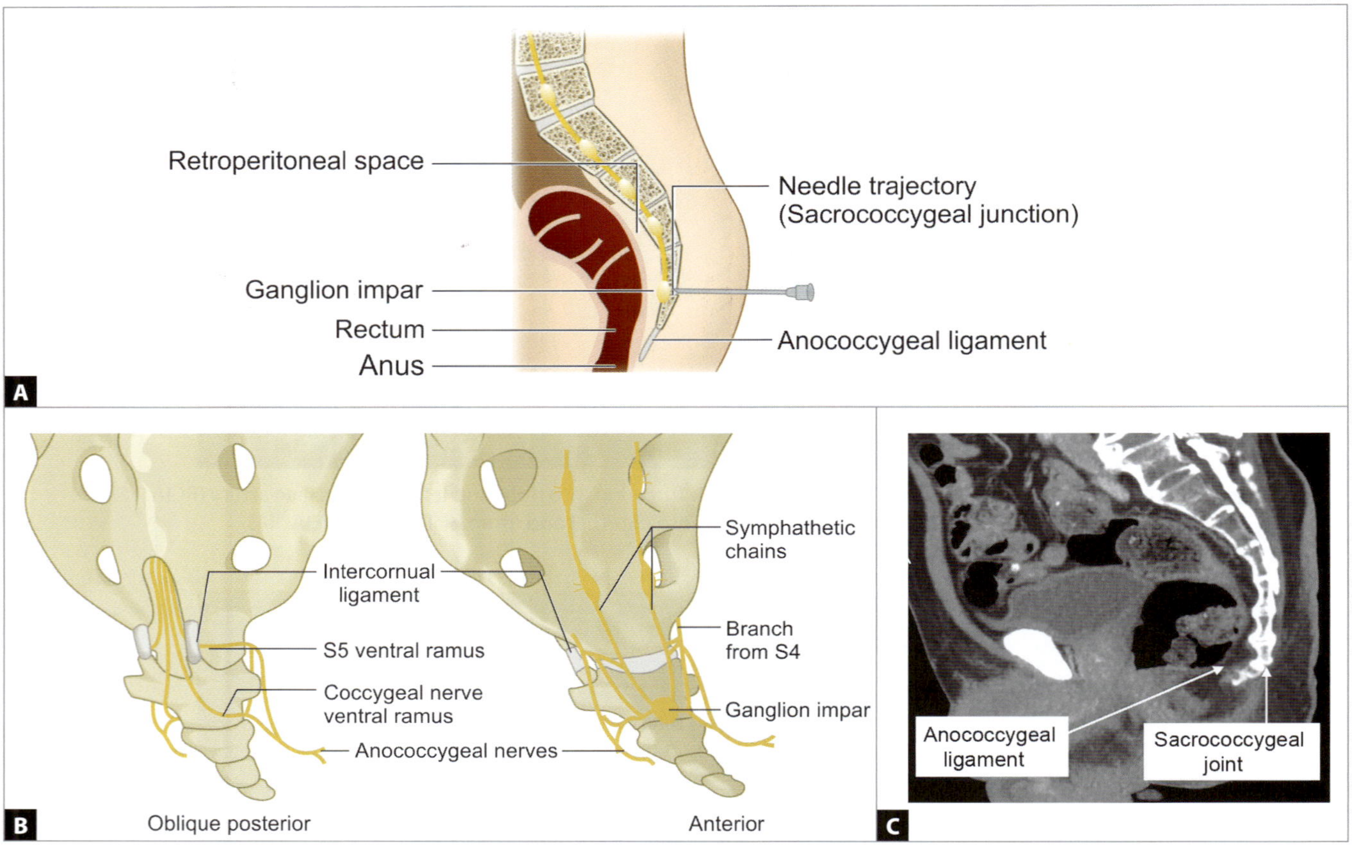

Retroperitoneal space
Needle trajectory (Sacrococcygeal junction)
Ganglion impar
Rectum
Anus
Anococcygeal ligament
A

Intercornual ligament
S5 ventral ramus
Coccygeal nerve ventral ramus
Anococcygeal nerves
Symphathetic chains
Branch from S4
Ganglion impar
Oblique posterior
Anterior
B

Anococcygeal ligament
Sacrococcygeal joint
C

Figs. 21A to C: (A and B) Anatomy of ganglion impar; (C) Computed tomography (CT) Sagittal view showing the landmarks for the Ganglion impar block.

localized, and often associated with sensations of burning and urgency.

Clinical candidates for a ganglion impar block often present with symptoms such as perineal and perianal burning pain, urinary or rectal urgency, and tenesmus. Indications for the procedure include pain in the sacral, rectal, anal, genital, vulva, and perineal regions that are sympathetically mediated (i.e., neuropathic or postherpetic neuralgia), coccydynia, or pain secondary to endometriosis or proctalgia fugax.[35]

The procedure is performed under fluoroscopy guidance. Plancarte originally described the *anococcygeal approach* in 1990, which involves positioning the patient laterally and advancing a curved needle through the anococcygeal membrane while using a finger in the rectum to guide the needle and mitigate the risk of rectal injury.[36] Alternative techniques have since been developed, including the *transsacrococcygeal* and *transdiscal approaches*. The transsacrococcygeal method for administering a ganglion impar block was first detailed by Wemm and Saberski.[37]

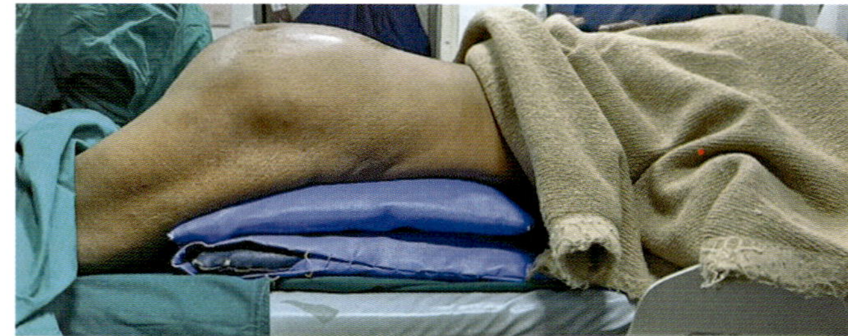

Fig. 22: The patient is placed in a prone or jackknife position for Ganglion impar block.

The transsacrococcygeal approach is performed with the patient in the prone position, with a pillow placed under the lower abdomen to optimize positioning **(Fig. 22)**. The site of needle insertion is identified by palpating the

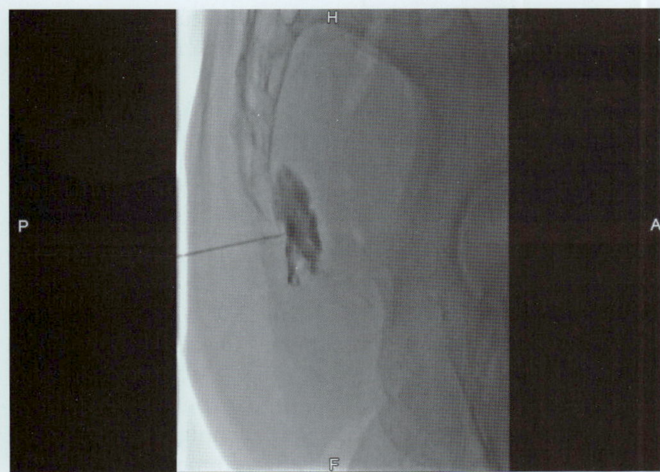

Fig. 23: Ganglion impar contrast spread in transsacrococcygeal approach.

sacral cornu and using a fluoroscope under complete aseptic preparation. A wheal of local anesthesia is created at the insertion site. With fluoroscopic C-arm guidance in a lateral position, a 22–25G needle is inserted through the skin, piercing the dorsal sacrococcygeal ligament at the midline. The needle is carefully advanced to the precoccygeal space, just anterior to the sacrococcygeal junction.[38]

To confirm proper needle placement, 1–2 mL of contrast is injected. The ideal contrast spread appears in the form of a "comma" shape as is seen in **Figure 23**. For a diagnostic block, 1–2 mL of local anesthetic, such as lignocaine or bupivacaine, is administered. If further intervention is required, a neurolytic agent, typically 6% phenol (2–8 mL), can be injected.

While the procedure is relatively safe, there is a risk of rectal injury and neuritis. Additionally, RFA of the ganglion impar has been described as an alternative technique for long-term pain relief.

Ultrasound has also been utilized for performing ganglion impar block via the transanococcygeal approach as well as the transsacrococcygeal approach.[39,40] However, ultrasound cannot reliably assess needle depth or injectate distribution due to artifacts caused by the sacral and coccygeal bones. Therefore, it is recommended to use a lateral fluoroscopic view to monitor needle depth, particularly for neurolytic injections.

CONCLUSION

Interventional techniques play an important role in the comprehensive management of cancer-related pain by addressing complex pain syndromes through a multimodal approach. The evolving paradigm emphasizes early implementation of interventional techniques for managing pain rather than using them as a last-resort option. With a broad spectrum of neuroablative and neuromodulation approaches along with a greater understanding of the pathophysiological basis of cancer-related pain, these interventions provide effective pain relief, particularly when conventional analgesics prove insufficient. Integrating interventional procedures alongside pharmacological therapies enhances patient outcomes, improving quality of life and optimizing the overall care trajectory for individuals suffering from refractory cancer pain.

REFERENCES

1. Pugh TM, Squarize F, Kiser AL. A comprehensive strategy to pain management for cancer patients in an inpatient rehabilitation facility. Front Pain Res (Lausanne). 2021: 2:688511.
2. Swerdlow M. The history of neurolytic block. In Techniques of neurolysis. Boston, MA: Springer; 1989. pp. 1-11.
3. Tuffer T. Anesthésie médullaire chirurgicale par injection sous-arachnoïdienne lombaire de cocaïne; technique et résultats. La Semaine Médicale. 1900;20:167.
4. Vig S, Bhan S, Bhatnagar S. Celiac plexus block–an old technique with new developments. Pain Physician. 2021;24(5):379-98.
5. Robechhi A, Capra R. Hydrocortisone (compound F); first clinical experiments in the field of rheumatology. Minerva Med. 1952;43(98):1259-63.
6. Lievre JA, Bloch-Mechel H, Pean G. L'hydrocortisone en injection locale. Rev Rhum. 1953;20:310-11.
7. Epstein JB, Wilkie DJ, Fisher DJ, Kim YO, Villines D. Neuropathic and nociceptive pain in head and neck cancer patients receiving radiation therapy. Head Neck Oncol. 2009;1:26.
8. Dennis J, Patin MD. Pain control in head and neck cancer. Curr Opin Otolaryngol Head Neck Surg. 1998;86(2):85-9.
9. Narouze S. Ultrasound-guided stellate ganglion block: safety and efficacy. Curr Pain Headache Rep. 2014;18(6):424.
10. Bhatia A, Flamer D, Peng PW. Evaluation of sonoanatomy relevant to performing stellate ganglion blocks using anterior and lateral simulated approaches: an observational study. Can J Anaesth. 2012;59(11):1040-7.
11. Rose KR, Stone JJ, Ren Z, Wang H, Jahromi BS. Percutaneous trigeminal rhizotomy in a biplane angiosuite: technical assessment J Neurointerv Surg. 2014;6(9):699-703.
12. Waldman SD. Atlas of Interventional Pain Management, 4th edition. Philadelphia: Elsevier; 2014.
13. Windsor RE, Jahnke S. Sphenopalatine ganglion blockade: a review and proposed modification of the transnasal technique. Pain Physician. 2004;7(2):283-6.

14. Tolba R, Weiss AL, Denis DJ. Sphenopalatine ganglion block and radiofrequency ablation: technical notes and efficacy. Ochsner J. 2019 Spring;19(1):32-7.
15. Pani N, Kumar Rath S. Regional & topical anaesthesia of upper airways. Indian J Anaesth. 2009;53(6):641-8.
16. Ažman J, Stopar Pintaric T, Cvetko E, Vlassakov K. Ultrasound-guided glossopharyngeal nerve block: a cadaver and a volunteer sonoanatomy study. Reg Anesth Pain Med. 2017;42(2):252-8.
17. Punj J, Sundaram S. Ultrasound-guided glossopharyngeal nerve block: description of a new technique. J Anaesthesiol Clin Pharmacol. 2021;37(3):483-5.
18. Aggarwal A, Suresh V, Gupta B, Sonthalia S. Post-herpetic Neuralgia: a systematic review of current interventional pain management strategies. J Cutan Aesthet Surg. 2020; 13(4):265-74.
19. Kambadakone A, Thabet A, Gervais DA, Mueller PR, Arellano RS. CT-guided celiac plexus neurolysis: a review of anatomy, indications, technique, and tips for successful treatment. Radiographics. 2011;31(6):1599-621.
20. Fujita Y, Sari A. Max Kappis and the celiac plexus block. Anesthesiology. 1997;86(2):508.
21. Lieberman RP, Waldman SD. Celiac plexus neurolysis with the modified transaortic approach. Radiology. 1990;175(1):274-6.
22. Ischia S, Luzzani A, Ischia A, Faggion S. A new approach to the neurolytic block of the coeliac plexus: the transaortic technique. Pain. 1983;16(4):333-41.
23. Ina H, Kitoh T, Kobayashi M, Imai S, Ofusa Y, Goto H. New technique for the neurolytic celiac plexus block: the transintervertebral disc approach. Anesthesiology. 1996;85(1):212-7.
24. In: Warfield CA, Bajwa ZH (Eds). Principles & Practice of Pain Medicine, 2nd edition. New York, NY: McGraw-Hill; 2004.
25. Seicean A. Celiac plexus neurolysis in pancreatic cancer: the endoscopic ultrasound approach. World J Gastroenterol. 2014;20(1):110-7.
26. Sakamoto H, Kitano M, Komaki T, Imai H, Kamata K, Kudo M. Endoscopic ultrasound-guided neurolysis in pancreatic cancer. Pancreatology. 2011;11:52-8.
27. Hochberg U, Ingelmo P, Solé E, Miró J, Rivera G, Perez J. Early Interventional Treatments for Patients with Cancer Pain: A Narrative Review. J Pain Res. 2023;16:1663-71.
28. Bhatnagar S, Joshi S, Rana SP, Mishra S, Garg R, Ahmed SM. Bedside ultrasound-guided celiac plexus neurolysis in upper abdominal cancer patients: a randomized, prospective study for comparison of percutaneous bilateral paramedian vs. unilateral paramedian needle-insertion technique. Pain Pract. 2014;14(2):E63-8.
29. Urits I, Schwartz R, Herman J, Berger AA, Lee D, Lee C, et al. A comprehensive update of the superior hypogastric block for the management of chronic pelvic pain. Curr Pain Headache Rep. 2021;25(3):13.
30. Plancarte R, Amescua C, Patt RB, Aldrete JA. Superior hypogastric plexus block for pelvic cancer pain. Anesthesiology. 1990;73(2):236-9.
31. Gofeld M, Shankar H, Benzon HT. Fluoroscopy and ultrasound-guided sympathetic blocks. Essentials Pain Med Elsevier. 2018;789-804.e2.
32. Turker G, Basagan-Mogol E, Gurbet A, Ozturk C, Uckunkaya N, Sahin S. A new technique for superior hypogastric plexus block: the posteromedian transdiscal approach. Tohoku J Exp Med. 2005;206(3):277-81.
33. Mishra S, Bhatnagar S, Rana SPS, Khurana D, Thulkar S. Efficacy of the anterior ultrasound-guided superior hypogastric plexus neurolysis in pelvic cancer pain in advanced gynecological cancer patients. Pain Med (United States). 2013;14(6):837-42.
34. Wallace MS, Leung AY, McBeth MD. Malignant Pain. In: Raj P (Ed). Textbook of Regional Anesthesia. Pennsylvania: Churchill Livingstone Publishers; 2002. p. 585.
35. Asmaranto, Susila D. Ganglion Impar Block and Neurolysis for Perineal Pain in Anal Adenocarcinoma: A Case Report. Pharmacogn J. 2024;16(3):711-5.
36. Plancarte R, Amescua C, Patt RB, Allende S. Presacral blockade of the ganglion of Walter (ganglion imp-ar). Anesthesiology. 1990;73(3A):A751.
37. Wemm K Jr, Saberski L. Modified approach to block the ganglion impar (Ganglion of Walther). Reg Anesth. 1995;20(6):544.
38. Toshniwal GR, Dureja GP, Prashanth SM. Transsacrococcygeal approach to ganglion impar block for management of chronic perineal pain: a prospective observational study. Pain Physician. 2007;10(5):661-6.
39. Bhatnagar S, Khanna S, Roshni S, Goyal GN, Mishra S, Rana SP, et al. Early Ultrasound-Guided Neurolysis for Pain Management in Gastrointestinal and Pelvic Malignancies: An Observational Study in a Tertiary Care Center of Urban India. Pain Pract. 2012;12(1):23-32.
40. Lin CS, Cheng JK, Hsu YW, Chen CC, Lao HC, Huang CJ, et al. Ultrasound-guided ganglion impar block: a technical report. Pain Med. 2010;11(3):390-4.

Palliative Care Medicine

60

CHAPTER

Principles of Palliative Care

Kalpana Balakrishnan, Meenakshi V Venketeswaran, Thendral Ramasamy

INTRODUCTION

This chapter briefly traces the history of palliative care from its origins to its evolution from belonging in a hospice to an entirely independent medical specialty. It describes the tenets of palliative care in the context of cancer and other life-limiting illnesses. It includes an overview of the symptomatology and treatment strategies in palliative care. A framework on communication and ethics is also provided.

HISTORY[1]

Though the origins of hospice (Latin word hospitium: hospitality) and palliative care (Latin word pallium: to cloak) go back many centuries, the catalyst for the modern hospice movement was Dame Cicely Saunders **(Fig. 1)**. Cicely started as a nurse, she later trained as a social worker and doctor, researching pain management.[2] She set up the St. Christopher's Hospice in London in 1967. She introduced the theory of "Total Pain" emphasizing the need to assess physical, psychosocial, and spiritual aspects of pain.[3] This philosophy of holistic care underpins the practice of palliative care.

- The World Health Organization defines palliative care (PC)[4] as an approach that improves the quality of life of patients and their families facing the problems associated with life-threatening illness, through the prevention and relief of suffering by means of early identification and impeccable assessment and treatment of pain and other problems, physical, psychosocial, and spiritual. Various international organizations agree that palliative care is suitable for all patients with serious illnesses, irrespective of their age, disease progression, or prognosis.
- *Palliative care:*
  - Provides relief from pain and other distressing symptoms
  - Affirms life and regards dying as a normal process
  - Intends neither to hasten nor postpone death

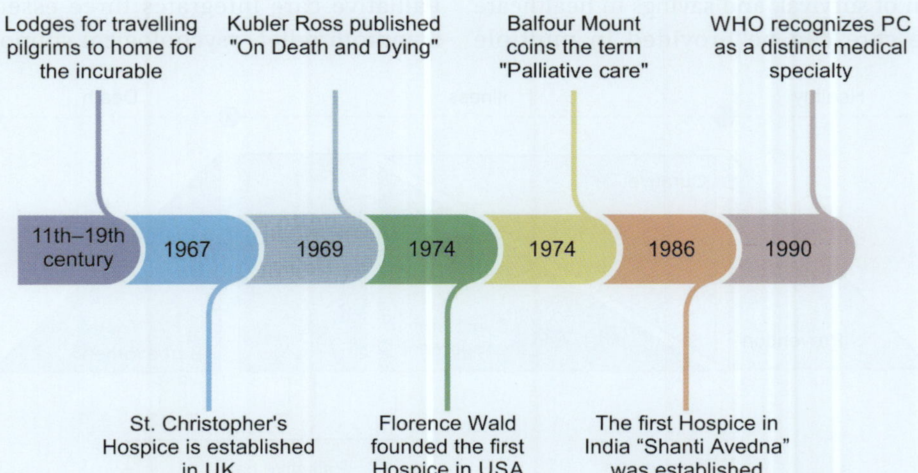

Fig. 1: Key timelines in the development of palliative care. (WHO: World Health Organization)
Source: NEJM Group (2020, December 30), Brief History of Palliative Care. NEJM Resident 360.

- Integrates the psychological and spiritual aspects of patient care
- Offers a support system to help patients live as actively as possible until death
- Offers a support system to help the family cope during the patient's illness and in their own bereavement
- Uses a team approach to address the needs of patients and their families, including bereavement counseling, if indicated
- Will enhance the quality of life, and may also positively influence the course of illness
- Is applicable early in the course of illness **(Fig. 2)**, in conjunction with other therapies that are intended to prolong life, such as chemotherapy or radiation therapy, and includes those investigations needed to better understand and manage distressing clinical complications[4]

While advanced cancer was the prototypical example for palliative care, it is now recognized that palliative care is just as essential for alleviating suffering due to advanced cardiovascular diseases, major organ failure, human immunodeficiency virus (HIV) and drug-resistant tuberculosis, severe burns, chronic respiratory and neurological illness, acute trauma, extreme birth prematurity, or extreme frailty of old age.[5,6] Integration of palliative care into the healthcare system has now become a global health imperative.[5] In addition, there is evidence supporting early integration of palliative care in the disease trajectory of patients clearly demonstrating reduction in the symptom burden, improvement in quality of life, prolongation of survival, and savings in healthcare costs.[7-10] Palliative care can be provided in multiple settings, e.g., the outpatient department, in-patient, home, and hospice.

Ritu, a 28-year-old mother, was diagnosed with advanced pancreatic cancer. Her husband frequently took leave to support her hospital visits. She endured severe pain, fatigue, and vomiting during chemotherapy. She was very anxious and wondered if she would be around for her daughter's birthday. The palliative care team managed her alongside the cancer therapy with analgesics and supportive counseling. Unfortunately, Ritu's disease spread to her lymph nodes, and she was prescribed radiation. She had started attending religious gatherings and practicing meditation. Psychological and spiritual guidance kept her going, and she made it to most of the radiotherapy sessions on her own. 2 months after her daughter's birthday, her condition worsened with jaundice and ascites. Too sick to travel to the hospital, the PC team made home visits to manage her symptoms. The family was counseled as well and actively supported her daughter. Ritu passed away at home. A month later, the PC team checked on her husband, who expressed gratitude for the support during their toughest times.

In this case vignette, we can appreciate that there was timely provision of holistic care for not only the patient but also the caregivers from the diagnosis of the disease till bereavement in the setting of their preference.

PALLIATIVE CARE COMPONENTS AND SYMPTOM MANAGEMENT

Overview

Palliative care integrates three essential components: Symptom relief, psychological support, and teamwork.

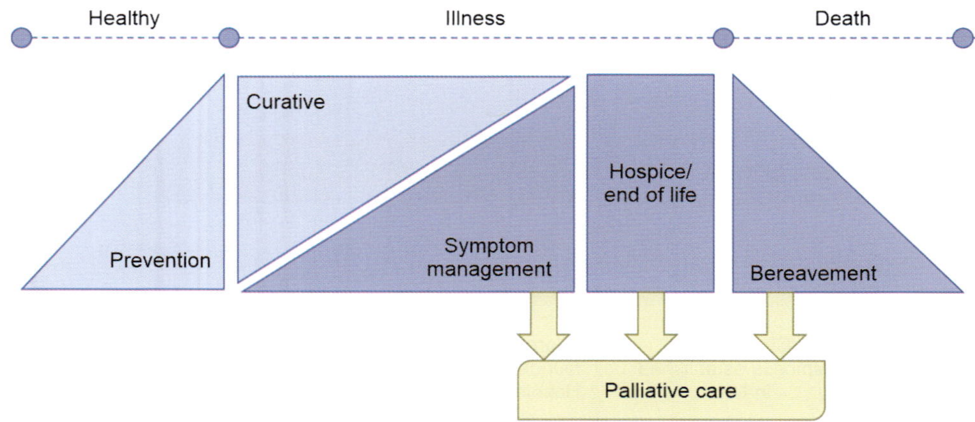

Fig. 2: The palliative care continuum.
Source: Adapted from Palliative Care 101: A Complete Guide to End-of-Life Care—Homage.

Patients experience increased symptom prevalence due to the disease, treatments, and disease progression, which is common across advanced chronic illnesses.[11] Pain and fatigue are the most frequent symptoms, followed by anorexia, breathlessness, and anxiety, indicating a common symptom pathway in palliative care patients.[12] Poor symptom control leads to increased suffering, noncompliance with therapy, functional decline, and poor quality of life, underscoring the need for a systematic approach to symptom identification and assessment.[13]

SYMPTOM ASSESSMENT AND MANAGEMENT

Assessment

Thorough assessment begins with history taking. Self-reporting of symptoms is preferred, but proxy reporting by carers is used when patients are too weak.[14] Mnemonics like "OPQRSTU" (Onset, Precipitating/Palliating factors, Quality, Severity, Temporal nature, Understanding) help detail symptoms like pain. Palliative care assessments cover physical, psychosocial, financial, and spiritual aspects, using a multidisciplinary team and validated tools **(Table 1)** to ensure holistic, patient-centered care, and capture under-reported symptoms.[15,16]

Management of common palliative care symptoms:

General principles include:

- Correcting reversible underlying causes
- Setting realistic goals for symptom optimization
- Explaining the reason for prescriptions
- Educating on the correct use of medication
- Utilizing both pharmacological and nonpharmacological interventions
- Addressing psychosomatic symptoms through psychological assessment
- Monitoring side effects and treatment responses
- *Pain:* Pain is the most common symptom prompting palliative care consultation. Successful pain management depends on understanding the etiology, classification, and severity of pain to formulate treatment plans. The WHO analgesic ladder is universally followed, with a modified fourth step for interventional pain methods **(Fig. 3)**.[17] Principles in chronic pain management include the use of the oral route, round-the-clock dosage instead of as needed, and access to rescue doses for breakthrough pain. Pharmacological management consists of nonopioids, opioids, and adjuvants.[18]

- *Nonopioids:* Acetaminophen and nonsteroidal anti-inflammatory drugs (NSAIDs) manage mild to moderate pain. Paracetamol is safe up to 3 g/day, with a reduced dose in cirrhotic patients. NSAIDs are chosen based on patient risk stratification.
- *Opioids:*
    - *Weak opioids:* Tramadol, codeine, and dihydrocodeine are used for moderate pain, often combined with paracetamol. Tramadol by its triple action of mu-opioid agonism, inhibition of noradrenergic reuptake, and serotonergic inhibition is useful in both nociceptive and neuropathic pain. The maximum daily recommended dose of tramadol is 400 mg. Being a prodrug, tramadol causes inadequate analgesia in poor metabolizers as a result of CYP2D6 polymorphism. Tramadol lowers seizure threshold, may cause serotonin toxicity, and is avoided in those who are at risk.
    - *Strong opioids:* Morphine, fentanyl, buprenorphine, methadone, and tapentadol are used for severe pain.
        - Morphine is the opioid of choice due to its low cost, oral formulation, and availability. Morphine is usually started at 5 mg every 4 hours for opioid-naive patients, with dose titration every 24–48 hours. Stable pain control allows a switch to sustained-release formulations.
        - Methadone is unique by its antagonistic effect on NMDA receptors and serotonin reuptake inhibition in addition to opioid agonism. The pharmacokinetic variability requires a careful dose titration and its potential for QT prolongation and drug interaction demands special training for its routine clinical use.[19] Methadone is used when morphine is poorly tolerated. The gastrointestinal route of elimination makes it safe in renal failure.
        - Tapentadol by its dual action on both mu opioid receptors and noradrenergic reuptake inhibition is useful in both nociceptive and neuropathic pain. The lower affinity for opioid receptor and lack of drug interaction have improved the safety of tapentadol.[20]
        - Fentanyl and buprenorphine are available as transdermal patches and are used when the

TABLE 1: Symptom assessment tools in palliative care.

S. No.	*Domain*	*Type of tool*	*Name of tool*
1.	PHYSICAL	Unidimensional tool (e.g., pain, nausea, breathlessness, and lack of appetite)	• Visual analog scale • Numerical rating scale • Categorical scale • Faces scale • Edmonton symptom assessment system
		Multidimensional tool for pain	• Brief pain inventory (BPI) • Mcgill pain questionnaire (MPQ) • Leeds assessment of neuropathic signs and symptoms (LANSS)
			• Pain Assessment in Advanced Dementia (PAINAD) Scale • Behavioral Pain Scale (BPS) • Adult Nonverbal Pain Scale (NVPS)
		Breathlessness	• Borg scale • Modified Medical Research Council; Dyspnea Scale (mMRC dyspnea scale) • Respiratory Distress Observation Scale (RDOS)
		Constipation	• Constipation Assessment Scale • Bowel Function Index • Bristol stool chart
		Fatigue	• Brief Fatigue Inventory (BFI) • Functional Assessment of Cancer Therapy-Fatigue (FACT-F) • EORTC QLQ-C30
		Delirium	• The Confusion Assessment Method (CAM) • Memorial Delirium Assessment Scale (MDAS) • Bedside Confusion Scale (BCS) • Communication Capacity Scale (CCS) • Agitation Distress Scale (ADS)
	Physical and psychological	Patient-reported outcome measures (PROMs)	• Edmonton symptom assessment scale • Memorial symptom assessment scale • Rotterdam symptom checklist
2.	Psychological	Unidimensional	• Distress thermometer
		Multidimensional Anxiety and depression	• National comprehensive cancer Network Distress scale (NCCN distress scale) • PHQ9 • Hospital anxiety and distress scale (HADS)
3.	Spiritual	Spiritual assessment tools	• FICA • HOPE questionnaire

oral route is unavailable. The time for onset is between 12 and 16 hours and reaches its peak effect by 24–36 hours. Hence, the initial 12–24 hours need supplemental analgesia with oral, intravenous, or subcutaneous opioids on its first application. The active drug remains in the subdermal layer for 24 hours after removal and helps sustain analgesia till the onset of action of the next patch. Transdermal fentanyl patches are available in various strengths and are changed once in 72 hours, while Buprenorphine patches are available for varying duration from 3 to 10 days. Local application of heat over the patch and fever are known to increase drug release and can cause overdose. Due to its extensive first-pass metabolism, buprenorphine is used as buccal film and sublingually.

- Side effects of opioids, such as nausea, vomiting, and constipation, are managed

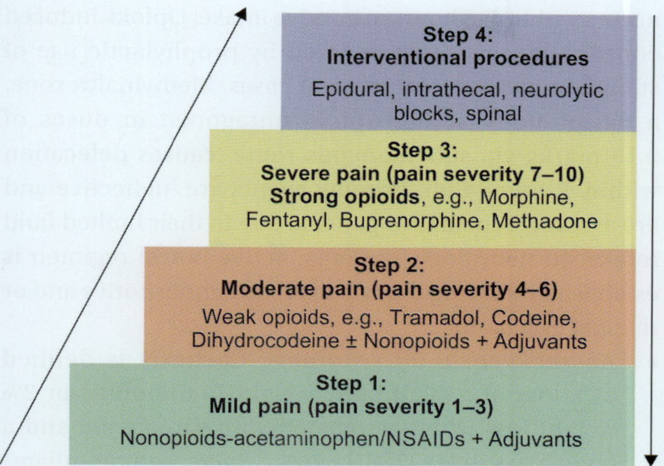

Fig. 3: Modified WHO analgesic ladder. (NSAIDs: nonsteroidal anti-inflammatory drugs; WHO: World Health Organization)

with prophylactic antiemetics and laxatives. Confusion, visual hallucinations, and myoclonus are less common neurotoxic effects managed with dose reduction and hydration. Pruritus is another rare side effect. Respiratory depression is very rare when opioids are carefully titrated to response. Opioid rotation is done when side effects are intolerable.[21]

- Breakthrough pain (BTP) is transient episodic pain occurring in a background of stable pain. Even though routine management is with an extra dose of regular opioid, transmucosal fentanyl with its quick onset of action in <15 minutes is preferred. Fentanyl is administered in a dose range of 50–1,600 µg via intranasal, buccal, transoral, and sublingual formulations for BTP.[22]
- *Special considerations:* In liver disease, fentanyl is the drug of choice, however low-dose morphine at longer intervals/as-needed dose is an alternative when fentanyl is unavailable. Methadone is avoided in end-stage liver disease. Due to renal elimination, active metabolites of strong opioids necessitate caution in end-stage renal failure. Fentanyl, Buprenorphine, and Methadone are safer due to the lack of active metabolites.

Subcutaneous route is a preferred alternative route when the oral route is unavailable for medicine administration. One half of the oral opioid dose is given for subcutaneous use and one third dose for intravenous use.

- *Adjuvants:* These are a group of drugs whose primary indication is for a medical condition with the secondary effect of analgesia. Adjuvants include anticonvulsants, antidepressants, steroids, Alpha-2 agonists, ketamine, lignocaine, anticholinergics, muscle relaxants, bisphosphonates, and calcitonin.[23] Adjuvants play a major role in neuropathic pain, musculoskeletal, malignant spinal cord compression, and malignant bowel obstruction.

- *Nausea and vomiting:* Both are distressing symptoms with various causes, including gastrointestinal issues, metabolic imbalances, toxins, vestibular, and cortical.[24] Constipation should be ruled out before using antiemetics. Treatment is based on the underlying cause and pathway.[25] Medications include metoclopramide and domperidone for gastric stasis, haloperidol for metabolic causes, steroids for intracranial pressure, and neurokinin-1 NK1 receptor antagonists like fosaprepitant and 5-hydroxytryptamine3 (5HT3) antagonists for chemotherapy. Levomepromazine and olanzapine serve as broad-spectrum antiemetics, while medical cannabinoid nabilone is used for chemotherapy. Octreotide helps with malignant bowel obstruction. Nonpharmacological measures include avoiding food and smells, nasogastric drainage, stenting, acupressure, acupuncture, and psychological interventions. Combining different classes of antiemetics, anticipatory prescription, and using the parenteral route can improve effectiveness.
- *Breathlessness:* It is another distressing symptom presenting as varying levels of breathing discomfort. Management starts with screening to gauge its presence, severity, and functional impact, followed by a detailed assessment using multidimensional tools to evaluate physical and emotional impact. Management includes:
  - Treat all reversible underlying conditions—anemia correction, use of diuretics, antibiotics, bronchodilators, etc.
  - Nonpharmacological measures include strategies for reducing perception, adopting diaphragmatic-friendly postures, energy conservation techniques, effective breathing methods like pursed lip breathing and "blow as you go," cognitive and

behavioral techniques, use of Breathlessness Aid services. The use of handheld fans positioned 15–20 cm from the face to direct airflow to the nasal area helps reduce perception by limiting sensory input from trigeminal areas.
  - Medical management in refractory breathlessness with sustained or immediate-release morphine, up to 30 mg/day, is safe and effective in chronic obstructive pulmonary disease (COPD). Benzodiazepines are not recommended as first-line management. Oxygen is advocated only for hypoxia-induced breathlessness, and noninvasive ventilation is beneficial for COPD patients with hypercapnia. High-grade evidence exists only for "use of handheld fan" and "opioids."[26]
- *Fatigue*: It is defined as "a subjective sensation of weakness, tiredness or lack of energy" disproportional to recent activity. This is often under-recognized and unreported. Pathophysiology is complex. Treatment begins with the correction of secondary causes such as fever, anemia, dyselectrolytemia, endocrine disorders, dehydration, and poor sleep hygiene.[27] Pharmacological management with short-course steroids, methylphenidate, and modafinil has inconsistent evidence. Aerobic exercise, resistance training, energy conservation, and energy restoration are effective in cancer-related fatigue. Fatigue in end-of-life situations actually helps conserve energy.
- *Constipation:* The causes can be organic, functional, and drug induced. Restricted mobility, food and water consumption, and medications are other contributory factors in patients with serious illness. Bloating, distension, and vomiting as a sequel to constipation have a significant impact on the quality of life of palliative care patients. After ruling out secondary causes and "complete bowel obstruction," laxatives are used in the treatment of constipation.[28] Laxatives are broadly classified into:
  - Osmotic laxatives—macrogol, lactulose, sorbitol, mannitol, saline, etc.
  - Stimulant laxatives—bisacodyl, senna and sodium picosulfate
  - Lubricant laxatives—liquid paraffin and docusate
  - Sorbitol and glycerol used as suppositories promote defecation reflex

  Laxatives are chosen based on their mechanism of action and underlying cause. The onset of defecation occurs within 5–8 hours of laxative intake. Opioid-induced constipation can be prevented by prophylactic use of stimulant laxatives. In resistant cases, Methylnaltrexone, a peripherally acting opioid antagonist in doses of 0.15 mg/kg via subcutaneous route, causes defecation within 4 hours. Bulk-forming agents are ineffective and are avoided in palliative patients due to their limited fluid intake. In neurologic patients, active bowel regimen is established with regular use of rectal suppositories and or manual evacuation.
- *Anorexia-cachexia syndrome:* Cachexia is defined as a loss of >5% of body weight in 6 months or 2% weight loss when associated with sarcopenia and a body mass index (BMI) <20%.[29] Increased proinflammatory cytokine production with resultant loss of appetite, fatigue, and reduced physical activity underscores significant weight loss and muscle wasting. Management begins with the correction of secondary causes such as nausea, vomiting, oral candidiasis, gastritis, dehydration, pain, weakness, and depression. Nonpharmacological measures include dietary counseling, nutritional supplementation, and physical activity. Pharmacological interventions to improve appetite include short course of steroids like prednisolone, dexamethasone, and methylprednisolone. Megestrol acetate 160–800 mg/day, tetrahydrocannabinol, mirtazapine 15 mg once a day, and olanzapine 2.5 mg once daily. Nutritional interventions like tube feeding with nasogastric tube (<4 weeks) or percutaneous endoscopic gastrostomy (PEG) are recommended in those with dysphagia and life expectancy >6 months.
- *Delirium* is a neurocognitive and neuropsychiatric condition characterized by inattention and impaired awareness with fluctuating severity. It may be hyperactive, hypoactive, or mixed. It is most common in the elderly, advanced cancer, and those with terminal illnesses. This is distressing to both patients and their caregivers and is a reason for hospitalization at the end of life. Hypothetical explanation for pathophysiology includes alterations in the neurotransmitter levels with decreased acetylcholine and elevated dopamine resulting in impaired neuronal network connectivity. Treatment is directed at looking for the underlying cause and correction of reversible factors like dehydration, constipation, infection, etc., before medical management.[30] Antipsychotics by their

dopaminergic antagonistic effects are used to control delirium. These include haloperidol, chlorpromazine, second-generation antipsychotics risperidone, olanzapine, and quetiapine, and third-generation drugs such as aripiprazole. Extrapyramidal side effects are common with antipsychotics. Care should be taken to prevent the recurrence or precipitation of delirium by aiding the perception of patients with the use of visual or hearing aids, orientation to day and night time, regular bowel regime, etc. In those with refractory agitated delirium, continuous palliative sedation with benzodiazepines or propofol or dexmedetomidine is considered after getting informed consent with the family. Benzodiazepines are useful in reversing refractory delirium due to alcohol withdrawal.

- *Anxiety and depression* contribute to psychological distress in patients with life-limiting illnesses.[31] Prevalence is estimated to be 24–50%. Older age, lack of family support, poor symptom control, diminished cognitive, and functional performance are all factors influencing anxiety and depression. Psychotherapeutic interventions include psychoeducation, mindfulness-based therapy, cognitive behavioral therapy, counseling, clinical hypnosis, dignity therapy, guided imagery, short-term life review, and progressive muscle relaxation. Pharmacotherapy for anxiety includes the use of benzodiazepines and antidepressants such as sertraline, bupropion, mirtazapine, olanzapine, and gabapentin. Antidepressants in combination with psychostimulant Methylphenidate are more effective in severe depression.
- *Spiritual distress*: "Spirituality is the dimension of human life that relates to the way people/community experience, express and/or seek meaning, purpose, and transcendence, and the way they connect to the moment, to self, to others, to nature, to the significant, and/or the sacred."[32] Patients with life-threatening illness with threat to future experience "no meaning and purpose in life" resulting in spiritual suffering and distress. "Being there," giving attention to hope of patients and families, addressing existential fears, music therapy, and dance movement therapy are interventions used in spiritual care.

COMMUNICATION IN PALLIATIVE CARE

Communication (Latin word communicatio: sharing) fundamentally refers to the process by which the sender conveys a message to a receiver. It is a dynamic process through which shared meaning is generated by the use of verbal, nonverbal, and listening cues.[33] In healthcare, situations are ongoing, high-contact, and emotionally charged, making effective communication critical for superior outcomes. Physicians and patients constantly exchange relevant information, which contributes to building rapport and trust and enables patients to make informed choices about their health and the treatments that they receive. There are challenges as well. For the clinicians, negotiating the patient's anxiety, health illiteracy, and unrealistic expectations has to be balanced with biological uncertainty.[34] While the patient has to maintain a balance between the complex processes, medical jargon, information overdose, power dynamics, and their own perceived knowledge, fears, and hopes.[33] But good communication can help in navigating this fragile space and improve patient experiences.

Communication is part art but also part science that can be learned. It consists of two components, verbal, i.e., transmission of information through spoken words, and nonverbal, which includes the reactions of the face, body, and voice.[35] Approximately 60–65% of communication is conveyed through nonverbal behaviors. Nonverbal behaviors are unconscious and reflect the person's attitude and emotions.[36]

Nonverbal communication can be classified into kinesics, haptics, vocalics, proxemics, and listening. Kinesics refers to body language, which could be facial expressions, posture, gestures, gait, or obvious body movements. For example, leaning forward, nodding, and maintaining eye contact during a patient interaction demonstrate that the clinician is keenly listening. Haptics is communicating through touch. In certain situations when words fail, touch has the capacity to express care, compassion, and comfort.[37] Vocalics is the paralanguage that accompanies the verbal content, i.e., the pitch, volume, rate, and vocal quality.[33] For example, a speaker with a pleasant voice is likely to be persuasive while a fast speaker is difficult to follow. Proxemics is communication through the use of space.[38] For example, serious conversations usually take place within the personal zone of individuals.

Active listening plays an elemental role in healthcare communication. While hearing is an automatic cerebral response, listening is an active, purposeful action directed at understanding the meaning of a conversation and connecting with the speaker. In the therapeutic setting, listening means being nonjudgmental, giving full attention, and observing both verbal and nonverbal cues. It also involves asking empathic questions (e.g., can you tell me more about how you are feeling?), allowing silence, paraphrasing for understanding, and ensuring the speaker has shared everything they need to. The purpose is to acknowledge the patient's story replete with experience and feelings to be able to effectively engage in the difficult conversations that occur in healthcare.[33,39]

Verbal communication is through the spoken words, which convey information. The words used by clinicians often consist of metaphors, labels, and jargon. Metaphors such as "waging a war on cancer" imply that patients need to fight the cancer. While labels such as "smoker" or "alcoholic" can carry stigma. The use of medical jargon, e.g., "Stage IV disease" or "metastatic" is to be avoided in patients with lower health literacy. Careful selection of words, which convey precise information in a respectful and sensitive manner without ambiguity in a language that the patient understands, is essential. Language should aid in comprehension and decision-making.[33,40]

Communication in palliative care frequently involves delivering "bad news" to patients and their family. *Bad news* is defined as "any information which adversely and seriously affects an individual's view of his or her future." Bad news may include a diagnosis of a life-limiting illness, disease recurrence, or treatment failure, as well as irreversible side effects, positive genetic test results, and discussions about hospice care and resuscitation when no further treatments are available. These conversations are more than just giving information, the challenge lies in managing the emotions of the patient and family while maintaining realistic hope. *SPIKES* protocol is one of the communication strategies that can be used to disclose unfavorable clinical information.[41] It consists of six steps, namely:

1. Step 1—*Setting* up the meeting: Schedule an appointment with the patient along with a family member of their preference, allot some privacy and uninterrupted time, adequate seating, apprise yourself with the medical history of the patient and establish a connect with the patient by identifying yourself, your role and using eye contact and or touch.
2. Step 2—Assessing the patients' *Perception*: Asking the patient what they already know about their condition helps gauge their understanding, health literacy, and language. This forms the guide to decide what information is to be shared. Example: "What have you been told about your condition so far?"
3. Step 3—Obtaining the patient's *Invitation*: Asking the patient how they would like to receive the information. Example: "Would you like to know everything about your illness or only basic information and then go to the treatment plan?" The step assesses the readiness of the patient to engage in knowledge sharing.
4. Step 4—Giving *Knowledge* and information: After a warning to the patient that some unexpected news is about to be revealed, the news is delivered in small chunks. Keep asking the patient at each stage if they have understood and want to go on further. Give them adequate time to process the information and avoid medical jargon.
5. Step 5-Addressing *Emotions* with *Empathic* responses: Patients will respond to the news with varying emotions such as anger, disbelief, sadness, crying, etc. The challenge is to support them in this phase using empathic responses for, e.g., "I see that this news has upset you, can I know more about what you are thinking right now?" "*NURSE*" is a useful mnemonic for responding to patient or family's emotion. It stands for naming, understanding, respecting, supporting, and exploring.[42] Naming the emotion reduces the intensity of the emotion, while saying that you understand is an acknowledgment of their distress, showing respect for them, providing support shows commitment, and exploring further gives the clinician insight into the patient's story.
6. *Summary and strategy:* Once the emotions have cleared, it is necessary to summarize what has been discussed in this conversation and make a follow-up plan. Clear plans for the future will allay the patient's distress to a certain extent.

While the SPIKES protocol provides a rough framework for breaking bad news, it is up to the clinician to tailor each conversation with the patient's understanding, preference, and values. Communication in palliative care is patient-centered and is a bidirectional exchange of information that is contextual, culture specific, and empathic. It aspires to engage the patient and family in actively participating in decision-making and receive goal concordant care.

ETHICS IN PALLIATIVE CARE

The goal of palliative care is to ensure patients' dignity and quality of life while striving for the best possible medical therapy for the disease.[43]

Ethics refers to the rules or standards governing the conduct of individuals or members of a profession and comes into play whenever a decision has to be made on a patient's treatment, especially in palliative care where decisions are made keeping the patient's request or quality of life in mind. Ethical issues in palliative care surface because of concerns about the quantum and the type of care that should be offered for someone with a chronic disease with likely limited life expectancy.[44]

The oncologist and the palliative care consultant face many conflicting ethical dilemmas when deciding treatment strategies for cancer patients. A clear knowledge of the ethical principles governing care, coupled with good communication skills, help in shared decision-making.

The four principles of medical ethics are as follows:

1. Autonomy
2. Beneficence
3. Nonmaleficence
4. Justice

Two more added aspects include (5) dignity and (6) truthfulness and honesty.

These six values should always be kept in mind while discussing and deciding on patients' treatment.[45]

- Autonomy is about the supreme self and states that a patient has the right to make informed choices. They can consent or not to a procedure or treatment after clearly understanding the implications of both options.
- Beneficence is always doing good to the patient, i.e., the clinician has the best interest of the patient in mind while making decisions.
- Nonmaleficence implies no harm to the patient while treatment is ongoing.
- Justice requires that all patients are treated well and fairly and also includes equitable use of available resources and balancing individual needs with those of society.

Applying ethical principles in practice often leads to conflict making it challenging to arrive at the correct course of action.

Autonomy (Collusion)

A 70-year-old male Mr M with oropharyngeal cancer treated with surgery and radiotherapy, now has local recurrence, the family requests that the patient not be told the prognosis: The patient has a right to know the diagnosis. The collusion that exists has to be skillfully negotiated by communicating the importance of sharing the truth. The fact that the patient will lose confidence as the disease progresses, and he realizes the truth has to be explained to the family.[46]

Autonomy and Beneficence

Mr M is posted for PEG insertion under sedation, on inquiry, while doing a preanesthesia assessment, you realize that the patient does not want the PEG but the family is insisting as it was an option given by the treating oncologist. This is a conflict between patients' autonomy and beneficence as his nutrition will likely improve with PEG. However, despite understanding the benefits, if the patient refuses PEG, his autonomy should be respected and the patient can refuse to consent for PEG.

Nonmaleficence with Beneficence

A 54-year-old lady with carcinoma cervix is posted for brachytherapy but refuses anesthesia as she is scared of the radiotherapy. This is a conflict of nonmaleficence with beneficence.

Obviously having the procedure and treatment is likely to be beneficial (likely curative) and not having the treatment would be harmful. Good communication should ensure the patient's fears are addressed and she undergoes treatment. Doctor insisting that the treatment is the better choice will lead to paternalism and can be avoided by communicating the benefits of treatment and ensuring that the patient understands the outcomes in either scenario.

Justice and Beneficence

Mr N, an 80-year-old patient with sepsis, is on triple inotropes and on ventilator. He is occupying an ICU bed while a young 34-year-old patient with schwannoma in the thoracolumbar region with vascular involvement requiring major vascular resection during surgery is awaiting surgery and cannot be accommodated in the surgical list due to lack of ICU beds. This is a conflict between justice and beneficence. Mr N on the ventilator could become better: a dilemma that is difficult to manage. Often there is no clear solution. What about the dignity and quality of life of Mr N in case he comes off the ventilator?

However, if Mr N has multiorgan failure and cannot be salvaged—should we withdraw support? Withholding and withdrawing support is often a big dilemma to the physicians both legally and morally, and will be dealt with in the end-of-life care chapter.

TABLE 2: Clinical decision-making based on Jonsen's four-box model.

Clinical indications (Based on principles of beneficence and nonmaleficence)	***Family and patient preferences (Autonomy of the patient)***
• What is the patient's medical diagnosis? History? problems? Prognosis? • Is the problem acute? Chronic? Critical? Emergent? Reversible? • Are the goals of treatment clear? • What are the probabilities of success? • Any plan B in case of therapeutic failure? • Essentially, how can this patient be benefited by medical and nursing care, and how can harm be avoided?	• Is the patient mentally and legally competent? Is there evidence of incapacity? • If mentally capable, what are the patient's preferences for treatment? • Has the patient understood the benefits and risks and given consent? • If not mentally capable, who is the appropriate surrogate? Is the surrogate aware of decision making? • Are there any patient expressed prior preferences, e.g., Advanced Directives? • If the patient is not in a position to cooperate with medical treatment? Enquire why? • Is the patient's autonomy being respected to the extent possible?
Quality of life (Principles of beneficence, nonmaleficence and justice)	***Related factors (Principle of justice)***
• What are the chances with or without treatment for a return to normal life? • What physical, mental, and social deficits are likely if treatment succeeds • Are there likely biases that may affect the provider's evaluation of the patient's quality of life? • Is the patient's present or future condition such that his or her continued life might be judged undesirable? • Is there any plan or reason to forego treatment? • Is supportive and palliative care planned?	• Are family issues likely to influence treatment decisions? • Are there treating team issues that might influence treatment decisions? • Any financial or economic factor? • Any religious or cultural factors? • Any limits on confidentiality? • Any problems of equal allocation of resources? • Any legal implications that may affect treatment decisions? • Is there any conflict of interest on the part of the treating team?

Source: Adapted from Jonsen A, Siegler M, Winslade W. Clinical Ethics: A Practical Approach to Ethical Decisions in Clinical Medicine, 6th edition. New York, NY: McGraw-Hill; 2006.

Most of these ethical dilemmas need to be managed by good communication and a clear understanding of the law and guidelines available.

The Jonsen model (or "four-box method" depicted in **Table 2**) is often used for decision-making[47] and helps in bringing the focus to the problem at hand. The purpose of the four boxes is simply to sort out data and get clarity on what is central to the discussion and what is merely interesting. Breaking down the boxes step by step highlights areas of confusion or disagreement. Once these are resolved, decision-making becomes much easier.

Intended and Foreseen Effects—the Doctrine of Double Effect

As the disease trajectory progresses toward the end of life, some medications used may have a potential for adverse effects that could be blamed for the causation of death. This could lead to a situation of avoiding a potentially useful drug, fearing the consequences.

The doctrine of double effect gives justification for the treatment.[48] *The doctrine of double effect states "a single act having two possible foreseeable effects, one good and one harmful, is not always morally prohibited if the harmful effect is not intended."*

As per the doctrine, so long as the intention of choosing a medicine is not to hasten death, the prescribing doctor is not guilty of the outcome even if that effect was foreseeable. Giving a sedative to provide comfort if it results in respiratory arrest and death, the doctor is not liable, as the intention was to assure comfort and improve quality of life.

Other areas where ethical principles and dilemmas come into play are in end-of-life care where decisions on withholding or withdrawing life support must be made.

There is a need to clearly understand the issues at hand by using the four-box model followed by clear and empathic communication to help resolve the many ethical conflicts that the palliative care physician confronts.

CONCLUSION

Palliative care is the specialized care of patients with the help of a multidisciplinary team, using empathic communication within an ethical framework.

REFERENCES

1. Saunders C. The evolution of palliative care. J R Soc Med. 2001;94(9):430-2.
2. Richmond C. Dame Cicely Saunders. BMJ. 2005; 331(7510):238.
3. Greenstreet W. The concept of total pain: a focused patient care study. Br J Nurs. 2001;10(19):1248-55.
4. Palliative care—1990, 2002 and 2023 WHO definitions. IAHPC Pallipedia. [online] Available from https://pallipedia.org/palliative-care-1990-2002-and-2023-who-definitions/. [Last accessed March, 2025].
5. Sleeman KE, de Brito M, Etkind S, Nkhoma K, Guo P, Higginson IJ, et al. The escalating global burden of serious health-related suffering: projections to 2060 by world regions, age groups, and health conditions. Lancet Glob Health. 2019;7(7):e883-92.
6. Mounsey L, Ferres M, Eastman P. Palliative care for the patient without cancer. Aust J Gen Pract. 2018;47(11):765-9.
7. Temel JS, Greer JA, Muzikansky A, Gallagher ER, Admane S, Jackson VA, et al. Early palliative care for patients with metastatic non-small-cell lung cancer. N Engl J Med. 2010; 363(8):733-42.
8. May P, Garrido MM, Cassel JB, Kelley AS, Meier DE, Normand C, et al. Prospective cohort study of hospital palliative care teams for inpatients with advanced cancer: earlier consultation is associated with larger cost-saving effect. J Clin Oncol. 2015;33(25):2745-52.
9. Yarra P, Annangi S. Early integration of palliative care in chronic obstructive pulmonary disease (COPD) is warranted based on symptom burden and quality of life. Evid-Based Nurs 2021;24:130.
10. Chiu HH, Murphy-Burke DM, Thomas SA, Melnyk Y, Kruthaup-Harper AL, Dong JJ, et al; BC Renal Palliative Care Committee. Advancing palliative care in patients with CKD: from ideas to practice. Am J Kidney Dis. 2021;77(3):420-6.
11. Solano JP, Gomes B, Higginson IJ. A comparison of symptom prevalence in far advanced cancer, AIDS, heart disease, chronic obstructive pulmonary disease and renal disease. J Pain Symptom Manage. 2006;31(1):58-69.
12. Moens K, Higginson IJ, Harding R; EURO IMPACT. Are there differences in the prevalence of palliative care-related problems in people living with advanced cancer and eight non-cancer conditions? A systematic review. J Pain Symptom Manage. 2014;48(4):660-77.
13. Cheville AL, Alberts SR, Rummans TA, Basford JR, Lapid MI, Sloan JA, et al. Improving adherence to cancer treatment by addressing quality of life in patients with advanced gastrointestinal cancers. J Pain Symptom Manage. 2015; 50:321-7.
14. Laugsand EA, Sprangers MA, Bjordal K, Skorpen F, Kaasa S, Klepstad P. Health care providers underestimate symptom intensities of cancer patients: a multicenter European study. Health Qual Life Outcomes. 2010;8:104.
15. Homsi J, Walsh D, Rivera N, Rybicki LA, Nelson KA, Legrand SB, et al. Symptom evaluation in palliative medicine: patient report vs systematic assessment. Support Care Cancer. 2006;14(5):444-53.
16. Fallon M, Walker J, Colvin L, Rodriguez A, Murray G, Sharpe M; Edinburgh Pain Assessment and Management Tool Study Group. Pain management in cancer center inpatients: a cluster randomized trial to evaluate a systematic integrated approach—the Edinburgh Pain Assessment and Management Tool. J Clin Oncol. 2018;36(13):1284-90.
17. Yang J, Bauer BA, Wahner-Roedler DL, Chon TY, Xiao L. The modified WHO analgesic ladder: is it appropriate for chronic non-cancer pain? J Pain Res. 2020;13:411-7.
18. Fallon M, Giusti R, Aielli F, Hoskin P, Rolke R, Sharma M, et al. Management of cancer pain in adult patients: ESMO Clinical Practice Guidelines. Ann Oncol. 2018;29(Suppl 4):iv166-91.
19. McPherson ML, Walker KA, Davis MP, Bruera E, Reddy A, Paice J, et al. Safe and appropriate use of methadone in hospice and palliative care: expert consensus white paper. J Pain Symptom Manage. 2019;57:635-45.e4.
20. Singh DR, Nag K, Shetti AN, Krishnaveni N. Tapentadol hydrochloride: a novel analgesic. Saudi J Anaesth. 2013;7(3):322-6.
21. Mercadante S, Caraceni A. Conversion ratios for opioid switching in the treatment of cancer pain: a systematic review. Palliat Med. 2011;25(5):504-15.
22. Abdel Shaheed C, Hayes C, Maher CG, Ballantyne JC, Underwood M, McLachlan AJ, et al. Opioid analgesics for nociceptive cancer pain: a comprehensive review. CA Cancer J Clin. 2024;74(3):286-313.
23. Mitra R, Jones S. Adjuvant analgesics in cancer pain: a review. Am J Hosp Palliat Care. 2012;29(1):70-9.
24. Stephenson J, Davies A. An assessment of aetiology-based guidelines for the management of nausea and vomiting in patients with advanced cancer. Support Care Cancer. 2006;14:348-53.
25. Keeley P. Nausea and vomiting in palliative care. Medicine. 2019;48:14-7.
26. Chin C, Booth S. Managing breathlessness: a palliative care approach. Postgrad Med J. 2016;92(1089):393-400.
27. Radbruch L, Strasser F, Elsner F, Gonçalves JF, Løge J, Kaasa S, et al. Fatigue in palliative care patients—an EAPC approach. Palliat Med. 2008;22(1):13-32.
28. Clemens KE, Klaschik E. Management of constipation in palliative care patients. Curr Opin Support Palliat Care. 2008;2(1):22-7.

29. Pandey S, Bradley L, Del Fabbro E. Updates in cancer cachexia: clinical management and pharmacologic interventions. Cancers (Basel). 2024;16(9):1696.
30. Bramati P, Bruera E. Delirium in palliative care. Cancers (Basel). 2021;13(23):5893.
31. Grassi L, Caruso R, Riba MB, et al. Anxiety and depression in adult cancer patients: ESMO Clinical Practice Guideline. ESMO Open. 2023;8(2):101155.
32. Nolan S, Saltmarsh P, Leget C. Spiritual care in palliative care: working towards an EAPC Task Force. Eur J Palliat Care. 2011;18:86-9.
33. Danaher TS, Berry LL, Howard C, Moore SG, Attai DJ. Improving how clinicians communicate with patients: an integrative review and framework. J Serv Res. 2023;26(4):493-510.
34. Dickinson JK, Guzman SJ, Maryniuk MD, O'Brian CA, Kadohiro JK, Jackson RA, et al. The use of language in diabetes care and education. Diabetes Care. 2017;40(12):1790-9.
35. Wanko Keutchafo EL, Kerr J, Baloyi OB. A model for effective nonverbal communication between nurses and older patients: a grounded theory inquiry. Healthcare (Basel). 2022;10(11):2119.
36. Foley GN, Gentile JP. Nonverbal communication in psychotherapy. Psychiatry (Edgmont). 2010;7(6):38-44.
37. Singh C, Leder D. Touch in the consultation. Br J Gen Pract. 2012;62(596):147-8.
38. Anjali H, Emmanuel H. Kinesics, haptics and proxemics: aspects of non-verbal communication. IOSR J Hum Soc Sci. 2015;20(2):47-52.
39. Shigeaki W, Fran TM, Ruth L. Therapeutic listening. In: Ruth L, Mariah S, Fran TM, (Eds). Complementary and Alternative Therapies in Nursing. New York: Springer Publishing Company; 2014.
40. Hui D, Zhukovsky DS, Bruera E. Serious illness conversations: paving the road with metaphors. Oncologist. 2018;23(6):730-3.
41. Baile WF, Buckman R, Lenzi R, Glober G, Beale EA, Kudelka AP. SPIKES—A six-step protocol for delivering bad news: application to the patient with cancer. Oncologist. 2000;5(4):302-11.
42. Back AL, Arnold RM, Baile WF, Tulsky JA, Fryer-Edwards K. Approaching difficult communication tasks in oncology. CA Cancer J Clin. 2005;55:164-77.
43. Rastogi P, Rastogi P. Ethics in palliative care. Highlights on several underestimated topics in palliative care. [online] Available from https://www.intechopen.com/chapters/56799. [Last accessed March, 2025].
44. Ethical issues in palliative care—UpToDate. [online] Available from: https://www.uptodate.com/contents/ethical-issues-in-palliative-care. [Last accessed March, 2025].
45. Mohanti BK. Ethics in palliative care. Indian J Palliat Carenet. 2009;15(2):89.
46. Fallowfield LJ, Jenkins VA, Beveridge HA. Truth may hurt but deceit hurts more: communication in palliative care. Palliat Medt. 2002;16(4):297-303.
47. Jonsen AR, Siegler M, Winslade WJ, Mishra R (Eds). Clinical Ethics: A Practical Approach to Ethical Decisions in Clinical Medicine. McGraw Hill; 2022. p. 262.
48. Quill TE, Dresser R, Brock DW. The rule of double effect—a critique of its role in end-of-life decision making. N Engl J Med. 1997;337(24):1768-71.

61 CHAPTER

Interventions in Palliative Care

Yogendra Singhal, Vikas Gupta, Surendra Kumar Pingoliya

Palliative care interventions are a crucial component of comprehensive healthcare for individuals facing serious illnesses. These interventions are designed to alleviate symptoms, manage pain, and address the emotional, social, and spiritual concerns of patients and their families. The primary goal is to enhance the quality of life by providing comfort and support, rather than focusing solely on curing the disease.[1] This approach involves a multidisciplinary team of healthcare providers who work together to offer comprehensive support. Palliative care can be provided alongside curative treatments at any stage of illness and is tailored to meet the unique needs of each individual, ensuring compassionate and personalized care that honors the patient's values and preferences.

Palliative care interventions can include medication management for pain and other distressing symptoms, counseling and psychological support, assistance with daily activities, and coordination of care among different healthcare providers. These interventions are personalized, taking into account the patient's values, preferences, and overall goals, and can be integrated at any stage of illness. By offering a holistic approach, palliative care interventions help patients navigate their healthcare journey with dignity and improved well-being.

This chapter delivers various interventions in palliative care, focusing on symptom management, psychosocial interventions, spiritual care, and legal and ethical aspects.

SYMPTOM MANAGEMENT

Effective symptom management is foundational in palliative care, aiming to alleviate physical discomfort and enhance patients' quality of life.

PAIN MANAGEMENT

Managing cancer pain effectively requires a comprehensive, multimodal approach, combining pharmacological and nonpharmacological interventions, interventional procedures, and supportive care. Here is a concise overview of the key strategies:

Pharmacological Interventions

Nonopioid analgesics:

- Acetaminophen is useful for mild-to-moderate pain and can be used alone or in combination with other medications.
- Nonsteroidal anti-inflammatory drugs (NSAIDs) are effective for pain associated with inflammation, such as bone pain, though they must be used cautiously due to potential gastrointestinal (GI), renal, and cardiovascular side effects.

Opioid analgesics:

- Weak opioids like tramadol and codeine should be used to treat moderate pain.
- Strong opioids such as morphine, oxycodone, hydromorphone, fentanyl, and methadone are standard treatments for moderate-to-severe pain, available in various forms (oral, intravenous, and patches). These medications help manage baseline pain.
- Breakthrough pain characterized by sudden, intense episodic pain should be managed by rapid-onset opioids like fentanyl.

Adjuvant analgesics:

- Antidepressants (e.g., amitriptyline, nortriptyline, and duloxetine) and gabapentinoids (e.g., gabapentin and pregabalin) are beneficial for neuropathic pain.
- Corticosteroids help with pain due to inflammation or nerve compression. Dexamethasone is a commonly prescribed steroid due to its lesser mineralocorticoid effects.
- Bisphosphonates (e.g., pamidronate and zoledronic acid) are used for bone pain from metastatic cancer.[2]

Nonpharmacological Interventions

- *Physical therapy and exercise:* Regular physical activity and specific exercises can help manage pain.
- *Acupuncture:* This traditional Chinese medicine technique has shown benefits in pain relief.
- *Cognitive behavioral therapy (CBT):* This helps patients manage pain by altering pain-related thoughts and behaviors.
- *Counseling:* This technique provides emotional support and coping strategies.
- *Relaxation techniques:* Methods such as guided imagery, meditation, and deep breathing can reduce pain perception.

Interventional Procedures

- *Nerve blocks:*
  - Epidural or spinal analgesia delivers medication directly into the spinal cord for significant pain relief.
  - Peripheral nerve blocks use local anesthetics or steroids near nerves to block pain signals from specific areas.
  - Nerve blocks can be performed by:
    - *Chemical neurolytic blocks:* Alcohol or phenol (6–10%) injections destroy nerve fibers transmitting pain signals, providing long-term relief.
    - *Radiofrequency ablation:* This technique uses heat to destroy nerve tissues responsible for pain transmission.
- *Vertebroplasty/kyphoplasty:* This is a minimally invasive procedure to stabilize fractured vertebrae caused by metastatic bone disease, offering pain relief.[3]
- *Intrathecal pumps:* These deliver pain medication directly into the spinal fluid, providing effective pain control with lower doses and fewer side effects.[4]
- *Radiation therapy and surgical interventions:*
  - Radiation therapy can shrink tumors causing pain, such as in bone metastases or spinal cord compression.
  - Surgical interventions may be necessary to remove or reduce the size of tumors causing pain by compressing nerves or other structures.

Regular pain assessments using standardized tools (numeric rating scale and visual analog scale) are essential for evaluating the effectiveness of interventions and making necessary adjustments to ensure optimal pain relief and minimal side effects. Therefore, effective cancer pain management requires a multifaceted approach combining medications, physical therapies, psychosocial support, interventional procedures, and education, facilitated by a multidisciplinary team.

DYSPNEA

Managing dyspnea (difficulty in breathing) in palliative care involves various interventions aimed at alleviating symptoms and improving the patient's quality of life. Here are some common approaches:

Pharmacological interventions:

- *Bronchodilators and corticosteroids:* These are used for patients with underlying lung conditions, such as chronic obstructive pulmonary disease (COPD) or asthma. Corticosteroids also help reduce tumor edema and thus relieve the compression effect of tumors on lung parenchyma.
- *Diuretics:* In patients with heart failure, diuretics can reduce fluid overload and ease breathing.
- *Benzodiazepines:* Medications such as lorazepam can help manage anxiety-associated dyspnea.[5]
- *Opioids:* If the patient is refractory to all medications, small doses of opioids (e.g., morphine) can alleviate the sensation of breathlessness.[6,7]
- *Oxygen therapy:* Supplemental oxygen can help if the patient is hypoxic, although its effectiveness in nonhypoxic patients is debated.

Nonpharmacological interventions:

- *Positioning and breathing techniques:* Encouraging patients to sit up or lean forward can help ease breathing. Diaphragmatic breathing and pursed lip breathing are frequently used techniques in COPD patients.[8]
- *Fan therapy:* A cool draft of air from a fan directed at the face can reduce the sensation of breathlessness.[9]
- *Relaxation techniques:* Guided imagery, breathing exercises, and progressive muscle relaxation can help manage anxiety and improve breathing.
- *Physical therapy:* Gentle exercises and techniques to clear secretions can be beneficial.
- *Psychological support:* Counseling and support groups can help patients cope with the emotional aspects of dyspnea.
- *Acupuncture and acupressure:* A systemic review examining the effect of acupuncture on breathless patients suffering from advanced disease demonstrated that breathlessness severity decreased significantly.[10]

Interventions for specific conditions:

- *Thoracocentesis*: For patients with pleural effusion, removing excess fluid from the pleural space can provide significant relief.
- *Paracentesis*: In cases of ascites, draining the fluid can reduce abdominal pressure and ease breathing.
- *Noninvasive ventilation (NIV)*: Techniques like continuous positive airway pressure (CPAP) or bi-level positive airway pressure (BiPAP) can support breathing in certain cases.

Patient and caregiver education:

- *Teach breathing techniques:* Educate patients and caregivers on techniques like pursed-lip breathing and diaphragmatic breathing.
- *Symptom monitoring:* Encourage regular monitoring of symptoms to adjust treatments as needed.
- *Emergency plan:* Develop a plan for managing acute episodes of dyspnea, including when to seek emergency care.

These interventions should be tailored to the individual patient's needs, taking into account the underlying cause of dyspnea, the patient's overall health status, and their preferences and goals for care. Interdisciplinary teams, including doctors, nurses, respiratory therapists, and palliative care specialists, can work together to provide comprehensive management of dyspnea and improve patients' quality of life.

NAUSEA AND VOMITING

Managing nausea and vomiting in palliative care requires a multifaceted approach tailored to the individual patient's needs and underlying causes. Here are some common interventions:

Pharmacological interventions:

- *Antiemetics:*
    - *5-HT3 receptor antagonists:* Ondansetron, granisetron, etc.
    - *Dopamine antagonists:* Metoclopramide, haloperidol, prochlorperazine, etc.
    - *Antihistamines:* Promethazine, cyclizine, etc.
    - *Anticholinergics:* Scopolamine.
    - *Neurokinin-1 (NK-1) receptor antagonists:* Aprepitant
- *Steroids:* Dexamethasone can be effective in reducing nausea associated with increased intracranial pressure.[11]
- *Proton pump inhibitors (PPIs) or H2 blockers:* These are effective in treating nausea related to GI issues, such as acid reflux or ulcers.
- *Cannabinoids:* Dronabinol or medical marijuana may help in some cases.[12]

Nonpharmacological interventions:

- *Dietary modifications:*
    - Small, frequent meals
    - Avoiding spicy, fatty, or strong-smelling foods
    - Encouraging bland, easy-to-digest foods
- Control malodor from colostomy, fungating tumor of decubitus ulcer.
- *Hydration:* Sips of water, ice chips, or clear fluids can help maintain hydration and reduce nausea.
- *Ginger:* Ginger tea, ginger ale, or ginger supplements can help alleviate nausea.[13]
- *Acupressure and acupuncture:* These complementary therapies can be effective for some patients.
- *Aromatherapy:* Essential oils like peppermint or lavender may help reduce nausea in some individuals.
- *Patient and caregiver education:* Identifying and avoiding known triggers of nausea, keeping a symptom diary to track patterns and identify effective interventions, and developing a plan for managing severe or sudden episodes of nausea and vomiting help patients suffering from nausea and vomiting.

Interventions for specific causes:

- *GI obstruction:*
    - *Nasogastric tube (NGT):* To relieve gastric distention
    - *Octreotide:* To reduce GI secretions
- *Chemotherapy-induced nausea:* Pretreatment with anti-emetics and adherence to protocols designed to minimize side effects

CONSTIPATION

Managing constipation in palliative care requires a combination of pharmacological, nonpharmacological, and lifestyle interventions tailored to the individual patient's needs.

Pharmacological interventions:

- *Laxatives:*
    - *Stool softeners:* Docusate can ease stool passage by softening it.
    - *Osmotic laxatives:* Polyethylene glycol and lactulose increase water content in the bowel, making stool passage easier.

  - *Stimulant laxatives:* Stimulant laxatives (e.g., senna and bisacodyl) can help stimulate bowel movements.
  - *Lubricant laxatives:* Mineral oil.
- *Suppositories:* Glycerin or bisacodyl suppositories stimulate bowel movements.
- *Enemas:* Sodium phosphate or mineral oil enemas may provide relief from impacted stool.

Nonpharmacological interventions:
- *Dietary modifications:* Increase dietary fiber through fruits, vegetables, and whole grains and ensure adequate fluid intake.
- *Physical activity:* Encourage as much activity as possible to stimulate bowel movements.
- *Regular toileting schedule:* Encourage regular toileting, especially after meals.
- *Abdominal massage:* Gentle massage can help increase GI motility and secretions as well as relax sphincters and decrease GI transit time.[14]
- *Patient and caregiver education:* Educate on signs of constipation, such as infrequent bowel movements, hard stools, and difficulty during defecation, and develop a plan for managing severe constipation and knowing when to seek medical attention. Address anxiety or psychological factors contributing to constipation and educate on maintaining regular bowel habits.

Interventions for specific causes:
- *Opioid-induced constipation:* Use stool softeners (docusate) and stimulant laxatives (bisacodyl and senna) together. If the patient is not responsive, add milk of magnesia, polyethylene glycol, and lactulose. If still nonresponsive, go for opioid rotation or peripherally acting opioid receptor antagonists like methylnaltrexone or naloxegol, which counteract opioid effects without affecting pain relief.[15]
- *Obstruction or tumor-related constipation:* Determine if surgical interventions are needed.
- *Neurological causes:* Tailored bowel regimens and possibly suppositories or enemas if there is impaired mobility or neurological impairment.

FATIGUE

Managing fatigue in palliative care involves a holistic approach, combining pharmacological, nonpharmacological, and supportive interventions tailored to the individual patient's needs.

Pharmacological interventions:
- *Stimulants:* Medications like methylphenidate or modafinil can help increase alertness and reduce fatigue.
- *Antidepressants:* Selective serotonin reuptake inhibitors (SSRIs) or serotonin-norepinephrine reuptake inhibitors (SNRIs) can help if the fatigue is related to depression.
- *Corticosteroids:* Short-term use of steroids like dexamethasone can provide an energy boost by reducing inflammatory cytokines.
- *Anemia management:* Erythropoiesis-stimulating agents (ESAs) or blood transfusions if the fatigue is due to anemia.

Nonpharmacological interventions:
- *Energy conservation techniques:* Educate on prioritizing tasks, planning activities, and taking regular breaks.
- *Exercise:* Gentle, regular exercise such as walking, yoga, or stretching can help improve energy levels.[16]
- *Nutrition:* Ensure a balanced diet with adequate calories and nutrients to prevent fatigue related to malnutrition.
- *Sleep hygiene:* Promote good sleep practices, such as maintaining a regular sleep schedule, creating a restful environment, and avoiding stimulants before bedtime.
- *Complementary therapies:* Techniques such as massage, acupuncture, and relaxation exercises can reduce fatigue and improve well-being.
- *Patient and caregiver education:* Identify and manage factors that exacerbate fatigue, such as stress, overexertion, or poor nutrition. Regularly assess fatigue levels and adjust interventions as needed.

Specific interventions for underlying causes:
- *Pain management:* Effective pain control can reduce fatigue.
- *Managing symptoms of chronic illnesses:* Control symptoms of conditions such as heart failure, COPD, or renal failure that contribute to fatigue.

These interventions, coordinated by an interdisciplinary team, can help manage fatigue, enhancing the patient's quality of life in palliative care settings.

ANOREXIA AND CACHEXIA

Cachexia–anorexia syndrome (CAS) is a multifactorial syndrome characterized by an involuntary loss of skeletal muscles and fat, reduced quality of life, and decreased survival. Managing anorexia–cachexia syndrome (ACS) in palliative care involves a comprehensive approach aimed at improving appetite, nutritional intake, and overall quality of life. Here are some key interventions.

Pharmacological interventions:

- *Appetite stimulants:*
  - *Corticosteroids:* Dexamethasone or prednisone can stimulate appetite and improve well-being.
  - *Progestogens:* Megestrol acetate can increase appetite and help in weight gain.
  - *Mirtazapine:* This is particularly useful in depression-related anorexia.
  - *Cannabinoids:* Dronabinol may help improve appetite in patients with acquired immunodeficiency syndrome (AIDS).[17]
- *Anabolic agents:*
  - *Androgens:* Oxandrolone or testosterone can help in some cases to increase muscle mass.
- *Anti-inflammatory agents:*
  - *Omega-3 fatty acids:* Fish oil supplements may have anti-inflammatory effects and improve appetite.
- *Prokinetic agents:*
  - *Metoclopramide:* It can help with gastric emptying and reducing early satiety.

Nonpharmacological interventions:

- *Nutritional support:*
  - *Dietary counseling:* Dietitians can provide tailored advice to meet patients' nutritional needs.
  - *High-calorie, high-protein diets:* Small, frequent meals with nutrient-dense foods.
  - *Small, frequent meals:* Eating small, nutrient-dense meals throughout the day can help manage anorexia.
  - *Enjoyable foods:* Encouraging patients to eat their favorite foods can improve intake and enjoyment.
- *Physical activity:* Gentle exercises, as tolerated, to maintain muscle mass and stimulate appetite.
- *Patient and caregiver education:* Create a pleasant eating environment, encourage eating with family, avoid stress during meal, and address symptoms such as pain, nausea, and constipation that can affect appetite.

PSYCHOSOCIAL INTERVENTIONS

Psychosocial interventions in palliative care are integral to addressing the comprehensive needs of patients facing life-limiting illnesses. These interventions encompass a range of therapeutic activities designed to support the emotional, social, and psychological well-being of patients and their families. They aim to alleviate distress, enhance coping mechanisms, and improve the quality of life by addressing issues, such as anxiety, depression, and grief. By incorporating techniques from counseling, support groups, CBT, and spiritual care, psychosocial interventions help create a holistic approach that respects the dignity and individual needs of each patient, fostering a supportive environment during the challenging end-of-life journey.

- *Cognitive behavioral therapy:* It involves structured sessions with a therapist to identify negative thought patterns and replace them with more balanced, realistic thoughts. It includes cognitive restructuring, behavioral activation (engaging in activities that improve mood), and skills training (e.g., relaxation techniques). Thus, it reduces the symptoms of depression and anxiety, improves coping skills, and enhances overall well-being.[18]
- *Mindfulness-based stress reduction (MBSR):* It is typically an 8-week program involving weekly group sessions and daily home practice of mindfulness meditation and gentle yoga. It includes mindfulness meditation (focused attention on the present moment), body scan exercises, and mindful movements. It lowers stress, reduces the symptoms of anxiety and depression, improves the quality of *life, and enhances emotional regulation.*[19]
- *Acceptance and commitment therapy (ACT):* ACT is a type of psychotherapy that emphasizes acceptance to deal with negative thoughts, feelings, symptoms, or circumstances. This therapy encourages increased commitment to healthy, constructive activities that uphold values and goals. It focuses on helping people accept difficult thoughts, feelings, sensations, and internal experiences while guiding them to commit to value-based actions. ACT therapists operate under a theory that suggests that increasing acceptance can lead to increased psychological flexibility. This approach may help people stop habitually avoiding specific thoughts or emotional experiences, which can lead to further psychological problems.[20]
- *Psychoeducation:* It is an evidence-based therapeutic intervention for patients and their loved ones that provides information and support to better understand and cope with illnesses. It is more often associated with serious mental illnesses, including dementia, clinical depression, anxiety disorder, eating disorder,

and bipolar and personality disorder. Psychoeducation offered to patients and family members teaches problem-solving and communication skills and provides education and resources in an empathetic and supportive environment that can take place in one-on-one discussions or in groups by qualified personnel. Many studies indicate that psychoeducation improves family well-being, lowers the rate of relapses and improves recovery, empowers patients with knowledge, reduces feelings of helplessness, and promotes proactive management of mental health.[21]

- *Bibliotherapy:* Bibliotherapy is a supportive psychotherapy, a brief self-help intervention, where through the reading of a chosen standard manual, emotion regulation skills are acquired through either behavioral therapy or cognitive therapy technique. The main advantage of this psychotherapy is its cost-effectiveness. It has been shown to be effective in the treatment of mild-to-moderate depression.[22]

Social Support Interventions

- *Support groups:* It emphasizes regular meetings (in-person or virtual) where patients share experiences and support each other under the guidance of a trained facilitator. It can be general cancer support groups or specific to certain types of cancer or stages of illness. It benefits patients by providing emotional support, reduces feelings of isolation, and fosters a sense of community.
- *Family counseling:* It includes sessions involving patients and their family members to address communication issues, emotional support, and family dynamics. Techniques involve family therapy sessions, communication skills training, and conflict resolution strategies. Thus, it improves family cohesion, enhances support systems, and reduces caregiver burden.
- *Peer support programs:* It connects patients with trained peer supporters who have experienced similar journeys. Techniques involve one-on-one meetings, phone calls, or online chats with peer supporters. It provides practical advice, emotional support from someone with shared experiences, and hope through seeing others who have successfully managed their condition.

Behavioral Interventions

- *Exercise and physical activities:* It includes the development of tailored exercise programs by healthcare professionals, considering the patient's physical condition and treatment side effects. It includes aerobic exercise, strength training, flexibility exercises, and balance training. It produces improved mood, reduces symptoms of depression and anxiety, enhances physical function, and boosts the overall quality of life.
- *Relaxation techniques:* Teaching patients methods to induce relaxation and reduce stress. It includes progressive muscle relaxation, deep breathing exercises, guided imagery, and biofeedback. It reduces anxiety, promotes relaxation, improves sleep, and enhances overall well-being.[23]

Pharmacological Interventions

Medication management:

- Prescribing and managing medications, such as antidepressants or antianxiety drugs.
- *Coordination:* Close monitoring by the oncology team to manage side effects and interactions with cancer treatments.
- It reduces severe symptoms of depression and anxiety, improves emotional stability, and complements psychosocial interventions.

SPIRITUAL INTERVENTIONS IN PALLIATIVE CARE

Spiritual distress in palliative care refers to the suffering that can occur when an individual experiences a disruption in their belief system, values, or sense of meaning and purpose in life, especially when facing a serious illness, the prospect of death, or significant losses. It is an important aspect to address in palliative care as it can significantly impact a patient's overall well-being and quality of life. When spiritual needs and spiritual distress are not addressed, patients are at risk of:

- *Emotional symptoms:* Anxiety, depression, guilt, anger, or despair
- *Behavioral symptoms:* Withdrawal from social interactions, changes in behavior or routines
- *Cognitive symptoms:* Confusion, difficulty making decisions, and questioning the meaning of life
- *Physical symptoms:* Pain and other physical symptoms can sometimes be exacerbated by spiritual distress.

Thus, spiritual care in palliative care enhances patient well-being by reducing anxiety, depression, and spiritual distress. It provides holistic support, improving the quality of life by fostering hope and resilience. Addressing spiritual needs aids in symptom management, strengthens relationships, and enhances communication. Spiritual care helps patients find meaning and purpose, respects cultural and religious values, and supports end-of-life transitions. It reduces isolation and empowers patients in decision-making. Additionally, it benefits healthcare providers by enhancing compassion and reducing burnout. Overall, spiritual care is crucial for comprehensive, dignified, and personalized patient support. Various interventions are practiced:

- *Understanding spiritual care in palliative settings:* Spirituality in palliative care encompasses the search for meaning, purpose, and connection amidst suffering and uncertainty. It acknowledges the diversity of spiritual beliefs and practices among patients and respects their individual journeys. Spiritual care aims to support patients in finding peace, reconciling conflicts, and addressing existential questions that arise during illness and end-of-life stages.
- *Chaplaincy services:* Chaplains play a central role in providing spiritual support within palliative care teams. They offer pastoral care, prayer, and religious rituals according to the patient's faith tradition or spiritual preferences. Chaplains are trained to listen empathetically, facilitate spiritual conversations, and provide comfort and guidance based on religious teachings and spiritual principles.[24]
- *Meaning-making and life review:* Life review and meaning-making interventions help patients reflect on their life experiences, relationships, and accomplishments. These interventions encourage patients to find significance and purpose in their lives, fostering acceptance and facilitating emotional and spiritual healing. Life review may involve storytelling, reminiscence therapy, and guided reflection sessions facilitated by trained professionals or volunteers. Using a life review can help patients with advanced cancer by providing an opportunity to discern and increase personal meaning from life, promote greater self-worth and internal well-being, and help with coping.[25]
- *Meditation and mindfulness practices:* Meditation and mindfulness techniques promote spiritual well-being by cultivating present-moment awareness, acceptance, and inner peace. These practices help patients manage stress, anxiety, and existential distress, enhancing emotional resilience and improving the overall quality of life. Mindfulness-based interventions may include guided meditation, breath awareness, and relaxation exercises tailored to individual preferences.[26]
- *Rituals and symbolic practices:* Rituals and symbolic practices hold profound meaning in spiritual care, providing comfort, solace, and a sense of continuity during times of transition and loss. These practices vary widely across cultures and traditions, encompassing rituals, such as prayer, blessings, anointing, sacred readings, and commemorative ceremonies. Rituals honor spiritual beliefs, mark significant milestones, and facilitate spiritual expression and connection.
- *Dignity therapy:* It is an evidence-based and clinically effective psychotherapeutic modality for patients who are classified as terminally ill. Illnesses that are irreversible may lead to loss of autonomy, severe physical pain, and challenging existential and spiritual experience, all of which contribute to the disintegration of a patient's sense of self and sometimes social ideation for a hastened death. It involves patients with life-limiting illnesses to express their most significant memories, moments of pride, and meaningful roles and requests for remembrance, which are documented by their surviving family members. It affords a means to address existential despair and erosion of personhood among patients with end-stage conditions.[27,28]
- *Integrating spirituality into multidisciplinary care:* Spiritual care is integrated into multidisciplinary palliative care teams to provide comprehensive support to patients and families. Collaboration among chaplains, healthcare providers, social workers, and counselors ensures holistic care that addresses the physical, emotional, social, and spiritual dimensions of suffering. Team-based approaches promote the coordination of spiritual interventions with medical treatment and psychosocial support, enhancing overall patient-centered care.
- *Cultural sensitivity and diversity:* Cultural sensitivity is essential in providing spiritual care and respecting diverse beliefs, practices, and traditions among patients from different cultural backgrounds. Healthcare providers receive training in cultural competence to understand and accommodate cultural preferences related to spirituality, ensuring that spiritual interventions are respectful, inclusive, and aligned with the patient's cultural identity.

ETHICAL INTERVENTIONS

Medical ethics in palliative care focuses on providing compassionate, patient-centered care aimed at alleviating suffering and enhancing the quality of life for patients with serious, often terminal illnesses. The core ethical principles include autonomy, beneficence, nonmaleficence, and justice.

- *Autonomy:* Respect for patient autonomy is fundamental. Patients should have the right to make informed decisions about their own care, including the acceptance or refusal of treatments. Advance directives and living wills are tools to ensure patients' wishes are respected even if they become unable to communicate them.
- *Beneficence:* Healthcare providers have an ethical duty to act in the best interest of the patient, aiming to provide benefits and balance against the risks and burdens of treatment.
- *Nonmaleficence:* "Do no harm" is a core principle. Interventions should not cause unnecessary suffering or harm to the patient.
- *Justice:* Fairness in the distribution of healthcare resources and ensuring all patients have access to palliative care regardless of their background or economic status.

COMMUNICATION

Communication in palliative care is crucial for ensuring that patients receive compassionate, effective, and patient-centered care. It involves clear, empathetic, and honest interactions between healthcare providers, patients, and their families. Effective communication helps in understanding the patient's values, preferences, and goals, which guides the care plan and decision-making process. It includes discussing prognosis, treatment options, and advance care planning, as well as addressing emotional, psychological, and spiritual needs. Good communication fosters trust, reduces anxiety, and supports patients and families in making informed decisions, ultimately enhancing the quality of life and care experience in palliative care settings.[29] Here are some key methods:

- *Active listening:* Pay close attention to what the patient and family members are saying without interrupting. This shows respect and understanding.
- *Empathy and compassion:* Show genuine concern and empathy for the patient's situation. Acknowledge their emotions and provide comfort through kind words and actions.
- *Clear and honest communication:* Provide information in a straightforward and honest manner, avoiding medical jargon. Ensure that the patient and family understand the information being shared.
- *Open-ended questions:* Use questions that encourage patients to express their thoughts and feelings fully. For example, "How are you feeling about your treatment options?"
- *Body language:* Maintain appropriate eye contact, nod, and use other body language cues to show attentiveness and understanding.
- *Regular updates:* Keep patients and their families informed about any changes in the patient's condition and treatment plans. Regular updates help in managing expectations and reducing anxiety.
- *Cultural sensitivity:* Be aware of and respect cultural differences in communication styles, beliefs, and practices related to illnesses and death.
- *Family meetings:* Conduct regular family meetings to discuss the patient's condition, treatment options, and care preferences. This ensures everyone is on the same page.
- *Advance care planning:* Discuss advance care directives and end-of-life care preferences early and regularly. This helps ensure that the patient's wishes are known and respected.
- *Emotional support:* Provide emotional support by acknowledging feelings, offering reassurance, and connecting patients and families with counseling services if needed.
- *Use of technology:* Utilize technology such as video calls to maintain communication with patients and families, especially when in-person visits are not possible.

LEGAL INTERVENTIONS

Legal interventions in palliative care are crucial for ensuring that patients' rights are protected, their wishes are respected, and care is provided within a framework of ethical and legal guidelines. Key legal interventions include the following:

- *Advance directives:* Advance care planning is the process by which patients, together with their families and healthcare providers, consider their values and goals and articulate preferences for future care. Advance directives are legal documents that allow patients to outline their preferences for medical treatment in case they become unable to communicate their decisions.[30]

Examples include living wills and power of attorney for healthcare.

- *Do not resuscitate (DNR) orders:* Legal orders indicating that a patient does not wish to undergo cardiopulmonary resuscitation (CPR) in the event of cardiac or respiratory arrest.
- *Guardianship and conservatorship:* Legal processes to appoint a person (guardian or conservator) to make healthcare decisions on behalf of a patient who is deemed incapable of making informed decisions.
- *Informed consent:* The legal requirement that healthcare providers must obtain voluntarily informed consent from patients or their legal surrogates before administering treatments or procedures, ensuring that patients understand the risks, benefits, and alternatives.
- *Palliative sedation:* Legal considerations surrounding the use of sedation to relieve intractable suffering in terminally ill patients, ensuring that it is administered ethically and with proper consent.
- *Euthanasia and physician-assisted suicide:* Legal in some jurisdictions, these practices involve intentionally ending a patient's life to relieve suffering, with strict regulations and ethical guidelines to prevent abuse and ensure informed consent.
- *State-specific laws:* Various states may have specific laws and regulations governing palliative and end-of-life care, such as Physician Orders for Life-Sustaining Treatment (POLST) forms that complement advance directives by providing medical orders based on a patient's preferences.
- *Confidentiality:* Legal and ethical duty to protect patient information. Exceptions may occur when there is a risk of harm to the patient or others.

CONCLUSION

Interventions in palliative care are essential for providing comprehensive support to patients with life-limiting illnesses. These interventions, including medical, psychosocial, and spiritual care, aim to enhance the quality of life by addressing physical discomfort, emotional distress, and existential concerns. The interdisciplinary approach ensures that care is tailored to each patient's unique needs, respecting their dignity and preferences. By fostering open communication and offering holistic support, palliative care interventions help reduce suffering, provide comfort, and support families through the end-of-life process and bereavement. This compassionate care improves overall well-being during challenging times.

REFERENCES

1. WHO Expert Committee on Cancer Pain Relief and Active Supportive Care & World Health Organization. (1990). Cancer pain relief and palliative care: report of a WHO expert committee [meeting held in Geneva from 3 to 10 July 1989]. World Health Organization. [online] Available from https://iris.who.int/handle/10665/39524 [Last accessed March, 2025].
2. Porta-Sales J, Garzon-Rodriguez C, Llorens-Torrome S, Brunelli C, Pigni A, Caraceni A. Evidence on the analgesic role of bisphosphonates and denosumab in the treatment of pain due to bone metastases: a systematic review within the European Association for Palliative Care guidelines project. Palliat Med. 2017;31(1):5-25.
3. Tseng YY, Yang ST, Tu PH, Yang TC, Lo YL. Minimally invasive vertebroplasty in the treatment of pain induced by spinal metastatic tumor. Minim Invasive Neurosurg. 2008;51(5):280-84.
4. Stearns L, Boortz-Marx R, Du Pen S, Friehs G, Gordon M, Halyard M, et al. Intrathecal drug delivery for the management of cancer pain: a multidisciplinary consensus of best clinical practices. J Support Oncol. 2005;3(6):399-408.
5. Yasuda S, Sugano S, Matsuda Y, Kako J, Takagi Y, Watanab H, et al. Systematic review and meta-analysis of the efficacy of benzodiazepines for dyspnea in patients with cancer. Jpn J Clin Oncol. 2023;53(4):327-34.
6. Barnes H, McDonald J, Smallwood N, Manser R. Opioids for the palliation of refractory breathlessness in adults with advanced disease and terminal illness. Cochrane Database Syst Rev. 2016;3(3):CD011008.
7. Ekstrom M, Bajwah S, Bland JM, Currow DC, Hussain J, Johnson MJ. One evidence base; three stories: do opioids relieve chronic breathlessness? Thorax. 2018;73(1):88-90.
8. Bott J, Blumenthal S, Buxton M, Ellum S, Falconer C, Garrod R, et al. Guidelines for the physiotherapy management of the adult, medical, spontaneously breathing patient. Thorax. 2009;64(Suppl 1):i1-i52.
9. Swan F, Newey A, Bland M, Allgar V, Booth S, Bausewein C, et al. Airflow relieves chronic breathlessness in people with advanced disease: an exploratory systematic review and meta-analyses. Palliat Med. 2019;33(6):618-33.
10. Von Trott P, Oei SL, Ramsenthaler C. Acupuncture for breathlessness in advanced diseases: a systematic review and meta-analysis. J Pain Symptom Manage. 2020;59(2):327-38.
11. Twycross R, Back I. Nausea and vomiting in advanced cancer. Eur J Palliat Care. 1998;5:39-45.
12. Walsh D, Nelson KA, Mahomoud FA. Established and potential therapeutic applications of cannabinoids in oncology. Support Care Cancer. 2003;11(3):137-43.

13. Arslan M, Ozdemir L. Oral intake of ginger for chemotherapy-induced nausea and vomiting among women with breast cancer. Clin J Oncol Nurs. 2015;19(5):E92-7.
14. Wickham RJ. Managing constipation in adults with cancer. J Adv Pract Oncol. 2017;8(2):149-61.
15. Thomas J, Karver S, Cooney GA, Chamberlain BH, Watt CK, Slatkin NE, et al. Methylnaltrexone for opioid-induced constipation in advanced illness. N Engl J Med. 2008;358(22):2332-43.
16. Cramp F. Daniel J. Exercise for the management of cancer-related fatigue in adults. Cochrane Database Syst Rev. 2008;16(2):CD006145.
17. Beal JE, Olson R, Laubenstein L, Morales JO, Bellman P, Yangco B, et al. Dronabinol as a treatment for anorexia associated with weight loss in patients with AIDS. J Pain Symptom Manage. 1995;10(2):89-97.
18. Thoma N, Pilecki B, McKay D. Contemporary cognitive behavior therapy: a review of theory, history, and evidence. Psychodyn Psychiatry. 2015;43(3):423-61.
19. Shennan C, Payne S, Fenlon D. What is the evidence for the use of mindfulness-based interventions in cancer care? A review. Psychooncology. 2011;20(7):681-97.
20. Hayes SC, Strosahl KD, Wilson KG. Acceptance and Commitment Therapy: the Process and Practice of Mindful Change, 2nd edition. New York, NY: Guilford Press; 2012.
21. Tay KCP, Seow CCD, Xiao C, Lee HMJ, Chiu HFK, Chan SWC. Structured interviews examining the burden, coping, self-efficacy, and quality of life among family caregivers of persons with dementia in Singapore. Dementia (London). 2016;15(2):204-20.
22. Lenkowsky RS. Bibliotherapy: a review and analysis of the literature. J Spec Educ. 1987;21(2):123-132.
23. Norelli SK, Long A, Krepps JM. Relaxation Techniques. (2024). Treasure Island (FL): StatPearls Publishing. [online] Available from https://www.ncbi.nlm.nih.gov/books/NBK513238/ [Last accessed March, 2025].
24. Lo R. The use of prayer in spiritual care. Aust J Holist Nurs. 2003;10(1):22-9.
25. Wang CW, Chow AY, Chan CL. The effects of life review interventions on spiritual well-being, psychological distress, and quality of life in patients with terminal or advanced cancer: a systematic review and meta-analysis of randomized controlled trials. Palliat Med. 2017;31(10):883-94.
26. Piderman KM, Breitkopf CR, Jenkins SM, Lapid MI, Kwete GM, Sytsma TT, et al. The impact of a spiritual legacy intervention in patients with brain cancers and other neurologic illnesses and their support persons. Psychooncology. 2017;26(3):346-53.
27. Chochinov HM, Hack T, Hassard T, Kristjanson LJ, McClement S, Harlos M. Dignity therapy: a novel psychotherapeutic intervention for patients near the end of life. J Clin Oncol. 2005;23(24):5520-5.
28. Martínez M, Arantzamendi M, Belar A, Carrasco JM, Carvajal A, Rullán M, et al. 'Dignity therapy,' a promising intervention in palliative care: a comprehensive systematic literature review. Palliat Med. 2017;31(6):492-509.
29. Back, AL. Patient–clinician communication issues in palliative care for patients with advanced cancer. J Clin Onco. 2020;38(9):866-76.
30. Pérez MdV, Macchi MJ, Agranatti AF. Advance directives in the context of end-of-life palliative care. Curr Opin Support Palliat Care. 2013;7(4):406-10.

62 CHAPTER

End-of-Life Care and Hospice

Anjum Shabbar Khan Joad, Minhaj Akhter, Manisha Hemrajani

I have got my leave. Bid me farewell, my brothers! I bow to you all and take my departure. Here I give back the keys of my door-and I give up all claims to my house. I only ask for last kind words from you. We were neighbors for long, but I received more than I could give. Now the day has dawned and the lamp that lit my dark corner is out. A summons has come and I am ready for my journey.

—Rabindranath Tagore, Gitanjali, XCIII[1]

INTRODUCTION

The number of patients with a cancer diagnosis requiring palliative care (PC) in India is estimated at 70–140 per 1,00,000 population.[2] The emphasis is gradually shifting toward integrating PC earlier during cancer treatment and employing a multidisciplinary approach to deliver holistic care. The PC and hospice model aims to improve the quality of life through the cancer trajectory and address the quality of death. The unit of care is the patient and caregivers. Despite significant progress, challenges persist in ensuring equitable access to high-quality end-of-life care (EOLC). India is ranked among the worst countries to die in, with a place of 59 out of 81 in the Quality of Death Index Report released in 2021.[3] EOLC encompasses the comprehensive management of individuals who are in the final stages of a terminal illness.

The scope of this chapter is to give an overview of the PC needs of a patient with advanced cancer. This will include the management of common symptoms and care of the patient during the dying phase.

DEFINITIONS

Palliative care is defined as "an approach that improves the quality of life of patients and that of their families who are facing challenges associated with life-limiting illnesses, whether physical, psychological, social, or spiritual."[4]

End-of-Life Care

The Indian Council of Medical Research (ICMR)[5] defines EOLC as "when the focus of care shifts from curative and life-prolonging treatment to symptom control, comfort, dignity, quality of life, and quality of dying instead of options aimed at cure or prolongation of life." According to the General Medical Council, UK patients are "approaching the end of life" when they are likely to die within a year.[6]

Terminally ill: Terminal care period has been described as ranging from 3–6 to 12 months.[7]

Hospice is a specific clinical program or approach that provides specialist PC. Hospice care is commonly perceived as PC for patients with advanced cancer and a short prognosis in a home-like setting.[8] In some settings, "hospice" describes services providing a long-term inpatient facility, or day hospice, or home hospice to patients near the end of life.

Total pain is a term described by Dame Cicely Saunders as the multidimensional nature of pain in patients with advanced cancer where physical pathology and psychological and emotional distress, social isolation, and spiritual disturbances lead to the total pain experience.[9]

ASSESSMENT OF PATIENTS NEEDS

The physical, psychological, social, spiritual, practical, and information needs must be assessed, addressed, and reviewed regularly. A comprehensive care plan helps to check all domains of care. The multidisciplinary team is instrumental in delivering quality PC.

COMMON SYMPTOMS AND MANAGEMENT

Pain, breathlessness, vomiting and nausea, fatigue, delirium, and anorexia are frequently seen in advanced cancer. The basic approach toward the management of all the symptoms is similar **(Box 1)**. Constipation, urinary complaints, pruritus, and oral ulcers can also increase symptom burden. It is also necessary to prevent complications, for instance, pressure sores or maggots.

Pain

Pain is one of the most distressing symptoms in advanced cancer.

Management

Comprehensive assessment is the first step **(Box 1)**. Treatment is determined by the etiopathogenesis of the pain **(Box 2)**.

Treat the Cause

Potentially reversible causes of pain need to be evaluated and addressed, e.g., abscesses, mucositis, and gastritis. Oncologic emergencies like malignant spinal cord compression, fractures, and thromboembolism must be kept in mind. Radiotherapy can alleviate the pain arising from bone metastases, spinal cord compression, and brain metastases. Radioactive isotopes may have a role in widespread sclerotic bone metastases.

BOX 1: Approach to symptom management.

- Comprehensive assessment, stage of disease, cancer-directed therapy, comorbid conditions, investigations, patient goals, values, and preferences
- Discuss management plan with patients and their family members
- Treat the cause, e.g., thoracocentesis in dyspnea due to pleural effusion
- Pharmacological treatment to palliate the symptom
- Nonpharmacological treatment, e.g., positioning in breathlessness
- Management of practical, psychological, social, and spiritual issues
- Caregiver support
- *Review:* Monitor response and modify treatment

BOX 2: The etiology of pain in cancer.

- *Cancer:* Invasion or metastases, e.g., pain due to a large bone tumor, painful bone metastases, or fracture
- Cancer-directed therapy, e.g., pain due to chemotherapy-induced peripheral neuropathy
- Unrelated to cancer, e.g., diabetic neuropathy in a patient with cancer
- Related to debility, e.g., pain due to pressure sores

Pharmacological Management

The World Health Organization (WHO) Analgesic Ladder[10] recommends a stepwise approach for managing cancer-related pain. The three-step model focuses on the individualized use of oral analgesics "by the clock," tailored to the individual **(Fig. 1)**.

Step 1: Nonsteroidal anti-inflammatory drugs and acetaminophen

Nonsteroidal anti-inflammatory drugs (NSAIDs) and acetaminophen **(Table 1)** are used to treat and alleviate somatic nociceptive pains, e.g., bone pain, inflammatory pain, and soft tissue inflammation, and have opioid-sparing effects. The lowest effective dose is prescribed for short periods to minimize gastrointestinal and renal toxicity. Selective COX-2 inhibitors are associated with lower gastrointestinal morbidity but, when used for a prolonged duration, are associated with cardiovascular accidents.[11]

Step 2: Moderate pain

Progression to opioids for moderate pain (e.g., tramadol and codeine), combined with nonopioids.

Step 3: Severe pain

Use of strong opioids, e.g., morphine, methadone, fentanyl, and buprenorphine. Opioids **(Table 2)** are the cornerstone of the management of moderate-to-severe pain in patients with cancer.[12]

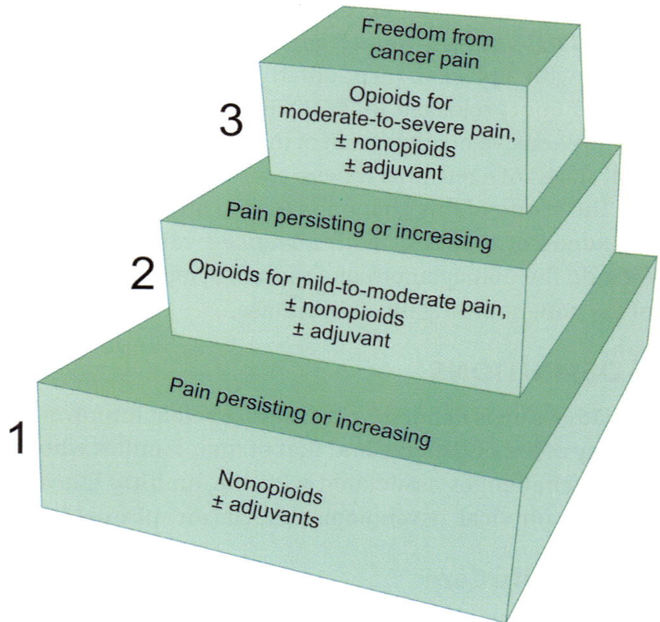

Fig. 1: The three-step analgesic ladder.

Adjuvant analgesics (e.g., antidepressants, anticonvulsants, and antispasmodics) can be added at any step to address specific pain, such as neuropathic pain. Prevention of opioid-induced nausea and vomiting and constipation is central to effective opioid therapy.

Neuropathic Pain

The prevalence of pain with a neuropathic mechanism ranged from a conservative estimate of 18.7–21.4% of all recorded cancer pains[13] but has been reported as high as 54% in a study conducted in tertiary cancer centers in North India.[14]

The pharmacological management of neuropathic pain is detailed in **Table 3**.

Nonpharmacological Techniques

Massage, acupuncture, transcutaneous electrical nerve stimulation, relaxation, guided imagery, art or music therapy, and mindfulness are useful techniques where expertise is available.[16] Interventional pain management is a key component in addressing cancer pain, offering advanced methods for patients with refractory pain. Interventions including the superior hypogastric block for pelvic cancer pain[17] provide significant pain relief by targeting specific nerve groups and reducing nociceptive input. Chemical neurolysis, with agents like alcohol or phenol, is used when diagnostic nerve blocks achieve significant relief. Radiofrequency ablation (RFA) is particularly effective for localized cancer pain, such as bone metastases.[18] Neuromodulation techniques, including spinal cord stimulation (SCS) and peripheral nerve stimulation (PNS), are employed to manage neuropathic pain through electrical modulation of the pain pathways. Intrathecal drug delivery systems, using very low doses of opioids like morphine, are effective for severe pain, allowing for lower doses and systemic side effects while providing targeted relief.[19]

TABLE 1: Step 1: Analgesics.

Drug	*Dose*	*Route*
Diclofenac	50–100 mg twice daily (max 150 mg/day)	Oral, intravenous, transdermal patch
Ibuprofen	200–400 mg every 4–6 hours (max 2,400 mg/day)	Oral
Naproxen	250–500 mg twice daily (max 1,000 mg/day)	Oral
Etoricoxib	60–120 mg once daily	Oral
Celecoxib	100–200 mg twice daily	Oral
Aspirin	325–650 mg every 4–6 hours (max 4 g/day)	Oral
Meloxicam	7.5–15 mg once daily	Oral
Acetaminophen	500 mg–1 g every 4–6 hours (max 3 g/day)	Oral, intravenous

TABLE 2: The opioids available in India.

Opioid	*Starting dose*	*Maximum dose*	*Route*	*Indication*
Tramadol	37.5–50 mg every 4–6 hours	400 mg/day	Oral, intravenous, subcutaneous	Moderate pain, neuropathic pain
Codeine	15 mg every 4–6 hours	240 mg/day	Oral	Mild-to-moderate pain, often combined with nonopioids
Morphine	2.5–10 mg every 4 hours, titrate based on response	Based on titration	Oral, intravenous, subcutaneous	Severe pain, including bone and visceral pain
Tapentadol	50–100 mg every 4–6 hours	500 mg/day	Oral	Moderate-to-severe pain
Buprenorphine	5–20 µg/h (transdermal patch)	Based on titration	Transdermal patch, sublingual	• Moderate-to-severe cancer pain • Expensive
Fentanyl	12–25 µg/hour (transdermal patch), titrate as needed	Based on titration	Transdermal patch, intravenous	• Severe chronic cancer pain • Expensive
Methadone	2.5–10 mg every 8–12 hours	Based on titration	Oral	• Neuropathic and severe cancer pain, opioid rotation • Needs specialist training and experience

TABLE 3: Drugs used in neuropathic pain.[15]

Drug	*MOA*	*Dose*	*Route*
Gabapentin	Modulates voltage-gated calcium channels to reduce neurotransmitter release	300 mg daily, up to 3,600 mg/day	Oral
Pregabalin	Binds to the alpha-2-delta subunit of voltage-gated calcium channels to decrease pain transmission	75 mg twice daily, up to 300 mg twice daily	Oral
Amitriptyline	Inhibits the reuptake of norepinephrine and serotonin	10–25 mg daily, up to 75–150 mg/day	Oral
Duloxetine	Inhibits the reuptake of serotonin and norepinephrine	30–60 mg once daily, up to 120 mg/day	Oral
Lidocaine	Blocks sodium channels to prevent nerve signal transmission	5% patch applied for up to 12 h/day	Topical postherpetic neuralgia
Capsaicin | topical |	Depletes substance P from sensory neurons to reduce pain signals	0.025–0.075% cream, applied up to four times daily	Topical
Ketamine	NMDA receptor antagonist reduces opioid tolerance and sensitization	0.1–0.5 mg/kg/h infusion	Intravenous

(MOA: mechanism of action; NMDA: *N*-methyl-d-aspartate)

BOX 3: Goals of pain management (5 As).

- *Analgesia:* Optimize analgesia
- *Activities:* Optimize activities of daily living
- *Adverse effects:* Minimize adverse effects, including financial toxicity
- *Aberrant behavior:* Keep in mind opioid use disorder
- *Affect:* Relationship between pain and mood

Multimodal strategies help achieve the goals of pain management **(Box 3)**.

Dyspnea

The prevalence of dyspnea in cancer is 16–77%, with a prevalence of up to 75–87% in patients with lung cancer.[20]

Management of Dyspnea

Treat the Cause

The correctable causes include pleural effusion, pulmonary edema or airflow obstruction in chronic obstructive pulmonary disease (COPD), and heart failure. Anxiety, anemia, muscle weakness, and infection can exacerbate breathlessness. Thoracocentesis and paracentesis may be considered if the prognosis is from weeks to months. Diuretics, antibiotics, transfusions, noninvasive ventilation, and anticoagulants (pulmonary emboli) have a role in selected patients.[21,22] Radiotherapy may be considered for superior vena cava syndrome.

Pharmacological Management

- *Opioids:* Morphine reduces the perception of breathlessness. Oral doses typically begin at 2.5–5 mg every 6 hours, adjusted to the patient's comfort. The upper limit of morphine for this indication is 30 mg in 24 hours.
- *Benzodiazepines:* Anxiety exacerbates dyspnea, and lorazepam (0.5–2 mg) calms the patient and mitigates panic.
- *Corticosteroids:* Dexamethasone (4–8 mg/day) is useful when inflammation or airway obstruction contributes to dyspnea, especially in cases of lymphangitic carcinomatosis or lung cancer.
- *Bronchodilators:* Nebulized salbutamol and ipratropium are prescribed for patients with bronchospasm to improve airflow.
- *Oxygen therapy:* Supplemental oxygen is recommended for patients with documented hypoxemia. Its effectiveness in nonhypoxemic dyspnea remains controversial.

Nonpharmacological Management[21,22]

- *Positioning:* Upright positioning or a high Fowler's position promotes better lung expansion.
- *Fan:* A handheld fan directed toward the face reduces the perception of dyspnea.
- Pacing activities and movements with a bronchodilator, morphine, and oxygen support.

- *Psychosocial support*: Counseling and relaxation techniques play an important role in reducing the emotional burden of breathlessness, particularly when anxiety is a contributing factor.

Delirium and Agitation

Delirium is a neurocognitive disorder characterized by an acute onset of confusion, fluctuating levels of consciousness, impaired attention, and altered cognition. It is reversible, but at the end of life, delirium tends to be persistent and is associated with significant distress for both patients and their families. Agitation refers to heightened physical and emotional restlessness, which can be a symptom of delirium, anxiety, or unresolved physical or emotional issues. Delirium is a frequent complication in terminally ill patients, with a prevalence ranging from 30% to 80% in those nearing the end of life, depending on the stage of illness and the setting of care.[23] The clinical presentation can vary **(Box 4)**.

Treat the Cause

Correctable causes of delirium and agitation include metabolic disturbances, such as hypercalcemia, hypoxia, or electrolyte imbalances. Medications like opioids, benzodiazepines, and corticosteroids may contribute to confusion and agitation through their central nervous system effects. Hepatic, renal, or respiratory dysfunction can further complicate the clinical picture by altering drug metabolism and exacerbating symptoms. Infection, dehydration, malnutrition, and sleep deprivation also play significant roles in the development of delirium, while neurological complications, particularly in patients with primary or metastatic brain cancer, can directly affect cognitive function and exacerbate agitation and confusion.[23]

The pharmacological management of delirium and agitation is detailed in **Table 4**.

BOX 4: Types of delirium.

- *Hyperactive delirium:* Characterized by restlessness, agitation, and sometimes aggressive behavior. Patients may experience hallucinations or paranoia
- *Hypoactive delirium:* Features lethargy, drowsiness, and decreased responsiveness. This type can be more challenging to diagnose but is associated with worse outcomes
- *Mixed delirium:* Patients fluctuate between hyperactive and hypoactive states, often within short periods

Nonpharmacological Management

- *Environmental modifications*: A calm, quiet environment with familiar objects and the presence of family members can reduce anxiety and confusion.
- *Orientation aids*: Using clocks and calendars and ensuring good lighting during daylight hours can reduce disorientation.
- Hydration and nutrition.
- *Sleep hygiene:* Promoting restful sleep and reducing nighttime disturbances can prevent the exacerbation of delirium.
- *Family support, education, and communication:* Involving family members in care and providing emotional support can reduce distress for both patients and families.[23,24]

Nausea and Vomiting

Nausea and vomiting are common, with a prevalence ranging from 40% to 70%, in advanced cancer. The etiology is often multifactorial. Nausea and vomiting can occur due to cancer or its treatment. Opioids and chemotherapy can also contribute to nausea by affecting the central

TABLE 4: Management of delirium and agitation.[23]

Drug	*Dose*	*Route*	*Indication*
Haloperidol	• *Oral:* 1–5 mg every 6–8 hours • *IV:* 0.5–2 mg every 4–6 hours	Oral/IV	Hyperactive delirium; first-line treatment for severe agitation
Olanzapine	*Oral:* 5–10 mg once daily	Oral	Delirium when haloperidol is ineffective or contraindicated
Quetiapine	*Oral:* 25 mg 12 hourly or once a day	Oral	
Lorazepam	*Oral/IV:* 0.5–2 mg every 4–6 hours	Oral/IV	Anxiety and severe distress; adjunct therapy
Midazolam	*SC/IV:* 2.5–5 mg every 2–4 hours	SC/IV	Severe terminal agitation; short-acting benzodiazepine

(IV: intravenous; SC: subcutaneous)

nervous system and gastrointestinal motility. Hypercalcemia, obstruction and infection of the gastrointestinal tract, uremia, liver dysfunction, sepsis, and electrolyte imbalances can cause nausea. Increased intracranial pressure, because of brain metastases or primary brain tumors, can cause vomiting. Psychological factors such as anxiety, fear, and emotional distress can manifest as physical symptoms, including nausea.[25,26]

Treat the Cause

Correctable causes such as severe constipation or fecal impaction, gastroparesis, gastroesophageal reflux disease (GERD), hypercalcemia, dehydration, uremia, and dyselectrolytemia need to be addressed. Radiation therapy can effectively palliate brain metastases. Endoscopic stenting can bypass selected gastrointestinal obstructions. In upper gastrointestinal obstruction, some patients will need a venting nasogastric tube or venting gastrostomy.

Pharmacological Management (Table 5)[26,27]

Pharmacological management can be mechanistic (based on the cause) or empirical (use of broad-spectrum antiemetics). Opioid rotation may be required. In severe vomiting, oral administration may not be possible, and sublingual, intravenous, subcutaneous, or rectal routes may be necessary.

Nonpharmacological Management

Dietary adjustments, such as small, frequent meals and avoiding foods that may trigger nausea, like fatty or spicy foods, can help reduce the frequency of symptoms. Maintaining proper hydration is also essential, as dehydration itself can exacerbate nausea. Positioning the patient with the head of the bed elevated can provide relief, particularly in cases of nausea caused by increased intracranial pressure or gastrointestinal reflux. Addressing psychological factors such as anxiety and emotional distress through counseling or relaxation techniques can play a role in managing nausea.[25-28]

Nutrition

Oral intake is decreased in most cancer patients approaching the terminal phase due to anorexia, nausea, vomiting, dysphagia, and intestinal obstruction. This often creates emotional distress and fear of death due to starvation among the family members and the caregivers. Nutritional advice depends on the position of the patient along the cancer trajectory. For patients who have an expected survival of a few months and are not receiving anticancer treatment, frequent small meals and nutritional supplements may be appropriate. The National Comprehensive Cancer Network[29] and the American Society for Parenteral and Enteral Network[30] guidelines recommend against the routine use of parenteral nutrition for advanced cancer patients. In a small subset of patients with gastrointestinal malignancy, obstruction, or malabsorption syndrome with an estimated survival of few months, or more, parenteral nutrition can be initiated. This intervention needs to be reviewed regularly to weigh the benefits and burdens. For patients with limited survival of a few weeks to a few months, aggressive nutritional interventions are likely to negatively impact the quality of life and do not improve survival.[31]

Fatigue

Fatigue and asthenia can be debilitating and profoundly affect patients' quality of life by reducing their ability to carry out daily activities and increasing emotional distress.

Cancer-related fatigue: A subjective sensation of tiredness or exhaustion that is not proportional to activity levels and is not relieved by rest or sleep. Asthenia is often described as a generalized weakness or lack of strength when even minimal exertion is overwhelming.[32]

TABLE 5: Pharmacological management of vomiting.[26,27]

Drug	*Dose*	*Route*	*Indication*
Metoclopramide	10 mg every 6–8 hours	Oral/subcutaneous	Nausea due to reduced gastric motility
Haloperidol	0.5–2 mg every 4–6 hours	Oral/subcutaneous	Opioid-induced nausea
Ondansetron	4–8 mg every 8 hours	Oral/intravenous	Nausea caused by chemotherapy or increased intracranial pressure or complete bowel obstruction
Dexamethasone	4–8 mg once daily	Oral/intravenous	Nausea related to intracranial pressure or inflammation
Cyclizine	50 mg every 6–8 hours	Oral	Motion sickness or vestibular-related nausea

TABLE 6: Pharmacological management of fatigue.[34]

Pharmacological management	***Details***
Corticosteroids	*Dexamethasone:* 4–8 mg daily boosts energy levels but limited by long-term side effects
Psychostimulants	*Methylphenidate:* 5–10 mg twice daily
Antidepressants	Have a role if there is concomitant depression

Management of Fatigue

The assessment should be comprehensive, combining subjective self-reports with objective clinical findings.

Treat the Cause

Cancer chemotherapy and radiotherapy contribute to systemic inflammation, can disrupt metabolism, affect oral intake, and cause anemia, dehydration, and electrolyte imbalance.[32] Immobilization and poor nutrition can lead to deconditioning, muscle wasting, and fatigue. Depression and anxiety often present with somatic symptoms like fatigue. Depression and fatigue are closely linked, and treating one can improve the other. Medications such as beta-blockers may cause bradycardia and subsequent fatigue. Combinations of medications (such as narcotics, antihistamines, antidepressants, and antiemetics) may lead to drowsiness and increased fatigue. Adjustment of the dose or timing may help decrease fatigue.

Anemia, dehydration, and infection can be corrected. Compromised intake because of disease-related dysphagia can be countered to some extent by calorie-dense, pureed feeds. Prevention and slowing of muscle wasting may need the input of rehabilitation and physiotherapy professionals.[32,33]

The pharmacological management of fatigue is detailed in **Table 6**.

Nonpharmacological Management

Exercises must be prescribed with caution in patients with bone metastases, risk of falls, and thrombocytopenia **(Table 7)**.

TABLE 7: Nonpharmacological management of fatigue.[35]

Nonpharmacological management	***Details***
Energy conservation	• Prioritize activities, schedule activities at times of peak energy • Postpone nonessential activities, one activity at a time • Use labor-saving assistive devices
Exercise	Yoga and light exercises improve strength, endurance, and mood
Nutritional support	Nutritionist's input, adequate intake, and supplements may play a role in early cachexia
Psychological support	CBT and counseling help manage psychological fatigue; caregiver support is key. Mindfulness based stress reduction
Sleep hygiene	Structured daily routine: Limit daytime naps (to not compromise with night-sleep quality), CBT for insomnia

(CBT: cognitive behavioral therapy)

Communication

The PC team needs to communicate empathetically with the patient and caregivers about end-of-life (EoL) symptoms, goals of care, prognostication, resuscitation, and life support. Despite extensive research about prognosis and life expectancy, the best estimates carry a degree of uncertainty. The expected life span may be broadly expressed in terms of months, weeks to months, and days to weeks. This can help the family and the patient plan goals of care. Effective communication with the family of a dying patient is important to ensure a "good death." All discussions must be documented in the patient records. This will ensure continuity of care and appropriate after-hours care.

THE TERMINAL PHASE: RECOGNITION OF DYING

Recognition of the terminal phase is crucial to ensure that a patient receives care that aligns with their EoL needs. This phase signals the transition from curative or life-prolonging interventions to comfort-focused care, prioritizing symptom management and patient dignity. The last weeks and days of life have been called the terminal phase of life or active dying. This is the period when uncertainty regarding prognosis diminishes, and death is imminent. The EOLC policy published by the Indian Association of Palliative Care (IAPC)[36] and the Indian Society of Critical Care Medicine (ISCCM)[37] elaborates on the care of the patient and their family through the dying process and the period after the death.

The following changes signal the beginning of the dying phase:

- *Rapid functional decline:* A decrease in the ability to perform daily tasks, increased bedbound periods, and loss of independence in activities, such as walking, eating, and personal hygiene. Patients may also become more withdrawn and spend more time sleeping. Functional declines are often accompanied by cognitive impairments, confusion, or disorientation.[38]
- *Vital sign changes:* Hypotension, tachycardia, bradycardia, or an irregular pulse can indicate imminent death. Patients may also exhibit abnormal respiratory patterns such as Cheyne-Stokes breathing, where periods of deep, rapid breathing alternate with slower, shallower breaths and pauses in breathing.
- *Appetite and nutritional decline:* A loss of appetite, decreased intake of food and fluids, and weight loss are other common signs. As the body's metabolic demands decrease, the patient may no longer feel hungry or thirsty.
- Families may notice significant changes in the patient's physical appearance as they become frail and gaunt.

The characteristic clinical signs and symptoms include a bedbound state, dysphagia of liquids, changes in the respiratory rate and pattern, pooling of airway secretions, tachycardia, peripheral cooling, oliguria, and mental changes, including delirium, disorientation, and hallucinations.

In a multicenter study of 357 cancer patients, Hui et al.[39] observed that five clinical signs had a high specificity (95%) and positive likelihood ratios for death within 3 days, including pulselessness of the radial artery, death rattle, oliguria (<100 mL in 12 hours), Cheyne-Stokes breathing, and respiration with mandibular movements.

The 10 principles for the best care for the dying person underpin the core elements of management at this stage.[40] These principles apply irrespective of the setting of care and preferred place of death **(Box 5)**.

BOX 5: The 10 principles for the best care for the dying person.

1. Recognition of dying by a multidisciplinary team (MDT) and documentation by the senior doctor
2. Communication regarding the condition with the person (where possible and appropriate) and the significant others
3. The dying person and those important to them should have the opportunity to discuss their concerns, feelings, faith, beliefs, values, and preferences with a person trained to handle this conversation
4. Anticipatory prescriptions for symptoms that can be expected (e.g., haloperidol for agitation)
5. All clinical interventions must be reviewed in the best interest of that individual
6. *Review of hydration needs:* Initiation, continuation, or cessation of artificial hydration
7. *Review of nutritional needs:* Continuation or cessation of artificial nutrition
8. A full discussion of the plan of care with the patient and their family
9. Regular reassessments of the dying person at least every 6 hours and an MDT daily review
10. Dignity in death. Care of the significant others after death

Symptom Control in the Actively Dying Patient

The control of symptoms at this stage is of paramount importance. Patients may not be able to express discomfort due to altered consciousness. Opioids play a key role in relieving the sensation of breathlessness, and benzodiazepines are useful in addressing terminal agitation. Repositioning and limiting fluids can also help reduce secretions and improve respiratory comfort in the final hours **(Table 8)**.

"Death rattle" occurs in the final stages of life when patients experience labored, noisy breathing due to the accumulation of respiratory secretions. This can be distressing for families, though patients are usually unaware of the sound. Management focuses on comfort measures, positioning, and medications.

Terminal delirium refers to delirium that occurs in the final hours or days of life, often as a precursor to death. It is typically irreversible and may present with heightened agitation, restlessness, or even hallucinations. The management goal shifts toward reducing suffering. The care and memory of an agitated, restless dying person can have a significant negative impact on families and healthcare professionals. As Dame Cicely Saunders said, "How people die remains in the memory of those who live on."[41]

Multidisciplinary Team

The patient and their family would benefit from the team approach, including the doctor, the nurse, the mental health professional, the volunteer, the social worker, and the spiritual counselor. Excellent nursing is a critical aspect of EOLC. Attention needs to be paid to the site(s) of pain, eyes/oral cavity, pressure sores, bowel and bladder disturbances, and other symptoms suggested either by verbal/nonverbal means. The use of alternative routes

TABLE 8: Symptom control in the actively dying patient.

Symptom	*Drug, doses, routes of administration*
• Pain • Titrate to optimal comfort • Need to balance pain relief against reduced level of consciousness where possible or desired	• Morphine or its equivalent: Maintain regular dosing • For dose escalations repeat every 1 hour orally or every 30 minutes for IV or SC routes of administration: as needed (PO, IV, rectal, subcutaneous, transdermal) • Adjuvants for neuropathic pain may be continued or if needed (be replaced by lignocaine/ketamine SC/IV)
Dyspnea	• Morphine or its equivalent: Morphine (1–2.5 mg SC every 4 hourly in the opioid naïve) • Terminal dyspnea with anxiety: Lorazepam—0.25–1 mg SL 8th hourly
• Nausea and vomiting • Consider change in route of administration if severe	• Gastroparesis: Metoclopramide—10–20 mg SC/IV 8th hourly/6th hourly • Central cause: Haloperidol—0.5–1.5 mg, SC/IV 12 hourly/8th hourly • Ondansetron (4 mg 8th hourly oral/IV) • Olanzapine (2.5 mg oral 12th hourly)
Gastric outlet obstruction	• Refractory vomiting: Ranitidine—50 mg 8th hourly, IV/SC, Octeotride—100–300 µg IV/SC 8th hourly • Colicky abdominal pain: Buscopan (hyoscine butylbromide) 20–40 mg IV/SC 6th hourly
Respiratory secretions	• Glycopyrrolate—0.2–0.4 mg 2–4 hourly, SC • Hyoscine butyl bromide—0.4 mg 2–4 hourly, SC
• Delirium with psychomotor agitation/terminal restlessness • Rule out fecal impaction, urinary tract infection (UTI), or distended bladder as causes of delirium • Decrease doses of drugs dependent upon liver or kidney function	• Antipsychotics • 0Haloperidol—1.5–5 mg SC/IV every 8 hours • 50% decrease in older/frail patients • Olanzapine—2.5–10 mg 12th hourly • Chlorpromazine—50–100 mg PO/PR/IV • Benzodiazepines Midazolam—2.5–5 mg 4th hourly, SC/IV
Seizures	Midazolam—2.5 mg stat SC/IV 10–20 mg maintenance for prevention

of medication can be initiated as the oral route may be more difficult. In the hospital setting a syringe pump and in the home setting a syringe driver for continuous infusions are convenient infusion options. Treatment plans should define anticipatory medications in the event of a breakthrough symptom. Decisions about the patient's preference of the place of death and allowing a natural death (AND) or do not resuscitate (DNR) need to be documented. Liberal visiting hours may be necessary in hospital settings.

Palliative Sedation

Sedation is commonly seen as an unintended adverse effect of medications used for symptom control. Proportionate palliative sedation has been defined as "intentional lowering of a dying patient's level of consciousness via careful, progressive increase of one or more sedating medicines that are titrated to provide relief of intolerable suffering from refractory symptoms to a degree acceptable to the patient using the minimum amount of sedation needed to achieve this goal."[42]

Refractory symptoms at the EoL lead to suffering. Uncontrolled suffering due to pain, breathlessness, and delirium at the EoL must be addressed as an emergency. For instance, excruciating pain that is not relieved after a trial of all aggressive measures would be termed refractory pain. The challenge is achieving symptom relief while maintaining consciousness.

Proportionate sedation is the minimum level of sedation necessary to achieve adequate relief of the refractory symptom. Initial titration for relief is followed by maintenance dosing or infusions. Many patients experience "conscious sedation" and respond to verbal stimuli, and can interact with family, and some patients need deeper sedation.

Benzodiazepines, neuroleptics, and general anesthetics are used for palliative sedation. Midazolam is administered generally by continuous infusion (intravenous/subcutaneous) for a sustained effect. (Starting dose: 0.5–1 mg/h, dose range from 1 to 20 mg/h.) Neuroleptics are used when there are signs and symptoms of delirium. Phenobarbital and propofol are also used for palliative sedation in combination with opioids.

"Good Death"

The concept of a "good death" or the "least bad death" or a peaceful death has been discussed and debated in the PC literature across physical, philosophical, and spiritual dimensions. The four core principles are alleviation of physical symptoms, support for psychosocial, spiritual, and social needs, individualized care sensitive to the cultural context, and service that meets the needs of the patient and their family. Individualized goal setting depends on the person, as values and preferences vary. For instance, every individual may not wish for death at home. A sense of completion of life may include for some, enough time to say goodbye, leave behind a legacy, and accept death. Others may prioritize control over the treatment and costs.

GUIDELINES TO SUPPORT A "NATURAL DEATH" IN THE HOSPITAL SETTING

Lack of knowledge about legal and constitutional support for EOLC, especially withholding aggressive treatments, has led to defensive practice and expensive, futile critical care. The lack of clarity about the withdrawal of inappropriate, life-sustaining measures has also resulted in prolonged unnecessary ventilatory support and vasopressor therapy. Consensus statements from professional societies of intensivists and PC physicians[36,37] paved the way for the stepwise initiation of comfort care. Advance care planning (ACP)[43] is the process that enables individuals who have decision-making capacity to deliberate over stage of cancer, treatment options, and prognosis with family and healthcare providers keeping in mind their personal values, disease stage, and prognosis and define and document goals and choices for future treatment. The record of these goals in the form of a legal document are advance directives (ADs).

Advance care planning is possible at any stage of cancer. It would be appropriate for the treating oncologist or PC professional to start the conversations regarding ACP when treating advanced or metastatic cancer. The Supreme Court (SC) of India, through landmark decisions in 2018[44] and 2023,[45] has recognized the right of a citizen to execute an AD, including the right to refuse treatment, if terminally ill. The ICMR (2020)[46] consensus statement describes an algorithm for "Do Not attempt resuscitation" orders. The joint statement of IAPC and ISCCM[47] describes the process to implement the recommendations of the 2023 SC judgment.

ETHICS OF END-OF-LIFE CARE

Euthanasia "is the intentional act of killing a terminally ill patient on voluntary request, by the direct intervention of a doctor for the purpose of the good of the patient."[5]

Euthanasia is illegal in India.

Withholding of life-sustaining treatment is a decision to not initiate or escalate aggressive life-sustaining measures in a terminally ill patient in keeping with the expressed wishes of the patient or surrogate.[5]

Withdrawal of life-sustaining treatment: "A decision made to cease or remove a life-sustaining intervention in terminal illness in accordance with the expressed wishes of the patient or surrogate."[5] Withholding and withdrawal of support are legal and ethical in India as specified in the AD.

The four pillars of ethics are respect for patient autonomy, beneficence, nonmaleficence, and justice. Withholding or withdrawing of the life support is an approach of "allowing natural death." In this setting, death because of an advanced incurable illness is in keeping with patients' wishes (patient autonomy) with symptoms well controlled (principle of beneficence) and prevents needless suffering (principle of nonmaleficence).

CAREGIVER AND BEREAVEMENT SUPPORT

Caregivers need considerable support during the last year of care[48] and after the death of the patient. The needs may vary according to the place of care. For instance, before transitioning to a compassionate discharge for death at home, families may need training for nursing issues like feeding through nasogastric tubes, prevention of bed sores and dressing of wounds, and practical issues about mortuary services. Bereavement support begins with identifying individuals/families at risk much before the death, e.g., death of a child or a young person. Anxiety, depression, somatic symptoms, and emotional distress should be identified and addressed. Mental health professionals can help bereaved family members through counseling and psychotherapy.

FUTURE DIRECTIONS IN END-OF-LIFE CARE

Early integration of PC into oncology, and awareness of ACP may help in achieving dignity in dying for cancer patients. ADs will with time be incorporated in electronic medical records.

The integration of artificial intelligence (AI) decision support tools into EOLC planning holds promising potential for the future. AI-based "nudges" can enhance the timing and quality of EoL conversations between clinicians and patients by identifying those at a high risk of short-term mortality through machine learning algorithms embedded in electronic health records. The early identification of patients who may benefit from PC and EoL planning could lead to improved patient outcomes, better alignment of treatment with patient preferences, and reduced unnecessary aggressive treatments near the EoL.[49]

CONCLUSION

This chapter provides an overview of practices that deliver a compassionate, dignified death and supports the family throughout the process and during bereavement. The efficient use of pharmacological and nonpharmacological therapy significantly alleviates symptoms in the hospital, hospice and home care setting. Timely advance care planning with patients and their healthcare power of attorney will limit the inappropriate use of life-sustaining treatments and critical resources. EOLC is an integral part of accreditation for quality medical care.

REFERENCES

1. Rabindranath Tagore. Gitanjali (Song Offerings); 1913.
2. Connor SR. Cecilia Sepulveda Bermedo M, Baxter S, et al. Senior Adviser Cancer Control, Chronic Diseases Prevention and Management, Chronic Diseases and Health Promotion. World Health Organization. 2014;7:11-8.
3. Finkelstein EA, Bhadelia A, Goh C, Baid D, Singh R, Bhatnagar S, et al. Cross country comparison of expert assessments of the quality of death and dying 2021. J Pain Symptom Manage. 2022;63(4):e419-29.
4. World Health Organization. (2002). National Cancer Control Programmes: Policies and Managerial Guidelines, 2nd edition. [online] Available from https://iris.who.int/handle/10665/42494. [Last accessed March, 2025].
5. Salins N, Gursahani R, Mathur R, Iyer S, Macaden S, Simha N, et al. Definition of terms used in limitation of treatment and providing palliative care at the end of life: the Indian Council of Medical Research Commission Report. Indian J Crit Care Med. 2018;22(4):249-62.
6. General Medical Council. (2010). Treatment and Care Towards the End of Life: Good Practice in Decision Making. London: General Medical Council. [online] Available from https://www.gmc-uk.org/ethical-guidance/ethical-guidance-for-doctors/treatment-and-care-towards-the-end-of-life. [Last accessed March, 2025].
7. Hui D, Mori M, Parsons HA, Kim SH, Li Z, Damani S, et al. The lack of standard definitions in the supportive and palliative oncology literature. J Pain Symptom Manage. 2012;43(3):582-92.
8. Hui D, Bruera E. Models of palliative care delivery for patients with cancer. J Clin Oncol. 2020;38(9):852-65.
9. Ong CK, Forbes D. Embracing Cicely Saunders's concept of total pain. BMJ. 2005;331(7516):576.
10. World Health Organization. Cancer Pain Relief: With a Guide to Opioid Availability. 2nd edition. Geneva: World Health Organization; 1996. pp. 7-8.
11. Sjøgren P, Elsner F, Kaasa S. Non-opioid analgesics. In: Cherny NI, Fallon M, Kaasa S, Portenoy RK, Currow DC (Eds). Oxford Textbook of Palliative Medicine, 6th edition. Oxford: Oxford University Press; 2021. pp. 424-33.
12. World Health Organization. (2019). WHO Guidelines for the Pharmacological and Radiotherapeutic Management of Cancer Pain in Adults and Adolescents. [online] Available from https://www.who.int/publications/i/item/9789241550390. [Last accessed March 2025].
13. Bennett MI, Rayment C, Hjermstad M, Aass N, Caraceni A, Kaasa S. Prevalence and aetiology of neuropathic pain in cancer patients: a systematic review. Pain. 2012;153(2):359-65.
14. Satija A, Joad AK, Rana SPS, Bhatnagar S. The burden of cancer-related neuropathic pain: a multi-centric cross-sectional observational study from North India. Indian J Palliat Care. 2021;27(1):104-8.
15. National Institute for Health and Care Excellence (NICE). (2013). Neuropathic pain in adults: pharmacological management in non-specialist settings [CG173]. London: NICE; 2013. [online] Available from https://www.nice.org.uk/guidance/cg173. [Last accessed March, 2025].
16. Tick H, Nielsen A, Pelletier KR, Bonakdar R, Simmons S, Glick R, et al. Evidence-based nonpharmacologic strategies for comprehensive pain care: the Consortium Pain Task Force White Paper. Explore (NY). 2018;14(3):177-211.
17. Rocha A, Plancarte R, Nataren RGR, Carrera IHS, Pacheco VALR, Hernandez-Porras BC. Effectiveness of superior hypogastric plexus neurolysis for pelvic cancer pain. Pain Physician. 2020;23(2):203-8.
18. Goetz MP, Callstrom MR, Charboneau JW, Farrell MA, Maus TP, Welch TJ, et al. Percutaneous image-guided radiofrequency ablation of painful metastases involving bone: a multicenter study. J Clin Oncol. 2004;22(2):300-6.

19. Aman MM, Mahmoud A, Deer T, Sayed D, Hagedorn JM, Brogan SE, et al. The American Society of Pain and Neuroscience (ASPN) best practices and guidelines for the interventional management of cancer-associated pain. J Pain Res. 2021;14:2139-64.
20. Johnson MJ, Currow DC. Breathlessness and other respiratory symptoms in palliative care. In: Cherny NI, Fallon M, Kaasa S, Portenoy RK, Currow DC (Eds). Oxford Textbook of Palliative Medicine, 6th edition. Oxford: Oxford University Press; 2021. pp. 589-603.
21. Mahler DA, Selecky PA, Harrod CG, Benditt JO, Carrieri-Kohlman V, Curtis JR, et al. American College of Chest Physicians consensus statement on the management of dyspnea in patients with advanced lung or heart disease. Chest. 2010;137(3):674-91.
22. Crombeen AM, Lilly EJ. Management of dyspnea in palliative care. Curr Oncol. 2020;27(3):142-5.
23. Bush SH, Lawlor PG, Ryan K, Centeno C, Lucchesi M, Kanji S, et al.; ESMO Guidelines Committee. Delirium in adult cancer patients: ESMO Clinical Practice Guidelines. Ann Oncol. 2018;29(Suppl 4):iv143-65.
24. Davis D, Searle SD, Tsui A. The Scottish Intercollegiate Guidelines Network: risk reduction and management of delirium. Age Ageing. 2019;48(4):485-8.
25. Glare P, Miller J, Nikolova T, Tickoo R. Treating nausea and vomiting in palliative care: a review. Clin Interv Aging. 2011;6:243-59.
26. Dorman S. Nausea and vomiting. In: Cherny NI, Fallon M, Kaasa S, Portenoy RK, Currow DC (Eds). Oxford Textbook of Palliative Medicine, 6th edition. Oxford: Oxford University Press; 2021. pp. 534-44.
27. Management of nausea and vomiting. In: Bruera E, Higginson IJ, von Gunten CF, Morita T (Eds). Textbook of Palliative Medicine and Supportive Care, 2nd edition. CRC Press; 2015.
28. Davis MP, Hallerberg G; Palliative Medicine Study Group of the Multinational Association of Supportive Care in Cancer. A systematic review of the treatment of nausea and/or vomiting in cancer unrelated to chemotherapy or radiation. J Pain Symptom Manage. 2010;39(4):756-67.
29. National Comprehensive Cancer Network (NCCN). Palliative Care. Version 1.2023. NCCN Clinical Practice Guidelines in Oncology. 2023. [online] Available from https://www.nccn.org/guidelines/category_3. [Last accessed March, 2025].
30. American Society for Parenteral and Enteral Nutrition. Guidelines for the use of parenteral and enteral nutrition in adult and pediatric patients. JPEN. 2002;26:1SA-38SA.
31 Bouleuc C, Anota A, Cornet C, Grodard G, Thiery-Vuillemin A, Dubroeucq O, et al. Impact on health-related quality of life of parenteral nutrition for patients with advanced cancer cachexia: results from a randomized controlled trial. Oncologist. 2020;25(5):e843-51.
32. Scialla SJ, Cole RP, Bednarz L. Redefining cancer-related asthenia-fatigue syndrome. J Palliat Med. 2006;9(4):866-72.
33. Gentile D, Beeler D, Wang XS, Ben-Arye E, Zick SM, Bao T, et al. Cancer-related fatigue outcome measures in integrative oncology: evidence for practice and research recommendations. Oncology (Williston Park). 2022;36(5):276-87.
34. Mustian KM, Alfano CM, Heckler C, Kleckner AS, Kleckner IR, Leach CR, et al. Comparison of pharmaceutical, psychological, and exercise treatments for cancer-related fatigue: a meta-analysis. JAMA Oncol. 2017;3(7):961-8.
35. Mustian KM, Sprod LK, Janelsins M, Peppone LJ, Mohile S. Exercise recommendations for cancer-related fatigue, cognitive impairment, sleep problems, depression, pain, anxiety, and physical dysfunction: a review. Oncol Hematol Rev. 2012;8(2):81-8
36. Macaden SC, Salins N, Muckaden M, Kulkarni P, Joad A, Nirabhawane V, et al. End of life care policy for the dying: consensus position statement of Indian association of palliative care. Indian J Palliat Care. 2014;20(3):171-81.
37. Myatra SN, Salins N, Iyer S, Macaden SC, Divatia JV, Muckaden M, et al. End-of-life care policy: an integrated care plan for the dying: a Joint Position Statement of the Indian Society of Critical Care Medicine (ISCCM) and the Indian Association of Palliative Care (IAPC). Indian J Crit Care Med. 2014;18(9):615-35.
38. Muhandiramge J, Orchard SG, Warner ET, van Londen GJ, Zalcberg JR. Functional decline in the cancer patient: a review. Cancers (Basel). 2022;14(6):1368.
39. Hui D, dos Santos R, Chisholm G, Bansal S, Silva TB, Kilgore K, et al. Clinical signs of impending death in cancer patients. Oncologist. 2014;19(6):681-7.
40. Ellershaw JE, Lakhani M. Best care for the dying patient. BMJ (Clin Res Ed). 2013;347:f4428.
41. Cicely Saunders Quotes. [online] Available from https://www.azquotes.com/author/20332-Cicely_Saunders. [Last accessed March, 2025].
42. Krakauer EL. Medical and ethical considerations in palliative sedation at the end-of-life 1180 In: Cherny NI, Fallon M, Kaasa S, Portenoy RK, Currow DC (Eds). Oxford Textbook of Palliative Medicine, 6th edition. Oxford: Oxford University Press; 2021. pp. 1180-90.
43. Mani RK, Simha SN, Gursahani R. The advance directives and foregoing of life support: where do we stand now? Indian J Crit Care Med. 2018;22(3):135-7.
44. Supreme Court of India. Common Cause (A Registered Society) v. Union of India & Another. Writ Petition (Civil) No. 215 of 2005. Judgment dated 9 March 2018. [cited 2025 Mar 15]. Available from https://digiscr.sci.gov.in/admin/judgement_file/judgement_pdf/2018/volume%206/Part%20I/common%20cause%20(%20

a%20regd.%20society)_union%20of%20india%20&%20another_1698658984.pdf [Last accessed April, 2025]

45. Supreme Court of India. Common Cause v. Union of India. Miscellaneous Application No. 1699 of 2019 in Writ Petition (Civil) No. 215 of 2005. Order dated 24 January 2023. [cited 2025 Mar 15]. Available from: https://digiscr.sci.gov.in/admin/judgement_file/judgement_pdf/2023/volume%201/Part%20I/2023_1_1137-1168_1702877638.pdf [Last accessed April, 2025]
46. Mathur R. (2020). ICMR Consensus Guidelines on 'Do Not Attempt Resuscitation'. Indian J Med Res. 2020;151(4):303-10.
47. Mani RK, Bhatnagar S, Butola S, Gursahani R, Mehta D, Simha S, et al. (2024). Indian Society of Critical Care Medicine and Indian Association of Palliative Care Expert Consensus and Position Statements for End-of-life and Palliative Care in the Intensive Care Unit. Indian J Crit Care Med. 2024;28(3):200-50.
48. Joad ASK, Mayamol TR, Chaturvedi M. What does the informal caregiver of a terminally ill cancer patient need? A study from a cancer centre. Indian JPalliat Care. 2011; 17(3):191-6.
49. Manz CR, Parikh RB, Small DS, Evans CN, Chivers C, Regli SH, et al. Effect of integrating machine learning mortality estimates with behavioral nudges to clinicians on serious illness conversations among patients with cancer: a stepped-wedge cluster randomized clinical trial. JAMA Oncol. 2020;6(12):e204759.

SECTION

Miscellaneous

63 CHAPTER

Anesthesia and Cancer Recurrence

Basanth Kumar Rayani, Anne Poornachand, Nitya Reddy R

INTRODUCTION

The term "neoplasm" refers to an abnormal proliferation of the cells or tissues in the body. Most of the neoplasms in humans are benign, which grow slowly and do not spread. The lethal characteristic feature of a malignant tumor is its ability to invade the surrounding structures and disseminate to distant organs leading to 90% of the cancer related deaths.[1] The treatment modalities for cancer include surgery, radiotherapy, and/or chemotherapy. It is often believed that the invisible micrometastases are already present at the time of cancer diagnosis. Tumor handling during surgery can lead to seeding of cancer cells, creating the circulating tumor cells (CTC). These CTCs disseminate to the distant organs and in a favorable microenvironment evolve into an evident metastasis. It is crucial to identify factors that may create a favorable microenvironment for seeding and survival of the CTC and growth of existing invisible micrometastases. Research is ongoing in this area on how the anesthetic agents or drugs influence the cancer outcome in terms of disease-free survival.

TUMOR MICROENVIRONMENT

The concepts of cancer biology are beyond the scope of this chapter, but a brief overview of the tumor microenvironment (TME) is illustrated in **Figure 1**. Malignant tissues secrete a variety of chemical mediators, including danger-associated molecular patterns (DAMPs), cytokines, and chemokines. These mediators recruit various cell types such as fibroblasts, myofibroblasts, immune inflammatory cells, vascular endothelial cells, and mesenchymal stem and progenitor cells. Malignant cells along with these recruited cells, create a stroma rich in inflammatory mediators that promote tumor survival. In addition, chronic inflammation in the TME transforms immunocompetent cells into an immunosuppressive phenotype, thereby enabling tumor cells to evade the immune system.[2] Data suggest that a lower number and an impaired function of natural killer (NK) cells are associated with local recurrence and metastasis.[3] The tumor stroma exhibits an abundant expression of beta-adrenergic receptors. The dense sympathetic innervation of malignant tissue and elevated circulating catecholamines, through their action on these adrenergic receptors, remodel the TME, and promote tumor growth and progression.[4] Inflammation resulting from a surgical wound is comparable to inflammation caused by neoplastic and recruited stromal cells, leading to a favorable microenvironment for tumor survival, growth, and dissemination.

Angiogenesis is a crucial component of tumor survival and metastasis. Vascular endothelial growth factor A (VEGF-A), hypoxia inducible factor (HIF-1), proangiogenic factors such as platelet-derived growth factor (PDGF), fibroblast growth factor (FGF), and matrix metalloproteinase (MMP) play significant roles in promoting angiogenesis and metastasis.[5,6] Tumor cells undergo epithelial mesenchymal transformation (EMT), which allows them to disseminate and invade the surrounding tissues.[7] The proteolytic enzymes secreted by these cells, particularly MMPs, help in the degradation of the extracellular matrix and the vascular endothelial basement membrane, facilitating tumor spread.

MECHANISMS OF METASTASIS

As previously discussed, tumor cells are shredded and released into systemic circulation during surgery, forming CTCs. The CTCs surge in the postoperative period, and their levels have been identified as a prognostic factor for recurrence.[7] The activated neutrophils and the chromatin extruded from them, form the neutrophil extracellular traps (NETs). The NETs and platelets engulf CTCs forming

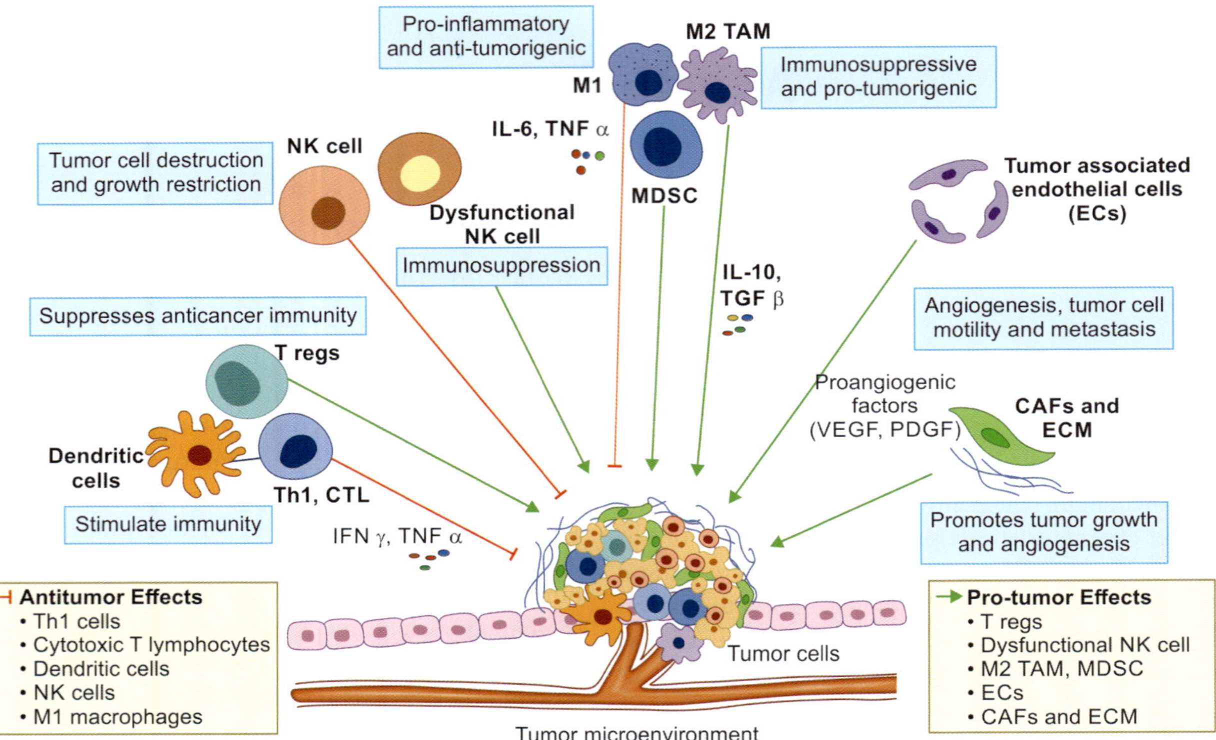

Fig. 1: The schematic diagram details the interactions within the tumor microenvironment (TME), highlighting the roles of various cellular components and chemical mediators in tumor growth, invasion, and metastasis. The green arrows indicate protumor effects, emphasizing the roles of T regulatory cells (T regs), dysfunctional natural killer (NK) cells, M2 tumor-associated macrophages (TAMs), myeloid-derived suppressor cells (MDSCs), endothelial cells (ECs), cancer-associated fibroblasts (CAFs), and the extracellular matrix (ECM). These elements together result in immunosuppression, angiogenesis, tumor cell motility, and metastasis. For example, M2 TAMs and MDSCs release immunosuppressive cytokines such as IL-10, and transforming growth factor beta (TGF-β), while ECs and CAFs promote angiogenesis through factors such as VEGF and PDGF (platelet-derived growth factor). Red arrows indicate antitumor effects, highlighting the roles of Th1 cells, cytotoxic T lymphocytes (CTLs), dendritic cells, NK cells, and M1 macrophages. These components enhance antitumor immunity and tumor cell destruction. Th1 cells and CTLs secrete cytokines such as IFN-γ and TNF-α, boosting immune responses against tumor cells.

the CTC-NET-platelet complex protecting the tumor cells from the physical stress of passing through capillaries and destruction by NK cells.[8] These complexes travel to distant organs and in areas of sluggish flow, they adhere and penetrate the capillary wall to form a premetastatic niche. The role of NETs in perioperative oncopathophysiology is well recognized and is an intermediate link between surgical stress and metastasis.

The perioperative period is characterized by a significant increase in CTCs during surgical manipulation. The ensuing inflammation and immunosuppression favor CTC survival, sequestration, and colonization **(Fig. 2)**. In the following text, we shall discuss how the choice of anesthesia technique and anesthetic drugs affect cancer recurrence, with relevant evidence from recent studies.

GENERAL ANESTHESIA

Effect of Inhalational Anesthetics on Cancer Recurrence[9]

Inhalational anesthetics are commonly used to maintain a balanced anesthesia. Laboratory and animal studies have shown an association between inhalational anesthetics and increased tumor spread. The above findings are supported by a retrospective study by Wigmore TJ et al., who found worse survival outcomes in cancer patients subjected to inhalation anesthesia than those who were subjected to intravenous (IV) anesthesia.[10] In certain cancer cell lines, inhalation anesthetics have been found to promote tumor cell proliferation, invasion, and migration by inducing protumor factors such as HIF-1α,

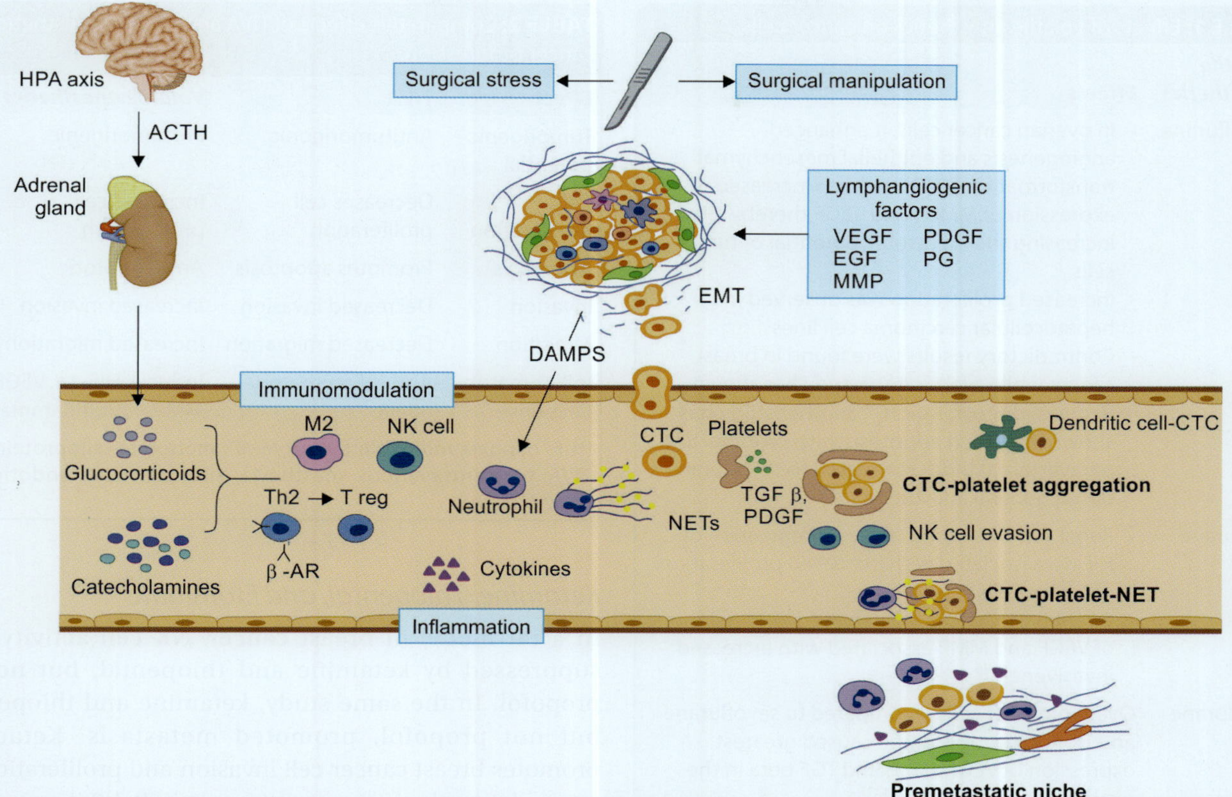

Fig. 2: Illustration of the Mechanisms for perioperative metastasis: Surgical stress activates the HPA (hypothalamo-pituitary-adrenal axis) axis, releasing glucocorticoids and catecholamines that modulate immune response resulting in reduced NK cell activity and increased T reg cell numbers. Surgical manipulation induces the release of circulating tumor cells (CTCs). NETs (neutrophil extracellular traps) and platelets aggregate with CTCs to form a complex that further supports tumor cell survival and the formation of a premetastatic niche. (ACTH: adrenocorticotropic hormone; EMT: epithelial mesenchymal transition; VEGF: vascular endothelial growth factor; PDGF: platelet-derived growth factor; EGF: endothelial growth factor; PG: prostaglandin; MMP: matrix metalloproteinases)

VEGF, and MMPs. Volatile agents have proinflammatory and immunosuppressive effects resulting in NK cell dysfunction. However, contrasting effects have been observed with different volatile agents in different cancer cell lines. **Table 1** summarizes the evidence from laboratory studies on the effects of inhalational anesthetics on cancer cells.

Nitrous Oxide

There is very limited data on nitrous oxide with respect to cancer recurrence. However, routine use of nitrous oxide is not recommended because of its effect on personnel health and environmental concerns.

Conclusion

Volatile anesthetics have been suggested to exhibit protumorigenic effects owing to their proinflammatory and immunosuppressive actions. However, there is conflicting evidence from both in vitro and in vivo studies. Evidence from large prospective randomized studies comparing volatile anesthesia with total intravenous anesthesia (TIVA) is needed to suggest any change in the current practice of anesthesia for preventing cancer recurrence.

Role of Intravenous Anesthetics in Cancer Recurrence

The role of IV anesthetics in cancer recurrence is an area of ongoing research and of considerable interest. Although various studies have investigated the impact of different anesthetic techniques on cancer outcomes, the evidence remains inconclusive. Some studies have suggested the potential benefits of IV anesthetics, particularly propofol, over volatile anesthetics.

TABLE 1: Effects of volatile anesthetics on cancer cells.

Volatile anesthetics	*Effects*
Sevoflurane	• In ovarian cancer cells, it enhanced angiogenesis and epithelial mesenchymal transformation (EMT) through increased expression of MMP's and VEGF thereby increasing the metastatic potential of tumor cells[11] • Increased proliferation was observed in hepatocellular carcinoma cell lines[12] • Contradictory results were found in breast cancer while a laboratory study has shown decreased proliferation,[13] another study has shown increased apoptosis with propofol and paravertebral block compared to sevoflurane-based general anesthesia[14]
Isoflurane	• Renal cell carcinoma cells—upregulation of HIF-1α associated with increased proliferation of tumor cells[15] • Ovarian cancer cells—increased expression of VEGF and MMP associated with increased invasiveness[16]
Desflurane	Ovarian cancer cells—compared to sevoflurane and isoflurane, desflurane caused greatest expression of VEGF, MMP, and TGF beta in the ovarian cancer tumor cells[11]

(MMP: matrix metalloproteinase; TGF: transforming growth factor; VEGF: vascular endothelial growth factor)

Propofol[7,17]

It is widely used in anesthesia induction, TIVA, and sedation in ICU. Most of the preclinical studies have shown that propofol exhibits antitumor properties. Propofol mitigates perioperative immunosuppression through its anti-inflammatory and antioxidant properties. Laboratory and animal studies have shown propofol to be associated with preserved and enhanced NK cell activity. Propofol suppressed the migration and invasion of nonsmall cell lung cancer (NSCLC) cells by decreasing HIF-1α expression. It promoted apoptosis in breast cancer cell lines via downregulation of miR-24 expression and upregulation of p27. In vitro, it decreased the expression of MMPs by inhibiting NF-kB pathway. It decreased the expression of neuroepithelial transforming gene-1 in breast cancer cell lines resulting in decreased migration. It has an inhibitory effect on tumor metastasis by decreasing the expression of adhesion molecules on tumor endothelial cells. Propofol decreased NETs formation which are known to protect the CTC.

TABLE 2: Comparative effects of TIVA and volatile anesthetics on cancer progression.

Effect	*TIVA*	*Volatile anesthetics*
Tumorigenic potential	Antitumorigenic	Protumorigenic
Cell proliferation	Decreases cell proliferation	Increases cell proliferation
Apoptosis	Promotes apoptosis	Anti-apoptotic
Invasion	Decreased invasion	Increased invasion
Migration	Decreased migration	Increased migration
Inflammatory Response	Anti-inflammatory effect	Induces HIF-1α, VEGF, MMP—proinflammatory

(HIF: hypoxia inducible factor; MMP: matrix metalloproteinase; TIVA: total intravenous anesthesia; VEGF: vascular endothelial growth factor)

Ketamine, Thiopental, and Etomidate[7,18,19]

In a rat model of breast cancer, NK cell activity was suppressed by ketamine and thiopental, but not by propofol. In the same study, ketamine and thiopental, but not propofol, promoted metastasis. Ketamine promotes breast cancer cell invasion and proliferation by upregulating the antiapoptotic protein Bcl-2. In contrast, ketamine inhibited proliferation of pancreatic cancer cell lines. In an in vitro study, etomidate suppressed cell proliferation and promoted apoptosis in NSCLC cells.[20] Etomidate was shown to have less of an effect on immune function than propofol in patients with lung adenocarcinoma.

Volatile Anesthetics versus Total Intravenous Anesthesia (Propofol)

Most data on the effect of volatile agents and IV anesthetics on cancer recurrence are from laboratory and animal studies **(Table 2)**. Clinical studies comparing with placebo may not possible for ethical reasons. Therefore, the available clinical evidence comes from the comparison between different anesthesia techniques, most of which are retrospective studies **(Table 3)**.

Conclusion

Laboratory and animal studies have shown that propofol exhibits antitumor properties, and volatile anesthetics can be protumorigenic. However, clinical evidence from retrospective studies and meta-analyses has shown inconsistent results with improved overall survival and

TABLE 3: Evidence from studies comparing the impact of TIVA (propofol) versus volatile anesthesia on cancer recurrence.

Cancer	*Study design*	*Author*	*Interpretation*
Glioblastoma	Retrospective (propofol vs. desflurane)	Huang YH et al.[21]	Improved OS and less recurrence in TIVA
	Retrospective (isoflurane/desflurane vs. isoflurane/desflurane + propofol)	Cata JP et al.[22]	No difference in OS and PFS between the groups
Gastric	Retrospective (TIVA vs. inhalation)	Wu WW et al.[23]	Increased OS in TIVA group
	Retrospective (propofol TIVA vs. desflurane)	Huang NC et al.[24]	Increased OS and reduced recurrence in TIVA group
	Retrospective (propofol TIVA vs. inhalation)	Zheng X et al.[25]	Increased OS in the TIVA group
Major cancer surgery	Retrospective (propofol TIVA vs. inhalation)	Oh TK et al.[26]	Better survival outcomes with propofol-based TIVA (major cancer surgeries)
Breast	Randomized trial (PVB + propofol vs. volatile + opioids)	Sessler DI et al.[27]	No difference in cancer recurrence between the groups
	Retrospective (TIVA vs. inhalation)	Yoo S et al.[28]	No difference in OS or RFS
Breast, gastric, colon, liver, glioma, and lung	• Systematic review and meta-analysis (propofol TIVA vs. inhalation) • 19 retrospective observational studies were included	Chang CY et al.[29]	Increased overall survival in the TIVA group but no difference in RFS between the groups
Breast, esophagus, and lung	Meta-analysis (Propofol TIVA vs. inhalation) 10 studies were included	Yap A et al.[30]	Increased OS and RFS in the TIVA group

(PFS: progression free survival; RFS: recurrence free survival; TIVA: total intravenous anesthesia; OS: overall survival)

recurrence-free survival in the TIVA group or no difference in recurrence-free survival between the groups. A large multicenter RCT comparing paravertebral block with propofol and volatile anesthesia with opioids in breast cancer surgeries showed no difference in recurrence-free survival between the groups. More prospective, adequately powered randomized studies are needed to draw any conclusion on preferring a particular anesthesia technique over the other, to prevent cancer recurrence.

Regional Anesthesia and Cancer Recurrence

Regional anesthesia involves the administration of local anesthetic drugs around a nerve plexus or in the fascial plane through which nerves pass, to anesthetize the distal area. Regional anesthesia may be performed as sole anesthesia or as an adjunct to general anesthesia, thereby reducing the opioid requirements. One of the many benefits of regional anesthesia, which is believed to play a protective role in cancer recurrence or metastasis, is the inhibition of the surgical stress response **(Flowchart 1)**.

Flowchart 1: Regional anesthesia and its effects.

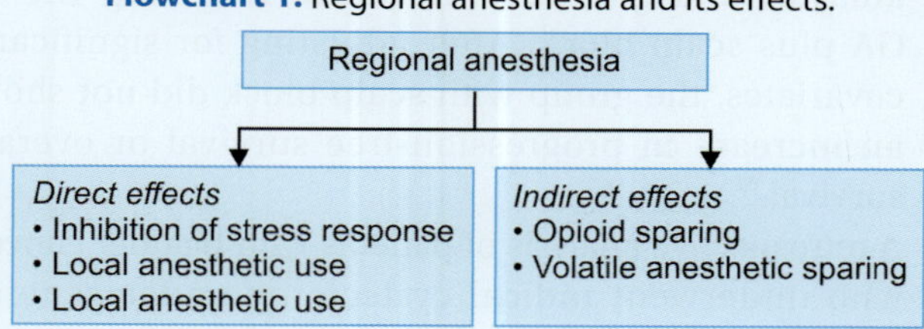

- *Effects of surgical stress response:* The stress response to surgery leads to increased circulating levels of cortisol and catecholamines through activation of the hypothalamic-pituitary-adrenal (HPA) axis. Catecholamines exert their action on cancer cells through adrenoreceptors, leading to the secretion of VEGF, interleukin 6 (IL-6), and MMP enzymes, all of which provide a favorable environment for cancer cells to invade and multiply.[31] The stress response negatively affects the NK cells, which are believed to kill residual tumor cells and CTCs during the perioperative period.
- Amide local anesthetics exert antitumor effects through various mechanisms of action (discussed under the section local anesthetics).
- Perioperative blood transfusion may be associated with cancer recurrence. An indirect beneficial effect of

regional anesthesia on cancer recurrence is conferred by lower blood loss and blood transfusion requirement.

- Opioids and volatile anesthetics have been implicated in cancer recurrence (discussed in the sections on Opioids and Volatile Anesthetics). Although the association is currently controversial and uncertain, regional anesthesia provides superior pain relief and decreases or obviates the need for opioids or volatile anesthetics.

Evidence from the Studies

- *Recurrence of breast cancer after regional or general anesthesia:* 2,132 women were enrolled in a multi-center randomized control trial (RCT) conducted by Sessler DI et al. between 2007 and 2018. Patients undergoing breast cancer resection were randomized into two groups of paravertebral block with propofol or sevoflurane with opioids. They concluded that propofol with paravertebral block did not reduce breast cancer recurrence compared to sevoflurane with opioids over a median follow-up of 36 months.[27]
- A retrospective study by Cata JP et al. (2018) observed the effect of scalp block on progression-free survival following craniotomies for malignant brain tumors. A total of 808 adult patients were included in the analysis and grouped into those receiving GA or GA plus scalp block. After adjusting for significant covariates, the group with scalp block did not show an increase in progression-free survival or overall survival.[32]
- A retrospective analysis of patients with bladder cancer who underwent radical cystectomy under general anesthesia with epidural versus general anesthesia alone was performed by Chipollini J et al. (2018) and they looked at recurrence-free and cancer-specific survival. The recurrence-free and cancer-specific survival were worse in the epidural group. The authors opined that this may be due to epidural sufentanil and higher morphine equivalents of this drug.[33] Doiron RC et al. (2016) could not demonstrate an association between thoracic epidural and short-term outcomes or long-term survival in their retrospective study on bladder cancer patients undergoing cystectomy.[34]
- Koumpan Y et al. (2018) retrospectively analyzed patients with bladder cancer who underwent transurethral resection of bladder tumor under spinal or general anesthesia and found a lower incidence of cancer recurrence in the spinal group.[35]
- Meta-analyses by Lee BM et al. (2015) and Weng M et al. (2016) have shown improved overall survival in the regional anesthesia group whereas the meta-analysis by Grandhi RK et al. (2017) showed no significant benefit in the regional anesthesia group.[36-38]

Conclusion

While in theory, regional anesthesia seems to be beneficial with respect to cancer recurrence as discussed, there is no conclusive evidence available to recommend regional anesthesia over GA for the same. Most clinical data available are from retrospective studies with conflicting results, and the same has been observed in meta-analyses. One large prospective multicenter RCT on breast cancer surgery did not show any benefit of regional anesthesia for improved recurrence-free survival.

Local Anesthetics, Oncophysiology and Cancer Recurrence

The various routes of administration of local anesthetics during the perioperative period include regional anesthesia, IV lidocaine, intraperitoneal installation, or peritumoral infiltration. The potential theoretical benefits of regional anesthesia in mitigating the spread of cancer have been discussed above. In addition, local anesthetics exert direct effects on cancer cells through voltage-gated sodium channels (VGSCs).[18] Upregulated VGSCs are present on cancer cells suggesting their possible role in oncophysiology and cancer progression, although the mechanism of action is still unclear. Perioperative systemic lidocaine infusion is known to decrease analgesic requirements, thereby reducing opioid consumption and conferring a possible indirect benefit of lower cancer metastasis. NK cells exposed to clinically relevant concentrations of lidocaine have shown enhanced activity in in-vitro studies.[39] The anti-inflammatory action of lidocaine may also reduce immunosuppression. In vitro and in vivo B-16 melanoma mouse model studies have shown lidocaine to be an inhibitor of angiogenesis, providing preclinical evidence that lidocaine may inhibit tumor growth and metastasis.[40] Studies have shown that lidocaine could act as a chemosensitizer, sensitizing certain tumors to chemotherapeutic agents such as cisplatin, 5-fluorouracil (5-FU), mitomycin C, and pirarubicin.[41]

Evidence from the Studies

- Research by Liu C et al. (2020) on ovarian cell cultures and a murine metastatic ovarian model concluded that lidocaine reduces the metastatic potential of ovarian cancer by inhibiting the NaV1.5-mediated EMT and FAK/Paxillin signaling pathway.[42]

- An in vitro study by YJ C et al. (2019) indicated that lidocaine suppressed the proliferation, migration, and invasion of human gastric cancer cells and induced apoptosis associated with decreased expression of bcl-2 and an increased Bax expression.[43]
- An in vivo study by Wall TP et al. (2019) using a mouse model of breast cancer surgery confirmed the beneficial effect of perioperative lidocaine in reducing pulmonary metastasis. Reduced MMP-2 levels were found in lidocaine-treated animals, a probable reason for the antimetastatic effect.[44]
- Badwe RA et al. (2023) conducted a multicenter randomized trial on 1,583 patients with early breast cancer and concluded that peritumoral infiltration of lidocaine before breast cancer surgery significantly increased disease-free survival and overall survival.[45]

Conclusion

Perioperative IV lidocaine provides analgesia, decreasing the requirement for opioids. It is also a safe and an inexpensive drug that can be used in regular clinical practice. Although many in vitro and animal model studies have shown the beneficial effects of perioperative lidocaine on cancer biology, evidence from further clinical trials in humans is required to support this.

OPIOIDS AND CANCER RECURRENCE

Perioperative pain through the activation of the hypothalamo-pituitary-adrenal (HPA) axis causes immunosuppression and thereby promotes cancer cell survival and proliferation **(Fig. 2)**. Good pain control could blunt the HPA response and in addition to early recovery and better patient experience may also result in lower cancer recurrence. Opioids are commonly used to control the pain associated with cancer and surgery. Evidence shows that opioids can modulate the TME through direct and indirect effects, as described in **Table 4**. However, the overall effects of opioids on cancer recurrence are still unclear, with inconsistent and conflicting results from available studies.

TABLE 4: The influence of opioids on tumor biology.

Direct effects	*Indirect effects*
• Tumor proliferation and apoptosis • Tumor cell invasion, migration, and metastasis	• Immunosuppression • Inflammation • Angiogenesis

- *Tumor proliferation and apoptosis:* Opioids are proposed to exert proliferative effects through the mu opioid receptor (MOR)[46] and antiproliferative effects via the opioid growth factor receptor (OGFR).[47]
- *Tumor cell invasion, migration, and metastasis:* Morphine has been proposed to both increase and decrease tumor migration. Increased vascular permeability is attributed to its proinvasive effects, whereas decreased MMP production results in anti-invasive effects.[48]
- *Immunosuppression:* Opioids have immunosuppressive effects either by directly acting on the immune cells through the MOR and toll-like receptor-4 or via central mechanisms suppressing splenic lymphocyte proliferation and NK cell cytotoxicity. In addition, HPA axis activity is increased with chronic opioid use resulting in elevated glucocorticoid levels and immunosuppression.[49]
- *Inflammation:* The effects of morphine on inflammation are complex, with kappa opioid receptor activation leading to anti-inflammatory responses and MOR activation promoting proinflammatory responses.[50]
- *Angiogenesis:* Morphine has both inhibitory and stimulatory effects on angiogenesis. At clinically relevant doses in a mouse model, it inhibited angiogenesis and tumor growth.[51] However, breast cancer cells exposed to morphine led to endothelial cell proliferation and angiogenesis[52]
  Most opioids are known to suppress NK cell activity but tramadol enhances NK cell activity and buprenorphine has no definite immunosuppressive effect.[53]

Conclusion

Laboratory studies have indicated that opioids may affect metastasis and tumor growth. However, the evidence is inconsistent and varies depending on the opioid used. Current clinical data on the perioperative effects of opioids are limited and remain inconclusive **(Table 5)**.

NSAIDs AND COX-2 INHIBITORS

Nonsteroidal anti-inflammatory drugs (NSAIDs), particularly cyclooxygenase 2 (COX-2) inhibitors, have been proposed to reduce cancer progression by inhibiting cyclooxygenase enzymes, thus decreasing prostaglandin E2 (PGE2) synthesis. PGE2 is linked to enhanced tumor

TABLE 5: Impact of opioid-sparing techniques versus opioid-based general anesthesia on cancer recurrence and survival.

Cancer	*Study design*	*Author*	*Interpretation*
Breast	Randomized trial (regional anesthesia vs. general anesthesia)	Sessler DI et al.[27]	Regional anesthesia-analgesia (paravertebral block and propofol) did not reduce breast cancer recurrence after potentially curative surgery compared with volatile anesthesia (sevoflurane) and opioids
	Systematic review	Lucia M et al.[54]	Inconclusive
	Retrospective analysis of prospectively maintained data	Montagna G et al.[55]	Intraoperative opioids have protective effect on recurrence-free survival (RFS) in triple negative breast cancer
	Prospective observational Cohort study	Cronin-Fenton DP et al.[56]	No clinical relevance
Prostate	Randomized trial (opioid free anesthesia vs. opioid based analgesia)	Rangel FP et al.[57]	Based on prostate specific antigen levels (PSA), intraoperative opioid use did not affect biochemical recurrence free survival
Kidney	Retrospective analysis	Silagy AW et al.[58]	Reduced use of intraoperative opioid was associated with improved RFS and Overall survival (OS)
Lung	Retrospective review of prospectively managed data (intraoperative opioid exposure on tumor genomic alterations)	Connolly JG et al.[59]	Intraoperative opioid exposure is associated with worse overall outcomes

(RFS: recurrence free survival OS: overall survival)

proliferation, angiogenesis, invasion, and immune suppression.[60] NSAIDs, due to their opioid-sparing properties, play a crucial role in multimodal analgesia, thereby reducing opioid-related complications and facilitating early recovery. Several trials have demonstrated the potential benefits of NSAIDs in cancer recurrence and disease-free survival. A retrospective study with 720 breast cancer patients showed that intraoperative administration of ketorolac or diclofenac was associated with improved overall and disease-free survival.[61] A cohort study of 2,308 colorectal cancer patients found that perioperative NSAIDs use reduced cancer recurrence risk, but there was no significant effect on disease-free survival.[62] In summary, NSAIDs and COX-2 inhibitors offer not only effective pain relief but also have the potential to prevent the recurrence of cancer due to their antitumorigenic properties.

BETA-BLOCKERS

Beta-blockers are used to treat anxiety, hypertension, and ischemic heart disease, and may also have protective effects against cancer progression. Preclinical studies have suggested that beta-blockers inhibit β-adrenoceptor signaling in cancer and immune cells there by reducing tumor cell invasion, associated inflammation, and vascular remodeling. A meta-analysis (2018) of 27 studies reported that beta-blocker use had no effect on the overall cancer recurrence. However, the effect is variable in cancer subgroups with low quality of evidence.[63] A phase 2 randomized controlled trial in breast cancer patients found that 1 week of preoperative propranolol administration reduced prometastatic biomarkers.[64] In triple negative breast cancer patients, regular β-blocker use at diagnosis was associated with reduced mortality and improved survival.[65] Another study in patients with prostate cancer found that incidental users of nonselective rather than selective β-blockers had a lower risk of cancer recurrence following radical prostatectomy.[66]

GLUCOCORTICOIDS

Glucocorticoids, particularly dexamethasone, are widely administered during the perioperative period owing to its anti-inflammatory, antiemetic, and analgesic properties. Evidence from laboratory studies on the role of dexamethasone in cancer recurrence is inconsistent and retrospective studies have shown heterogeneous effects. There was no significant impact observed in ovarian or endometrial cancer surgeries, while improved survival was noted in patients undergoing surgeries for NSCLC and reduced disease-free survival in patients undergoing surgery for rectal cancer. Despite these findings, current evidence does not support altering the perioperative use of dexamethasone to prevent cancer recurrence.[19]

OXYGEN

As previously discussed, the hypoxic environment in a tumor increases the expression of HIF-1α, which in turn promotes angiogenesis and has a protumorigenic effect. Hyperoxia also stimulates tumor cell growth by promoting angiogenesis.[67] An in vitro study by Crowley PD et al. reported that breast cancer cells exposed to high concentrations of oxygen showed increased migration and secretion of angiogenic factors.[68] In a posthoc analysis of 1,377 from 1,386 recruited patients in the PROXI trial, patients who underwent elective or emergency laparotomy were randomly assigned to receive 80% or 30% fraction of inspired oxygen (FiO_2) during surgery and 2-h postoperatively. They concluded that the occurrence of new or recurrent cancer was similar.[69] Therefore, it is advisable to adjust the fractional inspired oxygen concentration based on the patient's clinical condition and requirements rather than focusing on the likelihood of cancer recurrence.

PARACETAMOL

Paracetamol is used in the perioperative period as a component of multimodal analgesia and as an antipyretic. There is scant evidence regarding the association between paracetamol and cancer recurrence. However, epidemiological studies have shown an increased incidence of urinary tract cancers and a decreased risk of ovarian cancers among chronic paracetamol users; however, the overall results are inconsistent.[17]

ALPHA-2 ADRENOCEPTOR AGONISTS

Alpha-2 adrenergic receptor agonists, including dexmedetomidine and clonidine, are increasingly used during the perioperative period as part of multimodal analgesia, owing to their sedative, analgesic, and sympatholytic properties. Research indicates that dexmedetomidine promotes the migration, invasion, and proliferation of human breast cancer cell lines and enhances tumor growth in mice with breast cancer. However, evidence is inconclusive for other cancers, and randomized studies in humans are lacking. In a review article by Nair AS et al.,[70] the authors suggested that dexmedetomidine should be used cautiously in breast cancer surgery until more robust evidence is available.

CONCLUSION

Preclinical studies indicate that anesthetic agents and adjuvants may affect cancer progression. However the intricate nature of tumor biology, variable patient and surgical factors necessitate caution in interpreting the existing data and the application of these findings to clinical practice. Evidence from further randomized control trials and meta-analysis may provide future direction. Individualized anesthetic management of cancer patients presently, should be based on clinical status and safety of the patient.

REFERENCES

1. Lambert AW, Pattabiraman DR, Weinberg RA. Emerging biological principles of metastasis. Cell. 2017;168(4):670-91.
2. Böttcher JP, Bonavita E, Chakravarty P, Blees H, Cabeza-Cabrerizo M, Sammicheli S, et al. NK cells stimulate recruitment of cDC1 into the tumor microenvironment promoting cancer immune control. Cell. 2018;172(5):1022-37.
3. Barry KC, Hsu J, Broz ML, Cueto FJ, Binnewies M, Combes AJ, et al. A natural killer–dendritic cell axis defines checkpoint therapy–responsive tumor microenvironments. Nat Med. 2018;24(8):1178-91.
4. Zahalka AH, Arnal-Estapé A, Maryanovich M, Nakahara F, Cruz CD, Finley LW, et al. Adrenergic nerves activate an angio-metabolic switch in prostate cancer. Science. 2017; 358(6361):321-6.
5. Apte RS, Chen DS, Ferrara N. VEGF in signaling and disease: Beyond discovery and development. Cell. 2019;176(6):1248-64.
6. LaGory EL, Giaccia AJ. The ever-expanding role of HIF in tumour and stromal biology. Nature cell biology. 2016;18(4):356-65.
7. Xia SH, Zhou D, Ge F, Sun M, Chen X, Zhang H, et al. Influence of perioperative anesthesia on cancer recurrence: from basic science to clinical practice. Curr Oncol Rep. 2023;25(2):63-81.
8. Cools-Lartigue J, Spicer J, McDonald B, Gowing S, Chow S, Giannias B, et al. Neutrophil extracellular traps sequester circulating tumor cells and promote metastasis. J Clin Investig. 2013;123(8):3446-58.
9. Jing Y, Zhang Y, Pan R, Ding K, Chen R, Meng Q. Effect of inhalation anesthetics on tumor metastasis. Technology in Cancer Research & Treatment. 2022;21:15330338221121092.
10. Wigmore TJ, Mohammed K, Jhanjki S. Long-term survival for patients undergoing volatile versus IV anesthesia for cancer surgery: a retrospective analysis. Anesthesiology. 2016;124(1):69-79.

11. Iwasaki M, Zhao H, Jaffer T, Unwith S, Benzonana L, Lian Q, et al. Volatile anaesthetics enhance the metastasis related cellular signalling including CXCR2 of ovarian cancer cells. Oncotarget. 2016;7(18):26042.
12. Nishiwada T, Kawaraguchi Y, Uemura K, Sugimoto H, Kawaguchi M. Effect of sevoflurane on human hepatocellular carcinoma $HepG_2$ cells under conditions of high glucose and insulin. J Anesth. 2015;29:805-8.
13. Liu J, Yang L, Guo X, Jin G, Wang Q, Lv D, et al. Sevoflurane suppresses proliferation by upregulating microRNA-203 in breast cancer cells. Mol Med Rep. 2018;18(1):455-60.
14. Dubowitz JA, Rampes S, Enlund M, Ma D. Volatile and intravenous anesthetics and cancer. In: Hagberg CA, Nates JL, Riedel BP, Gottumukkala VNR, Buggy D (Eds). Perioperative Care of the Cancer Patient. Netherlands: Elsevier; 2023. pp. 128-39.
15. Benzonana LL, Perry NJ, Watts HR, Yang B, Perry IA, Coombes C, et al. Isoflurane, a commonly used volatile anesthetic, enhances renal cancer growth and malignant potential via the hypoxia-inducible factor cellular signaling pathway in vitro. Anesthesiology. 2013;119(3):593-605.
16. Luo X, Zhao H, Hennah L, Ning J, Liu J, Tu H, et al. Impact of isoflurane on malignant capability of ovarian cancer in vitro. Br J Anaesthesia. 2015;114(5):831-9.
17. Brogi E, Forfori F. Anesthesia and cancer recurrence: an overview. J Anesth Analg Crit Care. 2022;2(1):33.
18. Yang W, Cai J, Zabkiewicz C, Zhang H, Ruge F, Jiang WG. The effects of anesthetics on recurrence and metastasis of cancer, and clinical implications. World J Oncol. 2017;8(3):63.
19. Ahn HJ. Anesthesia and cancer recurrence: a narrative review. Anesth Pain Med. 2024;19(2):94-108.
20. Li D, Zhang J, Yin L, Jin Z, Chen X, Meng X. Etomidate inhibits cell proliferation and induces apoptosis in A549 nonsmall cell lung cancer cells via downregulating WWP2. Exp Ther Med. 2021;22(5):1-9.
21. Huang YH, Wu ZF, Lee MS, Lou YS, Wu KL, Cheng KI, et al. Propofol-based total intravenous anesthesia is associated with better survival than desflurane anesthesia in glioblastoma surgery. PLOS One. 2021;16(8):e0255627.
22. Cata JP, Hagan KB, Bhavsar SD, Arunkumar R, Grasu R, Dang A, et al. The use of isoflurane and desflurane as inhalational agents for glioblastoma surgery. A survival analysis. J Clin Neurosci. 2017;35:82-7.
23. Wu WW, Zhang WH, Zhang WY, Liu K, Chen XZ, Zhou ZG, et al. The long-term survival outcomes of gastric cancer patients with total intravenous anesthesia or inhalation anesthesia: a single-center retrospective cohort study. BMC Cancer. 2021;21:1-2.
24. Huang NC, Lee MS, Lai HC, Lin HT, Huang YH, Lu CH, et al. Propofol-based total intravenous anesthesia improves survival compared to desflurane anesthesia in gastric cancer surgery: a retrospective analysis. Medicine (Baltimore). 2020;99(25):e20714.
25. Zheng X, Wang Y, Dong L, Zhao S, Wang L, Chen H, et al. Effects of propofol-based total intravenous anesthesia on gastric cancer: a retrospective study. Onco Targets Ther. 2018;11:1141-8.
26. Oh TK, Jo H, Song IA. Propofol-based intravenous anesthesia is associated with improved survival outcomes after major cancer surgery: a nationwide cohort study in South Korea. Korean J Anesthesiol. 2023;76(5):461-70.
27. Sessler DI, Pei L, Huang Y, Fleischmann E, Marhofer P, Kurz A, et al. (2019) Recurrence of breast cancer after regional or general anesthesia: a randomized controlled trial. Lancet. 2019;394:1807-15.
28. Yoo S, Lee HB, Han W, Noh DY, Park SK, Kim WH, et al. Total Intravenous Anesthesia versus Inhalation Anesthesia for Breast Cancer Surgery: A Retrospective Cohort Study. Anesthesiology. 2019;130(1):31-40.
29. Chang CY, Wu MY, Chien YJ, Su IM, Wang SC, Kao MC. Anesthesia and long-term oncological outcomes: a systematic review and meta-analysis. Anesth Analg. 2021; 132(3):623-34.
30. Yap A, Lopez-Olivo MA, Dubowitz J, Hiller J, Riedel B. Anesthetic technique and cancer outcomes: a meta-analysis of total intravenous versus volatile anesthesia. Can J Anesth. 2019;5(66):546-61.
31. Neeman E, Ben-Eliyahu S. Surgery and stress promote cancer metastasis: new outlooks on perioperative mediating mechanisms and immune involvement. Brain Behav Immu. 2013;30:S32-40.
32. Cata JP, Bhavsar S, Hagan KB, Arunkumar R, Shi T, Grasu R, et al. Scalp blocks for brain tumor craniotomies: a retrospective survival analysis of a propensity match cohort of patients. J Clin Neurosci. 2018;51:46-51.
33. Chipollini J, Alford B, Boulware DC, Forget P, Gilbert SM, Lockhart JL, et al. Epidural anesthesia and cancer outcomes in bladder cancer patients: is it the technique or the medication? A matched-cohort analysis from a tertiary referral center. BMC Anesthesiol. 2018;18:1-9.
34. Doiron RC, Jaeger M, Booth CM, Wei X, Siemens DR. Is there a measurable association of epidural use at cystectomy and postoperative outcomes? A population-based study. Can Urol Assoc J. 2016;10(9-10):321.
35. Koumpan Y, Jaeger M, Mizubuti GB, Tanzola R, Jain K, Hosier G, et al. Spinal anesthesia is associated with lower recurrence rates after resection of nonmuscle invasive bladder cancer. J Urol. 2018;199(4):940-6.
36. Lee BM, Singh Ghotra V, Karam JA, Hernandez M, Pratt G, Cata JP. Regional anesthesia/analgesia and the risk of cancer recurrence and mortality after prostatectomy: a meta-analysis. Pain Manag. 2015;5(5):387-95.
37. Weng M, Chen W, Hou W, Li L, Ding M, Miao C. The effect of neuraxial anesthesia on cancer recurrence and survival

after cancer surgery: an updated meta-analysis. Oncotarget. 2016;7(12):15262.

38. Grandhi RK, Lee S, Abd-Elsayed A. The relationship between regional anesthesia and cancer: a meta-analysis. Ochsner J. 2017;17(4):345-61.
39. Cata JP, Ramirez MF, Velasquez JF, Di AI, Popat KU, Gottumukkala V, et al. Lidocaine stimulates the function of natural killer cells in different experimental settings. Anticancer Res. 2017;37(9):4727-32.
40. Gao J, Hu H, Wang X. Clinically relevant concentrations of lidocaine inhibit tumor angiogenesis through suppressing VEGF/VEGFR2 signaling. Cancer Chemother Pharmacol. 2019;83:1007-15.
41. Zhou D, Wang L, Cui Q, Iftikhar R, Xia Y, Xu P. Repositioning lidocaine as an anticancer drug: the role beyond anesthesia. Front Cell Dev Biol. 2020;8:565.
42. Liu C, Yu M, Li Y, Wang H, Xu C, Zhang X, et al. Lidocaine inhibits the metastatic potential of ovarian cancer by blocking NaV1. 5-mediated EMT and FAK/Paxillin signaling pathway. Cancer Med. 2021;10(1):337-49.
43. Ye L, Zhang Y, Chen YJ, Liu Q. Anti-tumor effects of lidocaine on human gastric cancer cells in vitro. Bratisl Lek Listy. 2019;120(3):212-7.
44. Wall TP, Crowley PD, Sherwin A, Foley AG, Buggy DJ. Effects of lidocaine and src inhibition on metastasis in a murine model of breast cancer surgery. Cancers. 2019;11(10):1414.
45. Badwe RA, Parmar V, Nair N, Joshi S, Hawaldar R, Pawar S, et al. Effect of peritumoral infiltration of local anesthetic before surgery on survival in early breast cancer. J Clin Oncol. 2023;41(18):3318-28.
46. Li Y, Li G, Tao T, Kang X, Liu C, Zhang X, et al. The μ-opioid receptor (MOR) promotes tumor initiation in hepatocellular carcinoma. Cancer Letters. 2019;453:1-9.
47. Kim JY, Ahn HJ, Kim JK, Kim J, Lee SH, Chae HB. Morphine suppresses lung cancer cell proliferation through the interaction with opioid growth factor receptor: an in vitro and human lung tissue study. Anesth Analg. 2016;123(6):1429-36.
48. Shariftabrizi A, Nifli AP, Ansari M, Saadat F, Ebrahimkhani MR, Alizadeh N, et al. Matrix metalloproteinase 2 secretion in WEHI 164 fibrosarcoma cells is nitric oxide-related and modified by morphine. Eur J Pharmacol. 2006;530(1-2):33-9.
49. Boland JW, Pockley AG. Influence of opioids on immune function in patients with cancer pain: from bench to bedside. Br J Pharmacol. 2018;175(14):2726-36.
50. Finley MJ, Happel CM, Kaminsky DE, Rogers T. Opioid and nociceptin receptors regulate cytokine and cytokine receptor expression. Cellular Immunol. 2008;252(1-2):146-54.
51. Koodie L, Ramakrishnan S, Roy S. Morphine suppresses tumor angiogenesis through a HIF-1α/p38MAPK pathway. Am J Pathol. 2010;177(2):984-97.
52. Gupta K, Kshirsagar S, Chang L, Schwartz R, Law PY, Yee D, et al. Morphine stimulates angiogenesis by activating proangiogenic and survival-promoting signaling and promotes breast tumor growth. Cancer Res. 2002; 62(15):4491-8.
53. Wang W, Xiao J, Shen S, Wang S, Chen M, Hu Y. Emerging effect of anesthesia on post-operative tumor recurrence and metastasis. J Int Med Res. 2019;47(8):3550-8.
54. Lucia M, Luca T, Federica DP, Cecilia G, Chiara M, Laura DM, et al. Opioids and breast cancer recurrence: a systematic review. Cancers. 2021;13(21):5499.
55. Montagna G, Gupta HV, Hannum M, Tan KS, Lee J, Scarpa JR, et al. Intraoperative opioids are associated with improved recurrence-free survival in triple-negative breast cancer. Br J Anaesth. 2021;126(2):367-76.
56. Cronin-Fenton DP, Heide-Jørgensen U, Ahern TP, Lash TL, Christiansen PM, Ejlertsen B, et al. Opioids and breast cancer recurrence: a Danish population-based cohort study. Cancer. 2015;121(19):3507-14.
57. Rangel FP, Auler Jr JO, Carmona MJ, Cordeiro MD, Nahas WC, Coelho RF, et al. Opioids and premature biochemical recurrence of prostate cancer: a randomised prospective clinical trial. Br J Anaesth. 2021;126(5):931-9.
58. Silagy AW, Hannum ML, Mano R, Attalla K, Scarpa JR, DiNatale RG, et al. Impact of intraoperative opioid and adjunct analgesic use on renal cell carcinoma recurrence: role for onco-anaesthesia. Br J Anaesth. 2020;125(5):e402-4.
59. Connolly JG, Tan KS, Mastrogiacomo B, Dycoco J, Caso R, Jones GD, et al. Intraoperative opioid exposure, tumour genomic alterations, and survival differences in people with lung adenocarcinoma. Br J Anaesth. 2021;127(1):75-84.
60. Farooqui M, Li Y, Rogers T, Poonawala T, Griffin RJ, Song CW, et al. COX-2 inhibitor celecoxib prevents chronic morphine-induced promotion of angiogenesis, tumour growth, metastasis and mortality, without compromising analgesia. Br J Cancer. 2007;97(11):1523-31.
61. Forget P, Bentin C, Machiels JP, Berlière M, Coulie PG, De Kock M. Intraoperative use of ketorolac or diclofenac is associated with improved disease-free survival and overall survival in conservative breast cancer surgery. Br J Anaesth. 2014;113(suppl_1):i82-7.
62. Schack A, Fransgaard T, Klein MF, Gögenur I. Perioperative use of nonsteroidal anti-inflammatory drugs decreases the risk of recurrence of cancer after colorectal resection: a cohort study based on prospective data. Ann Surg Oncol. 2019;26:3826-37.
63. Yap A, Lopez-Olivo MA, Dubowitz J, Pratt G, Hiller J, Gottumukkala V, et al. Effect of beta-blockers on cancer recurrence and survival: a meta-analysis of epidemiological and perioperative studies. Br J Anaesth. 2018;121(1):45-57.
64. Hiller JG, Cole SW, Crone EM, Byrne DJ, Shackleford DM, Pang JM, et al. Preoperative β-blockade with propranolol

reduces biomarkers of metastasis in breast cancer: a phase II randomized trial. Clin Cancer Res. 2020;26(8):1803-11.
65. Løfling LL, Støer NC, Sloan EK, Chang A, Gandini S, Ursin G, et al. β-blockers and breast cancer survival by molecular subtypes: a population-based cohort study and meta-analysis. Br J Cancer. 2022;127(6):1086-96.
66. Sivanesan S, Taskén KA, Grytli HH. Association of β-blocker use at time of Radical prostatectomy with rate of treatment for prostate cancer recurrence. JAMA Netw Open. 2022; 5(1):e2145230.
67. Tertil M, Jozkowicz A, Dulak J. Oxidative stress in tumor angiogenesis-therapeutic targets. Current pharmaceutical design. 2010;16(35):3877-94.
68. Crowley PD, Stuttgen V, O'Carroll E, Ash SA, Buggy DJ, Gallagher HC. Exposure to 60% oxygen promotes migration and upregulates angiogenesis factor secretion in breast cancer cells. Med Gas Res. 2017;7(4):226-35.
69. Meyhoff CS, Jorgensen LN, Wetterslev J, Siersma VD, Rasmussen LS, PROXI Trial Group. Risk of new or recurrent cancer after a high perioperative inspiratory oxygen fraction during abdominal surgery. Br J Anaesth. 2014;113(suppl_1):i74-81.
70. Nair AS, Saifuddin MS, Naik V, Rayani BK. Dexmedetomidine in cancer surgeries: present status and consequences with its use. Indian J Cancer. 2020;57(3):234-8.

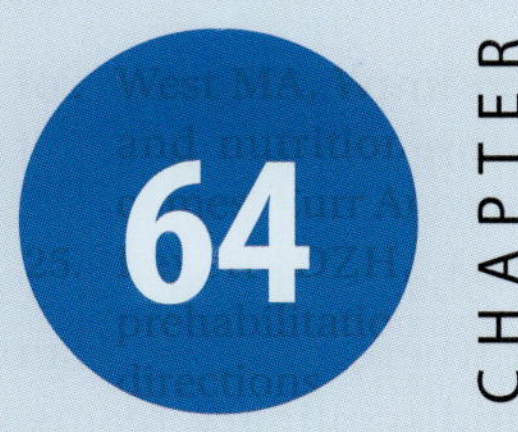

CHAPTER

Perioperative Management and Return to Intended Oncological Therapy after Major Cancer Surgeries

Sohan Lal Solanki, Divya Dabholkar

INTRODUCTION

The incidence of cancer cases is rising throughout the world. The International Agency for Research on Cancer (IARC) published the 2022 report providing a comprehensive overview of the global cancer burden surveyed in 115 countries. The report concluded with a mortality of 9.7 million in 2022 (9.96 million had been recorded in 2020) and 20 million new oncological cases (19.6 million in 2020). Death due to cancer is expected in 1 in 9 men and 1 in 12 women.[1] Since at least 60% of cancer patients require surgery during the course of their treatment,[2] there is an increasing demand to optimize perioperative care of cancer patients undergoing major surgical interventions.[3] 1-year survival outcomes may be improved by reducing early postoperative complications, thereby decreasing morbidity in oncological patients.[4,5]

Surgical interventions in cancer patients often require one or a combination of adjuvant therapies such as radiotherapy, chemotherapy, or immunotherapy. It is imperative that the patient be as physiologically optimized as possible while undergoing the adjuvant therapies as they are associated with significant adverse effects. In order to prevent recurrence and improve survival, it is important to assess the appropriate duration between postoperative recovery and initiation of planned adjuvant therapy.[6]

Return to intended oncologic therapy (RIOT) was first coined in 2014 as a novel metric in an observational study in patients undergoing liver resection, which demonstrated that chemotherapeutic regimen could be initiated 10 days earlier when enhanced recovery after surgery (ERAS) pathways were implemented.[5] It is observed that early implementation of adjuvant therapy improved overall survival.[7] Postoperative recovery after cancer surgery may be assessed with RIOT as a measurable standard.

Current definitions of RIOT include the interval to resume neoadjuvant therapy after surgery or the initiation of planned oncological therapy after surgery or the ratio of the number of patients who underwent planned adjuvant therapy postoperatively and the total number of postoperative patients for whom oncologic therapy was planned, both of which are in unspecified duration.

APPLICATIONS OF RETURN TO INTENDED ONCOLOGIC THERAPY

A retrospective study demonstrated survival benefits in patients with advanced ovarian carcinoma who received early chemotherapy (<28 days) *versus* late chemotherapy (>28 days) while observing the association between RIOT interval and subsequent oncological outcomes.[6] However, the survival benefit was noted only in women who underwent suboptimal debulking with subsequent residual tumor. Comparably, another study including women with advanced cancer of the ovary demonstrated a survival benefit with early chemotherapy (<19 days) in women who lacked residual tumor, whereas women with residual tumor showed no benefit from early chemotherapy.[8]

A retrospective analysis concluded decreased cancer recurrence or progression in patients whose chemotherapy had been delayed beyond 6 weeks after a surgical intervention but no impact on overall survival was noted.[9]

In contrast, lack of any association between RIOT and overall survival in ovarian cancer[10-13] has been observed in an array of studies. Indeed, initiating postoperative chemotherapy hastily may be associated with a number of adverse outcomes.[7,14]

Hayden et al.[15] reported a prospective randomized controlled trial of 40 women who underwent surgical debulking in ovarian carcinoma. RIOT interval reduced by 29 days in patients in whom 40 mL of 0.1% ropivacaine was infiltrated intraperitoneally accompanied by an intermittent infusion for 72 hours postsurgery.

Aloia et al.[5] evaluated patients with hepatocellular carcinoma to establish risk factors associated with the inability to RIOT, the RIOT rate, and its association with overall survival. A homogeneous cohort of 223 patients undergoing open surgery for colorectal liver metastases and 27 liver tumor patients treated with MIS hepatectomy were studied. Among open-approach surgery patients, 167 patients were given adjuvant therapy after surgery, thereby yielding a RIOT rate of 75%. Due to surgical complications 29 patients could not be given further intended treatment while 27 patients on account of poor performance status. Inability to RIOT was associated with risk factors such as hypertension, multiple preoperative chemotherapy regimens, and postoperative complications. Inability to RIOT correlated with shorter disease-free and overall survival. In comparison to the group of patients that underwent open surgery, 100% of minimally invasive surgery (MIS)-approach patients were able to initiate postoperative adjuvant therapy within a shorter time period, i.e., 15 days in MIS approach versus 42 days in open approach. The study concluded that RIOT rates should be routinely implemented as a quality indicator for both MIS and open-approach oncological surgical interventions.[5]

Nelson et al.[16] demonstrated how the application of enhanced recovery pathways (ERP) for patients with early-stage nonsmall cell lung cancer (NSCLC) at MD Anderson Cancer Centre yielded higher rates of adjuvant chemotherapy use, thereby demonstrating that ERP aided patients with early-stage NSCLC to RIOT.

Kim et al. reported similar observations about ERP and its association with RIOT in pancreatic and breast surgery patients.[17]

Pointer et al.[18] studied 15,132 open colectomies and 14,107 minimally invasive colectomies. 2-days shorter median length of stay (LOS) 4 versus 6 days was observed in minimally invasive colectomy patients with 1-week shorter median time to RIOT 6 versus 7 weeks. As compared to open colectomies, minimally invasive colectomies in colon cancer were found to be associated with a faster RIOT.

Garcia-Nebreda et al.[19] observed 70 patients with stomach cancer (35 in pre- and post-ERAS period each). 14 of the pre-ERAS and 22 patients of post-ERAS period received intended adjuvant treatment. Interval to RIOT was shorter in the post-ERAS period by 12 days compared to the pre-ERAS period. LOS was reduced in the ERAS group. The study concluded that the implementation of ERAS pathway for gastric carcinoma surgery demonstrated faster RIOT with reduced LOS.

Antunes et al.[20] conducted an observational study with 40 patients having colon cancer where an action plan was made with the hospital's multidisciplinary teams, surgical, and administrative departments to optimize the scheduling of appointments and minimize postoperative complications (paralytic ileus and fistula), through the Improvement Science methodology of the Institute for Healthcare Improvement (IHI). The actions include nutritional and physical therapy assessment in the pre and postoperative period, stringent control over glycemic status in the perioperative period, and an innovative anesthesia management protocol with the goal to reduce the use of opioids. The median time from surgery to the beginning of adjuvant treatment (RIOT) reduced from 46 days to 42 days and 100% of patients started adjuvant chemotherapy within 56 days.[21]

FACTORS AFFECTING RETURN TO INTENDED ONCOLOGIC THERAPY

Factors affecting RIOT are as follows ***(Fig. 1)****:*

- Open surgical approach
- Length of hospital stay
- Surgical complications
- Preexisting comorbidities
- Multiple preoperative chemotherapeutic regimens
- Adherence to ERAS pathways[22]

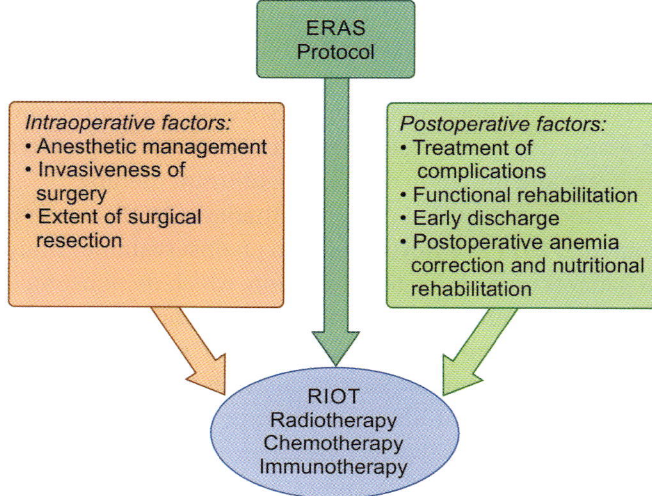

Fig. 1: Factors affecting RIOT. (ERAS: enhanced recovery after surgery; RIOT: return to intended oncologic therapy)

LIMITATIONS OF RETURN TO INTENDED ONCOLOGIC THERAPY

Return to intended oncologic therapy has numerous limitations as evident from clinical trials examining the impact of perioperative interventions on patient outcomes and overall survival.

- *No standardization:* An international group of anesthesiologists has identified standard endpoints for use in oncoanesthesia.[23] RIOT did not qualify as a metric for final consensus on criteria.
- *No information on chemotherapy regimen:* It lacks details regarding the tolerability of intended chemotherapeutic regimen, a requirement for dose reduction and termination of treatment due to adverse effects, all of which are observed in routine clinical practice. Any delay or dose reduction may impact overall survival.[24,25] RIOT interval fails to provide information on the given clinical decisions.
- *Lack of clear definition:* A minimum important clinical difference (MICD) is not defined for RIOT and may be different for different tumors or presence or absence of residual disease. Widely varying definitions ranging from 15 days to 12 weeks postsurgery of early and late chemotherapy have been applied.
- *Degree of subjectivity:* No evidence-based guideline currently directs when to initiate adjunctive therapy, the decision is in most cases made by the oncologist and surgeon, which is often guided by experience and institutional practice. This brings a degree of subjectivity to the interval between surgery and initiation of adjuvant therapy.
- *Conflicting evidence:* There is conflicting evidence on whether beneficial outcomes are seen with initiation of adjuvant therapy.
- *Difference in interpretation:* Cautious interpretation of RIOT intervals across different countries is required as institutional practices may differ. For instance, some institutes may prefer initiation of chemotherapy in hospitalized patients while others may do so as outpatients.
- *Logistic difficulties:* Resource shortcomings or administrative difficulties rather than patient-oriented factors may be observed in some countries influencing the initiation of therapy.
- *Limited knowledge:* As oncoanesthesia mainly focuses on the intraoperative period, the ability to influence RIOT with interventions during intraoperative period and ERAS programs may be limited.

Perhaps the focus should instead be on optimization of preoperative comorbidities if we are to positively impact RIOT interval. More studies need to focus on factors influencing the metric RIOT such as prehabilitation, including nutrition,[24] psychological support,[25] and preoperative exercise training and their impact on RIOT.

At present, the long-term correlation of RIOT with morbidity and survival remains unclear; however, it may be a useful yardstick to assess recovery after surgery.

ROLE OF PERIOPERATIVE PHYSICIAN IN RETURN TO INTENDED ONCOLOGIC THERAPY

Surgery elicits the surgical stress response, which is a physiological response given by the body to surgical injury. The activation of hypothalamic–pituitary–adrenal axis and sympathetic nervous system due to stimulation of afferent nerves and release of cytokines produce an integrated endocrine, hemodynamic, and immune response to restore body's dynamic steady state.[26,27] The endocrine response is catabolic in nature and results in a breakdown of body protein for energy production and synthesis of inflammatory proteins such as C-reactive protein, fibrinogen, and albumin. The endocrine response is clinically seen as raised blood glucose levels and protein breakdown.[27] This hemodynamic response maintains euvolemic status for cardiovascular stability, ensures end-organ perfusion, and meets the elevated oxygen demand by the peripheral tissues of the body; clinically, it may manifest as raised blood pressure, elevated heart rate, edema, and water retention. The immune response involves inflammatory pathways, mediated by a complex interaction of both pro and anti-inflammatory cytokines, with the goal to minimize tissue injury, eliminate infections, and promote the process of healing.[26]

Recent perioperative interventions aim to attenuate the adverse effects of the surgical stress response, such as prolonged catabolic states, while retaining its ability to restore homeostasis, which is the inherent purpose of the stress response.[28]

The ERAS protocols comprise multimodal, multidisciplinary perioperative elements that can improve outcomes[29,30] **(Fig. 2)**. A number of ERAS components are known to minimize stress response to surgery, e.g., preoperatively avoid fasting while intraoperative use of

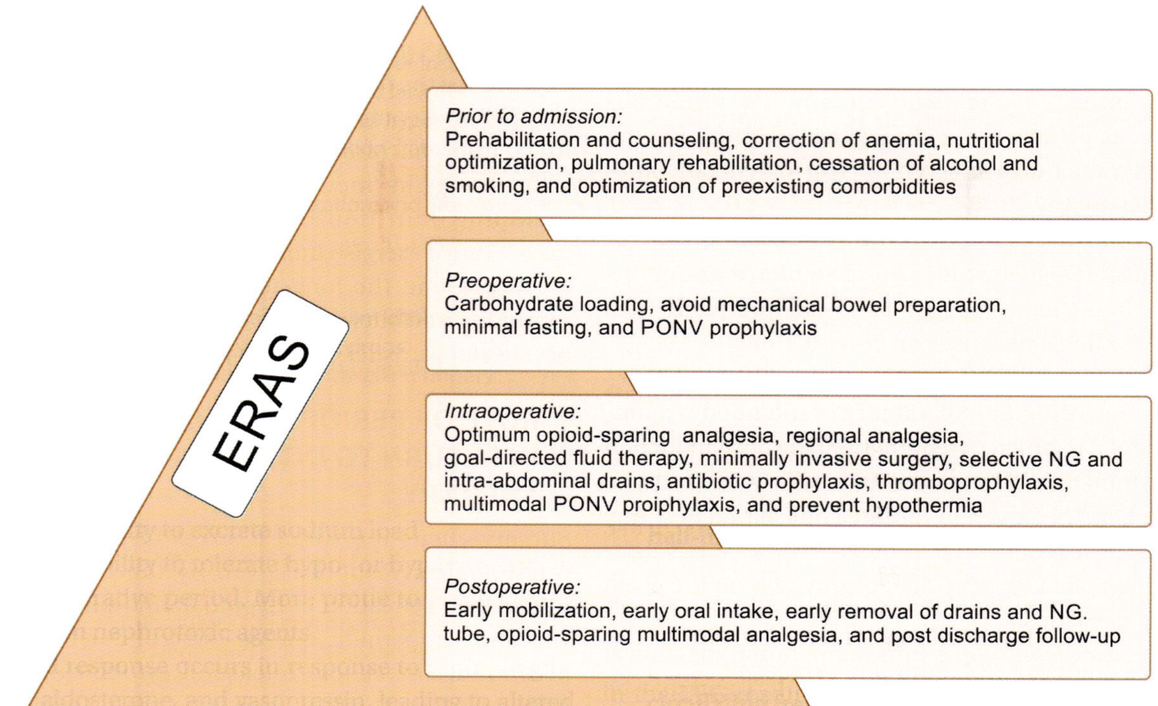

Fig. 2: Components of ERAS pathway. (ERAS: enhanced recovery after surgery; NG: nasogastric; PONV: postoperative nausea and vomiting)

minimally invasive surgical methods[31] so as to prevent excessive catabolism and reduce body protein loss while restoring strength and function.[32]

Cardiopulmonary exercise testing serves as an objective assessment of the cardiorespiratory endurance of the body under stress by means of the measurement of turnover of oxygen utilization in peripheral tissues at progressively increasing levels of physical work (i.e., exercise capacity).[33] Poor exercise capacity is the inability to perform physical exertion as expected (also known as exercise intolerance[33]) and may be attributed to insufficient cardiac reserve, myocardial ischemia, age- or disease-related deconditioning, and/or poor pulmonary reserve. Assessment of cardiorespiratory performance is thus an important evaluating factor to stratify those patients who are at elevated risk of complications in early postoperative period and those patients who are likely to suffer a postoperative functional decline. Measures of exercise capacity derived from cardiopulmonary exercise testing[31] can predict all-cause postoperative morbidity and mortality,[34] prolonged length of hospital stay,[35] and predict mortality after major surgery[36,37] **(Flowchart 1)**.

Prehabilitation and Functional Capacity

Prehabilitation programs aim to prepare patients physically and emotionally to withstand the stress of surgery.[38] Although there is no single definition for prehabilitation and these programs may vary as per patient's requirements,[39] the mainstay of this chapter is on multimodal prehabilitation programs, including nutrition, exercise, and psychological strategies that aim to enhance functional capacity before surgery and facilitate return of functional capacity after surgery.

Functional Capacity

An integration of cardiovascular, skeletal, and pulmonary health is required for unimpaired physiological reserve,[40] which is influenced by exercise,[40] nutritional,[41] and cognitive/psychological[42] reserve status.

Exercise

The exercise aspect of prehabilitation aims to augment physiological reserve and functional capacity of the cardiopulmonary and musculoskeletal systems.[43] Habitual

Flowchart 1: Efficacy of ERAS pathways to influence RIOT.

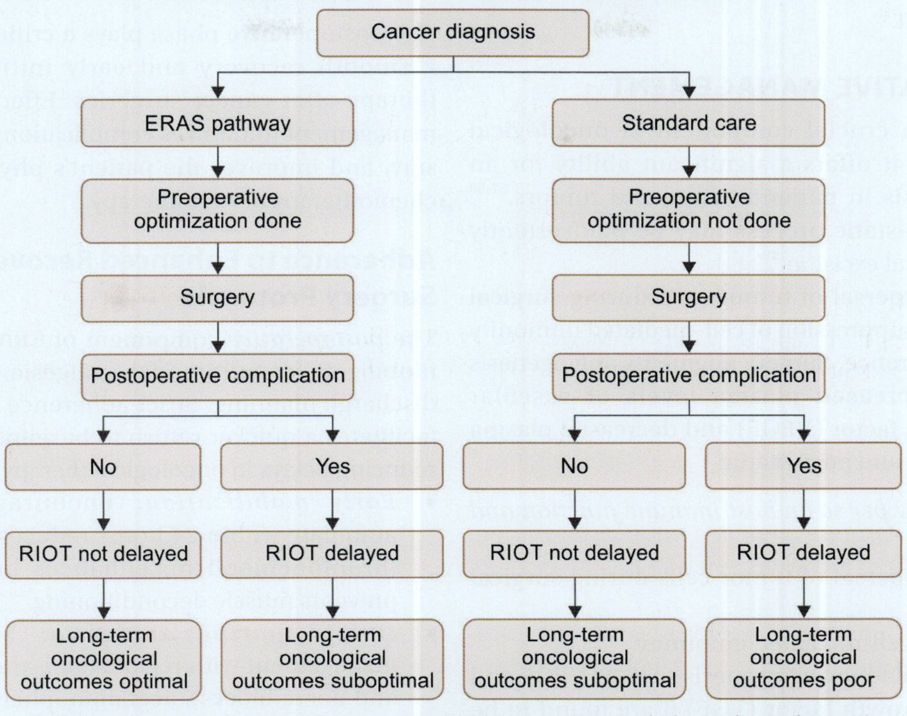

(ERAS: enhanced recovery after surgery; RIOT: return to intended oncologic therapy)

sustained physical activity and exercise contribute to preservation of physiological reserve,[44] and thereby enhance functional capacity.[45,46]

Nutritional Status

Provision of key anabolic nutrients, including dietary protein, supports anabolic gains.[47] Dietary protein provides the supply of amino acids to aid in building body's protein reserve. Advanced cancer is known to reduce anabolic potential; however, anabolic failure may be overcome with an adequate dose of amino acids.[47,48] Although amino acids may be supplied through dietary protein (i.e., substrate), many micronutrients such as vitamins and minerals serve as essential micronutrients for carbohydrate and protein metabolism. Pyridoxine (vitamin B_6) is a coenzyme that plays a role in protein metabolism. A micronutrient deficiency would inhibit anabolic potential of the dietary protein consumed, and thus provides rationale for nutrition provision/correction of malnutrition.[49] An overview of 55 systematic reviews of cancer prehabilitation highlighted low-to-very-low certainty evidence that nutritional prehabilitation minimizes the risk of complications, length of hospital stay, and mortality.[50]

Psychosocial Status

Few observational studies demonstrate that extreme levels of psychological stress, as seen in patients with significant anxiety or depression, may mount an exaggerated stress response even before surgery due to a dysregulated hypothalamic–pituitary–adrenal axis response, which may subsequently disrupt immune function in postoperative period and affect healing.[51] Preoperative anxiety, fear, and depression are associated with worse surgical outcomes, including increased length of hospital stay.[52,25] Depressed patients are less active preoperatively, have lower exercise capacity,[53] and anxious patients are observed to have higher opioid and inhalational anesthetic agent requirements than less distressed patients,[54,55] thus augmenting opioid-related adverse effects, including nausea and paralytic ileus,[52] that subsequently increases length of hospital stay.

The psychological aspect of prehabilitation aims to promote behavioral change (i.e., reinforce the importance of exercise and nutrition optimization) and psychological wellbeing preoperatively[25] with aim to reduce postoperative delirium as well.[56]

INTRAOPERATIVE MANAGEMENT

Surgery is often a crucial component of oncological management and it offers a significant ability for an improved prognosis in patients with solid tumors.[57,58] However, the metastatic process may be inadvertently facilitated by surgical excision.[59]

Inadvertent dispersal of tumor cells during surgical manipulation and suppression of cell-mediated immunity contribute to recurrence. Surgery augments angiogenesis by promoting increased plasma levels of vascular endothelial growth factor (VEGF) and decreased plasma levels of endostatin and angiostatin.

The effect of surgery per se on host immune function and metastasis:

- Inadvertent dispersal of tumor cells during surgical manipulation
- Suppression of cell-mediated immunity
- Cytokines stimulating angiogenesis such as VEGF and transforming growth factor (TGF) β are found to be increased after surgery.

Effect of anesthesia per se on host immune function and cancer:

- In a recent randomized controlled trial, the effect of low-dose ketamine on immune function in patients undergoing elective abdominal surgery indicated that it suppressed the natural killer (NK) cell cytotoxicity after surgery along with a reduced production of the proinflammatory cytokines, interleukin-6 (IL-6), and tumor necrosis factor-alpha (TNF-α).[60]
- Opioid analgesia and intrathecal bupivacaine use demonstrated the effectiveness of perioperative analgesia in preventing metastatic progression.[61]
- Regional anesthesia has proven to attenuate the neuro-humoral-endocrine stress response to surgery, thereby reducing the use of opioids as analgesic and minimizing intraoperative volatile anesthetic agent requirements.[62] These factors may allow early restoration of postoperative immune function and possibly impact recurrence.
- In a recent meta-analysis, 5,378 patients were studied to determine the effect of transfusion on disease recurrence, disease-free interval, and overall survival. An association between transfusion and reduction of cancer-free survival was noted.[62]

POSTOPERATIVE MANAGEMENT

The postoperative phase plays a critical role in ensuring a smooth recovery and early initiation of adjuvant therapy after cancer surgeries. Effective postoperative management minimizes complications, shortens hospital stay, and improves the patient's physical readiness for chemotherapy or radiotherapy.

Adherence to Enhanced Recovery after Surgery Protocols

The *postoperative* component of ERAS focuses on early mobilization, multimodal analgesia, gut recovery, and discharge planning. Strict adherence to these principles facilitates a quicker return to baseline functional status, reducing delays in oncological therapy.

- *Early mobilization:* Encouraging patients to ambulate within 24 hours reduces the risk of venous thromboembolism, enhances lung function, and prevents muscle deconditioning.
- *Opioid-sparing analgesia:* Multimodal pain management with regional anesthesia (e.g., epidurals and nerve blocks), acetaminophen, and nonsteroidal anti-inflammatory drugs (NSAIDs) minimizes opioid-related complications like ileus, nausea, and respiratory depression.
- *Early enteral nutrition:* Resuming oral intake as soon as possible supports gut integrity, prevents bacterial translocation, and enhances immune recovery.
- *Optimized fluid management:* Avoiding excessive intravenous fluids helps prevent postoperative complications such as pulmonary edema, anastomotic leaks, and prolonged ileus.

Reduced Incidence of Postoperative Complications

Postoperative complications can significantly delay chemotherapy or radiotherapy, affecting long-term oncological outcomes. Targeted interventions to reduce complications include:

- *Prevention of surgical site infections (SSI):* Maintaining aseptic dressing techniques and ensuring early drain removal reduces the risk of SSIs.
- *Respiratory optimization:* Incentive spirometry, breathing exercises, and early ambulation reduce the incidence of postoperative pneumonia.
- *Prevention of venous thromboembolism (VTE):* Pharmacologic prophylaxis (low-molecular-weight heparin) and mechanical prophylaxis (compression

stockings and sequential compression devices) help prevent deep vein thrombosis and pulmonary embolism.

- *Anastomotic leak surveillance:* Close monitoring for early signs of anastomotic leaks (tachycardia, fever, and abdominal distension) enables timely intervention, reducing the need for reoperation and prolonged hospitalization.
- *Avoiding postoperative ileus:* Strategies such as early oral feeding, chewing gum, and minimizing opioid use promote gastrointestinal motility and reduce the risk of prolonged ileus.

By preventing and managing these complications proactively, patients can recover faster and resume their oncological therapy without unnecessary delays.

Early Discharge

A structured discharge plan ensures that patients transition smoothly from the hospital to home, reducing healthcare-associated risks and expediting their return to chemotherapy or radiotherapy.

- *Criteria for early discharge:*
    - Pain control achieved with oral medications
    - Resumption of normal bowel function (passing flatus/stool)
    - Ability to ambulate independently
    - Stable vital signs and no evidence of postoperative complications
- *Post-discharge follow-up:*
    - Regular outpatient monitoring to assess wound healing, nutritional status, and functional recovery
    - Coordination with the oncology team to schedule chemotherapy or radiotherapy sessions
    - Home-based physiotherapy and nutritional counseling to optimize recovery.

Early discharge, when done with proper planning, minimizes hospital-related risks while ensuring that patients are fit for timely RIOT.

Correction of Anemia and Nutritional Rehabilitation

Anemia and malnutrition are common barriers to timely chemotherapy initiation postsurgery. Addressing these issues promptly improves functional recovery and chemotherapy tolerance.

- *Anemia correction:*
    - Early assessment and supplementation of iron, vitamin B_{12}, and folic acid
    - Blood transfusions when hemoglobin levels are critically low (<8 g/dL) to maintain adequate oxygen delivery
    - Erythropoiesis-stimulating agents in select patients undergoing chemotherapy
- *Nutritional rehabilitation:*
    - Early enteral feeding with high-protein, calorie-dense diets to promote wound healing
    - Nutritional supplements, including omega-3 fatty acids and micronutrients (zinc and vitamin C) to support immune function
    - Dietitian-guided interventions to correct deficiencies and enhance recovery.

Nutritional and hematological optimization significantly improves physical readiness for chemotherapy and minimizes the risk of treatment delays.

Early Removal of Nasogastric Tube and Intraperitoneal Drains

Prolonged use of nasogastric tubes and intraperitoneal drains increases infection risk, delays gut function recovery, and prolongs hospitalization. Early removal enhances patient comfort and supports faster rehabilitation.

- *Nasogastric tube management:*
    - Avoidance of routine nasogastric tube insertion in elective surgeries
    - Early removal (preferably within 24–48 hours) to facilitate oral feeding and gut motility
    - Encouragement of chewing gum therapy to stimulate bowel function
- *Drain removal strategy:*
    - Use of selective drain placement rather than routine usage
    - Monitoring drain output trends to determine safe removal timing
    - Removal as early as possible to minimize infection risk and improve mobility.

Early removal of these invasive devices allows for better ambulation, reduces discomfort, and expedites hospital discharge, ensuring patients are fit for timely oncological therapy.

CONCLUSION

While RIOT serves as a valuable metric to assess postoperative recovery, its role in improving long-term oncologic outcomes remains unclear. Standardization of RIOT definitions, optimization of perioperative care, and further research into prehabilitation strategies are crucial to improving cancer survival rates.

REFERENCES

1. Finnerty DT, Buggy DJ. Return to intended oncologic therapy: a potentially valuable endpoint for perioperative research in cancer patients? Br J Anaesth. 2020;124(5):508-10.
2. Alkire BC, Raykar NP, Shrime MG, Weiser TG, Bickler SW, Rose JA, et al. Global access to surgical care: a modelling study. Lancet Glob Health. 2015;3(6):e316-23.
3. Thota RS, Garg R, Ramkiran S, Divatia JV. Onco-anaesthesiology as an emerging sub-speciality domain: Need of the hour! Indian J Anaesth. 2020;64(1):69-71.
4. Lillemoe HA, Marcus RK, Kim BJ, Narula N, Davis CH, Shi Q, et al. Severe preoperative symptoms delay readiness to return to intended oncologic therapy (RIOT) after liver resection. Ann Surg Oncol. 2019;26(13):4548-55.
5. Aloia TA, Zimmitti G, Conrad C, Gottumukalla V, Kopetz S, Vauthey JN. Return to intended oncologic treatment (RIOT): A novel metric for evaluating the quality of oncosurgical therapy for malignancy. J Surg Oncol. 2014;110(2):107-14.
6. Hofstetter G, Concin N, Braicu I, Chekerov R, Sehouli J, Cadron I, et al. The time interval from surgery to start of chemotherapy significantly impacts prognosis in patients with advanced serous ovarian carcinoma-analysis of patient data in the prospective OVCAD study. Gynecol Oncol. 2013;131(1):15-20.
7. Flynn PM, Paul J, Cruickshank DJ; Scottish Gynaecological Cancer Trials Group. Does the interval from primary surgery to chemotherapy influence progression-free survival in ovarian cancer? Gynecol Oncol. 2002;86(3):354-7.
8. Mahner S, Eulenburg C, Staehle A, Wegscheider K, Reuss A, Pujade-Lauraine E, et al. Prognostic impact of the time interval between surgery and chemotherapy in advanced ovarian cancer: analysis of prospective randomised phase III trials. Eur J Cancer. 2013;49(1):142-9.
9. Singh S, Guetzko M, Resnick K. Preoperative predictors of delay in initiation of adjuvant chemotherapy in patients undergoing primary debulking surgery for ovarian cancer. Gynecol Oncol. 2016;143(2):241-5.
10. Rosa DD, Clamp A, Mullamitha S, Ton NC, Lau S, Byrd L, et al. The interval from surgery to chemotherapy in the treatment of advanced epithelial ovarian carcinoma. Eur J Surg Oncol. 2006;32(5):588-91.
11. Gadducci A, Sartori E, Landoni F, Zola P, Maggino T, Maggioni A, et al. Relationship between time interval from primary surgery to the start of taxane-plus platinum-based chemotherapy and clinical outcome of patients with advanced epithelial ovarian cancer: results of a multicenter retrospective Italian study. J Clinical Onc. 2005;23(4):751-8.
12. Aletti GD, Long HJ, Podratz KC, Cliby WA. Is time to chemotherapy a determinant of prognosis in advanced-stage ovarian cancer? Gynecol Oncol. 2007;104(1):212-6.
13. Paulsen T, Kaern J, Kjaerheim K, Haldorsen T, Tropé C. Influence of interval between primary surgery and chemotherapy on short-term survival of patients with advanced ovarian, tubal or peritoneal cancer. Gynecol Oncol. 2006;102(3):447-52.
14. Sorbe B. Prognostic importance of the time interval from surgery to chemotherapy in treatment of ovarian carcinoma. Int J Gynecol Cancer. 2004;14(5):788-93.
15. Hayden JM, Oras J, Block L, Thörn SE, Palmqvist C, Salehi S, et al. Intraperitoneal ropivacaine reduces time interval to initiation of chemotherapy after surgery for advanced ovarian cancer: randomised controlled double-blind pilot study. Br J Anaesth. 2020;124(5):562-70.
16. Nelson DB, Mehran RJ, Mitchell KG, Correa AM, Sepesi B, Antonoff MB, et al. Enhanced recovery after thoracic surgery is associated with improved adjuvant chemotherapy completion for non–small cell lung cancer. J Thorac Cardiovasc Surg. 2019;158(1):279-86.e1.
17. Kim BJ, Caudle AS, Gottumukkala V, Aloia TA. The Impact of postoperative complications on a timely return to intended oncologic therapy (RIOT): The role of enhanced recovery in the cancer journey. Int Anesthesiol Clin. 2016; 54(4):e33-46.
18. Pointer DT Jr, Felder SI, Powers BD, Dessureault S, Sanchez JA, Imanirad I, et al. Return to intended oncologic therapy after colectomy for stage III colon adenocarcinoma: does surgical approach matter? Colorectal Dis. 2023; 25(9):1760-70.
19. Garcia-Nebreda M, Zorrilla-Vaca A, Ripollés-Melchor J, Abad-Motos A, Alvaro Cifuentes E, Abad-Gurumeta A, et al. Early return to intended oncologic therapy after implementation of an enhanced recovery after surgery pathway for gastric cancer surgery. Langenbecks Arch Surg. 2022;407(6):2293-300.
20. Antunes C, Chibana A, Mello C, Riechelmann R. de Andrade V, Aguiar S Jr. P-319 How coordinated and integrated multidisciplinary work improved the return to intended oncologic treatment in colon cancer. Ann Onc. 2020;31(3):S193
21. Hanna RK, Poniewierski MS, Laskey RA, Lopez MA, Shafer A, Van Le L, Get al. Predictors of reduced relative dose intensity and its relationship to mortality in women receiving multi-agent chemotherapy for epithelial ovarian cancer. Gynecol Oncol. 2013;129(1):74-80.
22. Joseph N, Clark RM, Dizon DS, Lee MS, Goodman A, Boruta D Jr, et al. Delay in chemotherapy administration impacts survival in elderly patients with epithelial ovarian cancer. Gynecol Oncol. 2015;137(3):401-5.
23. Buggy DJ, Freeman J, Johnson MZ, Leslie K, Riedel B, Sessler DI, et al.; StEP-COMPAC Group. Systematic review and consensus definitions for standardised endpoints in perioperative medicine: postoperative cancer outcomes. Br J Anaesth. 2018;121(1):38-44.

24. West MA, Wischmeyer PE, Grocott MPW. Prehabilitation and nutritional support to improve perioperative outcomes. Curr Anesthesiol Rep. 2017;7(4):340-9.
25. Levett DZH, Grimmett C. Psychological factors, prehabilitation and surgical outcomes: Evidence and future directions. Anaesthesia. 2019;74(Suppl 1):36-42.
26. Weissman C. The metabolic response to stress: an overview and update. Anesthesiology. 1990;73(2):308-27.
27. Dobson GP. Addressing the global burden of trauma in major surgery. Front Surg. 2015;2:43.
28. Soeters PB, Grimble RF. Dangers, and benefits of the cytokine mediated response to injury and infection. Clin Nutr. 2009;28(6):583-96.
29. Ljungqvist O, de Boer HD, Balfour A, Fawcett WJ, Lobo DN, Nelson G, et al. Opportunities and challenges for the next phase of enhanced recovery after surgery: a review. JAMA Surg. 2021;156(8):775-84.
30. Amer MA, Smith MD, Herbison GP, Plank LD, McCall JL. Network meta-analysis of the effect of preoperative carbohydrate loading on recovery after elective surgery. Br J Surg. 2017;104(3):187-97.
31. Gillis C, Ljungqvist O, Carli F. Prehabilitation, enhanced recovery after surgery, or both? A narrative review. Br J Anaesth. 2022;128(3):434-48.
32. Basse L, Raskov HH, Hjort Jakobsen D, Sonne E, Billesbølle P, Hendel HW, et al. Accelerated postoperative recovery programme after colonic resection improves physical performance, pulmonary function and body composition. Br J Surg. 2002;89(4):446-53.
33. Older PO, Levett DZH. Cardiopulmonary exercise testing and surgery. Ann Am Thorac Soc. 2017;14 (Supplement_1):S74-83.
34. Wilson RJ, Davies S, Yates D, Redman J, Stone M. Impaired functional capacity is associated with all-cause mortality after major elective intra-abdominal surgery. Br J Anaesth. 2010;105(3):297-303.
35. Lai CW, Minto G, Challand CP, Hosie KB, Sneyd JR, Creanor S, et al. Patients' inability to perform a preoperative cardiopulmonary exercise test or demonstrate an anaerobic threshold is associated with inferior outcomes after major colorectal surgery. Br J Anaesth. 2013;111(4):607-11.
36. Colson M, Baglin J, Bolsin S, Grocott MP. Cardiopulmonary exercise testing predicts 5 yr survival after major surgery. Br J Anaesth. 2012;109(5):735-41
37. Moran J, Wilson F, Guinan E, McCormick P, Hussey J, Moriarty J. Role of cardiopulmonary exercise testing as a risk-assessment method in patients undergoing intra-abdominal surgery: a systematic review. Br J Anaesth. 2016;116(2):177-91.
38. Carli F, Gillis C, Scheede-Bergdahl C. Promoting a culture of prehabilitation for the surgical cancer patient. Acta Oncol. 2017;56(2):128-33.
39. Santa Mina D, Brahmbhatt P, Lopez C, Baima J, Gillis C, Trachtenberg L, et al. The case for prehabilitation prior to breast cancer treatment. PM R. 2017;9(9S2):S305-16.
40. Arnett SW, Laity JH, Agrawal SK, Cress ME. Aerobic reserve and physical functional performance in older adults. Age Ageing. 2008;37(4):384-9
41. Jetté M, Sidney K, Blümchen G. Metabolic equivalents (METS) in exercise testing, exercise prescription, and evaluation of functional capacity. Clin Cardiol. 1990;13(8):555-65.
42. Kelaiditi E, Cesari M, Canevelli M, van Kan GA, Ousset PJ, Gillette-Guyonnet S, et al.; IANA/IAGG. Cognitive frailty: Rational and definition from an (I.A.N.A./I.A.G.G.) international consensus group. J Nutr Health Aging. 2013;17(9):726-34.
43. Scheede-Bergdahl C, Minnella EM, Carli F. Multi-modal prehabilitation: Addressing the why, when, what, how, who and where next? anaesthesia. 2019;74 Suppl 1:20-6.
44. Goldspink DF. Ageing and activity: their effects on the functional reserve capacities of the heart and vascular smooth and skeletal muscles. Ergonomics. 2005;48(11-14):1334-51.
45. Peterson MD, Rhea MR, Sen A, Gordon PM. Resistance exercise for muscular strength in older adults: a meta-analysis. Ageing Res Rev. 2010;9(3):226-37.
46. Chou CH, Hwang CL, Wu YT. Effect of exercise on physical function, daily living activities, and quality of life in the frail older adults: a meta-analysis. Arch Phys Med Rehabil. 2012;93(2):237-44.
47. Deutz NE, Safar A, Schutzler S, Memelink R, Ferrando A, Spencer H, et al. Muscle protein synthesis in cancer patients can be stimulated with a specially formulated medical food. Clin Nutr. 2011;30(6):759-68.
48. Winter A, MacAdams J, Chevalier S. Normal protein anabolic response to hyperaminoacidemia in insulin-resistant patients with lung cancer cachexia. Clin Nutr. 2012;31(5):765-73.
49. Gillis C, Phillips SM. Protein for the pre-surgical cancer patient: a narrative review. Current Anesthesiology Reports. 2022:1-0.
50. McIsaac DI, Gill M, Boland L, Hutton B, Branje K, Shaw J, et al. Prehabilitation in adult patients undergoing surgery: an umbrella review of systematic reviews. Br J Anaesth. 2022;128(2):244-57.
51. Manou-Stathopoulou V, Korbonits M, Ackland GL. Redefining the perioperative stress response: a narrative review. Br J Anaesth. 2019;123(5):570-83.
52. Kiecolt-Glaser JK, Page GG, Marucha PT, MacCallum RC, Glaser R. Psychological influences on surgical recovery. Perspectives from psychoneuroimmunology. Am Psychol. 1998;53(11):1209-18.
53. Barrett-Bernstein M, Carli F, Gamsa A, Scheede-Bergdahl C, Minnella E, Ramanakumar AV, et al. Depression and

functional status in colorectal cancer patients awaiting surgery: impact of a multimodal prehabilitation program. Health Psychol. 2019;38(10):900-9.

54. Maranets I, Kain ZN. Preoperative anxiety and intraoperative anesthetic requirements. Anesth Analg. 1999;89(6):1346-51.
55. Kil HK, Kim WO, Chung WY, Kim GH, Seo H, Hong JY. Preoperative anxiety and pain sensitivity are independent predictors of propofol and sevoflurane requirements in general anaesthesia. Br J Anaesth. 2012;108(1):119-25.
56. Vlisides PE, Das AR, Thompson AM, Kunkler B, Zierau M, Cantley MJ, et al. Home-based cognitive prehabilitation in older surgical patients: a feasibility study. J Neurosurg Anesthesiol. 2019;31(2):212-7.
57. Snyder GL, Greenberg S. Effect of anaesthetic technique and other perioperative factors on cancer recurrence. Br J Anaesth. 2010;105(2):106-15.
58. Kavanagh T, Buggy DJ. Can anaesthetic technique effect postoperative outcome? Curr Opin Anaesthesiol. 2012;25(2):185-98.
59. Neeman E, Ben-Eliyahu S. Surgery and stress promote cancer metastasis: new outlooks on perioperative mediating mechanisms and immune involvement. Brain Behav Immun. 2013;30 Suppl:S32-40.
60. Beilin B, Rusabrov Y, Shapira Y, Roytblat L, Greemberg L, Yardeni IZ, et al. Low-dose ketamine affects immune responses in humans during the early postoperative period. Br J Anaesth. 2007;99(4):522-7.
61. Page GG, Blakely WP, Ben-Eliyahu S. Evidence that postoperative pain is a mediator of the tumor-promoting effects of surgery in rats. Pain. 2001;90(1-2):191-9.
62. Churchhouse AM, Mathews TJ, McBride OM, Dunning J. Does blood transfusion increase the chance of recurrence in patients undergoing surgery for lung cancer? Interact Cardiovasc Thorac Surg. 2012;14(1):85-90.

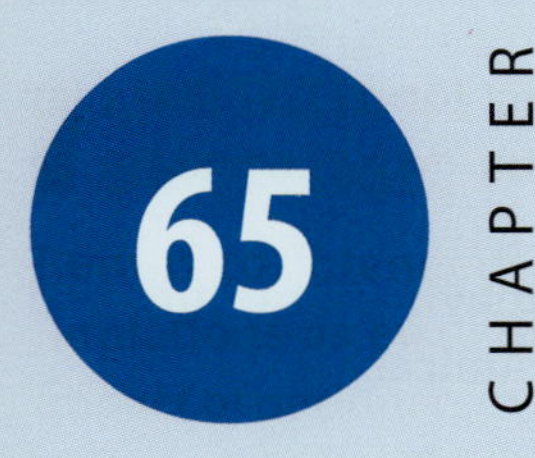

CHAPTER

Major Cancer Surgery for Geriatric Patients

Malini P Joshi, Akankshya Sarangi, Shilpushp J Bhosale

INTRODUCTION

An increasing life expectancy and an aging global population have led to a rise in elderly cancer patients, posing unique challenges in oncology and surgical care. Older adults have comorbidities, decreased physiological reserve, and psychosocial issues, which can complicate surgical interventions and affect outcomes. Due to the increased likelihood of these older patients having malignant rather than benign tumors, surgery remains the only option for a complete cure.

Understanding a geriatric patient's physiology is crucial for forming a safe and effective strategy for managing these patients.[1]

AGE-RELATED PHYSIOLOGICAL EFFECTS[2]

Cardiovascular System

- Larger pulse and blood pressure (BP) variations, hemodynamic instability, and postoperative hypertension occur due to:
  - Decreased beta response to hypotension
  - Increased systemic vascular resistance
  - Decreased vessel compliance due to calcification and vascular rigidity
- Increased myocardial oxygen demand, decreased coronary perfusion, and a higher risk of perioperative coronary ischemia
- Older patients have prolonged hypertension causing left ventricular strain and hypertrophy, aortic stenosis, and an aging conduction system manifesting as ectopic beats, heart block, and arrhythmias, especially atrial fibrillation
- Downregulation of myocardial catecholamine receptors, reduced responsiveness to sympathomimetic agents, and decreased heart rate and cardiac output

Respiratory System

- Decreased respiratory function and reserves due to stiff chest wall, flattened diaphragm, and weakened intercostal muscles
- Aging causes emphysematous changes with an increased alveolar surface area, decreased respiratory gas exchange, and ventilation–perfusion (V/Q) mismatch.
- Decreased functional residual capacity (FRC) and increased closing capacity (CC) cause airway closure prematurely.
- Blunted central responses to hypoxia and hypercarbia, with decreased respiratory drive

Neurological System

- Aging affects the central and peripheral nervous systems, increasing drug susceptibility, memory loss, cognitive decline, depression, decreased neuroplasticity, and delirium
- Cerebral perfusion and oxygenation need to be maintained in patients who have a high risk of cognitive dysfunction occurring postoperatively
- *Cognitive dysfunction:* Neuronal cell death, demyelination, and decline in neurotransmitters like dopamine and acetylcholine can all contribute to cognitive impairment.

  The risk factors for delirium are included in **Box 1**.
- Autonomic neuropathy is associated with aging and long-standing diabetes. The baroreceptor responses are affected, manifesting as perioperative hemodynamic instability, delayed gastric emptying, and aspiration risk.

Renal System

- Reduced cortical mass and blood flow and decreased glomerular filtration rate (GFR) worsened by diabetes, hypertension, and vasculopathy

BOX 1: Risk factors causing delirium.

- Dementia and cognitive disorder, untreated or insufficiently managed pain, depression, alcoholism, and lack of sleep
- *Disease:* Severe comorbidities, anemia, and hypoxia
- *Metabolic factors:* Malnutrition, dehydration status, and dyselectrolytemia
- Reduced functional status, immobilization, and impaired vision or hearing
- Surgery
- ICU admission
- *Polypharmacy:* Use of benzodiazepines, anticholinergics, antihistamines, and other psychotropic drugs
- Urinary retention, constipation, and indwelling urinary catheter

(ICU: intensive care unit)

- Decreased ability to excrete sodium load
- Decreased ability to tolerate hypo- or hypervolemia in the perioperative period. More prone to acute kidney injury from nephrotoxic agents
- Reduced response occurs in response to renin, angiotensin, aldosterone, and vasopressin, leading to altered volume status, electrolyte abnormalities, and increased effects of lipophilic agents

Gastrointestinal System

- Decreased esophageal motility and prolonged gastric emptying time increase the risk of aspiration.
- The synthesis of coagulation factors is affected causing an increased risk of bleeding.

Other systemic changes with implications for the anesthetist are as follows:

- Malnutrition associated with aging and cancer requires evaluation and management by the geriatrician.
- Hypothermia occurs due to an age-related decrease in muscle mass, reduced metabolic rate, and vascular hyporeactivity, leading to decreased heat production and reduced thermoregulation. Maintaining normothermia is important in avoiding complications, such as arrhythmias, cardiac events, infection, impaired coagulation function, reduced drug metabolism, and delayed wound healing.
- Older adults with diabetes mellitus are more likely to develop ischemia and peripheral artery disease, chronic renal failure, end-stage renal disease, peripheral neuropathy, autonomic dysfunction resulting in neurogenic bladder, and delayed gastric emptying.
- Visual impairment due to cataract formation, macular degeneration, and glaucoma can occur in older age groups.
- Sensorineural loss of hearing may lead to impaired cognition and difficulty in communication.

Drug pharmacokinetics and pharmacodynamics:

- The loading drug dose should be decreased due to a decrease in total body water and decreased central compartment.
- *Lipophilic drugs:* Increased volume of distribution occurs due to decreased plasma and intracellular volume with increased adipose tissue.
- Decreased hepatic mass and function, reduced hepatic blood flow, and hepatic microsomal enzyme activity cause reduced drug metabolism with a prolonged half-life of anesthetic drugs, thus leading to decreased dosage in this population.
- Decreased albumin levels with increased α1-acid glycoprotein affect protein-bound acidic drugs (i.e., benzodiazepines and propofol), resulting in increased circulating free drug concentrations.
- Changes in gastric motility, decreased peristalsis, and an increased gastric emptying time can all affect the absorption of medications in the gastrointestinal (GI) tract in a geriatric patient. A decrease in gastric blood flow and secretion of acids may prevent an effective ionization and uptake of drugs.
- Reduced gaseous exchange across the alveolar membrane in an older patient alters the translocation of inhaled anesthetic agents, affecting both induction and emergence and causing decreased minimum alveolar concentration.
- Decreased renal blood flow and GFR prolong the half-life of drugs excreted renally, warranting dose reduction in the elderly. Medication dosage should be based on the patient's estimated GFR to prevent renal dysfunction as they are prone to impaired renal function and chronic kidney disease.
- Increased opioid sensitivity should result in decreased dosage in this population.

Frailty

- Frailty is commonly associated with age more than 65 years although it is not synonymous with it. It is associated with increased vulnerability to stressors due to a decline in physiological reserves and impaired ability to maintain homeostasis.

- It is characterized by decreased function and balance with difficulty in performing activities of daily living (ADL). Decreased functional capacity, inability to perform social roles, inflammation, neuroendocrine dysregulation, sarcopenia, decreased memory function, and performance deficits in executive functions and speed processing may be associated with it.
- Frail patients are more susceptible to perioperative complications. They are evaluated by two main screening tests:
  1. The Fried Phenotypic Model includes factors such as unintentional weight loss, exhaustion, lower expenditure of energy, slower gait speed, and weakened grip strength.
  2. The cumulative deficit model takes into account all deficits in health and thus, a cumulative score is determined by: Present number of deficits divided by total number of deficits.
     - Frailty assessment is important for better evaluation and coordination of care for high-risk surgical patients. It helps assist in the formulation of an individualized clinical care plan and is an independent prognostic indicator.
     - Sarcopenia is associated with decreased muscle and subcutaneous fat loss and thinned-out skin layers, causing frequent bruising and pressure-related injuries, increased heat loss and ineffective shivering due to decreased muscle mass, and impaired thermoregulation.
- Osteoarthritis leads to pain, decreased mobility, fragility fractures, and reduced bone healing, thus affecting the quality of life.

Preoperative preparation: The population undergoing cancer surgery requires a thorough evaluation in view of decreased physiological functions, presence of comorbidities, and effects of chemotherapy and radiotherapy.

The multidisciplinary team involves a team of specialists who ensure a holistic approach to preoperative assessment and optimization:

- *Geriatrician:* To oversee the overall health and manage comorbidities
- *Oncologist:* For cancer-specific evaluation and treatment planning
- *Anesthesiologist:* To assess anesthesia risk and plan perioperative care
- *Nutritionist:* For dietary assessment and planning
- *Physiotherapist:* Create and monitor exercise programs

TABLE 1: Components of CGA.

Medical components	• Comorbidities and severity • Review drugs • Review patients' nutritional status
Mental status	• Cognition function • Review of patients' fears, mood, and anxiety
Functional status	• Performing basic daily living activities and tasks • Patients' gait with balance is affected • Performance status of exercise and activity • Performance of instrumental activities of daily living (IADLs)
Social factors	Presence of support from family and friends and social activities
Environmental factors	• Home comfort, facilities, and safety • Effective facilities for transport • Accessibility to local resources

(CGA: Comprehensive Geriatric Assessment)

It bears the responsibility of planning the course of treatment by weighing all available options (including whether to treat or not to treat, as well as whether to use surgery or less noninvasive methods), and when necessary, considering other surgical options (such as minimally invasive procedures), if possible.

Comprehensive Geriatric Assessment (CGA):[3,4] An elderly patient's functional capacity, physical health, cognitive status, and social environment are evaluated by CGA **(Table 1)**. In a study by Partridge et al., it decreased complications in the postoperative period and total length of hospital stay after elective vascular surgery.

Preoperative evaluation—functional status:[5-7]

- *Activities of daily living:* Assess the performance of basic self-care tasks (e.g., able to take bath, dressing, and eating).
- *Instrumental activities of daily living (IADLs):* Evaluate complex and precise activities (e.g., medication management and handling finances).
- *Performance status scales:* The performance status can be assessed by screening tools, such as the prolonged Timed Up and Go Test (TUG test) >15 seconds, Karnofsky Performance Status, or the Eastern Cooperative Oncology Group (ECOG) scale.
- Inquire about the history of falls and identify the risk. Assess for restrictions in walking and movement.

Cognitive functions:

- A preoperative previously existing cognitive impairment is an important predictor of delirium occurring postoperatively and possibly postoperative cognitive dysfunction (POCD).

- Baseline cognitive status should be assessed in all patients aged above 65 years as per the American Society of Anesthesiologists (ASA)-Brain Health Initiative guidelines and also the American College of Surgeons (ACS)-National Surgical Quality Improvement Program (NSQIP) guidelines.
- *Screening tools:* Mini-Cog test, Mini-Mental State Examination (MMSE), or Montreal Cognitive Assessment (MoCA)
- *Delirium assessment:* It is done by the Confusion Assessment Method (CAM) for baseline status and to evaluate the risk of having postoperative delirium.
- Implement strategies to prevent delirium, such as maintaining a regular sleep–wake cycle, ensuring adequate hydration, and minimizing the use of sedatives.
- *Anesthetic implications:* Avoid anticholinergic drugs as patients with dementia are sensitive to their adverse effects and are prone to develop neuroleptic malignant syndrome and impaired consciousness. Benzodiazepines and antihistaminics should be avoided or cautiously used in these patients.

Nutritional status: Poor perioperative outcomes have been associated with poor nutritional status in geriatric patients. It can be assessed by various screening tools such as Mini Nutritional Assessment, Malnutrition Universal Screening Tool (MUST), or Subjective Global Assessment (SGA) and by anthropometrical measurements, i.e., body mass index (BMI), unintentional weight loss, and serum albumin and prealbumin levels.

Patients at risk of severe malnutrition, as mentioned in **Box 2**, should be considered for nutritional support.

Comorbidities and polypharmacy:

- Assessment should be done to quantify the number and severity of comorbid conditions. Several screening scales, i.e., Charlson Comorbidity Index, are available to assess comorbidities.

BOX 2: Factors associated with severe nutritional risk (ESPEN guidelines).

- Body mass index (BMI) <18.5 kg/m^2
- S. albumin level <3.0 g/dL (and having no liver or kidney dysfunction)
- Unintentional weight loss >10–15% (happened within 6 months)

- Look for the effects of chemotherapy and radiotherapy.
- *Medication review:* A comprehensive review of current medications should be done to identify polypharmacy and potential drug interactions. Polypharmacy can increase the risk of adverse drug-related events. Therefore, a detailed and accurate medication history taking is vital.
- Drugs to be avoided and discontinued in the geriatric age group in the preoperative period are listed in **Box 3**.

Social support: Assessment of the living situations, availability of caregivers, and social network with the identification of community resources and support systems for geriatric patients is essential.

Risk stratification:[8,9]

- Risk stratification tools help predict perioperative morbidity and mortality, guide in decision-making, and help in patient counseling. It involves identification of high-risk older patients and the development of individualized and effective perioperative plan, thus improving patient outcomes. An emphasis on the assessment of cognition, functional status, and frailty is consistently prioritized in all the assessment tools
- *American Society of Anesthesiologists Physical Status:* It evaluates overall health status and anesthesia risk. Some studies have suggested that higher ASA scores are associated with poor postoperative outcomes, but this is subjective and subject to high interobserver variability.[9]
- Frailty has been used for assessing the perioperative risk status in older patients posted for surgery. Due to the lack of a universal and standard frailty screening tool, a standardized assessment of patient status is often lacking.

BOX 3: Drugs to be avoided and discontinued in the geriatric age group in the preoperative period.

- Nonessential drugs increasing surgical risk and drugs likely to have interactions should be discontinued or substituted
- Stop herbal medications at least 7 days before surgery
- Avoid benzodiazepines and consider reducing dosage, when possible, in the geriatric age group
- Avoid meperidine for analgesia. Ensure effective analgesia to reduce the risk of postoperative delirium
- Antihistaminic H1 antagonists (such as diphenhydramine) with strong anticholinergic effects should be cautiously used

- CGA assessment is time-consuming and thus might not be appropriate in the preoperative period.
- *Preoperative Assessment of Cancer in Elderly (PACE)*: It is a scoring system used to evaluate eligibility for surgery in the oncogeriatric population.[10]

Cardiovascular and respiratory evaluation: Older patients often have cardiovascular and respiratory comorbidities that need a thorough evaluation and optimization.

- *Cardiovascular assessment:* According to the American College of Cardiology–American Heart Association (ACC-AHA) guidelines, electrocardiogram, echocardiography, and cardiac stress testing should be done if indicated. Look for the side effects of chemotherapy, especially anthracyclines.
- *Pulmonary function tests (PFTs):* Lung functions should be evaluated, especially in patients with a history of smoking, chronic respiratory disease, or prior chemotherapy, which can cause lung problems.

Laboratory and imaging studies:

- Routine preoperative laboratory tests and imaging studies done to identify any underlying conditions that may impact surgical outcomes
- *Laboratory tests:* Complete blood count (CBC), liver and renal function tests, coagulation profile, and electrolytes
- *Imaging studies:* Chest X-rays, computed tomography (CT) scans, and other relevant imaging depending on the disease type and location

Preoperative optimization:

Multidisciplinary team involvement: By conducting a thorough preoperative assessment, healthcare providers can better prepare major cancer surgery for geriatric patients, reducing the risk of complications and improving recovery. Based on the assessment, interventions may be required to optimize patient's condition before surgery. Preoperative optimization in geriatric patients undergoing major cancer surgery involves multiple strategies to enhance patient's physical and mental health, thus reducing surgical risks and improving outcomes.

- *Medical optimization:* Management and stabilization of chronic medical conditions
- *Nutritional support:* Addressing deficiencies and optimizing nutritional status
- Prehabilitation

Prehabilitation programs start from the time of diagnosis to treatment, in which functional capacity can be improved by a variety of means, including optimization of comorbidities, improved nutritional status, and cardiopulmonary function.

Management of comorbidities:

- *Cardiovascular diseases:* Control hypertension, heart failure, and arrhythmias. Consider cardiology consultation for patients with significant cardiac history.
- *Respiratory diseases:* Older patients are more prone to pulmonary complications. Risk reduction will involve medically optimizing the treatment of preexisting pulmonary disease, smoking reduction, pulmonary rehabilitation, with preoperative respiratory muscle training, and having selective chest imaging and pulmonary function testing.
- *Diabetes management:* Achieve optimal blood glucose control. Consult an endocrinologist, if necessary.
- *Renal function:* Ensure proper hydration, monitor renal function, and adjust medications as needed.

Cognitive and psychological support:

- *Cognitive training:* Engage in cognitive exercises and activities to maintain or improve cognitive function.
- *Delirium prevention:* Identify and mitigate risk factors for postoperative delirium **(Box 1)**.

Nutritional support: Nutritional assessment and intervention:

- *Assessment:* Use screening tools like MUST, Nutritional Risk Index (NRI index), or SGA to identify malnutrition.
- *Dietary counseling:* Provide personalized dietary advice to improve caloric and protein intake.
- *Supplements:* Consider oral nutritional supplements for patients with poor dietary intake and immunonutrition in selected patients.
- *Feeding support:* Consider enteral or parenteral nutrition in patients who are unable to maintain sufficient oral intake.

Physical conditioning:

- *Exercise training:* Implement an individualized structured exercise program focusing on strength, endurance, and flexibility, according to patient's ability and medical conditions.
- *Physical therapy:* Work with a physical therapist to improve mobility, balance, and functional status.
- *Nutritional optimization:* Protein supplementation (1.5 g/kg/day).
- Identify iron-deficiency anemia and management.

Optimization of functional status:
ADL training: An occupational therapist can improve ADLs and IADLs.

Social support assessment:
- *Caregiver support:* Identify and involve family members or caregivers in the preoperative and postoperative care plan.
- *Community resources:* Connect patients with community resources, such as home health services, transportation, and meal delivery programs.

Education and informed consent—patient and family education:
- *Surgery education:* Provide detailed information about the surgical procedure, potential risks, and expected outcomes.
- *Recovery expectations:* Educate patients and caregivers about the recovery process, including potential complications and signs to watch for.

Informed consent:
- *Discussion:* Assess patient's decision-making capacity. Ensure that patients with cognitive dysfunction have a healthcare proxy. It is important that the patient understands the risks, advantages, and availability of other nonsurgical alternatives. Obtain informed consent considering the patient's cognitive and emotional state.

Anesthetic and pain management planning:
Anesthetic evaluation:
- *Preoperative consultation:* Consult with the anesthesiologist to discuss anesthesia options and plan perioperative care tailored to the patient's health status.
- *Regional anesthesia:* Consider regional anesthesia techniques to reduce the need for general anesthesia and improve postoperative pain.

Pain management:
- *Multimodal analgesia:* Develop a pain management plan using a combination of medications and techniques to minimize opioid use and manage pain effectively.

A collaborative approach of the multidisciplinary team is required to ensure comprehensive preoperative optimization. Healthcare providers can enhance the readiness of major cancer surgery for geriatric patients, aiming to reduce complications and improve overall outcomes. Intraoperative management requires meticulous planning and execution to address the unique physiological challenges posed by advanced age. The goal is to ensure hemodynamic stability, minimize surgical stress, and reduce the risk of complications.

Preoperative anesthetic evaluation:
- *Comprehensive assessment:* Review the patient's medical history, comorbidities, medications, and preoperative optimization measures.
- *Anesthesia plan:* Develop an individualized anesthesia plan considering the patient's own physiological status and his surgical requirements.

Choice of anesthesia:
- *General anesthesia:* Carefully titrate anesthetic agents to avoid hemodynamic instability. Consider using short-acting agents to facilitate rapid recovery.
- *Regional anesthesia:* Use regional techniques (e.g., epidural, spinal, and nerve blocks) when appropriate to reduce the need for general anesthesia and provide better postoperative pain control.
- *Combined techniques:* General and regional anesthesia combined techniques may be beneficial in reducing the risk of pulmonary complications.
- *Monitored anesthesia care:* Considered in some patients undergoing appropriate surgeries with doses of sedation drugs adjusted.
- *Medication dose adjustment:* Evaluate all prescription and nonprescription medications for potential interactions and side effects. Adjust dosages, discontinue nonessential drugs, and address polypharmacy.
- Succinylcholine-prolonged duration with reduced plasma cholinesterase levels in Alzheimer's disease and dementia patients who are being treated concomitantly with cholinesterase inhibitors.
- Monoamine oxidase inhibitors can cause potentially fatal cholinergic interactions with meperidine.
- Withhold angiotensin-converting enzyme inhibitors on the day of surgery to avoid significant hypotension during anesthesia induction.
- Preoperative review of anticoagulants ensuring adherence to guidelines before regional procedures so that surgery can be performed safely
- Opioids increase the risk of hypoventilation due to increased brain sensitivity and decreased clearance of opioids exaggerated by the synergistic use of benzodiazepines, which can result in adverse respiratory events.
- Etomidate, dexmedetomidine, and ketamine reduce the incidence of cardiorespiratory depression as compared to propofol or benzodiazepine.

- Nondepolarizing muscle relaxants (vecuronium and rocuronium) should be used cautiously as they have a prolonged duration of action. Cisatracurium or atracurium is mostly preferred, as its metabolism is independent of kidney or liver function.
- Drug reconciliation should be done with the surgical team to ensure patient safety.

Hemodynamic monitoring and management:
Invasive monitoring:
- *Arterial line:* Continuous BP monitoring is considered in high-risk surgeries for accurate hemodynamic assessment and management.
- *Central venous catheter:* Used for central venous pressure (CVP) monitoring and medications or fluid administration as needed.

Fluid management:
Restrictive or goal-directed fluid strategies are preferred.
- *Goal-directed therapy:* Use goal-directed fluid therapy with vasoactive medications to maintain optimal fluid balance and tissue perfusion, avoiding both hypovolemia and fluid overload in high-risk surgeries.

 While considering the fluid strategy, the effects of age, comorbidities, anesthetic agents, patient's volume status, and tissue perfusion all need to be considered and should be individualized.
- *Blood products:* Blood products should be administered if necessary, considering patient's age and comorbidities.

Respiratory management:
Ventilation strategies:
- *Lung-protective ventilation:* Use lower tidal volumes and positive end-expiratory pressure (PEEP) to minimize the risk of lung injury associated with mechanical ventilation.
- *Adequate oxygenation:* Ensure adequate oxygenation and ventilation, adjusting settings based on blood gas analysis and pulse oximeter readings.

Temperature management (maintain normothermia):
- *Continuous monitoring:* Monitor core body temperature throughout surgery.
- *Active warming:* Prevent perioperative hypothermia.

Positioning: Geriatric patients have more intraoperative injuries to pressure points due to poor circulatory flow and decreased skin integrity. Proper positioning and padding of bony prominences should be ensured perioperatively.

Intraoperative pain management:
Multimodal analgesia: Pain management planning should include a mix of medications and techniques so as to minimize the usage of opioids.

Regional anesthesia: Utilize epidural or spinal anesthesia for intraoperative and postoperative pain control.
- *Intravenous analgesics:* Administer opioids judiciously, supplemented with nonopioid analgesics [e.g., acetaminophen and nonsteroidal anti-inflammatory drugs (NSAIDs)] to minimize opioid use. NSAIDs should be used judiciously in older patients to avoid renal injury.
- *Local anesthetics:* Infiltrate local anesthetics at the surgical site to provide additional pain relief.

Blood glucose management:
- *Monitoring:* Regularly monitor blood glucose levels to maintain optimal glycemic control and avoid both hyperglycemia and hypoglycemia. Insulin therapy can be used as needed to manage blood glucose levels, considering patient's diabetic status and stress response to surgery.

Minimizing surgical stress:
Surgical technique:
- *Minimally invasive surgery:* Prefer minimally invasive techniques (e.g., laparoscopy and robotic) when feasible to reduce surgical trauma and facilitate faster recovery.
- *Gentle handling:* Careful tissue handling and hemostasis to minimize intraoperative bleeding and tissue damage.

Reduced operative time:
- *Efficiency:* Aim to minimize operative time without compromising the quality of the surgical procedure, reducing the duration of anesthesia and exposure to surgical stress.

Postoperative period: Postoperative care for geriatric patients following major cancer surgery is crucial for enhancing recovery, minimizing complications, and ensuring a return to baseline functional status.

The essential components of postoperative care include the following:
- *Extubation planning:* Assess readiness for extubation based on respiratory function and overall status of the patient.

- *Noninvasive ventilation:* Consider noninvasive ventilation [e.g., continuous positive airway pressure (CPAP) and bi-level continuous positive airway pressure (BiPAP)] postoperatively if needed to support respiratory function.

Monitoring and early detection of complications:
Intensive care: Patients with higher postoperative complications risk are admitted to intensive care units (ICUs) or high-dependency units (HDUs) for monitoring. Continuous monitoring of BP, heart rate, respiratory rate, and oxygen saturation is necessary in the postoperative period.

Laboratory tests:
- *Regular labs:* Monitor CBC, electrolytes, renal function, and blood glucose levels to detect abnormalities.
- *Arterial blood gases (ABGs):* Assess respiratory function and acid–base balance postoperatively, especially in patients with pre-existing respiratory conditions.

Respiratory complications: Atelectasis, pneumonia, and respiratory failure.

Care for respiratory hygiene includes the following:
- Chest physical therapy, incentive spirometry with deep breathing exercises prevents atelectasis and pneumonia, provides lung support. Usage of aspiration prophylaxis precautions and intraoperative regional anesthesia techniques is preferred in these patients.
- Supplemental oxygen maintains adequate oxygenation if needed.
- *Noninvasive ventilation:* CPAP or BiPAP for patients with respiratory insufficiency.

Postoperative nausea and vomiting: Although advanced age is not a risk factor, prophylactic interventions should be applied to elderly adults at moderate or high risk of postoperative nausea and vomiting. Appropriate risk stratification is important in the geriatric population to avoid medications, such as scopolamine, that may precipitate confusion and postoperative delirium.

Postoperative pain management: It is challenging as patients have a reduced perception of pain and are often undertreated for it. Therefore, a multimodal analgesic plan should be designed for this patient cohort.
- *Acetaminophen:* Given for milder intensity pain, via several routes—oral, intravenous, or rectal.
- Nonopioid alternatives include NSAIDs (judiciously given due to nephrotoxic effects), adjuvants like gabapentin or pregabalin, and other modalities, such as music, acupuncture, and massage therapy.
- Regional techniques (neuraxial or nerve blocks) reduce the requirement for systemic opioids.
- *Opioids:* Reduce dose if indicated, and patients require monitoring in the recovery room or ICU.
- Patient-controlled analgesia (PCA) for unsettled pain leads to improved patient satisfaction.

Prophylaxis and preventive measures:
Thromboembolism prevention:
- *Pharmacologic prophylaxis:* Administer anticoagulants (e.g., low-molecular-weight heparin) as recommended to reduce the risk of developing deep vein thrombosis and pulmonary embolism.
- *Mechanical prophylaxis:* Use graduated compression stockings or intermittent pneumatic compression devices.

Infection prevention:
- *Antibiotic prophylaxis:* Prophylactic antibiotics should be administered based on the surgical site and type of surgery to prevent surgical site infections.
- *Aseptic technique:* Strict aseptic techniques should be adhered to throughout the surgical procedure.

Hemodynamic support:
- *Fluid management:* Maintain optimal fluid balance with careful monitoring of fluid intake and output to maintain effective volume status and avoid inadequate tissue perfusion.
- *Medications:* Administer antihypertensives, diuretics, or inotropes as needed to manage BP and cardiac output.

Thromboembolism prevention:
- *Pharmacologic prophylaxis:* Continue anticoagulants (e.g., low-molecular-weight heparin) as per guidelines.
- *Mechanical prophylaxis:* Use intermittent pneumatic compression devices and encourage early mobilization.

Gastrointestinal care:
- *Early oral or enteral feeds:* As soon as feasible to promote healing and recovery.
- *Diet progression:* Gradually advance the diet from clear liquids to full liquids and then to solid foods based on tolerance level.

Bowel function:
- *Laxatives:* Use stool softeners or mild laxatives to prevent constipation, particularly in patients on opioids.
- *Monitoring:* Monitor for signs of ileus or bowel obstruction.

Wound care:

Surgical-site management:

- *Dressing changes:* Perform regular dressing changes using aseptic technique.
- *Monitoring:* Watch for signs of infection, dehiscence, or other complications.

Infection prevention:

Continue prophylactic antibiotics as per protocol and monitor for signs of infection while maintaining strict hygiene and aseptic techniques during wound care.

Mobilization and rehabilitation:

Early mobilization:

- *Ambulation:* Encourage patients to get out of bed and walk as soon as safe to do so.
- *Physical therapy:* Engage physical therapists to develop individualized exercise programs to improve strength, balance, and mobility.

Postoperative delirium:

- It is associated with increased mortality and longer ICU care and hospital stay and thus poor outcomes. Early screening for postoperative delirium in high-risk patients using screening tools can lead to optimal and effective early treatment.
- *Management:* Treat underlying causes, followed by multicomponent nonpharmacologic interventions. Pharmacologic treatment should be considered only for highly agitated, hyperactive behavior in patients who are likely to harm themselves or others.

Cognitive monitoring:

- *Cognitive stimulation:* Provide cognitive activities to engage the patient and prevent cognitive decline.

Psychological support: Psychological counseling or psychiatric support should be offered to address anxiety, depression, or other mental health concerns with support groups for emotional and social support.

Communication and coordination:

- *Multidisciplinary involvement and team communication:* Maintain communication with the entire surgical team, including anesthesiologists, surgeons, nurses, and other specialists with postoperative debriefings done to ensure all team members are informed about the patient's status and intraoperative events.

By implementing these strategies, the entire team can effectively manage the perioperative care of geriatric patients undergoing major cancer surgery, aiming to optimize outcomes and enhance recovery.

To summarize, the ACS-NSQIP guidelines have recommended preoperative assessment of surgical geriatric patients **(Box 4)**.[7]

BOX 4: ACS-NSQIP guidelines for preoperative assessment of surgical geriatric patients.

- Evaluation of patient's cognition and mental state and comprehension of the impending surgery
- Check for depressive episodes
- Identify risk factors for developing delirium in the postoperative period
- Screen for alcoholism and other likelihood of substance abuse or dependence
- For patients undergoing noncardiac surgery, perform a preoperative cardiac examination according to the American College of Cardiology/American Heart Association (ACC/AHA) criteria
- Determine factors that increase the risk of postoperative respiratory complications. Implement measures to avoid these complications
- Proper documentation of physical functional condition and any prior history of falls
- Document frailty score prior to surgery
- Document patient's preoperative nutritional status. If the patient is at severe nutritional risk, carry out appropriate interventions
- A detailed medication history should be taken to make appropriate perioperative adjustments in drug dosage. Avoid polypharmacy
- Ensure patient's treatment goals and expectations are met with the possible treatment outcomes
- Family and social support system should be looked into in the preoperative period
- Ask for appropriate diagnostic tests for elderly patients

CONCLUSION

Anesthesia for geriatric patients is challenging and complex due to their vulnerability to the stresses of hospitalization, anesthesia, and surgical procedures. Anesthesiologists should have a knowledge of the physiological, pharmacokinetic, and pharmacodynamic differences in these patients prior to subjecting these patients for surgery. A holistic, patient-centered approach involving a multidisciplinary team of surgeons, geriatricians, oncologists, anesthesiologists, physical therapists, nutritionists, and social workers and a careful perioperative management plan is needed to have the best outcomes for these patients.

REFERENCES

1. Amornyotin S. Anesthetic consideration for geriatric patients. In: Amornyotin S (Ed). Update in Geriatrics. London: Intechopen Limited; 2021 .p. 510.
2. Staheli B, Rondeau B. Anesthetic considerations in the geriatric population. In: StatPearls [Internet]. Treasure Island (FL): StatPearls Publishing; 2025.
3. Eamer G, Taheri A, Chen SS, Daviduck Q, Chambers T, Shi X, et al. Comprehensive geriatric assessment for older people admitted to a surgical service. Cochrane Database Syst Rev. 2018;1(1):CD012485.
4. Partridge JS, Harari D, Martin FC, Peacock JL, Bell R, Mohammed A, et al. Randomized clinical trial of comprehensive geriatric assessment and optimization in vascular surgery. Br J Surg. 2017;104(6):679-87.
5. Pang CL, Gooneratne M, Partridge JSL. Preoperative assessment of the older patient. BJA Educ. 2021;21(8):314-20.
6. Aceto P, Incalzi RA, Bettelli G, Carron M, Chiumiento F, Corcione A, et al. Perioperative Management of Elderly patients (PriME): recommendations from an Italian intersociety consensus. Aging Clin Exp Res. 2020;32(9):1647-73.
7. Chow WB, Cho CY, Rosenthal RA, Esnaola NF. ACS NSQIP/AGS Best Practice Guidelines: Optimal Preoperative Assessment of the Geriatric Surgical Patient; 2012.
8. Cook DJ. Geriatric anesthesia. In: New Frontiers in Geriatrics Research. American Geriatrics Association; 2004. pp. 9-14.
9. Aitken R, Harun NS, Maier AB. Which preoperative screening tool should be applied to older patients undergoing elective surgery to predict short-term postoperative outcomes? Lessons from systematic reviews, meta-analyses and guidelines. Intern Emerg Med. 2021;16(1):37-48.
10. Pope D, Ramesh H, Gennari R, Corsini G, Maffezzini M, Hoekstra HJ, et al. Pre-operative assessment of cancer in the elderly (PACE): a comprehensive assessment of underlying characteristics of elderly cancer patients prior to elective surgery. Surg Oncol. 2006;15(4):189-97.

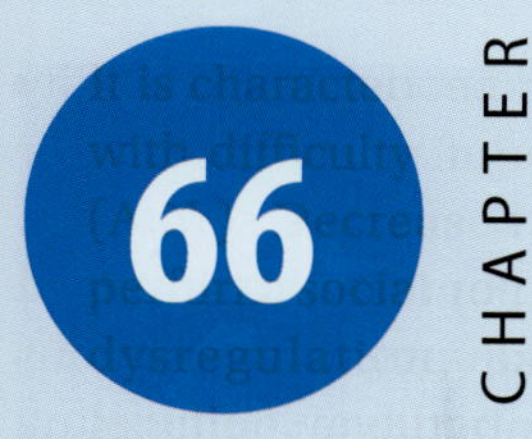

CHAPTER

Opioid-sparing and Opioid-free Onco-Anesthesia

Sohan Lal Solanki, Ankita Kadam

INTRODUCTION

Pain is a predictable consequence of surgery. Managing pain effectively poses a significant challenge for anesthesiologists, as poorly managed pain can lead to undesirable outcomes in the postoperative period.[1]

Opioids have long been considered the cornerstone for managing intraoperative and postoperative pain.[2] They are an integral part of balanced general anesthesia and remain a critical element of modern perioperative care. However, the use of opioids is associated with a range of short- and long-term adverse effects.[3,4]

To address these challenges, anesthesiologists and surgeons have increasingly adopted opioid-sparing analgesic techniques. These techniques involve the use of adjuncts to manage perioperative pain while minimizing opioid-related side effects.[5,6] OFA is a multimodal antinociception technique that relies exclusively on nonopioid agents during the perioperative period, avoiding the systemic, neuraxial, or intracavitary administration of opioids.[7,8]

HISTORY OF OPIOIDS

The medicinal use of natural opiates, such as opium derived from poppy juice, dates back to at least 300 BCE.[9,10] Opiates are a group of drugs derived from opium. Morphine, the most well-known opiate, was isolated in 1803, followed by codeine in 1832 and papaverine in 1848.[11]

The history of synthetic opioids began in the mid-20th century, with fentanyl synthesized in 1960 and first described for anesthesia use in 1962. The development of synthetic drugs with morphine-like properties expanded the definition of "opioid" to encompass all exogenous substances—natural and synthetic—that bind to opioid receptors and produce morphine-like effects.[12,13] Opioids are unique in providing analgesia without impairing touch, proprioception, or consciousness.

CHANGING TRENDS IN ANESTHESIA PRACTICE

On October 16, 1846, the first public demonstration of ether anesthesia took place, marking a turning point in surgical care.[14] Ether was initially used as a single anesthetic agent, but high doses often led to complications, including hemodynamic instability.

To address these issues, the concept of balanced general anesthesia was introduced by John Lundy in 1926. This approach involves the use of multiple drugs to achieve clinical goals such as unconsciousness, immobility, and muscle relaxation.[15]

The introduction of potent synthetic opioids, such as fentanyl, further advanced balanced general anesthesia, providing hemodynamic stability by inhibiting sympathetic responses without cardiovascular collapse or histamine release.[16] Opioids also mimic endogenous analgesic mechanisms, enhancing patient comfort and safety.

However, over the past two decades, concerns about opioid-related side effects have driven the development of opioid-sparing and OFA techniques.[17]

OPIOID SIDE EFFECTS

While opioids remain the most potent analgesics for managing acute perioperative pain,[18] their intraoperative use is associated with a range of complications, including postoperative sedation, nausea, and vomiting; respiratory depression and airway complications; paralytic ileus and urinary retention; prolonged hospital stays; increased healthcare costs; and decreased patient satisfaction.[19]

Opioid-induced hyperalgesia (OIH) is another significant concern, characterized by heightened sensitivity to pain due to nociceptive sensitization. OIH can occur after a single opioid dose or prolonged use, complicating postoperative pain management.[20]

OPIOID IMMUNOMODULATION AND CANCER RECURRENCE

Pain is a prevalent symptom among cancer patients, and opioids are commonly used for perioperative and chronic pain management. However, opioid-induced immunosuppression may contribute to cancer recurrence.

Opioids can alter immunity via neuroendocrine pathways or direct effects on immune cells, including the suppression of natural killer cell activity, which is critical for tumor surveillance. While prolonged opioid exposure is more likely to cause immunosuppression, the role of opioids in cancer progression remains controversial, with conflicting evidence from existing studies.[21-23]

BENEFITS OF OPIOID-FREE ANESTHESIA

Opioid-free anesthesia has demonstrated safety and efficacy in patients with conditions such as obstructive sleep apnea, obesity, asthma, and chronic obstructive pulmonary disease (COPD). It is particularly beneficial in oncologic surgeries.[24]

Opioid-free anesthesia strategies align with enhanced recovery after surgery (ERAS) protocols, facilitating early recovery with the following advantages: Faster ambulation and early oral hydration. Minimal parental fluid requirements. Reduced opioid-related side effects. Improved overall safety and patient outcomes.[25]

RATIONALE BEHIND THE USE OF NONOPIOID ADJUNCTS

The International Association for the Study of Pain defines pain as "an unpleasant sensory or emotional experience associated with actual or potential tissue damage or described in terms of such damage."[26] The unpleasant sensory and emotional nature of pain requires conscious awareness, making pain a conscious and distressing perception of noxious stimuli. This leads to hemodynamic changes such as tachycardia, hypertension, hyperventilation, and withdrawal responses, accompanied by discomfort. During surgery under general anesthesia, the patient is unconscious with adequate hypnosis [bispectral index (BIS) 40–60] and paralysis, preventing the conscious experience of pain. In such cases, only nociception is experienced. Surgical tissue insult activates nociceptive pathways, triggering autonomic reactions like tachycardia and hypertension. These responses are common clinical indicators of inadequate antinociception. The primary intraoperative objective, therefore, is to achieve hemodynamic stability by suppressing the consequences of noxious receptor stimulation. Numerous mediators, such as serotonin, norepinephrine, enkephalins, and peptides, are involved in the pain pathway. Nonopioid adjuncts target various components of the nociceptive pathway, inhibiting cardiovascular and neuroendocrine stress responses and thereby achieving hemodynamic stability.

COMPONENTS OF OPIOID-FREE ANESTHESIA

Opioid-free anesthesia interventions target peripheral, afferent, efferent, and central neural pathways. Analgesic strategies may interfere with one or multiple sites along the pain pathway. The following drugs are commonly employed to manage acute postoperative pain:

- Acetaminophen
- *Alpha-2 agonists:* Clonidine, Dexmedetomidine
- *Gabapentinoids:* Gabapentin, Pregabalin
- Ketamine
- Lidocaine
- Magnesium sulfate
- Nonsteroidal anti-inflammatory drugs (NSAIDs)
- Local anesthetics

PRE-EMPTIVE ANALGESIA

Pre-emptive analgesia is a proactive approach where treatment begins before surgery to prevent the central sensitization caused by incisional and inflammatory injuries during surgery and the early postoperative period.[27] This protective effect on the nociceptive system may make pre-emptive analgesia more effective than initiating similar treatments postoperatively. Commonly used agents include NSAIDs, ketamine, systemic antiepileptics (e.g., pregabalin and gabapentin), and local anesthetics via neuraxial administration, peripheral nerve blocks, or wound infiltrations.[28] Each drug class offers unique advantages and disadvantages.

NONSTEROIDAL ANTI-INFLAMMATORY DRUGS

Nonsteroidal anti-inflammatory drugs are a diverse group of analgesics with varying pharmacokinetic properties. Despite these differences, NSAIDs share several general characteristics. They are Food and Drugs Administration (FDA)-approved for antipyretic, anti-inflammatory, and analgesic purposes,[29] making them a first-line therapy in OFA for mild to moderate pain. However, their use is limited due to risks such as gastrointestinal and surgical site bleeding, as well as renal toxicity.

Acetaminophen

Acetaminophen, a nonopioid analgesic and antipyretic agent, is used to treat mild to moderate pain. It is frequently recommended for postsurgical pain management alongside NSAIDs.[30] Acetaminophen is integral to ERAS protocols. Intravenous administration bypasses liver metabolism, enhancing its safety profile. Its lack of effect on platelet function makes it suitable for use throughout surgical procedures.

Ketamine

Ketamine is an *N*-methyl-d-aspartate (NMDA) receptor antagonist with analgesic, amnesic, and opioid-sparing properties. It modulates pain transmission by acting on NMDA receptors in the brain and spinal cord and enhancing endogenous antinociceptive systems.[31] Perioperative ketamine use reduces postoperative pain scores and opioid consumption.[32]

Intravenous Lidocaine

Lidocaine, an amide local anesthetic, is administered intravenously during surgery to provide postoperative analgesia and reduce opioid consumption. Its analgesic and anti-inflammatory properties are well-documented, although its exact mechanism remains unclear.[33] A loading dose of 1–2 mg/kg, followed by an infusion at 1–2 mg/kg/h, is recommended, with administration ceasing within 1 hour post surgery to avoid local anesthetic systemic toxicity (LAST). Intravenous lidocaine is particularly beneficial in abdominal and spine surgeries.[34]

Magnesium

Magnesium has diverse actions, including bronchodilation, antiarrhythmic effects, antihypertensive properties, and neuroprotection in pre-eclampsia. It is a noncompetitive NMDA receptor antagonist that inhibits calcium influx.[35,36] Intraoperative magnesium administration has opioid-sparing effects, reduces pain scores, and decreases postoperative pain and opioid requirements. The recommended loading dose is 30–50 mg/kg over 10–15 minutes, followed by an infusion of 6–25 mg/kg/h. Close monitoring is essential to prevent magnesium toxicity.[37]

Gabapentinoids

Gabapentin and pregabalin bind to the $\alpha 2\delta 2$ subunit of presynaptic voltage-gated calcium channels, modulating excitatory neurotransmitter release in the dorsal horn and activating descending antinociceptive pathways.[38,39] Gabapentinoids produce significant opioid-sparing effects and reduce postoperative pain scores.[40] However, side effects such as sedation, dizziness, and neurocognitive dysfunction limit their use. Research is ongoing to optimize their perioperative application.

Alpha-2 Agonists

Alpha-2 agonists, such as dexmedetomidine and clonidine, stimulate $\alpha 2$-adrenergic receptors in the dorsal horn of the spinal cord and the locus coeruleus, exhibiting sedative, hypnotic, and analgesic properties.[41] Dexmedetomidine is 7–10 times more potent than clonidine.[42] It induces conscious sedation akin to natural sleep but may cause bradycardia and hypotension, even with single doses.

GENERAL CONSIDERATIONS FOR PERIOPERATIVE USE OF OPIOIDS

An expert committee from the Society of Onco-Anesthesia and Perioperative Care (SOAPC) has compiled best-practice evidence and expert opinions to draft perioperative consensus practice guidelines on the safe use of opioids in oncologic surgeries. Anesthesiologists and surgeons must balance three key considerations to optimize perioperative analgesia: The first is antinociception—ensuring adequate pain relief. The second is to minimize opioid-related adverse drug events (ORADEs)—reducing the risk of side effects associated with opioids, and the third is to limit opioid prescriptions at discharge—minimizing potential opioid-related adverse effects and the risk of misuse or abuse.[43]

Regional analgesia techniques, coupled with the judicious use of nonopioid agents such as NSAIDs, can significantly reduce or eliminate the need for opioids during the perioperative period.[44,45] A patient- and procedure-specific perioperative analgesia plan is essential, encompassing pain management strategies throughout the surgical journey from preoperative to postoperative phases.

Perioperative Strategies

- *Regional techniques:* For intraoperative and post-operative analgesia, preoperative placement of an

TABLE 1: Opioid-free anesthesia options in cancer surgeries.

Type of cancer surgery	*OFA techniques and medications*	*Bolus dose*	*Infusion dose*	*Advantages*	*Disadvantages*
Neurological cancer surgery	• Propofol infusion (TIVA) • Dexmedetomidine infusion • Magnesium sulfate • Ketamine (low dose for NMDA antagonism) • Scalp nerve blocks (e.g., supraorbital, auriculotemporal)	• *Propofol:* 1–2 mg/kg • *Dexmedetomidine:* 1 µg/kg over 10 min • *Magnesium sulfate:* 30–50 mg/kg	• *Propofol:* 50–150 µg/kg/min • *Dexmedetomidine:* 0.2–0.7 µg/kg/h • *Magnesium:* 5–15 mg/kg/h	• Stable hemodynamics • Reduced ICP • Neuroprotection	• Risk of sedation or delayed recovery • Monitoring required for magnesium and propofol infusions
Head and neck cancer surgeries (including free flap)	• TIVA with propofol • Dexmedetomidine infusion • Local anesthetic infiltration • Lidocaine infusion • Magnesium sulfate	• *Dexmedetomidine:* 1 µg/kg over 10 min • *Lidocaine:* 1–1.5 mg/kg	• *Dexmedetomidine:* 0.2–0.7 µg/kg/h • *Lidocaine:* 1–2 mg/min	• Effective hemodynamic stability • Reduced pain scores • Improved graft outcomes	• Risk of sedation • Requires meticulous monitoring
Thoracic cancer surgery	• Thoracic epidural analgesia (local anesthetics) • Paravertebral blocks • Serratus anterior plane block • Ketamine infusion • Lidocaine infusion • Magnesium sulfate	• *Ketamine:* 0.5 mg/kg • *Lidocaine:* 1–1.5 mg/kg • *Magnesium:* 30–50 mg/kg	• *Ketamine:* 0.1–0.3 mg/kg/h • *Lidocaine:* 1–2 mg/min • *Magnesium:* 5–15 mg/kg/h	• Excellent analgesia • Reduced opioid-related side effects • Improved respiratory outcomes	• Risk of local anesthetic toxicity • Potential bradycardia with magnesium
Breast cancer surgeries	• Pectoral nerve blocks (Pecs I and II) • Serratus anterior plane block • Dexmedetomidine infusion • Magnesium sulfate • TIVA with propofol and lidocaine	• *Dexmedetomidine:* 1 µg/kg over 10 minutes • *Lidocaine:* 1–1.5 mg/kg	• *Dexmedetomidine:* 0.2–0.7 µg/kg/h • *Lidocaine:* 1–2 mg/min	• Effective pain relief • Early recovery • Minimal systemic side effects	• Risk of block failure • Dexmedetomidine may cause bradycardia or hypotension
Gastrointestinal and HPB cancer surgeries	• Thoracic epidural or spinal analgesia • Transversus abdominis plane (TAP) block • Rectus sheath block • Ketamine infusion • Lidocaine infusion • Dexmedetomidine	• *Ketamine:* 0.5 mg/kg • *Lidocaine:* 1–1.5 mg/kg • *Dexmedetomidine:* 1 µg/kg over 10 minutes	• *Ketamine:* 0.1–0.3 mg/kg/h • *Lidocaine:* 1–2 mg/min • *Dexmedetomidine:* 0.2–0.7 µg/kg/h	• Multimodal pain relief • Faster bowel recovery • Reduced opioid-related complications	• Risk of hemodynamic instability with epidurals • Monitoring required for lidocaine infusion

Contd...

Contd...

Type of cancer surgery	***OFA techniques and medications***	***Bolus dose***	***Infusion dose***	***Advantages***	***Disadvantages***
Gynecological cancer surgeries	• Epidural analgesia • Quadratus lumborum block • TAP block • Magnesium sulfate • Ketamine infusion • Dexmedetomidine	• *Magnesium:* 30–50 mg/kg • *Ketamine:* 0.5 mg/kg • *Dexmedetomidine:* 1 µg/kg over 10 minutes	• *Magnesium:* 5–15 mg/kg/h • *Ketamine:* 0.1–0.3 mg/kg/h • *Dexmedetomidine:* 0.2–0.7 µg/kg/h	• Effective analgesia for open and laparoscopic procedures • Early mobilization	• Risk of block failure • Hypotension or sedation with magnesium or dexmedetomidine infusions
Urological cancer surgeries	• Thoracic epidural analgesia • Quadratus lumborum block • Lidocaine infusion • Ketamine infusion • Magnesium sulfate	• *Ketamine:* 0.5 mg/kg • *Lidocaine:* 1–1.5 mg/kg • *Magnesium:* 30–50 mg/kg	• *Ketamine:* 0.1–0.3 mg/kg/h • *Lidocaine:* 1–2 mg/min • *Magnesium:* 5–15 mg/kg/h	• Optimized pain control • Reduced postoperative complications	• Potential for toxicity with lidocaine • Monitoring required for magnesium and ketamine infusions
Bone and soft-tissue cancer surgeries	• Regional nerve blocks (e.g., brachial plexus, femoral, or sciatic blocks) • TIVA with propofol • Ketamine infusion • Dexmedetomidine infusion	• *Ketamine:* 0.5 mg/kg • *Dexmedetomidine:* 1 µg/kg over 10 minutes	• *Ketamine:* 0.1–0.3 mg/kg/h • *Dexmedetomidine:* 0.2–0.7 µg/kg/h	• Superior regional pain relief • Enhanced functional recovery • Minimized systemic side effects	• Risk of block failure • Hemodynamic effects of dexmedetomidine or ketamine infusions
Pediatric cancer surgeries	• Thoracic epidural analgesia • Caudal epidural block • Peripheral nerve blocks • Dexmedetomidine infusion • Ketamine infusion • Paracetamol and NSAIDs for adjunctive analgesia	• *Ketamine:* 0.5 mg/kg • *Dexmedetomidine:* 0.5–1 µg/kg	• *Ketamine:* 0.1–0.3 mg/kg/h • *Dexmedetomidine:* 0.2–0.7 µg/kg/h	• Superior pain control • Reduced opioid side effects • Safe for children	• Risk of sedation or hemodynamic effects • Requires weight-based dose adjustments

(HPB: hepato-pancreato-biliary; NMDA: *N*-methyl-d-aspartate; ICP: intracranial pressure; NSAIDs: nonsteroidal anti-inflammatory drugs; OFA: opioid-free anesthesia; TIVA: total intravenous anesthesia) epidural catheter, regional nerve blocks, or fascial plane catheters is recommended wherever feasible. Local anesthetics such as bupivacaine or ropivacaine should be used in these techniques.

- *Avoiding opioids in regional blocks:* Adjuvants like α-2 agonists (dexmedetomidine or clonidine) may be used to prolong the analgesic effects of local anesthetics without adding opioids.
- *Nonopioid adjuvants:* Intraoperative analgesia may include nonopioid agents such as acetaminophen (paracetamol), NSAIDs, α-2 agonists, lidocaine, or ketamine, either alone or in combination.
- *Postoperative analgesia:* Acetaminophen and NSAIDs can continue to provide pain relief. When opioids are used in the postoperative period for acute pain management, they should be transitioned to nonopioid medications once the acute phase resolves. Strong opioid prescriptions should not be issued for home use upon discharge.

Currently, there is no robust evidence favoring one analgesic technique or combination of nonopioid adjuncts over another. Each plan should be individualized to the patient and surgical procedure.

OPIOID-FREE ANESTHESIA PROTOCOLS

According to studies in clinical practice, the most commonly modified OFA techniques are those described by Mulier.[46] SOAPC also described the multimodal opioid-sparing oncoanesthesia techniques for cancer surgical patients.[47] OFA protocols typically include the following steps:

- *Preoperative premedication:* Intravenous pregabalin, gabapentin, or midazolam is administered at least 1 hour before surgery.[46-48]
- *Induction of OFA:* Dexmedetomidine is initiated 10–20 minutes before intubation to achieve a sympathetic block.[46-49] For adequate sympatholysis, analgesia, and anesthesia, coinduction with low doses of ketamine or lidocaine infusion is recommended, starting 10 minutes before intubation. Since intubation is a strong noxious stimulus, additional bolus doses of intravenous propofol and muscle relaxants, calculated based on ideal body weight (IBW), are used.
- *Maintenance of OFA:* Dexmedetomidine, lidocaine, or ketamine is used in combination with an inhalation agent [minimum alveolar concentration (MAC) of 0.5–1.0%] and neuromuscular blocking drugs if required for surgery. Magnesium infusion may be added as a coanalgesic if needed.
- *Discontinuation:* OFA agents are usually stopped 20 minutes before emergence.
- *Adjunctive measures:* Antiemetics, including dexamethasone boluses, are administered. Locoregional techniques for pain management, combined with nonopioid systemic analgesic medications, are employed as part of a patient- and procedure-specific multimodal opioid-sparing analgesia plan.
- Opioid-free anesthesia options in cancer surgeries are given in **Table 1**.

CONCLUSION

Opioid-free anesthesia represents the future of anesthesia practice, promising significant advancements in perioperative pain management. By replacing opioids with alternative analgesic strategies, OFA aims to reduce opioid-related side effects, facilitate earlier mobilization, enable faster discharge, and enhance patient satisfaction. The prescription of potent opioids for home use at discharge should be avoided. Clear instructions about the safe and judicious use of opioids, along with provisions for the return or disposal of unused medications, are essential. While laboratory investigations and low-quality human studies have raised concerns about the potential effects of opioids on cancer recurrence, current evidence remains inconclusive. Further high-quality research is required to substantiate these findings.

REFERENCES

1. Joshi GP, Kehlet H. Postoperative pain management in the era of ERAS: an overview. Best Pract Res Clin Anaesthesiol. 2019;33(3):259-67.
2. Yaksh TL, Wallace MS. Opioids, analgesia, and pain management. In: Brunton L, Chabner BA, Knollman B (Eds). Goodman and Gilman's: The Pharmacological Basis of Therapeutics. New York: McGraw Hill; 2011. pp. 481-526.
3. Oderda GM, Senagore AJ, Morland K, Iqbal SU, Kugel M, Liu S, et al. Opioid-related respiratory and gastrointestinal adverse events in patients with acute postoperative pain: prevalence, predictors, and burden. J Pain Palliative Care Pharmacother. 2019;33(3-4):82-97.
4. Gayer S, Palte H. Postoperative Nausea and Vomiting After Abdominal Surgery in Gastrointestinal and Colorectal Anaesthesia. CRC Press; 2016. pp. 403-16.
5. Kumar K, Kirksey MA, Duong S, Wu CL. A review of opioid-sparing modalities in perioperative pain management:

methods to decrease opioid use postoperatively. Anaesth Analg. 2017;125(5):1749-60.
6. Shanthanna H, Ladha KS, Kehlet H, Joshi GP. Perioperative opioid administration: a critical review of opioid-free versus opioid-sparing approaches. Anesthesiology. 2021;134(4):645-59.
7. Forget P. Opioid-free anaesthesia. Why and how? A contextual analysis. Anaesth Crit Care Pain Med. 2019;38(2):169-72.
8. Gupta L, Agarwal J, Saxena KN. Opioid-free anaesthesia: the conundrum and the solutions. Indian J Anaesth. 2022;66(Suppl 2):S91-4.
9. Kapoor L. Opium Poppy: Botany, Chemistry, and Pharmacology. CRC Press; 2020.
10. Kumar V. Handbook on Opium: History and Basis of Opioids in Therapeutics. Philadelphia: Elsevier; 2022.
11. Kaboudin B, Sohrabi M. Chemistry and synthesis of major opium alkaloids: a comprehensive review. J Iran Chem Soc. 2021;18(12):3177-218.
12. Nordal A. Natural and synthetic drugs with morphine-like effects considered from a pharmacognostic point of view. Bull Narcotics. 1956;8(1):18.
13. Eddy NB, Halbach H, Braenden OJ. Synthetic substances with morphine-like effect. Bull World Health Org. 1956;14(3):353-402.
14. Viets HR. The earliest printed references in newspapers and journals to the first public demonstration of ether anaesthesia in 1846. J Hist Med Allied Sci. 1949;4(2):149-69.
15. Ellis II TA, Narr BJ, Bacon DR. Developing a specialty: JS Lundy's three major contributions to anesthesiology. J Clin Anesth. 2004;16(3):226-9.
16. Stanley TH. The history of opioid use in anesthetic delivery. In: Eger EI II, Saidman LJ, Westhorpe RN (Eds) The Wondrous Story of Anesthesia. New York: Springer; 2014. pp. 641-59.
17. Siu EY, Moon TS. Opioid-free and opioid-sparing anesthesia. Int Anesthesiol Clin. 2020;58(2):34-41.
18. Egan TD. Are opioids indispensable for general anaesthesia? Br J Anaesth. 2019;122(6):e127-35.
19. Wheeler M, Oderda GM, Ashburn MA, Lipman AG. Adverse events associated with postoperative opioid analgesia: a systematic review. J Pain. 2002;3(3):159-80.
20. Yi P, Pryzbylkowski P. Opioid induced hyperalgesia. Pain Med. 2015;16(suppl_1):S32-6.
21. Rittner HL, Roewer N, Brack A. The clinical (ir) relevance of opioid-induced immune suppression. Curr Opin Anesthesiol. 2010;23(5):588-92.
22. Gundestrup S, Sjøgren P. Opioids can modulate the immune system. Ugeskrift for Laeger. 2014;176(5A):V08130516-.
23. Lucia M, Luca T, Federica DP, Cecilia G, Chiara M, Laura DM, Carlo DR, Grazia PM. Opioids and breast cancer recurrence: a systematic review. Cancers. 2021;13(21):5499.
24. Sultana A, Torres D, Schumann R. Special indications for opioid free anaesthesia and analgesia, patient and procedure related: including obesity, sleep apnoea, chronic obstructive pulmonary disease, complex regional pain syndromes, opioid addiction and cancer surgery. Best Pract Res Clin Anaesthesiol. 2017;31(4):547-60.
25. Echeverria-Villalobos M, Stoicea N, Todeschini AB, Fiorda-Diaz J, Uribe AA, Weaver T, et al. Enhanced recovery after surgery (ERAS): a perspective review of postoperative pain management under ERAS pathways and its role on opioid crisis in the United States. Clin J Pain. 2020;36(3):219-26.
26. Sneddon LU. Evolution of nociception and pain: evidence from fish models. Philos Trans R Soc B. 2019; 374(1785):37420190290.
27. Kissin I, Weiskopf RB. Preemptive analgesia. J Am Soc Anesthesiol. 2000;93(4):1138-43.
28. Mishra AK, Afzal M, Mookerjee SS, Bandyopadhyay KH, Paul A. Pre-emptive analgesia: recent trends and evidences. Indian J Pain. 2013;27(3):114.
29. Phillips WJ, Currier BL. Analgesic pharmacology: II. Specific analgesics. JAAOS-J Am Acad Orthop Surg. 2004;12(4):221-33.
30. Graham GG, Scott KF. Mechanisms of action of paracetamol and related analgesics. Inflammopharmacology. 2003; 11:401-13.
31. Sinner B, Graf BM. Ketamine. Handb Exp Pharmacol. 2008;(182):313-33.
32. Ramírez-Paesano C, Clarens CR, Mandujano JC, Bonev MB, Loaiza KS, Borghetti F, et al. Role of ketamine as part of the anti-hyperalgesic approach in opioid-free anaesthesia (OFA) and postoperative analgesia (OFAA).
33. Sun Y, Li T, Wang N, Yun Y, Gan TJ. Perioperative systemic lidocaine for postoperative analgesia and recovery after abdominal surgery: a meta-analysis of randomized controlled trials. Dis Colon Rectum. 2012;55(11):1183-94.
34. Dunn LK, Durieux ME. Perioperative use of intravenous lidocaine. Anesthesiology. 2017;126(4):729-37.
35. Monyer H, Sprengel R, Schoepfer R, Herb A, Higuchi M, Lomeli H, et al. Heteromeric NMDA receptors: molecular and functional distinction of subtypes. Science 1992; 256:1217-21.
36. Shimosawa T, Takano K, Ando K, Fujita T. Magnesium inhibits norepinephrine release by blocking N-type calcium channels at peripheral sympathetic nerve endings. Hypertension 2004; 44:897-902.
37. Forget P, Cata J. Stable anaesthesia with alternative to opioids: are ketamine and magnesium helpful in stabilizing hemodynamics during surgery? A systematic review and meta-analyses of randomized controlled trials. Best Pract Res Clin Anaesthesiol. 2017;31(4):523-31.
38. Arikkath J, Campbell KP. Auxiliary subunits: essential components of the voltage-gated calcium channel complex. Curr Opini Neurobiol. 2003;13(3):298-307.
39. Ho KY, Gan TJ, Habib AS. Gabapentin and postoperative pain—a systematic review of randomized controlled trials. Pain. 2006;126(1-3):91-101.

40. Tiippana EM, Hamunen K, Kontinen VK, Kalso E. Do surgical patients benefit from perioperative gabapentin/pregabalin? A systematic review of efficacy and safety. Anaesth Analg. 2007;104(6):1545-56.
41. Van Meel JC, De Jonge A, Timmermans PB, Van Zwieten PA. Selectivity of some alpha adrenoceptor agonists for peripheral alpha-1 and alpha-2 adrenoceptors in the normotensive rat. J Pharmacol Exp Ther. 1981;219(3): 760-7.
42. Gertler R, Brown HC, Mitchell DH, Silvius EN. Dexmedetomidine: a novel sedative-analgesic agent. In: Baylor University Medical Center Proceedings (Vol. 14, No. 1). Taylor & Francis; 2001. pp. 13-21.
43. Kharasch ED, Brunt LM. Perioperative opioids and public health. Anesthesiology. 2016;124(4):960-5.
44. Carmichael JC, Keller DS, Baldini G, Bordeianou L, Weiss E, Lee L, et al. Clinical practice guidelines for enhanced recovery after colon and rectal surgery from the American Society of Colon and Rectal Surgeons and Society of American Gastrointestinal and Endoscopic Surgeons. Dis Colon Rectum. 2017;60(8):761-84.
45. Meyer LA, Lasala J, Iniesta MD, Nick AM, Munsell MF, Shi Q, et al. Effect of an enhanced recovery after surgery program on opioid use and patient-reported outcomes. Obstet Gynecol. 2018;132(2):281-90.
46. Mulier JP. Is opioid-free general anaesthesia for breast and gynecological surgery a viable option? Curr Opin Anesthesiol. 2019;32(3):257-62.
47. Solanki SL, Thota RS, Rajan J, Gangakhedkar GR, Jain P, Gottumukkala V, et al. Multimodal opioid sparing onco-anesthesia: a consensus practice guideline from Society of Onco-Anesthesia and Perioperative Care (SOAPC). J Opioid Manag. 2021;17(5):417-37.
48. Soffin EM, Wetmore DS, Beckman JD, Sheha ED, Vaishnav AS, Albert TJ, et al. Opioid-free anaesthesia within an enhanced recovery after surgery pathway for minimally invasive lumbar spine surgery: a retrospective matched cohort study. Neurosurg Focus. 2019;46(4):E8.
49. Mauermann E, Ruppen W, Bandschapp O. Different protocols used today to achieve total opioid-free general anaesthesia without locoregional blocks. Best Pract Res Clin Anaesthesiol. 2017;31(4):533-45.

CHAPTER

Perioperative Point-of-care Investigations for Cancer Surgical Patients

Indubala Maurya, Ram Gopal Maurya, Sonali Banwait

INTRODUCTION

Anesthesiologists face several perioperative challenges during the management of patients undergoing cancer surgery, such as difficult airway, difficult cannulation, hemodynamic disturbances, metabolic abnormalities, and coagulation abnormalities. These perioperative challenges depend on the type of cancer, history of previous chemotherapy/radiotherapy, other comorbid conditions, and the specific procedure being performed. A comprehensive approach is required during perioperative management, which involves preoperative optimization and intraoperative and postoperative management tailored to the unique needs of cancer patients. Anesthesiologists can use various point-of-care (POC) investigations and interventions, which help in faster clinical decision-making during surgery, choosing appropriate treatment plans, and monitoring patients more effectively. Point-of-care investigations refer to rapid diagnostic tests that can be performed at the patient's bedside, thus allowing faster results and guided appropriate intervention. Various perioperative investigations and interventions that are easily applied in decision-making include point-of-care ultrasonography, blood gas analysis, coagulation monitoring, glucose measurements, hemoglobin/hematocrit analyses, urine analysis, etc.[1] Bedside investigation and intervention are indispensable in the preoperative, operating theater, and postoperative areas, including the intensive care unit (ICU), as rapid results and real-time insight contribute to better surgical outcomes. This chapter discusses various bedside diagnostic tests that can be used during the perioperative period for decision-making and guided intervention.

POINT-OF-CARE ULTRASOUND

Point-of-care ultrasound (POCUS) refers to using ultrasonography (USG) examinations at a patient's bedside by a primary healthcare provider to answer specific diagnostic questions and guide treatment and invasive procedures. It provides qualitative examination, which is simple, rapid, and goal-oriented, thus acting as a supplement to clinical evaluation. It is a safe, convenient, noninvasive, nonirradiating, and repeatable examination that can be used almost anywhere in the hospital. A variety of ultrasound machines are available for perioperative POCUS. Ultrasound use has been accelerated further with the availability and accessibility of small handheld to portable/cart-based ultrasound devices. Basic ultrasound machines provide B and M mode images with or without Doppler. However, more sophisticated USG machines have more advanced capabilities, such as continuous wave Doppler, pulsed wave Doppler, automated image optimization, etc., improving imaging appropriate for various diagnostic studies or interventions. Newer-generation USG machines have the feature of artificial intelligence (AI), which provides real-time image and quantitative tissue analysis.[2-4]

Perioperative POCUS includes USG examinations in the preoperative clinic, operating room, postoperative area, and the ICU. POCUS is an examination and intervention tool for elective and emergency indications, covering almost all body systems. This section will briefly cover common POCUS examinations, which can potentially help anesthesiologists in decision-making during preoperative examination on whether to advise further investigations; it would also assist in selecting the best anesthesia approach and can support perioperative and postoperative monitoring management.

Airway Ultrasonography

Point-of-care ultrasound is a promising tool for airway management, which can assist in the identification of important upper airway anatomy and airway parameters.

It can also guide airway interventions with real-time images[5] **(Table 1 and Fig. 1)**.

Anticipating a difficult airway is integral to preoperative evaluation to avoid adverse outcomes due to unanticipated deleterious situations. Traditionally, conventional clinical parameters, including obesity, mouth opening, Mallampati score, thyromental distance, neck extension, etc., are considered predictors for a difficult airway. Though the combination of these individual parameters, such as the Wilson score, etc., appears to have better predictive value, none of the examinations are proven to be ideal and valid for difficult airways. These clinical examinations assess the airway from the outside without any real-time view of the airway structures relevant for intubation. POCUS helps to predict the difficult airway and provides relevant anatomical information, which adds to airway assessment and management. The USG measurement of anterior neck soft tissue thickness at various points, such as the skin to the hyoid bone distance (SHBD), the skin to the epiglottis distance (DSE), skin to the anterior commissure of the vocal cords (DSAC), etc., has been studied for the prediction of difficult airway. Tongue thickness measured by USG also has the capacity to predict difficult tracheal intubation. Due to heterogeneous studies, the clinical use of various airway measurements is still debatable. However, the studies show the potential of POCUS to supplement traditional clinical airway assessment.[6-8]

TABLE 1: Perioperative use of airway ultrasonography (USG).

Use	*Indication*	*USG finding/measurement*
Preoperative	Anticipation of difficult airway	• Skin to the hyoid bone distance • Skin to the epiglottis distance • Skin to the anterior commissure of the vocal cords • Tongue thickness
	Identification and preprocedural marking of anatomical structures	Identification of cricothyroid membrane, tracheal rings, etc.
	Vocal cord examination	Vocal cord movement at the level of the thyroid cartilage in a transverse plane
	Prediction of the endotracheal tube/double lumen tube size	Tracheal diameter measurement above the sternoclavicular junction in the transverse section
Intraoperative	Confirmation of tracheal intubation	• Snowstorm sign • Bullet' sign • Double tract sign—Esophageal intubation • Lung sliding • Diaphragmatic movement
	Confirmation of one-lung ventilation	Lung sliding, diaphragmatic movement
	Airway blocks	Superior laryngeal nerve block, transtracheal injection
	Identification of cricothyroid membrane	Hyperechoic structure due to air–mucosal lining
Postoperative	Prediction of postextubation stridor	Laryngeal air column • Width <4.5 (0.8) mm • Shape of air column

Airway POCUS can also identify important airway structures, such as the thyroid cartilage, cricothyroid membrane (CTM), cricoid cartilage, and tracheal rings. It also helps during emergencies by showing structures that contribute to life-saving interventions, such as emergency front-of-neck access (FONA) in complete ventilation failure situations. It also assists in percutaneous tracheostomy and elective transtracheal cannulation. Ultrasound-guided CTM localization is especially beneficial if the landmarks cannot be palpated easily, e.g., obesity, history of radiotherapy, neck surgery, or abnormal neck anatomy. It is advisable to perform POCUS of the upper airway in a routine, nonemergency setting as a part of a preanesthetic checkup.[9,10]

The preoperative assessment of vocal cord dysfunction can be relevant for patients who are about to undergo procedures that endanger the superior or recurrent laryngeal nerve and already have a history of neck surgery, including thyroid or parathyroid surgery or lung surgery of the upper lobe. It has been proven that airway ultrasound has a very good correlation with endoscopic vocal cord examination. In addition to the noninvasiveness, the ultrasound can provide valuable information if an endoscopic examination is difficult, e.g., for mentally challenged patients and children.[11,12]

The tracheal diameter measured with POCUS correlates well with the tracheal diameters determined with computed tomography and helps to determine the correct size of the endotracheal tube or double-lumen

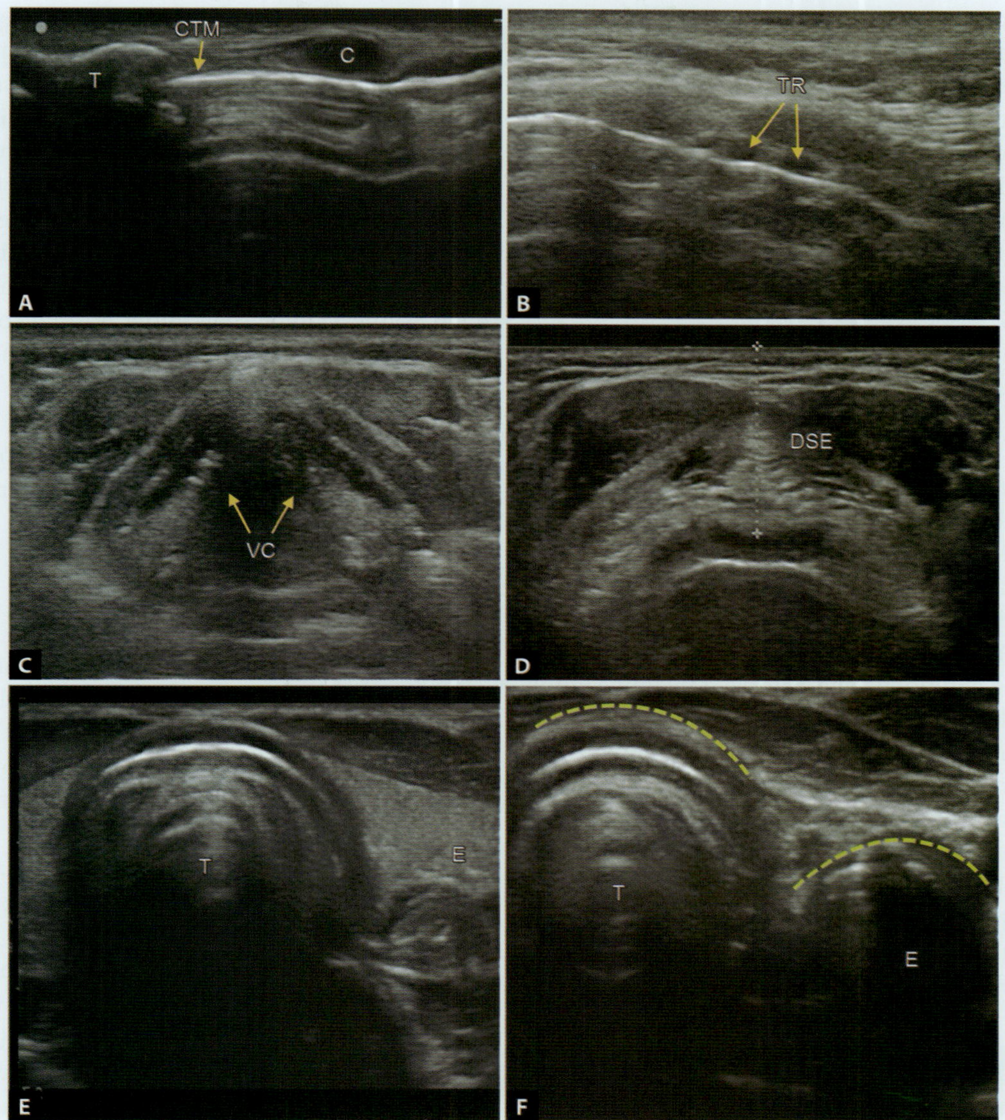

Figs. 1A to F: Airway USG. (CTM: cricothyroid membrane; C: cricoid cartilage; DSE: skin to epiglottic distance; E: esophagus; T: trachea, TR: tracheal ring; VC: vocal cord; USG: ultrasonography; Yellow dotted line: Shows double tract sign)

tube. The tracheal diameter is measured above the sternoclavicular junction perpendicular to the neck in the transverse section. Airway blocks for awake fiberoptic intubation can be performed under USG guidance, specifically for patients with difficult anatomy.[13-15]

After intubation, POCUS is helpful in confirmation of tracheal intubation, exclusion of esophageal intubation, and also for one-lung ventilation. POCUS provides real-time images of the neck during intubation and detects ventilation with signs of lung sliding or diaphragmatic movement. Although one-lung ventilation is typically assessed by direct visualization by flexible bronchoscopy, USG has also been shown to be superior to clinical exams alone. The USG sensitivity and specificity are 98 and 53%, superior to 85 and 41% with clinical assessment alone. POCUS is also useful in predicting postextubation stridor, which can be used as a surrogate or supplement to a cuff leak test.[16-18]

Lung Ultrasonography

Lung ultrasound (LUS) may be used as a primary tool for evaluating hypoxia, hypotension, and chest pain, along with clinical examination. Preoperatively, lung USG can be used to evaluate the degree of respiratory disease, such as pleural effusions, interstitial syndromes, and pulmonary edema. It also helps during the assessment and management of acute hemodynamic or respiratory disturbances during intraoperative and postoperative, e.g., pneumothorax, hemothorax, and acute pulmonary edema. Postprocedural lung complications such as pneumothorax after central line insertion can be ruled out using lung USG.[19]

Lung ultrasound involves the study of air–fluid interfaces in the lungs and the interpretation of ultrasound artifacts. Different transducers, such as phased array, convex, micro convex, or linear probes, are being used for LUS to optimize the artifacts, determine the lung pathology, and the patient's body habitus. For focused lung examinations, longitudinal scanning is done in six, eight, or twelve zones; transverse scanning is advised in areas of particular interest for a more thorough assessment of pathology **(Table 2)**.

Normal lung aeration is characterized by lung sliding, which is the sliding of the parietal and visceral pleura against each other at the pleural line (equivalent to a seashore sign on the M-mode). The A profile pattern of normal lung parenchyma is characterized by consistent, recurring horizontal reverberation artifacts that originate from the air below the pleural line. A-lines are reverberation artifacts that occur at an equal distance below the pleural line and become worse with depth. They are caused by ultrasonic waves bouncing between the probe and the visceral-parietal pleural interface. It appears during the insonation of an aerated lung. A-lines are normal findings found in healthy and aerated lungs; however, the absence of A-lines does not confirm pathology either. Also, the presence of A-lines does not rule out a pneumothorax. B-lines are hyperechoic vertical lines arising from the pleural line. They extend indefinitely, erase A-lines (when present), and move along lung sliding. B-lines are found in patients with alveolar-interstitial syndromes. However, a few B-lines can be seen under normal conditions when the patient is recumbent for a long time due to lung atelectasis **(Figs. 2A to D)**.

TABLE 2: Perioperative use of lung USG.

Common clinical condition	*USG findings*
Normal lung	Lung sliding (seashore sign on M mode), A-lines
Pneumothorax	Absent lung sliding on the affected side (barcode sign (M-mode) B-lines lung pulse identification of the lung point
Pleural effusion	Hypoechoic fluid around the lung base (spine sign, jellyfish sign)
Pulmonary edema	Confluent B-lines with increasing severity; lung sliding is present
Consolidation	Air bronchogram
ARDS	Bilateral or unilateral B-lines, lung sliding is present

(ARDS: acute respiratory distress syndrome; USG: ultrasonography)

Various LUS protocols, such as the Bedside Lung Ultrasound in Emergency (BLUE) protocol and Fluid Administration Limited by Lung Sonography (FALLS) protocol, are already well established.[20-22]

Gastric Ultrasonography

Point-of-care ultrasound can be used to check the adequacy of preoperative fasting by assessing the volume and character of gastric contents. It is primarily helpful for patients who are at risk, such as chronic opioid use, diabetes mellitus, patients with compliance and unknown fasting status, such as cognitive impairment and communication barriers.[23,24]

During USG, the antrum appears small and empty, with a "bull's eye" appearance. After ingestion of clear fluid, the antrum appears distended with hypoechoic or anechoic content with a "starry night" appearance. The antrum appears round and distended with increased echogenicity after ingestion of solid food ("frosted glass" appearance) **(Figs. 3A and B)**. In the presence of clear liquids, the approximate gastric volume can be estimated by measuring the cross-sectional area of the antrum measured at the level of the aorta. The volume of gastric contents (in milliliters) can be calculated as 27 + (14.6 * cross-sectional area of the antrum) – (1.28 * age). The risk of aspiration has been graded as per the gastric ultrasound **(Table 3)**.

Inferior Vena Cava Ultrasonography

Ultrasound examination of inferior vena cava (IVC) diameter and its variations with respiration [collapsibility index (CI)] can assess intravascular volume status and predict volume responsiveness. It can act as a dynamic parameter that reflects the interaction between the respiratory and cardiac cycles.

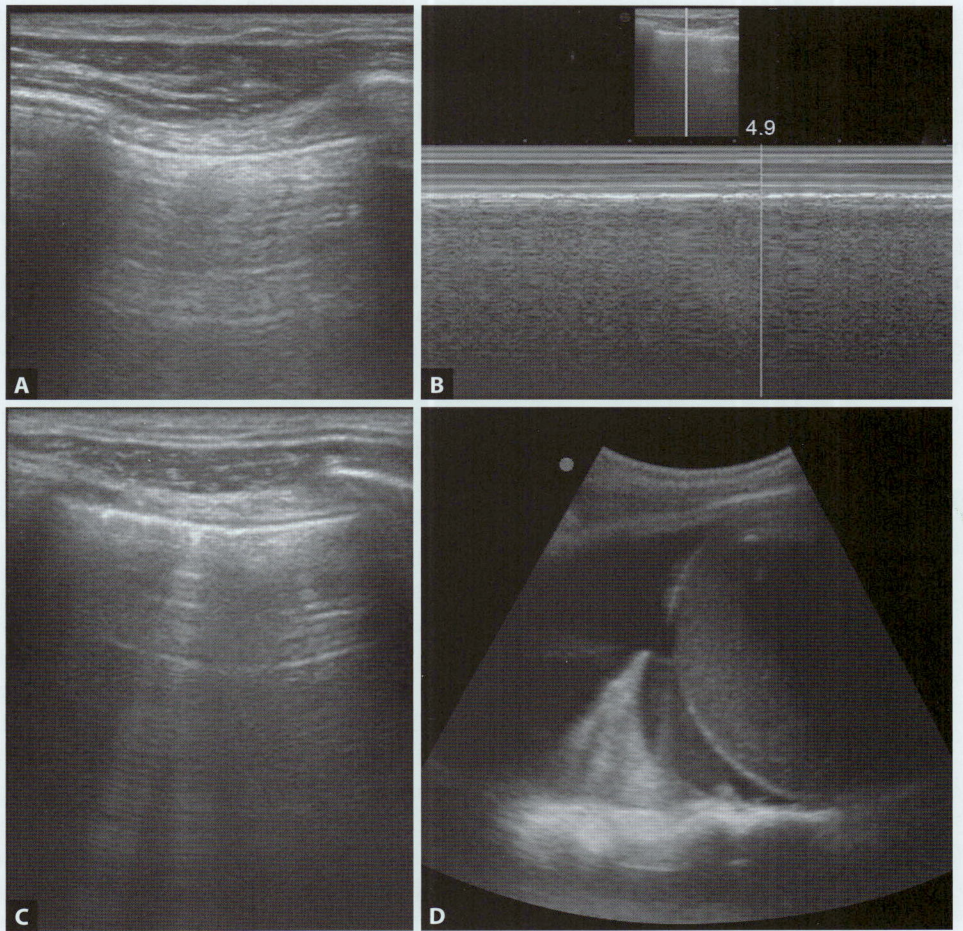

Figs. 2A to D: Lung ultrasonography (USG). (A) Normal lung on B mode; (B) Normal lung on M mode showing seashore sign; (C) B lines; (D) Pleural effusion (spine sign).

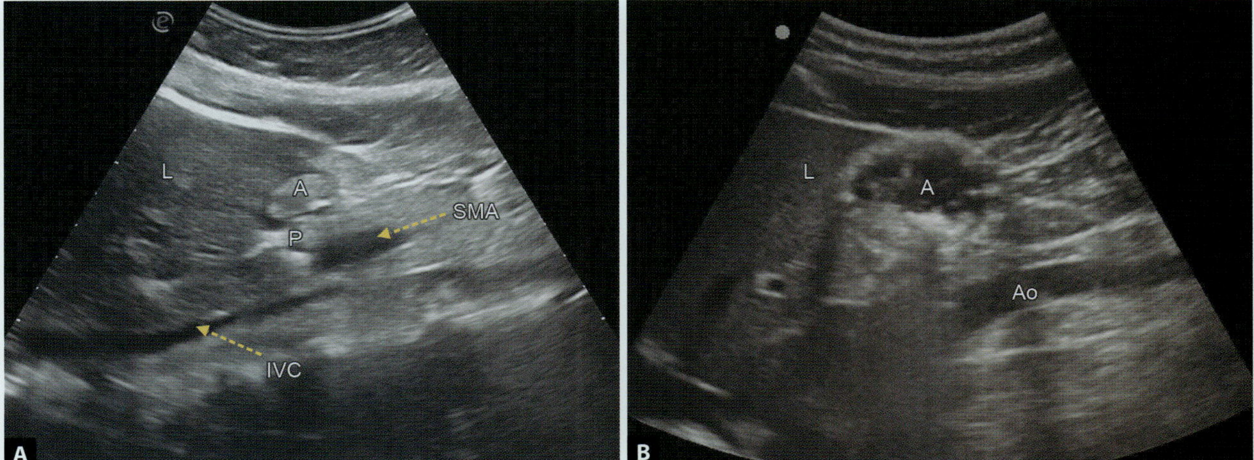

Figs. 3A and B: Gastric USG. (A) Empty gastric antrum; (B) Distended gastric antrum (mixture of solid and liquid food). (A: antrum; Ao: aorta; IVC: inferior vena cava; L: liver; P: pancreas, SMA: superior mesenteric artery; USG: ultrasonography)

A low-frequency convex or phased array transducer is used to assess the IVC from a subcostal view by a longitudinal scan, including the venoatrial junction. IVC examination can be repeated at frequent intervals during fluid resuscitation. It may complement ultrasound of the heart, lungs, and abdominal organs for hemodynamic assessment and management **(Figs. 4A and B)**. Although the physiology of IVC respiratory variations differs during mechanical ventilation and spontaneous breathing, the IVC CI and distensibility index are interconvertible. The equation calculates IVC variability: $(IVC_{max} - IVC_{min})/IVC_{max}$. Maximum IVC diameter ≤2.1 cm and collapsibility >50% suggest right atrial pressure (RAP) between 0 and 5 mm Hg, while a diameter >2.1 cm with <50% collapsibility indicates a high RAP of 10–20 mm Hg.[25,26]

However, various clinical factors can affect IVC diameter and collapsibility, such as tidal volume, positive end-expiratory pressure, respiratory effort, intrabdominal pressure, etc. Maximum IVC diameter predicts intravascular volume status at the extremes only. It has poor sensitivity and specificity in predicting volume responsiveness. IVC CI is profound in volume-responsive patients. Two recent meta-analyses have questioned its utility. IVC CI has potential biases while interpreting. IVC ultrasound must be interpreted in the context of the entire clinical situation.[27,28]

TABLE 3: Stratification of risk of aspiration as per gastric ultrasound.

Gastric volume grade	*USG findings*	*Risk of aspiration*
Grade 0	Antrum is empty in supine and right lateral decubitus positions	Low risk
Grade 1	Antrum is empty in the supine position, clear fluid is visible in the right lateral decubitus position, and gastric volume is estimated at <1.5 mL/kg	Low risk
Grade 2	Clear fluid is visible in the antrum in the supine and right lateral decubitus position, and volume >1.5 mL/kg	High risk

(USG: ultrasonography)

Abdominal Pelvic Ultrasonography

Focused assessment with sonography for trauma (FAST) is a well-established examination and commonly performed POCUS examinations in the emergency room, which detects free fluid suggestive of intra-abdominal bleeding and also looks for pericardial or pleural effusions. The FAST evaluates three potential spaces within the peritoneal cavity (hepatorenal recess, splenorenal recess, and suprapubic area) and the pericardium for any pathologic fluid **(Figs. 5A to E)**. Extended FAST (e-FAST) incorporated views of the right and left hemithorax to detect the presence of pneumothorax and pleural effusion.[29]

The same concepts of the FAST/eFAST examination can be utilized during the perioperative period for patients who deteriorate after abdominal procedures.

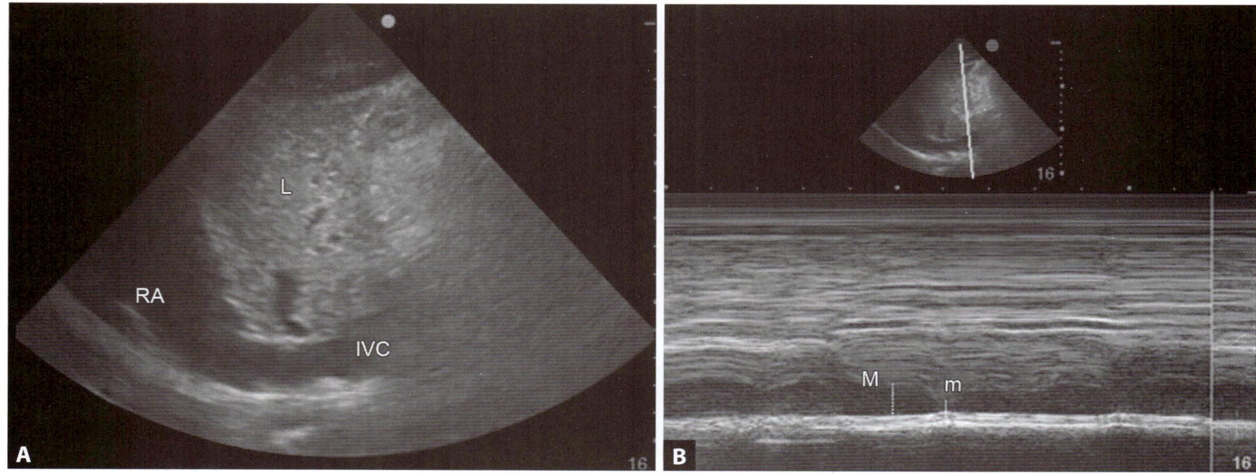

Figs. 4A and B: Inferior vena cava collapsibility. (IVC: inferior vena cava; L: liver; M: maximum diameter of IVC; m: minimum diameter of IVC; RA: right atrium)

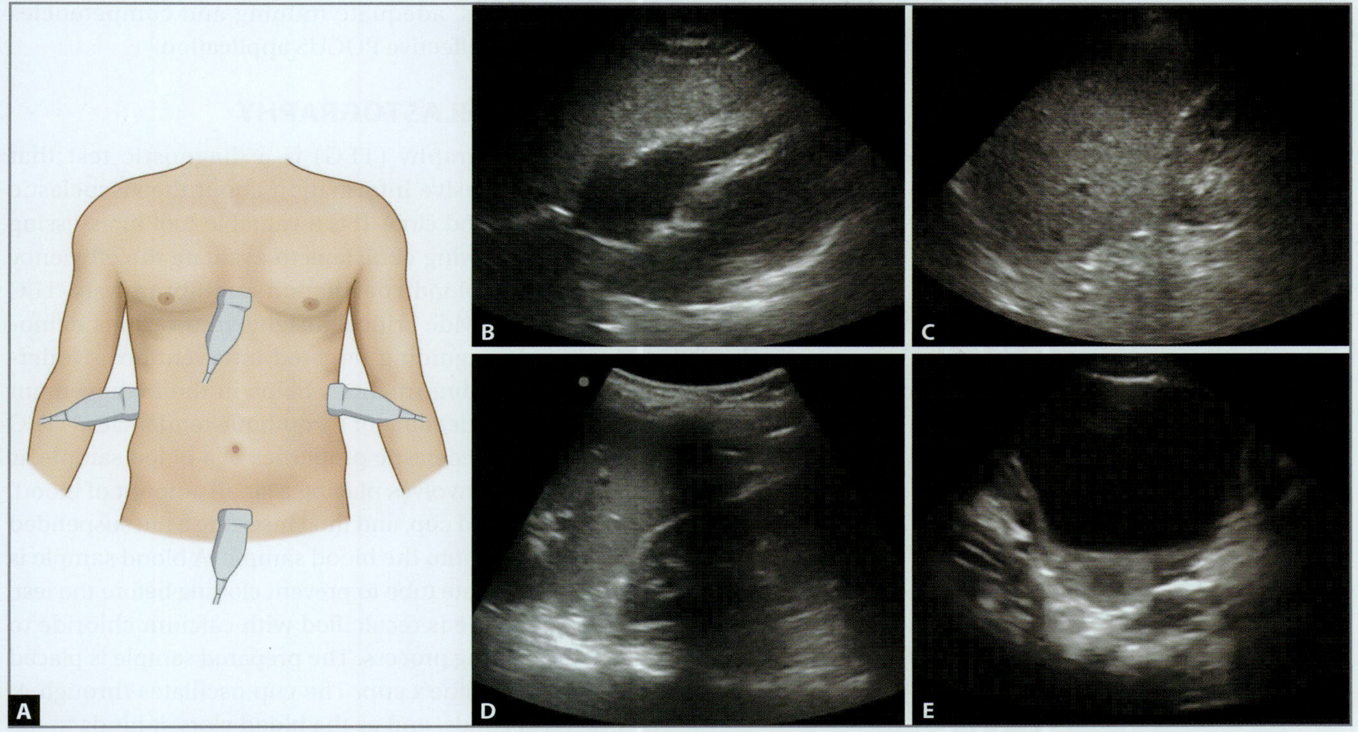

Figs. 5A to E: Focused assessment with sonography in trauma (FAST). (A) Probe position during FAST examination; (B) Right upper abdomen (Morison's space between liver and right kidney); (C) Left upper abdomen (perisplenic and left perirenal areas); (D) Suprapubic region (perivesical area); (E) Subxiphoid region (pericardium).

Rapid bedside diagnosis of postsurgical abdominal bleeding facilitates early transfer of the patients to the operating room for re-exploration. A suprapubic scan or urinary bladder evaluation can be helpful in assessing decreased urine output to rule out urine retention.

In combination with cardiac POCUS and IVC examination, FAST is utilized for rapid assessment and management of undifferentiated perioperative hypotension, known as the "Rapid Ultrasound in SHock (RUSH)" protocol. It has a sensitivity of 85% and specificity of 95% to identify the cause of undifferentiated hypotension.[30]

Other Perioperative Point-of-care Ultrasound

Point-of-care ultrasound is used for various elective and emergency procedures such as vascular cannulation, nerve blocks, pericardiocentesis, pleural effusion drainage, ascitic drainage, etc. **(Table 4)** Both venous and arterial cannulation have become routine during the perioperative period due to fewer procedural complications than landmark-guided procedures. Intravascular venous access to central and peripheral veins is facilitated with the use of ultrasound. POCUS imaging is done for vessel localization before puncture and also for guidance on needle, wire, and catheter placement. Many USG-guided nerve blocks for acute and chronic pain have been established. USG-guided neuraxial blocks are preferred in patients with difficult anatomy, such as morbid obesity.[31-34]

Point-of-care ultrasound is also utilized to screen deep vein thrombosis, evaluate raised intracranial pressure (optic nerve sheath diameter measurement), and assess sarcopenia **(Figs. 6 to 8)**.[35-37] Recent studies have shown the utility of POCUS during cardiopulmonary resuscitation (CPR). It helps to determine pulses by applying carotid artery compression and rapidly diagnosing reversible arrest causes.[38,39]

Limitations of Point-of-care Ultrasound

In clinical practice, it is important to understand the limitations of POCUS. Understanding its sensitivity and specificity in relation to other accepted diagnostic tests is a crucial factor in the effective use of perioperative POCUS for diagnostic purposes. Its usefulness also depends on the

TABLE 4: Other perioperative use of USG.

Other perioperative use	*Details*
Procedural use	• Peripheral nerve blocks (acute and chronic pain management) • Neuraxial anesthesia • Pericardiocentesis • Pleural effusion/ascitic fluid drainage • Vascular access
Assessment of intracranial pressure	• Measurement of optic nerve sheath diameter (ONSD) • It is measured 3 mm behind the eye globe • The upper limit of the normal ONSD is 5 mm in adults
Assessment of sarcopenia	Thickness of biceps/quadriceps femoris muscle
Deep vein thrombosis assessment	• Noncompressibility • Direct visualization of clot
Venous congestion assessment	• Venous Excess Ultrasound (VExUS) Score • Evaluates the severity of venous congestion in IVC, hepatic vein, portal vein, and renal veins
Cardiopulmonary resuscitation	• Check pulse by compression of the carotid artery in cardiac arrest patients • Diagnosis of reversible causes of arrest

(IVC: inferior vena cava; USG: ultrasonography)

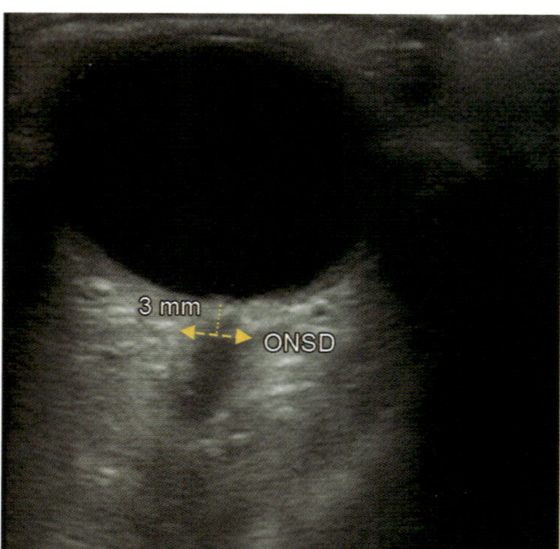

Fig. 6: Ultrasound measurement of optic nerve sheath diameter (ONSD). ONSD is measured 3 mm behind the eye globe.

anesthesiologist's experience in USG image acquisition and interpretation. Treating the acquired POCUS image is insufficient; the patient's clinical situation must be considered. Thus, adequate training and competencies are essential for effective POCUS application.

THROMBOELASTOGRAPHY

Thromboelastography (TEG) is a diagnostic test that gives comprehensive information about the viscoelastic properties of blood clots. It is a valuable tool in assessing hemostasis, allowing clinicians to evaluate the efficiency and kinetics of blood coagulation and fibrinolysis. TEG findings can provide critical insights into various hemostatic disorders, guiding targeted interventions. Understanding these abnormalities helps in the management of patients with bleeding or thrombotic tendencies.[40] TEG measures the viscoelastic properties of a blood sample as it clots. The test involves placing a small amount of blood, 340 μL, in a heated cup, and then inserting a pin suspended by a torsion wire into the blood sample. A blood sample is collected in a citrate tube to prevent clotting before the test. The blood sample is recalcified with calcium chloride to initiate the clotting process. The prepared sample is placed in the TEG machine's cup. The cup oscillates through 4° 45′ every 5 seconds, and as the blood clots, it binds to the pin, which causes the pin to oscillate. These oscillations are translated into a graphical representation known as a thromboelastogram, which displays the dynamic process of clot formation and breakdown to understand the patient's hemostatic status.[41]

Interpretation of Thromboelastogram

A normal TEG graph provides a visual representation of the blood clotting process and reflects normal hemostatic function. The graph typically consists of several key phases and parameters that describe the clotting process, from initiation to clot lysis[42] **(Figs. 9 and 10; Table 5)**.

Role of Thromboelastography During the Perioperative Period

Oncosurgeries are often associated with significant risks of both bleeding and hypercoagulable complications due to the complex interplay between cancer, surgery, and hemostatic function. Here are key aspects of the role of TEG in oncosurgeries:[43,44]

- *Assessment of coagulation status*: TEG provides a comprehensive picture of the coagulation process, including clot formation, strength, and dissolution. This detailed assessment allows clinicians to identify whether a patient is hypocoagulable (at risk of bleeding)

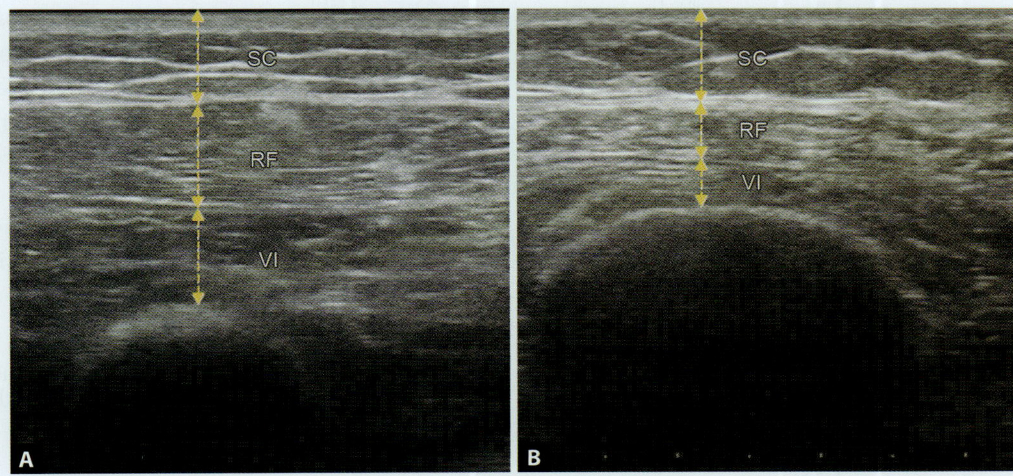

Figs. 7A and B: Ultrasound assessment of sarcopenia. (A) Healthy patient; (B) Sarcopenic patient. (RF: rectus femoris; SC: subcutaneous tissue; VI: vastus intermedius)

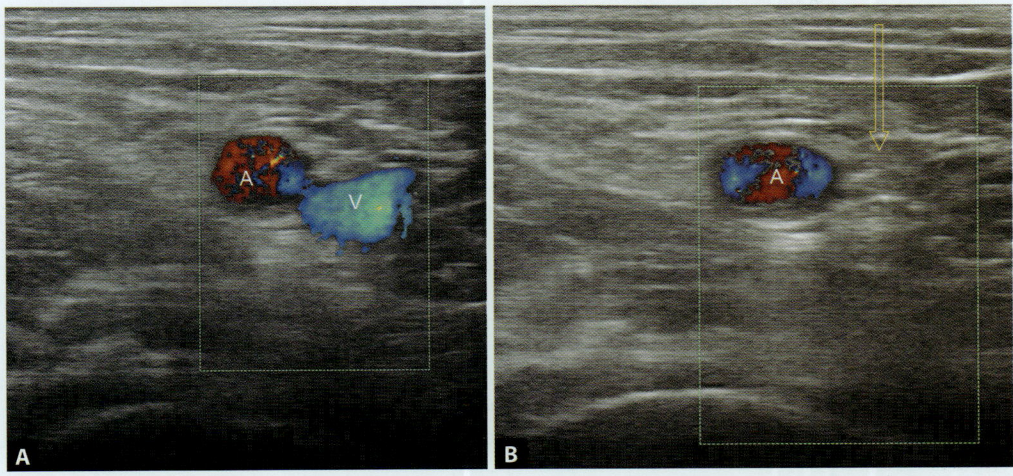

Figs. 8A and B: Deep vein thrombosis screening using compression ultrasound (color Doppler). (A) Without compression; (B) With compression. The yellow arrow depicts the direction of compression. (A: femoral artery; V: femoral vein)

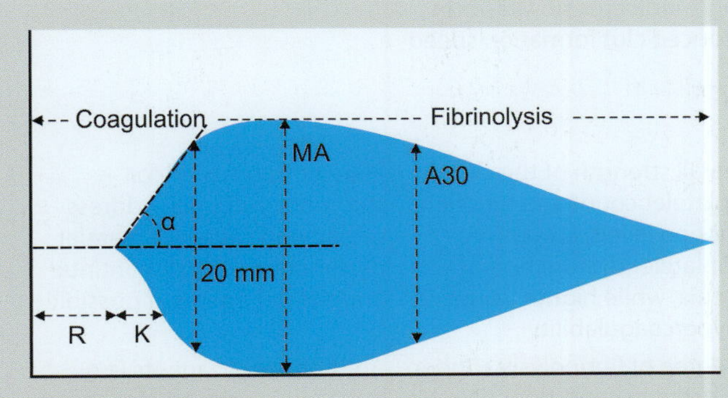

Fig. 9: Normal thromboelastogram. (A30: amplitude at 30 minutes; MA: maximum amplitude; R: reaction time; K: kinetics; α: alpha angle, i.e., slope between R and K)

or hypercoagulable (at risk of thrombosis), enabling tailored perioperative management strategies.

- *Guiding transfusion therapy*: During surgery, TEG helps guide the selection of blood products and hemostatic agents. By pinpointing specific coagulation deficiencies, such as platelet dysfunction or fibrinogen deficiency, TEG ensures that transfusion therapy is targeted and efficient. This precision reduces the need for unnecessary transfusions, minimizing risks such as transfusion-related acute lung injury (TRALI) and transfusion-associated circulatory overload (TACO).
- *Monitoring hemostatic therapy*: TEG's real-time monitoring capabilities are particularly useful in surgeries with high bleeding risks, such as cardiac and

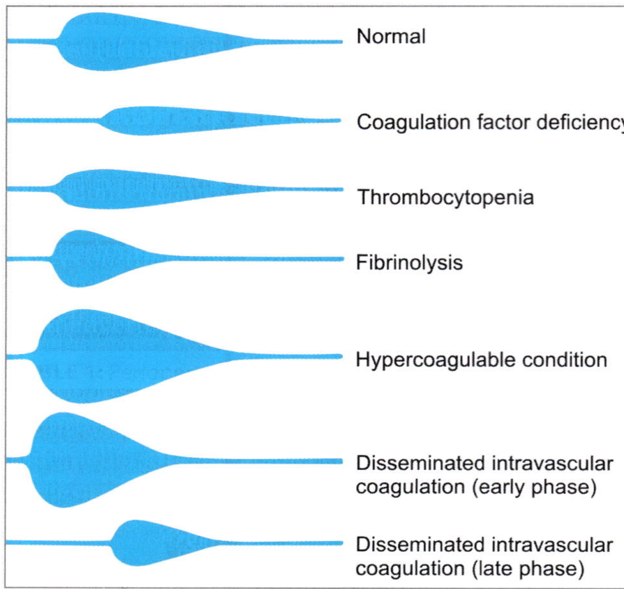

Fig. 10: Pathological thromboelastogram.

liver surgeries. It allows for the continuous assessment of the effectiveness of administered hemostatic agents and blood products, facilitating immediate adjustments to treatment protocols to maintain optimal hemostasis throughout the surgical procedure.

- *Reducing blood loss and improving outcome:* By enabling precise and timely interventions based on real-time data, TEG helps reduce both intraoperative and postoperative blood loss. This improves surgical outcomes, shortens recovery times, and reduces hospital stays. The use of TEG in the perioperative setting thus contributes to better overall patient care and resource utilization.

Advantages and Limitations of Thromboelastography

Thromboelastography can be easily performed at the bedside or in the operating room, offering POC

TABLE 5: Phases of thromboelastogram.

Parameter	*Description*	*Normal range*	*Significance*	*Management*
R-time (reaction time)	The time from the start of the test until the initial formation of a clot	5–10 minutes	• Indicates the time taken for the blood to begin forming a clot • Prolong R-time is often due to deficiencies in clotting factors (e.g., hemophilia) or anticoagulant therapy (e.g., warfarin, heparin), while a shorter R-time suggests a hypercoagulable state	*Prolonged R time:* Administer clotting factors (e.g., factor VIII or IX for hemophilia), fresh frozen plasma (FFP) and reversal of anticoagulation (e.g., vitamin K for warfarin, protamine sulfate for heparin)
K-time (kinetics)	The time from the end of the R-time until a fixed level of clot strength is reached (usually 20 mm of amplitude)	1–3 minutes	• Reflects the speed of clot formation • Prolonged K-time indicates slower clot formation, often due to fibrinogen deficiency or dysfunction	Administer cryoprecipitate or fibrinogen concentrate. FFP if fibrinogen concentrate is unavailable
Alpha angle (α)	The angle formed between the baseline and the tangent to the curve representing the rapid phase of fibrin build-up	53–72°	Represents the rate of clot formation. A lower alpha angle indicates slower fibrin buildup and reduced clot formation speed	—do—
MA (maximum amplitude)	The maximum vertical amplitude of the thromboelastography (TEG) trace	50–70 mm	Reflects the overall strength of the clot, influenced by platelet count and function, as well as fibrinogen levels. Lower MA values suggest platelet dysfunction or thrombocytopenia, while higher values may indicate hypercoagulability	Platelet transfusion for thrombocytopenia. Address underlying causes of platelet dysfunction (e.g., discontinue antiplatelet agents, if possible
LY30 (Lysis at 30 minutes)	The percentage decrease in amplitude 30 minutes after MA is reached	0–8%	Indicates the degree of fibrinolysis. Higher fibrinolysis can occur in conditions like disseminated intravascular coagulation (DIC), trauma, or liver disease	Antifibrinolytic agents (e.g., tranexamic acid, aminocaproic acid) inhibit excessive fibrinolysis. Treat underlying causes of hyperfibrinolysis (e.g., address DIC, manage liver disease)

testing. It provides a comprehensive real-time picture of clot formation and breakdown, thus allowing rapid decision-making. It reduces unnecessary transfusions by providing specific hemostatic information. However, TEG requires specialized equipment and trained personnel. Interpretation of results can be complex and may require expertise. It is more expensive than conventional laboratory coagulation tests like prothrombin time (PT), partial thromboplastin time (PTT), and international normalized ratio (INR).

ARTERIAL BLOOD GAS ANALYSIS

Arterial blood gas (ABG) is a diagnostic test that measures the levels of partial pressure of oxygen (PaO_2) and carbon dioxide ($PaCO_2$), as well as the pH (acidity or alkalinity) of blood drawn from an artery. Some blood gas analyzers also measure methemoglobin, carboxyhemoglobin, hemoglobin levels, and lactate levels. PaO_2 provides information about the oxygenation status, while $PaCO_2$ offers insight into the ventilation status, whether it is chronic or acute respiratory failure. $PaCO_2$ is influenced by the nature of ventilation and acid–base status.[45,46]

Specific Indications for Arterial Blood Gas in the Perioperative Intensive Care Unit Setting

The most common indication for ABG analysis in the perioperative period is to monitor and manage respiratory function and acid–base balance in patients who have undergone major surgery. These patients are often at risk for respiratory complications, such as hypoxemia (low blood oxygen levels), hypercapnia (elevated blood carbon dioxide levels), and acid–base imbalances due to various factors, including anesthesia, mechanical ventilation, and the surgical procedure itself **(Table 6)**. Variables in an ABG are shown in **Table 7**.

Common Causes of Arterial Blood Gas Reading Errors

It is important to remember that incorrect sample collection is a common cause of inaccurate ABG readings.

TABLE 6: Perioperative common indications of arterial blood gas (ABG).

Indications	*Clinical conditions*
Assessment of respiratory function	• Postoperative ventilation management • Detection of hypoxemia • Monitoring for hypercapnia
Evaluation of acid–base status	• Metabolic acidosis or alkalosis • Respiratory acidosis or alkalosis
Guiding therapeutic interventions	• Adjustment of mechanical ventilation • Titration of oxygen therapy • Management of electrolyte and fluid balance
Monitoring for cardiopulmonary complications	• Pulmonary complications • Cardiovascular complications

TABLE 7: Common variables in an arterial blood gas (ABG).

Variable	*Normal range*	*Units*	*Description*
pH	7.35–7.45		Indicates the acidity or alkalinity of the blood
Partial pressure of oxygen (PaO_2)	75–100	mm Hg	Measures the oxygen level in arterial blood
Partial pressure of carbon dioxide ($PaCO_2$)	35–45	mm Hg	Measures the carbon dioxide level in arterial blood
Bicarbonate (HCO_3^-)	22–26	mEq/L	Represents the metabolic component of the acid–base balance
Oxygen saturation (SaO_2)	95–100%	%	Percentage of hemoglobin saturated with oxygen
Base excess (BE)	−2 to +2	mEq/L	Indicates the amount of excess or insufficient level of bicarbonate in the system
Lactate	0.5–1.0	mmol/L	Measures the level of lactate, indicating tissue oxygenation and perfusion
Hemoglobin (Hb)	12–17	g/dL	Measures the concentration of hemoglobin in the blood
Carboxyhemoglobin (COHb)	<3	%	Measures the level of carbon monoxide bound to hemoglobin
Methemoglobin (MetHb)	<1.5	%	Measures the level of methemoglobin, a form of hemoglobin that cannot bind oxygen

TABLE 8: Types of primary acid–base disorder.

Type	*Primary disturbance*	*Compensation*	*Common causes*
Respiratory acidosis	Increased $PaCO_2$	Kidneys increase HCO_3^- reabsorption	COPD, severe asthma, respiratory muscle weakness, CNS depression (e.g., sedative overdose)
Respiratory alkalosis	Decreased $PaCO_2$	Kidneys decrease HCO_3^- reabsorption	Anxiety, fever, sepsis, high altitude, pulmonary embolism
Metabolic acidosis	Decreased HCO_3^-	Hyperventilation to decrease $PaCO_2$	Diabetic ketoacidosis, lactic acidosis, renal failure, toxin ingestion (methanol, ethylene glycol), diarrhea, renal tubular acidosis
Metabolic alkalosis	Increased HCO_3^-	Hypoventilation to increase $PaCO_2$	Vomiting, nasogastric suctioning, diuretic use, excessive bicarbonate intake, hypokalemia

(CNS: central nervous system; COPD: chronic obstructive pulmonary disease)

Air bubbles in the blood sample can lead to falsely low $PaCO_2$ and high PaO_2 levels. Inadequate mixing and venous contamination of the sample can also result in faulty readings. Delayed analysis and improper sample storage can contribute to inaccurate results.[47] Changes in ventilator parameters (such as over- or under-ventilation) and recent oxygen therapy during sampling can also affect ABG variables. Furthermore, equipment calibration and malfunctions are important factors to consider when encountering faulty readings. The use of heparin as the anticoagulant may cause a dilution of the sample. As a consequence, parameters such as pCO_2 and electrolytes are affected. Only 0.05 mL of heparin is required to anticoagulate 1 mL of blood. Plasma electrolytes decrease linearly with the dilution, along with pCO_2, cGlucose, and ctHb values. However, pH and pO_2 values are relatively unaffected by dilution.[48]

Acid–base Disorders

Acid–base disorders encountered during the perioperative period can be diagnosed by comprehensive situational analysis, assessment of clinical parameters and ABG analysis. The common acid–base disorders are as follows:[49,50]

- *Primary acid–base disorders* **(Table 8)**:
- *Other acid–base disorders:*
  - *High anion gap metabolic acidosis (HAGMA):* ("GOLD MARK")
    - Glycols (ethylene glycol, propylene glycol)
    - Oxoproline (pyroglutamic acid, the toxic metabolite of excessive acetaminophen or paracetamol)
    - l-Lactate (standard lactic acid seen in lactic acidosis)
    - d-Lactate (exogenous lactic acid produced by gut bacteria)
    - Methanol (this is inclusive of alcohols in general)
    - Aspirin (salicylic acid)
    - Renal failure (uremic acidosis)
    - Ketones (diabetic, alcoholic, and starvation ketosis)
  - *Nonanion gap metabolic acidosis:*
    - *Examples:* Diarrhea, renal tubular acidosis, ureteral diversion, excessive 0.9% saline infusion, treatment with carbonic anhydrase inhibitor.
  - *Mixed acid–base disorders:* Presence of two or more primary acid–base disturbances simultaneously.
    - *Examples:*
      - Chronic obstructive pulmonary disease (COPD) (respiratory acidosis) + vomiting (metabolic alkalosis)
      - Septic shock (lactic acidosis) + hyperventilation (respiratory alkalosis)

Basic Steps for Arterial Blood Gas Analysis

The following steps can be used for rapid interpretation of ABG.[51]

Normal values for calculation:

- Normal pH = 7.4, Normal $PaCO_2$ = 40 mm Hg, Normal HCO_3 = 24 mmol/L
- Normal AG = 12 mEq/L

Step 1: Check for the Validity of ABG

Check for the consistency of ABG of the report by using the modified Henderson equation.

$$[H^+] = \frac{24\,(PaCO_2)}{[HCO_3^-]}$$

TABLE 9: pH and corresponding H^+ (nmol/L).

pH	*Approximate [H⁺] (nmol/L)*
7.00	100
7.05	89
7.10	79
7.15	71
7.20	63
7.30	50
7.40	40
7.45	35
7.50	32
7.60	25

TABLE 10: Change in pH and $PaCO_2$ in acid–base disorder.

Disorder	*Primary*	*pH*	*$PaCO_2$*
Acidosis	Respiratory	pH ↓	$PaCO_2$ ↑
Acidosis	Metabolic	pH ↓	$PaCO_2$ ↓
Alkalosis	Respiratory	pH ↑	$PaCO_2$ ↓
Alkalosis	Metabolic	pH ↑	$PaCO_2$ ↑

The ABG is probably invalid if the pH and the $[H^+]$ are inconsistent **(Table 9)**.

Step 2: Look for Oxygenation and Ventilation Status

Patients' oxygenation and ventilation status can be assessed by assessment of PaO_2 and $PaCO_2$. Normal PaO_2 for age = 109 – (0.43 × age in years).[52] However, oxygenation status should be commented on considering the corresponding FiO_2.

Step 3: Look for pH

Is there alkalemia or acidemia present?

Look at pH; normal pH is 7.35–7.45. For calculation purposes, consider 7.4

- pH < 7.4 acidemia
- pH > 7.4 alkalemia

Step 4: Identify the Primary Disorder—Metabolic or Respiratory

In primary respiratory disorders, the pH and $PaCO_2$ change in opposite directions, while in metabolic disorders, they change in the *same* direction **(Table 10)**.

Step 5: Compensation

The human body maintains its acid–base balance through a buffer system. When one parameter is disrupted (primary disorder), the other parameter moves in the opposite direction to preserve the pH balance. This process is known as compensation. The compensatory response depends upon the adequate functioning of the lungs or kidneys and on the severity of the acid–base disturbance. Acute compensation occurs within 6–24 hours, while chronic compensation takes 1–4 days. Respiratory compensation occurs relatively faster than metabolic compensation. In clinical practice, complete compensation is rare.[53,54]

- *For primary respiratory disorder:*
  - Identify whether the primary respiratory disorder is acute or chronic
    - *For acute respiratory disorder:* Change in pH by 0.008 for every change in $PaCO_2$
    - *For chronic respiratory disorder:* Change in pH by 0.003 for every change in $PaCO_2$.
  - Compensation for a respiratory disorder:
    - *Acute respiratory acidosis:* $[HCO_3^-]$ increase by 1 mEq/L for every 10 mm Hg increase in $PaCO_2$ above 40.
    - *Chronic respiratory acidosis:* $[HCO_3^-]$ increase by 4 mEq/L for every 10 mm Hg increase in $PaCO_2$ above 40.
    - *Acute respiratory alkalosis:* $[HCO_3^-]$ decrease by 2 mEq/L for every 10 mm Hg fall in $PaCO_2$ below 40.
    - *Chronic respiratory alkalosis:* $[HCO_3^-]$ decrease by 5 mEq/L for every 10 mm Hg fall in $PaCO_2$ below 40.
- *For primary metabolic disorder:*
  - *Metabolic acidosis:* Expected $PaCO_2$ =1.5 × HCO_3 + 8 ± 2
  - *Metabolic alkalosis:* Expected $PaCO_2$ = 0.7 × HCO_3 + 20 ± 5

Step 6: Calculate the Anion Gap (If a Metabolic Acidosis Exists)

The anion gap is the difference between the measured cations and anions. Essentially, this represents the unmeasured anions in the blood. These unmeasured anions make up a significant portion of the total number of anions in the blood. Proteins predominantly contribute to this, including sulfates, phosphates, lactate, and ketones.

Normal anion gap = Na^{-} (Cl^{-} + HCO_3^{-})
= 12–14 mEq/L

Anion gap corrected (for albumin)
= Calculated anion gap + 2.5 × (Normal albumin g/dL – Observed albumin g/dL)

Step 7: Gap–Gap Ratio (Delta Ratio)

Mixed metabolic disturbances can be identified using the relationship between anion gap (AG) and HCO_3, which is called the gap-gap ratio.

Delta ratio = (Anion gap–12)/(24– [HCO_3])
= <0. 4→ Hyperchloremic normal AG acidosis (NAGMA)
= <1 → High AG acidosis (HAGMA) and NAGMA
= 1–2 → HAGMA
= >2 → Mixed acid–base abnormalities

VENOUS BLOOD GAS ANALYSIS

Clinical conditions in which a sample of arterial blood can be difficult to obtain due to diminished pulses or contraindicated, such as a negative Allen's test. A venous blood gas (VBG) can be considered to estimate systemic carbon dioxide and pH. Either a peripheral or central venous catheter can be considered for venous blood sampling. Central venous blood is preferred as it correlates better with ABG values. Venous measurements of PCO_2, pH, and HCO_3 can be interpreted with some minor adjustments. The central venous pH is approximately 0.03–0.05 lower than the arterial pH, and the PCO_2 is 4–5 mm Hg higher, with little or no rise in HCO_3. The peripheral venous pH is 0.03–0.04 lower than the arterial pH, the venous serum HCO_3 is 2–3 mEq/L higher, and PCO_2 is 3–8 mm Hg higher. VBG cannot be used for oxygenation assessment. Pulse oximetry along with VBGs can give some idea about the overall.[55]

DIGITAL HEMOGLOBINOMETER

Hemoglobin measurement remains important for perioperative transfusion-related decision-making. Hemoglobin level measurement by the central laboratory is the "gold standard"; however, it requires an adequate blood sample and time. Many a time, central laboratories are unable to provide real-time hemoglobin levels during an intraoperative acute phase where hemoglobin levels change rapidly due to bleeding and ongoing resuscitation. The availability of a number of POC investigations has revolutionized laboratory monitoring in perioperative settings. Hemoglobin levels can be obtained quickly and efficiently. Digital hemoglobinometers can be used during major surgeries with a high risk of blood loss. It facilitates decision-making and improves resuscitation efforts. HemoCue (HemoCue AB, Angelholm, Sweden) and I-Stat (Abbott Laboratories, Abbott Park, IL, USA) are the most common digital hemoglobinometers that provide mobile levels within minutes. HemoCue is based on absorption photometry, while I-Stat is on the conductometric method. A few drops of either capillary, venous, or arterial whole blood are needed for testing and providing rapid and accurate hemoglobin.

Previous studies have shown its clinical utility in emergency settings. However, whenever clinical conditions stabilize, blood samples for hemoglobin estimation should be sent to the central laboratory if possible.[56-58]

BLOOD GLUCOSE MONITORING

Perioperative hyperglycemia and hypoglycemia are associated with adverse outcomes such as cardiovascular events, short-term mortality, risk of surgical site infections, etc. Thus, it is imperative to keep perioperative blood glucose levels within the recommended range (glucose <180–200 mg/dL). Bedside blood glucose monitoring requires a drop of capillary blood and the use of a glucose meter. A large variety of blood glucose meters are available that are reasonably accurate. Incompatible test strips, noncalibrated meters, poor storage of the test strips, and use of expired strips can give erroneous glucose readings.

Many recent studies have shown the utility of continuous glucose monitoring (CGM) devices (e.g., MiniMed™ 770G System by Medtronic, USA) during the perioperative period. It measures glucose levels from interstitial fluid, assessed by an electrochemical enzymatic sensor inserted subcutaneously. Depending on the setting and device, glucose levels are reported every 5–15 minutes. CGM devices have alert systems for hypo- and hyperglycemia. The application of CGM devices with insulin pumps using a glucose control algorithm as closed-loop control (artificial pancreas) is now being studied during the perioperative period.[59]

OTHER POINT-OF-CARE INVESTIGATIONS

Many kit-based POC tests for troponin T, ketones, etc., are available, suitable for the perioperative period, including ICU settings. These commercially available kits are easy to handle and do not require special training.[60,61]

Some patients may sustain a myocardial injury during the perioperative period while undergoing noncardiac surgery, which is often difficult to diagnose using clinical criteria. Troponin T is a specific cardiac marker that indicates myocardial injury. A commercially available kit (Trop T kit) provides quick and reliable results. Thus, it can be valuable in decision-making, especially in cases of ST-elevation myocardial infarction.

Perioperative ketone levels are measured to identify diabetes ketoacidosis (DKA) due to insulin deficiency. The primary ketoacid found in the blood during ketoacidosis is beta-hydroxybutyrate. It can be measured by a POC blood testing kit. While the urine ketone analysis kit is a painless POC test that provides the average urine ketones' value since the last voided. It is relatively cheap, and no technical skill is required to use the equipment. The main ketone in urine is acetoacetic acid, which is a product of beta-hydroxybutyrate. POC urine ketone tests measure only acetoacetic acid but not beta-hydroxybutyrate, which may delay the early diagnosis of DKA. In DKA, the ratio of beta-hydroxybutyrate to acetoacetate ranges from 1:1 to 10:1. The delayed rise in acetoacetate during early DKA can underestimate the severity. Urine ketone strips also get affected by vitamin C.

CONCLUSION

A comprehensive approach including clinical judgment and appropriate investigation tailored to the individual patient, is required if perioperative challenge/crises arise during cancer surgeries. Various POC investigations and interventions, such as USG, ABG analysis, monitoring, thromboelastography, glucose measurements, hemoglobin/hematocrit analyses, and ketone analysis, may help in clinical decision-making. Point-of-care allows faster results and guided appropriate intervention. However, in clinical practice, it is essential to understand the limitations of every POC investigation. Understanding its sensitivity and specificity to gold standard diagnostic tests is critical.

REFERENCES

1. Gudaitytė J, Dvylys D, Šimeliūnaitė I. Anaesthetic challenges in cancer patients: current therapies and pain management. Acta Med Litu. 2017;24(2):121-7.
2. Gillman LM, Kirkpatrick AW. Portable bedside ultrasound: the visual stethoscope of the 21st century. Scand J Trauma Resusc Emerg Med. 2012;20:18.
3. Byrne M, Singleton M, Kalagara H, Haskins SC. Perioperative point-of-care ultrasound. Adv Anesth. 2021;39:189-213.
4. Kayarian F, Patel D, O'Brien JR, Schraft EK, Gottlieb M. Artificial intelligence and point-of-care ultrasound: benefits, limitations, and implications for the future. Am J Emerg Med. 2024;80:119-22.
5. You-Ten KE, Siddiqui N, Teoh WH, Kristensen MS. Point-of-care ultrasound (POCUS) of the upper airway. Can J Anaesth. 2018;65(4):473-84.
6. Carsetti A, Sorbello M, Adrario E, Donati A, Falcetta S. Airway ultrasound as predictor of difficult direct laryngoscopy: a systematic review and meta-analysis. Anesth Analg. 2022;134(4):740-50.
7. Daggupati H, Maurya I, Singh RD, Ravishankar M. Development of a scoring system for predicting difficult intubation using ultrasonography. Indian J Anaesth. 2020;64(3):187-92.
8. Yao W, Wang B. Can tongue thickness measured by ultrasonography predict difficult tracheal intubation? Br J Anaesth. 2017;118(4):601-9.
9. Rai Y, You-Ten E, Zasso F, De Castro C, Ye XY, Siddiqui N. The role of ultrasound in front-of-neck access for cricothyroid membrane identification: a systematic review. J Crit Care. 2020;60:161-8.
10. Rajajee V, Fletcher JJ, Rochlen LR, Jacobs TL. Real-time ultrasound-guided percutaneous dilatational tracheostomy: a feasibility study. Crit Care Lond Engl. 2011;15:R67.
11. Kumar A, Sinha C, Singh AK, Bhadani UK. Vocal cord dysfunction: ultrasonography-aided diagnosis during routine airway examination. Saudi J Anaesth. 2017; 11(3):370-1.
12. Kaneko T, Kato T, Shiko Y, Kawasaki Y, Koyama K. Assessment of pre-extubating recurrent laryngeal nerve palsy using ultrasound in postoperative patients with esophageal cancer: a prospective observational study. J Anesth. 2024;38(3):347-53.
13. Makireddy R, Cherian A, Elakkumanan LB, Bidkar PU, Kundra P. Correlation between correctly sized uncuffed endotracheal tube and ultrasonographically determined subglottic diameter in paediatric population. Indian J Anaesth. 2020;64(2):103-8.
14. Ahn JH, Park JH, Kim MS, Kang HC, Kim IS. Point of care airway ultrasound to select tracheal tube and determine insertion depth in cleft repair surgery. Sci Rep. 2021;11(1):4743.
15. Sustić A, Miletić D, Protić A, Ivancić A, Cicvarić T. Can ultrasound be useful for predicting the size of a left double-lumen bronchial tube? Tracheal width as measured by ultrasonography versus computed tomography. J Clin Anesth. 2008;20(4):247-52.
16. Das SK, Choupoo NS, Haldar R, Lahkar A. Transtracheal ultrasound for verification of endotracheal tube placement: a systematic review and meta-analysis. Can J Anaesth J 2015;62(4):413-23.
17. Álvarez-Díaz N, Amador-García I, Fuentes-Hernández M, Dorta-Guerra R. Comparison between transthoracic lung

ultrasound and a clinical method in confirming the position of double-lumen tube in thoracic anaesthesia. A pilot study. Rev Esp Anestesiol Reanim. 2015;62(6):305-12.
18. Venkategowda PM, Mahendrakar K, Rao SM, Mutkule DP, Shirodkar CG, Yogesh H. Laryngeal air column width ratio in predicting post extubation stridor. Indian J Crit Care Med. 2015;19(3):170-3.
19. Goffi A, Kruisselbrink R, Volpicelli G. The sound of air: point-of-care lung ultrasound in perioperative medicine. Can J Anaesth. 2018;65(4):399-416.
20. Lichtenstein DA. BLUE-protocol and FALLS-protocol: two applications of lung ultrasound in the critically ill. Chest. 2015;147(6):1659-70.
21. Asmara OD, Pitoyo CW, Wulani V, Harimurti K, Araminta AP. Accuracy of bedside lung ultrasound in emergency (BLUE) protocol to diagnose the cause of acute respiratory distress syndrome (ARDS): a meta-analysis. Acta Med Indones. 2022;54(2):266-82.
22. Northern T, Broyles MG, Nooli NP, Peirce A, Tuck BC, Coker BJ. Applications of perioperative lung ultrasound: from the clinic to the ICU. Int Anesthesiol Clin. 2022; 60(3):41-4.
23. Sharma G, Jacob R, Mahankali S, Ravindra MN. Preoperative assessment of gastric contents and volume using bedside ultrasound in adult patients: a prospective, observational, correlation study. Indian J Anaesth. 2018;62(10):753-8.
24. Meier I, Vogt AP, Meineri M, Kaiser HA, Luedi MM, Braun M. Point-of-care ultrasound in the preoperative setting. Best Pract Res Clin Anaesthesiol. 2020;34(2):315-24.
25. Kaptein EM, Kaptein MJ. Inferior vena cava ultrasound and other techniques for assessment of intravascular and extravascular volume: an update. Clin Kidney J. 2023; 16(11):1861-77.
26. Kaptein MJ, Kaptein EM. Inferior vena cava collapsibility index: clinical validation and application for assessment of relative intravascular volume. Adv Chronic Kidney Dis. 2021;28(3):218-26.
27. Orso D, Paoli I, Piani T, Cilenti FL, Cristiani L, Guglielmo N. Accuracy of ultrasonographic measurements of inferior vena cava to determine fluid responsiveness: a systematic review and meta-analysis. J Intensive Care Med. 2020; 35(4):354-63.
28. Long E, Oakley E, Duke T, Babl FE; Paediatric Research in Emergency Departments International Collaborative (PREDICT). Does respiratory variation in inferior vena cava diameter predict fluid responsiveness: a systematic review and meta-analysis. Shock. 2017;47(5):550-9.
29. de Haan JB, Sen S, Joo SS, Singleton M, Haskins SC. FAST exam for the anesthesiologist. Int Anesthesiol Clin. 2022;60(3):55-64.
30. Keikha M, Salehi-Marzijarani M, Soldoozi Nejat R, Sheikh Motahar Vahedi H, Mirrezaie SM. Diagnostic accuracy of rapid ultrasound in shock (RUSH) exam; A systematic review and meta-analysis. Bull Emerg Trauma. 2018;6(4):271-8.
31. Guay J, Suresh S, Kopp S. The use of ultrasound guidance for perioperative neuraxial and peripheral nerve blocks in children. Cochrane Database Syst Rev. 2019;2(2):CD011436.
32. Maitra S, Bhattacharjee S, Baidya DK. Comparison of long-, short-, and oblique-axis approaches for ultrasound-guided internal jugular vein cannulation: a network meta-analysis. J Vasc Access. 2020;21(2):204-9.
33. Bai B, Tian Y, Zhang Y, Yu C, Huang Y. Dynamic needle tip positioning versus the angle-distance technique for ultrasound-guided radial artery cannulation in adults: a randomized controlled trial. BMC Anesthesiol. 2020; 20(1):231.
34. Sharapi M, Afifi E, Al Mawla AM, Yassin MNA, Awwad SA, El-Samahy M. Ultrasound-based Accuro system versus traditional palpation technique for neuraxial anaesthesia: A systematic review and meta-analysis of randomised controlled trials. J Perioper Pract. 2023:17504589231215927.
35. Needleman L, Cronan JJ, Lilly MP, Merli GJ, Adhikari S, Hertzberg BS et al. Ultrasound for lower extremity deep venous thrombosis: multidisciplinary recommendations from the society of radiologists in ultrasound consensus conference. Circulation. 2018;137(14):1505-15.
36. Robba C, Santori G, Czosnyka M, Corradi F, Bragazzi N, Padayachy L, et al. Optic nerve sheath diameter measured sonographically as non-invasive estimator of intracranial pressure: a systematic review and meta-analysis. Intensive Care Med. 2018;44(8):1284-94.
37. Mueller N, Murthy S, Tainter CR, Lee J, Riddell K, Fintelmann FJ, et al. Can sarcopenia quantified by ultrasound of the rectus femoris muscle predict adverse outcome of surgical intensive care unit patients as well as frailty? A prospective, observational cohort study. Ann Surg. 2016;264(6):1116-24.
38. Kang SY, Jo IJ, Lee G, Park JE, Kim T, Lee SU et al. Point-of-care ultrasound compression of the carotid artery for pulse determination in cardiopulmonary resuscitation. Resuscitation. 2022;179:206-13.
39. Ávila-Reyes D, Acevedo-Cardona AO, Gómez-González JF, Echeverry-Piedrahita DR, Aguirre-Flórez M, Giraldo-Diaconeasa A. Point-of-care ultrasound in cardiorespiratory arrest (POCUS-CA): narrative review article. Ultrasound J. 2021;13(1):46.
40. Shaydakov ME, Sigmon DF, Blebea J. (2024). Thromboelastography. Treasure Island (FL): StatPearls Publishing. [online] Available from https://www.ncbi.nlm.nih.gov/books/NBK537061/. [Last accessed March, 2025].
41. Whiting D, DiNardo JA. TEG and ROTEM: technology and clinical applications. Am J Hematol. 2014;89(2):228-32.
42. Whitton TP, Healy WJ. Review of Thromboelastography (TEG): medical and surgical applications. Ther Adv Pulm Crit Care Med. 2023;18:29768675231208426.
43. Ramanujam V, DiMaria S, Varma V. Thromboelastography in the perioperative period: a literature review. Cureus. 2023;15(5):e39407.

44. Selby R. "TEG talk": expanding clinical roles for thromboelastography and rotational thromboelastometry. Hematol Am Soc Hematol Educ Prog. 2020;2020(1):67-75.
45. Cowley NJ, Owen A, Bion JF. Interpreting arterial blood gas results. BMJ. 2013;346:f16.
46. Larkin BG, Zimmanck RJ. Interpreting arterial blood gases successfully. AORN J. 2015;102(4):343-54; quiz 355-7.
47. Biswas CK, Ramos JM, Agroyannis B, Kerr DN. Blood gas analysis: effect of air bubbles in syringe and delay in estimation. Br Med J (Clin Res Ed). 1982;284(6320):923-7.
48. Börner U, Müller H, Höge R, Hempelmann G. The influence of anticoagulation on acid-base status and blood-gas analysis. Acta Anaesthesiol Scand.1984;28:277-9.
49. Hamilton PK, Morgan NA, Connolly GM, Maxwell AP. Understanding acid-base disorders. Ulster Med J. 2017; 86(3):161-6.
50. Brubaker RH, Vashisht R, Meseeha M. (2024). High anion gap metabolic acidosis. Treasure Island (FL): StatPearls Publishing. [online] Available from https://www.ncbi.nlm.nih.gov/books/NBK448090/. [Last accessed March, 2025].
51. Woodruff, David W. RN, CCRN, CNS, MSN. Six steps to ABG analysis. Nurs Crit Care. 2007;2(2):48-52.
52. Sorbini CA, Grassi V, Solinas E, Muiesan G. Arterial oxygen tension in relation to age in healthy subjects. Respiration. 1968;25(1):3-13.
53. Sood P, Paul G, Puri S. Interpreting arterial blood gas. Indian J Crit Care Med. 2010;14(2):57-64.
54. Neligan PJ, and Deutshman CS. Perioperative acid-base balance. In: Miller RD (Ed). Miller's Anesthesia, 8th edition. Philadelphia: Elsevier/Sauders; 2015. pp. 1811-30.
55. Schütz N, Roth D, Schwameis M, Röggla M, Domanovits H. Can venous blood gas be used as an alternative to arterial blood gas in intubated patients at admission to the emergency department? A retrospective study. Open Access Emerg Med. 2019;11:305-12.
56. Lamhaut L, Apriotesei R, Combes X, Lejay M, Carli P, Vivien B. Comparison of the accuracy of noninvasive hemoglobin monitoring by spectrophotometry (SpHb) and HemoCue® with automated laboratory hemoglobin measurement. Anesthesiology. 2011;115(3):548-54.
57. Kolotiniuk NV, Manecke GR, Pinsky MR, Banks D. Measures of blood hemoglobin and hematocrit during cardiac surgery: comparison of three point-of-care devices. J Cardiothorac Vasc Anesth. 2018;32(4):1638-41.
58. Morris BL, Hajduk J, Cheon EC, Ballard HA, Burjek NE. Comparison of two point-of-care measurements of hemoglobin against standard laboratory values during pediatric liver transplantation: a retrospective review. Paediatr Anaesth. 2022;32(10):1121-8.
59. Price CE, Fanelli JE, Aloi JA, Anzola SC, Vishneski SR, Saha AK, et al. Feasibility of intraoperative continuous glucose monitoring: an observational study in general surgery patients. J Clin Anesth. 2023;87:111090.
60. Huang J, Yeung AM, Bergenstal RM, Castorino K, Cengiz E, Dhatariya K, et al. Update on measuring ketones. J Diabetes Sci Technol. 2024;18(3):714-26.
61. Botto F, Alonso-Coello P, Chan MT, Villar JC, Xavier D, Srinathan S, et al. Myocardial injury after noncardiac surgery: a large, international, prospective cohort study establishing diagnostic criteria, characteristics, predictors, and 30-day outcomes. Anesthesiology. 2014;120(3):564-78.

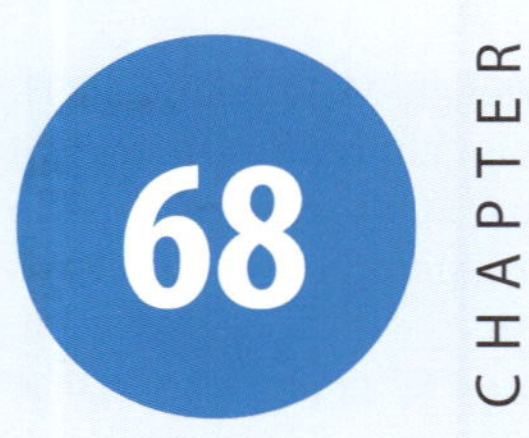

Perioperative Echocardiography for Major Cancer Surgeries

Pooja Natarajan, Arupratan Maiti, Muralidhar Kanchi

INTRODUCTION

Echocardiography is a highly sophisticated modality of diagnosis and monitoring that has revolutionized hemodynamic management in the modern era. It is an invaluable tool for troubleshooting multiple issues during the perioperative period.[1] Beginning with two-dimensional (2D) to currently three-dimensional (3D)/four-dimensional (4D) technology, echocardiography has now reached the artificial intelligence (AI) stage where computers aid in the analysis and interpretation of images. Many of the undiagnosed cardiac issues can preoperatively pose a problem during the intraoperative period, leading to morbidity and mortality of the patient.[2] Although transthoracic echocardiography (TTE) is relatively easy and can be done on an outpatient basis when the patient is awake, intraoperatively, it can be challenging and may not be feasible due to drapes, breach of sterility, and access to the chest wall. Nevertheless, the availability of transesophageal echocardiography (TEE) can be a good alternative for real-time hemodynamic monitoring during the intraoperative period. Hemodynamic monitoring during oncosurgery can be extremely challenging as we anticipate massive fluid shifts and cardiovascular stress. Multiple invasive hemodynamic monitoring tools are available in the market, such as continuous cardiac output (CCO) monitoring with pulmonary artery catheter (PAC), FloTrac® monitoring system, and Acumen Hypotension Prediction Index (HPI) software (by Edwards Lifesciences). Continuous echocardiography monitoring with TEE can be an indispensable tool for real-time cardiac function monitoring for anesthesiologists. TEE is considered a Category I indication for acute cardiovascular decompensation.[3] Cardiovascular diseases coexist with tumors or as a consequence of treatment with chemoradiation therapy.[4] The European Society of Cardiology (ESC) in 2022 brought out guidelines on cardio-oncology, which advocates for baseline risk assessment to identify high-risk oncology patients.[5] The knowledge of echocardiography for an anesthesiologist has become an integral part of the intraoperative and postoperative curriculum in the operation theater and intensive care unit (ICU).

TRANSESOPHAGEAL ECHOCARDIOGRAPHY

In 1971, the first esophageal ultrasound was reported to measure flow in the aortic arch.[6] From 1982 onward, the modern era of TEE began with phased-array transducers. TEE needs skill and training and has a long learning curve compared to TTE; hence, it is important to get familiar with the machine, knobology, and probe **(Figs. 1 and 2)**. It is performed under local anesthesia with sedation in the outpatient department or under general anesthesia in the operation theater. Absolute contraindications are patient refusal, esophageal injury/stricture/surgery/mass, and gastric bleed/ulcers. A few relative

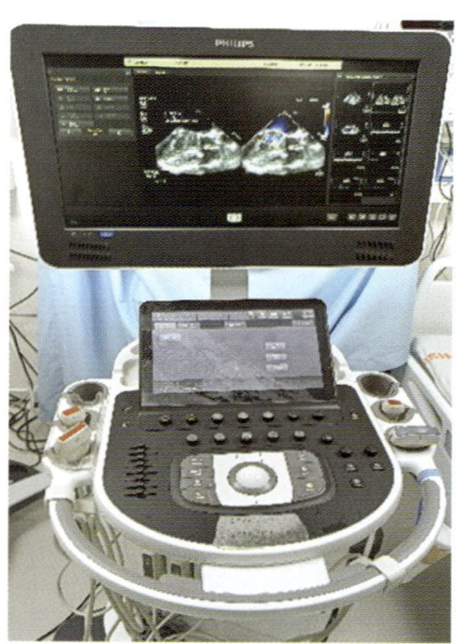

Fig. 1: TEE machine (Philips©, Massachusetts). (TEE: transesophageal echocardiography)

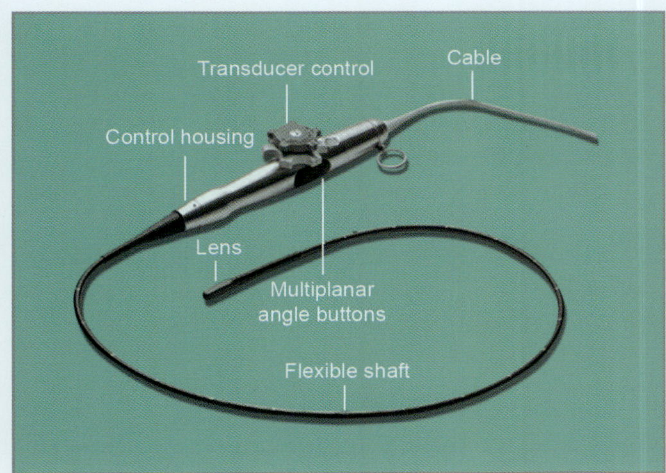

Fig. 2: Parts of the TEE probe (Philips©, Massachusetts). (TEE: transesophageal echocardiography)

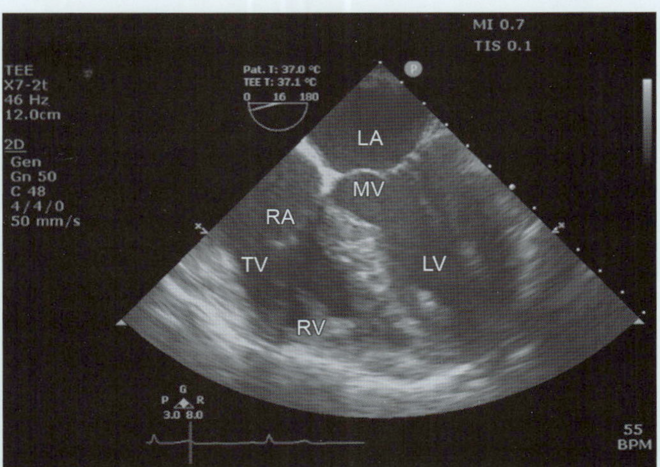

Fig. 3: TEE midesophageal four-chamber view at 0–20°. (LA: left atrium; MV: mitral valve; RA: right atrium; TV: tricuspid valve; LV: left ventricle; RV: right ventricle; TEE: transesophageal echocardiography)

contraindications are radiation to the neck/mediastinum, hiatus hernia, Barrett's esophagus, and coagulopathy.[6] Conventionally 20 original standard TEE views comprise a comprehensive TEE examination as described by the Society of Cardiovascular Anesthesiologists (SCA)/ American Society of Echocardiography (ASE) (1999).[6] Now, it has been augmented by eight additional views. Insertion of the TEE probe has to be done with extreme caution as upper airway injury/esophageal injury can be a catastrophic complication. There are four upper esophageal views at a distance of 25–30 cm from the incisor teeth: Upper-esophageal right pulmonary vein (UE RPV), upper-esophageal left pulmonary vein (UE LPV), upper-esophageal aortic arch long-axis, and upper-esophageal aortic arch short-axis. There are 16 midesophageal views around 30–35 cm from the incisor teeth: Midesophageal five-chamber (ME 5C), midesophageal four-chamber (ME 4C), midesophageal mitral commissural (ME MC), midesophageal two-chamber (ME 2C), midesophageal long-axis (ME LAX), midesophageal aortic valve long-axis (ME AV LAX), midesophageal ascending aortic long-axis (ME AA LAX), midesophageal ascending aortic short-axis (ME AA SAX), midesophageal aortic valve short-axis (ME AV SAX), midesophageal right ventricle inflow-outflow (ME RV IO), midesophageal right pulmonary vein (ME RPV), midesophageal modified bicaval tricuspid valve, midesophageal bicaval, midesophageal left atrial appendage (ME LAA), descending aortic short-axis (Desc Ao LAX), and descending aortic long-axis (Desc Ao LAX). There are eight transgastric views about 35–45 cm beyond the incisor teeth: Transgastric basal short-axis (TG Basal SAX), transgastric midpapillary short-axis, transgastric apical short-axis, transgastric right ventricular basal, transgastric right ventricular inflow–outflow, deep transgastric five-chamber (DTG 5C), transgastric two-chamber (TG2C), transgastric right ventricular inflow (TG RV I), transgastric long-axis (TG LAX), and transgastric inferior vena cava (TG IVC). For practical purposes, we will be concentrating on focused views for the diagnosis of challenging situations in the perioperative period.

The midesophageal four-chamber view **(Fig. 3)** obtained at 0–20° multiplane angle can visualize the chambers and valves of the heart, measure dimensions of the right atrium (RA), left atrium (LA), left ventricle (LV), right ventricle (RV), interatrial septum (IAS) for atrial septal defect (ASD), interventricular septum (IVS) for ventricular septal defect (VSD), mitral valve (MV) dysfunction like mitral stenosis (MS)/mitral regurgitation (MR), and tricuspid valve (TV) dysfunction like tricuspid stenosis (TS)/tricuspid regurgitation (TR). We can assess LV and RV systolic and diastolic function, regional wall motion abnormality (RWMA), color flow Doppler, and 2D spectral Doppler across valves to check gradients, pericardial/pleural effusion, and cardiac mass.

The midesophageal two-chamber view is obtained by increasing the transducer angle to 80–100° from the ME 4C view (0°); in this view, the LV function, RWMA, MV, and LAA can be assessed for clots **(Fig. 4)**.

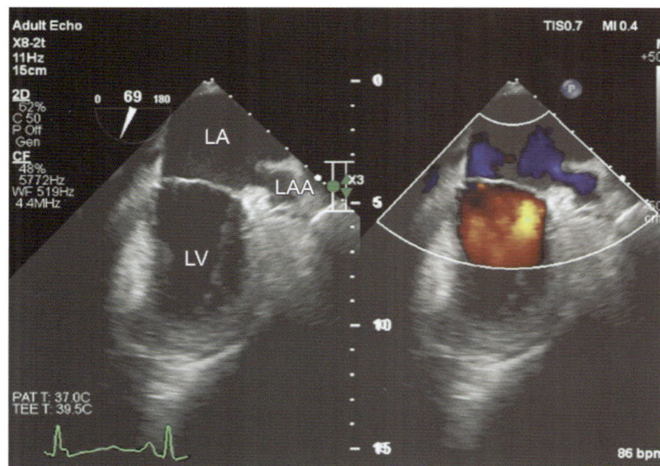

Fig. 4: TEE midesophageal two-chamber view at 80–100°. LA: left atrium; LV: left ventricle; LAA: left atrial appendage; TEE: transesophageal echocardiography)

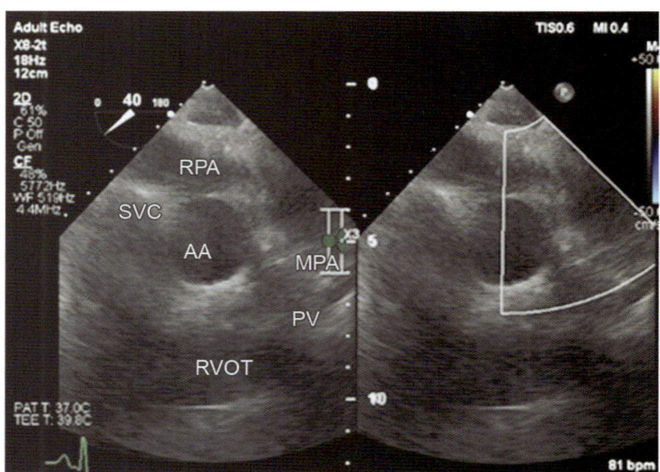

Fig. 6: TEE midesophageal ascending aorta short-axis view at 0–10°. (AA: ascending aorta; CE: contrast echocardiography; MPA: main pulmonary artery; PV: pulmonary valve; RPA: right pulmonary artery; RVOT: right ventricular outflow tract; SVC: superior vena cava; TEE: transesophageal echocardiography)

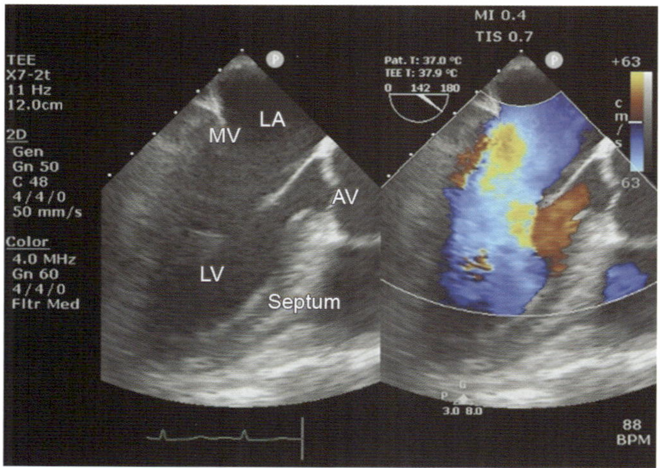

Fig. 5: TEE mid esophageal long axis view (ME LAX) view at 120–140°. (AV: aortic valve; LA: left atrium; LV: left ventricle; MV: mitral valve; TEE: transesophageal echocardiography)

The mid esophageal long axis view (ME LAX) is obtained by increasing the transducer angle from 120° to 140° from the ME 4C view (0°) **(Fig. 5)**. In this view, the LV can be assessed for its function, RWMA, MV pathology, hypertrophy of the septum, left ventricular outflow tract obstruction (LVOTO), AV, aortic root pathology, aneurysm, dissection, mass/thrombus, and VSD.

The midesophageal ascending aortic short-axis view (0–10°) is obtained by withdrawing the probe from the ME AV SAX view (30°) and rotating the transducer angle back to 0°. This view images the superior vena cava (SVC) in SAX, the ascending aorta (AA) in SAX, and the right and main pulmonary arteries in LAX **(Fig. 6)**.

The midesophageal bicaval view (90–110°) is obtained by turning the entire probe toward patients right from the ME 2C view (90°) **(Fig. 7)**. In this view, IVC, SVC, RA, IAS, and LA are visible and can diagnose patent foramen ovale (PFO), ASD, SVC collapsibility, catheter guidewires, effusion, and mass.

The midesophageal right ventricle inflow–outflow view is obtained from the ME AV SAX view (30°) by increasing the transducer angle to 50–75° **(Fig. 8)**. In this view, RA, RV, right ventricular outflow tract (RVOT), TV, pulmonary valve (PV), AV, LA, and main pulmonary artery (MPA) are visible. We can diagnose ASD, VSD, AV, TV, PV pathology, and the function of RV.

The transgastric midpapillary short-axis view is obtained by advancing the TEE probe in a neutral position into the stomach and anteflexing the probe tip **(Fig. 9)**. In this view, LV function, RWMA, LV wall thickness, VSD, and effusion can be diagnosed.

TRANSTHORACIC ECHOCARDIOGRAPHY

Transthoracic echocardiography is a bedside armamentarium for quick diagnosis and intervention of acute hemodynamic instability perioperatively. As an anesthesiologist, a basic knowledge of point-of-care

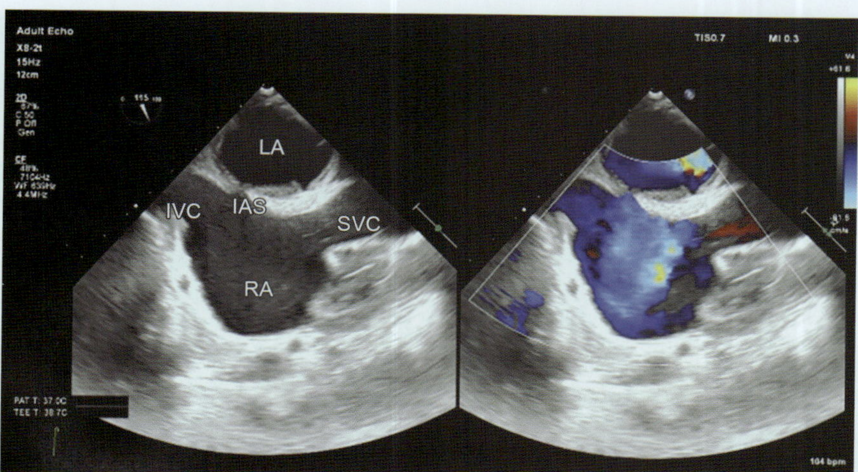

Fig. 7: TEE midesophageal bicaval view at 90°. (IAS: interatrial septum; IVC: inferior vena cava; LA: left atrium; RA: right atrium; SVC: superior vena cava; TEE: transesophageal echocardiography)

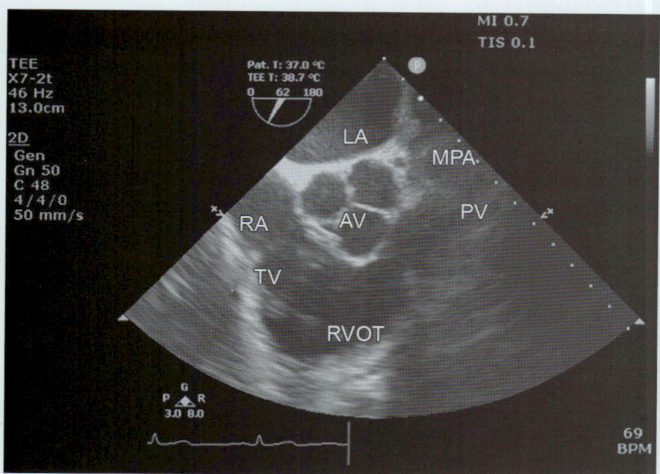

Fig. 8: TEE midesophageal right ventricular inflow–outflow view at 50–70°. (AV: aortic valve; LA: left atrium; MPA: main pulmonary artery; PV: pulmonary valve; RA: right atrium; RVOT: right ventricular outflow tract; TV: tricuspid valve; TEE: transesophageal echocardiography)

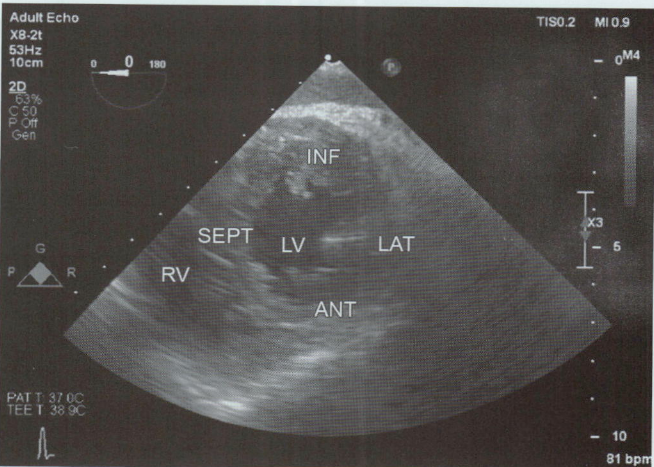

Fig. 9: TEE transgastric midpapillary short-axis view at 0°. (ANT: anterior; INF: inferior; LAT: lateral; LV: left ventricle; RV: right ventricle; SEPT: septum; TEE: transesophageal echocardiography)

ultrasound (POCUS) views in TTE can be lifesaving.[7] The burgeoning use of ultrasound technology has improved the speed of diagnosis and fastened the intervention and treatment process for better patient care. **Table 1** illustrates a few advantages and disadvantages of TTE.

Point-of-Care Views in Transthoracic Echocardiography

Point-of-care ultrasound consists of five focused views on TTE: The parasternal long axis (PLAX), the parasternal short axis (PSAX), the apical four-chamber (A4C), the subxiphoid (subcostal), and the IVC views.

In the parasternal long-axis view **(Fig. 10)**, the probe is placed on the left fourth intercostal space with the marker toward the left shoulder. In this view, we can assess the LV chamber size and morphology of valves and function. The functioning of MV, AV, shunts, effusion, and mass/thrombus can be assessed.

The parasternal short-axis view is obtained by rotating the probe 90° from the PLAX view with a marker pointing toward the right shoulder. From this view, we can get a midpapillary level view **(Fig. 11)**, MV level view (fish mouth

TABLE 1: Advantages and disadvantages of TTE.

Advantages	*Disadvantages*
• Easy access in awake patients • OPD basis/bedside • Noninvasive • Quick	• Thick chest wall poor echo window, obesity, poor patient cooperation • Difficult for intraoperative use due to sterility and drapes • Intermittent positive pressure ventilation • Difficult postoperative views in thoracic surgery, chest edema, pneumothorax, pneumopericardium, and drains • Severe chronic obstructive pulmonary disease

(OPD: outpatient department)

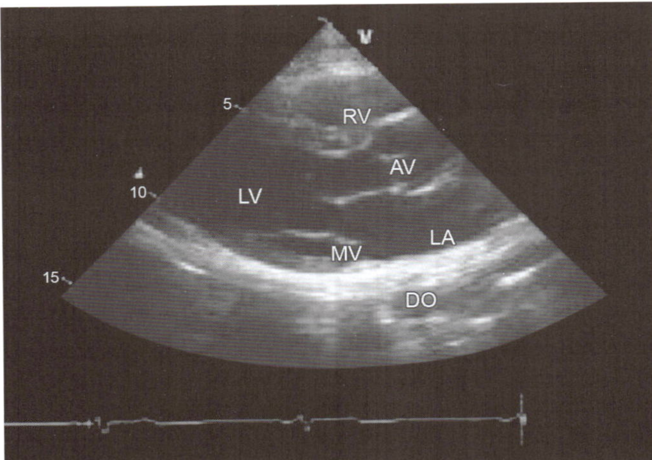

Fig. 10: TTE parasternal long-axis view. (AV: aortic valve; DO: descending aorta; LA: left atrium; LV: left ventricle; MV: mitral valve; RV: right ventricle; TTE: transthoracic echocardiography)

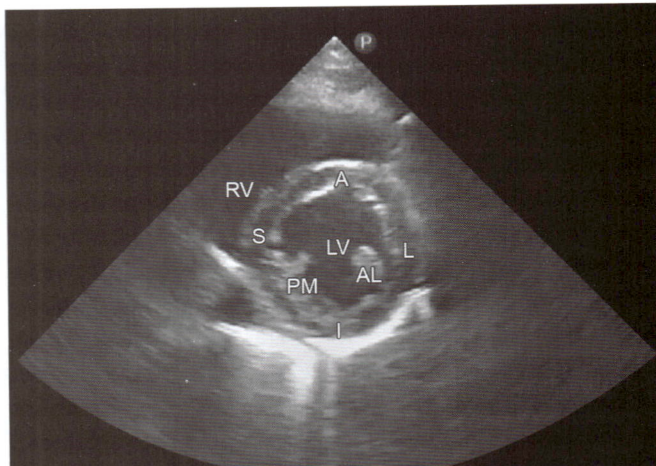

Fig. 11: TTE parasternal short-axis midpapillary view. (A: anterior; AL: anterolateral; I: inferior; L: lateral; PM: posteromedial; LV: left ventricle; RV: right ventricle; S: septal; TTE: transthoracic echocardiography)

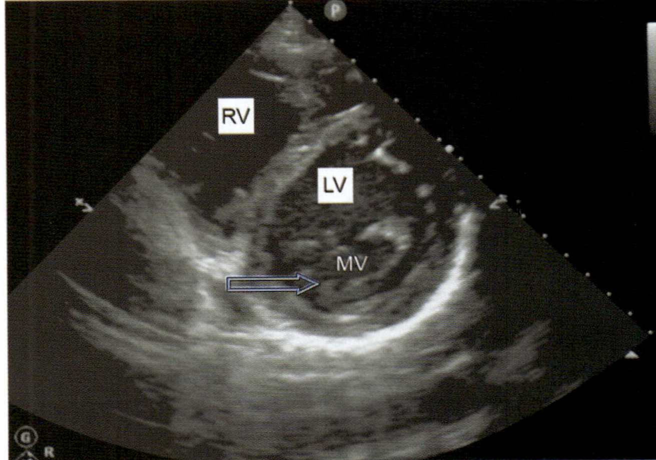

Fig. 12: TTE parasternal short-axis mitral valve (MV) view. (LV: left ventricle; RV: right ventricle; TTE: transthoracic echocardiography)

view) **(Fig. 12)**, and aortic valve level view (Mercedes Benz view) **(Fig. 13)**. The midpapillary level view gives LV ejection fraction (LVEF), RV dysfunction, and RWMA.

To obtain the PSAX AV view, tilt the probe inferiorly to visualize the AV in the center, LA, IAS, RA, TV, RV, RVOT, PV, and MPA.

For the apical four-chamber view, slide the transducer toward the apex from the PSAX view, with the marker pointing toward the patient's left **(Fig. 14)**. The subxiphoid or subcostal view is seen from a different viewpoint and shows the same structures as the A4C view. This view is useful when the A4C view is difficult to visualize.

The transthoracic echocardiography inferior vena cava view is obtained from a subcostal view rotate the probe 90 degrees counterclockwise (not clockwise) with the probe marker facing the patient's head (not the foot) **(Fig. 15)**. This view is good for assessing volume responsiveness and fluid status of the body with the estimation of central venous pressure (CVP).

PREOPERATIVE ASSESSMENT IN ONCOSURGICAL PATIENTS

It is vital to assess the cardiovascular reserve in oncosurgical patients before surgery as these are high-risk surgeries. The Revised Cardiac Risk Index (RCRI) is a reliable index to predict cardiac complications and mortality after major noncardiac surgery.[8] Heart failure

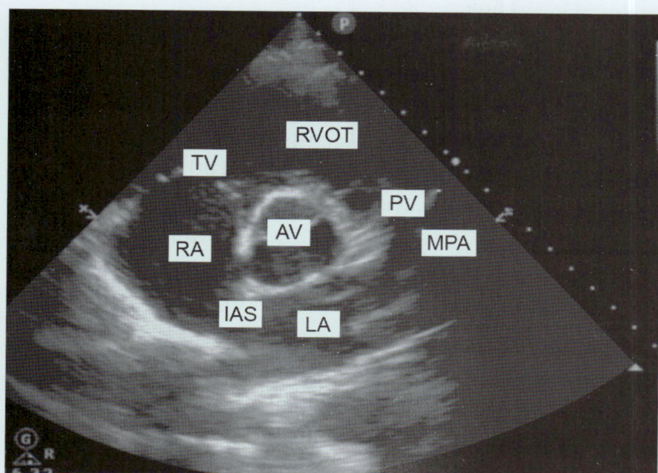

Fig. 13: TTE parasternal short-axis aortic valve (AV) view. (IAS: interatrial septum; LA: left atrium; MPA: main pulmonary artery; PV: pulmonary valve; RA: right atrium; RVOT: right ventricular outflow tract; TTE: transthoracic echocardiography; TV: tricuspid valve)

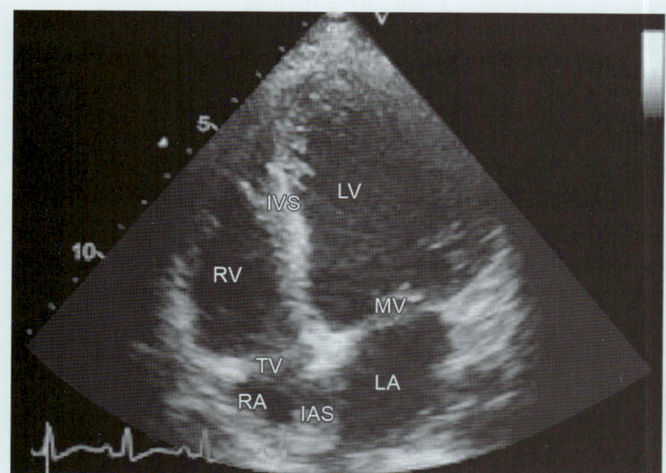

Fig. 14: TTE apical four-chamber view. (IAS: interatrial septum; IVS: interventricular septum; LA: left atrium; LV: left ventricle; MV: mitral valve; RA: right atrium; RV: right ventricle; TTE: transthoracic echocardiography; TV: tricuspid valve)

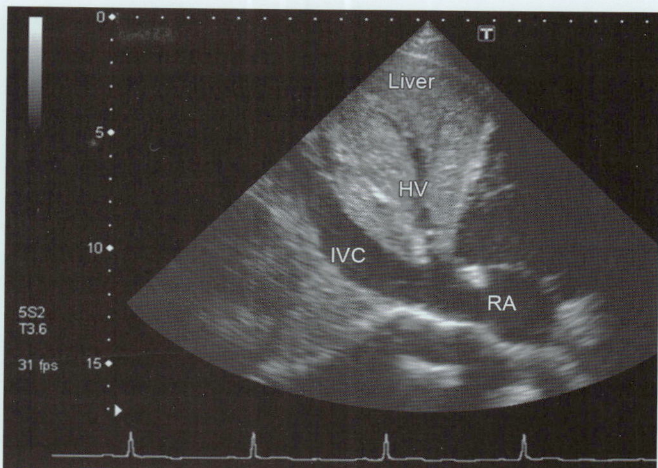

Fig. 15: TTE inferior vena cava (IVC) view. (HV: hepatic vein; RA: right atrium; TTE: transthoracic echocardiography)

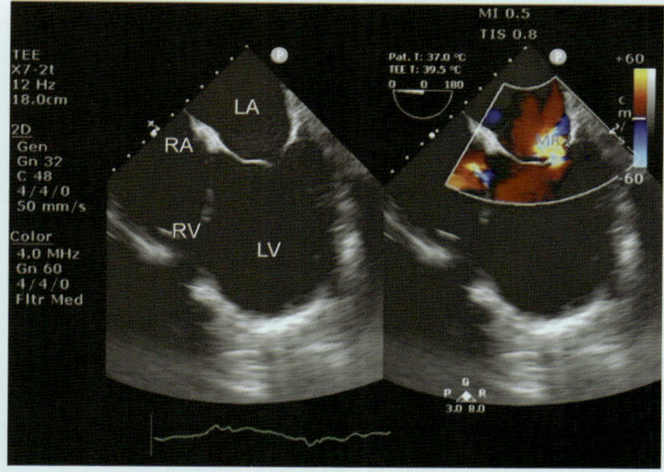

Fig. 16: TEE midesophageal four-chamber view showing dilated cardiomyopathy with mitral regurgitation. (LA: left atrium; LV: left ventricle; RA: right atrium; RV: right ventricle; TEE: transesophageal echocardiography)

(HF) due to oncology treatments has been shown to have a 2-year mortality rate as high as 60%.[9] Oncology treatment-induced cardiotoxicity is defined as a reduction in LVEF of more than 10% but less than 53% by the European Association of Cardiovascular Imaging (EACVI) and the ASE.[10]

Many of the chemotherapeutic agents like anthracycline derivatives (used in breast cancer), antimetabolite agents such as cytarabine or capecitabine, monoclonal antibodies, interleukins, alpha-interferon, 5-fluorouracil, and thyroxine kinase inhibitor drugs (used in thyroid cancer) cause cardiotoxicity.[11] Patients may develop cardiomyopathy and biventricular dysfunction **(Fig. 16)**. It is recommended to work up for the estimation of LVEF with 2D/3D, LV global longitudinal strain (GLS), right ventricular function, and any other lesions due to drug-induced cardiotoxicity.[12-14] Antivascular endothelial growth factor bevacizumab is known to cause pulmonary bleeding, edema, and embolism. Cyclophosphamide leads to pulmonary hypertension, and dasatinib causes pulmonary fibrosis, pulmonary hypertension, and right ventricular dysfunction.[15] Old age itself can be a risk factor due to hypertension, diabetes, and stiff connective tissue reducing the compliance of vasculature, leading to hypertension and increased afterload and myocardial strain. There is also a significantly reduced beta-receptor response, which hampers the normal physiological response to hypotension and could lead to vasoplegia. Postradiation therapy for mediastinal tumors causes constrictive pericarditis **(Fig. 17)** and fibrosis of the heart and lungs.[16]

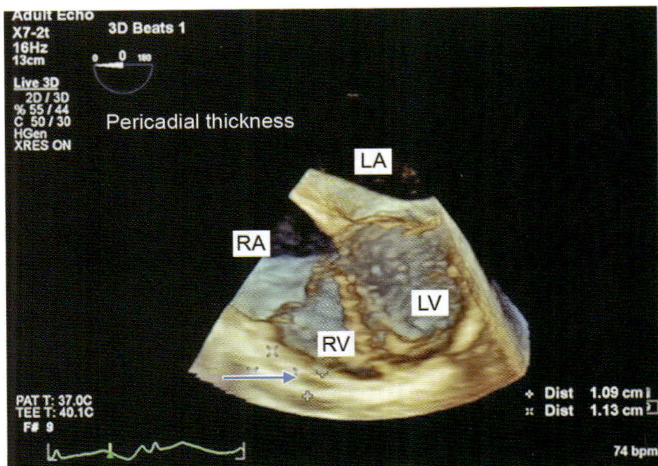

Fig. 17: 3D TEE midesophageal four-chamber view showing thickened pericardium in constrictive pericarditis postradiation therapy. Thickened pericardium >5 mm (blue arrow). (LA: left atrium; LV: left ventricle; RA: right atrium; RV: right ventricle; TEE: transesophageal echocardiography)

Assessment of Left Ventricular Function

The left ventricular ejection fraction calculation uses the modified Simpson's method **(Fig. 18)** in the ME 4C or ME 2C view. LVEF = End-diastolic volume (EDV) – end-systolic volume (ESV)/EDV × 100 calculates the LVEF. Normal values are 52–72%, and anything less than 30% is severe LV dysfunction. 3D volumetric analysis of LV is considered better than 2D. For early detection of subclinical LV dysfunction, when LVEF may be normal, LV GLS can be a good parameter to assess LV function[17] **(Fig. 19)**. It is always advisable to look for RWMA as few of the anticancer drugs aggravate ischemic heart disease.

Cardiac output (CO) calculation with left ventricular outflow tract (LVOT) diameter (d) and LVOT velocity time integral (VTI) can be done with spectral Doppler in TEE DTG view.

$$CO = \text{Stroke volume}\ (SV) \times \text{heart rate}\ (HR)$$

$$SV\,(\text{cm}^3) = \text{Cross-sectional area}\ (CSA)\ (\text{cm}^2) \times VTI\ (\text{cm})$$

$$CSA = \pi r^2 = 0.785d^2$$

Left ventricular diastolic dysfunction (LVDD) is common with radiotherapy drugs, with over 47% of patients showing HF even with normal LVEF.[18] In anthracycline therapy, 36% of the patients were diagnosed with asymptomatic diastolic dysfunction, within 1 week of starting therapy.[19] LV diastolic function can be measured using E and A values **(Fig. 20)** through inflow velocities across the MV with pulse wave Doppler, with normal values between 0.8 and 1.2, and values more than 2 predict

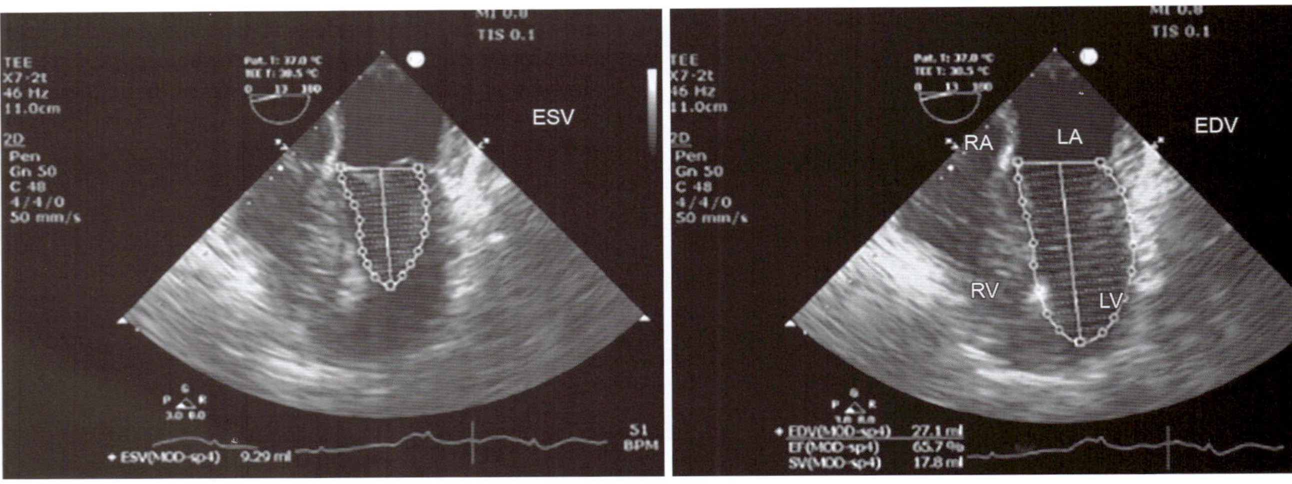

Fig. 18: TEE midesophageal four-chamber view showing modified Simpson's method for left ventricular ejection fraction calculation. (EDV: end-diastolic volume; ESV: end-systolic volume; LA: left atrium; LV: left ventricle; RA: right atrium; RV: right ventricle; TEE: transesophageal echocardiography)

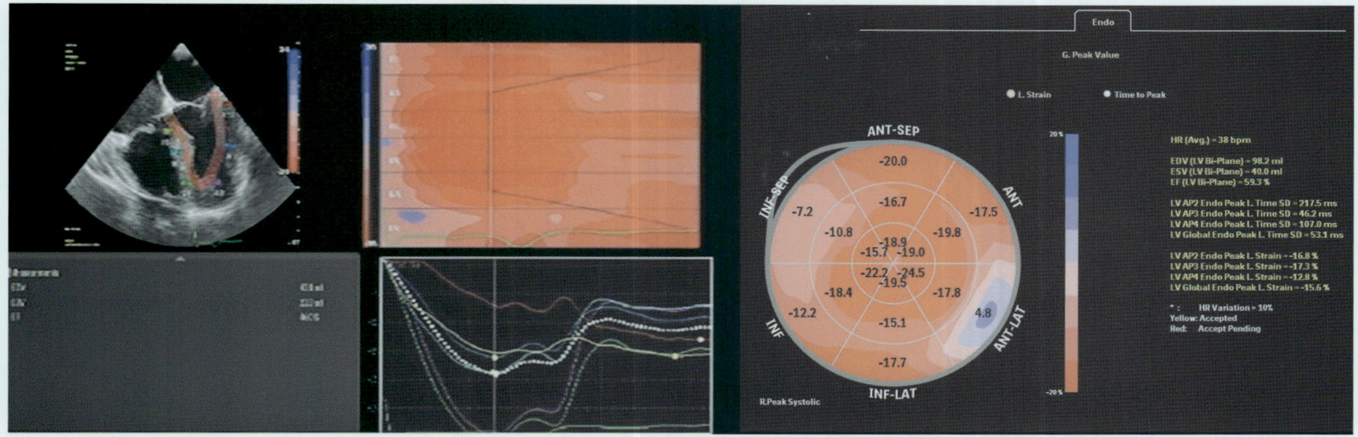

Fig. 19: Left ventricular strain measurement.

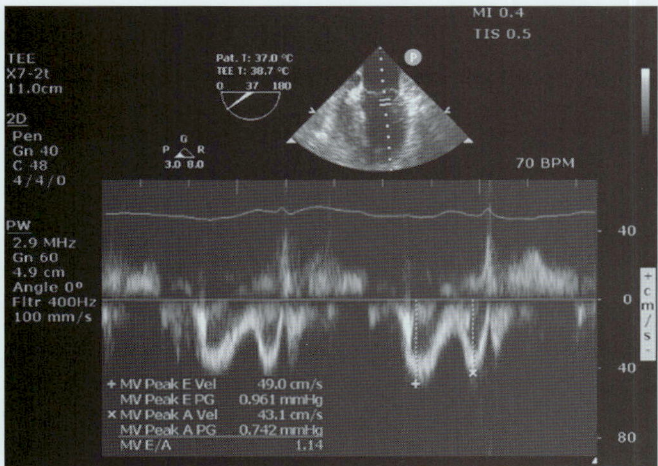

Fig. 20: TEE midesophageal four-chamber view with pulse wave (PW) Doppler of mitral inflow showing E and A waves. (TEE: transesophageal echocardiography)

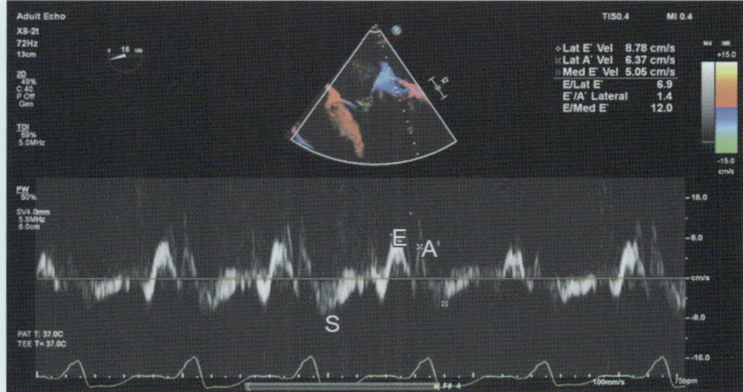

Fig. 21: TEE midesophageal four-chamber view with TDI measurement of lateral mitral annulus showing E′, A′, and S waves. (PW: pulsed wave; TDI: tissue Doppler imaging; TEE: transesophageal echocardiography)

grade III DD. Mitral annular tissue Doppler imaging (TDI) measures E′, A′, and S velocities from the medial and lateral mitral annulus **(Fig. 21)**. A ratio of E/E′ more than 14 predicts grade III DD (normal is <8).[20]

Assessment of Right Ventricular Function

Right ventricular dilatation **(Fig. 22)** can have various etiologies, including pulmonary embolism (PE), right-sided myocardial infarction, and lung pathologies (pulmonary hypertension, chronic obstructive pulmonary disease, and obstructive sleep apnea). RV dysfunction is diagnosed when tricuspid annular plane systolic excursion (TAPSE) is <17 mm, a fractional area change (FAC) is <35%, and tissue Doppler tricuspid annular systolic velocities

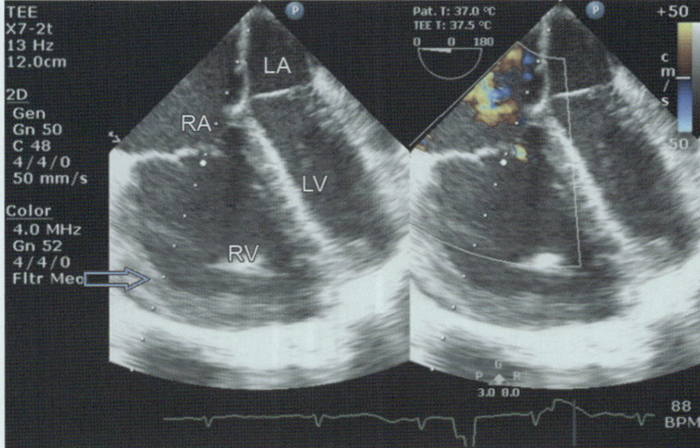

Fig. 22: TEE midesophageal four-chamber view showing dilated right atrium (RA) and right ventricle (RV) (blue arrow) with a shift of interatrial septum to the left and straightening of the interventricular septum in right ventricular failure. (LA: left atrium; LV: left ventricle; TEE: transesophageal echocardiography)

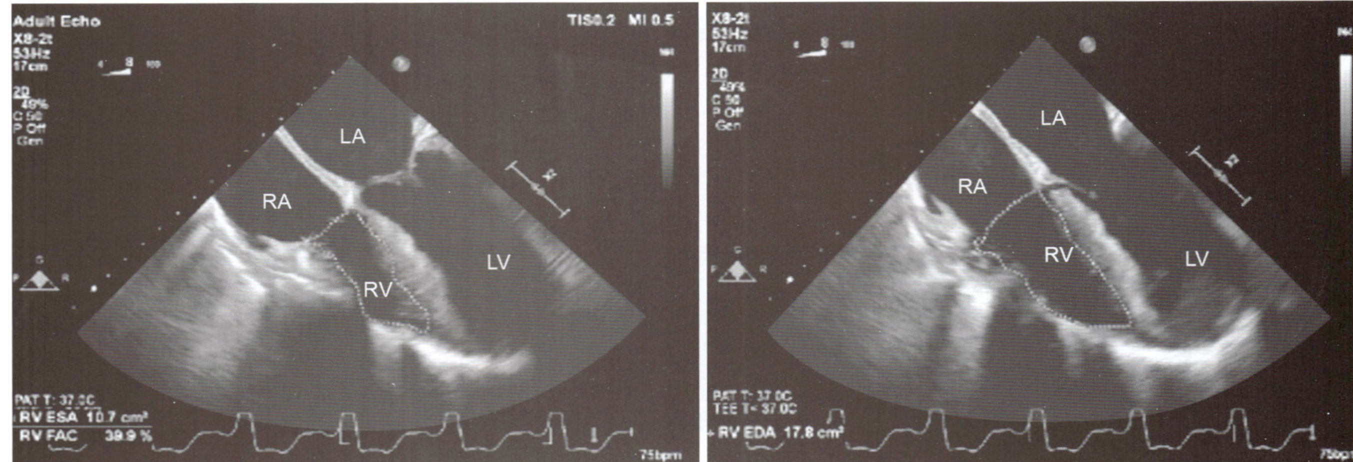

Fig. 23: TEE midesophageal four-chamber view showing measurements of right ventricular fractional area change (RV FAC). (LA: left atrium; LV: left ventricle; RA: right atrium; RV: right ventricle; RV ESA: right ventricular end-systolic area TEE: transesophageal echocardiography;)

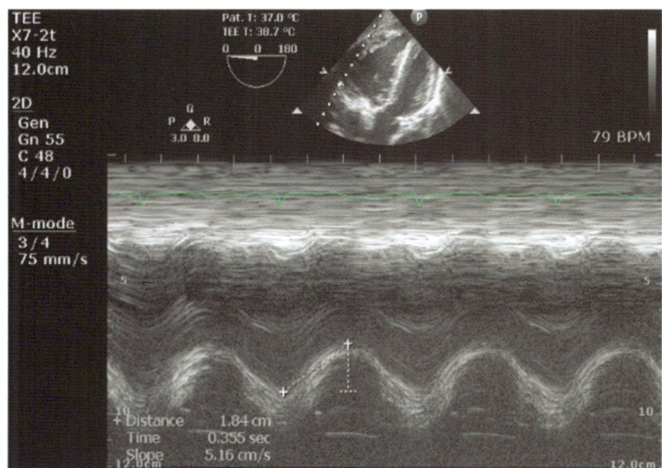

Fig. 24: TEE deep transgastric view showing tricuspid annular plane systolic excursion (TAPSE) measurement of the right ventricle with M-mode. (TEE: transesophageal echocardiography)

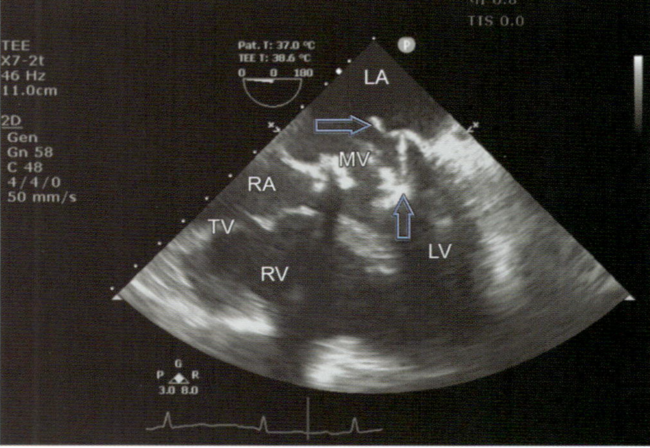

Fig. 25: TEE midesophageal four-chamber view showing vegetation on mitral valve (MV) (blue arrows). (LA: left atrium; LV: left ventricle; RA: right atrium; RV: right ventricle; TEE: transesophageal echocardiography; TV: tricuspid valve;)

(S') is <9 cm/s.[21] RVEF is best measured with 3D analysis due to its complex structure. TEE RV FAC can be measured in the ME 4C view **(Fig. 23)** by tracing the end diastolic area(EDA)- end systolic area(ESA)/EDA × 100 (normal value >42–56%),[22] and anything less than 35% is abnormal. TAPSE is the distance of systolic excursion of the lateral TV annulus measured in a longitudinal plane **(Fig. 24)**. It is a simple surrogate marker for global RV function (normal value >17 mm).

VALVULAR PATHOLOGY AND INFECTIVE ENDOCARDITIS

Although chemotherapy does not have any direct impact on the valves, indirect damage through secondary infectious endocarditis **(Fig. 25)** or thrombus formation can be observed.[23] Infection susceptibility due to immunosuppression state is common.

CARDIAC TUMORS

Cardiac tumors can be primarily benign (incidence 75%) and malignant (25%).[24] The most common benign tumors are myxoma (30% incidence in the LA > RA > RV = LV), lipoma (10% incidence LV > RA > IVS), papillary fibroelastoma (9% incidence AV > MV > TV), and fibroma (4% incidence LV > RV > IVS).

Primary malignant tumors of the heart (incidence 25%) are angiosarcoma, rhabdomyosarcoma, mesothelioma, and fibrosarcoma. Secondary metastatic tumors of the heart can be hematogenous, such as lymphoma, melanoma, or leukemia. Direct extension of the tumor from the lung, breast, or esophagus has to be dealt with caution: Intravascular extension into the IVC from the renal or hepatic tissue, and into the SVC from the bronchus or thyroid. Secondary to carcinoid heart or tumor infiltration, there is subendocardial fibrosis.

Clinical Implications with Cardiac Tumors

Preoperative evaluation is of utmost importance as there could be an extension into the airway, and anesthesia needs to be planned accordingly. Catastrophic bleeding and a difficult airway need to be anticipated. Ultrasonography can be helpful in evaluating tumor invasion into the airway, although computed tomography/magnetic resonance imaging (CT/MRI) is the gold standard. Postoperative hemodynamic compromise is common in SVC obstruction (SVCO) as there could be RV flow obstruction as well as reduced preload, and therefore vascular access is recommended to be inserted in the lower limbs for resuscitation. SVC syndrome can lead to backpressure changes and airway edema. It is wise to plan awake fiberoptic, rigid bronchoscopy, and surgical tracheostomy standby. A case like a calcific amorphous tumor of the heart in the right atrium **(Fig. 26)** can cause SVCO, which is seen in the ME-modified bicaval view on TEE **(Fig. 27)**. General anesthesia induction of patients with complete LV inflow obstruction **(Fig. 28)** and RV inflow obstruction **(Fig. 29)** can be very tricky, and one must be prepared for an emergency central cardiopulmonary bypass (CPB). Alternatively, elective peripheral CPB cannulation can be done under local anesthesia to be on the safer side.

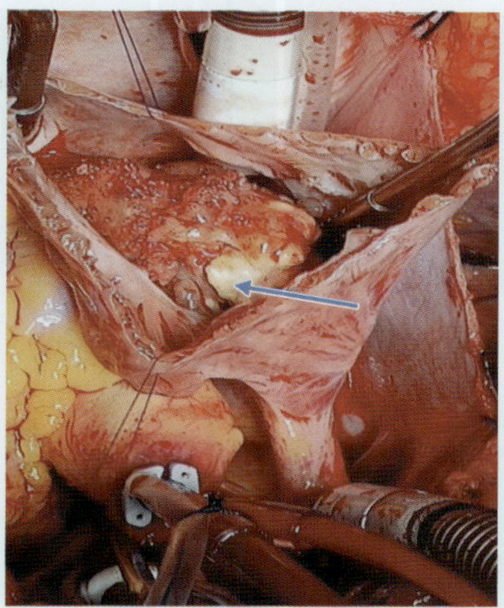

Fig. 26: Tumor of the right atrium showing calcification obstruction of the superior vena cava (blue arrow).

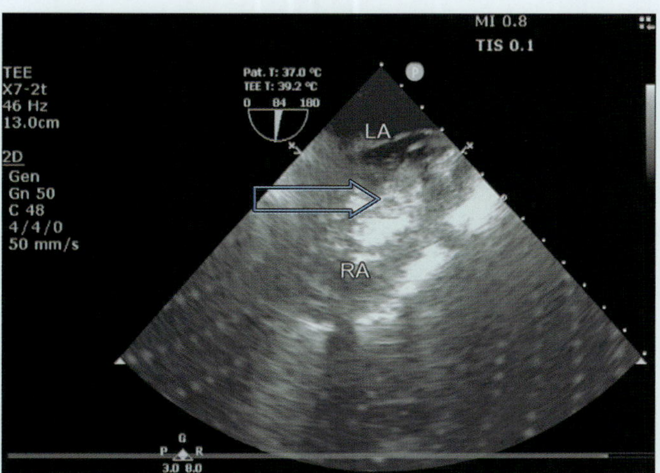

Fig. 27: TEE midesophageal bicaval view showing a right atrial mass extending to the superior vena cava causing an obstruction (blue arrow). (LA: left atrium; RA: right atrium; TEE: transesophageal echocardiography)

Clinical Implications of Thrombus in the Heart

One has to be extremely vigilant when there is a thrombus in the heart, especially on the left side of the heart as these could embolize and cause neurologic issues such as stroke and prolonged postoperative stay. Thrombus formation in the heart is widespread with dilated poor functional hearts as in dilated cardiomyopathy, ischemic cardiomyopathy, and aneurysm of the aorta/LV. Clots are commonly seen in MS, especially in LAA **(Fig. 30)**. Utmost caution is needed, especially when such patients have hemodynamically unstable arrhythmia (atrial fibrillation), which demands cardioversion to stabilize the situation. Neurological strokes due to embolization are common, with thrombus getting dislodged. Any spontaneous echo contrast in the heart needs further evaluation to look for a thrombus in the heart **(Fig. 31)**.

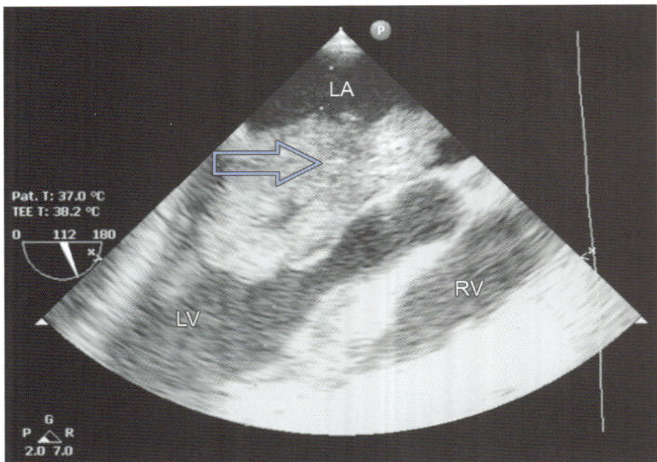

Fig. 28: TEE midesophageal left ventricular long-axis view showing large left atrial myxoma causing inflow obstruction of the left ventricle (LV) (blue arrow). (LA: left atrium; RV: right ventricle; TEE: transesophageal echocardiography)

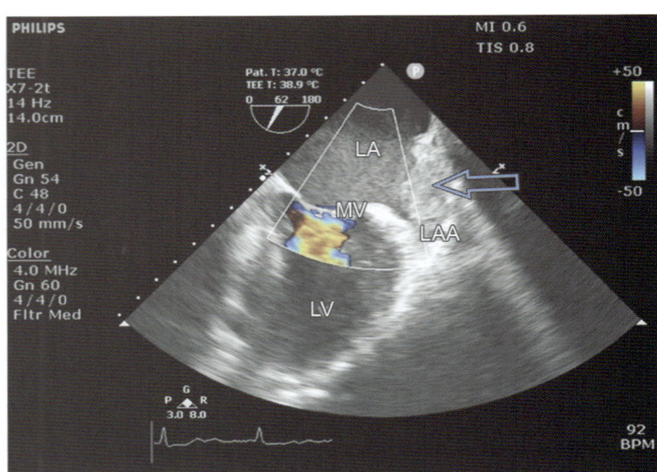

Fig. 30: TEE midesophageal two-chamber view showing left atrial appendage (LAA) clot (blue arrow) secondary to mitral stenosis. (LA: left atrium; LV: left ventricle; MV: mitral valve; TEE: transesophageal echocardiography)

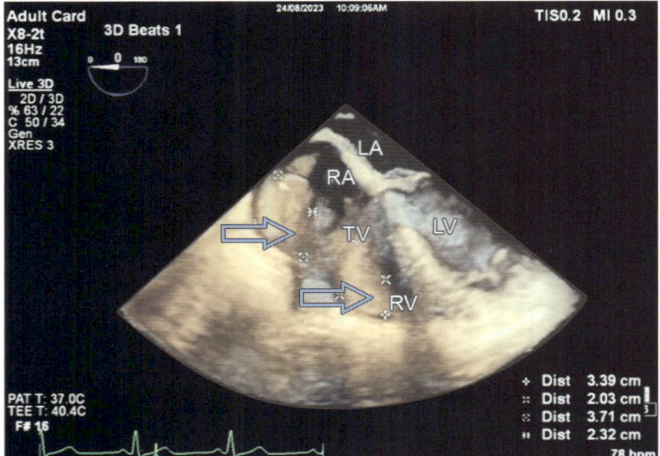

Fig. 29: 3D TEE image of midesophageal four-chamber view showing complete obstruction of the right side of the heart due to myxoma (blue arrows). (3D: three dimensional; LA: left atrium; LV: left ventricle; RA: right atrium; RV: right ventricle; TEE: transesophageal echocardiography; TV: tricuspid valve)

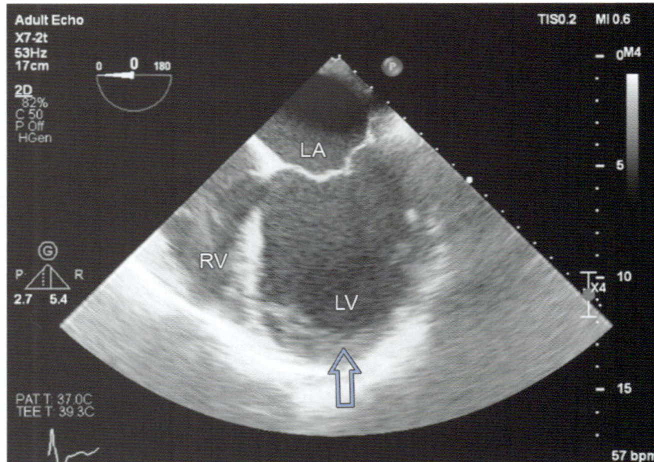

Fig. 31: TEE midesophageal four-chamber view showing a dilated left ventricle (LV) with spontaneous echo contrast with left ventricular apical thrombus (blue arrow). (LA: left atrium; RV: right ventricle; TEE: transesophageal echocardiography)

Clinical Implications of Tumor Extension in Inferior Vena Cava

Renal cell carcinomas are well known to invade the IVC **(Fig. 32)**, migrate to RA, and sometimes cause flow obstruction in the right heart **(Fig. 33)**. It is a combined team effort by the oncosurgeons and cardiac surgeons to address this issue, and TEE plays a vital role in real-time imaging and guiding the surgeon. Many a time, these tumors can cause paradoxical embolism in the presence of PFO/ASD.

Clinical Implications in Neurosurgery

Some of the neurosurgeries are done in the sitting position, and venous air embolism is a common occurence.[25] Echocardiography can identify air in the right heart, and it can be immediately aspirated via a central line. Around 25% of the patient population has PFO, which can cause

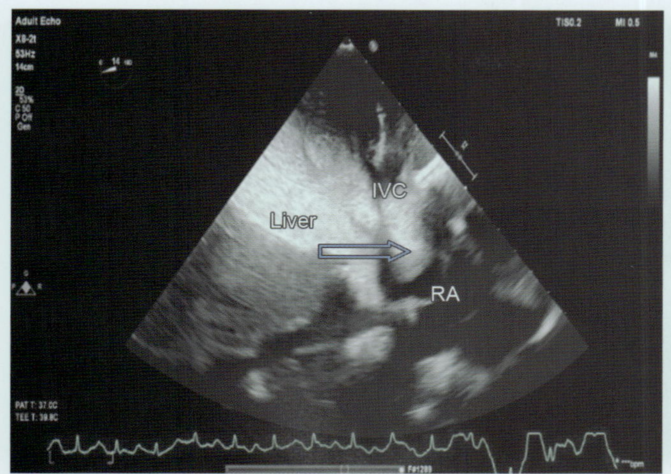

Fig. 32: TEE transgastric inferior vena cava (IVC) view showing renal cell carcinoma tumor extension into the IVC and the right atrium (RA) (blue arrow). (TEE: transesophageal echocardiography)

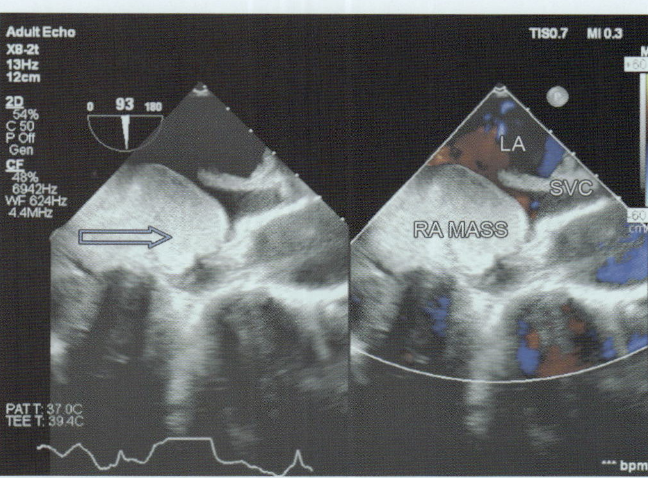

Fig. 33: TEE midesophageal bicaval view showing renal cell carcinoma tumor extension causing right heart obstruction (blue arrow). (LA: left atrium; RA MASS: right atrium mass; SVC: superior vena cava; TEE: transesophageal echocardiography)

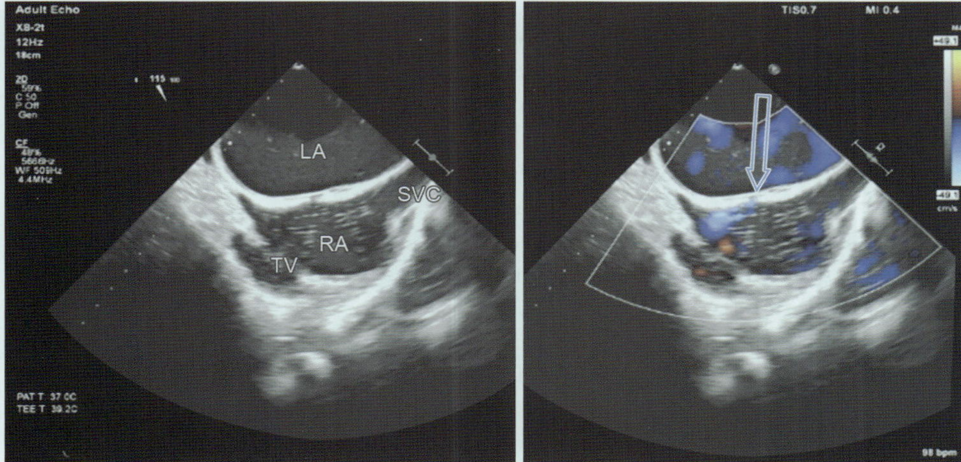

Fig. 34: TEE midesophageal bicaval view showing patent foramen ovale (blue arrow), and the white snowflakes seen in the right atrium are air bubbles. (LA: left atrium; SVC: superior vena cava; RA: right atrium; TEE: transesophageal echocardiography; TV: tricuspid valve)

paradoxical air embolism from the right atrium to the LA when the right heart pressures increase and can be a cause for thromboembolism and poor neurological outcome postoperatively. Intraoperatively, ME bicaval view on TEE with bubble test helps in identifying PFO **(Fig. 34)**.

Volume Assessment and Fluid Responsiveness

To achieve adequate delivery of oxygen (DO_2) to the cells and end-organ perfusion is the ultimate goal for fluid resuscitation. Major oncosurgeries have massive fluid shifts, and one has to prepare for the hemodynamic perturbances. One of them to mention would be cytoreductive surgery (CRS) with hyperthermic intraperitoneal chemotherapy (HIPEC). It is an extensive high-risk procedure for patients with peritoneal metastases with insensible fluid losses, fluid shifts, and acidosis. Tumors of the liver and bones have a high risk of bleeding, and one needs to keep a constant watch on the blood loss and

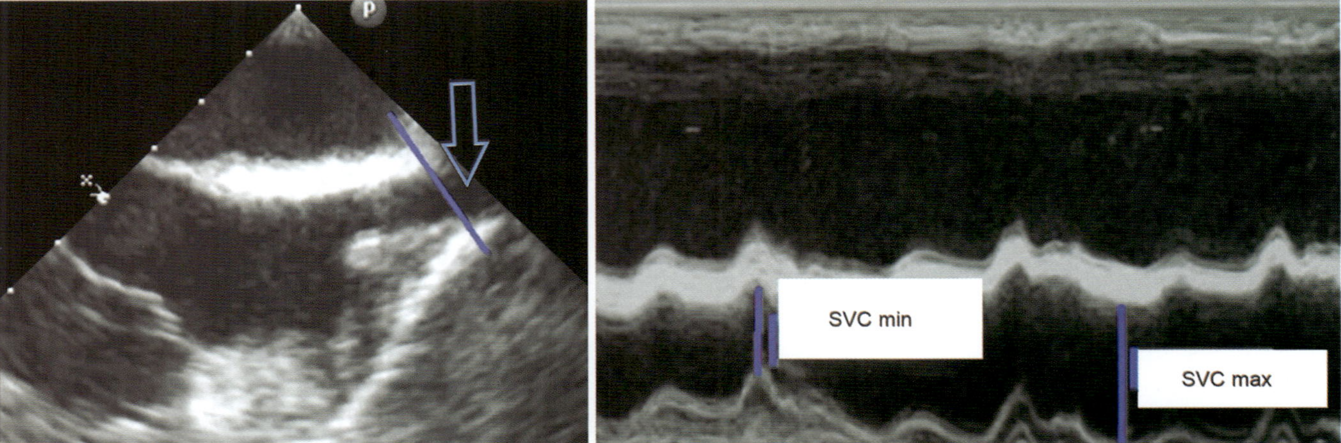

Fig. 35: TEE midesophageal bicaval view M-mode showing superior vena cava (SVC) collapsibility index measurements. (TEE: transesophageal echocardiography)

transfusion of blood products. Transfusion-associated circulatory overload (TACO) can be avoided with real-time monitoring of filling status with echocardiography. Several studies have shown that the right atrial pressures are connected to the respiratory diameter variation of great veins, and this in turn helps in assessing fluid responsiveness (FR).[26,27] Calculating FR in a patient is important as it is well known that the preload of the patient is dependent on the steep curve of the Frank–Starling curves, as the SV increases with preload, and once it reaches the flat portion of the curve, the SV does not change. In case we continue to administer fluid beyond this point, the patient could end up with pulmonary edema and HF.[28] To avoid fluid overload, we need to assess FR which is defined by a 15% increase in the stroke SV CO after fluid administration.[29] Stroke volume variation and pulse pressure variation are other dynamic indices that are proposed for predicting FR.[30,31] Aortic peak velocity and VTI variation (Ao-VTI) ≥10% during a passive leg-raising maneuver is another parameter that can be used as a discriminator for fluid responsiveness.

Superior Vena Cava Collapsibility Index

In mechanically ventilated patients, FR is seen with SVC M-mode measurements in the midesophageal bicaval view 90–110°, using the following formula[32] **(Fig. 35)**:

$$SVC - CI = (SVC_{max} - SVC_{min})/SVC_{max} \times 100\%.$$

Miniaturized transoesophageal echocardiography probe (hTEE) has been approved by the Food and Drug Administration (FDA) and can be left in situ for

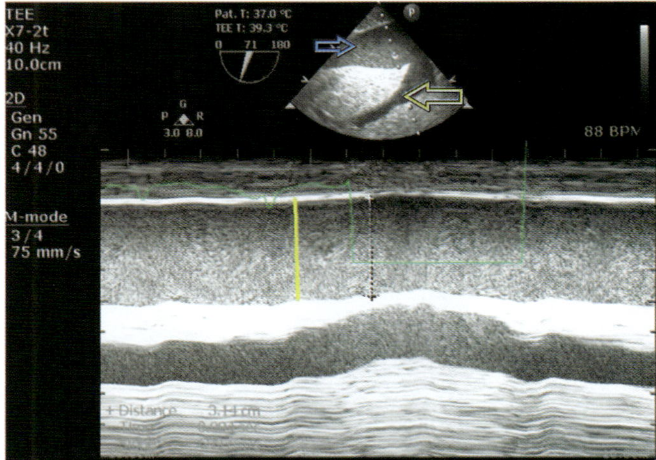

Fig. 36: TEE inferior vena cava view showing a dilated inferior vena cava (yellow line and blue arrows) and hepatic vein (yellow arrow) with no respiratory variation. (TEE: transesophageal echocardiography)

72 hours (ImaCor, Inc. Garden City, New Jersey). It is used for continuous monitoring of cardiac function in the ICU. Studies have shown that an superior vena cava collapsibility index (SVC-CI) of more than 37% predicted FR with a sensitivity of 90% and a specificity of 83%.[26]

Inferior Vena Cava Assessment

In patients who are spontaneously breathing, IVC collapsibility is measured (IVC collapse in inspiration), and in mechanically ventilated patients, IVC distensibility is measured (as intrathoracic pressure increases during ventilation) **(Fig. 36)**. Patients with an IVC diameter of more than 2.0 cm with no or minimal respiratory variations (<50%) are deemed to have elevated CVP (>15 mm Hg).

PERIOPERATIVE HYPOTENSION

Hypotension is a clinical nightmare in the perioperative period. Oncosurgeries are notorious for intraoperative bleeding and massive transfusion. Other common causes of hypotension and hemodynamic instability are sepsis, ventricular failure, pericardial effusion/tamponade, aortic dissection **(Fig. 37)** or aneurysm, and pneumothorax. Echocardiography helps determine the heart's size, volume, and function in fluid resuscitation, maintaining good preload and balancing the perfusion pressures. End-organ damage can be detrimental in the postoperative period, leading to acute kidney injury, bowel ischemia, and hepatic failure. Prolonged hypotension can also cause postoperative neurological issues, which need serious consideration in maintaining good hemodynamics intra-operatively. A hyperdynamic LV with an end-diastolic area of <10 cm^2 in the PSAX view or the papillary muscles opposing each other (kissing ventricles) is a strong indicator of hypovolemia.[33]

Pericardial effusion **(Fig. 38)** is one of the common causes of hypotension and elevated CVP. On echocardiography, RA systolic collapse and RV diastolic collapse are pathognomonic. It is an important finding in cardiac failure and bleeding disorders. Malignant pericardial effusion is most frequently observed in lung cancer, leukemia, breast cancer, lymphoma, and malignant melanoma.[34]

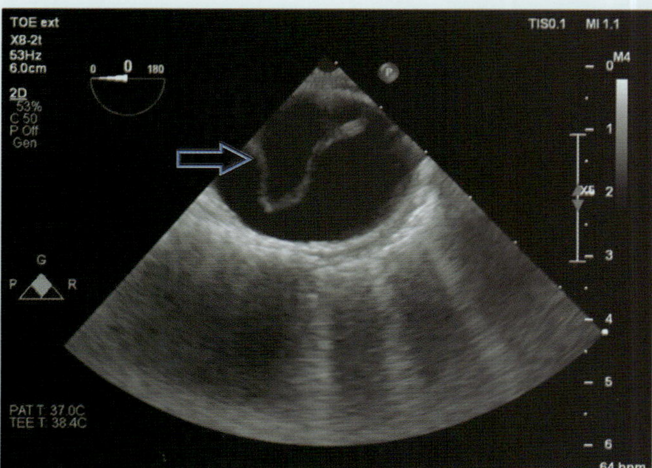

Fig. 37: TEE midesophageal descending aorta short-axis view showing aortic dissection flap (blue arrow). (TEE: transesophageal echocardiography)

Left ventricular hypertrophy can occur in chronic severe hypertension, aortic stenosis (AS), hypertrophic obstructive cardiomyopathy (HOCM), hyperdynamic states like sepsis, highly vasodilated states like vasoplegia, or high inotropes. The end-diastolic volume can be very low and might imitate a hypovolemic heart, and this needs to be treated with caution **(Fig. 39)**. Patients with HOCM have thickened septum, which causes systolic anterior motion (SAM) of the anterior MV leaflet **(Fig. 40)** during LV systole due to venturi effect and causes left LVOTO,

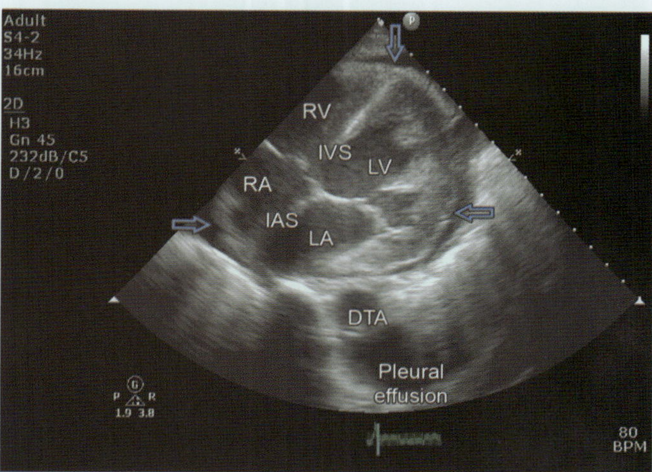

Fig. 38: TTE subcostal view showing pericardial effusion all around the heart (blue arrow). (DTA: descending thoracic aorta; IAS: interatrial septum; IVS: interventricular septum; LA: left atrium; LV: left ventricle; RA: right atrium; RV: right ventricle; TTE: transthoracic echocardiography)

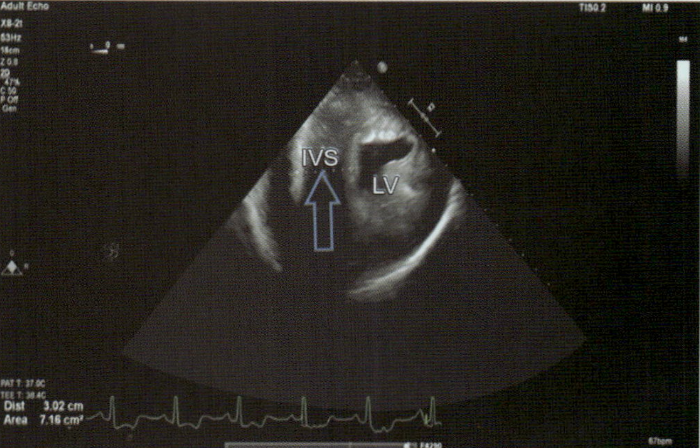

Fig. 39: TEE transgastric midpapillary short-axis view showing a thickened interventricular septum (IVS) (blue arrow) in a case of hypertrophic obstructive cardiomyopathy (HOCM). (LV: left ventricle; TEE: transesophageal echocardiography)

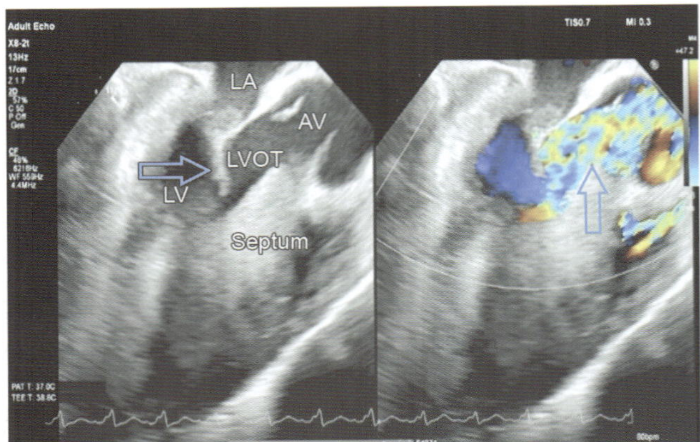

Fig. 40: TEE midesophageal left ventricular long-axis view showing a thickened interventricular septum with systolic anterior motion of the anterior mitral leaflet (blue arrow in the left image) and turbulence of flow in the left ventricular outflow tract (LVOT) (blue arrow in the right image) in a case of hypertrophic obstructive cardiomyopathy (HOCM). (AV: aortic valve; LA: left atrium; LV: left ventricle; TEE: transesophageal echocardiography)

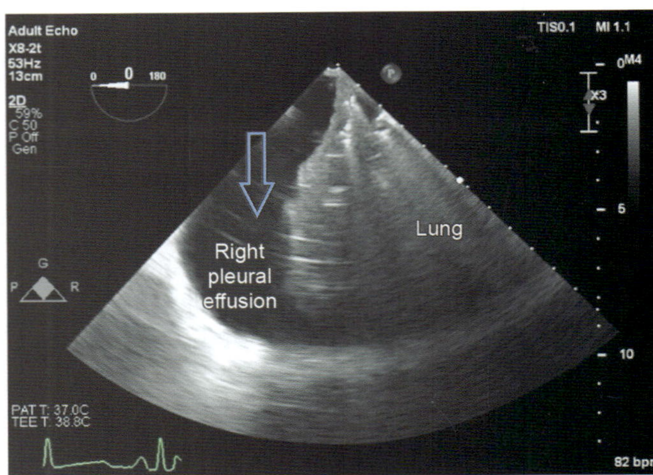

Fig. 42: TEE midesophageal view showing right pleural effusion (blue arrow). (TEE: transesophageal echocardiography)

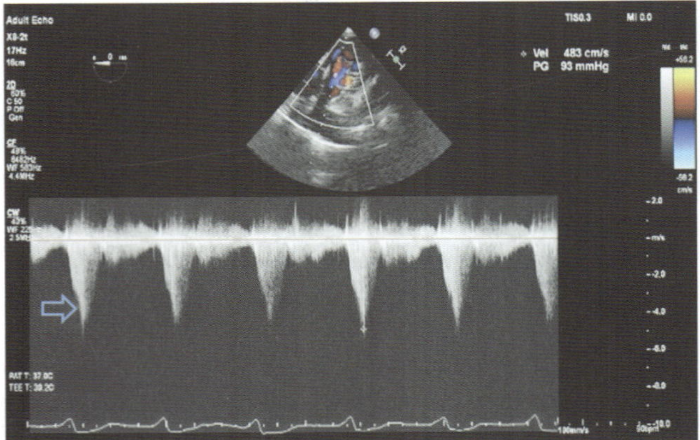

Fig. 41: TEE midesophageal deep transgastric view with continuous-wave Doppler of the left ventricular outflow tract (LVOT) showing dagger-shaped curve (blue arrow) in a case of hypertrophic obstructive cardiomyopathy (HOCM). (CW: continuous wave; TEE: transesophageal echocardiography)

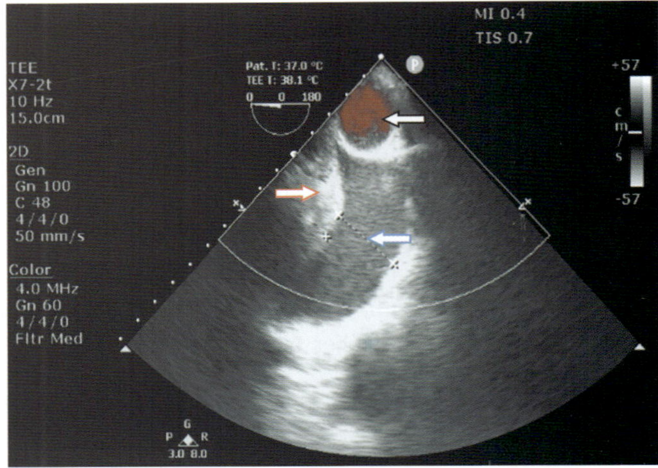

Fig. 43: TEE midesophageal descending aorta (white arrow) view showing left pleural effusion (blue arrow) and the collapsed lung (red arrow). (TEE: transesophageal echocardiography)

showing a classic dagger-shaped spectral Doppler when profiled **(Fig. 41)**. It is important to fill the patient and give vasopressors to maintain blood pressure in such conditions and not to administer inotropes as this can worsen the LVOTO.

HYPOXIA IN THE PERIOPERATIVE PERIOD

Acute hypoxia can occur due to pneumothorax, pleural effusion **(Figs. 42 and 43)**, lung collapse consolidation, acute PE, RV failure, and pulmonary edema due to LV failure.

Tension pneumothorax is a life-threatening complication if undiagnosed, and it is one of the causes of pulseless electrical activity, which needs to be ruled out during resuscitation. During thoracoscopic surgeries/robotic thoracic surgeries, there are high chances of injury to the contralateral lung either due to positive pressure ventilation, or rupture of the underlying bullae of the lung. As an anesthesiologist, intraoperatively, when we

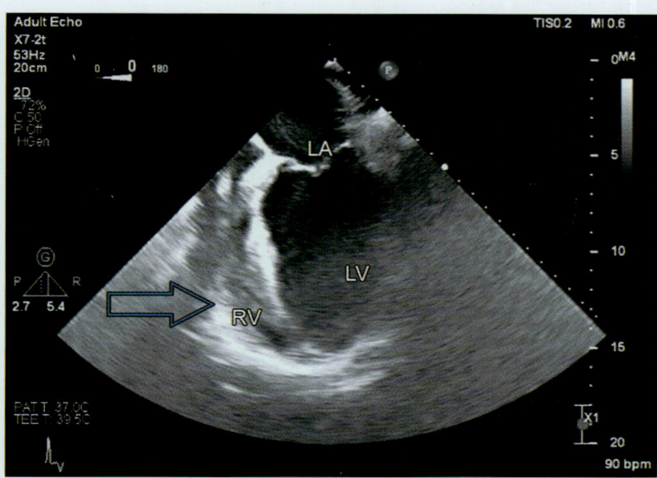

Fig. 44: TEE midesophageal four-chamber view showing compression of the right atrium and the right ventricle (RV) (blue arrow) and shift of the heart to the left due to right pneumothorax. (LA: left atrium; LV: left ventricle; TEE: transesophageal echocardiography)

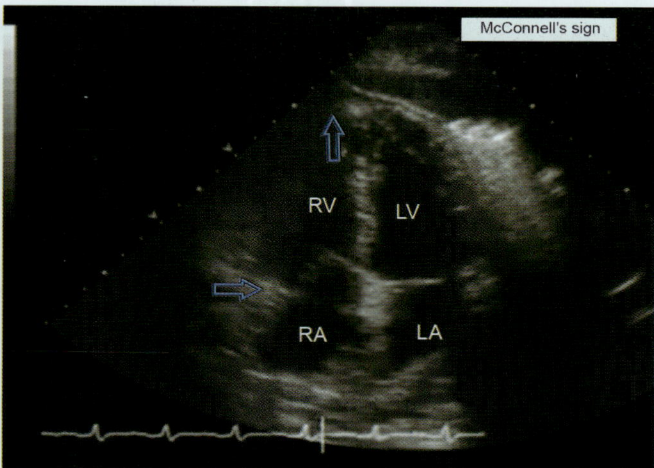

Fig. 45: TTE apical four-chamber view showing McConnell's sign, with the left ventricle (LV) showing a hyperkinetic apex (blue upward arrow) and basal hypokinesia (blue horizontal arrow). (LA: left atrium; RA: right atrium; RV: right ventricle; TTE: transthoracic echocardiography)

face situations with sudden desaturation during one-lung ventilation, reduced air entry, raised peak airway pressure, and hemodynamic instability, TEE could come to our rescue. On TEE in the ME 4C view, we can see compression of the RV and mass effect[35] **(Fig. 44)**. The movement of the parietal and visceral pleural over each other during respiration is responsible for the "gliding or sliding sign," which is absent in pneumothorax.

Acute pulmonary embolism is very common in patients with chronic diseases, and malignancy itself is a hypercoagulable state.[36] Deep vein thrombosis (DVT) in the perioperative period due to multiple factors could lead to acute PE and hypoxia with severe RV failure.[37,38] The McConnell sign is one of the sensitive as well as specific signs demonstrated with akinesis of the RV mid-free wall, with normal wall motion of the apex **(Fig. 45)**. Saddle thrombus can be life-threatening when thrombus is found obstructing the right pulmonary artery (RPA) and the left pulmonary artery (LPA) **(Fig. 46)**.

Chronic pulmonary thromboembolic pulmonary hypertension (CTEPH) secondary to antiphospholipid antibody (APLA) is another cause of recurrent DVT and PE.[39] Clots are present in the pulmonary arteries and cause hypoxia, severe RV dilation, and failure **(Fig. 47)**. In orthopedic surgeries, bone cement embolization is a known complication that can present as hypoxia and hypotension under regional anesthesia and requires conversion to general anesthesia. Echocardiography can

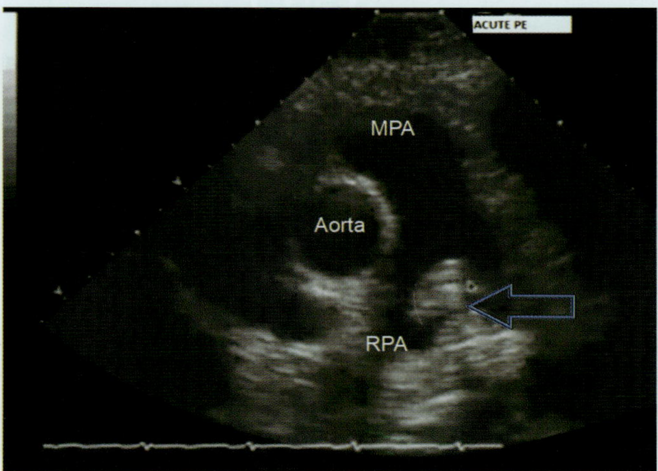

Fig. 46: TTE parasternal short-axis view of the bifurcation of the pulmonary arteries showing saddle thrombus (blue arrow). (MPA: main pulmonary artery; PE: pulmonary embolism RPA: right pulmonary artery; TTE: transthoracic echocardiography)

identify embolic floating in RA, RV, and acute PE, leading to RV failure.[40,41]

ECHOCARDIOGRAPHY FOR DEVICE INSERTION

Echocardiography plays a supportive role in the insertion and proper placement of CO monitoring devices like PAC in the heart **(Fig. 48)**. In situations leading to HF, rescue therapy with mechanical assist devices is essential, when

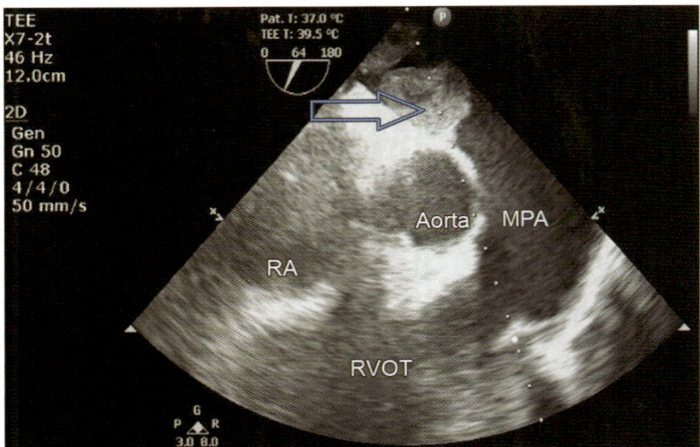

Fig. 47: TEE midesophageal ascending aorta short-axis view showing thrombus in the right pulmonary artery (blue arrow). (MPA: main pulmonary artery; RA: right atrium; RVOT: right ventricular outflow tract; TEE: transesophageal echocardiography)

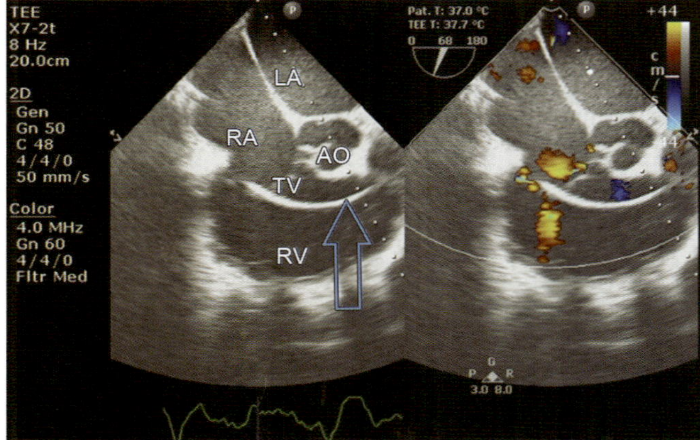

Fig. 48: TEE midesophageal right ventricular inflow–outflow view showing a pulmonary artery catheter (blue arrow). (AO: aorta; LA: left atrium; LV: left ventricle; RA: right atrium; RV: right ventricle; TEE: transesophageal echocardiography; TV: tricuspid valve)

inotropes fail to improve perfusion, and support is needed to preserve myocardium, further damage, and end-organ protection. TEE/TTE both play a vital role in the insertion of both veno-venous (VV) extracorporeal membrane oxygenation (ECMO) in acute lung injury and veno-arterial VA ECMO in cardiac failure. Guidance of SVC cannulation **(Fig. 49)** and femoral venous cannulation through IVC **(Fig. 50)** with echocardiography has led to safer and fewer complications.[42,43] Initiation of intra-aortic balloon pump (IABP) in HF through femoral arterial access, echocardiography-guided insertion of guidewire, and placement of IABP tip below the origin of the left subclavian artery is done under TEE guidance **(Fig. 51)**.

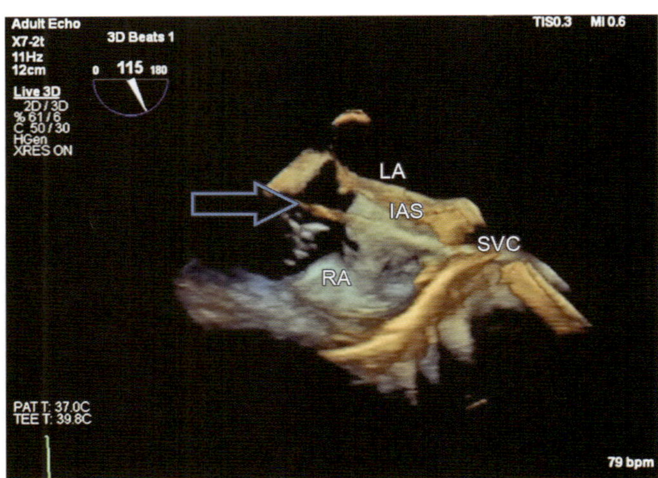

Fig. 49: 3D TEE midesophageal bicaval view showing a guidewire through the superior vena cava (SVC) into the right atrium (RA) for extracorporeal membrane oxygenation (ECMO) venous cannulation (blue arrow). (IAS: interatrial septum; LA: left atrium; TEE: transesophageal echocardiography)

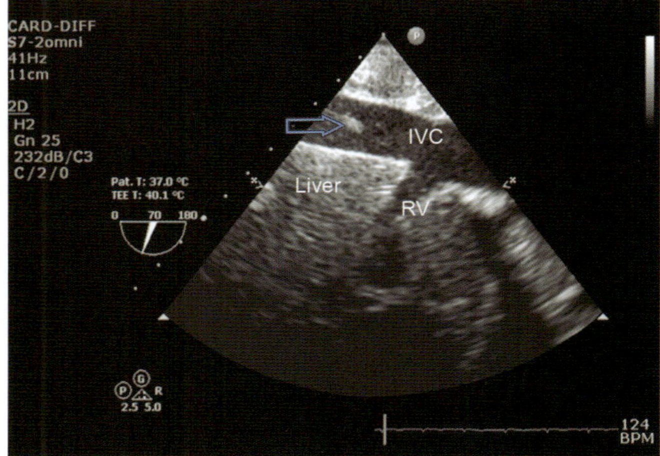

Fig. 50: TEE inferior vena cava view (IVC) with a guidewire for guiding venous cannulation in extracorporeal membrane oxygenation (ECMO) via femoral access (blue arrow). (RV: right ventricle; TEE: transesophageal echocardiography)

TEE helps in the positioning of Impella device (Abiomed, Massachusetts), in the case of cardiogenic shock.[44]

EVIDENCE FOR INTRAOPERATIVE ECHOCARDIOGRAPHY IN NONCARDIAC SURGERIES

Transesophageal echocardiography is an American Heart Association (AHA) and American College of Cardiology

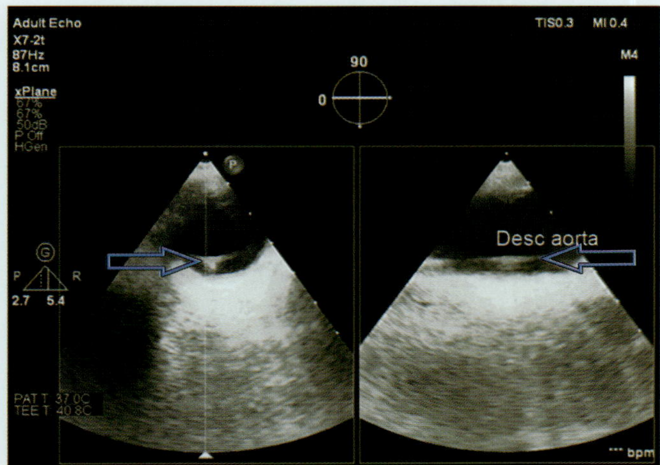

Fig. 51: TEE midesophageal descending aorta (DESC AORTA) X-plane view showing short- and long-axis with intra-aortic balloon pump (IABP) guidewire (blue arrows). (TEE: transesophageal echocardiography)

(ACC) class I recommendation (level B evidence) in MV repair surgery and in the surgical management of infective endocarditis.[45] TEE is a Class II recommendation (level B evidence) in all other types of cardiac surgery because its benefits remain unconfirmed.[46] The recent concept of rescue TEE for a large group of physicians is made available for emergency skills of focused TEE, and this could benefit patients with acute hemodynamic instability.[47]

STAGING OF CANCER

Schroder et al. used TEE for the evaluation of the invasion of the thoracic aorta in lung cancer patient staging.[48] Lung cancer staging can be done with mediastinal lymph nodes visualized on TEE.[49]

CONCLUSION

Echocardiography is one of the armamentariums during the hemodynamic monitoring of patients in the perioperative period, and its knowledge is of paramount importance for the better outcome of surgery.

REFERENCES

1. Cheitlin MD, Alpert JS, Armstrong WF, Aurigemma GP, Beller GA, Bierman FZ, et al. ACC/AHA guidelines for the clinical application of echocardiography: a report of the American College of Cardiology/American Heart Association Task Force on practice guidelines (Committee on Clinical Application of Echocardiography). Developed in collaboration with the American Society of Echocardiography. Circulation. 1997;95:1686-744.
2. Tank A, Hughey R, Ward RP, Nagele P, Rubin DS. Evaluation of appropriate use of preoperative echocardiography before major abdominal surgery: a retrospective cohort study. Anesthesiology. 2021;135(5):854-63.
3. Muralidhar K, Tempe D, Chakravarthy M, Shastry N, Kapoor PM, Tewari P, et al. Practice guidelines for perioperative transesophageal echocardiography: recommendations of the Indian association of cardiovascular thoracic anaesthesiologists. Ann Card Anaesth. 2013;16(4):268-78.
4. Paterson DI, Wiebe N, Cheung WY, Mackey JR, Pituskin E, Reiman A, et al. Incident cardiovascular disease among adults with cancer: a population-based cohort study. JACC CardioOncol. 2022;4(1):85-94.
5. Lyon AR, López-Fernández T, Couch LS, Asteggiano R, Aznar MC, Bergler-Klein J, et al.; ESC Scientific Document Group. 2022 ESC Guidelines on cardio oncology developed in collaboration with the European Haematology Association (EHA), the European Society for Therapeutic Radiology and Oncology (ESTRO) and the International Cardio-Oncology Society (IC-OS): Developed by the task force on cardio-oncology of the European Society of Cardiology (ESC). Eur Heart J. 2022;43(41):4229-361.
6. Hahn RT, Abraham T, Adams MS, Bruce CJ, Glas KE, Lang RM, et al. Guidelines for performing a comprehensive transesophageal echocardiographic examination: recommendations from the American Society of Echocardiography and the Society of Cardiovascular Anaesthesiologists. J Am Soc Echocardiogr. 2013;26(9):921-64.
7. Kalagara H, Coker B, Gerstein NS, Kukreja P, Deriy L, Pierce A, et al. Point-of-care ultrasound (POCUS) for the cardiothoracic anaesthesiologist. J Cardiothorac Vasc Anesth. 2022;36(4):1132-47.
8. Ford MK, Beattie WS, Wijeysundera DN. Systematic review: prediction of perioperative cardiac complications and mortality by the revised cardiac risk index. Ann Intern Med. 2010;152(1):26-35.
9. Fornaro A, Castelli G, Ciaccheri M, Tomberli B, Olivotto I, Gensini GF. Improving survival of chemotherapy-induced cardiomyopathy in the modern heart failure therapy era. Eur Heart J. 2013;34(suppl_1):2968.
10. Plana JC, Galderisi M, Barac A, Ewer MS, Ky B, Scherrer-Crosbie M, et al. Expert consensus for multimodality imaging evaluation of adult patients during and after cancer therapy: a report from the American Society of Echocardiography and the European Association of Cardiovascular Imaging. J Am Soc Echocardiogr. 2014;27(9):911-39.
11. Florescu M, Cinteza M, Vinereanu D. Chemotherapy-induced cardiotoxicity. Maedica (Bucur). 2013;8(1):59-67.
12. Liu JE, Barac A, Thavendiranathan P, Scherrer-Crosbie M. Strain imaging in cardio-oncology. JACC CardioOncol. 2020;2(5):677-89.

13. Dobson R, Ghosh AK, Ky B, Marwick T, Stout M, Harkness A, et al. BSE and BCOS guideline for transthoracic echocardiographic assessment of adult cancer patients receiving anthracyclines and/or trastuzumab. JACC CardioOncol. 2021;3(1):1-16.
14. Feng T, Guo Z, Su H, Zhang F, Zhu H, Wang A, et al. Progress in the use of echocardiography in patients with tumors. Rev Cardiovasc Med. 2024;25(1):22.
15. Tadic M, Cuspidi C, Hering D, Venneri L, Danylenko O. The influence of chemotherapy on the right ventricle: did we forget something? Clin Cardiol. 2017;40(7):437-43.
16. Nabiałek-Trojanowska I, Lewicka E, Wrona A, Kaleta AM, Lewicka-Potocka Z, Raczak G, et al. Cardiovascular complications after radiotherapy. Cardiol J. 2020; 27(6):836-47.
17. Medvedofsky D, Maffessanti F, Weinert L, Tehrani DM, Narang A, Addetia K, et al. 2D and 3D echocardiography-derived indices of left ventricular function and shape: relationship with mortality. JACC Cardiovasc Imaging. 2018;11(11):1569-79.
18. Owan TE, Hodge DO, Herges RM, Jacobsen SJ, Roger VL, Redfield MM. Trends in prevalence and outcome of heart failure with preserved ejection fraction. N Engl J Med. 2006;355(3):251-9.
19. Serrano JM, González I, Del Castillo S, Muñiz J, Morales LJ, Moreno F, et al. Diastolic dysfunction following anthracycline-based chemotherapy in breast cancer patients: incidence and predictors. Oncologist. 2015; 20(8):864-72.
20. Swaminathan M, Nicoara A, Phillips-Bute BG, Aeschlimann N, Milano CA, Mackensen GB, et al. Utility of a simple algorithm to grade diastolic dysfunction and predict outcome after coronary artery bypass graft surgery. Ann Thorac Surg. 2011;91(6):1844-50.
21. Galderisi M, Cosyns B, Edvardsen T, Cardim N, Delgado V, Di Salvo G, et al. Standardization of adult transthoracic echocardiography reporting in agreement with recent chamber quantification, diastolic function, and heart valve disease recommendations: an expert consensus document of the European Association of Cardiovascular Imaging. Eur Heart J Cardiovasc Imaging. 2017;18(12):1301-10.
22. Lang RM, Badano LP, Mor-Avi V, Afilalo J, Armstrong A, Ernande L, et al. Recommendations for cardiac chamber quantification by echocardiography in adults: an update from the American Society of Echocardiography and the European Association of Cardiovascular Imaging. J Am Soc Echocardiogr. 2015;28(1):1-39.e14.
23. Zamorano JL, Lancellotti P, Rodriguez Muñoz D, Aboyans V, Asteggiano R, Galderisi M, et al. 2016 ESC Position Paper on cancer treatments and cardiovascular toxicity developed under the auspices of the ESC Committee for Practice Guidelines: The Task Force for cancer treatments and cardiovascular toxicity of the European Society of Cardiology (ESC). Eur Heart J. 2016;37(36):2768-801.
24. Armstrong WF, Ryan T. Masses, tumours, and source of embolus. In: Feigenbaum H, Armstrong WF, Ryan T (Eds). Feigenbaum's Echocardiography. 7th edition. Philadelphia, PA: Lippincott Williams & Wilkins; 2010.
25. Rau TR, Plaschke K, Weigand MA, Maier C, Schramm C. Automatic detection of venous air embolism using trans-esophageal echocardiography in patients undergoing neurological surgery in the semi-sitting position: a pilot study. J Clin Monit Comput. 2021;35(5):1103-9.
26. Bubenek-Turconi ŞI, Hendy A, Băilă S, Drăgan A, Chioncel O, Văleanu L, et al. The value of a superior vena cava collapsibility index measured with a miniaturized transoesophageal monoplane continuous echocardiography probe to predict fluid responsiveness compared to stroke volume variations in open major vascular surgery: a prospective cohort study. J Clin Monit Comput. 2020;34(3):491-9.
27. Marik PE. Techniques for assessment of intravascular volume in critically ill patients. J Intensive Care Med. 2009;24(5):329-37.
28. Cecconi M, Hofer C, Teboul JL, Pettila V, Wilkman E, Molnar Z, et al.; Investigators F, Group ET. Erratum to: fluid challenges in intensive care: the FENICE study: a global inception cohort study. Intensive Care Med. 2015;41(9):1737-8.
29. Cecconi M, De Backer D, Antonelli M, Beale R, Bakker J, Hofer C, et al. Consensus on circulatory shock and hemodynamic monitoring. Task force of the European Society of Intensive Care Medicine. Intensive Care Med. 2014;40(12):1795-815.
30. Michard F, Teboul JL. Predicting fluid responsiveness in ICU patients: a critical analysis of the evidence. Chest. 2002;121(6):2000-8.
31. Cherpanath TGV, Hirsch A, Geerts BF, Lagrand WK, Leeflang MM, Schultz MJ, et al. Predicting fluid responsiveness by passive leg raising: a systematic review and meta-analysis of 23 clinical trials. Crit Care Med. 2016; 44(5):981-91.
32. Li Y, Jiang L, Wang L, Dou D, Feng Y. Evaluation of fluid responsiveness with dynamic superior vena cava collapsibility index in mechanically ventilated patients. Perioper Med (Lond). 2023;12(1):10.
33. Miller A, Mandeville J. Predicting and measuring fluid responsiveness with echocardiography. Echo Res Pract. 2016;3(2):G1-12.
34. Zito C, Longobardo L, Cadeddu C, Monte I, Novo G, Dell'Oglio S, et al. Cardiovascular imaging in the diagnosis and monitoring of cardiotoxicity: role of echocardiography. J Cardiovasc Med (Hagerstown). 2016;17(Suppl 1):e35-44.
35. Castro DM, Lung K, Douflé G. Straight curves: incidental diagnosis of pneumothorax on transesophageal echocardio-graphy. Am J Respir Crit Care Med. 2021;204(7):e88-91.
36. Caine GJ, Stonelake PS, Lip GYH, Kehoe ST. The hyper-coagulable state of malignancy: pathogenesis and current debate. Neoplasia. 2002;4(6):465-73.

37. Ribeiro A, Lindmaker P, Juhlin-Dannfelt A, Johnsson H, Jorfeldt L, et al. Echocardiography Doppler in pulmonary embolism: right ventricular dysfunction as a predictor of mortality rate. Am Heart J. 1997;134(3):479-87.
38. Grifoni S, Olivotto I, Cecchini P, Pieralli F, Camaiti A, Santoro G, et al. Short-term clinical outcome of patients with acute pulmonary embolism, normal blood pressure, and echocardiographic right ventricular dysfunction. Circulation. 2000;101(24):2817-22.
39. Zhu R, Cheng GY, Denas G, Pengo V. Antiphospholipid antibodies in chronic thromboembolic pulmonary hypertension. Eur J Intern Med. 2023;111:1-4.
40. Izumi Y, Ishihara S, Cammack I, Miyawaki I. Massive mass embolism detected by transesophageal echocardiography in bone cement implantation syndrome: a case report. JA Clin Rep. 2019;5(1):5.
41. Yang TH, Yang RS, Lin CP, Tseng TH. Bone cement implantation syndrome in bone tumor surgeries: incidence, risk factors, and clinical experience. Orthop Surg. 2021;13(1):109-15.
42. Hussey PT, von Mering G, Nanda NC, Ahmed MI, Addis DR. Echocardiography for extracorporeal membrane oxygenation. Echocardiography. 2022;39(2):339-70.
43. Castro DM, Abdelnour-Berchtold E, Urner M, Dragoi L, Cypel M, Fan E, et al. Transesophageal echocardiography-guided extracorporeal membrane oxygenation cannulation in COVID-19 patients. J Cardiothorac Vasc Anesth. 2022; 36(12):4296-304.
44. Khan H, Khan M, Munir A. TEE-guided bedside impella placement in refractory cardiogenic shock already supported with intra-aortic balloon pump. JACC. 2021; 77(18_Supplement_1);2580.
45. American Society of Anaesthesiologists and the Society of Cardiovascular Anaesthesiologists Task Force on Transesophageal Echocardiography. Anesthesiology. Practice guidelines for perioperative transesophageal echocardiography. An updated report by the American Society of Anaesthesiologists and the Society of Cardiovascular Anaesthesiologists Task Force on Transesophageal Echocardiography. Anesthesiology. 2010;112(5):1084-96.
46. Nishimura RA, Otto CM, Bonow RO, Carabello BA, Erwin JP 3rd, Guyton RA, et al. 2014 AHA/ACC guideline for the management of patients with valvular heart disease: a report of the American College of Cardiology/American Heart Association Task Force on Practice Guidelines. J Thorac Cardiovasc Surg. 2014;148:e1-132.
47. Efrimescu CI, Moorthy A, Griffin M. Rescue transesophageal echocardiography: a narrative review of current knowledge and practice. J Cardiothorac Vasc Anesth. 2023; 37(4):584-600.0
48. Schröder C, Schönhofer B, Vogel B. Transesophageal echographic determination of aortic invasion by lung cancer. Chest. 2005;127(2):438-42.
49. Jakob H, Lorenz J, Clement T, Börner N, Schweden F, Erbel R, et al. Mediastinal lymph node staging with transesophageal echography in cancer of the lung. Eur J Cardiothorac Surg. 1990;4(7);355-8.

69 CHAPTER

Oncological Emergencies

Pramila Madhu Chandan, Atul Prabhakar Kulkarni

INTRODUCTION

An oncologic emergency is a condition resulting from a metabolic or structural change caused by cancer or its therapy that requires urgent medical intervention to prevent morbidity and mortality.[1] Cancer patients are at risk for various life-threatening emergencies **(Table 1)**.

TABLE 1: Classification of oncological emergencies*.

Classification	*Oncologic emergencies*
Metabolic	• Tumor lysis syndrome (TLS) • Hypercalcemia • Hyponatremia • Hypoglycemia
Hematological	• Hyperleukocytosis • Hyperviscosity syndrome • Leukopenia • Anemia • Disseminated intravascular coagulation (DIC) • Hemophagocytic lymphohistiocytosis (HLH)
Structural	*Cardiovascular:* Malignant pericardial effusion and cardiac tamponade, superior vena cava (SVC) syndrome
	Neurological: Posterior reversible encephalopathy (PRES), raised intracranial pressure (ICP), malignant spinal cord compression (MSCC)
	Respiratory: Superior mediastinal syndrome, acute respiratory distress syndrome (ARDS), pulmonary embolism (PE)
Infections	• Febrile neutropenia (FN) • Septic shock
Treatment-related	• Chemotherapy extravasation • Chimeric antigen receptor-T-cell complications and toxicity • Immune checkpoint blockade-related adverse events

*Those highlighted in bold are discussed here.

Many are preventable and can be effectively managed, if promptly diagnosed. The first prerequisite for this is to have a high index of suspicion.

TUMOR LYSIS SYNDROME

Tumor lysis syndrome (TLS) is a life-threatening emergency occurring due to the rapid lysis of tumor cells and the abrupt release of their intracellular content (nucleic acids, proteins, and intracellular metabolites) into circulation exceeding renal excretory capacity, leading to hyperuricemia, hyperkalemia, and hyperphosphatemia **(Flowchart 1)**.[2] Due to hyperuricemia, uric acid secreted in the distal tubules and collecting ducts rises significantly, leading to an acidic pH and the formation of urate crystals, causing intraluminal tubular obstruction and acute renal dysfunction. Hyperphosphatemia gives rise to hypocalcemia by the formation of calcium phosphate crystals in the soft tissue and renal tract.[2]

Tumor lysis syndrome usually occurs after cytotoxic therapy; however, spontaneous TLS also occurs, particularly in patients with high tumor burden. It is most commonly seen in patients with hematological malignancies, particularly acute lymphoblastic leukemia (ALL) and Burkitt's lymphomas, although it can also occur less frequently in solid tumors. Malignancies with high tumor load, high proliferative rates, high chemosensitivity, and increased lactate dehydrogenase (LDH) levels are at risk of TLS, which usually occurs within 12–72 hours after the initiation of cytotoxic therapy.[2]

Cairo and Bishop's classification system for TLS is described in **Table 2**.

The key to the management of TLS includes close monitoring and prophylactic strategies for at-risk patients **(Table 3)** and early recognition and treatment of metabolic and renal complications. For high-risk cases, TLS parameters (potassium, phosphate, uric acid,

Flowchart 1: Pathophysiology of TLS and the mechanism of action of antihyperuricemic agents.

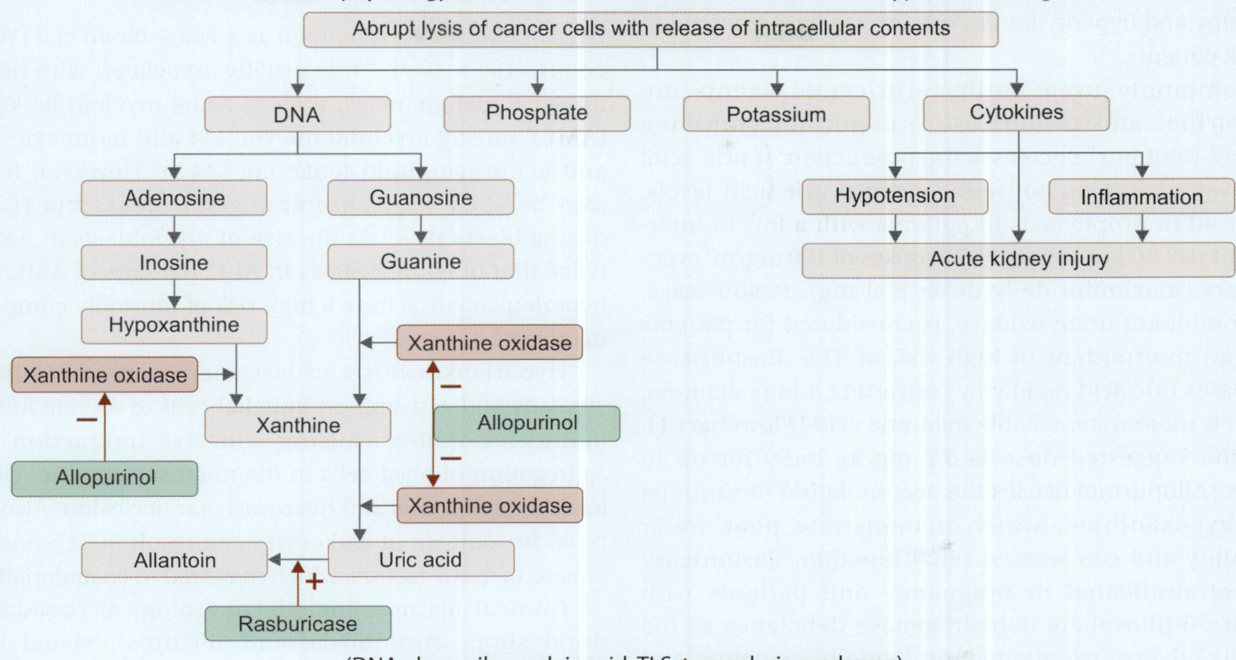

(DNA: deoxyribonucleic acid; TLS: tumor lysis syndrome)

TABLE 2: Lab definition of TLS (Cairo and Bishop's classification system).[2]

Laboratory TLS	*Clinical TLS*
The presence of two or more of the following blood abnormalities within 3 days before or 7 days after the initiation of therapy • Uric acid >8 mg/dL or 25% increase from baseline • Potassium >6 mEq/L (6 mmol/L) or 25% increase from baseline • Phosphorous >6.6 mg/dL (2.1 mmol/L) or 25% increase from baseline • Calcium <7 mg/dL (1.75 mmol/L) or 25% decrease from baseline	The presence of laboratory TLS with one or more of the following: • Acute renal failure (defined as a rise in creatinine to 1.5 times or more than the upper limit of normal that is not attributable to medications, decrease in urine output, uremia-related altered sensorium, or crystalline obstructive uropathy) • Cardiac arrhythmia or sudden death • Seizure

(TLS: tumor lysis syndrome)

calcium, creatinine, and LDH levels) should be monitored every 4–6 hours.[2]

Aggressive hydration (3–4 L/m^2/day) and sometimes diuresis to maintain an adequate urine output of ≥100 mL/m^2/h (3 mL/kg/h if ≤10 kg) is commonly considered in TLS.[2] Fluid balance should be meticulously

TABLE 3: Risk stratification in patients with TLS.

	Risk		
Type of cancer	*High*	*Intermediate*	*Low*
AML	WBC >50,000 Monoblastic	WBC: 10,000–50,000	WBC <10,000
ALL	WBC >100,000	WBC: 50,000–100,000	WBC <50,000
CLL		WBC 10,000–100,000 Treatment with fludarabine	WBC <10,000
NHL	Burkitt's lymphoblastic, B-ALL	DLBCL	Indolent NHL
Other hematological malignancies (including CML, multiple myeloma) and solid tumors		Rapid proliferation with expected rapid response to therapy	Remainder of patients

(ALL: acute lymphoblastic leukemia; AML: acute myeloid leukemia; B-ALL: Burkitt-type acute lymphoblastic; CLL: chronic lymphocytic leukemia; CML: chronic myeloid leukemia; DLBCL: diffuse large B-cell lymphoma; NHL: non-Hodgkin's lymphoma; TLS: tumor lysis syndrome; WBC: white blood cell)

monitored as TLS could lead to oliguria due to obstructive uropathy and hyperhydration can lead to fluid overload in at-risk patients.

Commonly used antihyperuricemic agents are allopurinol and rasburicase. Allopurinol (xanthine oxidase inhibitor) decreases the production of uric acid; however, as it does not reduce serum uric acid levels, it is used in prophylaxis in patients with a low to intermittent risk of developing TLS at doses of 100 mg/m^2 every 8 hours (maximum daily dose: 800 mg). Rasburicase, a recombinant urate oxidase, is considered for patients with an intermittent to high risk of TLS. Rasburicase decreases uric acid rapidly by converting it into allantoin, which is more water-soluble than uric acid **(Flowchart 1)**, and the suggested dose is 0.2 mg/kg daily for up to 5 days. Allopurinol causes the accumulation of xanthine and hypoxanthine, which demonstrate poor water solubility and can worsen renal function. Rasburicase is contraindicated in pregnancy and patients with glucose-6-phosphate dehydrogenase deficiency as the serious adverse events include hemolytic anemia and methemoglobinemia. Febuxostat, another xanthine oxidase inhibitor, has recently become available in India and can be used in those with an inadequate response or intolerance to allopurinol.

Other treatment strategies for TLS include correcting electrolyte abnormalities and the use of renal replacement therapy in refractory electrolyte abnormalities, calcium-phosphate product >70, and acute renal failure.[2]

Urine alkalinization is currently not recommended as a treatment for TLS as alkalinization of the urine minimizes the risk of urate crystal precipitation within the genitourinary tract, but may increase calcium-phosphate crystallization **(Fig. 1)**.[2,3]

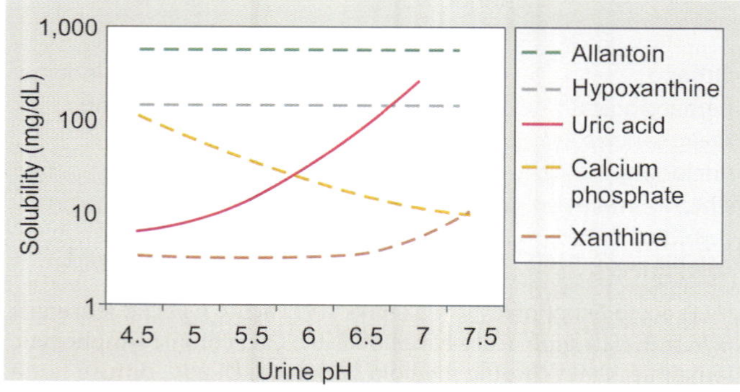

Fig. 1: Effect of urinary alkalization of solubility on various metabolites of xanthine.

HYPERLEUKOCYTOSIS

Hyperleukocytosis is defined as a white blood cell (WBC) count >100 × 10^9/L.[2] It is usually associated with hematological malignancies, such as acute myeloid leukemia (AML), mostly myelomonocytic M4 and monocytic M5, and acute lymphoid leukemia (ALL). However, it can also be seen with chronic myeloid leukemia (CML) during blast crisis.[4] As the size of myeloblasts in AML is twice that of lymphoblasts in ALL, patients of AML with hyperleukocytosis have a high risk of mortality compared to others.[2]

Hyperleukocytosis causes increased whole-blood viscosity and activates endothelial cells to secrete inflammatory cytokines, causing adhesive interaction and aggregation of blast cells in the microvasculature, which leads to leukostasis and microvascular occlusion. Also, the rapid breakdown of leukocytes can result in TLS and the release of tissue factors, which may lead to coagulopathy.[2,4]

Clinical features include neurological (headache, dural sinus thrombosis, and seizures), visual field changes (retinopathy and cortical infarction), respiratory distress, myocardial ischemia, disseminated intravascular coagulopathy (DIC), and multiorgan failure. Spuriously low PaO_2 levels can result from a high metabolic rate of blasts if the arterial blood gas sample is not processed in a timely fashion ("leukocyte larceny").[2]

Management of hyperleukocytosis includes hyperhydration to decrease whole-blood viscosity, prevention of TLS, correcting metabolic abnormalities, hydroxy urea (50–100 mg/kg/day), and early chemotherapy. Leukopheresis decreases the total WBC count by 20–50% and can be considered in symptomatic patients. Blood transfusion increases blood viscosity and thus should be avoided in hemodynamically stable patients.[2]

HYPERVISCOSITY SYNDROME

Hyperviscosity syndrome (HVS) refers to the clinical consequences of raised blood viscosity and can occur in a variety of malignancies including acute leukemias, monoclonal gammopathies such as Waldenstrom macroglobulinemia (WM), and multiple myeloma, wherein excessive amounts of circulating immunoglobulins are produced. The most common is immunoglobulin M (IgM) due to high molecular weight, but it can also occur with IgA molecules, as they tend to polymerize, or with the IgG3 subclass, as they undergo a concentration-dependent aggregation.[5]

These immunoglobulins then form aggregates and bind water (via their carbohydrate contents), which increases the osmotic pressure and resistance to blood flow. This causes impaired transit of blood cells, microvascular congestion, and reduced tissue perfusion. The normal range for serum viscosity (SV) is 1.2–2.8 centipoise (cP). Usually, patients will not become symptomatic unless SV goes above 3 cP.[5]

The classic triad of symptoms includes neurologic abnormalities (headache, altered mental status, ataxia, vertigo, or paresthesias), visual changes (blurring of vision, decreased visual acuity, and eventually blindness), and bleeding (gingival, uterus, and gastrointestinal tract), etc. The hyponatremia seen in HVS is pseudo-hyponatremia due to an artifact from the hyperproteinemia. Visual changes can be detected early at lower SV (2.1 cP), starting in the periphery of the retina, which then progresses to central retinal hemorrhages and vascular dilatation as the viscosity increases.[5] Mucosal bleeding is another common manifestation of HVS as the proteins coat the platelets and hinder their clot formation ability. Other clinical consequences of HVS include congestive heart failure, pulmonary edema, ischemic acute tubular necrosis, multiorgan system failure, and death if treatment is not promptly initiated.[5]

The mainstay of therapy is plasmapheresis, which is the fastest and most effective method to reduce blood viscosity, especially in IgM-related cases (as most IgM is intravascular). In cases of IgA- or IgG-related HVS, it may take multiple sessions to achieve the same result. Phlebotomy is another alternative if plasmapheresis is not available to reduce acute symptoms. The definitive treatment depends on diagnosis and often involves chemotherapeutic agents (alkylating agents or nucleoside analogs). Red-cell transfusions should be avoided unless critical, as this can increase SV, thus worsening HVS.[5]

DISSEMINATED INTRAVASCULAR COAGULATION

Disseminated intravascular coagulation (DIC) is an acquired condition, leading to the consumption of clotting factors and platelets followed by the intravascular deposition of fibrins. The two most important causes of DIC are sepsis and disseminated malignancies. It is estimated that 10–15% of patients with solid tumors and 15% of acute leukemia patients have some degree of DIC, in particular those with acute promyelocytic leukemia (APML).[2]

The clinical presentation of DIC can be classified into three distinct groups:[2]

1. *Subclinical:* The effect of thrombin and plasmin produced can only be seen in the laboratory markers [prothrombin time (PT) prolonged, partial thromboplastin time (PTT) prolonged, platelets decreased, fibrinogen level decreased, and fibrin split products increased], more likely in solid tumors;
2. *Hyperfibrinolysis:* The main manifestation is bleeding (the activation of the fibrinolytic system dominates), more likely in APML;
3. *Hypercoagulation:* The predominant clinical symptom is thrombosis (caused by excess thrombin), more likely in pancreatic and lung adenocarcinoma.

The International Society on Thrombosis and Hemostasis has devised objective scoring criteria to diagnose DIC, which consists of a five-step diagnostic algorithm to calculate the DIC score based on four laboratory tests (platelet count, fibrin markers, PT, and fibrinogen level) **(Table 4)**.[2]

The treatment of DIC is directed toward the treatment of the underlying cause. Cancer-related DIC requires immediate and appropriate treatment for the underlying cancer. All-trans retinoic acid (ATRA) should be given as soon as APML is suspected, as it can downregulate the procoagulant activities of the promyelocytic blasts and endothelial cells, leading to rapid improvement in coagulopathies.

Other treatment consists of mainly supportive options with judicious use of blood products, including platelets,

TABLE 4: International Society on Thrombosis and Hemostasis scoring system for the diagnosis of DIC.

Parameter	*Result*	*Score*
Platelet count	• >100 × 10^9/L • <100 × 10^9/L • <50 × 10^9/L	• 0 • 1 • 2
PT	• <3 second prolonged • >3 second but <6 second • >6 second	• 0 • 1 • 2
Fibrinogen	• >1.0 g/L • <1.0 g/L	• 0 • 1
FDP/D-dimer	• No increase • Moderate increase • Strong increase	• 0 • 2 (250–5,000) • 3 (>5,000)

Interpretation: A score >5 suggests the diagnosis of DIC.
(DIC: disseminated intravascular coagulation; FDP: fibrin degradation product; PT: prothrombin time)

fibrinogen, and cryoprecipitate. Especially in cancer patients who are at risk of thrombosis as well as bleeding, a thorough assessment of clinical and laboratory parameters is mandatory. Transfusion of blood products should be reserved only for active bleeding or in patients at risk of bleeding (e.g., requiring surgery or invasive procedures). Prothrombin complex concentrate is preferred over fresh frozen plasma (FFP) in cases of fluid overload. Tranexamic acid may be considered in hyperfibrinolytic DIC.[2]

HEMOPHAGOCYTIC LYMPHOHISTIOCYTOSIS

Hemophagocytic lymphohistiocytosis (HLH) is a hyperinflammatory condition characterized by inappropriate and dysregulated activation of natural killer (NK) cells, CD8+ cytotoxic T-cells, and macrophages that results in multiorgan failure and death.

Hemophagocytic lymphohistiocytosis presents as two distinct clinical entities:[6]

1. Primary HLH usually manifests in early childhood and occurs due to genetic mutations that impair the interaction between NK cells, CD8+ cytotoxic T-cells, and antigen-presenting cells, causing ineffective and dysregulated production of proinflammatory cytokines.
2. Secondary HLH manifests in adulthood—in response to an acute illness trigger, e.g., infection {viruses [like Epstein–Barr virus (EBV), cytomegalovirus (CMV), parvoviruses, and measles] bacteria, parasites, and fungi}, malignancy, and autoimmune disorders [i.e., macrophage activation syndrome (MAS)].

Normally, NK cells and CD8+ cytotoxic T-cells produce two cytolytic enzymes: Perforin (which forms destabilizing pores in the target cell's membrane) and granzyme (a proteolytic enzyme that causes osmotic shifts and target cell degradation). In HLH, this process is either dysregulated through genetic mutations or acquired through some immunogenic stimulus (infection or malignant cells). The ineffective interaction between NK cells, CD8+ cytotoxic T-cells, and their targets leads to more and more cytotoxic cell recruitment and a massive increase in circulating cytokines, leading to the widespread activation of macrophages, hemophagocytosis, and excessive, organ-damaging inflammation.[6]

Hemophagocytic lymphohistiocytosis diagnostic criteria are described in **Table 5**. Biopsy of either lymph nodes, bone marrow (BM), or spleen in suspected cases of HLH shows histopathologic findings of hemophagocytosis (macrophages are captured engulfing BM cells). Although pathognomonic, this finding is not required for diagnosis.[6]

TABLE 5: HLH diagnostic criteria.[6]

The original HLH-94 criteria: All the five criteria must be present to establish a diagnosis	• Fever • Cytopenias (at a minimal two lineages) • Splenomegaly • Hypertriglyceridemia (fasting >265 mg/dL ± hypofibrinogenemia (<1.5 g/dL) • Biopsy-proven hemophagocytosis
HLH-2004 criteria: Three additional laboratory criteria were added. Diagnosis is now established by the presence of any 5 out of the 8 total criteria	• Ferritin >500 ng/mL • Low or absent NK-cell activity • Elevated soluble CD25 concentration (a chain of soluble interleukin-2 receptor) >2,400 U/mL

Note: As per the HLH-2004 criteria, a diagnosis no longer requires the presence of biopsy-proven hemophagocytosis.
(HLH: hemophagocytic lymphohistiocytosis; NK: natural killer)

The "HScore" takes into consideration the following nine criteria: Fever, organomegaly, presence of immunosuppression, elevation in triglyceride levels, ferritin levels, fibrinogen levels, aspartate aminotransferase/serum glutamic oxaloacetic transaminase levels, presence of cytopenias, and hemophagocytosis in BM samples. A higher score means a higher probability of HLH (range: 0–337). H score of 169 corresponds to a sensitivity of 93% and a specificity of 86% in diagnosing HLH.[7]

The mainstay of treatment of HLH focuses on immunosuppression and cytotoxic therapy, both of which are contraindicated in patients with severe infection; thus, it is important to arrive at a clear diagnosis before the initiation of therapy protocol.

Hemophagocytic Lymphohistiocytosis-94 Treatment Protocol[6,7]

This includes an initial 8-week therapeutic course of etoposide (150 mg/m^2 twice weekly for 2 weeks and then weekly) with dexamethasone (10 mg/m^2 slowly tapered over 8 weeks). Continuation therapy consists of pulses of dexamethasone (10 mg/m^2 for 3 days every second week) and etoposide (150 mg/m^2 every alternating second week) with daily oral cyclosporine. In the case of progressive neurologic symptoms or a persistently abnormal cerebrospinal fluid (CSF), intrathecal methotrexate can be administered.

Hemophagocytic Lymphohistiocytosis-2004 Treatment Protocol

Hemophagocytic lymphohistiocytosis-2004 protocol is derived from the HLH-94 protocol, with the dosage and frequency of administering etoposide and dexamethasone being the same. The major difference is the initiation of cyclosporine A at the beginning of the initial phase of treatment to oppose the action of interferon (IFN)-c and achieve increased immunosuppression.

Furthermore, the HLH-2004 protocol proposes performing hematopoietic stem cell transplant (HSCT) on patients as soon as a donor is available and administering intrathecal prednisone, in addition to intrathecal methotrexate, for HLH causing progressive neurologic symptoms. The 5-year survival post-HSCT, in patients who received the HLH-2004 treatment protocol, was 66%, which was not considerably better than in patients who received the HLH-94 treatment protocol. Thus, most oncologists still use the HLH-94 treatment protocol, as the current evidence shows no significant clinical advantage over the HLH-94 treatment protocol.[6,7]

MALIGNANT SUPERIOR VENA CAVA OBSTRUCTION

Superior vena cava obstruction (SVCO) occurs due to extrinsic compression of the superior vena cava (SVC) or direct invasion by a tumor, impairing venous return to the heart. Non-Hodgkin's lymphoma and lung cancers account for most cases of malignant SVCO. Thrombus formation due to indwelling central venous catheters can also put oncology patients at increased risk of SVCO. The most common presenting symptoms are due to venous congestion and include face, neck, and upper extremity swelling, dyspnea at rest, and dilated neck and chest veins. Symptoms classically worsen when the patient is supine, as flow through the SVC lumen may be compromised further.[8]

Typical X-ray scan findings include widening of the superior mediastinum. Contrast-enhanced computed tomography can identify the precise location and extent of obstruction and detect the presence of a thrombus.

Head-end elevation, lateral or prone position, can be considered to reduce the mediastinal mass effect. In patients with SVCO, it is necessary to optimize the fluid status to maintain sufficient venous return and thereby adequate cardiac output. Steroids and radiotherapy may be considered to reduce the size of the tumor. Chemotherapy can be considered for chemo-sensitive malignancies, such as lymphoma or small-cell lung cancer.[2] Insertion of an endovascular stent in eligible patients with acute SVCO is the most effective and immediate means of resolving symptoms **(Table 6)**. Thrombus removal and anticoagulation treatment should be considered in cases secondary to thrombus formation.[8] Extracorporeal membrane oxygenation (ECMO) might be sometimes required as a supportive or rescue therapy.[2]

TABLE 6: Kishi scoring system to assist in decision-making for stent placement.

Clinical signs	***Weighting***
Neurological signs	
Awareness disorders or coma	4
Visual disorders, headache, vertigo, or memory disorders	3
Mental disorders	2
Malaise	1
Thoracic/pharyngeal/laryngeal signs	
Orthopnea or laryngeal edema	3
Stridor, dysphagia, or dyspnea	2
Coughing or pleurisy	1
Facial signs	
Lip edema, nasal obstruction, or epistaxis	2
Facial edema	1
Vessel dilation	
Neck, face, or arms	1

Interpretation: A score >4 indicates a need for percutaneous stent placement.[9]

EXTRAVASATION INJURIES SECONDARY TO CHEMOTHERAPY

With toxic chemotherapies, various extravasation injuries are possible. Pain, erythema, and swelling that progress to blanching, blistering, discoloration, and necrosis of the skin can occur. Prompt diagnosis, team training, vigilance, and patient education are the goals. Early treatment is crucial and includes stopping the infusion immediately and leaving the cannula in place, while the next steps are determined along with a multidisciplinary oncologist, a dermatologist, and a plastic surgery consult.[10]

CHIMERIC ANTIGEN RECEPTOR T-CELLS' COMPLICATIONS AND TOXICITY

Chimeric antigen receptor T-cell (CAR-T-cell) therapy utilizes a patient's T cells that are genetically reprogrammed to target and kill cancer cells. In 2017, the Food and Drug Administration (FDA) approved the first CAR-T-cell therapy, tisagenlecleucel, for relapsed/refractory B-cell ALL[4] followed by axicabtagene ciloleucel for relapsed/refractory diffuse large B-cell lymphoma.[4] CAR-T-cell therapy is associated with a variety of specific and unique toxicities, of which two main are cytokine release syndrome (CRS) and neurotoxicity.

Cytokine release syndrome: Initially, the patient may develop constitutional symptoms, but this can progress rapidly to multiple organ dysfunction syndrome. Important differential diagnoses of CRS are septic shock and MAS/HLH, which are itself adverse reactions to CAR-T-cell therapy. Thus, usually, antimicrobials are generally started while awaiting sepsis workup results. The role of procalcitonin as a biomarker in CRS is not as well established as in that of sepsis. C-reactive protein levels were thought to estimate the severity of CRS toxicity as it correlated well with interleukin (IL)-6 levels; however, its utility in predicting the severity of CRS remains unknown. Cytokine release syndrome treatment primarily focuses on supportive intensive care unit (ICU) care and pharmacologic treatments that may be targeted (tocilizumab) or generalized (corticosteroids). Tocilizumab [an interleukin 6 (IL-6) receptor antagonist] is commonly used at a dose of 8 mg/kg intravenously (IV) given for patients >30 kg and can be repeated if there is no response within 6 hours. Steroids should be considered as second-line therapy for patients who have either no or inadequate response to tocilizumab.

CONCLUSION

There is an obvious increase in the number of patients presenting with oncological emergencies due to advancements in the field of oncology. Thus, healthcare professionals involved in the care of oncology patients must be vigilant as early recognition and prompt treatment can reduce the chances of potential complications and improve clinical outcomes.

REFERENCES

1. Tan SJ. Recognition and treatment of oncologic emergencies: J Infus Nurs. 2002;25(3):182-8.
2. Leung KKY, Hon KL, Hui WF, Leung AKC, Li CK. Therapeutics for pediatric oncological emergencies. Drugs Context. 2021;(10):1-12.
3. Lewis MA, Hendrickson AW, Moynihan TJ. Oncologic emergencies: pathophysiology, presentation, diagnosis, and treatment. CA Cancer J Clin. 2011;61(5):287-314.
4. Thandra K, Salah Z, Chawla S. Oncologic emergencies—the old, the new, and the deadly. J Intensive Care Med. 2020; 35(1):3-13.
5. Behl D, Hendrickson AW, Moynihan TJ. Oncologic emergencies. Crit Care Clin. 2010;26(1):181-205.
6. Konkol S, Rai M. Lymphohistiocytosis. (2024). Treasure Island (FL): StatPearls Publishing. Available from https://www.ncbi.nlm.nih.gov/books/NBK557776/ [Last accessed March, 2025].
7. Ponnatt TS, Lilley CM, Mirza KM. Hemophagocytic lymphohistiocytosis. Arch Pathol Lab Med. 2022;146(4):507-19.
8. Regnier L, Wilkinson AN. Common oncologic emergencies. Can Fam Physician. 2023;69(1):28-32.
9. Lanciego C, Pangua C, Chacón JI, Velasco J, Boy RC, Viana A, et al. Endovascular stenting as the first step in the overall management of malignant superior vena cava syndrome. Am J Roentgenol. 2009;193(2):549-58.
10. Higdon ML, Atkinson CJ, Lawrence KV. Oncologic emergencies: recognition and initial management. Am Fam Physician. 2018;97(11):741-8.

CHAPTER 70

Non-operating Room Anesthesia

Lalita Gouri Mitra, Jagdeep Sharma, Sofia Jaswal

INTRODUCTION

Non-operating room anesthesia (NORA) or anesthesia in the non-theater environment (ANTE), refers to providing anesthesia services outside of a central, high-acuity operating room (OR) suite.[1] With advancements in medicine, diagnostic and minimally invasive interventional techniques are emerging which require anesthesia services in various remote locations. Hence, NORA has emerged as a subspecialty of anesthesia practice which is evolving over time.

CHALLENGES IN PROVIDING NONOPERATIVE ROOM ANESTHESIA

While providing NORA, the anesthetist faces challenges in locations that are not as ideal as in the OR. The challenges faced are discussed here.[2,3]

- *Space:* Other than in newer institutions, the diagnostic or interventional suites where NORA services are required are built as an additional facility for which space is carved out in the existing infrastructure. The anesthesia machine, crash cart, difficult airways trolley, and other important equipment are adjusted within the limited space, with the equipment and medications being transported back and forth from the OR complex. In case of an emergency in these locations, appropriate medication or equipment may not be easily available or accessible.
- *Ergonomics:* The ergonomics of the diagnostic suite where anesthesia services are to be provided are not ideal as in the OR as there is limited space available due to the presence of bulky diagnostic equipment. Anesthetists should be involved in the planning of these diagnostic suites from inception to ensure there is dedicated anesthesia space.
- *Equipment:* The anesthesia equipment available in a NORA location may not be the same as the one in the OR. The unfamiliarity with the new equipment makes it challenging to work in these locations in an emergency scenario. In many hospitals, newer equipment is allocated to the main OR while the existing or outdated ones are moved to remote locations where NORA services are required.
- *Medications:* The anesthesia and emergency medications need to be checked regularly both for availability and expiry before every procedure as they might not be stored properly as remote locations tend to be more isolated.
    - *Staffing and unfamiliar team:* Unlike surgeons, the doctors performing the procedures and their team are not used to working with the anesthesia team. The proceduralist team, due to lack of exposure or due to limited staffing, may not be able to assist the anesthetist timely nor effectively in case of hemodynamic instability or during an emergency where the airway needs to be secured.

GOALS[2,3]

- To deliver safe anesthesia or sedation for various procedures
- To provide ideal working conditions for the proceduralists
- To ensure patient safety by adhering to the American Society of Anesthesiology (ASA) minimum standards of monitoring guidelines in all patients
- To identify the intraprocedure complications early and to treat them accordingly
- Early resuscitation if the patient becomes hemodynamically unstable during the procedure

PERIOPERATIVE PLANNING FOR PROCEDURES[2,3]

Anesthetists are known for their contingency planning to minimize complications and to treat the worst possible outcomes. Perioperative planning includes meticulous planning within the NORA suite, preoperative assessment, intraoperative management, anesthesia techniques, postoperative care, and discharge criteria.

Nonoperative Room Anesthesia Suite

According to the ASA statement of minimum requirements for providing care in NORA locations to ensure patient safety, the following are included:[1-3]

- A source of continuous oxygen supply as well as a backup. Oxygen delivery from a central oxygen source is preferred and a full type E cylinder should be present as a backup source.
- A suction (central or portable) with the desired suction pressure in a working condition.
- Scavenging system for anesthesia gases.
- A self-inflating resuscitator bag for positive pressure ventilation which can administer at least 21% O_2.
- Adequate and essential anesthesia equipment and drugs for providing safe anesthesia.
- Adequate monitoring equipment to comply with ASA Standards for basic anesthetic monitoring, for all cases involving either general anesthesia (GA), regional anesthesia (RA), or monitored anesthesia care (MAC) **(Table 1)**.
- A qualified anesthetist should be present throughout the procedure for the conduct of anesthesia.
- An anesthesia machine maintained to current OR standards should be used in any location where inhaled anesthetics are to be used.
- Sufficient electrical outlets that adhere to facility standards.
- Adequate light source for illumination of the patient and equipment.
- Sufficient space to accommodate necessary equipment and personnel.

TABLE 1: Monitoring for nonoperative room anesthesia (NORA) procedures.[3]

Oxygenation	*Ventilation*	*Circulation*	*Temperature*
• Oxygen analyzer • Pulse oximeter	• Chest excursion • Breath sounds • Capnography	• Electrocardiogram • Pulse oximetry • Blood pressure • Arterial blood pressure • Palpation of a pulse • Auscultation of heart sounds	Temperature probe

- An emergency cart with emergency drugs, defibrillator, and other equipment to provide cardiopulmonary resuscitation which is easily accessible.
- Adequate anesthesia support staff.
- Adequate postanesthesia recovery room with staffing, oxygen source, and monitoring.

Patient Assessment[4,5]

The ASA has developed an evidence-based guideline that outlines all aspects of preoperative assessment and testing. Pre-existing comorbidities, treatment history, medications, functional status, allergies, and airway should be assessed thoroughly as we do for any patient scheduled for surgery. Sometimes patients with severe comorbid conditions are offered percutaneous interventions requiring NORA instead of open surgical procedures.[6] A study by Nagrebetsky found that the mean age of patients undergoing NORA procedures was 3.5 years greater than those undergoing traditional OR procedures.[7] The older patients may have multiple comorbid conditions with frailty, making them poor candidates for surgery. In the same study, the number of sick patients with ASA status III–V receiving NORA was higher (37.6%) as compared to those for OR procedures (33.0%). This emphasizes the importance of detailed preoperative evaluation for these patients. For all the patients coming for NORA, there should be an integrated approach for risk stratification, prehabilitation, and optimization of preexisting comorbidities before giving anesthesia to these patients.

Anesthesia Management

Due to the complexity of procedures and increasing concerns for patient safety, NORA is emerging as a subspeciality, and anesthetists have to ensure patient safety and quality assurance in every setting. Management plans differ from one patient to another based on the procedure and the patient factors. It is very important to have a plan for each patient individually before the patient is taken for NORA.[8,9]

Anesthesia technique: The anesthesia plan may be either MAC, spinal/neuraxial anesthesia with or without MAC, or GA depending upon various factors. The factors affecting the choice of anesthesia plan are as follows:[10]

- *Patient-specific factors:*
    - *Age:* Pediatric patients may not lie supine for procedures, hence requiring MAC/GA for various diagnostic and interventional procedures.

- *Position:* Inability to lie supine due to acute or chronic pain, anxiety, or dyspnea.
- Hemodynamic instability.
- Altered level of consciousness with risk of aspiration in patients presenting for neurointerventions.
- History of difficult airway.
- History of obstructive sleep apnea (OSA) making these patients more prone to the risk of airway obstructions and the need of urgently securing the airway. OSA must be identified, risk-stratified with STOP-BANG scoring, and airway adequately optimized.
- Patient preferences.

▪ *Procedure-specific factors:*
  - Type, duration, and complexity of procedure
  - Need of an uncomfortable position for a long time
  - Requirement of apnea or no movement during the procedure
  - Potential for development of hemodynamic instability

Positioning: The positioning of the patient should be discussed with the proceduralist, and the plan of the anesthesia to be made accordingly.

Monitoring: ASA standards of basic anesthesia monitoring apply to all the patients receiving either MAC, GA, or RA. Monitoring as described in **Table 1** should be applicable to all the NORA cases. Despite the formulation of the guidelines, it has been seen in a study that an inconsistent application of basic monitoring principles by the nonanesthetists in the NORA setting.[11]

Monitored anesthesia care: Most of the procedures of NORA are done under MAC which requires moderate sedation with natural airway and maintenance of spontaneous unobstructed respiration. The drug selection may depend on the type of procedure, the anticipated pain expected, and the duration. Sometimes, MAC is provided to supplement RA. Maintenance of depth of sedation sufficient to prevent movement may be challenging. Hence, monitoring the depth of sedation and patency of the airway is very important throughout the procedure. Obese patients or patients with OSA may need their airway to be secured definitively intraprocedure for which the anesthetists will require access to the airway with a ramp position.

Medication: The various drugs that can be used in NORA are summarized in **Table 2**.

TABLE 2: Various drugs used in NORA.

Drug	*Route*	*Dose*
Midazolam	IV	0.025–0.05 mg/kg (max 10 mg)
	IM	0.1–0.15 mg/kg
	Per rectal	1 mg/kg
	Sublingual	0.5–0.75 mg/kg
	Intranasal	0.2–0.3 mg/kg
Propofol	IV (induction)	2–3 mg/kg
	IV infusion	125–150 μg/kg/min
Ketamine	IV (sedation)	0.5–2 mg/kg
	IV (analgesic)	0.1 mg/kg
	IV infusion (analgesic)	0.1–0.3 mg/kg/h
Etomidate	IV	0.1–0.3 mg/kg
Dexmedetomidine	IV infusion	1–2 μg/kg over 10 minutes, then 0.5–1 μg/kg/h
Fentanyl	IV	1–3 μg/kg
Remifentanil	IV (infusion)	0.5–1 μg/kg/min

(IM: intramuscular; IV: intravenous; NORA: nonoperative room anesthesia)

Postprocedure Recovery and Discharge Criteria[2,3,12]

The recovery and discharge criteria after NORA are the same as after anesthesia in OR. A patient's vitals should be monitored in the recovery area along with the pain scores and level of consciousness. As most of the NORA procedures are minimally invasive, the patient can be discharged home the same day. The modified Aldrete scoring system (postanesthesia recovery score) can be used to assess for the "readiness to discharge." The patient should be fully conscious, maintaining airway, and pain-free with stable vitals before discharge.

MEDICATION SAFETY IN NONOPERATIVE ROOM ANESTHESIA[2,3]

Anesthetists have a unique role and responsibility as they are the only medical personnel who prescribe, secure, prepare, administer, and document medications, a process that can take up to 41 steps which is usually within a very short time interval, occurring in real time, autonomously, often in a distracting environment, and typically without standardized protocols.

The five categories of medication errors are incorrect dose, omission, substitution, repetition, and insertion. The mechanisms of error identified are inadequate communication, incorrect patient weight, nonobservance of institution guidelines, poor supervision, poor or no labeling, and miscalculation of dose.

The specific challenges for medication safety during NORA are as follows:

- Different and limited availability of medication in the NORA setting.
- Challenges during preparation and administration of medication (e.g., away from patient/low lighting/ multiple instrumentation).
- The anesthetists may be unfamiliar with the medications being administered during procedures performed in NORA sites (e.g., intrathecal or intra-arterial chemotherapy).
- Space constraints might force placement of the medication cart in a nonstandard configuration restricting timely access.
- Location of pharmacy may be far from the NORA site.

Steps that must be put in place at NORA sites to avoid medication-related problems:

- Every NORA site should have a standardized list of anesthesia medications.
- Medication to treat rare events, such as dantrolene for malignant hyperthermia or intralipid for local anesthetic toxicity, should be available immediately and located in a designated area.
- Medication must be labeled immediately with the drug name, concentration, and expiry.
- Standardized colors for different drug classes should be adopted to reduce "syringe switch errors" to avoid selecting an incorrect syringe even though the syringes on the drug trolley are correctly labeled.
- Prefilled syringes can be used to reduce the errors in diluting and labeling. Barcode scanners add another layer of safety.
- Task lighting on the workstation should be available where lighting is dim as is often seen in NORA sites.

NONOPERATIVE ROOM ANESTHESIA AT SPECIFIC LOCATIONS

Endoscopy

Specific challenges with the administration of anesthesia in the endoscopy[13] suite include titrating the adequate depth of sedation with a largely unprotected airway, preserving spontaneous ventilation, suppressing the cough reflex, and high patient turnover. The main objective of administering sedation for gastrointestinal endoscopy procedures is to reduce patient anxiety, discomfort, and amnesia and improve the outcome of the examination. The endoscopic procedures are usually performed under moderate sedation; the patient provides a purposeful response to verbal or tactile stimulation and maintains ventilator and cardiovascular function.

Preprocedure Evaluation

These patients have an increased risk of periprocedural aspiration and hypoxemia. Patients with symptoms of achalasia, gastric outlet obstruction, upper gastrointestinal (GI) bleeding, bleeding varices, esophageal stricture, intestinal obstruction, or who have undergone Heller's myotomy are at increased risk of aspiration. Glucagon-like peptides (semaglutide and liraglutide) delay gastric emptying, thereby increasing the chance of aspiration. Careful evaluation of the airway must be done. These patients must be well evaluated for all the conditions that might increase (e.g., elderly patients, obstructive sleep apnea, and severe liver or kidney disease) or reduce (e.g., anxiety, use of opioids, or other recreational drugs) sensitivity to the usual routine dose of sedatives. Awake tracheal intubation might be required in select cases. Adequate starvation and informed consent explaining the potential risks involved should be taken.

Patients must undergo a complete preprocedure evaluation for identification and optimization of any associated comorbidities as per ASA Guidelines for Anesthesia provider assistance. The anesthetist must anticipate complications in the following circumstances:

- Patients undergoing prolonged or therapeutic endoscopic procedures requiring deep sedation
- Patients intolerant to standard sedative administration
- American Society of Anesthesiology IV or V patients with severe comorbidities
- Increased chances of airway compromise in patients with anatomic abnormalities

Recommendations for Monitoring and Medication During Endoscopy[13]

All patients are monitored as per ASA standards with regular assessment of the sedation and ventilatory status throughout the procedure.

The recommended regimen for use includes a combination of an opioid with benzodiazepine, along with an appropriate adjunct like diphenhydramine, promethazine, or droperidol in certain patients. Propofol-based sedation is to be used when it is expected to improve patient comfort, safety, and procedural efficiency.

Special Considerations for Advanced Gastrointestinal Endoscopy Procedures

- Endoscopic retrograde cholangiopancreatography (ERCP)[14] is usually done in moderate to deep sedation. The use of a large endoscope during the procedure increases the risk of airway obstruction. GA with tracheal intubation in patients with a high risk of aspiration; complex and prolonged procedures. Laryngeal mask airway (LMA) Gastro is commonly used as an alternative to intubation.
- Esophageal dilation for esophageal strictures. This procedure is done under deep sedation, but intubation is needed in patients with a high risk of aspiration.
- Peroral endoscopic myotomy (POEM) is an endoscopic procedure done for Achalasia. It is done under GA with intubation and needs good muscle relaxation, as the patient should be still. Common complications include pneumothorax, pneumomediastinum, and subcutaneous emphysema.
- *Bariatric procedures:* The placement of intragastric balloons and percutaneous gastrostomy tubes is done under sedation. Sleeve gastroplasty and duodenal-jejunal bypass procedures are done under GA with muscle relaxation.

Interventional Radiology

Percutaneous Radiofrequency Ablation[15]

It is the direct application of targeted thermal energy therapy to specific focal tumors to achieve eradication or substantial reduction in tumor size. It is a safe and effective technique associated with site-specific treatment, few complications, decreased morbidity, and outpatient use. Anesthetic management varies widely, ranging from patients receiving LA alone to MAC, to RA or GA. It depends on the tumor's location and the practitioner's experience. It presents site-specific challenges that need to be managed with accuracy and precision. All patients must undergo preoperative evaluation and adequate optimization.

Specific challenges associated with specific organs are discussed in **Table 3**:

Endovascular Procedures

Endovascular therapy (EVT) includes mechanical thrombectomy or targeted direct intra-arterial administration of thrombolytics.[16] It can be performed under MAC or GA. Preoperative evaluation and preparation must run parallel as the timeline of the therapeutic window is quite narrow.

TABLE 3: Specific challenges associated with specific organs during NORA.

Site	Anesthesia technique	Positioning	Specific concerns	Complications
Lung	• GA • LA+MAC • TPVB • TEA • ICNB	Lateral, supine, or prone	Difficulty in breathing, hemoptysis, coughing, need for apneic pause during the procedure, and airway management can be difficult i/v/o airway loss, especially in the prone position	Bleeding, pneumothorax, and hemothorax
Liver	• GA • LA+MAC • TPVB • TEA	Supine	Management of acute pain for the subglissonian or tumors near the parietal peritoneum	Injury to the bile duct, major bleeding, pneumothorax, and perforation injury of colon
Bone	• GA • LA+MAC	Supine, lateral, and prone	Difficult airway management i/v/o airway loss in the prone position, dyspnea while treatment of rib tumors	Injury to the structures adjacent to the ablation site, viz., nerves, major vessels, bowel, and liver
Kidney	• GA • LA+MAC	Lateral, semiprone, and prone	Require apneic pause, acute pain management for ureteric or visceral injury, and difficulty in airway management due to airway loss in prone position	Bleeding, pneumothorax, and colonic and ureteral injury

(GA: general anesthesia; ICNB: intercostal nerve block; LA: local anesthesia; MAC: monitored anesthesia care; NORA: nonoperative room anesthesia; TEA: thoracic epidural anesthesia; TPVB: thoracic paravertebral block)

It should be very focused and precise. It must specifically mention the neurologic and cervical spine status, diabetes mellitus, cardiovascular status, and complete airway examination. Monitoring is as per ASA standards. It is preferable to put in an arterial catheter for invasive blood pressure monitoring, but its placement must not delay the procedure.

The choice of anesthesia technique should be based on the patient, procedure, availability of resources, and in close communication with the interventionalist. GA is preferred in patients with poor neurological status, high risk of aspiration, and hemodynamic instability, who cannot lie stable for the procedure, and who are at high risk of airway compromise. MAC is preferred in patients who can lie stable, cooperate/communicate well, and are able to maintain a patent airway.

Special Considerations During Endovascular Procedures

- Secondary ischemic insult by hypoxemia, excessive hyperventilation, and hemodynamic instability must always be avoided during induction, maintenance, and reversal of anesthesia.
- Hemodynamic goals must be optimized, maintained, and discussed with the interventionalist. A systolic blood pressure between 140 and 180 mm Hg must be maintained before recanalization during the EVT procedure.
- Maintain oxygen saturation >94% (viz., partial pressure of oxygen >60 mm Hg), and partial pressure of carbon dioxide between 35 and 45 mm Hg.
- Maintain normothermia and adequate blood glucose levels between 140 and 180 mg/dL.
- Maintain moderate sedation during MAC, with the use of rapid and short-acting agents for titration to target sedation levels, and regularly assess the level of sedation and ventilatory status.
- If there is any arterial perforation during EVT, it might need emergent craniotomy. The systolic blood pressure should be maintained <140 mm Hg. Anticoagulants, thrombolytics, and antiplatelet therapy may need to be reversed.

Transjugular Intrahepatic Portosystemic Shunt[17]

Transjugular intrahepatic portosystemic shunt (TIPSS) is a minimally invasive procedure that helps reduce portal pressures, thus providing symptomatic relief and survival benefits. Portal hypertension is defined when the hepatic venous pressure gradient is ≥6 mm Hg, with clinical manifestations usually presenting with a pressure gradient of ≥10 mm Hg. Usually seen in patients with liver cirrhosis, it presents in the form of varices, ascites, hydrothorax, hepatorenal syndrome, or hepatopulmonary syndrome.

Preoperative workup: Child-Pugh scoring should be done for risk stratification. Rule out any form of heart failure, pulmonary hypertension, respiratory dysfunction due to massive ascites/hydrothorax, coagulopathy, thrombocytopenia, or hepatic encephalopathy. Adequate blood/blood products must be arranged before the procedure.

Anesthesia techniques for TIPSS include GA or conscious sedation. GA with tracheal intubation is a preferred technique, as a secured airway reduces complications. Secure a wide bore peripheral intravenous access and use the left internal jugular vein or femoral vein for central line insertion. Invasive blood pressure monitoring should be done in patients who are hemodynamically unstable. Administration of the drugs should be done with caution considering the pharmacokinetics and pharmacodynamics of liver dysfunction. Short-acting drugs are preferred, such as midazolam, propofol, fentanyl/remifentanil, succinylcholine, and atracurium. Volatile anesthesia or total intravenous anesthesia is recommended for the maintenance of anesthesia.

Postprocedure care: Increased venous return post-TIPSS may precipitate heart failure and hemodynamic instability. Coagulopathy must be managed with adequate transfusion of blood and blood products. Hemodynamic instability may persist in patients with significant blood loss even after the procedure. Hepatic encephalopathy can be managed with a combination of lactulose and nonabsorbable antibiotics (rifaximin). Postprocedural sepsis is usually caused by gram-negative organisms such as *Escherichia coli*, *Klebsiella*, and *Enterococcus* and must be managed with appropriate antibiotics, fluid resuscitation, and vasopressor support.

Percutaneous Transhepatic Biliary Drainage[14]

Percutaneous transhepatic biliary drainage (PTBD) is done to treat biliary obstruction caused by hepatobiliary, pancreatic, or advanced gastrointestinal malignancies. Symptomatology includes jaundice, pruritis, pain, and cholangitis with transaminitis. These tumors usually occur in elderly patients, and they present in an advanced state, where radical surgeries are usually not possible. So, symptomatic relief and optimization are done by drainage methods—first ERCP, followed by endoscopic ultrasound-guided biliary drainage, and last by PTBD. It helps in successful biliary decompression, with easy monitoring, and manipulation of the catheter in case of obstruction.

Preoperative evaluation should be done in detail with specific attention to deranged liver function tests, complete blood count, renal function tests, coagulation profiles, ascites, and encephalopathy. Bradycardia is usually present due to the negative inotropic effects of the bile salts. The maximum analgesic requirement is at the time of dilatation and stenting. Anesthesia techniques commonly used are LA, conscious sedation, or less commonly GA. Drugs commonly used include short-acting benzodiazepine (midazolam), remifentanil (opioid), propofol, and ketamine. Adequacy of ventilation and maintenance of protective airway reflexes must always be confirmed. Complications include bleeding, biliary peritonitis due to biliary leakage, pneumothorax, and liver abscess.

Irreversible Electroporation[18]

It is a nonthermal ablative technology that uses high-voltage, direct-current (3 kV) pulses with low energy to induce cell death. With the application of an electric field around the cell, pores are created; high voltage leads to cell death. It is available as a nano knife system. It can be performed under computed tomography (CT) scan or ultrasound guidance. Usual indications include locally advanced soft tissue tumors of the pancreas, liver, kidney, and retroperitoneal tumors. Preoperatively, a complete cardiology work-up is essential, as the history of cardiac arrhythmias/pacemakers is a contraindication, as IRE increases the risk of ventricular arrhythmias.

Anesthesia technique: GA, with endotracheal intubation and deep neuromuscular blockade, is required during the procedure. Adequate analgesia with remifentanil/epidural block must be provided.

Magnetic Resonance Imaging and Computed Tomography Suite[19]

Nonoperative room anesthesia in the MRI suite presents unique challenges as compared to other sites. The field strength used commonly in clinical MRI examinations varies from 0.05 to 3.0 T, with most diagnostic scanners currently operating at 1.5 T.

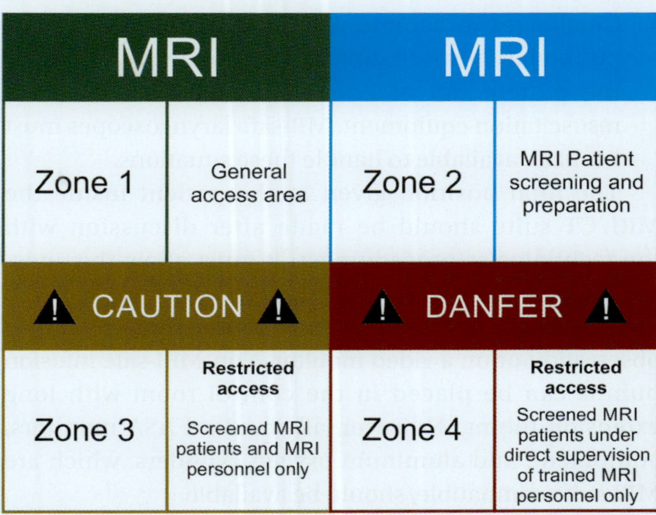

Fig. 1: Zones in MRI suite. (MRI: magnetic resonance imaging)

Various zones are **(Fig. 1)**:

- *Zone 1:* It is freely accessible to the general public.
- *Zone 2:* Itis a buffer area between Zone 1 and more restrictive Zone 3. Here, the patients are under the supervision of general MRI personnel.
- *Zone 3:* It should be restricted by a physical barrier. Only approved MRI personnel and patients that have undergone a medical questionnaire are allowed inside.
- *Zone 4:* It is strictly within the walls of the scanner room and must be accessed by passing through Zone 3.

The unique hazards include a strong magnetic field, radiofrequency, and loud acoustic noise. It is mandatory to use MRI-safe equipment for patient monitoring and delivery of anesthesia services.

Preanesthesia evaluation:

- Identification of the indications and type of anesthesia care required must be consulted with the radiologist regarding the patient's inability to lie supine, level of consciousness, or claustrophobia.
- To rule out pacemakers and implantable cardioverter defibrillators (ICDs) that are not MRI-safe, some of the transdermal patches (fentanyl, lignocaine) may contain aluminum or other metals increasing the risk of burns.
- The patients on continuous vasopressor requirement are at high risk due to the limited access to the patient and lack of resuscitation equipment in the scanner room. Specific care of linear gadolinium contrast must be taken as it is nephrotoxic.

- Challenges in communication and delayed cardiopulmonary resuscitation due to the need to relocate the patient out of Zone IV which has complete resuscitation equipment. MR-safe laryngoscopes must be made available to handle these situations.

The final position given to the patient inside the MRI/CT suite should be made after discussion with the technologist/proceduralist; it must allow the anesthesiologist to maintain an unobstructed view of the patient, anesthesia machine, and monitors, either by direct observation or on a video monitor. Non-MRI-safe infusion pumps can be placed in the control room with long extension tubing. However, all standard ASA monitors, equipment, and aluminum oxygen cylinders, which are MRI suite compatible, should be available.

In the CT suite, most of the issues are similar with the additional exposure to ionizing radiation. Staff must use protective equipment in the form of portable shields, lead aprons, thyroid collars, and eye protection.

Selection of anesthesia technique in MRI/CT suite:

- *Monitored anesthesia care:* Patients usually require light sedation for controlling anxiety/claustrophobia; moderate sedation might also be required in specific conditions to enable the patient to lie still for a prolonged period of time.
- *General anesthesia:* Induction is completed in the holding area or induction room; subsequently, the patient is shifted to the scanner room. It can be delivered via inhalational (MRI-safe sevoflurane vaporizer), or TIVA can be used as per patient requirement. MRI-safe infusion pumps must be available. A scavenging system must be in place to prevent anesthesia gas pollution in the MRI suite.

Interventional Cardiology

The cardiac catheter laboratory (CCL) is a claustrophobic environment.[20] Familiarization with the environment and close communication with cardiologists are the keys to the safe and successful delivery of anesthesia services in this zone. Various procedures done in the CCL include percutaneous closure of the septal defect, electrophysiologic procedures, percutaneous coronary intervention, percutaneous transcatheter aortic valve replacement, percutaneous transcatheter mitral valve replacement, and ICD.

The CCL consists of an anesthesia machine, a procedure workstation, a fluoroscope, equipment for dye injection, and catheters. Various challenges include unfamiliar environments, radiation exposure, limited equipment, and help from colleagues; the patient being far away requires long intravenous tubing and monitoring lines. As there is significant radiation exposure, all protective equipment must be used for the safety of the healthcare professionals. Ionic and nonionic dyes are used for cardiac imaging.

All patients must undergo a detailed preoperative evaluation before the procedure. Along with standard monitors, a radial arterial line for continuous beat-to-beat monitoring and central venous pressure monitoring in high-risk patients or patients undergoing complex procedures should be used. Transesophageal/transthoracic echocardiography can be used in select patients. Defibrillator pads must be placed to treat perioperative arrhythmias. At the time of induction, the fluoroscope must be moved away from the patient's head end, so that the airway can be secured. The anesthesia team, nursing staff, technologist, and cardiologist must always work in close synchrony.

Endobronchial Ultrasound[21]

Endobronchial ultrasound (EBUS) bronchoscopy is a procedure used to diagnose different types of lung disorders, including inflammation, infections, or cancer. The EBUS scope has a video camera with an ultrasound probe attached which is negotiated into the larynx, to create local images of the lungs and nearby lymph nodes to accurately locate and evaluate areas that need a closer look.

Preprocedure

Apart from routine bloodwork, the patient must get an X-ray chest and CT thorax. If the patient's effort tolerance is less, then a complete cardiopulmonary assessment should be done. Pulmonary function tests will need to be done only if clinical signs of respiratory compromise are present. Fasting timelines are as per guidelines. Preoperative 2% lignocaine nebulization should be done prior to taking the patient for the procedure. If the patient is on any bronchodilator or steroid nebulization, medication should be bought at the daycare center and taken before the procedure.

Intraoperative

The patient is positioned supine and all monitors as per ASA guidelines should be attached. The patient should be preoxygenated with 100% oxygen, and oxygen should be given via nasal prongs at the rate of 4–6 L/min during the procedure. Total intravenous anesthesia (TIVA) provides optimal conditions for EBUS, and it is preferred over volatile anesthetics because frequent suctioning of the airway by the bronchoscopist results in contamination of the room atmosphere by volatile anesthetics and in an inconsistent delivery of volatile anesthetic gas to the patient. Drugs commonly used are propofol, midazolam, fentanyl, remifentanil, etomidate, and ketamine. The airway can be secured by an LMA or endotracheal tube (ETT, minimum size 8). As the scope is introduced, 2% lignocaine should be sprayed intermittently to decrease cough due to the stimulus of the scope.

Laryngeal mask airway seems to be the most suitable device to secure the airway, as it provides adequate ventilation around the bronchoscope, and it allows access to higher mediastinal lymph node stations that would otherwise be obscured by the ETT. However, it may not be appropriate in obesity or untreated gastroesophageal reflux.

The disadvantage of an ETT is that the scope is directed in a central position by the tube, and it may be more difficult to get close to the tracheal wall with the tip of the scope and obtain adequate ultrasonographic imaging. It also has to be withdrawn to explore higher mediastinal nodes.

Postoperative

The patient may experience mild cough and sore throat. Complications include bleeding from the biopsy site, desaturation during or after the procedure, bronchospasm, infection, and a very small risk of lung collapse for which the patient will have to be treated and observed as an inpatient and not discharged. A postprocedure X-ray chest is recommended.

Brachytherapy Procedures

For brachytherapy, radioactive sources are placed within the body tissues or cavities close to the tumor. In low-dose-rate (LDR) brachytherapy, the implants are kept in situ for a prolonged period, and in high-dose-rate (HDR) brachytherapy is given repeatedly at weekly intervals. Perioperative challenges include immobility, good analgesia, and shifting of patients to the CT/MRI/radiation suite, where there is a lack of specialized staff/facilities, and the duration of these procedures varies. Indications include carcinoma of the breast, endometrium, cervix, head and neck, prostate, and penis.

Preoperative evaluation is done as routine for all other anesthesia procedures.

Anesthesia technique: The procedures can be done under LA, conscious sedation, RA, or GA depending upon the procedure. Brachytherapy procedures for the cervix and endometrium are usually done under neuraxial blocks, and for breast cancer, GA with/without erector spinae/serratus anterior plane block is recommended.

Pediatric Nonoperative Room Anesthesia

The combination of the remote nature of NORA and the diversity of patients in the pediatric population makes this population group especially challenging. Anesthetists must pay attention to age-dependent factors, pediatric comorbidities, and psychological development. Medication safety, radiation safety, risks of hypothermia, risks of contrast, and risks of airway compromise are even more pronounced in this patient group. Medication and contrast doses need to be recalculated to avoid incorrect dosing with catastrophic consequences. Pediatric patients may be more susceptible to DNA damage due to radiation exposure because of their higher cell mitotic rate.

Many NORA cases for children are diagnostic, necessitating the need for amnesia and immobility, though rarely analgesia. Medications, which have a minimal effect on respiratory drive (e.g., ketamine and dexmedetomidine), are popular choices in the NORA setting, as well as a propofol infusion titrated to amnesia while maintaining adequate ventilation.

Recognizing the risks of sedation on this population, several novel techniques have been proposed to reduce the use of pharmaceutical agents. Virtual reality technology can be used as a form of distraction to reduce pain and anxiety associated with procedures. Studies have shown that this modality can reduce or eliminate the need for anesthetics, thereby improving patient and parent satisfaction, reducing exposure to anesthetics, and improving efficiency. Another technique adopted with great success in infants is the “feed and wrap” technique. This technique induces natural sleep in an infant to obtain quality MRI images. Studies have demonstrated that the feed and wrap technique has been a primary technique in neonatal intensive care units across the USA and can be used successfully in infants undergoing MRI.

Specific Procedures[22-24]

Ophthalmic Artery Chemotherapy

Ophthalmic artery chemotherapy (OAC) is a relatively new procedure used as a primary treatment for advanced retinoblastoma or as a secondary treatment in recurrent cases, performed under GA. Using a sterile technique, a catheter is placed in the femoral artery and advanced through the ipsilateral internal carotid artery (ICA). The arterial anatomy is visualized with angiography and the catheter is then advanced into the ostium of the ophthalmic artery (OA). The chemotherapeutic agent is then injected there. This allows for the selective administration of the chemotherapeutic agent as close to the malignancy as possible. OAC is performed outside of the OR in interventional neuroradiology. There are unique challenges of NORA as discussed earlier in performing these procedures. Communication between the anesthesia provider and the proceduralist is of utmost concern to ensure the safety of the patient.

Concerns related to the OAC:

- Anaphylactoid reactions to contrast media usually occur within five minutes of exposure but a delayed reaction can also occur. Patients at risk for allergic reactions to contrast dye include those with asthma, ectopic tendencies, and history of reactions to contrast dye. All medications to treat such a reaction should be available in interventional radiology, including epinephrine and intravenous fluids.
- Intraoperative cardiorespiratory instability due to a severe decrease in lung compliance is reported in the literature that might occur due to an atypical form of bronchospasm. It is rapid in onset but has good recovery and excellent response to epinephrine. Other potential causes are anaphylactoid reaction and pulmonary edema leading to altered alveolar fluid content. It is preferred to ventilate the patients with pressure control ventilation, so that a small decrease in tidal volume is detected early.
- Patients sometimes may develop bradycardia and hypotension while manipulating the OA. The mechanism for the cardiopulmonary changes during catheter manipulation within ICA and OA is likely to be neural reflex as suggested by the abrupt onset and rapid resolution. While the precise mechanism is unclear, it may be related to one or more of the following reflexes. The oculocardiac reflex, triggered by traction on the eye, causes bradycardia. The afferent limb is the ophthalmic branch of the trigeminal nerve, and the efferent is the vagus nerve. Asystole triggered three times consecutively in an adult undergoing catheterization of the distal OA for attempted embolization of an arteriovenous fistula supplied by the ethmoid artery has been reported in the literature.
- *Oculorespiratory reflex (ORR):* This is bradypnea or apnea triggered by ocular traction. It is seen during strabismus surgery in spontaneously breathing patients. Trigeminal stimulation can cause apnea, bradycardia, and bronchoconstriction. Catheter manipulation of the ICA or OA may be stimulating trigeminal afferents in the blood vessel and causing a neural reflex-type response in the pulmonary and cardiovascular systems mediated at least in part by the vagus nerve.

Pediatric Radiotherapy[25]

Radiotherapy is an important modality in the curative and palliative management of many pediatric malignancies. 40–50% of children with amenable types of cancer receive radiotherapy as part of their initial treatment. Planning and delivering of the radiotherapy treatment modalities require anesthesia services in the treatment rooms. Precise positioning and immobilization of the patient during treatment is essential to ensure that high-energy radiation can be delivered to the tumor while minimizing exposure to healthy surrounding tissues. Anesthesia for pediatric radiotherapy poses its own unique set of challenges. Despite being a nonpainful procedure, anesthesia for anxiolysis and immobility in younger patients is often required for treatment planning and daily treatment. Before starting the treatment, a simulation CT scan is done, and a mold is prepared according to the part to be treated. This is prepared during treatment planning and is typically either a mask placed over the face or a cast into which the body area is placed. Molds hold the treatment area in a fixed position to facilitate patient setup and accuracy of treatment. Patients need sedation to ensure immobilization during this process. After treatment planning is done, most patients receive a series of daily outpatient treatments (Monday to Friday). The number of treatments varies but typically lasts 3–6 weeks depending on tumor type, stage, location, and size and goal of treatment (palliative versus curative). Treatment time (including setup) varies greatly from tens of minutes to several hours, depending on the area treated. Intravenous (IV) cannulation is done every week on Monday depending on the institution's protocols, sedation is given with that cannula for a week and is removed on Friday. IV cannulation can be a concern in those with difficult cannulation. Anesthetic technique varies from sedation to GA, depending on the age and cooperation of the child. Oxygen may be delivered via nasal tubing, face mask, or laryngeal mask. Most of the patients require MAC with intravenous sedation for the procedure. Another concern while delivering anesthesia to these patients is that patients need to be monitored from a distance with cameras and screens showing the patient and the monitor outside the treatment room. Care should be given to positioning the patient, ensuring adequate strapping so that the patient does not fall off the table, and securing the monitoring leads so that it does not interfere with the movement of the machine. Imaging may need to be repeated during the treatment course to monitor the tumor load and allow modification of the treatment plan, if required. The patient will require sedation/MAC for the same.

Nonoperative Room Anesthesia for Children with Mediastinal Masses[26]

Pediatric patients with leukemia and lymphoma may present with mediastinal masses. These patients require anesthesia for various diagnostic and therapeutic procedures during evaluation and treatment courses. These patients may present as a real challenge to the anesthetist as it is difficult to give sedation to these patients when there is no imaging done to know how big the mass is. The ideal way to proceed is to look for the signs and symptoms of airway compression. Any history of airway collapse during crying or waking up while sleeping may signify possible airway compression with the mass **(Table 4)**. These patients may present for diagnostic CT scans during evaluation. A baseline chest X-ray guides the size of the mediastinal mass and can be done without sedation. If there is no airway collapse suspected in history, sedation with maintenance of spontaneous ventilation is preferred. Spontaneous breathing techniques are recommended to avoid airway compression. A rigid bronchoscope should be present for backup in case any airway collapse with anesthesia happens. These mediastinal masses respond to the treatment modalities and decrease in size once the treatment (chemotherapy/steroids) is started.

Peak expiratory flow rate (PEFR) offers insights into the central airway diameter. A reduction of 50% or more in predicted PEFR in the supine position is associated with anesthetic complications. Shamberger developed a risk assessment box **(Table 5)** to aid in selecting the most appropriate anesthetic technique that can be used in older children and adults who can perform the PFT.

TABLE 4: Signs and symptoms of mediastinal mass*.

Common symptoms	*Common signs*
Dyspnea and cough	Tachypnea
Hoarseness	Stridor
New onset wheezing	Rhonchi, decreased breath sound
Syncope, chest pain, and night sweats	
Weight loss	
Dysphagia	
Superior vena cava obstruction	

**Cause of concern if they increase in supine posture.*

TABLE 5: Shamberger risk assessment box.

Group	*PEFR*	*Tracheal CSA (% of predicted)*	*Anesthetic technique*
A (moderate risk)	>50%	< 50%	LA/GA spontaneous ventilation, avoid muscle relaxation
B (low risk)	>50%	> 50%	GA
C (high risk)	<50%	< 50%	LA only
D (moderate risk)	<50%	> 50%	LA/GA spontaneous ventilation, avoid muscle relaxation

(CSA: cross-sectional area; GA: general anesthesia; LA: local anesthesia; PEFR: peak expiratory flow rate)

Nonoperative Room Anesthesia for Radiological Procedures

Pediatric patients require NORA for various diagnostic and therapeutic radiological procedures. Patients require MAC for undergoing CT, MRI, and interventional radiology procedures such as CT-guided biopsy. As mentioned earlier, radiation exposure is always a concern in children undergoing CT or any other intervention radiology procedure. Ensuring fasting of 2 hours for clear fluids in these children makes them less irritable when they come for the procedure. Immobilization and anxiolysis are targets while performing CT and MRI; however, analgesia is required when any diagnostic intervention is performed.

The choice of drugs always depends on the type of procedure being done. Sedation/MAC is preferred in most cases when a CT scan is to be done. Radiology procedures and MRI are done under MAC or GA depending on the type of procedure and the duration expected. Maintaining an adequate unobstructed airway is required while giving sedation to these children, and monitoring the same throughout the procedure is essential.

Nonoperative Room Anesthesia for Short Diagnostic or Therapeutic Procedures

Pediatric patients need NORA for various diagnostic and therapeutic procedures such as bone marrow aspiration, bone marrow biopsy, intrathecal chemotherapy injection, and insertion of difficult peripherally inserted central catheter (PICC). The patient needs immobilization and MAC or GA with bag and mask is mostly preferred in these procedures. For procedures like bone marrow biopsy and painful procedures, the patient needs analgesia for the same.

POSTPROCEDURE CARE[12]

The basic requirements for safe monitoring and recovery after anesthesia are the same for all patients as per ASA Practice Guidelines for postanesthetic care and the ASA standards for postanesthetic care; however, postoperative care of every patient receiving NORA will vary depending upon the procedure.

Challenges specific to post-NORA care include the following:

- There could be long transport times to a recovery unit.
- Recovery needs to be efficient so that the patient can be discharged timely to allow rapid patient turnover in a busy procedural site.
- The anesthetist should be able to recognize and react to a wide variety of postintervention complications and differentiate between patients who may safely recover near the NORA site and those who require shifting to a recovery unit.

Standards of practices that should be in place at any NORA site:[2,3]

- Transport to the recovery area should include supplemental oxygen and monitoring as appropriate to the patient's condition.
- Handover should be standardized through a checklist and a thorough handover should be given to the staff assuming care in the recovery area mentioning the specific procedure performed, and its associated risks and complications to ensure situational awareness for the recovery unit staff.
- Appropriate equipment and personnel must be available in any postanesthetic recovery location to ensure adequate respiratory and cardiovascular function monitoring and to provide cardiopulmonary resuscitation if the need arises.
- Standardized handover tools and scoring systems and well-planned "fast-track" recovery protocols aid in identifying patients who can be safely discharged in a high-volume NORA site.

ORGANIZATION, TRAINING, AND EDUCATION

Before undertaking anesthetic procedures in NORA sites, the standard recommendations for all anesthetists include the following:[1-3]

- It is essential to be familiar with the layout of the remote location and the location of emergency medication and equipment, be aware of the local guidelines, protocols, and standard of practice, and know how to call for additional assistance and help should the need arise.
- All training anesthetists who are providing NORA should be diligently supervised. The level of supervision will depend on the stage of their training, how familiar they are with the specific site and procedure, and how complex the case is.
- Regular multidisciplinary simulation training sessions should be conducted to improve the performance and outcomes of NORA services.
- Regular training, education, and upgradation regarding the safe delivery of sedation and ANTE should be undertaken by anesthetists, technicians, anesthesia nurses, and recovery room staff.
- In countries and institutes where nonanesthetic sedation practitioners are permitted to provide care for NORA procedures, hospitals should consider involving anesthetists in their training and in placing SOPs in place.
- The use of checklists and team briefings should be employed to encourage teamwork and communication. Discussions should include how to recognize a complication and to be prepared, e.g., bleeding and life-threating loss of the airway or cardiac arrest.

Every plan should involve the anesthetist and the proceduralist. Communication, teamwork, and planning go a long way in keeping the patient safe.

- Every center should have a system relating to the reporting and auditing of near misses and critical incidents.
- Offsite locations (e.g., psychiatric facility or day clinics) should have a plan in place to transfer a patient to a referral center if needed and one should do the procedure in an operating theater environment if the clinical status of the patient is not conducive to a NORA site.

TAKE-HOME POINTS

- *Definition of MAC:* During MAC, an anesthesia clinician continually monitors and supports the patient's vital functions; diagnoses and treats clinical problems that occur; administers sedative, anxiolytic, or analgesic medications if needed; and converts to GA if required.
- *Definition of NORA:* NORA refers to providing anesthesia services outside of the OR.
- *Preanesthetic evaluation:* Preanesthetic evaluation and preparation for NORA should be the same as for any patient who will undergo GA. Depending on the procedure, it is very essential to assess the patient's ability to lie still, cooperate, and communicate, if required.
- *Monitoring:* Standard physiologic monitoring should be done during NORA, as is done for GA. Capnography should be used for patients who receive moderate or deep sedation. To avoid oversedation, the level of sedation should be assessed continually during MAC/NORA. Any patient who is unarousable to a painful stimulus is, by definition, under GA.
- *Choice of medications:* To provide MAC/NORA, medications with rapid onset and short duration of action are recommended to allow rapid titration of the effect and quick recovery. Drugs commonly administered for MAC/NORA include the following:
    - *Midazolam:* A short-acting benzodiazepine with anxiolytic, amnesic, and sedative effects, without analgesic effects but can potentiate the effects of other sedatives and opioids and can cause respiratory depression when given in high doses or with other sedatives or opioids.
    - *Propofol:* A rapidly acting, short-acting sedative/hypnotic with modest amnestic and antiemetic properties at subhypnotic doses, without analgesic effects.
    - *Opioids:* More commonly used opioids for MAC/NORA are fentanyl and remifentanil. Fentanyl is a short-acting opioid that is usually administered by intermittent bolus. Remifentanil is an ultrashort-acting opioid that is often administered by infusion, with or without initial or supplemental bolus with a very rapid clinical recovery as the elimination half-life is approximately 3 minutes regardless of the duration of infusion.
    - *Dexmedetomidine:* It is a selective alpha2-adrenergic agonist, which acts like a sedative, an anxiolytic, and a modest analgesic. In doses used for sedation, it does not produce respiratory depression and maintains the normal ventilatory response to hypercarbia. Since its onset of action is slow, this drug is most useful for longer procedures and for patients who are at higher risk of respiratory depression or airway obstruction.
    - *Ketamine:* It produces a dissociative state accompanied by amnesia and intense analgesia with minimal respiratory depression at sedative doses. It can be administered as a supplement to other sedatives and analgesics to reduce the need for opioids.
- *Medication administration:* Sedatives and analgesics may be administered by intravenous bolus, continuous infusion, or by a computer-assisted administration system. Put checklists and guidelines in place to prevent drug errors in high-volume centers.
- *Strategy as per procedure:* SOPs should be in place and training is essential. It can be modified for patient factors and planned procedures.
    - *Procedures with minimal or no pain:* For short, painless diagnostic procedures (e.g., MRI and CT scans), one can use a bolus of midazolam (1–2 mg IV) followed by small, titrated supplemental doses (e.g., 0.5–1 mg IV). For patients with morbid obesity, obstructive sleep apnea, acute or chronic pain, or severe anxiety, dexmedetomidine (0.1–0.7 µg/kg/h IV infusion) can be used which may supplement with ketamine (0.5–1 mg/kg IV).
    - *Procedures with brief, initial pain:* For procedures that involve only an initial, brief painful stimulus (e.g., local anesthetic infiltration, peripheral nerve blocks, eye block, and diagnostic puncture) one can administer midazolam 1–2 mg IV with

fentanyl 50–100 μg IV, or propofol 0.5–1 mg/kg IV, or remifentanil 0.5–1 μg/kg IV.

- *Procedures with variable pain throughout:* For procedures that cause variable degrees of pain throughout one can use infusions or repeated boluses of hypnotics and analgesics. For example, in gastrointestinal endoscopy, one can administer propofol (initial bolus of 0.5–1 mg/kg followed by 25–75 μg/kg/min), supplemented as necessary with fentanyl 25–50 μg or ketamine 0.5–1 mg/kg IV. For a procedure involving the larynx (e.g., thyroplasty and arytenoid adduction), one can administer dexmedetomidine (0.3–0.7 μg/kg/h IV) with remifentanil (0.03–0.04 μg/kg/min IV). Alternatively, for patients who are at increased risk of airway obstruction or respiratory depression (e.g., patients with obstructive sleep apnea or morbid obesity), one can administer dexmedetomidine (0.1–0.7 μg/kg/h IV infusion) and may supplement with ketamine (0.5–1 mg/kg IV).

- *Postoperative care and complications:* The rate of serious complications during and after MAC/NORA appears to be like that seen with GA. The most frequent mechanism for injury is respiratory depression due to oversedation, and in many cases, the injury may be preventable with appropriate monitoring, vigilance, and anticipation.
- *Organization:* All checklists, SOPs, and standard monitoring techniques routinely used in the OR should be used in these remote locations as their safety record is proven beyond doubt. There should be open communication with all teams involved with regular team briefings and multidisciplinary team meetings to set expectations and discuss concerns before the procedure so that unanticipated situations and challenges can be dealt with.

CONCLUSION

The demand for anesthesia care outside of the theater environment is increasing and NORA is emerging as a subspecialty of anesthesiology practice. Ultimately, anesthesia care in NORA sites must meet the same standard of care as care provided in the OR for which a thorough appreciation of the unique challenges of a NORA environment is essential.

REFERENCES

1. Wahr JA, Abernathy JH, Lazarra EH, Keebler JR, Wall MH, Lynch I, et al. Medication safety in the operating room: literature and expert-based recommendations. Br J Anaesth. 2017;118(1):32-43.
2. Dabu-Bondoc SM. Standard procedures in nonoperating room anesthesia. Curr Opin Anesthesiol. 2020;33(4):539-47.
3. Routman J, Boggs SD. Patient monitoring in the nonoperating room anesthesia (NORA) setting: current advances in technology. Curr Opin Anaesthesiol. 2021;34(4):430-6.
4. American Society of Anesthesiologists. (2013) Statement on nonoperating room anesthetizing locations. [online] Available from http://www.asahq.org/quality-and-practicemanagement/standards-and-guidelines#. [Last accessed March, 2025].
5. American Society of Anesthesiologists. (2011) Standards for basic anesthetic monitoring. [online] Available from https://www.asahq.org/standards-and-practice-parameters/standards-for-basic-anesthetic-monitoring. [Last accessed March, 2025].
6. Apfelbaum JL, Connis RT, Nickinovich DG; American Society of Anesthesiologists Task Force on Preanesthesia Evaluation; Pasternak LR, Arens JF, et al. Practice advisory for preanesthesia evaluation: an updated report by the American Society of Anesthesiologists Task Force on Preanesthesia Evaluation. Anesthesiology. 2012;116(3):522-38.
7. Nagrebetsky A, Gabriel RA, Dutton RP, Urman RD. Growth of nonoperating room anesthesia care in the United States: a contemporary trends analysis. Anesth Analg. 2017;124:1261-7.
8. Wong T, Georgiadis PL, Urman RD, Tsai MH. Non-Operating Room Anesthesia: Patient Selection and Special Considerations. Local Reg Anesth. 2020;13:1-9.
9. Yeh T, Beutler SS, Urman RD. What we can learn from nonoperating room anesthesia registries: analysis of clinical outcomes and closed claims data. Curr Opin Anaesthesiol. 2020;33:527.
10. Faddoul A, Bonnet F. Is there a place for regional anesthesia in nonoperating room anesthesia? Curr Opin Anaesthesiol. 2020;33:561.
11. Fanning RM. Monitoring during sedation given by non-anaesthetic doctors. Anaesthesia. 2008;63(4):370-4.
12. Chung F, Ghan V, Ong D. A post-anesthetic discharge scoring system for home readiness after ambulatory surgery. J Clin Anesth. 1995;7:500-6.
13. Goudra B. (2024). Anaesthesia for gastrointestinal endoscopy in adults. [online] Available from https://www.uptodate.com/contents/anesthesia-for-gastrointestinal-endoscopy-in-adults. [Last accessed March, 2025].
14. Zerem E, Imširović B, Kunosić S, Zerem D, Zerem O. Percutaneous biliary drainage for obstructive jaundice in

patients with inoperable, malignant biliary obstruction. Clin Exp Hepatol. 2022;8(1):70-7.
15. Piccioni F, Poli A, Templeton LC, Templeton TW, Rispoli M, Vetrugno L, et al. Anesthesia for Percutaneous Radiofrequency Tumor Ablation (PRFA): A Review of Current Practice and Techniques. Local Reg Anesth. 2019;12:127-37.
16. Navarro JC. (2024). Anesthesia for endovascular therapy for acute ischemic stroke in adults. [online] Available from https://www.uptodate.com/contents/anesthesia-for-endovascular-therapy-for-acute-ischemic-stroke-in-adults. [Last accessed March, 2025].
17. Chana A, James M, Veale P. Anesthesia for transjugular intrahepatic portosystemic shunt insertion. BJA Educ. 2016;16:405-19.
18. Narayanan G. Irreversible Electroporation. Semin Intervent Radiol. 2015;32(4):349-55.
19. Ruskin KJ. (2024). Anesthesia for magnetic resonance imaging and computed tomography procedures. [online] Available from https://www.uptodate.com/contents/anesthesia-for-magnetic-resonance-imaging-and-computed-tomography-procedures. [Last accessed March, 2025].
20. Hulme APK, Tharion JG, Cordery RA. Anaesthesia in the cardiac catheterization laboratory. Anaesth Intensive Care Med. 2024;25(3):198-206.
21. Canneto B, Ferraroli G, Falezza G, Infante MV. Ideal conditions to perform EBUS-TBNA. J Thorac Dis. 2017;9(Suppl 5):S414-7.
22. Scharoun JH, Han JH, Gobin YP. Anesthesia for Ophthalmic Artery Chemosurgery. Anesthesiology. 2017;126:165-72.
23. Vaithialingam B, Gopal S, Chandrashekhar S, Malik D. Anesthetic management of super-selective intra-arterial Melphalan injection in an infant with retinoblastoma. Saudi J Anaesth. 2023;17(3):434-6.
24. Lewis H, James I. Update on anaesthesia for paediatric ophthalmic surgery. BJA Educ. 2021;21(1):32-8.
25. Fortney JT, Halperin EC, Hertz CM, Schulman SR. Anesthesia for pediatric external beam radiation therapy. Intern J Rad Onc. 1999;44(3):587-91.
26. Tan A, Nolan JA. Anesthesia for children with anterior mediastinal masses. Paediatr Anaesth. 2022;32(1):4-9.

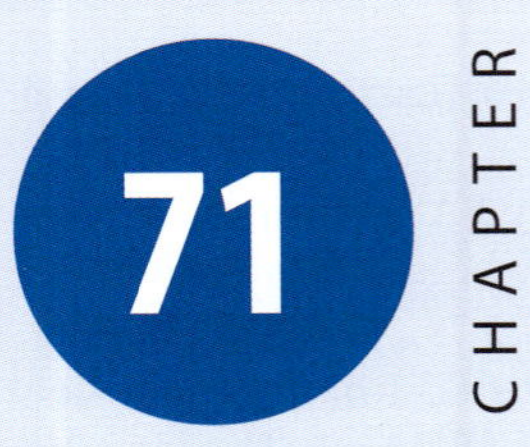

Perioperative Blood Management and Massive Blood Transfusion

Vijaya P Patil, Sagar Joshi

INTRODUCTION

Perioperative blood management and massive blood transfusion (MBT) are critical aspects of patient care in modern anesthesiology and surgery. These practices have evolved significantly in recent years, driven by advances in our understanding of coagulation, improvement in blood product availability and processing, and the development of evidence-based protocols. It aims to optimize patients; minimize blood loss and effectively use blood products to get the best possible outcomes. MBT protocols are integral to managing life-threatening hemorrhages, requiring a systematic, multidisciplinary approach to ensure timely and effective care. In this chapter, we will explore the latest developments in perioperative blood management strategies and MBT protocols with a focus on optimizing patient outcomes while minimizing unnecessary transfusions and associated risks.

PATIENT BLOOD MANAGEMENT

Patient blood management (PBM) is an evidence-based approach that uses both preoperative strategies to optimize a patient's hemoglobin status and surgical strategies to minimize the use of blood transfusion in a perioperative setting. Even though its main application is in the surgical population, its principles can be applied to nonsurgical conditions needing transfusion of blood and blood products.[1]

CORE PRINCIPLES OF PATIENT BLOOD MANAGEMENT

The core principles of PBM revolve around three main pillars:

- Perioperative optimizing erythropoiesis
- Minimizing blood loss and timely management of perioperative coagulopathy
- Tolerance to postoperative anemia by optimizing physiology

These principles are applied throughout the perioperative period from preoperative assessment to postoperative care for improved patient outcomes.[2]

PREOPERATIVE OPTIMIZATION

Detection and Management of Anemia

World Health Organization (WHO) has identified anemia as a major public health issue mainly in low- and middle-income countries, the main causes being iron deficiency, thalassemia, and malaria. Preoperative anemia is a significant risk factor for adverse outcomes and increased transfusion requirements. Early detection and management of anemia are crucial.[2-4]

Screening: All patients undergoing major surgery should be screened for anemia. WHO defines anemia as Hb <13 g/dL in males and <12 g/dL in females.[5,6] However, many recent guidelines suggest considering <13 g/dL as a universal cut-off for anemia in supramajor and major blood loss surgeries to start the necessary correction early.[7] Strategies to optimize hemoglobin should be started at least 3–4 weeks before the planned procedure. This allows time for investigating and treating underlying causes.[8,9]

Role of iron studies: Iron deficiency is a common cause of preoperative anemia. Identifying the cause of iron deficiency anemia helps in effective and timely optimization. Iron studies help differentiate iron deficiency anemia from anemia caused by chronic disease **(Table 1)**.

Intravenous (IV) iron therapy is more effective as compared to oral iron in increasing hemoglobin levels and reducing transfusion requirements for obvious reasons being 100% bioavailability and elimination of patient compliance factor.[8,10] The median rate of hemoglobin rise with oral iron is 0.23 g/dL in 14 days versus 0.58 g/dL with

TABLE 1: Iron studies pattern in iron deficiency anemia.

	Iron deficiency	Anemia of chronic disease
Ferritin	Low	Normal/high
TIBC/transferrin	High	Low
Transferrin saturation	Low	Low
Iron	Low	Low

(TIBC: total iron-binding capacity)

TABLE 2: National Blood Authority of Australia simplified formula for IV iron dose calculation based on weight.

National Blood Authority of Australia has given a simplified formula for IV iron dose calculation based on body weight and starting hemoglobin (Hb g/dL)[14]	Ideal Body weight >35 kg <70 kg	Ideal body weight ≥70 kg
<10 g/dL	1,500 mg	2,000 mg
≥10 g/dL	100 mg	1,500 mg

TABLE 3: Overview of different iron formulations.[15]

	Iron sucrose (IS)	Sodium ferric gluconate (SFG)	Low molecular weight iron dextran (ID)	Ferric carboxymaltose (FCM)	Ferric derisomaltose (FDI)	Ferumoxytol (FMX)
Maximal single dose	200 mg	125 mg	20 mg/kg	• 1,000 mg (EMA) • 750 mg (FDA)	• 20 mg/kg (EMA) • 1000 mg (FDA)	510 mg
Maximal weekly dose	500 mg	Not stated	Not stated	• 1,000 mg (EMA) • 750mg (FDA)	20 mg/kg (EMA)	1,020 mg (EMA, FDA)
Minimum administration time	• 30 minutes (EMA) • 15 minutes • (FDA)	60 minutes (FDA)	15 minutes then 100 mg/ 15 minutes (EMA)	15 minutes (EMA, FDA)	• 15 minutes (<1,000 mg), 30 minutes (>1,000 mg) EMA • 20 minutes (FDA)	15 minutes (EMA)

(EMA: European Medicines Agency, FDA: Food and Drug Administration)

IV iron. Whereas in 28 days, the rise in hemoglobin was 0.91–1.3 g/dL with oral iron as compared to 1.83–1.9 g/dL with IV iron.[11-13] There is enough evidence to suggest preoperative iron supplements help in increasing hemoglobin levels and reducing transfusion requirements.[8,10]

Management of Iron Deficiency Anemia

Oral iron: Current recommendations suggest 40–60 mg elemental iron daily or 80–100 mg elemental iron on alternate days in adolescents and adults, which amounts to 200 mg of ferrous fumarate or sulphate daily or 400 mg of ferrous fumarate or sulfate on alternate days. Oral iron gets absorbed in ferrous form and thus iron preparations containing ferrous form have better bioavailability as compared to ferric form. Gastric acid plays a key role in iron absorption and hence oral iron supplements should not be given with proton pump inhibitors (PPIs) or antacids but to be taken with citric foods to increase its absorption.

IV iron: Hypersensitivity reactions and anaphylactic reactions occurred most frequently with iron dextran. Current IV iron preparations are much safer and are well tolerated. However, every IV iron therapy should be given in a monitored area with a resuscitation facility.

To calculate the dose of IV Iron, one needs to know the whole-body iron deficit which is calculated using the Ganzoni formula which is as follows:

$$\text{Total iron dose} = [\text{Actual body weight} \times (\text{Target Hb} - \text{Actual Hb})] \times 2.4 + \text{iron depot (mg)}$$

where most studies mention that iron depot stores as 500 mg in the average adult. One can also choose a dose from product labels (a common practice) or based on local protocols **(Tables 2 and 3)**.

Erythropoiesis-stimulating agents: In cases of anemia not fully corrected by iron therapy, erythropoiesis-stimulating agents may be considered, particularly in patients at high risk for transfusion. For example, Epoetin—alpha, beta, and zeta, darbepoetin alpha, and methoxy polyethylene glycol-epoetin beta. Epoetin alpha initial dose is 50–100 U/kg thrice weekly. Darbepoetin alpha 0.45 µg/kg IV or SC weekly or 0.75µg/kg IV or SC every 2 weekly.[8,16]

Optimization of Coagulation

Preoperative assessment of coagulation status is essential, particularly in patients with known coagulation disorders or those on anticoagulant medications.[17]

Management of anticoagulants: Careful management of anticoagulant medications in the perioperative period is crucial. This may involve temporary discontinuation, bridging therapy, or the use of reversal agents as appropriate **(Table 4)**.[18]

Preoperative Autologous Donation

Patients can be considered for preoperative autologous donation (PAD) when they are scheduled for elective surgery and likely to receive transfusion. It is a process in which one or more units are collected before an elective procedure for reinfusion during or after the procedure. It decreases or eliminates complications from allogeneic blood transfusions such as transfusion reactions, and transmission of blood-borne diseases, decreases immunomodulation, and conserves blood resources. Patients should be at least 50 kg with hemoglobin of >11g%. Patients donate 1 unit of blood per week from a month before surgery with the last donation being at least 72 hours before surgery. It is labor intensive and needs good organization skills. It is indicated in patients with rare blood groups and patients who reject and do not consent to allogeneic blood transfusion. Patients can be treated with iron supplements and erythropoiesis-stimulating agents to increase RBC production. The main drawback of this strategy is high cost and wastage as the units need to be discarded if not used.

TABLE 4: Guidance for withholding anticoagulants before surgery.

Anticoagulants	*Number of days of cessation before surgery*
Aspirin	Continued
Clopidogrel	5 days
Direct oral anticoagulants	• 24 hours for low-risk procedures and normal renal function • 48 hours for high-risk procedures and normal renal function OR low-risk procedure and abnormal renal function (CrCl <30 mL/min) • 72–96 hours for high-risk procedure and abnormal renal function (CrCl <30 mL/min)
Warfarin	5 days

INTRAOPERATIVE STRATEGIES

Restrictive Transfusion Trigger

In patients without significant comorbidities, restrictive transfusion triggers are to be followed as per patient comorbidities, ongoing losses, and institutional protocols. It can vary from 7 to 9 mg/dL of hemoglobin.

Positioning

Circulatory changes induced by the perioperative positioning of patients can be used to reduce or increase blood loss by promoting or opposing venous drainage in a field.

Venous drainage axes should not be compressed, as this can lead to increased blood loss. Prone positioning, for example, can increase the inferior vena cava pressure and therefore lead to an increased risk of bleeding, so appropriate use of pillows under the chest and pelvis is essential to reduce intra-abdominal pressure.

Maintaining the surgical field above the heart where possible, for example, in head and neck surgery, gynecology and neurosurgery can also reduce bleeding at these sites.

Thermoregulation

Hypothermia can lead to altered enzyme function in the clotting cascade, including effects on fibrinolysis and reduced platelet function. The combination of these factors may result in abnormal hemostasis with an increased risk of intraoperative bleeding. Hypothermia also leads to an increase in Hb oxygen affinity, reduced cardiac output, and ultimately a reduction in tissue oxygenation.

Regional Nerve Blocks

Loss of sympathetic tone as a result of regional anesthesia may help reduce the arterial and peripheral venous blood pressure in the surgical field, resulting in less intraoperative blood loss. A meta-analysis of 66 studies in 2006 showed that spinal or epidural anesthesia was associated with a significant decrease in the estimated blood loss (at the end of the procedure) when compared with general anesthesia.[10,17]

Blood Pressure Management

Lowering the mean arterial pressure (MAP) in a controlled way reduces end-organ blood flow and may help decrease blood loss. The risks of inducing hypotension must be tailored for an individual patient and balanced to ensure appropriate vital organ perfusion. Several methods can be used to lower MAP, including deepening the anesthetic (volatile or total IV anesthetic) or using extra opioids. Additional antihypertensives can also be considered in a closely controlled manner, for example, beta-blockers such as labetalol or esmolol, a potent and titratable arteriovenous dilator such as sodium nitroprusside, or a primary venodilator such as glyceryl trinitrate. An infiltration of local anesthetic combined with vasoconstrictors such as adrenaline may be useful to help reduce blood loss in the area of local distribution.

Surgical Techniques

A proactive approach to managing bleeding and preventing ongoing loss is crucial to blood conservation. MIS techniques such as laparoscopic surgeries and robotic-assisted surgeries reduce tissue trauma and bleeding. Preventative measures such as the use of tourniquets when feasible, vascular control, laser, or harmonic scalpel usage also help in reducing blood loss. Vessel ligation should be proactive rather than reactive. Other methods to stop bleeding early include pressure, ligation, diathermy, and topical vasoconstrictors (e.g., the use of adrenaline-soaked swabs and the use of fibrin glues, gelatin sponges, and oxidized cellulose).[17]

Cell Salvage

The term intraoperative blood collection or cell salvage describes the technique of collecting, processing, and reinfusing blood lost by a patient during surgery. It may be acceptable for use in patients who do not consent to allogeneic or preoperative autologous blood transfusions. Intraoperative cell salvage is an effective technique for reducing allogeneic blood transfusion in eligible patients undergoing procedures with significant blood loss and is advocated in all surgeries with expected blood loss of >1,000 mL, especially trauma, cardiac, orthopedic, and obstetric scenarios.[19]

Pharmacological Strategies

- *Tranexamic acid:* The use of tranexamic acid has been shown to reduce blood loss and transfusion requirements in various surgical settings, including cardiac, orthopedic, and obstetric procedures. A single dose of 15 mg/kg is the most frequently used dose which has been shown to reduce perioperative blood loss and transfusion requirements across various surgical disciplines.[8,20,21]
- *Fibrinogen concentrate:* In cases of significant fibrinogen depletion, the use of fibrinogen concentrate can be more effective than fresh frozen plasma (FFP) in restoring fibrinogen levels quickly and improving clot stability. When the baseline fibrinogen is unknown a standard dose of 70 mg/kg body weight is recommended.[8,22,23]
- *Prothrombin complex concentrate (PCC):* In patients requiring urgent reversal of vitamin K antagonists, PCC is preferred over FFP due to its rapid action and reduced volume.[8] In patients with major ongoing blood loss, patients will also need volume and a combination of FFP and cryoprecipitate can be used. The standard dose of PCC is based on factor IX content and patient's international normalized ratio (INR).[24]
  - *INR 2.0–3.9:* 25 IU/kg
  - *INR 4.0–6.0:* 35 IU/kg
  - *INR >6.0:* 50 IU/kg
- *Recombinant factor VIIa (rFVIIa):* While controversial, rFVIIa may be considered as a rescue therapy in cases of refractory bleeding, though its use should be carefully weighed against the risk of thrombotic complications. It is used in a standard dose of 90–120 μg/kg as an IV bolus and can be repeated every 2–3 hourly until hemostasis is achieved.[25-27]

ACUTE NORMOVOLEMIC HEMODILUTION

Acute normovolemic hemodilution (ANH) is a procedure initiated before the start of significant blood loss, whole blood is removed from a patient while simultaneously restoring intravascular volume with either crystalloid (1.2 mL/1 mL of blood removed) or colloid (1 mL/1 mL of blood removed) solutions to maintain adequate hemodynamic. When major bleeding has stopped or when clinically appropriate, the collected blood is then reinfused into the patient in the reverse order of collection because the first unit collected has the highest concentration of coagulation factors and platelets and the highest Hb level. Benefits of ANH are:

- The patient's blood has enhanced oxygen-carrying capacity because of a higher hematocrit.
- Greater clotting ability owing to platelets and other coagulation factors.
- Fewer red blood cells (RBCs) are lost per mm of blood loss during surgery due to hemodilution.

POSTOPERATIVE MANAGEMENT

Monitoring and Management of Postoperative Anemia

Close monitoring of hemoglobin levels and symptoms of anemia are essential in the postoperative period. Management strategies include:

- Restrictive transfusion trigger
- Minimizing iatrogenic blood loss from laboratory testing by following proper indications—avoid unnecessary tests, collect minimum blood required for any test, use point of care technology, etc.
- Early detection and management of postoperative bleeding
- Optimizing ventilation (reducing work of breathing and O_2 consumption) and perfusion (use of vasopressors) when indicated
- Consideration of IV iron therapy for patients with iron deficiency anemia and major intraoperative blood loss.[8,10]

Thromboprophylaxis

Balancing the risk of thrombosis with the risk of bleeding is crucial in the postoperative period. Individualized thromboprophylaxis strategies should be implemented based on patient risk factors and the nature of the surgical procedure **(Table 5)**.[17]

MASSIVE BLOOD TRANSFUSION PROTOCOLS

Massive transfusion is typically defined as the replacement of:[29]

- 1 blood volume or 10 packed red blood cells (PRBCs) within 24 hours

TABLE 5: Patient blood management.[28]

Preoperative	• Detect anemia • Identify the cause of anemia and manage it • Refer for further evaluation • Treat suboptimal iron stores/iron deficiency/anemia of chronic disease • Treat other hematinic deficiencies • *Note:* Anemia is a contraindication for elective surgery	• Identify and manage bleeding risk • Minimize iatrogenic blood loss • Procedure planning and rehearsal • Preoperative autologous blood donation (in selected cases or when patient choice)	• Assess/optimize the patient's physiological reserve, and risk factors • Compare estimated blood loss with patient-specific tolerable blood loss • Restrictive transfusion threshold • Formulate patient-specific blood conservation modalities
Intraoperative	Timing surgery with hematological optimization	• Meticulous hemostasis and surgical techniques • Blood-sparing surgical techniques • Anesthetic blood-conserving strategies • Autologous blood options • Pharmacological/hemostatic agents	• Optimize cardiac output • Optimize ventilation and oxygenation • Restrictive transfusion thresholds
Postoperative	• Stimulate erythropoiesis • Be aware of drug interactions that increase anemia	• Vigilant monitoring and management of postoperative bleeding • Avoid secondary hemorrhage • Rapid warning/maintain normothermia (unless hypothermia specifically indicated) • Autologous blood salvage • Minimize iatrogenic blood loss • Hemostasis/anticoagulation management • Prophylaxis of upper GI hemorrhage • Avoid/treat infections properly • Be aware of adverse effects of medications	• Optimize anemia reserve • Maximize oxygen delivery • Minimize oxygen consumption • Avoid/treat infections promptly • Restrictive transfusion thresholds

- >50% of blood volume within 3 hours
- >4 RBC units within 1 hour, or bleeding >150 mL/min
- In children transfusion of >40 mL/kg

Massive transfusion protocols (MTPs) are designed to facilitate the rapid and coordinated delivery of blood products to critically bleeding patients.

Activation Criteria

Early recognition of patients who may require massive transfusion is crucial. The ABC score is a clinically useful and validated scoring system in trauma based on four variables, which include a pulse rate exceeding 120 bpm, a systolic blood pressure below 90 mm Hg, a positive result on the focused assessment with sonography for trauma (FAST) examination, and a penetrating torso injury. Each variable is assigned 1 point, and patients with a score of 2 or more points indicate the necessity to initiate an MTP. In nontrauma cases, there are no standard criteria for this and is based on clinical judgment. One can consider factors such as patient hemodynamic status, rapidity of blood loss, and expected blood loss.

Common activation criteria include:[29]

- Assessment of blood consumption (ABC) score ≥2
- Persistent hemodynamic instability
- Active bleeding requiring surgery or angioembolization
- Blood transfusion in the trauma bay

Pathophysiology of Massive Hemorrhage

Massive hemorrhage leads to a complex set of physiological derangements known as the "lethal triad":

- *Coagulopathy:* Dilution of coagulation factors, consumption of platelets and factors, and hyperfibrinolysis
- *Acidosis:* Tissue hypoperfusion leading to lactic acidosis
- *Hypothermia:* Loss of temperature homeostasis, cold fluid infusion, less area for surface warming, and heat loss from open coelomic cavities in major surgeries

These factors create a vicious cycle that can rapidly lead to irreversible shock and death if not promptly addressed.

MBT protocols should include massive blood loss scenarios that require team efforts for successful outcomes.

- *Predefined team roles:* Surgeons, anesthesiologists, transfusion medicine specialists, and nursing staff
- *Standardized ratios:* A common approach is a 1:1:1 ratio of RBCs, FFP, and platelets, however, this can vary based on institutional choice and practice.
- *Rapid communication:* Coordination with the blood bank for timely supply of products

Management Goals during Massive Transfusion

- Hemoglobin >7–9 g/dL (depending on patient factors and expected rate of loss)
- Platelet count >50,000/µL [>100,000/µL for central nervous system (CNS) injury]
- INR <1.5
- Fibrinogen >1.5–2.0 g/L
- Ionized calcium >1.0 mmol/L (4.0 mg/dL)
- pH >7.2
- Core temperature >36°C

Components of Massive Transfusion Protocol

Modern MTPs typically include:

- Rapid delivery of blood products in predefined ratios
- Point-of-care coagulation testing such as thromboelastography (TEG) and rotational thromboelastometry (ROTEM).[8,10]
- Targeted use of hemostatic agents
- Clear communication protocols between clinical teams and blood banks

A typical MTP pack may include:

- 6 units PRBCs
- 6 units FFP
- 1 unit apheresis platelets [single donor platelet (SDP)] or 6 units of pooled platelets [random donor platelet (RDP)]

Requirements during ongoing major blood loss scenario:

- 2–3 large bore IV access (14–18 G)
- Adequate manpower
- Effective communication with the blood bank
- Sufficient no of sample collection, investigations, transfusing, and procurement of blood and blood products
- A blood fluid warmer, surface warmer, and core temperature monitoring
- Invasive arterial pressure monitoring
- Adequate crystalloid and colloid supply
- Rapid infusion pumps and pressure bags
- Adequate calcium, magnesium, inotropes, vasopressors, and heparin
- Syringe pumps, pressure lines, syringes, blood sets, and vacutainers

Close monitoring is essential during massive transfusion to guide ongoing resuscitation efforts and prevent complications. Key parameters to monitor include:

- *Vital signs*: Beat-to-beat blood pressure, heart rate, oxygen saturation, and urine output
- *Laboratory values*: Hemoglobin, platelet count, prothrombin time (PT)/INR, activated partial thromboplastin time (aPTT), fibrinogen, and ionized calcium
- *Point-of-care coagulation tests*: TEG or ROTEM, point-of-care hemoglobin monitor, and point-of-care coagulation testing such as INR
- Core temperature
- Acid-base status and lactate levels

Special Considerations

- *Trauma:* Trauma-induced coagulopathy is a complex process involving tissue injury, shock, hemodilution, and consumption of coagulation factors. Early initiation of balanced transfusion protocols and use of tranexamic acid have been shown to improve outcomes in severely injured trauma patients.[10,30]
- *Obstetric hemorrhage:* Obstetric hemorrhage remains a leading cause of maternal mortality worldwide. Key considerations in managing obstetric hemorrhage include:
    - Early recognition and activation of MTPs
    - Aggressive management of uterine atony
    - Consideration of fibrinogen replacement, as fibrinogen levels tend to fall rapidly in obstetric hemorrhage.[10,31]
- *Cardiac surgery:* Cardiac surgery presents unique challenges due to the use of cardiopulmonary bypass and the need for systemic anticoagulation. Strategies to minimize blood loss and transfusion requirements in cardiac surgery include:
    - Meticulous surgical technique
    - Optimal heparin management and protamine reversal
    - Use of antifibrinolytic agents
    - Cell salvage
    - Point-of-care guided hemostatic management **(Table 6)**[18]
- *Hemolytic reactions:* Hemolysis of donor or recipient RBCs can result from ABO-Rh incompatibility, hemolyzed or fragile RBCs, or plasma antibodies. It is the most common transfusion reaction and can be acute or delayed. Hemolysis is intravascular and can cause hemoglobinuria, acute kidney injury (AKI), or even disseminated intravascular coagulation (DIC). Patients can develop shock. The transfusion should be stopped immediately and goal should be to maintain BP and high urine output.
- *Febrile reactions:* They can occur without hemolysis. It can be related to cytokines or antibodies directed toward the white blood cell human leukocyte antigen (WBC-HLA). There can be simultaneous allergic reactions, fever, chills, or rigors. It is more common in people receiving multiple transfusions. Most of these reactions are successfully treated with paracetamol. One can use leukoreduced packed cells or leukoreduction filters for transplant patients and patients with more than one febrile reaction history.
- *Transfusion-associated circulatory overload (TACO):* This is one of the leading causes of transfusion-related fatalities. According to the Annual Serious Hazards of Transfusion (SHOT) report in 2017, 44.1% of the reported transfusion-related fatalities were due to TACO. This typically happens in patients with poor adaptability to volume overload such as patients with cardiac and renal dysfunction and patients with positive fluid balance. Treatment is supportive in the form of oxygen supplementation, diuretics and endotracheal intubation, and mechanical ventilation in worst-case scenarios.

TABLE 6: Complications of blood transfusion.

Types of reactions	*Acute (onset <24 hours)*	*Delayed (onset >24 hours)*
Immune-mediated	• Acute hemolytic • Febrile nonhemolytic • Allergic/anaphylactic • Transfusion-related lung injury (TRALI)	• Delayed hemolytic reactions • Transfusion-associated graft vs. host disease (TAGVHD) • Post-transfusion purpura • Alloimmunization
Nonimmune mediated	• Transfusion-associated circulatory overload (TACO) • Nonimmune hemolysis • Air embolism • Hyperkalemia • Hypocalcemia • hypotension	• Iron overload • Malaria and infections

- *Transfusion-related lung injury (TRALI):* According to the National Blood Collection and Utilization Survey, the incidence of TRALI is around 0.08–15.1% per patient and 0.01–1.12% per product. According to the 2017 SHOT report, around 4% of the reported transfusion-related fatalities were due to TRALI. Patients with underlying inflammatory conditions such as chronic alcohol abuse, liver surgery, and trauma are more prone to get TRALI following transfusion of blood and blood products, mainly blood products with higher plasma components. Antigranulocyte and/or anti-HLA antibodies, agglutinate and degranulate in donor plasma within the lungs causing TRALI. There is ARDS with no cardiogenic pulmonary edema. Treatment is supportive in the form of oxygen supplementation, CPAP therapy, and in the worst scenarios endotracheal intubation and invasive mechanical ventilation.
- *Allergic reaction:* Allergic reactions can range from urticaria to anaphylaxis. Treatment is antihistaminic, hydrocortisone, and adrenaline.
- *Electrolyte imbalance:* Massive transfusion can cause hypocalcemia, hyperkalemia, and even citrate toxicity in rare occasions (patients with liver failure).

The most common symptoms of transfusion are chills, rigors, dyspnea, itching, urticaria, flank pain, and light-headedness. Early recognition of symptoms of transfusion reaction warrants immediate stoppage of the transfusion and prompt reporting to the blood bank.

EMERGING TRENDS AND FUTURE DIRECTIONS

Whole Blood Transfusion

There is renewed interest in the use of whole blood for the resuscitation of massively bleeding patients. Recent studies have shown potential benefits of whole blood transfusion in terms of improved hemostasis and reduced overall transfusion volumes.[30,32]

Artificial Oxygen Carriers

Development of artificial oxygen carriers, such as hemoglobin-based oxygen carriers and perfluorocarbon-based oxygen carriers, continues. Various other substances that carry or facilitate the transport of oxygen are labeled as Hb-based O_2 carriers (HBOCs). Polymerized hemoglobin products, perfluorocarbon emulsion. HBOCs have advantages over human blood by not requiring type and crossmatch and not transmitting infectious viruses, typical characteristics of most synthetic blood products focus only on the ability to carry O_2 not on other functions. Effective only for 12–24 hours, so good for short term till blood arrives. While not yet approved for routine clinical use, these products hold promise for situations where blood products are unavailable or contraindicated.[33]

Personalized Transfusion Medicine

Advances in genomics and proteomics are paving the way for more personalized approaches to transfusion medicine. This includes better matching of blood products to individual patients and tailored management of coagulation disorders.[33,34]

Machine Learning and Predictive Analytics

The application of machine learning algorithms to large datasets of patient information and transfusion outcomes holds promise for developing more accurate predictive models for transfusion requirements and patient outcomes.[35]

CONCLUSION

Perioperative blood management and MTPs have evolved significantly in recent years, driven by a growing body of evidence and technological advancements. The shift toward more conservative transfusion strategies, coupled with proactive measures to optimize patients' blood, has led to improved outcomes and reduced reliance on allogeneic blood products.

Key principles for optimal perioperative blood management include:

- Early identification and treatment of preoperative anemia
- Implementation of multimodal blood conservation strategies
- Use of point-of-care testing to guide targeted therapy
- Adherence to evidence-based transfusion triggers
- Rapid and coordinated response to massive hemorrhage through well-designed protocols

As research continues to refine our understanding of coagulation physiology and the impact of various blood management strategies, practices will likely continue to evolve. The future of perioperative blood management lies in increasingly personalized approaches, leveraging advanced technologies, and data analytics to optimize patient care and outcomes.

Anesthesiologists play a crucial role in perioperative blood management, from preoperative assessment and optimization to intraoperative conservation strategies and management of MTPs. By staying abreast of the latest evidence and guidelines in this rapidly evolving field, anesthesiologists can significantly contribute to improved patient outcomes and more efficient use of valuable blood resources.

REFERENCES

1. Auron M. Blood Management: A Current Opportunity in Perioperative Medicine. JMIR Perioper Med. 2024;7(1):e57012.
2. WFSA. (2025). Perioperative-Patient Blood Management (P-PBM). [online] Available from https://wfsahq.org/our-work/safety-quality/perioperative-patient-blood-management-p-pbm/ [Last accessed March, 2025].
3. Thakrar SV, Clevenger B, Mallett S. Patient blood management and perioperative anaemia. BJA Educ. 2017;17(1):28-34.
4. Shander A, Corwin HL, Meier J, Auerbach M, Bisbe E, Blitz J, et al. Recommendations From the International Consensus Conference on Anemia Management in Surgical Patients (ICCAMS). Ann Surg. 2023;277(4):581-90.
5. WHO. (2024). Guideline on haemoglobin cutoffs to define anaemia in individuals and populations. [online] Available from https://www.who.int/publications/i/item/9789240088542 [Last accessed March, 2025].
6. Khurana R, Kanvinde P, Mudaliar S. UPDATE Revised WHO Guidelines on Hemoglobin Cutoffs to Define Anemia in Individuals and Populations. Indian Pediatr. 2024; 61(7):671-4.
7. Lin Y. Preoperative anemia-screening clinics. Hematology. 2019;2019(1):570-6.
8. Theissen A, Folléa G, Garban F, Carlier M, Pontone S, Lassale B, et al. Perioperative Patient Blood Management (excluding obstetrics): Guidelines from the French National Authority for Health. Anaesth Crit Care Pain Med. 2024;43(5):101404.
9. Goodnough LT, Maniatis A, Earnshaw P, Benoni G, Beris P, Bisbe E, et al. Detection, evaluation, and management of preoperative anaemia in the elective orthopaedic surgical patient: NATA guidelines. Br J Anaesth.. 2011;106(1):13.
10. Krishna HM, Prasad MK, Mitragotri MV, Bipin GI, Gupta D, Sharma R. Recent advances in perioperative blood management. Indian J Anaesth. 2023;67(1):130.
11. Das SN, Devi A, Mohanta BB, Choudhury A, Swain A, Thatoi PK. Oral versus intravenous iron therapy in iron deficiency anemia: An observational study. J Family Med Prim Care. 2020;9(7):3619.
12. Md Shohail H, Kumar Taye M, Teron L, Ranjan Rajkhowa N, Ahmed M, Firdaus Khan M. Oral iron versus intravenous iron therapy in moderate iron deficiency anemia in pregnancy. J Family Med Prim Care. 2020;9(7):3619-22.
13. Amrane S, Skupski B, Prasad N, Tsai T. Intravenous Iron Infusion as an Alternative to Blood Transfusion in Severely Anemic Gynecologic Patients [5Q]. Obstet Gynecol. 2016;127(Supplement 1):140S.
14. Iron product choice and dose calculation guide for adults | National Blood Authority [Internet]. [cited 2025 Mar 25]. Available from: https://www.blood.gov.au/iron-product-choice-and-dose-calculation-guide-adults.
15. Schaefer B, Meindl E, Wagner S, Tilg H, Zoller H. Intravenous iron supplementation therapy. Mol Aspects Med. 2020;75:100862.
16. FDA. (2017). Information on Erythropoiesis-Stimulating Agents (ESA) Epoetin alfa (marketed as Procrit, Epogen), Darbepoetin alfa (marketed as Aranesp). [online] Available from https://www.fda.gov/drugs/postmarket-drug-safety-information-patients-and-providers/information-erythropoiesis-stimulating-agents-esa-epoetin-alfa-marketed-procrit-epogen-darbepoetin [Last accessed March, 2025].
17. Lenet T, McIsaac DI, Hallet JH, Jerath A, Lalu MM, Nicholls SG, et al. Intraoperative Blood Management Strategies for Patients Undergoing Noncardiac Surgery: The Ottawa Intraoperative Transfusion Consensus. JAMA Netw Open. 2023;6(12):E2349559.
18. Casselman FPA, Lance MD, Ahmed A, Ascari A, Blanco-Morillo J, Bolliger D, et al. 2024 EACTS/EACTAIC Guidelines on patient blood management in adult cardiac surgery in collaboration with EBCP. Eur J Cardiothorac Surg. 2024:ezae352
19. National Blood Authority. (2024). Patient blood management. [online] Available from https://www.blood.gov.au/clinical-guidance/patient-blood-management [Last accessed March, 2025].
20. American College of Surgeons. (2014). ACS TQIP Massive Transfusion in Trauma Guidelines. [online] Available from https://www.facs.org/media/zcjdtrd1/transfusion_guildelines.pdf [Last accessed March, 2025].
21. Heyns M, Knight P, Steve AK, Yeung JK. A Single Preoperative Dose of Tranexamic Acid Reduces Perioperative Blood Loss: A Meta-analysis. Ann Surg. 2021;273(1):75-81.
22. RiaSTAP. (2025). RiaSTAP Dosing and Administration. [online] Available from https://www.riastap.com/professional/about-riastap/dosing-and-administration.aspx [Last accessed March, 2025].
23. Drugs.com. (2025). Fibrinogen Dosage Guide + Max Dose, Adjustments.[online] . Available from https://www.drugs.com/dosage/fibrinogen.html [Last accessed March 2025].
24. EMed. Octaplex®-Prothrombin Complex Concentrate (PCC). (2024). [online] Available from https://emed.ie/Pharmacology/Haematol/Octaplex.php [Last accessed March, 2025].

25. Neal MD, Marsh A, Marino R, Kautza B, Raval JS, Forsythe RM, et al. Massive Transfusion: An Evidence-Based Review of Recent Developments. Arch Surg. 2012; 147(6):563-71.
26. Ranucci M, Isgrò G, Soro G, Conti D, De Toffol B. Efficacy and Safety of Recombinant Activated Factor VII in Major Surgical Procedures: Systematic Review and Meta-analysis of Randomized Clinical Trials. Arch Surg. 2008;143(3):296-304.
27. NovoSeven® RT. Recommended. (2020) Dosing for Treatment of Bleeding Episodes and Surgery. [online] Available from https://www.novomedlink.com/rare-bleeding-disorders/products/treatments/novosevenrt/dosing-administration/quick-reference.html [Last accessed, 2025].
28. International Foundation for Patient Blood Management. What is Patient Blood Management? [online] Available from https://patientbloodmanagement.org/learn/what-is-patient-blood-management/ [Last accessed March, 2025].
29. Jennings LK, Watson S. Massive Transfusion. Treasure Island (FL): StatPearls; 2025.
30. Lammers D, Hu P, Rokayak O, Baird EW, Betzold RD, Hashmi Z, et al. Preferential whole blood transfusion during the early resuscitation period is associated with decreased mortality and transfusion requirements in traumatically injured patients. Trauma Surg Acute Care Open. 2024;9(1):e001358.
31. Vaishnav SB, Pal R, Pandey S, Shinde M, Padaliya A. Massive Transfusion Protocol: A Boon for Salvaging Patients of Obstetric Hemorrhage. Asian Res J Gynaecol Obstet. 2024;7(1):236-48.
32. Morris FJD, Åhman R, Craswell A, Didriksson H, Jonsson C, Gisselgård M, et al. Effect of perioperative blood transfusion on preoperative haemoglobin levels as a risk factor for long-term outcomes in patients undergoing major noncardiac surgery: a prospective multicentre observational study. Br J Anaesth. 2024;133(6):1183-91.
33. Rabello G, Monteiro R, Meneghini B, Jatene FB. When innovation meets patient blood management – a new way to see bleeding. Hematol Transfus Cell Ther. 2025;47(1):103691.
34. Keltner NM, Cushing MM, Haas T, Spinella PC. Analyzing and modeling massive transfusion strategies and the role of fibrinogen-How much is the patient actually receiving? Transfusion (Paris). 2024;64 Suppl 2(S2):S136-45.
35. Pan Z, Charoenkwan K. Prediction Models for Perioperative Blood Transfusion in Patients Undergoing Gynecologic Surgery: A Systematic Review. Diagnostics. 2024;14(18):2018.

CHAPTER 72

Cancer and Venous Thromboembolism

Jyotirmay Kirtania, Shreyasi Ray, Uddalak Chattopadhyay

INTRODUCTION

Thrombosis remains a well-established complication in individuals with malignancy, significantly influencing morbidity, mortality, and therapeutic planning. Venous thromboembolism (VTE), encompassing deep vein thrombosis and pulmonary embolism, is historically recognized as the predominant manifestation of cancer-associated thrombosis. However, increasing evidence now implicates arterial thrombosis—including myocardial infarction and ischemic stroke—as important, albeit less frequently acknowledged, consequence of cancer and its treatment. The bidirectional relationship between cancer and thrombosis is rooted in a multifactorial pathophysiology involving tumor-derived procoagulant factors, endothelial activation, cytokine release, and aberrant platelet function.

Patients with cancer represent a hypercoagulable subset due to both intrinsic factors—such as tumor histology, stage, and location—and extrinsic triggers including surgery, chemotherapy, targeted agents, central venous catheters, and immobility. Notably, certain malignancies such as pancreatic, gastric, brain, and lung cancers confer disproportionately high thrombotic risk. The administration of agents such as platinum-based chemotherapies, antiangiogenic therapies, and immune checkpoint inhibitors further modulates this risk by promoting endothelial dysfunction, platelet activation, and inflammatory cytokine cascades.

Clinically, cancer-associated thrombosis poses diagnostic and therapeutic challenges. Symptoms often overlap with those of the underlying malignancy or its complications, and routine diagnostic imaging may be complicated by preexisting anatomical distortions or comorbid conditions. The management of thrombosis in this setting necessitates careful balancing of thrombotic and bleeding risks, particularly in the context of thrombocytopenia, gastrointestinal lesions, or recent surgical interventions. Anticoagulant selection is further influenced by drug-drug interactions, organ dysfunction, and evolving evidence regarding direct oral anticoagulants (DOACs) versus low-molecular-weight heparin.

This chapter explores the epidemiology, risk factors, pathophysiology, clinical manifestations, and management strategies of both arterial and venous thrombotic events in patients with cancer, emphasizing individualized risk assessment and evidence-informed decision-making.

OVERVIEW OF CANCER-ASSOCIATED THROMBOSIS

Patients with cancer face a significantly increased risk for both arterial and VTE, contributing to substantial morbidity and mortality.[1,2] VTE has been identified as the second leading cause of death among cancer patients.[2,3] Encompassing deep venous thrombosis (DVT) and pulmonary embolism (PE), VTE emerges as the most common thrombotic complication in cancer patients, predominantly affecting the elderly.[1]

The association between cancer and VTE has been recognized for over two centuries.[4] Cancer patients are at a nine to twelve-fold higher risk of developing VTE compared to the general population and exhibit significantly higher bleeding rates during anticoagulant therapy than noncancer VTE patients.[2] The occurrence of VTE in these patients often disrupts cancer treatment, reduces quality of life, and escalates morbidity and mortality.[5]

Furthermore, cancer patients with VTE experience shorter survival times than those without VTE.[6] However, most studies evaluating the mortality associated with VTE in cancer patients are dated, have small or selected sample sizes, or focus on short-term outcomes.[1]

Advancements in cancer therapies, including targeted treatments and immunotherapy, alongside improved diagnostic modalities, have significantly altered cancer management and patient outcomes. Despite these advancements, the incidence of VTE in cancer patients within 1 year has increased from 1% to over 3% in recent decades.[2] This rise may be attributed to the aging oncology population, frequent detection of asymptomatic clots during diagnostic imaging, and the use of prothrombotic cancer therapies.[7] Additionally, targeted therapies and immunotherapy have emerged as significant risk factors for VTE, alongside distant metastases and chemotherapy.[5,7]

PATHOPHYSIOLOGY AND RISK FACTORS FOR CANCER-ASSOCIATED THROMBOSIS

The development of VTE, including conditions such as DVT and PE, in cancer patients is multifactorial and closely linked to Virchow's triad: Venous stasis, vascular damage, and blood hypercoagulability.[8] The nuanced interplay of these elements, exacerbated by cancer and its treatment, predisposes patients to thrombotic events.[5]

Virchow's triad, comprising venous stasis, vascular damage, and hypercoagulability, underpins the pathophysiology of VTE. Despite extensive research, the precise mechanisms linking oncogenesis to VTE remain incompletely understood.[2] Identified risk factors include tumor-specific characteristics, therapeutic interventions, and patient-related elements.[9]

Among tumor-associated factors, tissue factor (TF), microparticles (MPs), proinflammatory cytokines, and cancer procoagulants (CP) significantly contribute to a prothrombotic state. Tumor-derived factors such as tumor necrosis factor-alpha (TNF-α), interleukin-1 beta (IL-1β), and vascular endothelial growth factor (VEGF) exacerbate this state by inducing TF expression on monocytes and other mechanisms.[4,10]

The risk of developing cancer-associated VTE is further modulated by tumor-specific attributes such as site, type, metastatic stage, histological diversity, and disease duration.[1] Treatment-related risk factors include surgical procedures, hospitalization, chemotherapy, hormonal therapies, and radiation treatments.[3] Additionally, patient demographics, performance status, comorbidities, prior history of thrombosis, and genetic predispositions toward hypercoagulability significantly influence the VTE risk profile.[9]

Biomarkers such as elevated D-dimer levels and prechemotherapy platelet counts have demonstrated prognostic utility in predicting VTE risk, underscoring the need for further research to optimize thromboprophylaxis strategies.[7,9] These biomarkers play a critical role in mitigating mortality and reducing thromboembolic events in this high-risk population[5] **(Figs. 1 and 2)**.

IMPACT OF VENOUS THROMBOEMBOLISM ON CANCER SURVIVAL

In oncological populations, the prevalence of VTE significantly surpasses that observed in noncancer cohorts.[1] The variance in incidence rates can be attributed to a spectrum of factors,[1] encompassing demographic attributes,[8] intrinsic patient risks,[2] oncological typology and developmental phase,[10] chemotherapeutic regimes and modalities,[4] utilization of CVCs, as well as the methodologies employed in VTE detection and documentation.[1]

Notably, the postponement or discontinuation of chemotherapy, alongside direct VTE sequelae, such as PE, amplifies mortality risks.[11] Particularly, the occurrence of VTE within a 2-year post-diagnosis window emerges as a critical determinant of heightened mortality, especially pronounced in cases involving localized malignancies.[6]

In the context of VTE prophylaxis within this high-risk demographic, low-molecular-weight heparin (LMWH), with a focus on dalteparin, is increasingly considered.[7] The necessity for additional research is underscored, aiming to elucidate the efficacy of thromboprophylaxis strategies in mitigating mortality and thromboembolic adverse outcomes among cancer patients.[12]

Of note, arterial thrombosis can account for a substantial number of deaths in individuals undergoing chemotherapy. A review of 4,466 ambulatory patients with cancer who were receiving chemotherapy reported that thrombosis was one of the three most common causes of death.[7] The majority of the deaths related to thromboembolic disease were due to arterial thrombosis (e.g., myocardial infarction and stroke) rather than VTE. Of the 141 deaths that occurred during chemotherapy administration (3.2%), the three leading causes of death were cancer progression (71%), infection (9%), and thromboembolic disease (9% total; 5.6% arterial and 3.5% venous).[7]

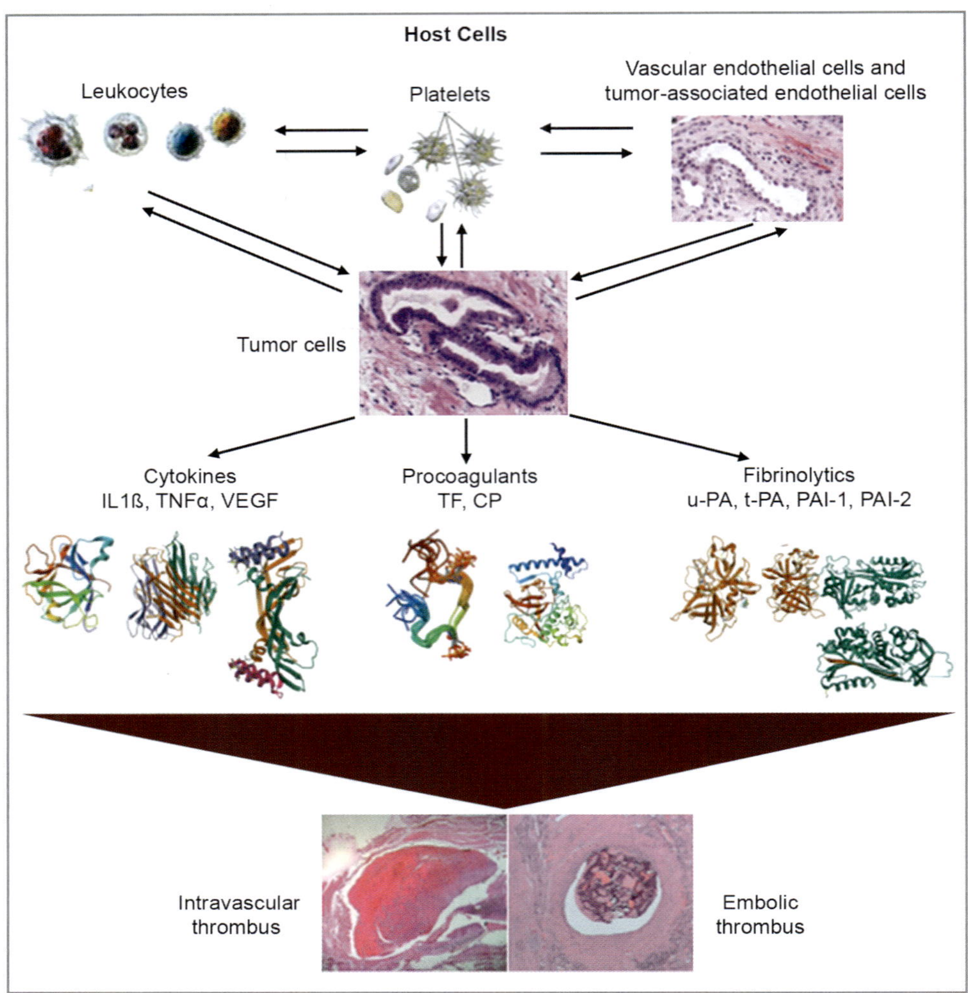

Fig. 1: Pathogenesis of cancer-induced venous thromboembolism. Interleukin 1 beta (IL-1β), tumor necrosis factor-alpha (TNFα), vascular endothelial growth factor (VEGF), tissue factor (TF), cancer procoagulant (CP), urokinase-type plasminogen activator (u-PA), tissue-type plasminogen activator (t-PA), plasminogen activator inhibitor type 1 (PAI-1), plasminogen activator inhibitor type 2 (PAI-2) are the key molecules in the process.[4]

CHEMOTHERAPY-INDUCED THROMBOSIS

Chemotherapeutic intervention represents an established, independent risk factor forVTE genesis and significantly amplifies the risk of VTE recurrence in oncological contexts by a factor of four.[13] The incidence of chemotherapy-associated VTE is modulated by several variables, including neoplasm typology and anatomical locale, chemotherapeutic regimen specifics, and the concurrent administration of hormonal and targeted therapeutic agents.[9] Chemotherapy exacerbates the prothrombotic milieu through diverse mechanistic pathways.[6,11]

To anticipate chemotherapy-associated VTE risk, scoring frameworks such as the Khorana score[14] are advocated. Prophylactic administration of LMWH has demonstrated efficacy in mitigating VTE risk in actively treated cancer cohorts.[7] Nevertheless, the empirical basis for employing direct oral anticoagulants in the prophylaxis of cancer-associated thrombosis remains scant,[12] necessitating further investigative endeavors.

CATHETER-RELATED THROMBOSIS IN CANCER

Central venous catheters, including peripherally inserted central catheters (PICCs), Hickman catheters,

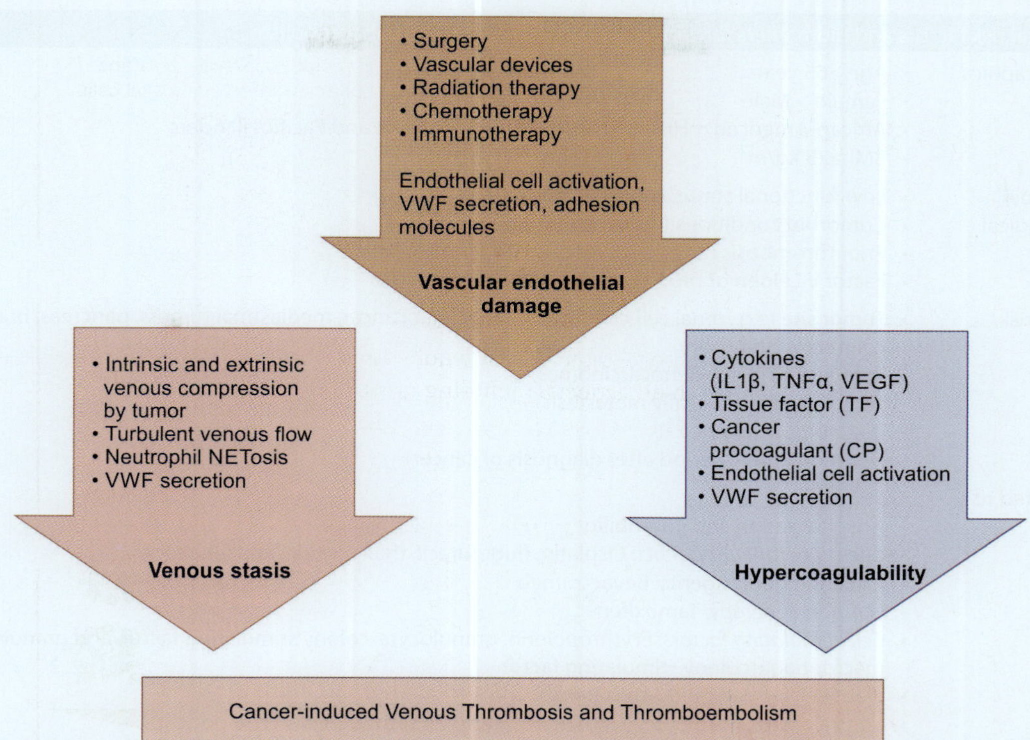

Fig. 2: Pathogenesis of tumor-induced local thrombi.[4] (IL: interleukin; TNFα: tumor necrosis factor alpha; VEGF: vascular endothelial growth factor; VWF: von Willebrand factor)

and chemoport catheters, serve as pivotal instruments for the administration of chemotherapy, intravenous medications, and blood transfusions in the oncological therapeutic landscape.[8] Catheter-related thrombosis (CRT), a prevalent complication among cancer patients, is significantly underreported, primarily due to the asymptomatic nature of numerous instances.[13]

The etiology of CRT is multifactorial, with risk factors spanning patient demographics, such as age, the anatomical specificity of venous structures, tumor histological characteristics, dimensions, and localization, in addition to the inherent properties of the catheter type employed **(Table 1)**.[14]

Diagnostic approaches to CRT face inherent limitations, with Doppler ultrasound constituting the initial investigative tool, albeit with potential for nondiagnostic outcomes.[10] In scenarios of Doppler ultrasound inadequacy yet persistent clinical suspicion, contrast venography is deployed, serving as the "gold standard" for CRT diagnosis.[11] Additionally, the advent of contrast-enhanced computed tomography (CT) and magnetic resonance imaging (MRI) offers promising, albeit occasionally utilized, alternative diagnostic modalities.[12]

MANAGEMENT OF CANCER-ASSOCIATED THROMBOSIS

Anticoagulant therapy remains a cornerstone for both prophylaxis and management of thrombotic events, irrespective of oncological status in individuals exhibiting a low hemorrhagic risk profile.[11] Contraindications to anticoagulation encompass scenarios of active hemorrhage, recent surgical interventions, established bleeding diathesis, coagulopathies, or a platelet count subthreshold of $<50,000/\mu L$.[6] Immediate therapeutic strategies entail the administration of LMWH or unfractionated heparin (UFH), transitioning to extended-duration management via LMWH, vitamin K antagonists (VKA), or direct oral anticoagulants (DOACs).[7]

In the context of acute VTE within oncological patients, the induction of anticoagulation for a period ranging from 5 to 10 days is advocated, with LMWH positioned as the preferred agent barring contraindications.[13] The selection

TABLE 1: Clinical risk factors and biomarkers for cancer-associated venous thromboembolism.[2,7]

Patient demographics	• Age ≥65 years • Female > Male • African-American > Hispanic and Caucasian > Asian and Pacific Islanders • BMI ≥25 kg/m^2
Functional status, and nononcological comorbidities	• Low functional status and immobility • Comorbid conditions (hypertension) • Prior thrombosis (arterial or venous) • Factor V Leiden or prothrombin (Factor II) mutations
Tumor-related risk factors	• Tumor site (e.g., renal cell cancer, hepatocellular cancer, mediastinal tumors, pancreas, brain, stomach, colorectal, and ovary) • Tumor type (e.g., adenocarcinomas) • Tumor stage (especially metastasis) • Histological variance • Duration (initial period after diagnosis of cancer)
Treatment-related risk factors	• Surgery • Hospitalization and immobility • *Chemotherapeutic agents:* Cisplatin, fluorouracil, thalidomide, and lenalidomide • Antiangiogenic agents: Bevacizumab • *Hormonal therapy:* Tamoxifen • *Cell-stimulating factors:* Erythropoietin, granulocyte-colony stimulating factor, and granulocyte macrophage-colony stimulating factor • Platelets and red blood cells transfusion • Central venous catheters (CVC) (PICC, Hickman's catheter, and chemoport) • *Immune checkpoint inhibitors (ICI):* PD1 inhibitors (nivolumab, pembrolizumab, and cemiplimab) or its ligands (atezolizumab, avelumab, and durvalumab); CTLA-4 inhibitors (ipilimumab)
Laboratory parameters and biomarkers	• Platelets ≥350,000/mm^3 • Leukocytes >11,000/mm^3 • Elevated tissue factor • Elevated D-dimer • Elevated fibrinogen (factor 1) • Elevated prothrombin (factor 2) • Elevated thrombin-antithrombin complex (TAT) • Elevated soluble P-selectin (CD62P) • Elevated C-reactive protein

(BMI: body mass index; CTLA: cytotoxic T-lymphocyte-associated; PICC: peripherally inserted central catheter)

of the anticoagulant regimen is contingent upon patient-specific parameters including renal function, adherence to treatment, and dietary compliance.[6] Fondaparinux and DOACs present viable initial treatment alternatives.[12] UFH is favored under circumstances necessitating prompt reversal of anticoagulation, such as renal insufficiency, elevated risk of hemorrhage, and procedural interventions.[7]

Factor Xa inhibitors, endorsed for the initiation of therapy in DVT and acute PE, obviate the requirement for anticoagulation efficacy monitoring.[11] For individuals contraindicated for sustained LMWH therapy, indirect oral anticoagulants, such as warfarin, are deemed acceptable for long-term management.[6] DOACs emerge as an alternative in scenarios precluding LMWH usage, attributed to factors such as renal compromise (creatinine clearance <30 mL/min), financial constraints, nonadherence, or needle aversion.[12] The prescribed duration for anticoagulation extends to a minimum of 3 months.[7]

In oncological patients with VTE presenting contraindications to pharmacological anticoagulation, mechanical prophylaxis, exemplified by the insertion of an inferior vena cava filter (IVCF), may represent the sole therapeutic avenue.[11]

SPECIAL CASES IN CANCER-ASSOCIATED THROMBOSIS

Thrombosis and thrombocytopenia frequently manifest in the oncological setting, attributable to microangiopathic anomalies such as thrombotic thrombocytopenic purpura (TTP), immune-mediated disorders, immune thrombocytopenic purpura (ITP), and heparin-induced thrombocytopenia (HIT), alongside the adverse effects of chemotherapy or the direct oncogenic impact.[6,13] Recurrence of VTE during anticoagulation therapy is notably prevalent, with metastatic disease, younger patient age, and a brief interval between cancer diagnosis, and the initial VTE episode delineated as significant risk factors.[7,15] VTE poses a substantial management obstacle in individuals with renal dysfunction.[11]

Incidental VTE, identified serendipitously during imaging evaluations for alternative clinical rationales, often traces back to underlying malignancy or chemotherapy-related adverse effects.[9] Furthermore, Philadelphia chromosome-negative myeloproliferative disorders, encompassing polycythemia vera (PV), essential thrombocythemia (ET), and primary myelofibrosis (PMF), are associated with an elevated risk for both venous and arterial thromboembolic events.[16]

The correlation between hematological malignancies and increased VTE incidence is also emerging, underscoring the intricate relationship between cancer and thrombotic complications.[17]

ANTITUMOR EFFECTS OF HEPARIN

Isolated from liver and heart tissues in 1916, heparin's anticoagulant properties were elucidated in conjunction with a plasma component, subsequently identified as heparin-cofactor.[18] Subsequent developments have yielded a diverse spectrum of heparin molecules, engineered to leverage their anti-tumor attributes.[19] Heparin sulfate, a pivotal constituent of the extracellular matrix, upon degradation by heparanase—an enzyme secreted by neoplastic cells—has been implicated in augmenting tumor invasiveness.[20,21]

The antiangiogenic properties of heparin are principally attributed to its capacity to diminish fibrin levels and inhibit thrombin genesis.[22] Furthermore, natural killer (NK) cells, instrumental in the eradication of circulating tumor entities, augment the antineoplastic potential of heparin, as substantiated by various investigative undertakings.[20]

Among the assorted heparin derivatives, butanoylated heparin emerges with notably diminished anticoagulative potency yet exhibits substantially enhanced antitumor efficacy relative to UFH at elevated dosages.[23] Comparative analysis concerning the antitumor efficacies between LMWH and butanoylated heparin remains to be undertaken, presenting an avenue for future research endeavors to delineate the optimal heparin formulation for antitumor applications.[24]

PROPHYLAXIS OF VENOUS THROMBOEMBOLISM IN CANCER

In the oncological patient cohort, the predisposition to VTE and its sequelae markedly escalates, underscoring the criticality of discerning patients at elevated risk.[25] The Khorana score, a stratification tool, delineates cancer patients into low- and high-risk categories based on neoplasm typology, chemotherapeutic protocols, hematologic parameters, and an aggregate of clinical and laboratory indices **(Table 2)**.[14]

For cancer patients experiencing hospitalization with concomitant limited ambulation, the prophylactic administration of LMWH or UFH is advocated.[2] In instances

TABLE 2: Khorana risk score of cancer-associated thrombosis.[14]

Characteristic	***Score***
Cancer type	
• Stomach and pancreas	2
• Lung, lymphoma, gynecologic, bladder, and testicular	1
• Other	0
Prechemotherapy platelet count ≥350 × 10^9/L	
• Yes	1
• No	0
Hemoglobin level <10 g/dL or using red blood cell or growth factors	
• Yes	1
• No	0
Prechemotherapy leukocyte count >11 × 10^9/L	
• Yes	1
• No	0
Body mass index ≥35 kg/m^2	
• Yes	1
• No	0
Total score: 0 = low risk for thrombosis 1–2 = Intermediate risk for thrombosis ≥3 = High risk for thrombosis	

where anticoagulation presents contraindications, mechanical prophylaxis emerges as a viable alternative.[7]

Pertaining to oncological patients undergoing surgical interventions, the initiation of perioperative VTE prophylaxis via pharmacologic anticoagulation is advised, barring scenarios involving minor procedures or explicit anticoagulant contraindications.[2] For ambulatory patients, the American Society of Clinical Oncology (ASCO) does not endorse routine anticoagulant application barring circumstances typified by high risk, exemplified by a Khorana score ≥2, or in cases of multiple myeloma with thalidomide or lenalidomide therapy.[2]

Such individuals are candidates for VTE prophylaxis employing apixaban, rivaroxaban, or LMWH.[3] Furthermore, ASCO emphasizes the necessity for periodic VTE risk assessments among cancer patients and the imperative of patient education regarding the manifestations and indicators of VTE.[2]

General considerations for VTE prophylaxis among cancer patients:

- Assess VTE risk at initial diagnosis and periodically, especially when starting systemic therapy.[14]
- Educate patients about VTE risks, particularly during surgery, hospitalization, and systemic therapy.[2]

Thromboprophylaxis recommendations:

- Hospitalized cancer patients
    - LMWH prophylaxis is recommended for patients with active cancer, acute illness, or reduced mobility, excluding those with bleeding risks.[7]
    - Avoid routine thromboprophylaxis with LMWH, apixaban, rivaroxaban, and antiplatelets for minor procedures, chemotherapy infusion, or stem-cell transplantation.[2]
- Ambulatory cancer patients during chemotherapy
    - Routine thromboprophylaxis is not recommended for all outpatient cancer patients.[3]
    - Give thromboprophylaxis with apixaban, rivaroxaban, or LMWH in high-risk outpatients (Khorana score ≥2).[14]
    - Give thromboprophylaxis with aspirin or LMWH in multiple myeloma patients on thalidomide or lenalidomide.[2]
- Cancer surgery
- Give thromboprophylaxis with UFH or LMWH for major surgeries, unless contraindicated, such as active bleeding or high bleeding risk surgeries[2]
- Start prophylaxis preoperatively (24–12 hours prior to surgery) unless contraindicated.[3]
- Combine pharmacologic with mechanical thromboprophylaxis methods unless contraindicated, particularly in high-risk patients.[7]
- Continue thromboprophylaxis postoperatively for 7–10 days, extend to 4 weeks for high-risk abdominal or pelvic surgeries[2]

Treatment of Established Venous Thromboembolism in Cancer Patients

- LMWH is preferred for initial 5–10 days of anticoagulation for newly diagnosed VTE.[13]
- For long-term anticoagulation, prefer LMWH, apixaban, or rivaroxaban over VKA (e.g., warfarin or acenocoumarol).[7]
- Continue anticoagulation beyond 6 months for patients with ongoing cancer treatment or metastatic disease.[3]
- Vena cava filter insertion is not recommended except in specific acute conditions.[12]
- Consider vena cava filter as an adjunct in recurrent thrombosis despite anticoagulation.[11]
- Treat central nervous system (CNS) malignancy patients with VTE as other cancer patients.[2]
- Treat incidental PE and DVT as symptomatic VTE.[7]
- Treatment of isolated subsegmental PE or visceral vein thrombosis should be individualized.[3]
- Anticoagulants are not recommended as therapy to improve survival in cancer without established VTE. [2,3]

Note: LMWH (enoxaparin and fondaparinux) and DOAC (apixaban and rivaroxaban) doses should be individualized. Read the up-to-date official version of prescribing information (PI) of these drugs before prescribing.

MODIFICATION OF ANTICOAGULANT AND ANTIPLATELET THERAPY FOR CANCER SURGERIES

Anticoagulation and antiplatelet therapy in cancer patients with thrombocytopenia: Thrombocytopenia is associated with adverse outcomes in arterial or venous thrombosis. Anticoagulation should be modified or withheld when platelets are <50×10^9/L, but scientific data are scarce. The thrombotic risk is lower in nonacute VTE, catheter-related VTE, and atrial fibrillation. Use aspirin in acute coronary syndrome when platelets are >30×10^9/L.[26] Heparin bridging therapy in patients receiving VKA therapy increases perioperative bleeding risk.[11]

Perioperative heparin bridging therapy is not recommended in:

- In patients receiving VKA therapy for atrial fibrillation who require VKA interruption for an elective cancer surgery/procedure[11]
- In patients receiving VKA therapy for a mechanical heart valve or VTE who require VKA interruption for an elective cancer surgery/procedure[11]
- In patients receiving VKA therapy who require VKA interruption for a colonoscopy with anticipated polypectomy[11]

Perioperative heparin bridging therapy is recommended in: In patients receiving a DOAC (apixaban, rivaroxaban, and dabigatran) who require an elective cancer surgery/procedure, stop the DOAC for 1–2 days (1–4 days for dabigatran) before the surgery/procedure. Bridge the perioperative period with LMWH. Postoperatively, restart the DOAC about 24 hours after a low/moderate-bleed-risk surgery/procedure and 48–72 hours after a high-bleed-risk surgery/procedure **(Table 3)**.[11]

In patients receiving low-dose aspirin who are undergoing elective cancer surgeries aspirin may be continued.[11] Exception being intracranial surgeries and cancer surgeries with anticipated major blood loss.

Patients with malignancy may have tumor-specific factors that lead to an unacceptably high bleeding risk with anticoagulation. These include active major bleeding, severe uncompensated coagulopathy, thrombocytopenia or severe platelet dysfunction, uncontrolled hypertension, and recent or planned surgery or invasive procedure (e.g., neuraxial anesthesia and placement of central venous or arterial catheters).[11]

CHALLENGING CASE REPORTS: ANESTHETIC MANAGEMENT OF CANCER-ASSOCIATED THROMBOSIS

Case 1

Background: This case involves a patient with advanced renal cell carcinoma, where the tumor thrombus extended from the inferior vena cava (IVC) into the right atrium and pulmonary artery, presenting significant challenges for surgical and anesthetic management.

Clinical challenge: The patient, a 50-year-old male, was admitted with a diagnosis of right renal cell carcinoma and a tumor thrombus that had progressed into the IVC and pulmonary artery, causing severe symptoms including poor appetite, abdominal distension, and vomiting, accompanied by wheezing and progressive exacerbation.

Anesthetic Management

Preoperative preparation: The patient was prepared by correction of malnutrition and anemia. Due to anticipated intraoperative major blood loss, 20 units of packed red blood cells (RBCs), 2,000 mL of fresh frozen plasma, and 3 units of platelets were reserved.

Operative details: Anesthesia was induced and maintained with a combination of etomidate, sufentanil, and sevoflurane. The complexities of managing such a patient included maintaining hemodynamic stability during the removal of a large tumor thrombus under cardiopulmonary bypass.

TABLE 3: Guidance recommendations regarding perioperative management of antithrombotic and antiplatelet agents.[27]

Antithrombotic therapies	Vitamin K antagonists (VKA)	Direct oral anticoagulant (DOAC)		COX1 inhibitor	$P2Y_{12}$ inhibitors			
					Cardiac surgery	Noncardiac surgery		
	Warfarin and acenocoumarol	Apixaban, edoxaban, and rivaroxaban	Dabigatran	Aspirin	Any $P2Y_{12}$ inhibitor	Clopidogrel	Prasugrel	Ticagrelor
Time to stop before elective surgeries	5 days before	1–2 days before	1–4 days before	3–7 days before	Stop, continue Aspirin	5 days before	7 days before	3–5 days
Time to restart after surgery	Within 24 hours	After 24 hours	Within 24 hours	Within 24 hours	Continue aspirin	Within 24 hours	Within 24 hours	Within 24 hours

(COX: cyclooxygenase)

Surgical procedure: The surgery involved a radical nephrectomy with the removal of the tumor thrombus using cardiopulmonary bypass, which took 396 minutes with a total surgical time of 724 minutes. Significant challenges during surgery included managing massive intraoperative blood loss (22,000 mL) and ensuring adequate organ perfusion and oxygenation.

Postoperative care: The patient required extensive monitoring and management in the intensive care unit (ICU), including mechanical ventilation for 39 hours postsurgery and careful management of fluid and electrolyte balance.

Outcome: The patient was discharged in good health and was doing well at 1 year follow-up after surgery.

Reference: Chen S, Lu L, Zheng X, Lin Y, Bao L, Zhang B, et al. (2024)[27]

Case 2

Background: 46-year-old female diagnosed with a malignant ovarian tumor and concurrent deep venous thrombosis (Trousseau's syndrome)

Clinical challenge: Developed a massive cerebral infarction despite ongoing anticoagulation therapy, complicating surgical intervention.

Anesthetic approach: Utilized general anesthesia with desflurane and remifentanil. Strategically placed a temporary IVCF and transitioned from oral anticoagulants to intravenous UFH preoperatively.

Surgical and postoperative management: Performed successful semi-radical gynecological surgery 1 month post cerebral infarction. Postoperatively, managed pain with a peripheral nerve block and continuous intravenous fentanyl, leading to a stable recovery without further complications.

Reference: Watanabe Y, Matsunuma K, Kaneda T. (2020).[28]

Case 3

Background: 39-year-old female undergoing craniotomy for high-grade astrocytoma

Clinical challenge: Experienced a sudden intraoperative decrease in end-tidal CO_2 and O_2 saturation, indicative of pulmonary embolism.

Anesthetic management: Initiated immediate resuscitative measures, including central venous aspiration, administration of 100% oxygen, ephedrine, and intravenous fluids, along with heparin for acute management.

Outcome: Postevent, placed an IVC filter and started on long-term anticoagulation with enoxaparin. The patient subsequently underwent successful tumor resection, continuing anticoagulation therapy.

Reference: Khraise WN, Allouh MZ, Hiasat MY, Said RS. (2016)[29]

CONCLUSION

Thrombotic complications, both venous and arterial, are integral to the natural history and treatment of malignancy. Their incidence reflects a dynamic interplay of cancer biology, host response, and iatrogenic factors. Prompt recognition and appropriate management are essential, given the prognostic implications and potential therapeutic interruptions that may arise. Advancements in anticoagulant therapies and risk stratification tools have broadened the scope for personalized prophylaxis and treatment.

REFERENCES

1. Timp JF, Braekkan SK, Versteeg HH, Cannegieter SC. Epidemiology of cancer-associated venous thrombosis. Blood. 2013;122(10):1712-23.
2. Farge D, Frere C, Connors JM, Ay C, Khorana AA, Munoz A, et al. 2019 international clinical practice guidelines for the treatment and prophylaxis of venous thromboembolism in patients with cancer. Lancet Oncol. 2019;20(10):e566-81.
3. Key NS, Khorana AA, Kuderer NM, Bohlke K, Lee AYY, Arcelus JI, et al. Venous thromboembolism prophylaxis and treatment in patients with cancer: ASCO Clinical Practice Guideline Update. J Clin Oncol. 2020;38(5):496-520.
4. Varki A. Trousseau's syndrome: Multiple definitions and multiple mechanisms. Blood. 2007;110(6):1723-9.
5. Chew HK, Wun T, Harvey D, Zhou H, White RH. Incidence of venous thromboembolism and its effect on survival among patients with common cancers. Arch Intern Med. 2006;166(4):458-64.
6. Khorana AA, Connolly GC. Assessing risk of venous thromboembolism in the patient with cancer. J Clin Oncol. 2009;27(29):4839-47.
7. Prandoni P, Lensing AW, Piccioli A, Bernardi E, Simioni P, Girolami B, et al. Recurrent venous thromboembolism and bleeding complications during anticoagulant treatment in patients with cancer and venous thrombosis. Blood. 2002;100(10):3484-8.
8. Lyman GH, Carrier M, Ay C, Di Nisio M, Hicks LK, Khorana AA, et al. American Society of Hematology 2021 guidelines for management of venous thromboembolism: Prevention

and treatment in patients with cancer. Blood Adv. 2021; 5(4):927-74.

9. Connors JM. Thrombophilia testing and venous thrombosis. N Engl J Med. 2017;377(12):1177-87.
10. Ay C, Dunkler D, Marosi C, Chiriac AL, Vormittag R, Simanek, et al. Prediction of venous thromboembolism in cancer patients. Blood. 2010;116(24):5377-82.
11. Verso M, Agnelli G. Venous thromboembolism associated with long-term use of central venous catheters in cancer patients. Blood. 2003;102(3):966-72.
12. Kasthuri RS, Taubman MB, Mackman N. Role of tissue factor in cancer. J Clin Oncol. 2009;27(29):4834-8.
13. Khorana AA, Francis CW, Culakova E, Fisher RI, Kuderer NM, Lyman GH. Thromboembolism in hospitalized neutropenic cancer patients. Blood. 2008;111(10):4902-7.
14. Kasthuri RS, Mackman N. Tissue factor and cancer. Semin Thromb Hemost. 2012;38(2):123-9.
15. Di Nisio M, Lee AYY, Carrier M, Liebman HA, Khorana AA; Subcommittee on Haemostasis and Malignancy. Diagnosis and treatment of incidental venous thromboembolism in cancer patients: Guidance from the SSC of the ISTH. Thromb Haemost. 2015;13(5):880-3.
16. Tefferi A, Barbui T. Polycythemia vera and essential thrombocythemia: 2019 update on diagnosis, risk-stratification and management. Am J Hematol. 2019;94(1): 133-43.
17. McLean J. The discovery of heparin. Circulation. 1959; 19(1):75-8.
18. Linhardt RJ, Gunay NS. Production and applications of microbial heparinases. Nat Rev Cancer. 2008;8(11):865-73.
19. Vlodavsky I, Ilan N, Sanderson RD. Heparanase: Biology, function, and clinical applications. Crit Rev Oncol Hematol. 2007;62(1):3-18.
20. Pisano C, Vlodavsky I, Ilan N, Zunino F. The potential of heparanase as a therapeutic target in cancer. Biochem Pharmacol. 2014;89(1):12-9.
21. Casu B, Lindahl U. Structure and biological interactions of heparin and heparan sulfate. J Biol Chem. 2001;57:159-206.
22. Napolitano M, Cosmi B, Lip GYH. Butanoylated heparin: A promising antitumoral agent with reduced anticoagulant activity. Thromb Res. 2004;114(2):85-92.
23. Yu L, Garg HG, Li B, Linhardt RJ, Hales CA. Antitumor effect of butanoylated heparin with low anticoagulant activity on lung cancer growth in mice and rats. Curr Cancer Drug Targets. 2010;10(2):229-41.
24. Leader A, Gurevich-Shapiro A, Spectre G. Anticoagulant and antiplatelet treatment in cancer patients with thrombocytopenia. Thromb Res. 2020;191 (Suppl 1):S68-73.
25. Douketis JD, Spyropoulos AC, Murad MH, Arcelus JI, Dager WE, Dunn AS, et al. Perioperative management of antithrombotic therapy: An American College of Chest Physicians clinical practice guideline. Chest. 2022;162(5):e207-43.
26. Chhaya VY, Kibbe MR. What surgeons need to know about the recent updates to the chest guidelines on antithrombotic therapy for venous thromboembolic disease and perioperative management of antithrombotic therapy. Ann Surg. 2023;278(4):e695-7.
27. Chen S, Lu L, Zheng X, Lin Y, Bao L, Zhang B, et al. Case report: Anesthetic management for removal of tumor thrombus in the inferior vena cava and pulmonary artery in renal cell carcinoma. Front Oncol. 2024;14:1372625.
28. Watanabe Y, Matsunuma K, Kaneda T. A case of successful anesthetic management in a patient with Trousseau's syndrome who underwent surgery for malignant ovarian tumor. JA Clin Rep. 2020;6:32.
29. Khraise WN, Allouh MZ, Hiasat MY, Said RS. Successful management of intraoperative acute bilateral pulmonary embolism in a high-grade astrocytoma patient. Am J Case Rep. 2016;17:632-6.

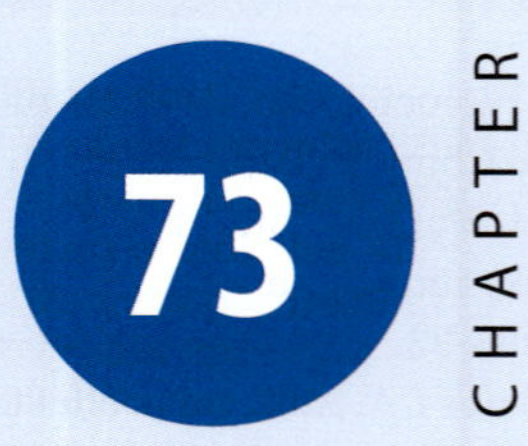

Perioperative Management of Cancer Surgeries During Pregnancy

Aditi Suri, Usha Yadav, Rupesh Yadav

INTRODUCTION

Cancer that occurs during pregnancy or within 1 year of delivery is termed gestational cancer. The incidence of gestational cancers has risen over the past decade. Cancers of the breast, thyroid, gynecological, and hematological malignancies are the most common cancers that occur during pregnancy. An international study on 1,170 pregnant women found breast cancer to be the most common type of cancer during pregnancy (39%) and cervical (13%), lymphoma, and leukemia among others.[1]

The etiological factors for pregnancy-related cancers are deemed as increased age at pregnancy with higher incidence seen in pregnancies above the age of 40 years compared to those below the age of 30 years.

Another study on 1,798 pregnant women observed an incidence of 137.2 per 100,000 pregnancies **(Table 1)**. They also observed that around 23% of women in their study were above the age of 35 years.

The diagnosis of cancer during pregnancy requires a meticulous management approach that involves the expertise of multidisciplinary teams for diagnostic and therapeutic reasons. The treatment goals should keep in mind not only the pregnant patient but also the growing fetus. The gestational age of the fetus and its associated characteristic physiological changes must be borne in mind. The patient's preference is the primary guiding principle that is combined with the best available evidence.

TABLE 1: Incidence of various common cancers in pregnancy.[1,2]

Type of cancer	*Incidence during pregnancy (per 100,00 women)*
Breast	268
Ovary	5.7
Cervix	9.5
Melanoma	12
Hematological	11.2

PHYSIOLOGICAL MATERNAL CHANGES DURING PREGNANCY AND DIAGNOSIS OF CANCER

The diagnosis of cancer can often be obscured by physiological changes of pregnancy **(Table 2)**. The presence of breast or abdominal discomfort, anemia, and fatigue may be overlooked as symptoms of pregnancy, thus delaying the evaluation and treatment of cancer. The gravid uterus can hinder the examination of the abdomen.

Being a rare condition, there may be a delay on the part of the physician in advising imaging that may involve the use of radiation or contrast agents. Many diagnostic tests may provide inaccurate false positive or false negative results in pregnancy, causing a diagnostic dilemma and delay in diagnosis and treatment.[3,4]

DIAGNOSTIC MODALITIES FOR CANCER WORKUP DURING PREGNANCY

Imaging

Exposure to ionizing radiation from imaging modalities poses a serious risk of teratogenicity, fetal growth retardation, or death. The gestational age of the fetus determines the extent of risk to the fetus. The first trimester being the period of organogenesis carries a high risk of radiation-related major malformations. Cumulated doses higher than 100 mGy are associated with severe harm to the fetus. Detrimental effects of radiation on the fetus can be prevented by preferring imaging modalities such as magnetic resonance imaging (MRI) or ultrasound. Computed tomography (CT) scans and fluoroscopic procedures should be avoided. The protective abdominal shield can be used wherever necessary.

TABLE 2: Fetal and maternal physiological changes in normal pregnancy.[1,5]

	First trimester (till 12 weeks)	***Second trimester (12–28 weeks)***	***Third trimester (>28)***
Fetal growth	• Rapid organogenesis • Most drugs cross the placenta	• Developing organ systems • Surfactant develops viability threshold 20–24 weeks	Fetal neural development and weight gain
Placenta	• *Factors affecting transplacental transfer:* Lipid solubility, protein binding, tissue binding, pKa, pH, blood flow, and small molecular size <600 Daltons • *Drugs that undergo placental transfer:* Atropine, benzodiazepine, IV induction agents, local anesthetics, and opioids • *Drugs that do not undergo placental transfer:* Depolarizing and nondepolarizing muscle relaxants		
Maternal changes	High risk of miscarriage	Suitable time for surgical intervention	Risk of preterm labor with surgical intervention
	• *CVS*: ↑ CO, SV HR, blood volume (30–45%), clotting factors increased • *RS*: ↑ oxygen consumption, ↓ FRC (20–40%), faster desaturation • *Airway*: Higher Mallampati grading, presence of short neck, mucosal capillary engorgement and swelling, large breasts. High risk for difficult intubation • *Hemodynamic changes*: ↓ hematocrit, anemia of pregnancy, hypercoagulable state with risk of venous thromboembolism. Intraoperative hemodynamic stability is important to maintain adequate uteroplacental circulation • *Gastrointestinal system*: ↓ tone of lower esophageal sphincter increases the risk of gastric aspiration • *Pharmacokinetics*: ↑ Vd of drugs, increased free fraction of drugs, increased hepatic and renal clearance • *Breast changes*: Enlarged, engorged breasts, tenderness, and breast lump		
Trimester	***First***	***Second***	***Third***
Treatment for cancer Chemotherapy	Avoided due effect to organogenesis	Can be administered provided safe drug regime	Avoided near the end of pregnancy
Radiotherapy	Avoided	Given in dose <100 mGy	Given in dose <100 mGy
Surgery	Avoided	Safest time for surgery	Risk of preterm labor

(CO: cardiac output; CVS: cardiovascular system; FRC: functional residual capacity; HR: heart rate; IV: intravenous; RS: respiratory system; SV: stroke volume; Vd: volume of distribution)

Contrast dyes like gadolinium, which have low molecular weight may cross the placenta and are generally not indicated in pregnancy due to paucity of literature on their effects on human fetus. Gadobenate and meglumine are viable alternatives. Iodinated contrast dyes can cause hypothyroidism in the neonate and should therefore be followed up. Iodine^{131} is thus contraindicated in pregnancy. tecgnetium^{99m} is preferred instead.

Different imaging techniques and their radiation dose to the fetus are tabulated in **Table 3**.[6-9]

Tumor Markers

The reliability of tumor markers can be questioned. Markers such as CA-125, alpha-fetoprotein (AFP), and CA15-3, which are normally elevated in pregnancy, are not reliable when evaluating for cancer in pregnancy. Others such as CA19-9, lactate dehydrogenase (LDH), and

TABLE 3: Irradiation dose of imaging modalities.[1,5]

Imaging technique	***Fetal irradiation dose (mGy)***
X-ray thorax	0.0005–0.01
X-ray extremity, cervical spine	<0.001
Mammography	0.001–0.01
X-ray abdomen	0.1–3.0
CT chest	0.01–0.66
CT abdomen	1.3–35
CT pelvis	10–50
^{18}FDG PET	10–50
USG	0
MRI	0

(Green: very low dose; orange: low moderate; red: high dose; CT: computed tomography; ^{18}FDG PET: 18F-fluorodeoxyglucose positron emission tomography; MRI: magnetic resonance imaging; USG: ultrasonography)

anti-Müllerian hormone (AMH) can be used because they are not normally elevated in pregnancy.[10-12]

Biopsy

A tissue or bone marrow biopsy is done to confirm the cancer diagnosis. The hyperestrogenic state of pregnancy may obscure the diagnosis. A core/excisional biopsy is more reliable than a fine needle aspirate cytology (FNAC).[13]

MANAGEMENT OF CANCER DURING PREGNANCY

Chemotherapy During Pregnancy[7,8]

Most chemotherapeutic agents are capable of crossing the placenta and reaching the fetus. Existing literature thus recommends against the use of chemotherapy during the first trimester. The rate of transplacental transfer is high with carboplatin and moderate with anthracyclines. Most agents are fit for use after a 12–14-week period of gestation (POG). Trastuzumab can cause fetal lung hypoplasia and decreased liquor and is thus contraindicated during pregnancy.

Suppression of the immune system and hematopoiesis can occur as a side effect of chemotherapy, which can lead to the risk of concurrent infection and deranged blood counts. Keeping this in mind, an elective delivery should be planned at least 3 weeks after chemotherapy. Also, chemotherapy should not be administered after 37 weeks POG in anticipation of the patient going into spontaneous labor.

Radiotherapy During Pregnancy[1,8,14,15]

Administration of radiotherapy to a pregnant patient with cancer carries a high risk of fetal harm depending on the period of gestation and radiation dose. The maximum adverse effects like congenital anomalies and growth retardation are seen with radiotherapy during the first 12–15 weeks POG.

Adverse effects due to radiotherapy can be categorized as deterministic or stochastic. Deterministic effects are seen above a threshold dose of 100 mGy, while stochastic effects are devoid of any threshold dose limit.

Mental functional disability is known to increase with RT doses of >100 mGy. Similar adverse effects such as mental retardation, microcephaly, sterility, and intrauterine growth retardation can occur in the second and third trimesters, although lower with doses <500 mGy.

Radiotherapy is, therefore, contraindicated for pelvic malignancies. For other tumors, it may be given whenever doses to the fetus are below 100 mGy at any POG. The estimated fetal dose exposure should be calculated as per the AAPM guidelines. The care plan should be customized for each patient by joint decision-making of a radiation oncologist, medical physicist, and the patient herself.

Surgery[16-18]

Surgery for malignant tumors can be performed in all trimesters, although the second trimester is preferred, especially for abdominal malignancies. Surgical intervention in the first trimester carries the risk of miscarriage, while the risk of preterm delivery should be explained in the third trimester.

Preanesthetic Evaluation

Detailed history of cancer as well as pregnancy-related symptoms and other comorbidities. Ongoing medications and neoadjuvant chemotherapy should be asked. Postchemotherapy two-dimensional (2D) ECHO can be done to rule out chemotherapy-related cardiac toxicity, especially when doxorubicin and cyclophosphamide have been administered. Preoperative examination by an obstetrician is mandatory. The risk–benefit ratio of undergoing cancer surgery is weighed with fetal and maternal well-being. The same is discussed with the patient and appropriate written informed consent is taken. Considering the risk of difficult airway and aspiration, preoperative aspiration prophylaxis using nonparticulate antacid should be given.

INTRAOPERATIVE MANAGEMENT

Premedication

Verbal reassurance instead of preanesthetic premedication can be given.

The following aspects should be borne in mind whenever caring for a pregnant patient undergoing surgery.

- *General anesthetic goals:* The general principle of avoiding hypoxia, hypercarbia, and acidosis, maintenance of normothermia, and adequate uteroplacental perfusion throughout the intraoperative period are important.
- *Fetal monitoring:* The American College of Obstetricians and Gynecologists (ACOG) recommends the fetal heart rate (FHR) measurement using the Doppler ultrasound

before and after any surgery irrespective of gestational age. They recommend monitoring of attraction also in a viable fetus.[19]

- *Multidisciplinary team:* A team of obstetricians and neonatologists should be notified to intervene in the event of abnormal intraoperative FHR. The plan of management in such a scenario arise, should be discussed with the patient as well in the preoperative period.
- *Preoperative fasting:* Standard preoperative fasting guidelines of 6–8 hours for solids and 2 hours for clear liquids. The administration of H2 antagonist and nonparticulate antacid should be individualized.[20]
- *Positioning:* A 30° left lateral tilt is preferred to the supine position.
- *Airway:* Preparedness for the possibility of a difficult airway in a pregnant patient needs no emphasis. The airway changes described in **Table 3** can cause intubation to become difficult and desaturation occurs sooner compared to nonpregnant individuals. So, a difficult airway cart with smaller endotracheal tubes (ETTs), airway adjuncts such as oropharyngeal, nasopharyngeal airway, stylet, bougie, and smaller-sized tubes is highly recommended. Preoxygenation with 100% oxygen for 5 minutes followed by rapid sequence induction and intubation with cricoid pressure is recommended.[21]
- *Intraoperative analgesia:* Analgesia can be provided using opioid analgesics such as fentanyl and morphine safely, especially when pregnancy is expected to continue. Nonsteroidal anti-inflammatory drugs (NSAIDs) although best avoided, may be used in sporadic doses with the exception of paracetamol, which is safe. Multimodal analgesia using systemic plus regional techniques is recommended.
- *Anesthetic drugs and placental transfer to fetus:* As previously stated in **Table 2**, transfer of anesthetic drugs to the fetus is impacted by the molecular weight of the drug, the extent of its protein binding, pKa (pH at which the drug is 50% ionized), and plasma protein binding. The transfer of drugs across the placenta can also be categorized in **Table 4**. The molecular and placental transfer characteristics of common anesthesia drugs are mentioned in **Table 5**.
- *Volatile anesthetic agents*: Pregnancy reduces the minimum alveolar concentration of volatile agents.

TABLE 4: Types of placental transfer of drugs.[22]

Type 1	*Complete transfer:* Rapidly crosses the placenta with high maternal and fetal concentrations	Thiopentone
Type 2	*Exceeding transfer:* They reach higher concentrations in fetal blood as compared to maternal blood	Ketamine
Type 3	*Incomplete transfer:* Achievement of greater concentration in maternal blood than fetal blood due to their inability to cross placenta	Succinylcholine

TABLE 5: Molecular and placental transfer characteristics of common anesthetic drugs.[22]

Drug	***Molecule characteristics***	***Placental transfer***
Induction agents: • Propofol • Thiopentone	 • Lipid soluble • Lipid soluble, weak acid, and 75% albumin bound	 • Yes • Yes
Opioids: • Fentanyl • Morphine	 • Lipid soluble • Less lipid soluble, low protein binding	 • Yes • Yes
Neuromuscular blockers	Poorly lipid soluble, large ionized molecules	No
Volatile agents	Low molecular weight, highly lipid soluble	Yes
Local anesthetic agents • Lignocaine • Bupivacaine	 • Low protein binding, less lipid soluble • More lipid soluble, more protein binding • Both lignocaine and bupivacaine can cause "ion trapping" in fetus in the presence of acidosis	 • Yes • Yes
Benzodiazepines	Lipid soluble, unionized	Yes
Neostigmine	Quaternary compound, small molecule	Yes
• Glycopyrrolate	• Quaternary compound, fully ionized	• No
• Atropine	• Lipid-soluble tertiary amine	• Yes

They augment uterine relaxation, and high MAC levels can cause hypotension.

- *Neuromuscular blocking agents (NMBs):* NMBs can cross the placenta in small amounts. There may be reduced levels of plasma cholinesterase and thus use of neuromuscular monitoring to guide the muscle relaxant dose is recommended.
- *Regional anesthesia techniques* like epidural analgesia and peripheral nerve blocks have the added advantage of better perioperative pain control and reduced requirement of systemic analgesics.
- *Extubation:* It is advisable to extubate the patient once fully awake and at a train of four ratio (TOF) > 0.9.
- *Deep venous thrombosis* (DVT)*:* Pregnancy being a hypercoagulable state predisposes to DVT and thromboembolism. This risk is augmented with immobility in the perioperative period. DVT prophylaxis can prevent this risk.

Perioperative Analgesia

Perioperative analgesia can be provided by the use of regional analgesia techniques like epidural or regional nerve block. The use of NSAIDs is avoided for fear of fetal adverse effects like the risk of neural tube defects, cleft lip/palate, or other structural limb defects when administered in the first trimester. Administering NSAIDs in the third trimester is associated with premature closure of ductus arteriosus and pulmonary hypertension.[23]

Laparoscopic Surgery Versus Laparotomy[24,25]

Laparotomy requires a midline vertical incision. The laparoscopic approach required careful placement of ports to avoid injury to the gravid uterus. Intra-abdominal pressure should be kept at 10–13 mm Hg with minimum procedure time with maximum expertise. It is technically challenging to perform laparoscopic surgery in a gravid uterus >26–28 weeks of gestation, so an open approach is preferred.

Surgery and Risk of Preterm Labor[21]

Surgical intervention in the third trimester and procedures involving manipulation of the uterus can predispose the patient to go into preterm labor. Prophylactic tocolytics are therefore advised for 48 hours in the above scenario. Other agents like volatile anesthetics, magnesium sulfate, and beta-agonist agents also relax the uterus.

SPECIFIC CANCERS IN PREGNANCY

Breast Cancer[1,16,18,26]

Pregnancy-associated breast cancer (PABC) is the most common among pregnancy-associated cancers and accounts for 0.2–3.8% of breast cancers. It is seen to occur in 1 in 3,000 to 1 in 10,000 pregnant women. The age of presentation is usually around 20 weeks POG. Owing to pregnancy-related breast changes, the condition is often diagnosed late and at an advanced stage. These tumors are usually hormone receptor negative and HER2 positive indicative of a bad prognosis. Anthracycline-based regimes that include adriamycin, epirubicin, cyclophosphamide, and fluorouracil can be used safely, whereas trastuzumab is contraindicated. Patients may come for modified radical mastectomy, breast-conservative therapy, or mastectomy with breast reconstruction surgery.

Ovarian Cancer[5,8,13,27]

Around 1–3% of adnexal masses of pregnancy are malignant. Among these, germ cell tumors are most common. Diagnosis is usually made by abdominal or transvaginal ultrasound. Tumor markers such as CA 125, AFP, and beta-hCG are unreliable in pregnancy. Both chemotherapy with carboplatin or paclitaxel and surgery are recommended in the second trimester and before 37 weeks of gestation. Disease prognosis is the same as that of nonpregnant females.

Cervical Cancer[27,28]

The management of cervical cancer differs from that in nonpregnant patients because radical surgery and radiotherapy to the pelvis are not possible during pregnancy. Early-stage cancers can be treated after delivery while radical surgery if needed can be done in the same setting as the cesarean section.

Ovarian Cancer

Germ cell tumors and sex cord stromal tumors are the tumor types commonly encountered during pregnancy. Early stages can be offered surgical treatment in the second or third trimesters via laparoscopic or open approach. Paclitaxel/carboplatin chemotherapy is recommended. Vaginal delivery is preferred in early-stage cancers. Oncological outcomes are similar to nonpregnant women.

Lymphoma[10,29]

Hodgkin's lymphoma (HL) and non-Hodgkin's lymphoma (NHL) form 6% and 5% of cancers occurring during pregnancy. The outcome is usually favorable for both mother and fetus, with a rare need to terminate the pregnancy. Classical HL (cHL) is the most common subtype diagnosed during pregnancy. HL is managed with the ABVD (adriamycin, bleomycin, vinblastine, and dacarbazine) regime that can be used safely during the second and third trimesters. Chemotherapy regime R-CHOP (rituximab, cyclophosphamide, doxorubicin, vincristine, and prednisone) is the standard of care for NHL.

Melanoma[30,31]

Melanomas are aggressive skin cancers. It has been suggested that melanomas associated with pregnancy may have a worse prognosis. Melanomas may be mistaken for normal pregnancy-related increased pigmentation causing a delay in diagnosis. There is increased lymphangiogenesis, increased pregnancy-associated plasma protein A (PAPP-A), and increased levels of growth factors of pregnancy all of which may interact and promote the growth and metastases of melanomas in pregnancy. Surgical intervention can be safely performed in the second trimester.

CONCLUSION

The diagnosis and management of cancer during pregnancy require a multidisciplinary team approach keeping in mind that the patient's preference should be the primary guiding principle for management.

REFERENCES

1. Sorouri K, Loren AW, Amant F, Partridge AH. Patient-centered care in the management of cancer during pregnancy. Am Soc Clin Oncol Educ Book. 2023;43:e100037.
2. Cottreau CM, Dashevsky I, Andrade SE, Li DK, Nekhlyudov L, Raebel MA, et al. Pregnancy-Associated Cancer: A U.S. Population-Based Study. J Womens Health (Larchmt). 2019;28(2):250-257. doi: 10.1089/jwh.2018.6962.
3. Andersson TM, Johansson AL, Fredriksson I, Lambe M. Cancer during pregnancy and the postpartum period: a population-based study. Cancer. 2015;121(12):2072-7.
4. de Haan J, Vandecaveye V, Han SN, Van de Vijver KK, Amant F. Difficulties with diagnosis of malignancies in pregnancy. Best Pract Res Clin Obstet Gynaecol. 2016; 33:19-32.
5. Hepner A, Negrini D, Hase EA, Exman P, Testa L, Trinconi AF, et al. Cancer during pregnancy: the oncologist overview. World J Oncol. 2019;10(1):28-34.
6. Frisch A, Walter TC, Hamm B, Denecke T. Efficacy of oral contrast agents for upper gastrointestinal signal suppression in MRCP: a systematic review of the literature. Acta Radiol Open. 2017;6(9):2058460117727315.
7. Amant F, Han SN, Gziri MM, Vandenbroucke T, Verheecke M, Van Calsteren K. Management of cancer in pregnancy. Best Prac Res Clin Obstet Gynaecol. 2015;29(5):741-53.
8. Cubillo A, Morales S, Goñi E, Matute F, Muñoz JL, Pérez-Díaz D, et al. Multidisciplinary consensus on cancer management during pregnancy. Clin Transl Oncol. 2021;23(6):1054-66.
9. Bourjeily G, Chalhoub M, Phornphutkul C, Alleyne TC, Woodfield CA, Chen KK. Neonatal thyroid function: effect of a single exposure to iodinated contrast medium in utero. Radiology. 2010;256(3):744-50.
10. Maggen C, Wolters VERA, Van Calsteren K, Cardonick E, Laenen A, Heimovaara JH, et al; International Network on Cancer, Infertility and Pregnancy (INCIP). Impact of chemotherapy during pregnancy on fetal growth. J Matern Fetal Neonatal Med. 2022;35(26):10314-23.
11. Kruer MC, Steiner RD. The role of evidence-based medicine and clinical trials in rare genetic disorders. Clin Genet. 2008;74(3):197-207.
12. van Gerwen M, Maggen C, Cardonick E, Verwaaijen EJ, van den Heuvel-Eibrink M, Shmakov RG, et al; International Network on Cancer, Infertility and Pregnancy. Association of chemotherapy timing in pregnancy with congenital malformation. JAMA Netw Open. 2021;4(6):e2113180.
13. Mukhopadhyay A, Shinde A, Naik R. Ovarian cysts and cancer in pregnancy. Best Pract Res Clin Obstet Gynaecol. 2016;33:58-72.
14. Fagerstrom JM. Radiation oncology department policy development for patients who may become pregnant. J Appl Clin Med Phys. 2024;25:e14256.
15. Yoon I, Slesinger TL. (2024). Radiation exposure in pregnancy. Treasure Island (FL): StatPearls Publishing. [online] Available from https://www.ncbi.nlm.nih.gov/books/NBK551690/ [Last accessed March, 2025].
16. Eskandari A, Alipour S. Aspects of anesthesia for breast surgery during pregnancy. In: Alipour S, Omranipour R (Eds). Diseases of the Breast during Pregnancy and Lactation [Internet]. Cham: Springer International Publishing; 2020. pp. 107-14. (Advances in Experimental Medicine and Biology; vol. 1252). Available from http://link.springer.com/10.1007/978-3-030-41596-9_14 [Last accessed March, 2025].
17. Auron M, Duran Castillo MY, Garcia OFD. Perioperative management of pregnant women undergoing nonobstetric surgery. CCJM. 2021;88(1):27-34.
18. Sawada A, Sotome S, Kusakai M, Yamakage M. Successful anesthetic management for total mastectomy in a pregnant woman using general anesthesia combined with continuous erector spinae plane block: a case report. JA Clin Rep. 2019;5(1):23.

19. ACOG Committee. Opinion No. 775: nonobstetric surgery during pregnancy. Obstet Gynecol. 2019;133:e285e6.
20. Brakke BD, Sviggum HP. Anaesthesia for non-obstetric surgery during pregnancy. BJA Educ. 2023;23(3):78-83.
21. Upadya M, Saneesh PJ. Anaesthesia for non-obstetric surgery during pregnancy. Indian J Anaesth. 2016;60(4):234-41.
22. Griffiths SK, Campbell JP. Placental structure, function and drug transfer. Contin Edu Anaesth Crit Care Pain. 2015;15(2):84-9.
23. Koren G, Florescu A, Costei AM, Boskovic R, Moretti ME. Nonsteroidal antiinflammatory drugs during third trimester and the risk of premature closure of the ductus arteriosus: a meta-analysis. Ann Pharmacother. 2006;40(5):824-9.
24. Michos G, Dagklis T, Papanikolaou E, Peitsidis NI, Kalogiannidis IA, Mamopoulos AM, et al. Laparoscopy in pregnancy: a comparative review of national guidelines. Cureus. 2023;15(5):e38904.
25. Haggerty E, Daly J. Anaesthesia and non-obstetric surgery in pregnancy. BJA Educ. 2021;21(2):42-3.
26. Liberale V, Tripodi E, Ottino L, Biglia N. Surgery on breast cancer in pregnancy. Transl Cancer Res. 2019;8(S5):S493-502.
27. Zagouri F, Dimitrakakis C, Marinopoulos S, Tsigginou A, Dimopoulos MA. Cancer in pregnancy: disentangling treatment modalities. ESMO Open. 2016;1(3):e000016.
28. Peccatori FA, Azim HA Jr, Orecchia R, Hoekstra HJ, Pavlidis N, Kesic V, et al.; ESMO Guidelines Working Group. Cancer, pregnancy and fertility: ESMO Clinical Practice Guidelines for diagnosis, treatment and follow-up. Ann Oncol. 2013;24 Suppl 6:vi160-70.
29. Pinnix CC, Andraos TY, Milgrom S, Fanale MA. The management of lymphoma in the setting of pregnancy. Curr Hematol Malig Rep. 2017;12(3):251-6.
30. Still R, Brennecke S. Melanoma in pregnancy. Obstet Med. 2017;10(3):107-12.
31. Carter TJ, George C, Harwood C, Nathan P. Melanoma in pregnancy: diagnosis and management in early-stage and advanced disease. Eur J Cancer. 2022;166:240-53.

CHAPTER 74

Artificial Intelligence in Onco-Anesthesia and Critical Care

Sohan Lal Solanki, Ashwini Rane

INTRODUCTION

Artificial intelligence (AI) is a field of computer science focused on creating systems or machines that can perform tasks typically requiring human intelligence. These tasks include reasoning, problem-solving, understanding natural language, recognizing patterns, and decision-making. The renowned computer scientist John McCarthy created the field of AI in 1956, defining it as science and engineering of making intelligent machines.[1] Since the advent of AI technologies, their utility has been demonstrated across multiple domains, including modern medicine. Current medical practice increasingly relies on advanced mathematical techniques and computational analyses, encompassing data mining, decision support systems, evidence-based practices, robotic interventions, and diagnostic processes. The complexity of AI can affect physicians' comprehension and interpretation of the results.[2] Therefore, it is important to educate physicians. Physicians should also be involved while applying machine learning (ML) algorithms.

Artificial intelligence systems use various techniques, including ML (where systems learn from data and improve over time), deep learning (a subset of ML involving neural networks with many layers), and natural language processing (NLP; which focuses on the interaction between computers and human languages).[3]

Machine learning is a subset of AI, which provides machines the ability to learn automatically and improve from the data pattern analysis. It is a computer program that can learn how to produce behavior not explicitly programmed by the author. Deep learning is a subset of ML, which uses a multilayer neural network to solve complex problems. Deep learning utilizes unstructured data to learn[4] **(Fig. 1)**.

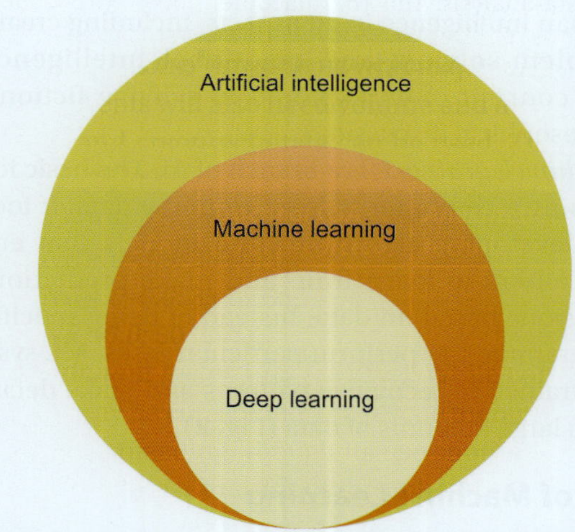

Fig. 1: Hierarchical representation of artificial intelligence, machine learning, and deep learning.

The application of AI within the medical field spans from diagnostic tasks in radiology[5] and pathology[6] to therapeutic and interventional procedures in cardiology. In the field of anesthesiology, AI holds promise for significantly improving various facets of patient care, including preoperative assessment, intraoperative management, postoperative recovery, and critical care.[7]

Onco-anesthesia presents unique challenges due to the complexity and variability of cancer-related conditions and treatments. The integration of AI in anesthesiology marks its importance in terms of optimization of patient's outcomes through enhanced predictive analytics, real-time monitoring, and personalized treatment strategies.

Incorporating AI into anesthesia not only enhances patient safety and care but also supports anesthesiologists by providing valuable insights, improving decision-making, and optimizing workflows. As the technology continues to advance, the integration of AI in anesthesia is likely to become increasingly sophisticated and beneficial. Therefore, basic knowledge of AI is necessary in this modern era of ML.

STAGES OF ARTIFICIAL INTELLIGENCE

- *Narrow AI:* This is the most common type of AI. It is designed to perform a specific task. Common examples include Siri, Alexa, and face recognition in computer and mobile.
- *General AI:* This is a theoretical form of AI that would have the ability to understand, learn, and apply intelligence across a wide range of tasks, similar to human capabilities. General AI does not exist yet and is a topic of ongoing research.
- *Super AI:* This is a hypothetical AI that would surpass human intelligence in all aspects, including creativity, problem-solving, and emotional intelligence. It is a concept often explored in science fiction and philosophical discussions.
- *Machine learning:* It is a branch of AI. The basic idea is training a computer to learn from the data. It focuses on developing algorithms and models that enable computers to learn from and make predictions or decisions based on data. Instead of being specifically programmed to perform particular tasks, ML systems are trained to recognize patterns and make decisions from large amounts of data **(Fig. 2)**.[8]

Types of Machine Learning

Based on the data submitted to the computer, ML is divided into the following types:

- *Supervised:* The machine is fed with labeled data. It involves training data set and test data set. The machine analyzes the training data and relates it to the given outcome. Based on the available data, the machine creates the algorithms to map the labeled input to the given output. Test data is used to validate the algorithm's performance. An example includes Kendale et al.[9] who conducted a supervised learning study on electronic health record data with the goal of identifying patients who experienced postinduction hypotension with a target mean BP of 50 mm Hg. The training data set included 70% of the patients with variables such as the American Society of Anesthesiologists (ASA) physical status, age, body mass index, comorbidities, and medications as well as the blood pressures of the patients. The test data set of 30% was used to analyze to assess how accurately the algorithm could predict postinduction hypotension. Further external validation can also be done by using a new set of data from other sources.
- *Unsupervised:* The system is supplied with unlabeled data without a predetermined objective. The machine tries to find patterns or groupings. The machine analyzes the data to understand and discover the output. This type of learning is useful to classify the data.
- *Reinforcement:* Based on the trial-and-error method, the system is placed in the environment and learns how to behave in the surroundings, by performing certain actions. It is a reward-based learning, e.g., to deliver the intravenous (IV) propofol based on the patient's bispectral index (BIS) and mean arterial pressure (MAP).

Machine Learning Problem

Machine learning includes a wide range of problems that can be addressed using various algorithms and techniques. Common ML problems can be classification, regression, clustering, NLP, image recognition, and recommendation systems. Each of these ML problems requires specific algorithms and techniques tailored to the nature of the data and the task at hand. Solutions typically involve selecting the right model, training it with relevant data, and evaluating its performance to ensure that it meets the desired goals.[10]

Deep Learning

Deep learning involves training neural networks with multiple layers to learn from data. These models are designed to automatically learn and improve from experience without particular instruction for every task. The core concept of deep learning involves neural network. It consists of multiple layers of interconnected neurons where each node processes the information and passes it to the subsequent node (neuron).[4,10]

Layers of Deep Learning

- *Input layer:* Receives the raw data

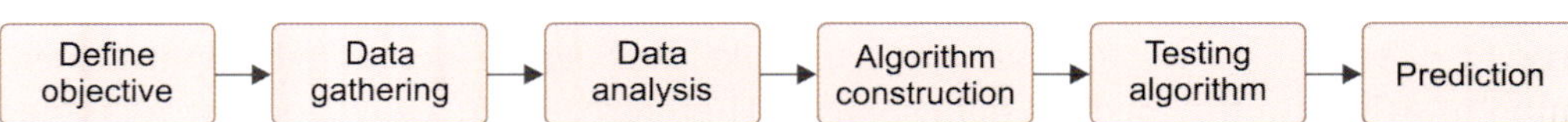

Fig. 2: Steps involved in machine learning.

- *Hidden layers:* Intermediate layers where computations are performed. Each hidden layer extracts increasingly abstract features from the data.
- *Output layer:* Produces the final prediction or classification

Models of Deep Learning

- *Convolutional neural networks (CNNs):* These can analyze imaging data related to anesthesia procedures, such as identifying anatomical landmarks or assessing the quality of ultrasound images used for nerve block guidance.
- *Recurrent neural networks (RNNs):* Time series data: RNNs, particularly with long short-term memory (LSTM) cells, can analyze time series data from patient monitoring systems. This includes predicting anesthesia-related events or complications by analyzing sequences of vital signs and other continuous monitoring data.
- *LSTM networks:* These are used to predict patient responses to anesthesia by modeling temporal dependencies in vital signs and drug administration data. This can help in predicting adverse events or optimizing drug dosages over time and forecasting potential complications or changes in patient condition during surgery based on historical data.
- *NLP:* Extracting relevant information from unstructured clinical notes and reports related to anesthesia and perioperative care

APPLICATION OF ARTIFICIAL INTELLIGENCE IN ANESTHESIA

It can be divided into three main domains:

1. Preoperative anesthesia
2. Intraoperative management
3. Risk prediction and prediction of events, e.g., predict surgery length or postoperative complications

Preoperative Anesthesia

- *Preoperative anesthesia checkup:* The preoperative assessment is a crucial aspect of onco-anesthesia management. With the recent developments in AI, it can now play a significant role in the preoperative evaluation process. AI technologies can aid anesthesiologists in screening, risk assessment, and creating patient-specific anesthesia plans. One such application is a smart anesthesia tool, powered by AI, which analyzes patient data, identifies potential preoperative concerns, and provides an ASA classification along with up-to-date recommendations for further assessment.[11]

  Additionally, airway assessment using AI involves evaluating facial features, speech features, and body habitus.[12]
- *Preoperative investigations:* The integration of AI into the imaging of tumor pathology aids in determining the operability of tumors. For example, AI-driven imaging of the biliary system and hepatic tumors can help predict postoperative liver function impairment.[13]
- *Risk prediction in the preoperative period:* Recently, the ML model has been developed to predict postoperative in-hospital mortality by evaluating the preoperative risk factor.[14] It includes large data from the hospital record from preoperative comorbidities, investigations, type of surgery, postoperative course, and investigations.

Intraoperative Management

- *Induction:* Mechanical robots are being developed for a range of medical procedures, including intubation, ventilation, and nerve blocks, though these applications are still being evaluated. While numerous mechanical robots have been tested on mannequins, multicenter trials are essential to fully assess their clinical effectiveness. The integration of AI into anesthesia induction and maintenance dates back to the 1990s with the creation of the "Diprifusor" system, which utilizes AI for the target-controlled infusion of propofol.[15]
- *Anesthesia drug delivery:* AI has the potential to enhance anesthesia delivery by optimizing the dosage and administration of anesthetic agents tailored to individual patient characteristics and surgical needs. Examples of AI applications in anesthesia include personalized anesthetic plans, automated dose adjustments, closed-loop anesthesia delivery systems, and automated drug administration.[16] These automated anesthesia systems require two key inputs:
  1. A measurement of the depth of anesthesia, which can be assessed using scores or surrogate measures based on EEG or other clinical parameters
  2. A target sedation level set by the user

  Several studies have explored methods to control drug delivery to achieve a specific BIS value, utilizing either simple pharmacokinetic

TABLE 1: Examples of AI mode and their functions in medical applications.

AI system	*Function*
McSleepy[15]	Simultaneously balances hypnosis, analgesia, and neuromuscular block
SEDASYS[17]	Propofol infusion for mild-to-moderate sedation
Models for vasopressor titration[18]	Automatic titration of vasopressor according to NIBP, SV, and SVV
Da Vinci surgical system[19]	First to be used for fiberoptic intubations
Kepler intubation system[20]	Robotic arm-guided intubation
IntuBot[21]	Audio–visual-based navigation system for intubation

(AI: artificial intelligence; NIBP: noninvasive blood pressure; SV: stroke volume; SVV: stroke volume variation)

models or advanced ML techniques, including reinforcement learning.[22,23] Additionally, ML-based control systems have been developed to automate neuromuscular blockade delivery.[24]

Several other pharmacological models using AI have been introduced for delivering anesthesia and other drugs, as shown in **Table 1**.

- *Monitoring of depth of anesthesia:* Maintaining adequate depth of anesthesia is crucial as it may lead to either awareness or hemodynamic instability. The BIS was the first index approved by the FDA to measure the depth of anesthesia.[25] AI offers a comprehensive assessment of the depth of anesthesia and level of consciousness through sophisticated data analysis and integration of multiple physiological signals. While most studies have focused on the BIS and electroencephalography (EEG), other clinical signals have also been explored in the context of anesthesia depth monitoring such as midlatency auditory evoked potential.[26] The heart rate variability is used to assess the sedation level in critical care.[27] However, while AI's potential is significant, the evidence supporting its benefits in clinical outcomes is still evolving. Ramaswamy et al. evaluated the clinical utility of ML to assess the level of sedation, and they found that it gives a clinically useful, unbiased estimation of the level of sedation with low interindividual variability.[28]
- *Automated fluid therapy:* Fluid therapy poses unique challenges when compared to other measures such as heart rate or blood pressure, as the "optimal" fluid status is not clearly defined or easily assessed.[24] Despite these difficulties, algorithms can be developed to closely replicate how clinicians administer fluids, especially when guided by established protocols.[29] Numerous human trials utilizing a closed-loop, goal-directed fluid therapy algorithm have demonstrated increased adherence to protocols, reduced hospital stays, and fewer postoperative complications in major surgery patients.[30,31] Various teams worldwide are actively developing closed-loop fluid resuscitation algorithms. Additionally, early efforts are underway to integrate fluid resuscitation with other common resuscitation drugs, such as vasopressors. Currently, two commercially available devices, Concert and NeuroWave, are on the market.
- *Automated titration of vasopressors:* Closed-loop vasopressor controllers have also been studied in patients undergoing major abdominal surgeries. They found that events of intraoperative hypotension were less with the automated system as compared to doctors managing hemodynamic.[32] Another randomized controlled trial (RCT) of intraoperative hypotension in patients undergoing abdominal and orthopedic surgeries was divided into a computer-assisted individualized hemodynamic group and a manually adjusted goal-directed fluid therapy group. The incidence of hypotension was lower in the computer-assisted group than in the manually adjusted group.[33] Both studies included small sample sizes and were single-centered; results were difficult to extrapolate to other surgeries. Evidence for automated vasopressor titration in clinical stings is very few. Management of intraoperative hemodynamic also includes cardiac output monitoring with simultaneous fluid management. Libert and colleagues developed and tested a closed-loop system that can coadminister vasopressors and fluids with good performance metrics.[34] Arterial pressure management, while complex and multifactorial, has great promise as a subject for automated management because of the known link to poor outcomes.

Risk and Event Prediction

The "reactive, proactive, and predictive levels approach" is an innovative risk management model in ML that was proposed recently to apply in anesthesia. It introduces distinct practices that can be tailored to manage patient

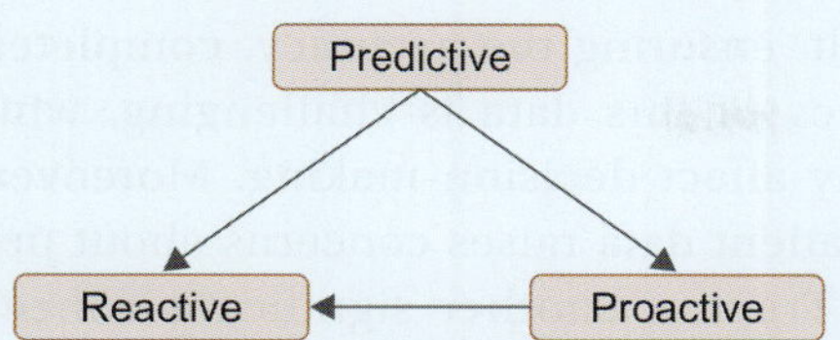

Fig. 3: Patient risk management practice.

risks effectively at every stage of care.[35] By incorporating ML, this approach enhances anesthesia practice through continuous risk assessment **(Fig. 3)**.

- In the *reactive phase*, ML helps anesthesiologists respond to immediate complications as they arise during anesthesia.
- In the *proactive phase*, ML tools anticipate potential risks before they manifest, allowing the anesthesiologist to take preventive action.
- In the *predictive phase*, the advanced data analysis predicts potential complications before they occur, helping the medical team act pre-emptively with more precision. By combining these three phases—reactive, proactive, and predictive—along with the power of ML, anesthesiologists can continuously adapt their strategies to safeguard patient's well-being, ensuring that risks are minimized throughout the perioperative journey. This integrated approach ultimately leads to safer anesthesia practices and better patient outcomes.
    - A hypotension prediction algorithm generates a "hypotension prediction index" (HPI), which assigns a value from 0 to 100 based on the severity of the risk. It can effectively forecast hypotension 10–15 minutes before it becomes clinically evident by analyzing subtle hemodynamic changes in arterial waveforms that precede the onset of hypotension. This concept was introduced by Hatib and colleagues.[36] Various studies have been conducted to validate this algorithm.[37,38] Gangakhedkar et al. reported on the use of HPI in patients undergoing oncological surgeries, such as cytoreductive surgery (CRS) combined with hyperthermic intraperitoneal chemotherapy (HIPEC), finding it beneficial.[39] Additionally, Lee et al. performed a retrospective observational analysis involving data from 3,301 patients. They employed deep learning algorithms to make real-time predictions of imminent intraoperative hypotensive events at 5, 10, and 15 minutes by utilizing biosignal waveforms in noncardiac surgical contexts.[40]
    - *Other perioperative events:* Various AI models have been developed to predict perioperative event prediction, such as perioperative cardiovascular complications risk, pulmonary complications, intraoperative hypoxemia,[41] renal complications such as acute kidney injury (AKI), postoperative mortality,[42] and 30-day postoperative mortality.[43]

ARTIFICIAL INTELLIGENCE IN CRITICAL CARE

The application of AI in critical care is still under evaluation due to the "black box" nature of ML. The "black box" nature in AI refers to the lack of transparency in how ML models, especially complex ones such as deep learning, make decisions. In these systems, the decision-making process is not easily understandable or interpretable by humans. While there have been small-scale studies incorporating AI in the monitoring of critically ill patients, several AI applications in critical care include disease diagnosis, mortality risk prediction, disease progression forecasting, length of hospital stay prediction, and assisting in clinical decision-making.

Diagnosis in Critical Care

Brown et al. considered automated endotracheal tube placement check with the use of deep neural network (DNN) as a point of care in the intensive care unit (ICU). This study confirms the verification of endotracheal tube placement and appropriate placement of the tube, making it a promising development for clinical practice, especially in high-pressure environments where accurate tube placement is crucial.[44]

Artificial intelligence helps clinicians to diagnose conditions for which the patient has landed up in critical care, by utilizing investigations and images provided for ML. CNN has been evolved to evaluate the patient with head injury which is otherwise difficult to evaluate by a manual method from computed tomography of the brain.[45] Application of ML by the reinforcement learning approach in critical care has been used to develop an algorithm that helps to identify electrolyte abnormalities, guides whether the correction is needed, and how it should be done.[46]

Prediction of Critical Events and Mortality

Machine learning can be used to predict critical events in health care, helping to prevent them and reduce their adverse effects. For example, a study demonstrated that

AI and ML could predict tachycardia occurring up to 75 minutes before the onset of shock.[47] Prediction of hypotension in critical care patients has been already discovered by using the random forest model and logistic regression in ML with almost 92.7% sensitivity.[48] Another study applies the random forest model of ML in critical care which predicts cardiorespiratory instability 90 minutes before the actual occurrence.[49] Several other studies have been published in recent years to predict acute renal failure in burn patients[50] and general population in critical care,[51] populations at risk of developing *Clostridium difficile* infections,[52] and fluid responsiveness after fluid administration.[53]

Several models have been introduced to predict critical care mortality which are more accurate than the standard scoring system in ICU (APACHE, SOFA).[54,55] The design of these models is complex to understand and yet to be studied prospectively; therefore, they are not in clinical use.

Mechanical Ventilation

Several studies have shown that the ML model can detect patient–ventilator asynchrony by observing changes in pressure and flow signals.[56] Ventilator asynchrony can be predicted by monitoring airway signals with the help of Hidden Markov models.[57] Hidden Markov model is a statistical model, which analyze the unobserved (hidden) data and develops the predictive system.

Complex Decision-Making in Critical Care

Reinforcement learning in ML can be utilized to offer individualized treatment to the diverse nature of septic shock and varying host response.[58] AI can also monitor a series of electrocardiograms (ECGs) and help in the diagnosis of coronary events in critical care.[59]

To predict the length of ICU stay and readmission, several large-scale studies have been performed to create an algorithm that will predict the length of hospital stay with accuracy.[60] The model for risk of readmission to the ICU was developed from the MIMIC III (Medical Information Mart for Intensive Care) database.[61]

Limitations of Artificial Intelligence

While AI shows promise and innovation in the fields of anesthesia and critical care, it is not without its challenges. One major issue is that its effectiveness relies heavily on data, which can be difficult to manage and maintain. As a result, ensuring the accuracy, completeness, and consistency of this data is challenging, which could potentially affect decision-making. Moreover, feeding AI with patient data raises concerns about privacy and security. Trust is another significant concern, given the "black box" nature of AI and the possibility of AI hallucinations.

Furthermore, over-reliance on AI could lead to skill degradation in anesthesiologists, making it more difficult for them to respond effectively when AI systems fail or are faced with situations beyond their capabilities. Accountability for incorrect recommendations could lead to harm to patients. There are substantial risks and unknowns involved. To fully leverage the benefits of AI while safeguarding both patient and clinician safety, more research is needed—especially focusing on human factors and qualitative aspects of AI tool design and integration into clinical workflows.

CONCLUSION

Artificial intelligence has great potential to improve care in both onco-anesthesia and critical care. It can help tailor anesthesia plans for cancer patients more accurately and improve decision-making in critical situations. AI can also predict risks and detect problems early in critical care, allowing for quicker interventions and better outcomes. While challenges remain, such as understanding how AI makes its decisions, continued research and testing will help unlock its full potential. As AI technology advances, it will become a valuable tool in improving patient care in these important areas.

REFERENCES

1. McCarthy J. Applications of circumscription to formalizing common-sense knowledge. Artif Intell. 1986;28(1):89-116.
2. Azar AT, El-Metwally SM. Decision tree classifiers for automated medical diagnosis. Neural Comput Appl. 2013;23:2387-403.
3. Mitchell TM. Machine Learning, Vol. 1. New York: McGraw Hill; 1997.
4. Bini SA. Artificial intelligence, machine learning, deep learning, and cognitive computing: what do these terms mean and how will they impact health care? J Arthroplasty. 2018;33(8):2358-61.
5. Huang P, Lin CT, Li Y, Tammemagi MC, Brock MV, Atkar-Khattra S, et al. Prediction of lung cancer risk at follow-up screening with low-dose CT: a training and validation study of a deep learning method. Lancet Digit Heal. 2019;1(7):e353-62.

6. Bera K, Schalper KA, Rimm DL, Velcheti V, Madabhushi A. Artificial intelligence in digital pathology—new tools for diagnosis and precision oncology. Nat Rev Clin Oncol. 2019;16(11):703-15.
7. Hashimoto DA, Witkowski E, Gao L, Meireles O, Rosman G. Artificial intelligence in anesthesiology: current techniques, clinical applications, and limitations. Anesthesiology. 2020;132(2):379-94.
8. He J, Baxter SL, Xu J, Xu J, Zhou X, Zhang K. The practical implementation of artificial intelligence technologies in medicine. Nat Med. 2019;25(1):30-6.
9. Kendale S, Kulkarni P, Rosenberg AD, Wang J. Supervised machine-learning predictive analytics for prediction of postinduction hypotension. Anesthesiology. 2018;129(4): 675-88.
10. Sarker IH. Machine learning: algorithms, real-world applications and research directions. SN Comput Sci. 2021;2(3):160.
11. Alekberli T, Alekberli FR, Mimouni C, Muhammed AA. Smart-anesthesia application with artificial intelligence for a preoperative evaluation of patients. J Res Innov Anesth. 2020;5(1):21-2.
12. Xia M. Artificial intelligence in airway management. In: Xia M, Jiang H (Eds). Artificial Intelligence in Anesthesiology. Singapore: Springer; 2023. pp. 41-54.
13. Xie A, Fang C, Huang Y, Fan Y, Pan J, Peng F. Application of three-dimensional reconstruction and visible simulation technique in reoperation of hepatolithiasis. J Gastroenterol Hepatol. 2013;28(2):248-54.
14. Graeßner M, Jungwirth B, Frank E, Schaller SJ, Kochs E, Ulm K, et al. Enabling personalized perioperative risk prediction by using a machine-learning model based on preoperative data. Sci Rep. 2023;13(1):7128.
15. Glen JB. The development of 'Diprifusor': a TCI system for propofol. Anaesthesia. 1998;53:13-21.
16. Liberman MY, Ching S, Chemali J, Brown EN. A closed-loop anesthetic delivery system for real-time control of burst suppression. J Neural Eng. 2013;10(4):46004.
17. Hoskins SL, Elgjo GI, Lu J, Ying H, Grady JJ, Herndon DN, et al. Closed-loop resuscitation of burn shock. J Burn Care Res. 2006;27(3):377-85.
18. Joosten A, Delaporte A, Alexander B, Su F, Creteur J, Vincent JL, et al. Automated titration of vasopressor infusion using a closed-loop controller: in vivo feasibility study using a swine model. Anesthesiology. 2019;130(3): 394-403.
19. Tighe PJ, Badiyan SJ, Luria I, Lampotang S, Parekattil S. Robot-assisted airway support: a simulated case. Anesth Analg. 2010;111(4):929-31.
20. Hemmerling TM, Wehbe M, Zaouter C, Taddei R, Morse J. The Kepler intubation system. Anesth Analg. 2012; 114(3):590-4.
21. Cheng X, Jiang G, Lee K, Laker YN. Intubot: design and prototyping of a robotic intubation device. In: 2018 IEEE International Conference on Robotics and Automation (ICRA). IEEE; 2018. pp. 1482-7.
22. Schamberg G, Badgeley M, Meschede-Krasa B, Kwon O, Brown EN. Continuous action deep reinforcement learning for propofol dosing during general anesthesia. Artif Intell Med. 2022;123:102227.
23. Liu N, Lory C, Assenzo V, Cocard V, Chazot T, Le Guen M, et al. Feasibility of closed-loop co-administration of propofol and remifentanil guided by the bispectral index in obese patients: a prospective cohort comparison. Br J Anaesth. 2015;114(4):605-14.
24. Rinehart J, Liu N, Alexander B, Cannesson M. Closed-loop systems in anesthesia: is there a potential for closed-loop fluid management and hemodynamic optimization? Anesth Analg. 2012;114(1):130-43.
25. Hwang E, Park HS, Kim HS, Kim JY, Jeong H, Kim J, et al. Development of a bispectral index score prediction model based on an interpretable deep learning algorithm. Artif Intell Med. 2023;143:102569.
26. Zhang XS, Roy RJ, Schwender D, Daunderer M. Discrimination of anesthetic states using mid-latency auditory evoked potential and artificial neural networks. Ann Biomed Eng. 2001;29:446-53.
27. Nagaraj SB, Biswal S, Boyle EJ, Zhou DW, McClain LM, Bajwa EK, et al. Patient-specific classification of ICU sedation levels from heart rate variability. Crit Care Med. 2017;45(7):e683-90.
28. Ramaswamy SM, Kuizenga MH, Weerink MAS, Vereecke HEM, Struys MMRF, Nagaraj SB. Novel drug-independent sedation level estimation based on machine learning of quantitative frontal electroencephalogram features in healthy volunteers. Br J Anaesth. 2019; 123(4):479-87.
29. Avital G, Snider EJ, Berard D, Vega SJ, Hernandez Torres SI, Convertino VA, et al. Closed-loop controlled fluid administration systems: a comprehensive scoping review. J Pers Med. 2022;12(7):1168.
30. Rollins KE, Lobo DN. Intraoperative goal-directed fluid therapy in elective major abdominal surgery: a meta-analysis of randomized controlled trials. Ann Surg. 2016;263(3):465-76.
31. Joosten A, Hafiane R, Pustetto M, Van Obbergh L, Quackels T, Buggenhout A, et al. Practical impact of a decision support for goal-directed fluid therapy on protocol adherence: a clinical implementation study in patients undergoing major abdominal surgery. J Clin Monit Comput. 2019;33:15-24.
32. Joosten A, Chirnoaga D, Van der Linden P, Barvais L, Alexander B, Duranteau J, et al. Automated closed-loop versus manually controlled norepinephrine infusion in patients undergoing intermediate-to high-risk abdominal surgery: a randomised controlled trial. Br J Anaesth. 2021;126(1):210-8.

33. Joosten A, Rinehart J, Van der Linden P, Alexander B, Penna C, De Montblanc J, et al. Computer-assisted individualized hemodynamic management reduces intraoperative hypotension in intermediate-and high-risk surgery: a randomized controlled trial. Anesthesiology. 2021;135(2):258-72.
34. Libert N, Chenegros G, Harrois A, Baudry N, Cordurie G, Benosman R, et al. Performance of closed-loop resuscitation of haemorrhagic shock with fluid alone or in combination with norepinephrine: an experimental study. Ann Intensive Care. 2018;8:1-10.
35. Gambus PL, Jaramillo S. Machine learning in anaesthesia: reactive, proactive... predictive! Br J Anaesth. 2019; 123(4):401-3.
36. Hatib F, Jian Z, Buddi S, Lee C, Settels J, Sibert K, et al. Machine-learning algorithm to predict hypotension based on high-fidelity arterial pressure waveform analysis. Anesthesiology. 2018;129(4):663-74.
37. Davies SJ, Vistisen ST, Jian Z, Hatib F, Scheeren TWL. Ability of an arterial waveform analysis–derived hypotension prediction index to predict future hypotensive events in surgical patients. Anesth Analg. 2020;130(2):352-9.
38. Ranucci M, Barile L, Ambrogi F, Pistuddi V. Discrimination and calibration properties of the hypotension probability indicator during cardiac and vascular surgery. Minerva Anestesiol. 2018;85(7):724-30.
39. Gangakhedkar GR, Solanki SL, Divatia JV. The use of Hypotension Prediction Index in cytoreductive surgery (CRS) with hyperthermic intraperitoneal chemotherapy (HIPEC). Indian J Anaesth. 2022;66(4):294-8.
40. Lee S, Lee HC, Chu YS, Song SW, Ahn GJ, Lee H, et al. Deep learning models for the prediction of intraoperative hypotension. Br J Anaesth. 2021;126(4):808-17.
41. Lundberg SM, Nair B, Vavilala MS, Horibe M, Eisses MJ, Adams T, et al. Explainable machine-learning predictions for the prevention of hypoxaemia during surgery. Nat Biomed Eng. 2018;2(10):749-60.
42. Fritz BA, Cui Z, Zhang M, He Y, Chen Y, Kronzer A, et al. Deep-learning model for predicting 30-day postoperative mortality. Br J Anaesth. 2019;123(5):688-95.
43. Lee CK, Hofer I, Gabel E, Baldi P, Cannesson M. Development and validation of a deep neural network model for prediction of postoperative in-hospital mortality. Anesthesiology. 2018;129(4):649-62.
44. Brown MS, Wong K-P, Shrestha L, Wahi-Anwar M, Daly M, Foster G, et al. Automated endotracheal tube placement check using semantically embedded deep neural networks. Acad Radiol. 2023;30(3):412-20.
45. Monteiro M, Newcombe VFJ, Mathieu F, Adatia K, Kamnitsas K, Ferrante E, et al. Multiclass semantic segmentation and quantification of traumatic brain injury lesions on head CT using deep learning: an algorithm development and multicentre validation study. Lancet Digit Heal. 2020;2(6):e314-22.
46. Prasad N, Mandyam A, Chivers C, Draugelis M, Hanson III CW, Engelhardt BE, et al. Guiding efficient, effective, and patient-oriented electrolyte replacement in critical care: an artificial intelligence reinforcement learning approach. J Pers Med. 2022;12(5):661.
47. Davoudi A, Malhotra KR, Shickel B, Siegel S, Williams S, Ruppert M, et al. Intelligent ICU for autonomous patient monitoring using pervasive sensing and deep learning. Sci Rep. 2019;9(1):8020.
48. Yoon JH, Jeanselme V, Dubrawski A, Hravnak M, Pinsky MR, Clermont G. Prediction of hypotension events with physiologic vital sign signatures in the intensive care unit. Crit Care. 2020;24:1-9.
49. Yoon JH, Pinsky MR. Predicting adverse hemodynamic events in critically ill patients. Curr Opin Crit Care. 2018; 24(3):196-203.
50. Tran NK, Sen S, Palmieri TL, Lima K, Falwell S, Wajda J, et al. Artificial intelligence and machine learning for predicting acute kidney injury in severely burned patients: a proof of concept. Burns. 2019;45(6):1350-8.
51. Flechet M, Falini S, Bonetti C, Güiza F, Schetz M, Van den Berghe G, et al. Machine learning versus physicians' prediction of acute kidney injury in critically ill adults: a prospective evaluation of the AKIpredictor. Crit Care. 2019;23:1-10.
52. Li BY, Oh J, Young VB, Rao K, Wiens J. Using machine learning and the electronic health record to predict complicated *Clostridium difficile* infection. In: Open forum infectious diseases. Oxford University Press. US; 2019. p. ofz186.
53. Zhang Z, Ho KM, Hong Y. Machine learning for the prediction of volume responsiveness in patients with oliguric acute kidney injury in critical care. Crit Care. 2019;23:1-10.
54. Awad A, Bader-El-Den M, McNicholas J, Briggs J. Early hospital mortality prediction of intensive care unit patients using an ensemble learning approach. Int J Med Inform. 2017;108:185-95.
55. Holmgren G, Andersson P, Jakobsson A, Frigyesi A. Artificial neural networks improve and simplify intensive care mortality prognostication: a national cohort study of 217,289 first-time intensive care unit admissions. J Intensive Care. 2019;7:1-8.
56. Blanch L, Sales B, Montanya J, Lucangelo U, Garcia-Esquirol O, Villagra A, et al. Validation of the Better Care® system to detect ineffective efforts during expiration in mechanically ventilated patients: a pilot study. Intensive Care Med. 2012;38:772-80.
57. Marchuk Y, Magrans R, Sales B, Montanya J, López-Aguilar J, De Haro C, et al. Predicting patient-ventilator asynchronies with hidden Markov models. Scientific reports. 2018;8(1):17614.

58. Komorowski M, Celi LA, Badawi O, Gordon AC, Faisal AA. The artificial intelligence clinician learns optimal treatment strategies for sepsis in intensive care. Nat Med. 2018;24(11):1716-20.
59. Chen KW, Wang YC, Liu MH, Tsai BY, Wu MY, Hsieh PH, et al. Artificial intelligence-assisted remote detection of ST-elevation myocardial infarction using a mini-12-lead electrocardiogram device in prehospital ambulance care. Front Cardiovasc Med. 2022;9:1001982.
60. Houthooft R, Ruyssinck J, van der Herten J, Stijven S, Couckuyt I, Gadeyne B, et al. Predictive modelling of survival and length of stay in critically ill patients using sequential organ failure scores. Artif Intell Med. 2015;63(3): 191-207.
61. Lin YW, Zhou Y, Faghri F, Shaw MJ, Campbell RH. Analysis and prediction of unplanned intensive care unit readmission using recurrent neural networks with long short-term memory. PloS one. 2019;14(7):e0218942.

75 CHAPTER

Research in Onco-Anesthesia

Priya Ranganathan

INTRODUCTION

The burden of cancer is increasing exponentially, and more than two thirds of patients with cancer will need anesthesia for either diagnosis, treatment, or palliation.[1] Despite advances in surgery and perioperative care, cancer recurrence and metastasis remain a serious problem, compromising patient outcomes. It has been hypothesized that the surgical process itself promotes tumor spread through several mechanisms: Local and distal shedding of tumor cells, angiogenesis, inflammatory response, and immunosuppression.[2] This has raised questions about the role of antitumor anesthetic strategies in the perioperative period, and whether anesthetic interventions can be used to modify the perioperative environment to influence long-term cancer outcomes, the so-called window of opportunity.

Current Evidence on the Impact of Anesthetic Strategies and Perioperative Interventions on Oncological Outcomes

There has been a growing interest in the role of anesthetic strategies and perioperative interventions on oncological outcomes. The key areas of study include inhalation versus intravenous anesthetic techniques, the role of opioids and the concept of opioid-free anesthesia, and the impact of agents such as beta-blockers, alpha-adrenergic agonists, steroids, regional analgesia and local anesthetics, ketamine, and cyclo-oxygenase 2 (COX2) inhibitors.

Inhalation versus Intravenous Anesthetics

In preclinical studies, volatile anesthetics have been shown to have both pro- and antitumoral actions.[3] This spectrum of activity is possibly dependent on the type of cell line used, the incubation period, and the type, concentration, and duration of the administration of volatile agents. Inhalation agents have been postulated to cause proliferation, migration, invasion, and angiogenesis in cancer cells, as well as affect cell-mediated immunity and the stress response.[3] In contrast, propofol has predominantly antitumoral activity both through direct inhibition of tumor cells and indirectly through activation of natural killer (NK) cells and anti-inflammatory properties.[2]

In contrast, in vivo studies have been equivocal and been able to conclusively establish the superiority of one anesthetic technique over the other. Some in vivo studies have shown the superiority of intravenous over inhalation anesthesia with respect to cellular immunity and inflammatory markers.[4] In contrast, others have shown better immune profiles with general anesthesia (combined with epidural) compared to intravenous techniques.[5] A randomized controlled trial comparing intravenous and inhalation techniques for patients undergoing breast cancer surgery found no difference in recurrence rates.[6] A systematic review of studies comparing intravenous with inhalation anesthesia for oncological outcomes identified only retrospective cohort studies.[7] Propofol was superior to volatile agents (specifically desflurane) for overall survival but had no impact on recurrence-free survival. There was also substantial heterogeneity between studies. These paradoxical findings along with other limitations of retrospective data invalidated the findings of the review. This was also substantiated by a subsequent large retrospective study in patients undergoing surgery for digestive cancers that showed no difference in overall or recurrence-free survival between patients who received either volatile or intravenous anesthesia.[8] The results of other randomized studies on this topic are awaited.

Analgesia Techniques: Opioids, Regional Analgesia, and Local Anesthetics

Opioids: Since opioids are the mainstay in cancer anesthesia, used for induction, maintenance, and post-operative analgesia, there has been a lot of debate about the role of opioids in cancer recurrence. Data from preclinical studies suggest a negative impact based on immunosuppression and the inhibition of NK cell activity.[3] However, there are also contradicting reports of improved NK cell activity and inhibition of angiogenesis.[3] For patients undergoing surgery for breast cancer who received perioperative and postoperative opioids, there are conflicting reports with mixed results regarding the impact of opioid use on recurrence rates.[9] A systematic review of studies comparing opioid-free with opioid-based analgesia techniques found inadequate data to support the benefits of opioid-free techniques on either short- or long-term outcomes.[10] Opioid-free anesthesia typically requires the use of regional analgesia techniques and/or adjuncts like dexmedetomidine or ketamine for pain relief, which are also postulated to have protective effects on cancer recurrence. Therefore, it is unclear whether any observed effects can be conclusively attributed to the lack of opioids.

Local Anesthetics and Regional Analgesia

The impact of regional analgesia and local anesthetics on short- and long-term postoperative outcomes is multi-factorial through direct and indirect pathways. Regional analgesia techniques reduce the requirement for opioids and volatile anesthetics in the intra- and postoperative periods. They also decrease stress response and inhibit inflammatory markers. The use of regional anesthesia results in improved pain control, which in turn can affect levels of stress and inflammatory markers. Regional analgesia has also been associated with faster recovery and postoperative discharge from the hospital and can possibly hasten the time to return to intended oncologic therapy, which in turn will impact long-term oncological outcomes. Local anesthetics, especially lignocaine, have been shown to have a direct inhibitory effect on tumor cell proliferation through antiangiogenic and anti-inflammatory properties. A systematic review of preclinical studies showed that local anesthetics have antitumorigenic properties.[11] Retrospective data also suggest that intravenous lignocaine may improve survival in patients undergoing pancreatectomy.[12] However, there is a lack of high-quality clinical evidence to show better oncological outcomes in patients receiving local anesthesia or regional techniques.[3] A meta-analysis comparing the relationship between regional anesthesia and cancer found no impact on overall survival, recurrence-free survival, or biochemical recurrence-free survival, across a variety of cancers.[13]

Other Perioperative Strategies

Various other interventions in the perioperative period such as beta-blockers, COX-2 inhibitors, alpha-adrenergic agonists such as dexmedetomidine, steroids especially dexamethasone, ketamine, and avoidance of blood transfusion and hypothermia have also been hypothesized to have an impact on cancer outcomes but have been studied to a lesser extent; however, there is no conclusive evidence to support the use of any of these interventions.[14]

Problem with Existing Research Data

The key challenges in research in onco-anesthesia appear to be the failure of translation of in vitro findings into clinical evidence and the lack of good-quality data to establish causal relationships between perioperative anesthetic interventions and cancer outcomes. Most of the data that we have are preclinical from animal models and may not necessarily have similar applications in humans. The scarce clinical data available are restricted to retrospective studies, single-center studies, and small samples. There are dissimilarities between studies in terms of setting, population intervention, and outcome, leading to heterogeneity and the inability to pool the results of studies.

Many interventions tested in the perioperative period are multimodal, and it is difficult to separate the effect of individual components. For example, the perioperative use of regional analgesia results in opioid-sparing and reduces the requirement for volatile anesthetics. It is, therefore, unclear whether any benefits seen are due to those of regional anesthesia or the action of local anesthetic, or the avoidance of opioids or inhalation agents.

Another important limitation of current research is the heterogeneity and lack of standard outcome definitions across studies, making comparisons difficult. An important initiative is the STEP (Standardizing Endpoints in Perioperative) cancer outcomes initiative, which has identified six standardized endpoints for use in perioperative trials examining cancer outcomes, to support benchmarking and pooling of results.[15]

Finally, it has been argued that the "one-size-fits-all" approach may not be suitable for studying the effect of perioperative interventions. Just as oncological therapies are increasingly being modified to target individual patient and tumor characteristics (the precision oncology-based approach), it is possible that the response to perioperative interventions may vary depending on the patient, cancer, or tumor types.[16]

Examples of Ongoing Studies that Might Influence Practice

We need high-quality evidence to demonstrate a causal link between specific perioperative anesthetic strategies and cancer outcomes. There are several ongoing studies, the results of which are likely to influence practice in the near future.

The VAPOR C (Volatile Anesthesia and Perioperative Outcomes Related to Cancer) is a pragmatic, randomized controlled trial, with a two-by-two factorial design.[17] Two sets of interventions are being compared in this study: Inhalation anesthesia (sevoflurane) versus intravenous anesthesia (propofol) and intravenous lignocaine infusion versus no-lignocaine infusion. This trial includes patients undergoing colorectal or lung cancer surgery, with two primary hypotheses: Propofol total intravenous anesthesia (TIVA) and lidocaine increase disease-free survival compared with volatile anesthesia. The secondary endpoints include the impact of anesthesia on postoperative complications, quality of recovery, return to adjuvant therapies, and incidence of chronic pain. After an initial successful pilot and feasibility study, the trial commenced accrual but is currently on hold for a protocol amendment.[18]

The Cancer and Anaesthesia (CAN) study compares propofol- and sevoflurane-based techniques for the maintenance of anesthesia in patients undergoing surgery for breast or colorectal cancer.[19] The primary endpoints are 1-year and 5-year overall survival. Data from the breast cancer cohort have shown no difference in outcomes between the groups; the results from the colorectal cohort are awaited.[20]

The General Anesthetics in CAncer REsection Surgery (GA-CARES) is a pragmatic randomized multicenter trial of propofol versus volatile inhalational anesthesia for patients with eight types of cancer undergoing surgery.[21] The trial aims to look at all-cause mortality and recurrence-free survival.

The GAS TIVA study compares inhalational gas anesthesia (GAS) with intravenous anesthesia (TIVA) techniques for the maintenance of anesthesia in patients undergoing curative resection for lung cancer.[22] The hypothesis is that recurrence-free survival will be superior in patients receiving TIVA.

CONCLUSION

The perioperative period represents an important opportunity to manipulate the environment to improve short- and long-term outcomes after surgery for cancer. Several potential interventions that can be implemented in this period have been identified; however, currently, there is inadequate evidence to support the use of any of these strategies. There is, therefore, the need for large, well-designed randomized controlled trials focused on strategies in the perioperative period, using a personalized approach, to account for heterogeneity in response.

REFERENCES

1. Sullivan R, Alatise OI, Anderson BO, Audisio R, Autier P, Aggarwal A, et al. Global cancer surgery: delivering safe, affordable, and timely cancer surgery. Lancet Oncol. 2015;16(11):1193-224.
2. Ramirez MF, Cata JP. Anesthesia techniques and long-term oncological outcomes. Front Oncol. 2021;11:788918.
3. Xia SH, Zhou D, Ge F, Sun M, Chen X, Zhang H, et al. Influence of perioperative anesthesia on cancer recurrence: from basic science to clinical practice. Curr Oncol Rep. 2023;25(2):63-81.
4. Chen J, Luo F, Lei M, Chen Z. A study on cellular immune function of patients treated with radical resection of pulmonary carcinoma with two different methods of anesthesia and analgesia. J BUON. 2017;22(6):1416-21.
5. Xu Q, Shi NJ, Zhang H, Zhu YM. Effects of combined general-epidural anesthesia and total intravenous anesthesia on cellular immunity and prognosis in patients with non-small cell lung cancer: a comparative study. Mol Med Rep. 2017;16(4):4445-54.
6. Sessler DI, Pei L, Huang Y, Fleischmann E, Marhofer P, Kurz A, et al; Breast Cancer Recurrence Collaboration. Recurrence of breast cancer after regional or general anaesthesia: a randomised controlled trial. Lancet. 2019; 394(10211):1807-15.
7. Chang CY, Wu MY, Chien YJ, Su IM, Wang SC, Kao MC. Anesthesia and long-term oncological outcomes: a systematic review and meta-analysis. Anesth Analg. 2021;132(3):623-34.
8. Makito K, Matsui H, Fushimi K, Yasunaga H. Volatile versus total intravenous anesthesia for cancer prognosis in patients having digestive cancer surgery. Anesthesiology. 2020;133(4):764-73.

9. Thomas TE, Bowers K, Gomez D, Morgan O, Borowsky PA, Dutta R, et al. The association between perioperative opioids and breast cancer recurrence: a narrative review of the literature. Transl Breast Cancer Res. 2023;4:12.
10. Bugada D, Drotar M, Finazzi S, Real G, Lorini LF, Forget P. Opioid-free anesthesia and postoperative outcomes in cancer surgery: a systematic review. Cancers (Basel). 2022; 15(1):64.
11. Matos AC, Marques IA, Pires AS, Valentim A, Abrantes AM, Botelho MF. The potential effect of lidocaine, ropivacaine, levobupivacaine and morphine on breast cancer pre-clinical models: a systematic review. Int J Mol Sci. 2022; 23(3):1894.
12. Zhang H, Yang L, Zhu X, Zhu M, Sun Z, Cata JP, et al. Association between intraoperative intravenous lidocaine infusion and survival in patients undergoing pancreatectomy for pancreatic cancer: a retrospective study. Br J Anaesth. 2020;125(2):141-8.
13. Grandhi RK, Lee S, Abd-Elsayed A. The relationship between regional anesthesia and cancer: a metaanalysis. Ochsner J. 2017;17(4):345-61.
14. Wall T, Sherwin A, Ma D, Buggy DJ. Influence of perioperative anaesthetic and analgesic interventions on oncological outcomes: a narrative review. Br J Anaesth. 2019;123(2):135-50.
15. Buggy DJ, Freeman J, Johnson MZ, Leslie K, Riedel B, Sessler DI, et al; StEP-COMPAC Group. Systematic review and consensus definitions for standardised endpoints in perioperative medicine: postoperative cancer outcomes. Br J Anaesth. 2018;121(1):38-44.
16. Mincer JS, Buggy DJ. Anaesthesia, analgesia, and cancer outcomes: time to think like oncologists? Br J Anaesth. 2023;131(2):193-6.
17. Volatile anaesthesia and perioperative outcomes related to cancer [Internet]. Available from: https://www.anzca.edu.au/profiles/ctn-trials/underway/vapor-c-trial [Last accessed March, 2025].
18. Dubowitz JA, Cata JP, De Silva AP, Braat S, Shan D, Yee K, et al; the Global Onco-Anaesthesia Research Collaboration Group. Volatile anaesthesia and peri-operative outcomes related to cancer: a feasibility and pilot study for a large randomised control trial. Anaesthesia. 2021;76(9): 1198-206.
19. Enlund M, Enlund A, Berglund A, Bergkvist L. Rationale and design of the CAN study: an RCT of survival after propofol- or sevoflurane-based anesthesia for cancer surgery. Curr Pharm Des. 2019;25(28):3028-33.
20. Enlund M, Berglund A, Enlund A, Lundberg J, Wärnberg F, Wang DX, et al; CAN-study group. Impact of general anaesthesia on breast cancer survival: a 5-year follow up of a pragmatic, randomised, controlled trial, the CAN-study, comparing propofol and sevoflurane. EClinicalMedicine. 2023;60:102037.
21. Bennett-Guerrero E, Romeiser JL, DeMaria S, Nadler JW, Quinn TD, Ponnappan SK, et al. General Anesthetics in CAncer REsection Surgery (GA-CARES) randomized multicenter trial of propofol vs volatile inhalational anesthesia: protocol description. Perioper Med (Lond). 2023;12(1):2.
22. Kim J, Yoon S, Song IK, Lee K, Hwang W, Kim H, et al. Recurrence-free survival after curative resection of non-small cell lung cancer between inhalational gas anesthesia and propofol-based total intravenous anesthesia: a multicenter, randomized, clinical trial (GAS TIVA trial): protocol description. Perioper Med (Lond). 2024; 13(1):79.

Index

Page numbers followed by *b* refer to box, *f* refer to figure, *fc* refer to flowchart, and *t* refer to table.

A

B

F

G

H

J

M

N

Q

R

S

T

U

V